a LANGE medical book

MW00682271

CURRENT Care of Women: Diagnosis & Treatment

Edited by:

Dawn P. Lemcke, MD, FACP
Assistant Professor of Clinical Medicine
Director of Ambulatory Care Education
Southern Arizona Veterans Affairs Health Care System
Tucson, Arizona

Lorna A. Marshall, MD
Assistant Clinical Professor
Department of Obstetrics and Gynecology
University of Washington School of Medicine
Section Head, Reproductive Endocrinology
Department of Obstetrics and Gynecology
Virginia Mason Medical Center
Seattle, Washington

Julie Pattison, MD
Women's Health Clerkship Coordinator
Attending Physician
Department of General Internal Medicine
Virginia Mason Medical Center
Seattle, Washington

Deborah S. Cowley, MD
Professor and Director, Residency Training Program
Department of Psychiatry and Behavioral Sciences
University of Washington School of Medicine
Seattle, Washington

Lange Medical Books/McGraw-Hill
Medical Publishing Division

New York   Chicago   San Francisco   Lisbon   London   Madrid   Mexico City   Milan   New Delhi   San Juan   Seoul
Singapore   Sydney   Toronto

Tho McGraw-Hill Companies

2 3 4 5 6 7 8 9 0 DOC/DOC 0 9 8 7 6 5 4 3

ISBN: 0-07-138770-6
ISSN: 1082-1333

Notice

Medicine is an ever-changing science. As new research and clinical experience broaden our knowledge, changes in treatment and drug therapy are required. The editors and the publisher of this work have checked with sources believed to be reliable in their efforts to provide information that is complete and generally in accord with the standards accepted at the time of publication. However, in view of the possibility of human error or changes in medical sciences, neither the editors nor the publisher nor any other party who has been involved in the preparation or publication of this work warrants that the information contained herein is in every respect accurate or complete, and they disclaim all responsibility for any errors or omissions or for the results obtained from use of the information contained in this work. Readers are encouraged to confirm the information contained herein with other sources. For example and in particular, readers are advised to check the product information sheet included in the package of each drug they plan to administer to be certain that the information contained in this work is accurate and that changes have not been made in the recommended dose or in the contraindications for administration. This recommendation is of particular importance in connection with new or infrequently used drugs.

This book was set in Adobe Garamond by Pine Tree Composition, Inc.
The editors were Catherine Johnson and Karen Edmonson.
The production supervisor was Richard Ruzycka.
The index was prepared by Pamela Edwards.
RR Donnelley was the printer and binder.

This book is printed on acid-free paper.
INTERNATIONAL EDITION ISBN: 0-07-121977-3

Contents

Contributors

David M. Aboulafia, MD
Attending Hematologist-Oncologist
Virginia Mason Clinic
Seattle, Washington
Clinical Professor of Medicine
University of Washington
Seattle, Washington
Medical Director
Bailey-Boushay House
Seattle, Washington

Rita L. Bender, BA, JD
Attorney
Skellenger Bender, PS
Seattle, Washington

James W. Benson, Jr., MD
Clinical Associate Professor
Division of Endocrinology and Metabolism
Department of Medicine
University of Washington School of Medicine
Seattle, Washington
Endocrinologist and Director of Graduate Medical
Education
Division of Endocrinology
Department of Medicine
Virginia Mason Medical Center
Seattle, Washington

Jennifer D. Bolen, MD, PLLL
Department of Psychiatry
Swedish Medical Center
Seattle, Washington

Renee D. Boss, MD
Chief Resident
Department of Pediatrics
University of Arizona School of Medicine
Tucson, Arizona

James E. Bredfeldt, MD
Gastroenterologist/Hepatologist
Section of Gastroenterology
Virginia Mason Medical Center
Seattle, Washington

Dale Brown, JR, MD
Professor and Vice Chairman of Clinical Affairs
Department of Obstetrics and Gynecology
Baylor College of Medicine
Houston, Texas

Roger W. Bush, MD, FACP
Director, Internal Medicine Residency Program
Virginia Mason Medical Center
Seattle, Washington

Judy M. Cheng, MD, PhD
Division of Hematology-Oncology
University of California-San Francisco
San Francisco, California

Susan C. Conway, MD, MPH, MMSc
Reproductive Endocrinologist
Section of Fertility and Reproductive Endocrinology
Department of Surgery
Virginia Mason Medical Center
Seattle, Washington

Fanny Correa, MSW, CT
Practicum Instructor
School of Social Work
University of Washington
Seattle, Washington
Clinical Director, Separation and Loss Services
Virginia Mason Medical Center
Seattle, Washington

Bonnie Dattel, MD
Professor of Obstetrics and Gynecology
Associate Director, Division of Maternal-Fetal
Medicine
Assistant Dean, Eastern Virginia Medical School
Norfolk, Virginia

Roberta Haynes de Regt, MD
Clinical Assistant Professor
Division of Maternal Fetal Medicine
Department of Obstetrics and Gynecology
University of Washington School of Medicine
Seattle, Washington
Section Chief
Department of Obstetrics and Gynecology
Evergreen Hospital Medical Center
Kirkland, Washington

Mary Ann Draye, ARNP, MPH, FNP
Assistant Professor and Director
Division of Primary Care, FNP Program
Department of Psychosocial and Community Health
University of Washington School of Nursing
Seattle, Washington

Deborah A. Fuchs, MD
Hematopathology Fellow
Department of Pathology
University of Arizona Health Sciences Center
Tucson, Arizona

Edward F. Gibbons, MD, FACC, FACP
Deputy Chief, Cardiology Services
Department of Medicine
Virginia Mason Medical Center
Seattle, Washington

Barbara S. Giesser, MD
Associate Clinical Professor
Department of Neurology
Reed Neurological Research Center
University of California, Los Angeles School
of Medicine
Los Angeles, California

Fred E. Govier, MD
Head, Section of Urology
Virginia Mason Medical Center
Seattle, Washington

Beverly B. Green MD, MPH
Associate Director
Department of Preventive Care
Group Health Cooperative of Puget Sound
Seattle, Washington

Julia R. Heiman, PhD
Professor
Department of Psychiatry and Behavioral Sciences
University of Washington Psychiatry Outpatient
Center
Seattle, Washington

Jan L Hillson, MD
Head, Division of Rheumatology and Clinical
Immunology
Virginia Mason Medical Center
Seattle, Washington

William P. Johnson, MD
Associate Program Director
Department of Medicine
University of Arizona Health Sciences Center
Tucson, Arizona

Steven Juergens, MD
Assistant Clinical Professor of Psychiatry
Department of Psychiatry
University of Washington
Seattle, Washington
Section Head, Psychiatry
Medical Director, Virginia Mason Outpatient
Chemical Dependency Program
Virginia Mason Medical Center
Seattle, Washington

Raymond H. Kaufman, MD
Professor of Obstetrics and Gynecology and Pathology
Department of Obstetrics and Gynecology
Baylor College of Medicine
Houston, Texas

Kathleen C. Kobashi, MD
Co-Director, Continence Center at Virginia Mason
Section of Urology and Renal Transplantation
Virginia Mason Medical Center
Seattle, Washington

Susan Kupferman, MD
Section of Gynecology
Virginia Mason Medical Center
Seattle, Washington

Joyce Lammert MD, PhD
Clinical Assistant Professor
Department of Allergy and Immunology
University of Washington
Seattle, Washington
Section Head
Division of Asthma, Allergy, and Immunology
Virginia Mason Clinic
Seattle, Washington

Gerard S. Letterie, MD, FACOG, FACP
Associate Clinical Professor
Department of Obstetrics and Gynecology
University of Washington
Seattle, Washington
Medical Director
Center for Fertility and Reproductive Endocrinology
Virginia Mason Medical Center
Seattle, Washington

Mitchell R. Levy, MD
Acting Clinical Instructor
Department of Psychiatry and Behavioral Sciences
University of Washington Outpatient Psychiatry Clinic
Seattle, Washington

Donald Lieberman, MD
Department of Internal Medicine
University Health Care at North Hills
Tucson, Arizona

Richard S. Liebowitz, MD
Assistant Clinical Professor of Medicine
Division of General Internal Medicine
Department of Medicine
Duke University Medical Center
Durham, North Carolina
Medical Director
Duke Center for Integrative Medicine
Durham, North Carolina

David Likosky, MD
Clinical Instructor
University of Washington School of Medicine
Seattle, Washington
Hospitalist
Departments of Neurology and Internal Medicine
Chief, Department of Medicine
Evergreen Hospital
Kirkland, Washington

Michael Longo, MD
Deputy Section Chief
Division of Cardiology
Virginia Mason Medical Center
Seattle, Washington

Tim McAfee, MD, MPH
Executive Medical Director
Group Health Cooperative
Center for Health Promotion
Tukwila, Washington

Kathryn D. McGonigle, MD
Section of Gynecologic Oncology
Department of Obstetrics and Gynecology
Virginia Mason Medical Center
Seattle, Washington

Joan Miller, MD
Department of General Internal Medicine
Virginia Mason Medical Center
Seattle, Washington

Howard G. Muntz, MD
Clinical Associate Professor of Obstetrics and
Gynecology
University of Washington School of Medicine
Seattle, Washington
Section of Gynecologic Oncology
Virginia Mason Medical Center
Seattle, Washington

Paul Mystkowski, MD
Section of Endocrinology
Virginia Mason Medical Center
Seattle, Washington

Suseela Narra, MD
Virginia Mason Federal Way
Federal Way, Washington

Patricia L. Paddison, MD
Psychiatrist
Department of Psychiatry
Virginia Mason Medical Center
Seattle, Washington

Erica S. Pascarelli, MD
Resident Physician
Department of Internal Medicine
Virginia Mason Medical Center
Seattle, Washington

Margot Putukian, MD
Assistant Professor
Department of Orthopedics and Internal Medicine
Pennsylvania State University College of Medicine, and
Team Physician
Pennsylvania State University
University Park, Pennsylvania

Mandy D. Henderson Robertson, MD
Head, Division of Rheumatology and Clinical
Immunology
Virginia Mason Medical Center
Seattle, Washington

Patricia A. Robertson, MD
Professor of Clinical Obstetrics and Gynecology
Division of Perinatal Medicine and Genetics
Department of Obstetrics, Gynecology and
Reproductive Sciences
University of California, San Francisco
San Francisco, California

Alan B. Rothblatt, MD
Physician
Division of Reproductive Endocrinology & Infertility
Department of Obstetrics and Gynecology
Virginia Mason Medical Center
Seattle, Washington

Hope S. Rugo, MD
Associate Clinical Professor of Medicine
University of California San Francisco
Comprehensive Cancer Center
San Francisco, California

Edward K. Rynearson, MD
Clinical Professor
Department of Psychiatry
University of Washington
Medical Director
Division of Separation and Loss Services
Virginia Mason Medical Center
Seattle, Washington

Kian J. Samimi, MD, PhD
Assistant Professor and Section Chief
Section of Plastic Surgery
Department of Surgery
University of Arizona
Tucson, Arizona

Ali Sarram, MD
Fellow, Section of Urology
Virginia Mason Medical Center
Seattle, Washington

Paul Smith, MD
Clinical Assistant Professor of Medicine
University of Washington School of Medicine
Seattle, Washington
Department of General Internal Medicine
Virginia Mason Medical Center
Seattle, Washington

Karen Smith, MD
Section Head
Department of General Internal Medicine
Virginia Mason Federal Way
Federal Way, Washington

David E. Soper, MD
Vice Chairman of Business and Clinical Affairs
Director, Division of Gynecology
Department of Obstetrics and Gynecology
Medical University of South Carolina
Charleston, South Carolina

Alison Stopeck, MD
Associate Professor of Medicine
University of Arizona
Arizona Cancer Center
Tucson, Arizona

Naomi F. Sugar, MD
Clinical Associate Professor
Department of Pediatrics
University of Washington
Seattle, Washington

Nancy Sugg MD, MPH
Associate Professor of Medicine
Division of General Internal Medicine
Department of Medicine
University of Washington School of Medicine
Seattle, Washington
Medical Director
Pioneer Square Clinic
Seattle, Washington

Catherine S. Thompson, MD
Nephrologist
Section of Nephrology
Department of Internal Medicine
Virginia Mason Medical Center
Seattle, Washington

Joyce A. Tinsley, MD
Associate Professor of Psychiatry
University of Connecticut
Farmington, Connecticut

Richard A. Wahl, MD
Associate Professor of Clinical Pediatrics
Director of Adolescent Medicine
Director, Pediatric Clinic
Department of Pediatrics
University of Arizona
Tucson, Arizona

Kathe Wallace, PT
Women's Physical Therapy
Private Practice
Seattle, Washington

Debra G. Wechter, MD
Virginia Mason Medical Center
Seattle, Washington

Preface

In the last decade, research in the basic and clinical sciences has delved into gender differences—from the molecular level up to and including disease states and their outcomes.

From this research comes the realization that treatment of women's health may need to differ drastically from the treatment of men's health. In the very near future, clinicians may need to consider the sex of the patient in almost every decision they make, from deciding which medication to prescribe, to how to motivate a patient to make lifestyle changes.

Previously, clinical studies had failed to recruit women and men in equal numbers; now there is the realization that we can no longer generalize research from men to women. Therefore, studies actively seek adequate numbers of female participants to make gender-specific recommendations on both the therapeutic outcomes and safety issues. There is still progress to be made in reporting results separately for women and men so that gender-specific conclusions can be drawn. And finally, there has been the realization that outcomes of various disease states in women may differ from their male counterparts not because of the biology of being a woman but because of bias in treatments that are offered to women compared with men (eg, angiograms in suspected coronary disease, anticoagulation in atrial fibrillation, and carotid endarterectomies for carotid stenosis). Perhaps most importantly, outcomes may differ because women live their lives differently from men. Their disease courses are often different due to the responsibilities of family and children making it difficult to care for themselves when they are ill.

Eight years ago, we published *Primary Care of Women*. Women's health was in its infancy, and we could only allude to studies aimed specifically at women such as the Women's Health Initiative (WHI), the Heart and Estrogen/Progestin Replacement Study (HERS) trial, and so many more. In reading the Preface to *Primary Care of Women*, which has served as a foundation for *Current Care of Women: Diagnosis & Treatment*, we stated "Much of the material contained in this edition will change dramatically in the next decade with the increase in research regarding women's health."

As promised, it is with excitement that we present *Current Care of Women: Diagnosis & Treatment*. Any chapter that dealt with hormone replacement therapy has been completely revised based on the WHI and the HERS trial findings and recommendations. Chapters have been added to include complementary treatments, autoimmune diseases, breast augmentations and complications thereof, irritable bowel disease, multiple sclerosis, polycystic ovarian syndrome, dermatologic issues in women, and medicolegal issues.

Current Care of Women: Diagnosis & Treatment is multidisciplinary, incorporating general health topics relating to women such as prevention and health promotion. Other chapters deal with specific subsets of women such as adolescents and lesbians. And finally, most of the chapters deal with specific topics in internal medicine, obstetrics and gynecology, and mental health. The specific topics included are those that are unique to, more prevalent in, or present differently in women. It is not the intent of this book to provide an in-depth discussion of the topics but rather a clinically useful overview with references and Web sites to which the reader can turn for more details.

It is our hope that *Current Care of Women: Diagnosis & Treatment* will help the clinician begin to incorporate gender specifics into their care of women and begin asking questions about what we know and what we do not know about women's unique presentations and needs in health care. It is also our hope that each time this book is revised there will be more ways that women's health has been enhanced and made better.

INTENDED AUDIENCE

This book will be helpful for those providing primary care to women including internists, family physicians, obstetricians-gynecologists, allied health professionals, as well as medical students and residents.

ACKNOWLEDGEMENTS

The editors wish to thank the following persons for their help in this major undertaking: the authors for their time and knowledge of their topics, our patients from whom we learn how to be better doctors, and finally our families and children who remain ever supportive of our endeavors in medicine.

Dawn P. Lemcke, MD
Julie Pattison, MD
Lorna A. Marshall, MD
Deborah S. Cowley, MD

SECTION I

General Issues

Adolescent Medicine

1

Richard A. Wahl, MD, & Renee D. Boss, MD [1]

The primary care of adolescent girls is becoming an increasingly important aspect within the larger study of woman's health care. A recent text devoted to this topic provides an excellent introduction to the health needs of teens (Coupey, 2000). This chapter will provide background and structure for working with adolescents in a clinical setting.

Coupey SM: Primary Care of Adolescent Girls. Hanley & Belfus, 2000.

EPIDEMIOLOGY

The 2000 US census reported 19.6 million adolescent girls (defined as ages 10–19 years), representing 13.8% of the total US female population, with projections to reach 20.3 million adolescent girls in the United States by 2010.

The birth rate among adolescent mothers, aged 15–19 years, has dropped by 22% over the past decade, reaching a high in 1991 of 62 live births per 1000 girls, and descending to a low in 2000 of 48.7 births per 1000 girls. The United States still ranks as having the highest birth rate among adolescent girls in the developed world (Table 1–1).

In addition to unwanted pregnancies, high-risk behaviors place sexually active teenagers at risk for sexually transmitted diseases (STDs) and HIV infection. It is important to note that one of six teenagers will contract an STD each year, and 25% of AIDS cases involve young adults (people in their 20s) who probably were infected during adolescence, in most instances through unprotected heterosexual activity. In contrast to the United States, Western Europe and Scandinavia have a much lower rate of teenage pregnancy despite equivalent amounts of sexual activity among teenagers. Some authors attribute this difference to the nonjudgmental attitudes toward sex, easy access to contraceptive services for young people (including availability of contraceptives at low cost without the threat of parental notification), and comprehensive sex education programs.

The top three leading causes of death among US adolescents in 2000 were accidental trauma, responsible for half of all deaths; homicide, responsible for 15%; and suicide, responsible for 12% of all adolescent deaths. Motor vehicle accidents alone make up three fourths of all "accidental" deaths. These three causes accounted for a full 74% of all adolescent deaths. In comparison, the next two causes on the list (malignancy and heart disease) together caused only 8% of all adolescent deaths. Clearly, the vast majority of adolescent deaths are preventable.

The biennial Youth Risk Behavior Survey (YRBS) published by the Centers for Disease Control and Prevention accurately reflects the health risks to which these girls are exposed. Over 15,000 adolescents throughout the United States were interviewed. The survey results provide the most accurate picture available of adolescent health as well as of those behaviors that place adolescents at high risk.

The 1999 YRBS demonstrated many high-risk behaviors among high school students that contributed to the common causes of death: 1 of 6 students do not routinely wear a seat belt, 1 of 3 students rode in a car with a driver who was under the influence of alcohol, 1 of 6 students carried a weapon to school, half of all students consumed alcohol during the previous month, one quarter had smoked marijuana, and 1 of 12 high school students had attempted suicide during the previous year. Half of high school students are not virgins,

[1]The authors wish to gratefully acknowledge Dr. Jane L. Becker, author of the Adolescent Medicine chapter in *Primary Care of Women,* © 1995 by Appleton & Lange. Our work represents a revision of Dr. Becker's original chapter.

Table 1–1. Rates of birth, abortion, and pregnancy per year (per 1000 adolescents, 15–19 years).

Country	Birth rate	Abortion rate	Pregnancy rate
Japan	3.9	6.3	10.1
Italy	6.9	5.1	12.0
Sweden	7.7	17.2	24.9
Holland	8.2	4.0	12.2
Denmark	8.3	14.4	22.7
Belgium	9.1	5.0	14.1
Finland	9.9	10.7	20.5
France	10.0	10.2	20.2
Germany	12.5	3.6	16.1
Norway	13.5	18.7	32.3
Israel	18.0	9.8	27.9
Australia	19.8	23.8	43.7
Canada	24.2	21.2	45.4
United Kingdom	28.4	18.6	46.9
Belarus	39.0	34.3	73.3
Romania	42.0	32.0	74.0
Russia	45.6	56.1	101.7
Bulgaria	49.6	33.7	83.3
United States	54.4	29.2	83.6

(Adopted, with permission, from Singh S, Darroch JE. Adolescent pregnancy and childbearing: levels and trends in developed countries. *Fam Plann Perspect.* 2000;32(1):14–23. Available from http://www.agi-usa.org/.)

and of these more than half do not regularly use condoms.

In adults, two thirds of all deaths are caused by cancer and cardiovascular disease. These illnesses too have their roots in the adolescent years: 1 of 3 high school students smoke tobacco, 1 of 6 students are at high risk for adult obesity, and fewer than 1 of 4 adolescents reported a diet that contained appropriate portions of fruits and vegetables. Seven of 10 students do not take physical education classes in school.

Centers for Disease Control and Prevention: Youth Risk Behavior Surveillance—United States, 1999. MMWR Surveill Summ. 2000;49(SS05):1. Available from http://www.cdc.gov [PMID: 10981282]

Guyer B et al: Annual Summary of Vital Statistics: Trends in the Health of Americans During the 20th Century. Pediatrics 2000;106:1307. Available at http://www.pediatrics.org [PMID: 11099582]

Hoyert DL et al: Annual Summary of Vital Statistics: 2000. Pediatrics 2001;108:1241. Annual updates published each December, available at http://www.pediatrics.org [PMID: 11731644]

Singh S, Darroch JE: Adolescent pregnancy and childbearing: levels and trends in developed countries. Fam Plann Perspect 2000;32:14. Available from http://www.agi-usa.org [PMID: 10710702]

GROWTH & DEVELOPMENT

Puberty & Physical Development

The magnitude of physical growth and change during puberty is enormous. Growth in height during puberty accounts for 20–25% of final adult height, and pubertal weight gain accounts for 50% of an adult's ideal body weight. Most of the bone mineral content present throughout adult life is deposited during the adolescent years. Behaviors that interfere with bone mineralization during adolescence (such as eating disorders or strenuous exercise) may place the teen at increased risk for osteoporosis in later life.

The precise trigger of the onset of puberty is not completely understood. The trigger appears to be related to decreased sensitivity of the hypothalamus and pituitary to circulating sex hormones, resulting in an increase in levels of luteinizing hormone (LH) and follicle-stimulating hormone (FSH). The gonads respond to increased levels of LH and FSH by synthesizing and secreting more estrogen, progesterone, and testosterone, which leads to the estrogen-induced LH surge that ultimately results in regular menses and ova production. Adrenal androgens promote the acquisition and maintenance of sexual hair.

Physical evidence of female sexual development is present at an average age of 11.2 years, but the age of onset ranges from 9 to 13.4 years. The average length of time for completion of puberty is 4 years, with a range of 1.5–8 years. In most girls, breast budding is the first sign of puberty. Typically, thelarche (breast development) is followed by pubarche (pubic hair growth), followed by the growth spurt (peak height velocity), and finally, menarche. The average age for thelarche is 10.5–11 years, ranging from 8 to 13 years. Pubarche generally follows thelarche within 6 months to 1 year. On average, peak height velocity occurs at 12.1 years.

The mean age for menarche is 12.7 years, ranging from ages 9 to 16. Menarche predictably occurs within 30 months of the onset of breast budding, generally during Tanner stage 4. (Tanner stages are explained later in this section.) Menarche always occurs after peak height velocity has been attained; growth after menarche is limited to 2–5 cm. Generally, for the first year after menarche, 50% of the cycles are anovulatory, and often the menses remain irregular for the first 6–24 months.

The average growth spurt lasts approximately 24–36 months. Most often, linear bone growth is completed by 16 years of age, and height gain ranges from 5.4 to

11.2 cm. In general, an adolescent should be evaluated when her height falls within the lowest 2% or highest 98% of the population. It is important, given the strong genetic component to ultimate height attainment, that the health care provider consider the height of the parents before beginning a complete evaluation. A girl's final adult height can be estimated by subtracting 6.5 cm. (or 2.5") from the mid-parental height:

$$\text{Predicted adult height} = (\text{height of mother} + \text{height of father}) / 2 - (6.5 \text{ cm or } 2.5")$$

In 1962, Tanner developed a sexual maturity rating scale for male and female adolescents that is used widely in clinical practice. The Tanner staging system, depicted in Figures 1–1 and 1–2, divides pubertal development into five stages. Stage 1 represents the prepubescent girl, and stage 2 indicates early development. Stages 3 and 4 are intermediary stages reflecting increased maturity, while stage 5 indicates the completion of the development of secondary sex characteristics.

Variations in the timing of pubertal development may result from a number of factors, including genetics, nutrition, and chronic medical problems. Reassurance and education about the timing of development can be comforting to concerned teenagers. Variations that are outside the standard range require evaluation. An evaluation for abnormal development generally is indicated if there is no breast development by age 13, menses has not occurred by age 16, or menarche occurs before age 10.

Psychological Development

Adolescence is commonly divided into three stages: early adolescence (from 11 to 14 years), middle adolescence (15 to 18 years) and late adolescence (19 to 21+ years). These "stages" roughly correspond to junior high/middle school, high school, and post high school periods. While this is an artificial division, it is useful in following the changes in an adolescent's cognitive development.

Most early adolescents are functioning in Piaget's "concrete operational" level and have very concrete or literal thought processes. In talking with younger teens, it is important to be direct and "concrete." An early adolescent is likely to answer the question "What brought you here today" with "The bus."

Middle adolescence is a time of transition to "formal operational" thought processes, when a teen is better able to handle abstraction and takes a less literal approach to understanding her world. By late adolescence, most young adults have attained the formal op-

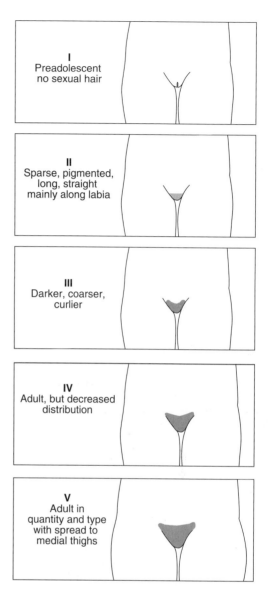

Figure 1–1. Tanner stages of pubic hair development. Stage 1 Preadolescent: No secondary sexual hair. Stage 2: Sparse, long, pigmented hair, straight or slightly curled, along labia. Stage 3: Darker, coarser, and curlier hair, spread more widely. Stage 4: Adult distribution, sparing medial thighs. Stage 5: Adult distribution, including medial thighs.

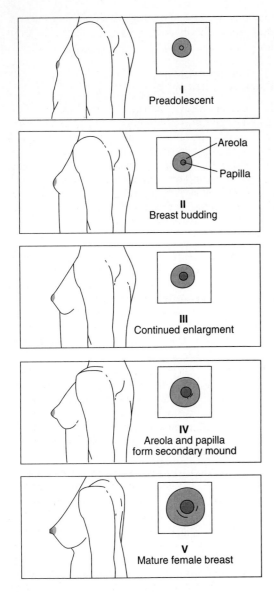

Figure 1–2. Tanner stages of breast development. Stage 1 Preadolescent: No secondary sexual development present, elevation of papilla only. Stage 2: Breast budding, with areola and papilla elevated over a discrete and palpable breast bud. Stage 3: Breast and areola continue to enlarge. Stage 4: Areola and papilla form a secondary mound, discrete from breast contour. Stage 5: Adult breast development. Areola no longer forms a separate mound.

erational level, although studies have demonstrated that many adults maintain a concrete operational interpretation of their world. Keeping these developmental stages in mind as you talk with your patients will help avoid misunderstanding, such as when a teen interprets your metaphoric statement literally.

Development Tasks

The four major developmental tasks of adolescence are (1) gaining independence from parents, (2) accepting body image, (3) establishing a peer group, and (4) developing an identity (including a sexual, moral, religious, and vocational identity).

A. EARLY ADOLESCENCE

During early adolescence (ages 11–14 years), the following changes are often seen: (1) decreased dependence on family, (eg, less family activity); (2) body image concerns resulting in a preoccupation with comparing oneself to others to answer the question, "Am I normal?"; (3) increased interest in the peer group (which usually involves same-sex friendships); and (4) early identity development with the first thoughts regarding future plans. Career plans at this stage are often unrealistic and may entail goals such as becoming a famous rock star.

B. MIDDLE ADOLESCENCE

The 4 developmental tasks are exhibited at this stage (ages 15–18) by (1) an escalation of parent-child conflict as the struggle for independence increases, (2) a new comfort with the body as the teenager begins to focus on the possibility of attracting a partner, (3) increasing involvement in peer culture and sexual experimentation, and (4) identity concerns that focus on the question, "Who am I?"

An increase in risk-taking behavior is seen during middle adolescence. The teenager is separating from her family and often feels powerful both physically and psychologically. The operative mode is the "myth of immunity," wherein the teenager believes that "it won't happen to me." These feelings, combined with her sense of being unique as well as the dramatic physical and psychological changes she experiences, are often manifested by a teen's increase in risk taking behavior.

C. LATE ADOLESCENCE

During late adolescence (ages 19–21+), there is (1) increasing autonomy from parents; (2) a greater comfort with the body, with puberty completed; (3) decreased importance of the peer group, with a shift in focus toward the achievement of intimacy with one person; and (4) development of practical career goals and plans.

Marshall WA, Tanner JM: Variations in pattern of pubertal changes in girls. Arch Dis Child 1969;44:291. [PMID: 5785179]

Neinstein LS: Adolescent Health Care: A Practical Guide. Lippincott Williams & Wilkins, 2002.

Orr DP: Helping adolescents toward adulthood. Contemp Pediatr 1998;15:55. Available from http://www.contemporarypediatrics.com/

HEALTH SCREENING GUIDELINES

The American Medical Association (AMA) responded to the need for specific advice on adolescent health screening with its "Guidelines for Adolescent Preventive Services" (GAPS). GAPS provides a framework for the organization and content of routine health care services for adolescents. Acknowledging the impact of the social morbidities on the health of today's adolescent population, the guidelines emphasize preventive service visits, which focus on health guidance screening and prevention of physical, emotional, and behavioral conditions that are a threat to the health of adolescents. Table 1–2 depicts the GAPS recommendations in the areas of health guidance, screening (including history, physical assessment, and laboratory tests), and immunizations for each age.

The AMA GAPS program also provides a useful collection of tracking forms and patient and parent questionnaires, available from the AMA's web site (http://www.ama-assn.org) in both English and Spanish.

American Medical Association, Department of Adolescent Health: Guidelines for Adolescent Preventive Services (GAPS): Recommendations Monograph. American Medical Association, 1997. Available from http://www.ama-assn.org

THE OFFICE VISIT

Adolescents come to a medical setting for a wide variety of reasons. They may present for a routine physical examination required by camp, school, an athletic team, or an employer, or at the request of their parents. Adolescent girls often present for routine gynecologic care (pelvic examination, Papanicolaou smear, and contraception), or for concerns about possible pregnancy or sexually transmitted infections. Teenagers often seek care for a multitude of minor acute medical problems. Frequently, an adolescent presents with a noncontroversial complaint to gain access to the clinician when she has a desire to speak about something else. Behavioral changes or somatic complaints may be secondary to a variety of emotional problems; for example, abdominal pain may be the presenting complaint for school avoidance, peer group issues, fear of pregnancy, or sexual abuse. The physician must ask the right questions to determine the true reason for the visit (see following section, The HEADS Interview). Younger teens may even feel that the physician should somehow already know why she is there, engaging in a bit of "magical" thinking.

Patient Consent

Before entering the examination room to see an adolescent patient, issues concerning consent for treatment must be considered. Most states define the legal age of majority as 18 years and do not permit minors to provide consent for their own medical care. The actual legal status of minors is much more complex, as each state has varied legislation permitting minors to provide their own consent in a variety of clinical and legal situations. These "exceptions" in each state may include the following:

1. **Emancipation:** A minor is usually considered emancipated if she is living free from parental care, custody, and support. Emancipated minors are usually able to give consent for their own medical care. A homeless teen is often considered emancipated without needing to meet other requirements. The exact definition of emancipation varies by state.

2. **Married:** A married teen is considered emancipated and can provide consent for her own care. Note that an unmarried mother is not necessarily considered emancipated, and thus while she may be able to provide consent for her infant's medical care, she may not necessarily be able to provide consent for her own.

3. **Military service:** Most states grant emancipation to minors who are in uniform in a military service.

4. **Mature minor:** Many states have a "mature minor" doctrine written into their statutes. If a teen, usually above a certain age, is considered by her physician to have sufficient intellectual and emotional maturity to be able to provide informed consent in a mature manner, she may do so. States usually require some form of attestation by the physician in the medical record to document the minor's "mature" status.

5. **STDs, drug abuse, sexual abuse:** Many states permit a teen, again often above a stated age, to provide consent for these concerns.

6. **Abortion:** Some states add further restrictions involving parental notification and consent for pregnancy termination, even if a teen meets other standards for consent. Such legislation has recently been challenged in some states and remains in flux.

7. **Contraception:** Title X of the US Public Health Service Act mandates that all clinics that receive

Table 1–2. AMA Guidelines for Adolescent Preventive Services (GAPS). Preventive health services by age and procedure.

Procedure	Early 11	Early 12	Early 13	Early 14	Middle 15	Middle 16	Middle 17	Late 18	Late 19	Late 20	Late 21
Health guidance											
Parenting*		•				•					
Development	•	•	•	•	•	•	•	•	•	•	•
Diet and physical activity	•	•	•	•	•	•	•	•	•	•	•
Healthy lifestyles**	•	•	•	•	•	•	•	•	•	•	•
Injury prevention	•	•	•	•	•	•	•	•	•	•	•
Screening history											
Eating disorders	•	•	•	•	•	•	•	•	•	•	•
Sexual activity***	•	•	•	•	•	•	•	•	•	•	•
Alcohol and other drug use	•	•	•	•	•	•	•	•	•	•	•
Tobacco use	•	•	•	•	•	•	•	•	•	•	•
Abuse	•	•	•	•	•	•	•	•	•	•	•
School performance	•	•	•	•	•	•	•	•	•	•	•
Depression	•	•	•	•	•	•	•	•	•	•	•
Risk for suicide	•	•	•	•	•	•	•	•	•	•	•
Physical assessment											
Blood pressure	•	•	•	•	•	•	•	•	•	•	•
BMI	•	•	•	•	•	•	•	•	•	•	•
Comprehensive exam		•				•			•		
Tests											
Cholesterol		1				1			1		
TB		2				2			2		
GC, Chalmydia, syphilis, HPV		3				3			3		
HIV		4				4			4		
Pap smear		5				5			5		
Immunizations											
MMR	•										
Td	•					0					
Hepatitis B	•					6			6		
Hepatitis A		7				7			7		
Varicella		8				8			8		

Adolescents and young adults have a unique set of health care needs. The recommendations for *Guidelines for Adolescent Preventive Services (GAPS)* emphasize annual clinical preventive services visits that address both the developmental and psychosocial aspects of health, in addition to traditional biomedical conditions. These recommendations were developed by the American Medical Association with contributions from a Scientific Advisory Panel, composed of national experts, as well as representatives of primary care medical organizations and the health insurance industry. The body of scientific evidence indicated that the periodicity and content of preventive services can be important in promoting the health and well-being of adolescents.

1. Screening test performed once if family history is positive for early cardiovascular disease or hyperlipidemia.
2. Screen if positive for exposure to active TB or lives/works in high-risk situation, (eg, homeless shelter, health care facility).
3. Screen at least annually if sexually active.
4. Screen if high-risk for infection.
5. Screen annually if sexually active or if 18 years or older.
6. Vaccinate if high risk for hepatitis B infection.
7. Vaccinate if at risk for hepatitis A infection.
8. Vaccinate if no reliable history of chicken pox.
*A parent health guidance visit is recommended during early and middle adolescence.
**Includes counseling regarding sexual behavior and avoidance of tobacco, alcohol, and other drug use.
***Includes history of unintended pregnancy and STD.
O Do not give if administered in last five years.

TB, tuberculosis; GC, gonorrhea; HPV, human papillomavirus; MMR, measles, mumps, and rubella (vaccine).
American Medical Association, Department of Adolescent Health. Guidelines for Adolescent preventive Services (GAPS): Recommendations Monograph. Chicago, IL: American Medical Association; 1997.

Title X funds must provide confidential family planning services to teens. If such service is to be confidential, it is implied that a teen can provide consent on her own, without the need for parental involvement. It is the opinion of many states' Attorneys General that in the absence of specific language in state statute covering provision of contraceptive services, Title X language applies to all teens who request confidential contraceptive services.

8. **HIV testing:** Many states have specific requirements on consent procedures for HIV testing. Unless specifically stated otherwise in local statute, HIV testing can be considered testing for an STD and, if permitted, a teen can provide her own consent.

It is important to learn the specific statutes that apply in your state. Speaking with an attorney is helpful, but remember that several situations are open to differences of opinion; the attorney's response may depend on who the client is—a hospital attorney will seek to reduce all risk for the hospital and may thus provide a more restrictive understanding of the law than that held by others. (See Chapter 4, Medicolegal Issues.)

Confidentiality

The reassurance to a teen that all communications between her and her physician will be kept in strictest confidence is vitally important to her; unfortunately, it cannot be given without some hedging. Much of the significant history that is obtained from teens involves very sensitive areas (see following section, The HEADS Interview). A strong bond of trust between the teen and physician is required. Every attempt must be made to safeguard that trust, but teens must also be informed that not all information will always be kept strictly confidential. While state statutes determine the specifics of consent by a minor, there are very few specific statutes that specifically protect a minor's medical record, especially from her parents. In most (if not all) states, parents can gain access to their minor child's medical record by requesting a copy. In addition, there will be specific instances when the physician must breach confidentiality to protect either the adolescent herself or others: suicidal or homicidal ideation is an obvious example and the presence of an infection that requires the notification of the local health department is another. Still, it is important to attempt to protect a teen's confidentiality to the extent possible.

If both the parent and the teenager enter the office together, it is helpful to begin by reviewing the ground rules of confidentiality and making sure that both parent and teen agree to them. It should be stated clearly that after the initial segment of the interview, the parent will be asked to step out of the examination room. (The teenager and her parents should not be offered the choice.) The teenager then has the remainder of the interview and the examination in privacy. It is important to state specifically to the parent and teenager that, except as noted above, the content of what she says is confidential unless she chooses to share it.

When a parent wishes to speak with the clinician alone, permission should be sought from the adolescent. Some parents feel that if they are paying the bill, they have a right to know what is discussed throughout the interview with their child. When the clinician explains the benefits derived from a confidential interview, namely, a complete and candid history, the parent generally acquiesces. Most parents have some awareness of the needs of their teenager and are grateful for the time spent by the clinician with their child. When appropriate, it is helpful to encourage the teenager to share information with her parents.

It is important not to place a teen in a situation where she feels forced to lie. If a parent refuses to leave the room, it is best not to ask questions that the teen may not wish to discuss in front of a parent.

Issues for the Male Clinician

The male clinician faces particular challenges with the female adolescent. The physician may have been the patient's doctor from infancy, may treat other family members, and may be surprised one day to find out that his 12- or 13-year-old patient now requests to see his female colleague. Sometimes this issue arises when the patient is as young as 8- or 9-years-old. This serves as a reminder that much of what physicians do involves potentially awkward and embarrassing situations. These situations can be particularly uncomfortable for a teenage girl, for whom gender and sexuality may be important preoccupations.

The adult literature reveals that a patient is more likely to receive a complete reproductive health history and examination if he or she sees a physician of the same sex; the explanation is patient and physician discomfort with male physician-female patient dyads and female physician-male patient dyads. This poses a particular risk for the adolescent girl who presents to the male clinician for anxiety-provoking experiences such as the first pelvic examination and Papanicolaou smear. The first pelvic examination is particularly important in a teen's health care because if it is not done with patience and reassurance, she may not return for another such examination. This would be very dangerous at the point in her life where she is at the greatest risk for STDs and unplanned pregnancy.

There are several steps that the male clinician can take to make his interaction with the adolescent female patient more comfortable. He should take care to maintain the patient's modesty with gowns and drapes. He should have a female chaperone present for any examination of the breasts or genitals. He should acknowledge any discomfort the patient may have in seeing a male physician and offer to recommend the patient to a female colleague for future examinations. Finally, he should make sure that he himself is very comfortable obtaining these histories and performing these physical examinations on teenage girls; this may require acknowledging what makes him uncomfortable and taking steps to enhance his skills and comfort level in those areas.

Interviewing Adolescents

A. THE JOINT INTERVIEW

After reviewing the confidentiality issue, the clinician may begin by asking the teenager why she is seeking medical attention. Directing questions to the teenager rather than the parent helps empower the young person. It is important for clinicians to establish themselves as the adolescent's advocate rather than as an agent of the parent; at the same time, physicians must avoid an adversarial relationship with the parent. If the clinician has previously gained knowledge of the adolescent's situation from any source, such as a school note or phone call, it makes good sense to mention this at the beginning of the interview, thereby avoiding a difficult situation later that may compromise the provider's or the teenager's credibility.

During this limited joint interview, it is useful to include the parent in the collection of data, gathering information regarding pertinent aspects of the adolescent's birth history, perinatal events, immunization history, family history, and history of allergies that the teenager may not know. This discussion is a practical way of educating the teenager about her childhood medical history. The joint interview also can be a time to observe family dynamics and to develop a rapport with the parent. Following this brief shared interview, a feedback session may be arranged for the summation when findings and recommendations can be reviewed with both the adolescent and the parent within the guidelines of confidentiality.

B. THE ADOLESCENT INTERVIEW

Teenagers often give a different reason for their visit once they are afforded privacy with the clinician. Communication may be facilitated by beginning this section of the interview with noncontroversial, open-ended questions. Data can be gathered via both verbal and nonverbal communication.

The interview technique must be tailored to the developmental stage of the adolescent; for example, young teenagers may have a difficult time with open-ended questions.

C. MEDICAL HISTORY

The medical history includes questions about past illnesses, past surgeries, medications, allergies, and immunizations, and includes a review of systems similar to that conducted for an adult. In the review of systems for adolescents, particular attention should be paid to questions concerning weight changes, exercise, abdominal pains, respiratory problems, genitourinary or menstrual problems, and visual changes. To screen for an eating disorder, the clinician might ask the teenager how she feels about her current weight, whether she has ever attempted to lose weight and if so, how—by restricting food intake; by using laxatives, diuretics, diet pills; or by purging. Two screening questions with sensitivity and specificity for eating disorders are "Do you ever eat in secret?" and "Are you satisfied with your eating patterns?" The menstrual history should include onset of menarche, length of time between periods, nature of flow, cramping, midcycle spotting, vaginal discharge, and breast symptoms.

D. PSYCHOSOCIAL HISTORY

Because the "social morbidities" (sexual behavior, substance abuse, and injury) are the most common causes of adolescent morbidity and mortality, the psychosocial interview is a major portion of the history gathered.

1. The HEADS Interview—The HEADS questions provide clinicians with an easy-to-use structure for assessing the high-risk behaviors of adolescents. Variations on the HEADS interview have been used in adolescent medicine for the last three decades; it continues to provide the best structure for the adolescent interview. A suggested version follows:

Home
Education/Employment
(Eating/Exercise)
Activities (Arrests)
Drugs
Depression/Suicide
Sexuality

The HEADS interview can be conducted in a few minutes, with one line written per item, or it can be an in-depth psychosocial interview requiring an hour of time and several pages of notes, depending on both the presenting complaint and the clinical situation. It is essential, however, to include some variation of these questions in every adolescent encounter. The answers to these questions will often be more significant than the identified chief complaint, and will often in fact be the unspoken reason for the office visit.

2. HEADS Questions—Following are some examples of questions that can be asked during the interview.

(1) **Home:** Who lives at home with you? (Presence/absence of father?) Is there anyone new in the household? Basic family medical history questions can also be included here.

(2) **Education/Employment:** What school do you go to? (Are you in school?) What grade are you in? (Is this the appropriate grade for age?) How is school going? Are you working? How many hours per week? (In addition to school?)

(3) **Eating/Exercise:** (Can be asked selectively.) Are you happy with your weight? Do you have any questions about your nutrition? What is the most you have ever weighed? What is the least? Have you ever tried to lose weight? How? How long do you exercise each day? What do you do? And how much?

(4) **Activities:** What do you like to do in your free time? What types of activities are you involved with? (Sports? Dance? Religious groups? Girl Scouts? Asking about supportive, positive activities is as important as asking about risk behaviors.) Selectively: Have you ever been arrested? Is there any gang activity at your school or in your neighborhood? Are any of your friends involved with gang activities? Wear gang colors?

(5) **Drugs:** Do you smoke (tobacco)? How many cigarettes a day? When did you start? (pack-years?) When did you last drink any alcohol? How much is "a lot" for you? How often do you drink that much? (selectively: **CAGE** questions – Felt the need to **C**ut down? Have others **A**nnoyed you by commenting on your use? Have you ever felt **G**uilt about your use? Have you ever needed an **E**ye-opener/alcohol first thing in the morning?) What drugs have you ever tried or experimented with? How often? IV drug use?

(6) **Depression/Suicide:** Do you ever feel sad or depressed? How often? Have you ever thought about injuring yourself or about suicide? Have you ever tried (or made a plan)? Did you tell anyone about this? Have you ever been in counseling?

(7) **Sexuality:** How old were you when you had your first menstrual period? When was your most recent period? Do you find yourself attracted to boys? girls? both? Have you ever had any sexual experiences with anyone? (Type of experiences, number of partners: male and/or female.) Have you ever been pregnant? Use of contraception? Condoms? Last pelvic examination? History of STDs? Current need for contraception? Have you ever felt threatened or been physically injured by a date or by someone you were going out with? Has anyone ever made you have sex when you did not want to?

Physical Examination

Most adolescents are extremely sensitive and concerned about their rapidly changing body. Reassurance during the physical examination that the findings are within the normal range can alleviate many unspoken fears and concerns. Reassurance can be as simple as telling the patient how strong her heart sounds or that her lungs sound clear. Physical variations noted during the examination that could cause body image anxiety, such as obesity, early or late pubertal development, or acne, should be mentioned and discussed. If the provider notices a physical problem, it is likely that the teenager has noticed it also and is concerned. Adolescents usually are grateful for the opportunity to discuss their concerns if the topics are approached sensitively. Often, education regarding the prevalence, natural history, and treatment options can relieve anxiety about a concern.

Yearly charting of height, weight, BMI (body mass index) if indicated, and pubertal development (Tanner stage) is useful as a means of tracking growth. Heights can be plotted on a height velocity curve so that the physician can evaluate whether the growth spurt has begun. Further evaluation may be necessary if a girl does not reach the growth spurt by age 12. Blood pressure should be measured. The need for dental referral should be assessed by examining her teeth for caries and malocclusion. Visual and auditory assessment are particularly important because deficits in these areas may be a source of embarrassment and may not be reported initially. Visual screening should be done at the initial visit and repeated every 2–3 years. Auditory testing should be done at least one time during adolescence. The thyroid should be examined for nodularity or enlargement. Examination of the skin should focus on the presence of acne or hirsutism.

Examination of the breasts allows for Tanner staging, evaluation for disparity in size, and introduction to breast self-examination for the older adolescent. Although breasts may begin to develop asynchronously, disparity in size often corrects itself.

The orthopedic examination should focus on problems that present during puberty. This would include an evaluation of gait to rule out slipped capital femoral epiphysis, of the tibial tubercle to rule out Osgood-Schlatter disease, and of the spine to evaluate for scoliosis. Scoliosis screening is important in early adolescence, as any detectible curvature may worsen during the growth spurt.

The timing of an adolescent's first pelvic examination remains somewhat controversial. A pelvic examination is not required for teenagers who have not yet had any sexual activity. Cervical cancer screening (Papanicolaou [Pap] smear) is needed within 3 years of the onset of vaginal intercourse and should probably be initiated (even in the absence of sexual activity) by age 21. Pelvic examinations are not necessary before initiating hormonal contraception but should be included in follow-up examinations. Once an adolescent girl begins to have vaginal intercouse, annual pelvic examinations should be done.

For a first pelvic examination, it is worthwhile to spend some time reviewing the normal female anatomy with a model or a drawing and explaining what the examination will entail. This exercise can help dispel any myths the teenager may have heard about pelvic examinations. Following this discussion with a review of the indications for a pelvic examination educates the adolescent as to what she can expect that day and on subsequent visits.

It may be helpful to acknowledge during the first pelvic examination that some girls worry about the examination being painful or embarrassing. Talking with the teenager about what she has heard about the examination and addressing those issues can be reassuring. Letting the teenager know that she is in control at all times and that the provider will stop the examination if she asks is a useful way to reframe a situation that may make the patient feel vulnerable.

A routine yearly pelvic examination is recommended beginning at age 18–21 in women who have never been active sexually. For teenagers who are currently active sexually, a pelvic examination is indicated every 6–12 months or with each new partner.

The routine pelvic examination in an adolescent includes a Pap smear and screening for STDs including gonorrhea, chlamydia, and trichomoniasis, as well as serologies for syhillis and HIV testing. In all adolescents, particular attention should be paid to inspection of the external genitalia, checking for nonambiguous genitalia, clitoral size (usually 2–4 mm wide), distribution and characteristics of pubic hair (for pubertal development), signs of mucosal estrogenization, and hymen patency. The cervix in adolescents often has an ectropion, which is a red and rough area surrounding the os that represents the endocervical columnar cells extending on to the exocervix. Ectropion is of concern only if it is very large or extends onto the lateral walls of the vagina.

At the end of the visit, a summary of the findings, the diagnosis, and the recommendations is discussed with the adolescent. Following this discussion, the parent may be brought back into the room for a joint summary of the findings and treatment plan within the boundaries of confidentiality.

Centers for Disease Control and Prevention. Sexually transmitted diseases treatment guidelines 2002. MMWR 2002;51(RR-6).

Cohen E, Mackenzie RG, Yates GL: HEADS, a psychosocial risk assessment instrument: implications for designing effective intervention programs for runaway youth. J Adolesc Health 1991;12:539. [PMID: 1772892]

ANTICIPATORY GUIDANCE

Adolescent Sexuality

Gender and sexuality are issues that are often very confusing for the preadolescent and adolescent. Developmental theory shows that children can identify themselves as a boy or a girl from a very young age and demonstrate understanding of gender roles. Children as young as 3- to 4-years-old exhibit stereotyped gender behavior, with girls choosing dolls and playing house and boys preferring to play with trucks. Gender, however, is not a quality that is simply attained and thereafter established. Much remains to be determined about how a person will accommodate to the internal and external pressures secondary to gender roles. Conflicts about what clothes one will wear, what games one will play, which playmates one will befriend, and who one will choose for romance require frequent rethinking and rearranging of one's concept of gender.

Questions and confusion about gender often reach a critical point during adolescence, a time when there are many pressures from peers to conform to norms of behavior and appearance. Dating and sexual exploration also become prominent developmental milestones. Many teens will have doubts about their sexuality, and they may find it difficult to admit that they find themselves attracted to the same sex partners. For some persons, these feelings will be transient, and they will ultimately choose partners of the opposite sex and will identify themselves as heterosexual. Other teens will continue to find themselves attracted to people of the same sex. All teens can benefit from the guidance of a sensitive physician.

The girl who is confused about her sexual orientation should be reassured that this is normal for an adolescent, and that she should not feel embarrassed or guilty about her feelings. She should be encouraged to allow the decision to happen over time, not to rush herself to feel something that she does not. Many of these girls will, over time, choose male partners and identify themselves as heterosexual. This is still not the final step in resolving confusion about sexuality and gender. The heterosexual teen may be faced with particular pressures; pressure to have sex, date rape, and partner violence are realities that a physician should discuss with teens.

Other teenage girls may continue their attraction to other girls and may ultimately define themselves as bisexual or homosexual. In addition to some of the risks that face heterosexual girls, lesbian and bisexual girls are at increased risk for depression, substance abuse, homelessness, and suicide. Gay and bisexual teens who come out to their parents may be punished, devalued, beaten, or disowned. Some parents do demonstrate tolerance and acceptance of their gay or bisexual teen and can become tremendously supportive of their children. Physicians can help the teen who is thinking about coming out to her parents by asking her to think about these questions: Are you sure about your sexual orientation? Do you have support in case your parents are angry with you? Are you financially dependent on your parents, and if so, what will you do if they withdraw that support? Can you be patient if it takes your parents months or years to accept what you have to say to them? The physician should help the teen to consider these issues before recommending that she come out to her parents. Physicians should also ask gay adolescent teens about any violence they have suffered because of their sexual orientation.

Physicians can foster trust in adolescent patients about these issues by using neutral language during the history and physical examination and never assuming that a patient is homosexual or heterosexual. An easy way to bring up the subject is to say, "Do you have a boyfriend or a girlfriend?" Most patients will find this direct question surprising, which gives the provider the chance to say, "Well, I have gay and straight patients, so I never assume anything," or some such variation with which you are comfortable. In fact, your own comfort level with discussing these issues is probably the most important factor that will determine whether a teen opens up to you with her questions of gender and sexuality. Most cities have a gay and lesbian community center where you can find information and handouts about resources available to teens in your community.

Sexual Activity

Most teens engage in some form of sexual activity by the time they reach their 21st birthday. Some persons begin as early as 10- and 11-years-old. This means that a physician cannot begin early enough to talk about puberty, sexual behavior, STDs, and pregnancy.

Details about the transmission, diagnosis, and treatment of individual STDs can be found in Chapter 34. It is important to remember that the risk for the teen patient of contracting an STD is very high because of the persistently low use of adequate protection. Nearly one third of sexually active adolescents do not regularly use contraception; even fewer regularly use a barrier method. The physician should strive to frequently discuss the risk of STDs and pregnancy with their teen patients, to increase the opportunities to educate the patient, and to provide access to contraception and barrier methods. Offer free condoms discreetly in the office to both male and female patients. Be knowledgeable about community resources for free testing and treatment of STDs. Encourage teen patients to discuss contraception and STD protection with their parents but remember that parental consent is not necessary for these prescriptions.

Adolescent Pregnancy

There are more than 1,225,000 teen pregnancies in the United States each year, resulting in 400,000 births per year. For every 100 pregnant teenaged girls in the United States, 55 will give birth to a live infant, 15 will miscarry, and 30 will have an induced abortion. Teen pregnancy poses a number of serious risks both for the baby and the mother. The infant is more likely to be premature, to have intrauterine growth retardation, and developmental disabilities. The child is also more likely to experience child neglect or abuse as it grows older. The teen mother is more likely to experience hypertension, anemia, and preterm labor than older mothers. They are at risk for not returning to school and are at increased risk for domestic violence. One quarter of teen mothers will have a second child within 2 years of their first childbirth. The physician should do his or her best to prevent unplanned teen pregnancy by acknowledging that it is a risk for all teenage girls and should be talked about openly and repeatedly. Methods of birth control are discussed in Chapter 52. It should be remembered that emergency contraception is an important adjunct to any form of contraception prescribed and is particularly relevant for teens who frequently fail to use contraception during intercourse.

If a pregnant teen patient comes to her physician for advice, be ready to discuss all options available. The clinician should explore the patient's support structure, the likelihood that her parents will be accepting and helpful, and the likelihood that the baby's father will be involved. The patient's level of maturity should be assessed, paying attention to the patient's plans for the future. The patient should be asked whether she wants to continue with the pregnancy or if she is planning an abortion. If she plans to continue with the pregnancy, refer her for her obstetric care but continue to see her for her other health issues and, if appropriate, offer to be the baby's physician as well. This continuity of care can be a support for the patient. If the teen chooses abortion, know what resources are available in your community. Be aware of cost and insurance issues, because if a teen delays the abortion by several weeks to find the necessary funds, she places herself at greater medical risk.

Substance Abuse

Substance abuse has reached epidemic proportions in the adolescent community. The first drug used is often nicotine. By the age of 11, one of five adolescents has smoked cigarettes, and by age 15, one of seven smokes

Table 1–3. Herbs and dietary supplements commonly used by adolescent girls.

Use	Supplement	Chemical Constituent	Scientific Evidence of Efficacy	Side Effects, Risks, Interactions
PMS	Chasteberry (*Vitex agnus-castus*)	Sex steroids, flavonoids, iridoid, glycosides	Several randomly controlled trials suggest possible benefit in PMS. No studies on long-term use or use by teens.	Stomach upset, itching, mild rash
	Evening primrose oil (EPO) (*Oenothera biennsis*)	Gamma lineolic acid (GLA)	Of five randomized placebo-controlled trials, most were of insufficient quality to draw a clear conclusion about EPO's efficacy. Two randomized, controlled studies suggest that EPO is helpful in treating PMS-associated breast pain.	GI distress, headache
	Dong quai root (*Angelica sinensis*)	Furocoumarins, β-sitosterol, flavonoids	Chinese case studies report benefits with menstrual irregularities. No controlled studies exist.	GI upset, rash, photo-sensitivity, enhanced effect of anticoagulants
UTI	Cranberry (*Vaccinium macrocarpon*)	Proanthocyanidin	Case-control study and double-blind controlled studies demonstrate utility of cranberry in UTI prophylaxis.	Those sensitive to the effects of sugar should use cranberry with caution
	Uva ursi/bearberry (*Areto-staphylos uva-ursi*)	Hydroquinones: arbutins and tannins	Case series and one randomized controlled trial support efficacy.	GI toxicity. Do not use with urine acidifiers
Weight loss	Dandelion (*Taraxacum officinale*)	Sesquiter-pene lac-tones (bitters), triterpenses and sterols, flavonoids, mucilage, and inulin	No human studies.	Rare allergic reaction in sensitive persons
	Senna (*Cassia senna*)	Anthraquinone glycosides	Controlled studies in humans show efficacy as a laxative.	Cramps, diarrhea. Chronic use can lead to dependency and low potassium levels
	Ma huang (*Ephedra sinica*)	Ephedrine, pseudoephedrine	Two randomized controlled studies show benefit; one shows no benefit.	Insomnia, restlessness, anxiety, irritability, tachycardia, cardiac arrhythmias, hypertension, dependence, and death. Contraindicated in patients with diabetes, glaucoma, and thyroid disease and those taking MAO inhibitors

PMS, premenstrual syndrome: UTI, urinary tract infection; GI, gastrointestinal; MAO, monoamine oxidase.
Reprinted with permission from Gardiner P, Conboy L, Kemper K. Herbs and adolescent girls: Avoiding the hazards of self-treatment. *Contemp Pediatr.* 2000;17(3):133–154.

daily. The mean age of onset for cigarette smoking is 12. Sixty percent of adults who smoke began by the time they were 14, and essentially all adult smokers began smoking when underage. The only population with increasing numbers of cigarette smokers is female adolescents. Besides the serious health risks posed by cigarette use itself, smoking may be the earliest sign of difficulties to come; cigarette smoking at a young age is a marker for children at increased risk for other unhealthy behaviors.

Alcohol is the most commonly abused substance among adolescents, with 39% of high school seniors reporting getting drunk within the past 2 weeks and at least 90% of high school seniors reporting some alcohol use. As many as 4.2% of high school seniors report daily use. The mean age of onset of alcohol consumption is 12.6. Alcohol-related injuries account for one of five deaths in teenagers between the ages of 15 and 20.

Marijuana is used daily by 9% of high school seniors. The average age of onset for marijuana use is 14.4 years. There are a multitude of other drugs that are used by teenagers with negative sequelae. Besides the dangers of the drugs themselves, poor judgment is the rule while under the influence. Adolescents who are intoxicated may engage in other high-risk activities, such as unsafe sex or riding in a motor vehicle with an intoxicated driver, that they would not engage in if they were sober.

Other substances are increasing in abuse. Reviews discussing inhalant abuse, Ecstasy (MDMA), GHB, and ketamine are listed in the references.

Graeme KA: New drugs of abuse. Emerg Med Clin North Am 2000;18:625. [PMID: 11130930]

Kurtzman TL, Otsuka KN, Wahl RA: Inhalant abuse by adolescents. J Adolesc Health 2001;28:170. Available at http://www.medicinedirect.com/journal/journal?sdid=5072 [PMID: 11226839]

COMPLEMENTARY & ALTERNATIVE APPROACHES

As adolescents seek increased independence in their daily lives, more teens look to complementary and alternative modalities in their self-treatment of common adolescent health concerns. The ready availability of over-the-counter supplements and the anticipated safety of "natural" products lead many teens to self-medicate with various herbal preparations. Herbs used by teens for weight loss, or to treat premenstrual symptoms and urinary tract infections are listed in Table 1–3.

Gardiner P, Conboy LA, Kemper KJ: Herbs and adolescent girls: avoiding the hazards of self-treatment. Contemp Pediatr 2000;17:133. Available from http://www.contemporarypediatrics.com [PMID: 10660631]

RELEVANT WEB SITES

Almost all teens in the United States now have access to the Internet, either at home, in school, or in a public library. Adolescents are often more proficient at computer use than are their parents or physicians and make great use of resources found on web pages. Much of this information is helpful, useful, and accurate but much of it is derived from very questionable sources.

The Internet sites listed below are likely to provide reliable information to the teen, her parents, and her physician. Please be advised that there is no guarantee about these sites, and some of the listed web addresses are very likely to be out of date by the time this book is in print. All sites were verified as of August 2002.

For Teens

[The Children's Hospital of Boston site for young women]
http://www.youngwomenshealth.org/
[American Social Health Association: I Wanna Know]
http://www.iwannaknow.org
[Kid's Health Site: Alfred I. duPont Hospital for Children in Wilmington, DE]
http://www.kidshealth.org
[TeenGrowth.com: well researched information aimed at adolescents]
http://www.teengrowth.com
Parents, Families, and Friends of Lesbians and Gays
http://www.pflag.org

For Physicians

[Society for Adolescent Medicine]
http://www.adolescenthealth.org/
[International Association for Adolescent Health]
http://www.iaah.org/index.html
[Guidelines for Adolescent Preventive Services (GAPS)—AMA]
http://www.ama-assn.org
[Sexuality Information and Education Council of the U.S. (SIECUS)]
http://www.siecus.org
[The National Campaign to Prevent Teen Pregnancy]
http://www.teenpregnancy.org
[Children Now and the Kaiser Family Foundation: Talking with Kids About Tough Issues]
http://www.talkingwithkids.org
[MedScout: Web hub for medical sites. Wide variety of adolescent links, some excellent, some not]
http://www.medscout.com/health/adolescent
[CDC Biennial Youth Risk Behavior Surveys]
http://www.cdc.gov/nccdphp/youthris.htm

Health Care for Lesbians

Patricia A. Robertson, MD

Approximately 5% of female patients are lesbian or women who have affection for or attraction to other women. Lesbians are diverse in terms of cultural background, ethnic or racial identity, age, education, income, and place of residence (although there is a higher prevalence of lesbians in urban rather than rural areas). When women identify themselves as lesbians, about 15% of them are sexually active with men as well as women. Some women identify themselves as bisexual, implying sexual activity with both genders.

The Institute of Medicine recently declared lesbians as an underserved minority by the medical care system in the United States because of access issues and concern by lesbians that if they seek care from traditional sources, they will experience discrimination based on sexual orientation. In general, lesbians and bisexual women have decreased access to care than heterosexual women. The epidemiologic issues in lesbian health care are just now being defined. However, some areas of lesbian health have been studied so far with case-control data, small quantitative studies, and some qualitative studies. Hopefully, research funding in the future will be available to identify areas of need for lesbians and bisexual women to improve their health care.

Diamant A et al: Health behaviors, health status and access to and use of health care: a population-based study of lesbians, bisexual and heterosexual women. Arch Fam Med 2000;9:1043.

Institute of Medicine, Lesbian Health: Current Assessment and Direction for the Future, National Academy Press, Washington DC, 1999.

DISCLOSURE OF SEXUAL ORIENTATION

Disclosure rates to physicians by their lesbian patients vary. Most lesbians prefer that their primary care provider know about their sexual orientation, but unless these patients are specifically asked about their sexual partners, most do not spontaneously disclose their sexual orientation.

Lesbians of color disclose even less frequently than white women. It is very important to have office forms that have additional options to "married," "single," or "divorced" on the initial paperwork, such as "domestic partner" or "other." When a history is taken by the practitioner, the question "Are you sexually active with men, women, both, or neither" is very appropriate for all patients and allows patients to realize that the practitioner's approach is inclusive. It is imperative that clinicians do not assume all female patients are heterosexual.

It is important to obtain patient permission before noting a sexual orientation in the medical record because some lesbians may face discrimination in the workplace if their employer sees their medical file (eg, for disability reasons). About 70% of lesbians are in monogamous same-sex relationships. If a lesbian patient is in a relationship with a woman who the patient would like to designate as the person who will make medical decisions if she becomes incapacitated, remind the patient that power of attorney forms need to be completed and kept up to date. It is very useful for the patient to give a copy to her primary practitioner for her office chart.

Because many lesbians have had difficult experiences with the health care system, there will often be a partner or friend present with the lesbian patient. If the partner is present for the initial history, it is important to have time to privately interview the patient to screen for domestic violence, drug and alcohol use, and so on.

PRIMARY CARE ISSUES/SCREENING

Recent studies have documented that self-identified lesbians have increased body mass index. In general, an increased body mass index increases the risk of cardiovascular disease, certain cancers, and orthopedic disabilities in later years. In this same study, it was noted that lesbians participate in more vigorous exercise than heterosexual women do; the relationship of this finding to any increased cardiovascular risks due to a high body mass index needs to be clarified in future research.

A study by Koh found that bisexual women were less likely than heterosexual women to have cholesterol screening (OD 0.29) or appropriate mammography (OD 0.33). A history of illicit substance use was higher in lesbians in this study compared with heterosexual women (OD 2.04), so appropriate screening for hepatitis C and B infections should be done. In a recent study in Australia, the hepatitis C antibody was found in more lesbians than heterosexual women attending a public clinic (OR 7.7).

Aaron D et al: Behavioral risk factors for disease and preventive health practices among lesbians. Am J Public Health 2001; 91:972.

Fethers K et al: Sexually transmitted infections and risk behaviors in women who have sex with women. Sex Transm Infect 2000;76:345.

Koh A: Use of preventive health behaviors by lesbian, bisexual, and heterosexual women: questionnaire survey. West J Med 2000; 172:379.

REPRODUCTIVE TRACT ISSUES

In general, lesbians have fewer sexually transmitted infections than heterosexual women, so screening should be done according to the individual history and risk factors. There may be an increased rate of bacterial vaginosis in lesbians, but the clinical significance is unclear at this time. There is a decreased incidence of genital warts in lesbians (OR 0.7), but a significant number of lesbians have been exposed to the human papillomavirus (13%).

All lesbians need Papanicolaou's (Pap) smears according to established guidelines for heterosexual women. The vast majority of lesbians have been heterosexually active in the past (about 90%), and in general, lesbians have a decreased frequency of Pap smears compared with heterosexual women. Cervical dysplasia can develop in lesbians who have never been sexually active with men. Lesbians should be routinely screened with Pap smears.

Compared with heterosexual women, lesbians may be at increased risk for HIV infection because of sexual contact with men who have an increased risk of being infected with HIV (gay men, for example). Lesbians as a group have approximately a 10% risk of having a history of injection drug use; thus, HIV screening for lesbians should be done according to the usual risk guidelines.

Increasing numbers of lesbians are becoming pregnant, either through donor insemination or intercourse with a friend. As with heterosexual women, it is important that lesbians of reproductive age consume daily multi-vitamins; vitamins need to be taken for 3 months before conception to decrease the rate of birth defects. If a lesbian patient requests information on resources such as sperm banks, infertility clinics, and so on, it is important to refer her appropriately. Currently, approximately 75% of Assisted Reproductive Technology practices offer services to lesbian patients.

Children raised in a family with lesbian parents have no significant differences from those children raised in families with heterosexual parents. The American Academy of Pediatricians recently released a Technical Bulletin emphasizing that children who grow up with 1 or 2 gay and/or lesbian parents fare as well in emotional, cognitive, social, and sexual functioning as do children whose parents are heterosexual.

Furthermore, it is very important that lesbians who are considering parenting consult a family attorney with specialized expertise in family law in the state where the lesbian lives. The current laws frequently do not cover these alternative families, and contracts may need to be put in place to safeguard the interests of all participating prospective parents.

Unintended pregnancies do occur in lesbians, especially in lesbian adolescents, so counseling about preventing unintended pregnancy is very important. In the 1987 Minnesota Adolescent Health Survey, bisexual (33%) and lesbian (29%) respondents were about as likely as heterosexual adolescents to have had intercourse. However, lesbian and bisexual respondents had a significantly higher prevalence of pregnancy (12%) and physical or sexual abuse (20%) than heterosexual or unsure adolescents.

Brewaeys A: Review: parent-child relationships and child development in donor insemination families: Hum Reprod Update 2001;7:38. [PMID: 11212073]

Fethers K et al: Sexually transmitted infections and risk behaviors in women who have sex with women. Sex Transm Infect 2000;76:345.

Marrazo J et al: Papanicolaou test screening and prevalence of genital human papillomavirus among women who have sex with women: Am J Public Health 2001;91:947.

Perrin E: Technical report: coparent or second-parent adoption by same-sex parents. Pediatrics 2002;109:341. [PMID: 11826220]

Saewyc E et al: Sexual intercourse, abuse, and pregnancy among adolescent women: does sexual orientation make a difference? Fam Plann Perspect 1999;31:127. [PMID: 10379429]

Stern J et al: Access to services at assisted reproductive technology clinics: a survey of policies and practices: Am J Obstet Gynecol 2001;184:591.

CANCER

Indirect evidence suggests that lesbians may have a higher incidence of cancer than heterosexual women—specifically colon cancer (risk factor of increased body mass index), breast cancer (risk factors of nulliparity and increased body mass index), lung cancer (risk factor of increased smoking), cervical cancer (risk factor of infrequent Pap smears), and ovarian cancer (risk factors of increased body mass index and decreased oral contraceptive use).

Dibble S, Roberts S, Robertson P: Risk factors for ovarian cancer: lesbian and heterosexual women. Oncol Nurs Forum 2002; 29:E1.

Roberts S et al: Differences in risk factors for breast cancer: lesbian and heterosexual women: Journal of the Gay and Lesbian Medical Association 1998;2:93.

MENTAL HEALTH ISSUES

There is a lack of methodologically sound epidemiologic data on the prevalence of mental disorders in lesbians. A higher frequency of the experience of discrimination may underlie some observations of greater psychiatric morbidity among lesbians. Certainly, depression has been underdiagnosed for years in all women, and lesbians may be at higher risk because of this experience of discrimination. Treatment of depression in lesbians mirrors that of heterosexual women, although there are some important differences of which primary care providers should be aware. Lesbians may be less accepting of medication and more accepting of psychotherapy as a treatment for depression. If psychotherapy is recommended, the primary care provider should be sure that the lesbian is being referred to either a lesbian therapist or someone experienced with lesbian clients. Unfortunately, many lesbian women have spent hours and money with a heterosexual therapist only to educate the therapist about lesbian issues but without getting what she needs out of the therapy.

When the sisters of lesbians are used for a control group in terms of mental health status, Rothblum found no differences except that the lesbians had higher self-esteem. She did find that bisexual women had significantly poorer mental health than did lesbians and their heterosexual sisters.

There is evidence that lesbian women are more likely than heterosexual women to meet the definition for childhood sexual abuse, which is associated with an increased incidence of lifetime alcohol abuse in both lesbian and heterosexual women.

Sexual assault is very common in both lesbians and heterosexual women, with the incidence being approximately 40% in surveys. The difference between lesbian and heterosexual assaults was that 0% of the lesbian women received follow-up counseling. Many lesbians attribute incidences of sexual assault with ongoing sexual problems in relationships.

Hughes T, Johnson T, Wilsnach C: Sexual assault and alcohol abuse: a comparison of lesbian and heterosexual women. J Subst Abuse 2001;13:515.

Mays V, Cochran S: Mental health correlates of perceived discrimination among lesbians, gay, and bisexual adults in the United States. Am J Public Health 2001;91:1869.

Rothblum E, Factor R: Lesbians and their sisters as a control group: demographic and mental health factors. Psychol Sci 200112: 63. [PMID: 11294230]

SUBSTANCE USE

Lesbian and bisexual women younger than 50-years-old are more likely to smoke and drink heavily than heterosexual women. Specifically, lesbian and bisexual women aged 20–34 report higher weekly alcohol consumption and less abstention compared with heterosexual women. Cigarette smoking is also increased in lesbian and bisexual women.

Fethers K et al: Sexually transmitted infections and risk behaviors in women who have sex with women. Sex Transm Infect 2000;76:345.

Gruskin E et al: Patterns of cigarette smoking and alcohol use among lesbian and bisexual women enrolled in a large health maintenance organization. Am J Public Health 2001;91:976.

DOMESTIC VIOLENCE

About 47% of lesbians have been victimized by a same-sex partner in the past. Many factors for lesbian battering are similar to those in the incidents of heterosexual partner abuse (eg, concurrent use of substances such as alcohol). Counseling resources and shelters are usually quite limited for battered lesbians, compounded by the problem of inadequate training of counselors in domestic violence in the lesbian community.

In one study, less than half of the counselors had coursework or practical experience pertaining to domestic violence and lesbian concerns. These counselors perceived heterosexual battering as more violent than lesbian battering, even though the presented scenarios were the same except for the difference in sexual orientation.

Burke L, Follingstad D: Violence in lesbian and gay relationships: theory, prevalence, and correlational factors: Clin Psychol Rev 1999;19:487. [PMID: 10467488]

Waldner-Haugrud L, Gratch L, Magruder B: Victimization and perpetuation rates of violence in gay and lesbian relationship: gender issues explored. Violence Vict 1997;12:173. [PMID: 9403987]

Wise A, Bowman S: Comparison of beginning counselors' responses to lesbian vs. heterosexual partner abuse. Violence Vict 1997;12:127. [PMID: 9403983]

TRANSSEXUAL HEALTH ISSUES

Transsexuals are persons who are biologically one gender but who identify themselves as members of the opposite gender. Transgendered is a broader term, referring to persons who are transsexual, as well as cross-dressers, biologically intersexed, or persons otherwise challenging strict gender norms.

The diagnosis of gender identity disorder should be established by a qualified and experienced mental health professional. Once a diagnosis has been established, hormones are usually prescribed (surgery is not always pursued). Because the doses of the hormones are higher than those prescribed for heterosexuals (eg, for menopausal replacement), a very careful history and physical examination needs to be done. An excellent summary article on the medical care of the transsexual patient with accompanying hormone regimens is available. A retrospective study compared mortality in 816 male-to-female and 293 female-to-male patients with age- and gender-matched standardized ratios from the Dutch population and found no increased mortality among the gender patients taking hormones; however, there was a 20-fold increase in thrombolic events in the patients taking estrogen and a significant increase in suicide. Transgendered people frequently seek hormones from nontraditional sources, fearing that they will be misunderstood by traditional medical practitioners. As with lesbian and bisexual women, it is important to be reassuring that treatment by traditional practitioners can be nonjudgmental and supportive.

Oriel K: Medical care of transsexual patients. Journal of the Gay and Lesbian Medical Association 2000;4:185.

When to Refer to a Specialist

When referring lesbians to subspecialists, it is important to consider, whenever possible, lesbian friendly providers. A resource that may be helpful to primary care providers is the Gay and Lesbian Medical Health Association, which maintains lists of friendly providers for these patients.

SUMMARY

Lesbian health issues regarding specific health risks and medical communications are just now beginning to be studied. The access and sensitivity practitioners can provide has a great impact on the health of lesbian patients because getting them into the office is the first step in addressing their health care needs. At this time, it is essential to carefully inquire about such health issues as past and present drug (including cigarettes) and alcohol use, depression, family planning, and prevention of sexually transmitted diseases including HIV, mammograms, cholesterol screening, domestic violence, and a history of sexual abuse. It is important that lesbian-friendly referrals are available for patients whose problems are outside the realm of the primary care practitioner. Primary practitioners should be an advocate for the nonjudgmental care of lesbian patients, whether that be in an office or a hospital setting.

Ethical Issues

3

Lorna A. Marshall, MD

Ethics is the formal study of moral behavior in which moral obligations are analyzed in terms of recognized values and principles of society. Ethics becomes important in health care when personal determinations about what is right and wrong become inadequate to reach resolution of conflicting values. A logical and disciplined approach to a complex ethical problem becomes necessary. A full discussion of the various theories and processes of ethics that can be used in clinical decision-making is beyond the scope of this chapter. Four basic ethical principles are used frequently in approaching clinical situations:

1. Autonomy—the respect for self-determination of the patient.
2. Beneficence—the duty to do what is good for the patient.
3. Nonmaleficence—the duty to avoid harming the patient.
4. Justice—the right of the patient to be treated fairly and to a fair allocation of society's resources.

Ethical issues that are specific to women often involve choices regarding sexuality and reproduction, including choices that involve obligations to the fetus. However, ethical issues can be identified in all stages of a woman's life and often focus on issues of gender equality and the right of women to equal consideration and just treatment.

CHILDHOOD

Parents are the recognized surrogate decision makers for their children. If the parents disagree about health care decisions, or if the health care provider believes that the parents are not acting in the best interest of the child, conflict may occur. Such disagreement may arise in cases of young women who have been victims of abuse or rape. One or both parents may refuse to give permission for health care, perhaps because of the involvement of a family member. The health care provider must consider whether the parent is acting in the best interest of the child; if it is believed that the parent is not acting in the child's interest, the court may be asked to appoint a guardian. Choices such as these should be made with careful consideration for all the facts of the case. The potential harm to children of causing a rift between their parents can be a compelling reason against proceeding further.

ADOLESCENCE

The identification of a surrogate decision maker for adolescents becomes especially difficult when decisions about contraceptive care and abortion are necessary. It is important for health care providers to know the laws in their state regarding parental notification or consent. Most states allow minors to give consent for treatment of sexually transmitted diseases. Most states also allow pregnant minors to give consent for procedures on themselves and usually on their offspring. However, the majority of states require parental consent or notification before a provider can perform an abortion on a minor, although many states do not enforce these laws (see Chapter 4, Medicolegal Issues).

In some cases, laws requiring parental permission may conflict with the health care provider's assessment of what is best for the patient. Identification of who is the patient—the adolescent or her parents—becomes problematic.

PREGNANCY

In obstetrics, the health care provider has the interests of two patients in view; these interests are interrelated and sometimes conflicting. In the past, obstetricians generally considered the welfare of the mother as the primary concern. In recent years, there have been changes in our perception of the fetus as a patient. For example, fetuses now can undergo surgery and other treatments for disorders in utero. The definition of the fetus as a patient is changing gradually. More than ever, the obstetrician must balance maternal health and maternal autonomy with the welfare of the fetus.

The mother generally has been considered the surrogate decision maker for the fetus, because decisions that affect the fetus almost always directly affect her. Usually, women are willing to accept considerable risk to themselves for the welfare of the fetus. When the mother refuses treatment that may be beneficial to the fetus, the obstetrician is faced with competing interests. To override the patient's wishes may be in the best interest of the fetus but also violates the patient's autonomy and right to refuse care. Recently, husbands or other, unrelated third parties have attempted to make decisions concerning the fetus, despite disagreement with the wishes of the mother.

Rarely, a court has ordered a cesarean section or other treatment to be performed on a pregnant woman, indicating that in rare circumstances concerns of the fetus may be as important as or more important than the interests of the mother. However, such choices may not be in the long-term interest of society if they discourage women from seeking care because of fear of loss of autonomy. In addition, some major professional groups have raised concerns that the involvement of the courts may criminalize the refusal of care by pregnant women. Most states do have statutes that explicitly forbid the withdrawal or withholding of life support from a pregnant patient, regardless of her advance directives. In this case, the therapeutic interests of the fetus are thought to be sufficient to limit the autonomy of the pregnant woman.

Mandatory screening for HIV infection in pregnant women has been considered in some jurisdictions and provides an example of a possible conflict between the interest of the mother and that of the fetus. If the mother is HIV-positive, therapy is now available antenatally that may benefit the health of the fetus. However, the identification of an HIV-positive woman in a nonconfidential screening may have significant economic and social consequences for the woman, such as social discrimination and denial of insurance coverage or employment.

ABORTION

Few topics in health care have received as much attention from society as the issue of abortion. The 1973 Supreme Court decision in *Roe v Wade* upheld the right of a woman to terminate her pregnancy until the time of fetal viability and thereafter when necessary to protect her own life or health. In 1992, the Supreme Court reaffirmed the decision in *Roe v Wade*. Considerable conflict still exists in the United States regarding this issue. Although the legal right to an abortion is ensured, abortions often are not publicly financed. Respect for women's wishes for health care becomes biased, therefore, on socioeconomic grounds. The issue of financing abortions as part of just health care reform has become a major source of conflict.

In general, the main ethical issue regarding abortion is the conflict between respect for a woman's autonomy and society's interest in the fetus. Central to the issue is the definition of life and whether or not to differentiate among the fertilized egg, embryo, fetus, and newborn infant in that definition. In one point of view, a fetus whose survival is contingent on using the woman's body could be assigned fewer rights than one who is able to survive independently. Whether and by what vehicle society should be involved in topics about which there is such strong moral disagreement are important questions.

The use of nonselective embryo reduction to reduce the number of gestations resulting from ovulation induction or reproductive technologies is considered by some to raise different ethical issues because the ultimate goal of the woman is to have a healthy child.

The potential use of prenatal diagnostic methods to determine the gender of a fetus, followed by abortion for gender selection, raises a myriad of ethical issues. Whereas in this country gender selection is rare, it is common in India and some other countries. Widespread use of abortion for gender selection may change the sex ratio of the population, as well as promote gender discrimination. In this case, can the potential for serious societal harm justifiably lead to restriction of the choices available to prospective parents? Is autonomy with regard to reproductive matters an absolute right?

REPRODUCTIVE TECHNOLOGIES

The advances and greater availability of the reproductive technologies have raised new ethical issues. In the United States, there is a strong presumptive right to reproductive freedom. It has been argued that procreative liberty should extend to any available reproductive technologies, as long as no tangible harm results. Whether, when, and how to limit procreative liberty is a subject of controversy.

Again, defining the beginning of life is central to an approach to this topic. Some people argue that the early embryo deserves special respect but not the full rights of an individual. Differing views on the moral status of the embryo affect debates on discard of embryos and embryo research, including the use of embryonic stem cells for research.

The introduction of a third party into reproduction, with sperm, egg, or embryo donation or with surrogate relationships has increased the number and complexity of ethical issues. Reports of large payments to egg donors raised concerns about exploitation of donors, as well as the devaluation of human life by treating eggs as commodities. In response, the ethics committee of the American Society for Reproductive Medicine has recommended limits on financial compensation to egg donors.

Finally, new definitions of reproduction continue to challenge the medical profession and society. Reproductive technology makes postmenopausal and posthumous conception possible and could result in procedures to enhance genetic attributes or even clone a human being. Ethical conflicts include the rights of an individual to choose such procedures versus the extent to which society wishes to limit these practices.

OTHER ETHICAL ISSUES OF ADULT WOMEN

Gender and sociocultural differences between patients and providers may subtly influence the style and content of physician-patient communication, how patients make choices, and the care they receive. Providers should be aware of bias in their judgments concerning patient choices.

In general, women consider themselves to be less powerful in society than men. When they are ill and in a hospital setting, they feel even less powerful. The task of consenting to treatment may be given to the "more powerful" person, with the patient incompletely informed. The health care provider must take pains to ensure that the patient is truly informed and that she feels she has the freedom to consent to or refuse care without coercion.

All patients should be encouraged to prepare advance directives and to appoint a durable power of attorney for health care. When no durable power of attorney has been appointed, each state has a hierarchy for surrogate decision-making. In some circumstances, such as regarding lesbian couples, states may not recognize the person most able to make surrogate decisions unless a durable power of attorney has been appointed. Patients should be encouraged to express their feelings about withdrawal and withholding of support to both her health care provider and her durable power of attorney or surrogate decision maker. It is the physician's responsibility to be sure that the surrogate does not make a decision that would be in conflict with the patient's previously stated wishes.

ELDERLY WOMEN & END-OF-LIFE ISSUES

Advance directives and other end-of-life issues become even more important when the patient is elderly. Because women are likely to outlive their spouse, arrangements for a durable power of attorney for health care other than the spouse need to be made.

An additional problem with the elderly is the determination of a patient's competence and her ability to make choices. When treatment is refused by the patient and competence is questioned, the provider may have to decide whether to follow the desires of the patient or of her surrogate. Providers should be aware that there is documentation of gender disparity in court decisions

surrounding the right to refuse life-sustaining treatment. In right-to-die cases, the previously stated wishes of men are much more likely to be honored than are those of women. Such evidence should motivate women to make their treatment decisions and advance directives as explicit as possible.

Because of limited economic resources, health care reform at the federal and state levels may have a dramatic impact on elderly women. For example, age-based rationing of expensive treatments such as kidney transplants has been discussed as a means to limit health care expenditure. Because women's life expectancy is greater than men's, such rationing may be unfairly applied to women who may otherwise have many years to live. Guidelines or mandates about the termination of care for chronically or terminally ill patients also would affect women disproportionately, for the same reason.

Annas GJ: The Supreme Court, privacy, and abortion. N Engl J Med 1989;321:1200. [PMID: 2677728]

American College of Obstetricians and Gynecologists: Ethics in Obstetrics and Gynecology. American College of Obstetricians and Gynecologists, 2002.

Beauchamp TL, Childress JF: *Principles of Biomedical Ethics,* 5th ed. Oxford University Press, 2001.

Draper H: Women, forced caesareans and antenatal responsibilities. J Med Ethics 1996;22:327. [PMID: 8961116]

Ethics Committee of the American Society for Reproductive Medicine: Financial incentives in recruitment of oocyte donors. Fertil Steril 2000;74:216. [PMID: 10970169]

Jonsen AR, Siegler M, Winslade WJ: *Clinical Ethics: A Practical Approach to Ethical Decisions in Clinical Medicine,* 4th ed. McGraw-Hill, 1998.

Mandatory parental consent to abortion. Council on Ethical and Judicial Affairs, American Medical Association. JAMA 1993; 269:82. [PMID: 8416412]

Miles SH, August A: Courts, gender and the "right to die." Law Med Health Care 1990;18:85. [PMID: 2374456]

Robertson JA: *Children of Choice: Freedom and the New Reproductive Technologies.* Princeton University Press, 1994.

Relevant Web Sites

[American Society for Reproductive Medicine] Ethical guidelines published since 1984 are available to nonmembers.

www.asrm.org

[National Bioethics Advisory Commission]

www.bioethics.gov

[National Reference Center for Bioethics Literature] Most comprehensive bioethics web site, including basic, educational and teaching resources.

www.georgetown.edu/research/nrcbl

[The Hastings Center]

www.thehastingscenter.org

Medicolegal Issues

4

Rita L. Bender, JD

There are a number of legal issues related to the health care of women, which—if not unique to women—tend to arise more often for them.

DIRECTIVE TO PHYSICIANS & POWER OF ATTORNEY

A patient is legally competent to make her own decisions about the nature and extent of health care as long as she is capable of understanding. In the event she becomes incapacitated, those decisions will need to be made by someone else. A health care provider may not disclose health care information about a competent patient to any other person without appropriate written authorization. However, such disclosures may be made to the person authorized to make medical decisions for an incompetent patient.

If a patient becomes incapacitated and has not executed a directive to physicians that outlines the extent of treatment she is willing to receive, family members may attempt to express her presumed wishes for her. This can be a nightmare for the treating physician, as family members may disagree among themselves or may have positions about the extent or duration of treatment that the doctor suspects to be contrary to the wishes of the patient.

The person who is authorized to consent to health care for the incompetent patient may exercise the rights of the patient. The surrogate decision makers under the Uniform Health Care Information Act are, in order of priority: legal guardian, holder of durable power of attorney, spouse, adult children, parents, and adult brothers and sisters. Unanimity is required when there is more than one person in the group of authorized decision-makers, such as multiple adult children. Therefore, a durable power of attorney is important because it designates the specific person authorized by the disabled patient to make decisions on her behalf.

Where there is no durable power of attorney, conflict regarding care, or even access to medical records, can result in the need to obtain a guardianship order pursuant to the law of the state where the patient resides or is hospitalized. Such court actions are both costly and time consuming. Even so, without a directive, the court is left to guess, based solely on the testimony of friends and family, the patient's actual intent regarding treatment, and how best to further that intent.

The directive to physicians and durable power of attorney are companion documents. The directive will give the physician instructions regarding the patient's treatment preferences; however, it may not be sufficient to avoid conflict among family members as to interpretation. The durable power of attorney designates a person who has the authority to make the decisions on behalf of the incapacitated patient. Thus, disputes about the patient's presumed intentions are resolved.

While a directive and power of attorney are important for all patients, and particularly those who are aging or facing end-of-life treatment, they are also legal instruments that are extremely important for same-sex couples. Whereas husbands and wives are treated by the law as next of kin, with authority for medical decisions about guardianship or durable power to the contrary, unmarried persons need a directive and power of attorney designating each other as the authorized person to make treatment decisions. Without those documents, unmarried partners may not be able to override a sibling or parent, the closest legal relative of the patient, and thus the person with legal authority to make treatment decisions. In such a scenario, the patient's partner can be isolated from the decision making, unable to assert the intentions of the patient. The power of attorney is the patient's way of ensuring that the person whom she wishes to vest with this important decision-making power is the one who holds it. It also avoids the need for a guardianship in the event of disagreeing relatives.

So too, an adult patient who has been emotionally controlled by a domineering parent, child, or spouse can use the power of attorney to designate the person who she most trusts to make important medical decisions.

Patients should be encouraged to create directives and durable powers and to leave copies of them in their medical files, available to treating physicians should the need arise. Many clinics and hospitals have forms available for their patients, consistent with the law of the state, which can be completed by the patient without an attorney.

ABORTION RIGHTS

One of the concepts with which some people have difficulty is the legal principal that only the pregnant woman has the right to make a decision to terminate or not to terminate her pregnancy, within the limitations of the time constraints imposed by state and federal law. While a father can be required to provide child support for his offspring, he can neither compel the mother to consent to an abortion nor can he prevent her from so doing. A father may be entitled to notice of the mother's plan to place the baby for adoption, but he is not entitled to notice of her planned abortion. (See the following sections on Surrogacy and Treatment of Minor Patients.)

Although no states' laws may ban abortion outright, there are 22 states that currently have laws by which women are required to delay some hours or days after receiving state-mandated information regarding abortion. As of July 2001, 17 of the 22 states are enforcing the laws.

The United States Supreme Court has permitted constraints upon abortion only as the fetus grows to such an age that it may be viable outside the womb. In the years since *Roe v Wade* was decided in 1973, medical technology has pushed back the point of independent viability somewhat, thus creating legal conundrums for some courts. However, the concept of an adult woman's right to control her own body remains core to the law of abortion rights and other medical issues regarding reproductive treatment.

Title X of the Public Health Service Act of 1970 and the Medicaid Statute, Title XIX of the Social Security Act of 1965, make provision for the funding of reproductive health services to low-income women. Title X funds currently cannot be used for abortion services. Service providers receiving these funds must provide pelvic examinations, Papanicolaou (Pap) smears, breast examinations, screening for sexually transmitted diseases, infertility screening, and referrals.

SURROGACY

The area of assisted reproduction has expanded with the medical technology, creating a variety of possible medical options for infertile couples. The law is not consistent throughout the country with regard to whether surrogacy is legal (if so, under what circumstances) and how the parental rights of the intended parents will be established. Some states have statutes that permit surrogacy or render it illegal. Some states have developed their law by litigation rather than legislation. Where surrogacy is permitted, the surrogate must be a mentally competent adult.

It is difficult to predict the outcome of potential disputes in this very new legal area. There is as yet little decisional case law, resolving the conflicts between the parties who may claim an interest in the genetic material, and those cases that exist are not consistent. The legal tangle is even more difficult when the surrogate and the intended parents live in different states or the implantation occurs in a different state than the birth or intended adoption, since the states' laws may conflict.

Surrogate as Genetic Parent

The first surrogates were women who became pregnant by artificial insemination, having agreed to gestate a fetus to term for intended parents. Sometimes the sperm donor was the partner of the intended mother. On other occasions, the donor was another man, and neither he nor the surrogate mother intended to parent. In either of these cases, the surrogate was the genetic parent of the child to whom she gave birth. The intended father might or might not be a genetic parent. The earliest of the litigated surrogacy cases, *In re Baby M*, recognized some custodial rights of a surrogate who was the genetic parent of the infant she claimed. The outcome in such cases varies with state law, where such law exists.

Gestational Host

Surrogacy has expanded past artificial insemination of a volunteer gestational mother. The surrogate may gestate an embryo that has been created in vitro from the egg and sperm of the intended parents. Or, she may be the gestational host for an embryo that develops from the donated sperm and donated egg of a man and woman neither of whom are the intended parents. While there is still no clear line of cases from state to state, the courts seem inclined to favor the rights of the intended parents to have the opportunity to parent, where the surrogate is not the genetic parent but rather a gestational host.

Creating Legal Parentage

In most states that permit surrogacy, the intended parents will have to adopt the newborn in order to establish their parentage. In California and Massachusetts, parentage may presently be established by a court finding of parentage by the intended parents, without an adoption by them of the child. This emerging legal concept has resulted in some states considering legislation that provides for a certification of parentage by the intended parents. (For instance, see Washington state version of the Uniform Parentage Act.) Where there can be such a declaration of the maternity of the intended mother, adoption will not be necessary.

When adoption is required, if the intended father is the genetic parent, the legal proceeding may resemble an adoption by a stepparent, in which the surrogate is relinquishing any parental rights she may have to the partner of the father. In the event that the surrogate were to change her mind before the adoption was completed, some state courts have refused to terminate her parental rights to the child, while others have sided with the intended parent(s). Even when the surrogate is not the genetic parent, most states do not yet permit a finding of parentage by the intended parents, absent an adoption. This sometimes results in the need for both biologic parents to adopt their own child.

Surrogate's Rights During Treatment & Pregnancy

The right to make decisions concerning her medical treatment and decisions to abandon the attempt at creating a pregnancy, belong to the patient alone. The right to decide on an abortion is vested in the woman carrying the pregnancy. Even in situations in which the developing fetus is the genetic child of both intended parents, the surrogate is the only person who has the legal right to terminate the pregnancy or to refuse to do so. It is important for persons considering surrogate pregnancy to understand that as intended parents, they cannot control these decisions. A surrogate, upon hearing that the fetus she carries has a genetic abnormality, might decide to abort, contrary to the wishes of the intended parents. She may determine to carry the fetus to term, in opposition to the desires of the intended parents. In the event of multiple fetuses, decisions about selective reduction belong to the surrogate as well.

Although the intended parents cannot determine whether or not there will be an abortion, they would likely be responsible for the costs of parenting a child born as the result of their surrogacy arrangements, most especially if the infant was the genetic offspring of one or both of them.

Rights of the Intended Parents

Although the intended parents cannot control the medical treatment of the donor or surrogate, as patients themselves, they can determine each of their own course of treatment. The surrogate has no say in those medical decisions.

However, there is the potential for legal conflict between intended parents. Although there is sometimes a surrogacy undertaken for a single person, usually the intended parents are a heterosexual or homosexual couple. At the onset, everyone's intention is the same: A pregnancy will be created, which the surrogate will carry to term; after the birth, the surrogate's rights will be terminated and the intended parents will assume all legal rights and responsibility for the child. There may be more eggs harvested, or early-stage embryos created, than are used in the implantation. The additional material may be cryopreserved.

If thereafter the intended parents disagree about the continuing preservation, disposition, or use of the material, a difficult legal quandary is created. The original donor of eggs or sperm may assert an interest. There are cases in several states. They provide little guidance. Some cases favor the wishes of the biologic progenitor, as between the intended parents. Some favor the wishes of the party who opposes destruction of the genetic material. Many states have not ruled yet on these questions.

All parties to a surrogacy should define in advance their agreements as to ownership of the genetic material and who among them will have the right to decide future use or disposition.

In the event that a child was born who had profound disabilities, and the intended parents did not want to assume the care of the child, it is likely that they would be financially liable for the costs of care. Should they be unwilling to assume parental responsibility for the child, and the surrogate also chose not to parent, the child would probably be surrendered to the care of the state and either placed for adoption with another willing family, or placed into foster care. Without adoption by another family, it is reasonable to anticipate that the intended parents' financial responsibility would continue.

There are numerous legal risks involved in surrogacy, and each of the parties should be fully informed. Many physicians who treat patients with regard to surrogacy require that the parties to the arrangement execute a contract that provides for the circumstances that can be contemplated. Patients should be encouraged to consult with a knowledgeable attorney before proceeding with the medical procedures. While the doctor is not responsible for the patient's judgment, ensuring that the patient gets necessary information may be a form of informed consent.

EGG & SPERM DONATION

The intended parent(s) of a child may be neither the producer of the sperm or ova.

Artificial Insemination

Each state has a uniform provision for artificial insemination, with minor variations. This statute provides that the donor of sperm shall not be treated in law as the father of a child who may be conceived, so long as the donation is made under the supervision of a physician, the donor is not the husband of the recipient, and the husband of the recipient consents to the insemination where recipient is married. Conversely, unmarried donor and recipient may consent to donor's recognition as the father. Consents must be in writing and the physician must certify the signatures and the date of the insemination. Physicians undertaking artificial insemination must document the source of the sperm (by code when anonymous donor) and date of insemination. A report of the insemination is filed with the state department of vital records.

Egg Donation

The donor clearly has the right to control her own treatment and to withdraw from participation at any time prior to the collection of the ova. However, egg donation is trickier than sperm donation as a legal matter. There is not yet a uniform statute that defines the rights of the recipient or donor to the genetic material, although the state of Washington has adopted statutory provisions in its version of the Uniform Parentage Act. A contract may provide for the ownership and right to use or dispose of the eggs following the harvesting. The donor may acknowledge that she will not have parental rights to any child that may result from the use of her donated ova. There are no reported cases in which the donor successfully has been able to assert a right to the material after fertilization; however, there are conflicting cases regarding rights, as between intended parents, to the disposition of the fertilized material.

Physicians would be wise to encourage patients to execute a contract. Many doctors require a signed contract in the patient's medical file before proceeding with any treatment directed toward stimulation and harvesting of ova. Such a contract can be a protection to donor and recipient as well as to the physician. There are two patients, the donor and the recipient, and each must be provided with detailed information about the course of her treatment, risks involved, and right to withdraw from further medication or procedures. Both women must be clear that each of them is the only person who may consent to the course of treatment, even though there are other persons who have an interest in the outcome.

ANONYMITY IN ASSISTED REPRODUCTION

Intended parents and sperm and egg donors often want anonymity from each other. In the case of sperm donors who contribute through donor bank or laboratory facilities as anonymous donors, their confidentiality is supposedly protected. The parties sign contractual agreements providing that anonymity will not be breached. The harvesting of eggs from anonymous donors, and implantation of the resultant embryos are also dealt with by contracts that are meant to protect the identity of the parties. However, there is a California case which held that in a negligence lawsuit against a sperm bank for failure to reveal genetic history of the sperm donor, the parents of the resulting child would be permitted to obtain the donor's medical records and depose him to obtain family history, although the court did not rule that the donor's name would be revealed. This case balances the interests of the child against those of the donor. It seems to indicate that under some circumstances, the assurance of privacy might not be fully protected.

RIGHTS OF SAME-SEX PARENTS

Because many same-sex couples achieve their parentage by way of artificial insemination or surrogacy, the legal issues are mostly the same for them as for heterosexual families who engage in assisted reproduction. However, once the child is born, the homosexual couple faces issues in ensuring their legal parentage.

The woman who did not birth the child will not be permitted to adopt her partner's child in many states, either by specific legislation prohibiting same-sex adoption, as in Florida and New Hampshire, or by case law in some other states. The states that will permit second parent adoption often do so without a specific statute or case law allowing it, but rather, on a case-by-case exercise of judicial interpretation by the trial court.

In states that do not permit adoption by a homosexual couple, the partner who does not bear the child will have to try to protect her rights by way of contract, which may or may not be enforceable. This will be the situation, as well, in cases in which a homosexual couple seeks to parent a "stranger" child, but reside in a state where they cannot be co-petitioners for the adoption of that child. One will adopt, the other will not have parental rights.

Gay men, whose child may be the result of a surrogacy in which only one of them is the biologic parent, also face the issue of second parent adoption. That is, the biologic father can be named on the birth certificate, but the surrogate may not be able to relinquish her parental rights to the father's partner. If neither man is the biologic father, it is possible that neither could be permitted to adopt in a state that bans any homosexual adoption. The current list of states that permit or prohibit homosexual or second parent adoption is to be found in the resource section.

TREATMENT OF MINORS

Persons under the age of 18 are minors. They do not have the legal capacity to consent to medical care or treatment. The consent of a parent or a legal guardian is necessary. However, there are some statutory exceptions, which vary somewhat state by state, to the requirement of parental consent in the treatment of minors.

Sexually Transmitted Diseases

In most states, an individual 14 years of age and older may consent to health care for any actual or suspected sexually transmitted disease. Title X funds are available for screening for sexually transmitted diseases, regardless of the age of the patient.

Abortion Procedure

The US Supreme Court has held that laws requiring the consent or notification of a minor's parent(s) or legal guardian prior to the provision of abortion services are constitutional only if they include a constitutionally sound "judicial bypass" procedure allowing the minor to request a court-issued waiver of the consent requirement.

For a judicial bypass provision to pass constitutional muster, it must not unduly burden the young woman's right to an abortion. The Supreme Court has held that a bypass provision must: (1) allow the minor to bypass the consent requirement if she establishes that she is mature enough and well enough informed to make the abortion decision independently; (2) allow the minor to bypass the consent requirement if she establishes that the abortion would be in her best interests; (3) ensure the minor's anonymity; and (4) provide for expeditious bypass procedures.

Litigation regarding the constitutionality of parental consent and notification laws is ongoing. As of July 2001, 43 states had laws requiring minors to obtain the consent of, or notify, one or both her parents before obtaining an abortion. Most include exceptions for medical emergencies.

States where parental consent laws are presently enforced include the following: Alabama, Idaho, Indiana, Kentucky, Louisiana, Maine, Massachusetts, Michigan, Mississippi, Missouri, North Carolina, North Dakota, Oklahoma, Pennsylvania, Rhode Island, South Carolina, Tennessee, Wisconsin, and Wyoming. Of these states, Mississippi and North Dakota require the consent of both parents. Maine, North Carolina, and South Carolina provide an alternative to parental consent, allowing the minor to obtain the consent of a grandparent or providing a doctor-authorized waiver

under certain circumstances. All states except Oklahoma have a judicial bypass procedure.

States where parental notification laws presently are enforced include the following: Arkansas, Delaware, Georgia, Iowa, Kansas, Maryland, Minnesota, Nebraska, Ohio, South Dakota, Texas, Utah, Virginia, and West Virginia. Arkansas, Minnesota, and Utah require the notification of both parents. Delaware, Iowa, Maryland, Ohio, and West Virginia provide an alternative to parental notification. All states except Utah have a judicial bypass procedure.

The following states' parental consent laws were enjoined or were not enforced as of July 2001: Alaska, Arizona, California, and New Mexico. Parental notification laws were enjoined or were not enforced in Colorado, Florida, Illinois, Montana, Nevada, and New Jersey.

As of July 2001, eight states had enacted no law regarding parental notification or consent: Connecticut, Hawaii, New Hampshire, New York, Oregon, Vermont, Washington, and the District of Columbia.

Oral Contraceptives

Federal law controls authorization for treatment of minors with regard to prescription of oral contraceptives. Title X and the Medicaid statute require the confidential provision of contraceptive services to recipients of these programs, regardless of their age. Courts have ruled that laws requiring parental notification or consent prior to the provision of contraceptives violate these statutes. In striking down parental notification laws, courts have emphasized the importance of confidentiality to the physician-patient relationship and recognized the important public policy interest in encouraging minors to obtain contraception.

Drug & Alcohol Treatment

Most states do not prohibit drug and alcohol screening and treatment of adolescent patients without parental involvement.

Voluntary Sterilization

Federal regulations require that a patient be competent and over the age of 21 in order to consent to voluntary sterilization.

Blood Transfusion

When a patient is a child, the parent or guardian can refuse under most states laws to permit a blood transfusion, if the refusal does not endanger life or threaten to result in serious impairment of bodily function. If such danger exists and the parent or guardian will not consent, the health care provider must notify the proper state authority in order that a petition can be brought before the court for permission to treat.

Immunizations

Childhood immunizations are enumerated in the National Immunization Guidelines. In most states, exemptions are permitted for medical, religious, philosophical or personal reasons. The National Childhood Vaccine Injury Act of 1986, Title III of Pub.L. 99–660 sets forth the requirements for providing informed consent about vaccine benefits and risks.

REFERENCE SOURCE DOCUMENTS

Statutes

Fla. Stat. Ann Sec. 63.042(3) (West 1985). Florida prohibits homosexual adoption.

N.H. Rev. Stat. Ann. Sec. 170-B:4 (1990). New Hampshire prohibits homosexual adoption.

National Childhood Vaccine Injury Act of 1986, Title III of Pub.L. 99-660. Informed consent requirements.

Public Health Service Act of 1970, Title X. Access to contraceptives; STD screening and treatment; infertility assessment.

Social Security Act of 1965, the Medicaid Statute, Title XIX. Reproductive health services for low-income women.

Uniform Health Care Information Act. Decision makers for incompetent persons.

Uniform Parentage Act, Section 5 Artificial Insemination statute.

WA. RCW 26.26 (2002), Washington version of Uniform Parentage Act, with provision for recognition of intended parents in donor and surrogacy.

Cases

Adoptions of BLVB and ELVB, 160 Vt. 368, 628 A2d 1271 (Supreme Ct. of Vermont 1993). Lesbian biological mother's rights will not be terminated by the adoption of her child by her partner, thus making both women the legal mothers of the child.

Adoption of Two Children by HNR, 285 NJ Super 1, 666 A2d 535 (Supreme Ct. App. Div. 1995). New Jersey permits the lesbian partner of biological mother to adopt, so that the couple is recognized as the legal parents.

Adoption of Tammy, 619 N.E. 2d 315 (Supreme Judicial Ct. of Massachusetts 1993). Same-sex couple may jointly adopt.

Bellotti v Baird, 443 U.S. 622 (1979). Consent for minor abortion; judicial bypass.

County of St. Charles, Mo. v Missouri Family Health Council, 107 F.3d 682 (8th Cir. 1997). No parental consent or notification for providing contraceptives to minors.

Hodgson v Minnesota, 497 US 417 (1990). Criteria for judicial bypass.

In re Adoption of Evan, 583 N.Y.S. 2d 997 (1992). New York permits the lesbian partner of a biological mother to adopt, so that the couple were both recognized as the legal parents.

Jane Does 1 through 4 v Utah Dept. of Health, 776 F.2d 253 (10th Cir. 1985). No parental consent or notification for providing contraceptives to minors.

Johnson v Superior Court of Los Angeles County; California Cryobank, Inc., 80 Cal. App. 4th 1050 (2000). Parents of child born as a result of anonymous sperm donation may depose donor and obtain medical records.

Jones v T.H., 425 US 986 (1976). No parental consent or notification for providing contraceptives to minors.

Lambert v Wicklund, 520 US 292 (1997). Criteria for judicial bypass.

MMD and BHM, 662 A2d 837 (D.C. Ct. of Appeals 1995). Same-sex couple may jointly adopt.

New York v Heckler, 719 F.2d 1191 (2nd Cir. 1983). No parental consent or notification for providing contraceptives to minors.

Ohio v Akron Center for Reproductive Health, 497 US 502 (1990) (*Akron II*). Consent for minor abortion.

Petition of *KM and DM to Adopt Olivia M.* 274 Ill. App 3d 189, 653 NE 2d 888 (Appellate Ct. of Ill 1995). Same-sex couple has standing to file joint adoption petition.

Planned Parenthood Affiliates of California v Van DeCamp, 181 Cal. App. 3d 245 (Ca. Ct. App. 1986). Physician-patient relationship preserved by confidential contraceptive provision to minors.

Planned Parenthood Ass'n v Dandoy, 810 F.2d 984 (10th Cir. 1987) No parental consent or notification for providing contraceptives to minors.

Planned Parenthood Fed'n v Heckler, 712 F.2d 650 (D.C. Cir. 1983). No parental consent or notification for providing contraceptives to minors.

Planned Parenthood of Southeastern Pennsylvania v Casey, 505 US 833 (1992). Criteria for judicial bypass.

Roe v Wade, 410 U.S.113 (1973). Legality of abortion.

Code of Federal Regulations

42 CFR sec. 59.11. Confidential provision of contraceptives.

42 CFR sec. 441.253, .257 & 258. Voluntary sterilization requirements.

Other Publications

Restrictions on Young Women's Access to Abortion Services. Center for Reproductive Law and Policy publication; July 2001.

SECTION II

Preventive Health Care

Preventive Services

5

Paul A. Smith, MD

Because clinicians often see women with medical problems that could have been avoided, it is easy for them to appreciate the importance of disease prevention. They also see patients with advanced stages of disease that may be difficult or impossible to treat successfully and for which the outcome would have been more favorable had the condition been recognized and treated earlier. The benefit from the application of preventive services can be seen readily in the prevention of poliomyelitis epidemics in the United States, the decline in stroke rate due to screening for and treatment of hypertension, and the marked reduction in deaths from cervical cancer.

Despite the benefits of preventive services, however, they should be selected with great care. Because all people are potential recipients of preventive services, the financial costs may be enormous. In choosing interventions for healthy women, clinicians must be certain that the benefit will be greater than any potential risk. Randomized prospective studies provide the most reliable evidence to support a recommendation of a preventive intervention. This type of study has shown that the use of mammography to detect breast cancer in women results in decreased mortality. Benefit can only be strongly suggested from well-done observational (eg, case-controlled) studies, such as decreased mortality from colon cancer through the use of sigmoidoscopy.

For other interventions, such as with self-examination of the breast, there may be insufficient data on clinical efficacy. There are many examples of screening tests or preventive treatments that looked promising on a theoretic basis but when studied in randomized trials were shown to have no benefit. Examples are routine chest radiographs to detect lung cancer in cigarette smokers and medical therapy for hyperlipidemia in young, healthy people without other risk factors for cardiovascular disease.

The Canadian Task Force (CTF) on the Periodic Health Examination, the United States Preventive Services Task Force (USPSTF), the American College of Physicians (ACP), and others have evaluated preventive services with exhaustive critical reviews, using explicit criteria to grade the evidence and link it with the strength of each recommendation. Many expert groups have also published guidelines. Selected recommendations are summarized in Table 5–1: the emphasis is on services for which the evidence is strongest or for which controversy exists.

Other published recommendations come from medical specialty societies, national governmental agencies such as the National Cholesterol Education Program (NCEP), professional and scientific societies such as the American Cancer Society (ACS), and individual experts; often there is not a clear consensus among reports.

TYPES OF PREVENTIVE SERVICES

Preventive services include screening for disease with physical examination, history taking, and testing; counseling about health behaviors; and providing immunizations and chemoprophylaxis. A critical review of the screening physical examination done for prevention has left little to be recommended universally other than blood pressure measurement. Some of the most effective interventions are recommendations that affect health behaviors such as tobacco use, physical activity, nutrition, alcohol and drug use, and accidental injury prevention. Conventional clinical activities—such as performing screening tests—may be less important than counseling and patient education in some instances.

There has been increasing recognition of the importance of selectivity in ordering screening tests and providing preventive services. Knowledge of a patient's in-

Table 5–1. Prevention and screening recommendations for women.

Intervention	Health Condition	Target Group	Recommendation
Physical Exam			
Blood Pressure	CHD, cerebrovascular disease, renal disease		
Routine		18 year+	Every 1–2 years and every visit for other reasons
High risk		18 year+, diastolic BP is 85–90 mm Hg, 1 or more CHD risk factors present	Every year
Clinician Breast Examination	Breast cancer		
Routine		19 year+ (ACOG), 40 year+ (ACS, USPSTF), 50 year+ (AAFP, CTF)	Every year
High risk		18 year+ (ACP), 35 year+ (CTF, USPSTF), history of premenopausal breast cancer in a first-degree family member	Every year
Laboratory Testing			
Mammography	Breast cancer		
Routine		40 year+ (ACS, USPSTF) 50 year+ (AAFP, CTF)	Every year (ACS, ACR) Every 1–2 years (AAFP, CTF, USPSTF)
High Risk		35–40 year+, history of premenopausal breast cancer in a first-degree family member, other risk factors (ACP)	Every year (CTF, USPSTF)
Papanicolaou Smear	Cervical cancer		
Routine		18 year+, no other risk factors (see text)	Every 1–3 years
		65 year+, low risk and regular negative screening throughout past 10 years	Discontinue
High risk		18 year+ or onset of intercourse, presence of risk factors	Every year
Sigmoidoscopy	Colorectal cancer		
Routine		50 year+ (ACP, AAFP, CTF, ACG, USPSTF, others)	Every 5 years (ACP)
High risk		50 year+ (USPSTF), hx one first-degree family member with colon cancer or personal hx of endometrial, ovarian, or breast cancer	Every 5 years
FOBT	Colorectal cancer		
Routine		50 year+ (Same as sigmoidoscopy)	Every year
High risk		Same as sigmoidoscopy	Every year
Colonoscopy	Colorectal cancer		
Routine		50 year+ (AAFP, ACS, ACG, ACOG)	Every 10 years
Very high risk		See text	Frequency depends on risk category
Nonfasting Cholesterol	CHD		
Routine		20 year+ (NCEP III), 35 year+ (USPSTF), 45 year+ (AAFP)	Every 5 years More frequently individual clinical judgment
Counseling			
Tobacco Use	Cardiovascular disease, some cancers, lung disease	All women (CTF, USPSTF, others)	Actively counsel smokers to quit, offer pharmacotherapy, primary prevention messages to adolescents

(continued)

Table 5–1. Prevention and screening recommendations for women. (continued)

Intervention	Health Condition	Target Group	Recommendation
Alcohol Use	Accidents, suicide, homicide, hypertension, heart and liver disease, etc.		
Routine		All women	Counsel alcohol moderation, abstention when driving and during pregnancy
High risk		Problem drinkers	Case finding strategy
Dietary Fat, Sodium, Fiber	CHD, hypertension	18 year+ (ACP, USPSTF), no comment (CTF)	Advise diet to maintain desirable weight, total fat < 30% of calories, saturated fat < 10% of calories, cholesterol < 300 mg/d, high fiber foods, limit salt
Calcium Intake	Osteoporosis	18 year+ (USPSTF, CTF)	Counsel to maintain adequate calcium intake by natural diet and supplements
Exercise	CHD, osteoporosis, other	18 year+ (USPSTF), 40 years+ (CTF)	Educate about the role of exercise in disease prevention (USPSTF), teach effect of immobility on bone mass (CTF)
Injury Prevention **Seat Belt Use**	Motor vehicle accidents	All women	Advise seat belt use (ACP, CTF, USPSTF)
Sexual Behavior	Unwanted pregnancy, sexually transmitted diseases	All women	Advise contraceptives (CTF, USPSTF), barrier methods and safe sexual practices to prevent STD (USPSTF)

dividual risk for a specific condition is essential to determine the likelihood of benefit. This requires consideration of the patient's past medical history, age, sex, family history, and personal health habits. Individual risk assessment with appropriate selection of services decreases adverse consequences of screening and increases absolute risk reduction.

Periodic Health Assessment

The evaluation of asymptomatic people has changed from the traditional complete history and physical examination. The periodic health examination focuses on history-taking to assess individual risk (eg, tobacco use, family history of colon or breast cancer, use of seat belts), directed physical examination, and counseling. Barriers to accomplishment of these measures include lack of payment to providers for screening visits and

other preventive services, uncertainty over which services are recommended, and lack of time or training on the part of clinicians to enable counseling or assessment of risk. Because most people in the United States see a physician at least once a year, these episodic visits can also be used as opportunities to provide preventive services.

Screening

Screening is performed to detect disease before symptoms are evident. Tests that are useful for helping diagnose disease in symptomatic patients or for monitoring patients with established disease may have no value in screening, eg, use of CA-125 for ovarian cancer. Whether or not a screening method leads to improved outcome depends on the characteristics of the disease, the screening test, and the patient population. The disease must cause significant morbidity and mortality. The natural history should include an asymptomatic period in which the diagnosis can be made, and the results of early treatment must be superior to those obtained after symptoms appear. The test must be sensitive and specific, with reasonable cost and patient acceptance. The condition must be prevalent enough in the population to justify screening. The patient must have sufficient life expectancy to warrant intervention and be willing to undergo the screening and potential treatment.

Counseling

Clinicians who use counseling interventions give patients information and advice regarding personal behaviors so that the risk of illness and injury can be reduced. For an intervention to be considered effective, evidence must show that clinicians can influence the personal behavior through counseling and that behavior change may improve outcome (see Chapter 7). A good example is cigarette smoking cessation.

Chemoprophylaxis & Immunizations

Chemoprophylaxis refers to prescribing medications for healthy people as primary preventive measures to decrease the risk of disease (eg, aspirin to prevent vascular disease or tamoxifen to prevent breast cancer). For chemoprophylaxis to be effective, morbidity or mortality from the disease in question must be reduced without other adverse effects and the patient must be able to comply.

Immunizations are given to prevent viral and bacterial illness. Risk assessment is required to guide individual recommendations (see Chapter 6, Immunizations).

Periodic Health Examinations: Summary of AAFP Policy Recommendations and Age Charts. http://www.aafp.org/exam.xml

Canadian Task Force on the Periodic Health Examination. http://www.ctfphc.org/index.html

Cancer Prevention and Early Detection 2002. American Cancer Society. http://www.cancer.org.

US Preventive Services Task Force. Guide to clinical preventive services. 2nd ed. Office of Disease Prevention and Health Promotion. US Government Printing Office, 1996.

US Preventive Services Task Force. Guide to clinical preventive services. 3rd ed. 2000–2002. Available online at http://www.ahrq.gov/clinic/cps3dix.htm.

CARDIOVASCULAR DISEASE

Cardiovascular disease (CVD) is the leading cause of death in American women, accounting for 45% of all deaths, primarily from coronary heart disease (CHD) and stroke. There has been an overall reduction in the death rate due to CVD in the United States over the past few decades, but the rate of decline has been less in women than in men. Because the risk of CVD increases with age, the absolute number of CVD deaths is increasing; in the year 2000, there were 30 million American women over age 50. Thirty-five percent of all deaths among women are caused by CHD, and 50% of all people who die of CHD are women. Although women have CHD as frequently as men do, disease generally develops 10–15 years later. The most effective strategy for disease reduction is primary prevention through risk factor modification. The modifiable risk factors are tobacco use, hypertension, hypercholesterolemia, and physical inactivity.

Tobacco Use

Currently, 11–30% of adult American women smoke cigarettes, with greater risk for tobacco use associated with younger age, rural geographic location, less education, and ethnicity. There is much evidence that smoking cessation reduces the risk of myocardial infarction in women as well as men. Benefit from stopping smoking is realized almost immediately; by 5 to 10 years, the risk of CHD in the ex-smoker approximates that of people who have never smoked. Brief office interventions, pharmacotherapy, and behavior modification programs have been shown to be effective in reducing smoking rates (see Chapter 7). All women should be asked about tobacco use at each clinical encounter, and current users should be counseled to stop and assisted when willing to do so.

Hypertension

The USPSTF, CTF, and the ACP all recommend measuring blood pressure at every clinical encounter and at least every 2 years in normotensive persons, yearly if diastolic pressure is 85–90 mmHg. The diagnosis of hypertension (systolic blood pressure greater than 140 mmHg, diastolic blood pressure greater than 90 mmHg) should not be made on the basis of one reading; it should be based on 3 separate visits with at least 2 measurements at each visit. Early detection and medical treatment of hypertension reduces cardiovascular events and mortality; this benefit is well established by randomized controlled trials in men. The higher the elevation in blood pressure, the greater the clinical improvement with treatment. Since 1972, a greater than 40% reduction in age-adjusted stroke mortality has been observed in women and is attributed largely to early detection and treatment of hypertension. Once hypertension has been diagnosed, patients should be counseled on lifestyle treatments that include dietary change (sodium and fat restriction), weight reduction if appropriate, physical activity, moderation of alcohol consumption, and reduction of other cardiovascular risk factors. Drug therapy should be advised in accordance with published guidelines.

Hypercholesterolemia

Hypercholesterolemia is associated with accelerated atherosclerosis and CHD in women as well as in men. The risk for CHD increases with higher levels of total cholesterol (TC) and lower levels of high-density (HDL) cholesterol in a continuous, graded fashion over most of the range of cholesterol values. This association appears to be stronger in older women; CHD develops later in women than in men. In primary prevention trials, cholesterol-lowering drug treatment decreased CHD events by 30% in people with high TC or with average TC and low HDL. In the 1 trial that included women, the benefit seen in postmenopausal women was equal to that in men. Controversy exists over who benefits from screening. The absolute benefit from treatment in women may be less than in men of similar ages because of their lower CHD rates. The USPSTF, the ACP, and the American Academy of Family Physicians (AAFP) recommend screening women with other CHD risk factors (eg, smoking, hypertension, diabetes, familial hyperlipidemia, and premature CHD) at age 20, and those at average risk beginning at ages 35 to 45. The NCEP recommends periodic screening in all adults beginning at age 20. The CTF recommends case finding in middle-aged men only. The rationale for screening low-risk women later is that nearly all those whose risk of CHD is as high as those in existing prevention trials will be identified. The primary goals for screening young women are to promote healthy lifestyles and to identify those with familial hyperlipidemia that would not be found by selective screening. Whether cholesterol screening is effective in achieving these goals is unknown. The optimal interval for screening is uncertain, with most recommending every 5 years, more frequently if lipids are near levels warranting therapy. The age to stop screening is also uncertain. Most CHD in women presents after age 65; however, those with persistently normal lipid levels are unlikely to change with further screening. Older women most likely to benefit from screening are those previously unscreened, especially with other CHD risk, who would be candidates for drug treatment. Screening by measuring non-fasting TC and HDL is most practical. The NCEP recommends a fasting lipoprotein profile (TC, HDL, low-density lipoprotein [LDL] cholesterol, and triglycerides), as the initial screen, with the rationale that interventions and goals are guided by LDL.

The benefit of secondary prevention by treating women with known CHD disease with drugs for hy-

perlipidemia is robust and well established. Identifying hypercholesterolemia in those similarly at risk, such as those with peripheral vascular disease, diabetes, and multiple risk factors is a high priority (see Chapter 29, Risk Factors for Coronary Artery Disease & Their Treatment).

Exercise

A sedentary lifestyle is increasingly pervasive in the United States, with half of all adults engaging in no regular leisure time physical activity, and a quarter entirely sedentary. Regular physical activity is associated with a decreased risk for development of cardiovascular disease, obesity, diabetes mellitus, and osteoporosis in women. Persons who are most sedentary benefit from even small increases in physical activity, such as walking. The effectiveness of counseling patients to change their exercise habits has been less certain; however, recent trials using structured behavior change interventions have shown sustained increases in physical activity and health measures (see Chapter 7).

Chemoprophylaxis

Routine use of aspirin in all women for the primary prevention of CHD events and stroke is not recommended. Aspirin has been shown to decrease the incidence of CHD in men who are at increased risk for heart disease, while increasing the incidence of gastrointestinal bleeding and hemorrhagic stroke. Whether aspirin prevents CHD events in women is unclear, although observational data suggests that it may. A potential reduced rate of myocardial infarction needs to be balanced against hemorrhagic complications. A practical approach is to calculate a woman's absolute risk for CHD using published or online tools based on Framingham data. Women with known coronary artery disease or diabetes mellitus are likely to benefit from aspirin.

A clinical practice guideline for treating tobacco use and dependence: A US Public Health Service report. The Tobacco Use and Dependence Clinical Practice Guideline Panel, Staff, and Consortium Representatives. JAMA 2000;283:3244. [PMID: 10866874]

Aspirin for the primary prevention of cardiovascular events: recommendation and rationale. Ann Intern Med 2002;136:157. [PMID: 11790071]

Aspirin for the Primary Prevention of Cardiovascular Events. Recommendations and Rationale. January 2002. Agency for Healthcare Research and Quality, Rockville, MD. http://www.ahrq.gov/clinic/3rduspstf/aspirin/asprr.htm.

Executive Summary of the Third Report of the National Cholesterol Education Program (NCEP) Expert Panel on the Detection, Evaluation, and Treatment of High Blood Cholesterol in Adults (Adult Treatment Panel III). JAMA 2001;285: 2486. http://www.nhlbi.nih.gov/guidelines/cholesterol/atp_iii.htm. [PMID: 11368702]

Garber AM, Browner WS, Hulley SB: Cholesterol screening in asymptomatic adults, revisited. Part 2. Ann Intern Med 1996;124:518. [PMID: 8602715]

Logan AG: Lowering the blood total cholesterol level to prevent coronary heart disease. In: *Canadian Task Force on the Periodic Health Examination. Canadian Guide to Clinical Preventive Health Care.* Ottawa: Health Canada; 1994:650.

Pate RR et al: Physical activity and public health: a recommendation from the Centers for Disease Control and Prevention and the American College of Sports Medicine. JAMA 1995;273:402. [PMID: 7823386]

Screening adults for lipid disorders: recommendations and rationale. Am J Prev Med 2001;20(3S):73. http://www.ahrq.gov/clinic/ajpmsuppl/lipidrr.htm. [PMID: 11306235]

The Sixth Report of the Joint National Committee on the Prevention, Detection, Evaluation, and Treatment of High Blood Pressure (JNC VI). NIH Publication No. 98-4080. http://www.nhlbi.nih.gov/guidelines/hypertension/jncintro.htm.

Treating Tobacco Use and Dependence. Quick Reference Guide for Clinicians, October 2000. US Public Health Service. http://www.surgeongeneral.gov/tobacco/tobaqrg.htm.

CANCER

Breast Cancer

Breast cancer is the second most common cause of cancer death in women in the United States, surpassed only by lung cancer. There will be approximately 203,500 new diagnoses of breast cancer accounting for an estimated 39,600 deaths in 2002. Since 1989, breast cancer mortality rates have declined on the average of 2.1% per year. This decline is largely attributed to early detection by screening mammography and effective adjuvant therapy. Lifetime risk of the development of breast cancer is estimated to be 12.5%. Age is the major risk factor for breast cancer in women, with 85% occurring in women over age 50, 10% in women in their 40s, and 5% in women younger than 40. Risk is increased with personal or family history of breast cancer, early menarche, late menopause, first child after age 30, and prior breast biopsy with atypical hyperplasia. Because tumors detected at an early stage have a favorable prognosis with treatment, screening is an attractive option.

A. MAMMOGRAPHY

Multiple randomized trials of mammography screening, with or without clinician breast examination, have shown a clear reduction in breast cancer mortality. The evidence is strongest in women aged 50–69, the age of most women who participated in trials. The benefit in women aged 40–49 is less certain. Most of the trials found a mortality benefit in this age group, but it was less than in older women. Absolute benefit is also smaller due to the lower incidence of breast cancer in younger women. Observed mortality reduction was delayed in women entering the trials in their 40s; this delay was sufficient so that some of the benefit could be attributed to screening after age 50. The optimal frequency of screening has not been established. Trials have demonstrated similar mortality benefit using mammograms at a frequency ranging from 12 to 33 months. The age at which the benefit of screening is lost is also uncertain. No trial has included women over age 74. Breast cancer mortality increases with age, but women are also more likely to die of other diseases. Women with limited life expectancy are unlikely to benefit from screening. The USPSTF found that the absolute benefit from screening mammography increases along a continuum from age 40 to age 70, whereas the potential risks of screening due to false-positive results, unnecessary procedures, and anxiety diminishes. The point at which the risk-benefit ratio favors screening is subject to choice. In a change from previous guidelines, the USPSTF now recommends screening mammography for women aged 40 and older. This is consistent with the recommendations of the American Medical Association, the ACS, the American College of Obstetrics and Gynecology (ACOG), the American College of Radiology (ACR), and the National Cancer Institute.

Although there are no large studies of screening high-risk groups using mammography, the recommendation is to examine women at greatest risk for breast cancer with annual mammograms beginning at age 35 or 40.

B. BREAST EXAMINATION BY A CLINICIAN

Physical examination of the breast by a clinician has not been studied as an independent intervention. From studies combining mammography and breast examination by a clinician, mammography detects 90% of cancers and examination by a physician detects 50%, with much overlap. Ten percent of cancers are detected by physician examination alone, and 40% by mammography alone, suggesting that the physical examination by a physician may be complementary.

C. SELF-EXAMINATION OF THE BREAST

Self-examination of the breast has not been shown to be effective, and there may be some risk of unnecessary procedures or false-positive results. Two randomized trials failed to show a mortality benefit from self-examination of the breast, although these trials were done in countries where mammography and breast examination by a clinician are not routinely performed and may not be applicable to American women. Some studies of self-examination of the breast have found increased rates of biopsy for benign disease.

D. Genetic Testing

Testing for BRCA1 and BRCA2 may be appropriate for some patients with one or more first-degree family members with premenopausal breast cancer. It is suggested that the decision for testing be coupled with expert counseling to achieve a clear plan if the test is positive (which could include observation, bilateral mastectomy, oophorectomy, or tamoxifen). Insurance and social implications should be considered.

E. Tamoxifen

Prophylaxis with tamoxifen has been shown to reduce breast cancer development but also has significant potential side effects such as thromboembolic disease and endometrial cancer. Risks and benefits of tamoxifen therapy should be discussed with all women at high risk for breast cancer (see Chapter 35, Breast Cancer).

Cervical Cancer

Cervical cancer is a common gynecologic malignant disease in the United States, with 13,000 new cases and 4100 deaths estimated to occur in 2002. Modifiable risk factors include cigarette smoking, multiple sexual partners, and not using a barrier method for birth control. Since the practice of routine Papanicolaou (Pap) testing has become widespread, mortality from cervical cancer has decreased by 70% in the United States. Observational studies have documented similar results in Canada and several European countries, with marked reduction in cervical cancer death rates temporally related to adoption of routine Pap smears. Randomized trials have not been performed; because of the strength of the evidence to date, they will not be done for ethical reasons.

There is consensus that all women should be screened beginning at the time of first intercourse or at age 18; more than 60% of women in the United States experience intercourse by the age of 18. Screening should occur every 1 to 3 years, with the frequency dependent on individual risk. Women who are at higher risk should receive annual Pap tests; risk factors include three or more lifetime partners, intercourse before age 21, evidence of human papillomavirus on previous Pap smears, prior cervical cancer or dysplasia, history of cigarette smoking, and low socioeconomic status. Increased risk is also associated with having a male partner who has had multiple previous partners—information rarely known to the clinician. With so many women in 1 or more of these categories, it may be easier for clinicians to perform annual Pap smears unless there is certainty of low risk. In women at low risk, testing every 3 years gives 96% of the benefit of annual testing. It has been recommended that women at low risk who have 3 consecutive negative Pap smears may, at the clinician's discretion, have longer intervals between Pap smears. It is not clear when Pap testing is no longer necessary. If a woman is at low risk and has had regular screening with consistently normal smears up to the age of 65 to 70 years, additional screening may not be necessary. Even if Pap smears are not deemed necessary, inspection of the genital tract to detect other malignant pelvic disease and gynecologic problems should continue.

Women who have not had any sexual partners are at very low risk for cervical cancer. Women with prior total hysterectomy for a benign condition, adequate histologic evidence that the cervix has been removed, and no previous abnormal Pap smears require no further screening for cervical cancer. Women who have had vaginal or cervical neoplasia at hysterectomy and those with prior endometrial cancer are at higher risk for developing vaginal neoplasia and need continued screening with vaginal smears. Women infected with HIV are at high risk for invasive cervical neoplasia. In this group, annual Pap testing after 2 normal tests 6 months apart is recommended by the Centers for Disease Control and Prevention. Women who have had in utero diethylstilbestrol (DES) exposure require annual Pap smears but no special screening.

Ovarian Cancer

Ovarian cancer is the leading cause of gynecologic cancer death and the fourth leading cause of all female cancer deaths in the United States, with an estimated 23,000 new cases and 13,900 deaths in 2002. For those at average risk, lifetime occurrence is 1.2%. Risk is increased with first- or second-degree family members with ovarian cancer, and it is decreased with oral contraception use, parity, and breast-feeding. Routine screening is not recommended. Bimanual pelvic examination, serum CA-125 testing, and transvaginal ultrasonography all lack sufficient sensitivity to detect cancers early enough to alter prognosis. Routine screening with CA-125 or ultrasonography in women older than 50 would result in more than 30 false-positive test results for each ovarian cancer detected. Women with false-positive test results would undergo undue stress and invasive testing, including laparotomy. Women from families who have the rare hereditary ovarian cancer syndrome should be referred to a gynecologic oncologist. For further discussion of ovarian cancer, see Chapter 50, Evaluation of Adnexal Masses & Screening for Ovarian Cancer.

Endometrial Uterine Cancer

Routine screening for endometrial cancer is not recommended. Women should be educated to report all abnormal uterine bleeding. Endometrial sampling or other diagnostic testing should be used to evaluate women with such symptoms (see Chapter 18, Menopause).

CANCER OF THE COLON & RECTUM

Colorectal cancer (CRC) is the third most common cause of cancer death among American women, with 77,900 new cases and 29,100 deaths estimated for 2002. The incidence is similar in men and women until age 50 and then becomes higher in men than in women. Because women live longer, there are more new cases and deaths in women. The average lifetime risk is 5%, and 90% of cancers occur after age 50. Modifiable risk factors for CRC include sedentary lifestyle, obesity, diet high in red meat and low in vegetables, and more than 1 drink of alcohol per day. At the time of diagnosis, more than half of CRCs are at an advanced stage. Surgical treatment is effective at an earlier stage. Because it is thought that most CRCs arise from polyps, screening strategies to identify localized cancers and find polyps for removal may decrease mortality. Special screening has been recommended for persons at high risk; risk factors include CRC in a first-degree family member, familial adenomatous polyposis (FAP) or hereditary nonpolyposis colon cancer (HNPCC), ulcerative colitis, and prior colon cancer or polyp.

Persons at average risk account for 80% of CRC, and fecal occult blood testing (FOBT), sigmoidoscopy, and colonoscopy as well as other emerging tests should be considered in this group.

A. FECAL OCCULT BLOOD TESTING

Of the 5 large randomized controlled trials of FOBT, 3 have shown a mortality benefit. The greatest benefit was seen in a study using 6 guaiac-impregnated rehydrated slides performed every year, every 2 years, or not at all. There were equal numbers of men and women in all 3 groups. After 13 years of follow-up study, a 33% reduction in mortality from CRC was found in the screened group compared with the unscreened control group. No difference in mortality was observed between the annually and the biannually screened groups. With the use of rehydrated slides, the number of false-positive results was greatly increased. In this study, the positivity rate of each screening was nearly 10%, with a positive predictive value for cancer of only 2.2%. All patients with positive results were referred for further study, usually colonoscopy; it has been estimated that half to one third of the screening benefit may have been caused by chance selection for colonoscopy. The sensitivity of FOBT for CRC is poor, about 30%. Given the modest mortality benefit, poor positive predictive value, and low sensitivity, FOBT is a less than ideal sole method for CRC screening.

B. SIGMOIDOSCOPY

There are no randomized trials of sigmoidoscopy, although a well-designed case-controlled study offers strong evidence for reduced mortality from CRC by about 30%. The mortality benefit for screening persisted for 10 years. Only about half of the currently diagnosed CRCs and polyps are within the view of the longer, 60-cm flexible sigmoidoscope however. Theoretically, there may be benefit from combining FOBT and sigmoidoscopy, but this has not been studied directly. All patients with polyps seen on sigmoidoscopy should be biopsied, and if an adenomatous polyp or cancer is found, they should be referred for colonoscopy.

C. COLONOSCOPY

Colonoscopy has become an increasingly popular choice for CRC screening in average risk persons, in addition to being the standard evaluation of those at high risk. Although not studied directly in screening trials, the colonoscope can be viewed as a very long sigmoidoscope, therefore benefit from the sigmoidoscopy trials can be inferred for colonoscopy. Approximately half of neoplasms occur in the proximal colon, beyond the reach of the sigmoidoscope. Half of these patients with proximal neoplasms have no distal polyps to prompt further investigation, and therefore the neoplasm would be missed by sigmoidoscopy alone. Colonoscopy has the additional advantage of removing polyps at the time of screening as well as a long interval (10 years) between recommended screenings in low risk persons.

The ACS, AAFP, American College of Gastroenterology (ACG), American College of Surgery, and USPSTF all recommend screening women age 50 or older using one of these strategies. According to the ACG, colonoscopy is the preferred method. The USPSTF states that it is unclear whether the increased accuracy of colonoscopy compared with alternative methods offsets the additional complications, costs, and inconvenience.

D. EMERGING TESTS

Virtual colonoscopy (computer-enhanced spiral computed tomography (CT) after bowel preparation and air insufflation) has shown promise. Limitations of virtual colonoscopy include high cost, false-positive results, limited expertise, and patient discomfort and embarrassment that may be worse than colonoscopy. Newer tests for FOBT and fecal genetic abnormalities have been insufficiently studied to be included as screening options.

E. SCREENING FOR HIGH-RISK PATIENTS

Patients at increased risk for CRC warrant different screening, depending on the reason for increased risk.

For those with a first-degree family member with CRC or adenomatous polyp occurring before age 60 or with multiple family members, with CRC, screening with colonoscopy should begin at age 40. Those with chronic ulcerative colitis should be screened with colonoscopy beginning 8 years after the onset of pancolitis or 15 years after the onset of disease limited to the left colon. Those with FAP and HNPCC should be referred to a specialist to consider genetic counseling and to begin early screening.

Lung Cancer

Lung cancer is the leading cause of cancer death in women in the United States, with an estimated 79,200 new cases and 65,700 deaths in 2002. Seventy-nine percent of lung cancers in women are attributed to cigarette smoking. Screening by chest roentgenogram and sputum cytology is ineffective. Screening by chest CT is being studied but is not recommended for routine care. Primary prevention by promoting smoking cessation is the most effective clinical intervention. All women who smoke should be advised of the cancer risk and be counseled to stop.

Barton MB, Harris R, Fletcher S: The rational clinical examination. Does this patient have breast cancer? The screening breast examination: should it be done? How? JAMA 1999;282:1270. [PMID: 10517431]

Baxter N: Preventive health care, 2001 update: should women be taught breast self-examination for breast cancer? CMAJ 2001;164:1837. [PMID: 11450279]

Canadian Task Force on the Periodic Health Examination. Ottawa (Canada): Health Canada; 1994:788 (reaffirmed by the CTFPHE 1999) http://www.ctfphc.org/index.html.

Carlson KJ, Skates SJ, Singer DE: Screening for ovarian cancer. Ann Intern Med 1994;121:124. [PMID: 8017726]

Committee on Gynecologic Practice. Recommendations on the frequency of Pap test screening. ACOG Committee Opinion 1995: p 152.

Eddy DM: Screening for cervical cancer. Ann Intern Med 1990; 113:214. [PMID: 2115753]

Feig SA et al: American College of Radiology guidelines for breast cancer screening. Am J Roentgenol 1998;171:29. [PMID: 9648758]

Pignone M et al: Screening for colorectal cancer in adults at average risk: a summary of the evidence for the US Preventive Services Task Force. Ann Intern Med 2002;137:132. [PMID: 12118972]

Screening for Breast Cancer. Recommendations and rationale, US Preventive Services Task Force March 2002. http:/www.ahcpr.gov/clinic/3rduspstf/breastcancer/brcanrr.htm.

Screening for colorectal cancer: recommendations and rationale. Ann Intern Med 2002;137:129. [PMID: 12118971]

US Preventive Services Task Force. Guide to clinical preventive services. 2nd ed. Washington, DC: Office of Disease Prevention and Health Promotion, U.S. Government Printing Office, 1996.

Winawer SJ et al: Colorectal cancer screening: clinical guidelines and rationale. Gastroenterology 1997;112:594. [PMID: 9024315]

COUNSELING TO PREVENT DISEASE & INJURY

All women should be encouraged to wear seat belts to prevent automobile injury and death. Also recommended is counseling on the use of motorcycle helmets, home fire safety precautions, and the danger of firearms.

There is consensus to advise patients who smoke to stop and to counsel nonsmokers to avoid tobacco use. All persons should be advised to limit their use of alcohol, stop alcohol consumption during pregnancy, and avoid driving after any alcohol use. Clinicians should use a case-finding strategy to identify problem drinkers (see Chapter 9, Chemical Dependency); they should educate patients about the dangers of illicit drugs and counsel against their use.

The USPSTF recommends safe sexual practices to reduce the risk of sexually transmitted disease and counseling to prevent unwanted pregnancy. Screening for cervical chlamydia should be routinely performed for sexually active women age 25 years and younger as well as other asymptomatic women at increased risk for infection (see Chapter 34, Sexually Transmitted Infections & Pelvic Inflammatory Disease).

Functional and cognitive assessment of the elderly is recommended.

When evaluating asymptomatic high-risk women for thyroid dysfunction, there is inadequate evidence supporting or refuting the value of screening thyroid-stimulating hormone levels. However, a high index of suspicion should be maintained because of the high prevalence of disease and the often subtle nature of the symptoms, especially in the elderly.

Periodic screening with fasting glucose for type 2 and gestational diabetes in high-risk populations is controversial.

Dietary counseling is discussed in Chapter 7.

Immunizations

6

Karen C. Smith, MD

Immunization guidelines in the United States are well standardized by the Advisory Committee on Immunization Practices (ACIP), and little controversy exists regarding their implementation. The general recommendations are presented here along with recent updates in practices. Special considerations that apply to women who are pregnant or may become so in the near future are also discussed.

THE CHALLENGE OF UNIVERSAL IMMUNIZATION

The most challenging issue facing health care providers is how to provide universal coverage effectively. It is incumbent on primary care specialists to review their patients' immunization needs periodically, to update services as appropriate, and to provide documentation in the patients' charts of services rendered.

Surveys of physicians' practice patterns and chart audits show only 12–24% compliance in appropriate tetanus vaccinations. Influenza vaccines in patients 65 years or older were given and documented in 12–68% of the charts.

In many primary care practices, compliance with guidelines is hampered by the lack of a consistent review process with patients, inadequate time to discuss the rationale for making the recommendations, and absence of a referenced chart documenting when immunizations are updated. The use of patient-held minirecords has been suggested as a means to increase patients' awareness of their need for receiving immunizations on schedule. Using these minirecords has shown an increasing compliance with children's immunizations. Providing printed guidelines concerning anticipated immunization requirements by age during routine office visits may also be helpful.

Dickey LL: Promoting preventive care with patient-held minirecords: a review. Patient Educ Couns 1993;20:37. [PMID: 8474946]

Kottke TE, Brekke ML, Solberg LI: Making "time" for preventive services. Mayo Clin Proc 1993;68:785. [PMID: 8331981]

Lewis CE: Disease prevention and health promotion practices of primary care physicians in the United States. Am J Prev Med 1988;4(4 Suppl):9. [PMID: 3079144]

Payne T et al: Development and validation of an immunization tracking system in a large health maintenance organization. Am J Prev Med 1993;9:96. [PMID: 8471277]

DIPHTHERIA & TETANUS

A diphtheria-tetanus (dT) combined vaccine may be updated every 10 years in adults. It appears that people over the age of 55, and especially over age 65, are frequently at risk for tetanus infections in the United States. Reasons for this statistic include the lack of primary immunization in some elderly patients and waning immunity to tetanus in people who have been immunized in the past. A careful history should be obtained regarding any past tetanus vaccines. If doubt exists as to the last booster date, the patient may be vaccinated without concern for significant side effects even if the previous vaccine was given within 10 years. The schedule for primary immunization includes 3 injections given at time zero, 4 weeks or longer after the first injection, and 6–12 months after the second dose. Local side effects such as itching or swelling at the injection site are common, but major side effects are extremely rare. An alternative strategy was recently advised by the Task Force on Adult Immunization (composed of representatives from American College of Physicians, Infectious Diseases Society of America, and Centers for Disease Control and Prevention). If a completed pediatrics series of primary immunization and an adolescent or adult booster can be documented, a single booster at age 50 provides lifelong protection. This new recommendation does not alter management of the injured patient. In the setting of a minor wound, a dT booster should be administered unless there is documentation of a booster within the last 10 years. When immunization status is doubtful or remote and a patient presents with a large, dirty wound, tetanus immune globulin should be given simultaneously with a dT booster.

Diphtheria is becoming more prevalent in poor urban populations in the United States and is seen increasingly in third-world populations. The vaccine is conjugated with tetanus so that compliance with the tetanus guidelines ensures immunity to diphtheria. The dT combination is preferred over a tetanus booster alone because of the continued need to protect patients from both diseases. Pregnancy is not a contraindication to use of the dT vaccine (Table 6–1).

Briggs GG et al: *Drugs in Pregnancy and Lactation: A Reference Guide to Fetal and Neonatal Risk,* 3rd ed. Williams & Wilkins, 1990.

Table 6–1. Immunization recommendations.

Immunization	Recommendations	Recommendations During Pregnancy
Diphtheria/tetanus	Complete primary series; booster every 10 years[1]	Not contraindicated
Influenza	Annually starting age 50 and in others who meet criteria[1]	Indicated in second and third trimesters but not first
Pneumococcal	Once at age 65 or older; once in younger women who meet criteria[1]	If otherwise indicated
Hepatitis A	*	Contraindicated
Hepatitis B	High-risk women*	If otherwise indicated
Measles, mumps, rubella	Once if born after 1956[1]	Contraindicated; pregnancy should be avoided for 3 months after receiving
Rubella	[1]	Contraindicated
Measles (Rubeola)	[1]	Contraindicated
Varicella	*	Contraindicated
Meningococcus	*	Not contraindicated

[1]See text for additional information.

Guide for Adult Immunization, 3rd ed. American College of Physicians, 1994.

Tetanus—United States, 1987 and 1988. MMWR 1990; 39 (No.3):37.

INFLUENZA

Influenza control is markedly improved by immunizing people who are at high risk for complications of infection as well as those who are at low risk but may have direct contact with high-risk persons. Persons who should be immunized because of higher risk include people age 50 and over as well as younger patients who have chronic cardiovascular or lung disease, kidney failure, liver disease, HIV infection, cancer, and diabetes. Women in their second and third trimesters of pregnancy during influenza season are advised to receive the vaccine. In addition, others who qualify are residents of long-term–care facilities, organ transplant recipients, and alcoholics. Low-risk people who should consider immunization are health care workers and others caring for high-risk patients, anyone with a high risk of exposure, and anyone who chooses prophylaxis to avoid potential loss of work time. Parents of children at risk for complications from influenza infection should consider immunization. The only contraindication is a history of anaphylaxis to eggs or other components of the vaccine. In high-risk people with a significant risk of allergic reaction to the vaccine, desensitization may be considered. Adults with acute febrile illnesses should wait until resolution of the acute infection before receiving the vaccine, but concurrent minor illnesses do not necessitate a delay in immunization.

Side effects are relatively uncommon. The most frequently reported symptom is soreness at the injection site, which lasts approximately 48 hours. Rarely, systemic reactions of fever, malaise, and myalgia appear 6–12 hours after injection and last 1–2 days. These symptoms occur most commonly in people who never have been exposed previously to any influenza virus or vaccine. A delayed-type local allergic reaction is induced occasionally by thimerosal, which is included in the vaccine. Finally, it should be noted that reports of Guillain-Barré sequelae related to the influenza vaccine have not increased since the 1976–1977 "swine flu" season. Influenza vaccine may be given concurrently at different sites with any one of the following vaccines: pneumococcal, measles-mumps-rubella (MMR), oral polio, *Haemophilus influenzae* group B (HIB), dT, and pertussis.

There are now a variety of antiviral drugs used to treat influenza symptoms. Newer preparations, including zanamivir and oseltamivir, have at least some activity against influenza A and B, whereas the older agents amantadine and rimantadine are active only against type A. Amantadine may be given concurrently with the influenza vaccine in patients exposed to influenza A and should be continued for 2 weeks after immunization. It also may be administered to patients who probably have acute influenza A infection; it is most valuable when started within 48 hours of the onset of symptoms. Finally, amantadine may be useful in patients who are at high risk throughout the flu season if the influenza vaccine is definitely contraindicated.

Administration of the influenza vaccine is not recommended during the first trimester of pregnancy. The vaccine is considered safe in lactating women. Amantadine is classified in pregnancy category C; it should be used, therefore, only when the benefits are believed to outweigh the potential complications of infection.

Briggs GG et al: *Drugs in Pregnancy and Lactation: A Reference Guide to Fetal and Neonatal Risk,* 3rd ed. Williams & Wilkins, 1990.

Bridges CB et al: Prevention and control of influenza: Recommendations of the Advisory Committee on Immunization Practices (ACIP). MMWR 2002;51(RR-3):1. [PMID: 1200217]

PNEUMOCOCCUS

There is general agreement that pneumococcal vaccine should be given once at age 65 for additional protection against otherwise life-threatening pneumococcal illness, which is common in this age group. Certain adults should receive the pneumococcal vaccine before age 65. This group is composed of people with the following medical illnesses: chronic cardiac or pulmonary disease, sickle cell anemia, any lymphoma or hematologic malignant condition, asplenia, diabetes mellitus, alcoholism, chronic liver disease (including cirrhosis), multiple myeloma, chronic renal disease (especially with the need for dialysis or with nephrotic syndrome), and other conditions associated with immunodeficiency (including HIV infection). People living in facilities where there is a greater risk of exposure also should be immunized. This vaccine may be given concurrently with influenza vaccine but at a different injection site. Boosters of the vaccine are usually not given because of the frequency of side effects associated with reimmunization. However, the Task Force on Adult Immunizations recommends a second pneumococcal vaccine after age 65, if initial immunization was given before that age. A minimum of 6 years should elapse between immunizations.

Pregnancy is not a contraindication to use of the pneumococcal vaccine in women who should be immunized based on the aforementioned criteria.

Centers for Disease Control and Prevention: Prevention of pneumococcal disease: recommendations of the Advisory Committee on Immunization Practices (ACIP). MMWR 1997; 46(RR-8):1. [PMID: 9132580]

Gardner P, et al: Adult immunizations. Ann Intern Med 1996; 12:35. [PMID: 7503476]

Guide for Adult Immunization, 3rd ed. American College of Physicians, 1994.

HEPATITIS B

The annual incidence of hepatitis B in the United States is approximately 200,000 to 300,000. Completion of a series of the hepatitis B vaccine is 85–90% effective in preventing clinical hepatitis and viral infection. If measurable hepatitis B surface antibody occurs in the vaccine recipient, protection from infection appears to be 100%. Hepatitis B vaccine currently is recommended only in adults at higher than average risk of exposure to the virus. Health professionals and others (eg, police officers) likely to have an occupational exposure to blood products are advised to receive the vaccine series. Other persons who appear to be at high risk for infection include patients undergoing dialysis, those who have hemophilia or for other reasons receive blood products regularly, some residents of long-term–care facilities, injection drug users, household contacts of hepatitis B carriers, sexually active persons with multiple partners, Alaskan Eskimos, Pacific Islanders, and homosexual and bisexual men. People in these categories should receive hepatitis B vaccine if they have negative serologic test results for hepatitis B surface antibody or antigen. Concurrent initiation of hepatitis B vaccine with passive immunization or hepatitis B immune globulin (HBIG) is advisable when a person is exposed to a needle or a splash of fluids contaminated with—or at high risk of containing—hepatitis B and when a person has had sexual contact with someone who may have acute hepatitis B infection. The recommended schedule for immunization is time 0, 1 month later, and 6–12 months later. If there is a delay in obtaining the second booster, it should be administered as soon as possible, and the third dose should be given no sooner than 2 months following the second dose. Completion of the immunization series confers 80–95% protection against clinical hepatitis and chronic hepatitis. When the recipient is known to have developed a hepatitis B surface antibody response to serologic testing, immunity is thought to be 100%.

Postvaccination assessment of immunity may be advisable in recipients older than 30 years because seroconversion rates may be lower in older individuals. Persons who are at greatest risk for exposure through daily activities or lifestyle (eg, patients undergoing dialysis and staff at dialysis units) or whose immunity response is likely to be low (eg, those taking immunosuppressive medications or who have immunosuppressive diseases) should consider testing for immunity within 6 months of completing the series. If antibody levels are below 10 mIU/mL, 1 or more boosters should be considered.

Side effects are limited to minor reactions. Between 3% and 29% of vaccinees have local pain. Between 1% and 6% have a fever above 37.7 °C and associated constitutional symptoms. Questions have been raised about a low incidence of associated Guillain-Barré syndrome, but this relationship appears to be doubtful.

Pregnant women considered at high risk for exposure to hepatitis B should be immunized. It is widely accepted that hepatitis B surface antigen testing is included in standard prenatal laboratory screenings.

Guide for Adult Immunization, 3rd ed. American College of Physicians, 1994.

US Preventive Services Task Force: *Guide to Preventive Services,* 2e. International Medical Publishing, 1996.

HEPATITIS A

Hepatitis A infection occurs in approximately 100,000 persons per year in the United States. It is contracted by the fecal-oral route, unlike the sexual and parenteral transmission of hepatitis B. There are an estimated 100 deaths annually from hepatitis A infection and the cost to the nation is greater than $200 million. The risk of hepatitis A infection for certain international travelers is even greater and leads to recommendations to use the vaccine for certain destinations.

Hepatitis A vaccine has been available since 1996 and is safe to use in women. Routine use is not recommended, however. Only women who have chronic liver disease of any type, injection drug users, women who receive clotting factor concentrates for clotting disorders, and women with high occupational exposure are targeted to receive the vaccine outside of travel situations. The relevant occupational exposures would be those in which handling fecal specimens is routine.

A previous infection with hepatitis A provides immunity to the disease. This can be determined by laboratory evaluation for hepatitis A antibodies (only the "total" antibody level needs to be checked unless acute hepatitis A is a possibility; in that case, IgM titers are requested to clarify the results). Recent data demonstrated that 33% of all US citizens are already immune to hepatitis A and would not need the vaccine if clinically indicated for work or travel. Older persons have an even higher likelihood of prior exposure. In the non-immune person receiving vaccine, the first dose leads to 80–90% immunity within 2 weeks and 96% immunity after 1 month. When the single booster is given 6–12 months later, seroconversion is thought to be 100%. The vaccine should be avoided when there is a known allergy to alum or 2-phenoxyethanol (only in the Havrix preparation), hypersensitivity reaction to the first dose, pregnancy (inadequate safety data), and in the setting of a concurrent acute illness.

Centers for Disease Control and Prevention: Prevention of hepatitis A through active or passive immunization. MMWR 1996;45(RR-15):1. [PMID: 9005304]

Gardner P, et al: Adult immunizations. Ann Intern Med 1996; 12:35. [PMID: 7503476]

MEASLES (RUBEOLA), MUMPS & RUBELLA

Women of child-bearing age born after 1956 should receive at least 1 vaccine containing MMR unless there is evidence from medical records indicating prior infection, immunization after age 12 months, or serologic documentation of immunity. Many adults born in the early 1960s or later have received this immunization, but documentation should be confirmed when possible, or serologic testing may be considered. Inadvertent repeat immunization is not likely to be harmful if immunization status cannot be determined easily. The two-dose childhood MMR vaccine currently administered is believed to give lifelong immunity; therefore, boosters are unnecessary.

Women who cannot document immunity to rubella during pregnancy should be immunized immediately after delivery, preferably with an MMR vaccine. Because immunity after a single measles vaccine has been noted to wane, women born after 1956 who have had only 1 documented vaccination and who have an increased risk of exposure to measles should receive a booster. This vaccine may be administered as attenuated measles virus or as a second MMR. Those who are thought to be at increased risk for exposure are students, health care workers, and travelers to areas where measles is prevalent.

Side effects associated with the rubella portion of the vaccine include rash, lymphadenopathy, and arthralgias or frank arthritis. Adult women appear to be more susceptible than others to these complications. Side effects of the measles vaccine include fever in 5–15% of recipients, beginning 5–12 days after the injection and lasting 48 hours. Women who have had anaphylaxis from gelatin or neomycin should not receive the vaccine. If the 3-component vaccine is not needed, vaccination with only rubella or rubeola vaccines are available to use individually.

Because MMR as well as rubella or measles vaccines are live-virus vaccines, they are contraindicated in immunocompromised persons and during pregnancy. With rubella vaccine, there is concern that a low incidence of congenital rubella syndrome (CRS) may result from vaccinating women in the first trimester of pregnancy. There are no substantial data, however, linking inadvertent vaccine administration during pregnancy to fetal abnormalities. Theoretic concerns about the possibility of CRS lead to the aforementioned recommendation but are not grounds for pregnancy termination. Women should be counseled to avoid becoming pregnant for 3 months after receiving the vaccine.

Cunningham FG et al: *Williams Obstetrics,* 19th ed. Appleton & Lange, 1993.

Gardner P, et al: Adult immunizations. Ann Intern Med 1996; 12:35. [PMID: 7503476]

VARICELLA

Varicella vaccine has been available since 1996 and effectively prevents or reduces the severity of primary varicella-zoster (chickenpox) infection. Greater than 90% of women are immune to this virus when tested. If a woman provides a convincing history of infection or immunization, no testing or vaccination is recommended. Of those who recall no varicella infection, over 70% have evidence of immunity on testing. The CDC advocates testing for immunity in women who are candidates to receive the vaccine, such as health care and other (eg, day care) workers who are likely to be exposed to the virus, household contacts of immunocompromised individuals, international travelers, and young women in college campus facilities or similar crowded living environments. Women of child-bearing age should also consider vaccination if not immune. Two doses of vaccine are indicated, 1–2 months apart. Seroconversion is 78% after the first dose and 99% after the second.

Side effects (such as fever) may appear up to 6 weeks after vaccination. Local effects also occur in 25–33% and include local swelling, tenderness, and erythema. In up to 8% of persons, a local or disseminated rash may appear. Contraindications include a known allergy to the vaccine or history of anaphylaxis to gelatin or neomycin.

The vaccine is contraindicated in pregnant women because it is a live virus. Women should avoid becoming pregnant for 1 month after vaccination. Its use in HIV infection is not studied.

Centers for Disease Control and Prevention: Prevention of varicella. Recommendations of the Advisory Committee on Immunization Practices (ACIP). MMWR 1996;45(RR-11):1. [PMID: 8668119]

Gardner P, et al: Adult immunizations. Ann Intern Med 1996; 12:35. [PMID: 7503476]

MENINGOCOCCUS

Neisseria meningitidis infection is fortunately rare in the United States. It is a devastating disease, with at least a 10% mortality rate. Most cases are sporadic, but recent studies have shown a higher susceptibility of college students in residential housing. College freshmen are statistically the highest at-risk population. The national rate of infection is 0.8 to 1.3 per 100,000; however the rate for college freshmen in dormitories rises to around 5 per 100,000. About two thirds of the infections would be covered by the 4 serotypes included in the vaccine (A, C, Y, and W-135). In 1997, the American College Health Association recommended that college students consider receiving this vaccine. It appears to be specifically beneficial for students entering residential living facilities on college campuses.

The vaccine is given in a single dose and is not contraindicated in pregnant women. Side effects are minimal and include pain and erythema at the injection site appearing within the first 48 hours. Fevers are present in 5%. A serious reaction such as anaphylaxis will occur in under 0.1 per 100,000 vaccinated persons.

Bruce MG et al: Risk factors for meningococcal disease in college students. JAMA 2001;286:288. [PMID: 11495618]

Centers for Disease Control and Prevention: Meningococcal disease and college students. Recommendations of the Advisory Committee on Immunization Practices (ACIP). MMWR 2000;49(RR-7):13. [PMID: 10902835]

Health Promotion: Tobacco Reduction & Improved Diet & Fitness

7

Tim McAfee, MD, MPH, & Beverly Green, MD, MPH

The largest causes of disease in women (and men) are tobacco use, poor nutrition, and reduced activity. Together they account for over 700,000 deaths/year in the United States alone. Analyses from a population-based perspective have demonstrated that helping people to stop smoking, exercise more, and lower cholesterol levels by 10% would prevent one third to half of all premature deaths. In the words of the US Preventive Services Task Force, which exhaustively reviewed the evidence for prevention screening and intervention effectiveness: "the most promising role for prevention in current medical practice may lie in changing the personal health behaviors of patients long before clinical disease develops."

There are very practical tools that clinicians can use to help their patients change their behaviors for the better. These tools have been demonstrated most definitively in the realm of tobacco use but are being applied as well to improving patient's nutrition and exercise habits.

GENERAL APPROACH TO THE PATIENT

General Considerations

Most smokers want to quit. Most sedentary people want to exercise more. However, most patients find it very difficult to actually change these behaviors. Similarly, most health care practitioners want to help their patients stop smoking, increase exercise, and eat more fruits and vegetables. However, clinicians often do not provide the type of advice and support that will result in a patient's success. For example, only 1 in 5 women who smoke recall being advised by their physician to quit smoking during the previous year. Fortunately, there are simple changes that clinicians can make to dramatically increase a patient's chance for success.

Brief Counseling Techniques

Most clinicians do not have the time or the expertise to engage in in-depth counseling. Fortunately, there are easily mastered brief counseling techniques that im-

prove the likelihood that patients will change their behavior for the better, especially when coupled with the office system changes discussed below. These techniques can be applied in as little as 3 minutes in an office or hospital visit. Use of these techniques also increases the satisfaction of the practitioner.

A. POSITIVE ADVICE

Providing consistent, brief advice to quit smoking during regular office visits is associated with a 1.6-fold increase in the quit rate in a clinical practice. The impact of clinician's advice about nutrition and exercise is less well-studied but appears promising. Advice is most effective if it is clear, personalized, and strong but non-judgmental. Advice may also be more effective if it is coupled with an offer of assistance or referral so that the patient understands the clinician wants to help, not harass. For example, a clinician may say "As your physician, I believe that starting an exercise program, such as walking for 30 minutes at least 5 days a week, will dramatically improve your health. I know this can be challenging to do, and if you decide you want to increase your exercise, we can discuss ways to make it easier."

B. STAGES OF CHANGE

The "stages of change" model provides a useful framework to help the busy clinician rapidly assess how to approach different patients. It proposes that patients benefit from different types of intervention based on how ready they are to make a change. There are 5 stages: precontemplative, contemplative, action, maintenance, and relapse.

Patients may be precontemplative (not planning on changing) for 2 reasons: (1) they may truly not want to change or (2) they may feel that it is impossible to change. Physicians can intervene by increasing motivation, rather than suggesting concrete ways to change. Explore what it would take to interest them in changing. It is up to the patient to decide what to do. It is okay to take "NO" for an answer! For people who feel it is impossible to change, try to create a sense of hope.

Patients who are contemplative are thinking about changing but do not yet have a concrete plan or date in mind. Clinicians can help by reinforcing the benefits of changing the behavior and formulating a plan.

The person who is in the action stage is actively planning or making a change. Physicians can offer their assistance and provide practical advice.

Patients in the maintenance stage (having successfully made the change) are at high risk for relapse, especially in the first year. Physicians should continue to reinforce the positive benefits and ask the patient if she feels confident about not relapsing. Look for telltale signs of potential relapse (such as depression in smokers).

Most patients who successfully change a behavior go through multiple cycles of attempts and relapse. Clinicians can help by encouraging the patient who relapses to begin preparing for another attempt. For example, the physician can advise the patient to view the attempt as a partial success, not a failure.

The stages of change approach is beneficial because it recognizes that people do not change a behavior all at once, and it encourages the clinician to support the patient no matter what the stage, leading to more satisfying interactions. Although the stages of change model provides a useful starting point, there is controversy and lack of clinical trial evidence about using detailed staging questions. The most important thing to ascertain is whether the patient wants to change the behavior.

C. SKILL-BUILDING

There are skills involved in changing behavior that can prove to be of enormous help to people. Patients can learn to eat healthier by reading nutrition labels, estimating appropriate portion size, and keeping a journal of caloric intake and exercise habits. If the goal is to quit smoking, patients can practice refusing a cigarette from a friend.

D. MOTIVATIONAL INTERVIEWING

Motivational interviewing is a direct, patient-centered counseling style that emphasizes helping patients explore and resolve ambivalence. Motivational interviewing identifies a series of assumptions healthcare practitioners often make that are inappropriate about behavior change: (1) this person ought to change, (2) this person wants to change, (3) this patient's health must be their prime motive for what they do, (4) unless the patient decides to change right now, the clinician has failed, (5) patients are either motivated to change or not, (6) I'm the expert; the patient must follow my advice. Rather, motivational interviewing is guided by several general principles: (1) using empathy or reflective listening, (2) avoiding arguing with patient; assume the patient is responsible for the decision to change,

and (3) supporting self-efficacy and optimism for change.

Opportunities for Counseling

Even if a practitioner is highly motivated, helping patients change a behavior can be very difficult to do. Using reminders in a patient's chart and taking the opportunity to counsel smokers to quit while they are hospitalized have been shown to help physicians effectively intervene with tobacco users and can also be considered for other health concerns.

During a regular office visit, tobacco status can be included as a "vital sign." The office staff member who escorts the patient to the examining room can be responsible for noting whether the patient is a current, former, or never smoker. This status should be recorded in the same area as blood pressure (Figure 7–1). Placing smoking-status stickers prominently on the chart (such as on a problem list) can also help. Electronic medical records can also incorporate smoking-status reminders.

For patients who have indicated they want to quit smoking, readily accessible follow-up is important. Having a health educator or nurse who is available to provide more detailed counseling to patients motivated to make a change in a health behavior has been shown to be very effective. This type of counseling can also be provided over the phone.

In addition to addressing health promotion during women's acute care visits, regularly scheduled visits every few years to review health status allows for more structured attention to lifestyle issues. Rather than framing such visits as primarily "physicals" or "Pap visits," it makes sense to include more focus on evaluating lifestyle practices and providing counseling and support for behavior change (see Chapter 5, Preventive Services).

Hospitalizations provide a potential "golden moment" for smoking cessation because most hospitalized smokers are more motivated to quit due to the increased awareness of the link between smoking and illness, unable to smoke due to confinement, and a "captive audience" for learning about how to quit long-term.

Skinner HA: Promoting Health Through Organizational Change. University of Toronto, 2002.

Miller W, Rollnick S: Motivational Interviewing: Preparing People to Change Addictive Behavior. The Guilford Press, 1991.

US Community Preventive Services Task Force 2002 www.thecommunityguide.org/home

US Preventive Services Task Force. Guide to clinical preventive services, 2nd ed. Williams & Wilkins, 1996. http://www.ahcpr.gov/clinic/uspstfix.htm

```
┌──────────────────────────────────────────────────────┐
│                    VITAL SIGN STAMP                    │
│                                                        │
│  Blood Pressure:_____   Pulse:_____   │
│                                                        │
│  Height: _____   Weight: _____          │
│                                                        │
│  Temperature:_____                              │
│                                                        │
│  Tobacco Use:   Current      Former (Quit date)_____ Never │
│                                                        │
│                 (circle one)                           │
└──────────────────────────────────────────────────────┘
```

Figure 7–1. Tobacco status as a "vital sign."

REDUCING TOBACCO USE & DEPENDENCE

 ## ESSENTIALS OF DIAGNOSIS

- *Self-reporting is usually as accurate as laboratory confirmation.*
- *Pregnant women may underreport tobacco use. (Laboratory confirmation possible by testing urine for cotinine.)*
- *Daily use of any amount is usually indicative of some dependence.*

General Considerations

Clinicians play a crucial role in helping women who smoke understand the negative impact continued smoking has on their health and the dramatic benefits to be gained by quitting. Although almost all women understand that smoking is "bad" for them, very few understand the magnitude of impact. Since 1973, there has been a 124% increase in lung cancer in women. Lung cancer has surpassed breast cancer as the number 1 cause of cancer mortality in women. This increase is entirely due to the marked increase in the prevalence of smoking among women during the past 50 years.

Women may be less likely than men to be successful during a specific quit attempt. Women are more likely than men to identify weight control as a reason to continue smoking. Current or past history of depression is more likely to complicate a quit attempt in women than in men.

Women should also be made aware of the dangers of environmental tobacco smoke (ETS), which is the third leading cause of preventable death in the United States (> 50,000 deaths per year). Women working as waitresses in restaurants and bars that allow smoking, or who live with partners who smoke, are particularly sus-

ceptible to increased incidences of lung cancer and heart disease. In addition, mothers may be motivated to quit by increasing their awareness of the impact of ETS on the health of their children. Asthma, chronic respiratory infection, and chronic otitis media are strongly correlated with ETS exposure.

Prevention

Every day in the United States, over 1000 girls begin smoking regularly. Substantial price increases in cigarettes and mass media campaigns may help decrease teenage initiation. Unfortunately, there is much less evidence for what clinicians can do to keep girls from starting to smoke.

Clinical Findings

Clinicians should not rely on the presence of objective clinical findings to diagnose tobacco use and dependence. Taking a good tobacco history is far more reliable than the "sniff" test, or hearing crackles at lung bases on auscultation, both of which are not sensitive.

Complications

Smoking is associated with several complications unique to women, including a 2-fold increase in cervical cancer and multiple negative pregnancy outcomes including low birth weight (2.1-fold increase), premature rupture of membranes, placental abruption and previa, and preterm delivery. Infants born to mothers who smoke have a higher perinatal mortality and are more prone to sudden infant death syndrome and developmental delay. Effects of smoking on breast cancer incidence are less clear.

Women who use tobacco are also susceptible to the same protean manifestations of tobacco use as men, including a 2-fold increase in cardiovascular disease, a 10-fold increase in chronic obstructive pulmonary disease, and up to a 20-fold increase in head and neck tumors. Tobacco use is responsible for almost a third of all fatal cancers.

Recent evidence review strongly supports the positive role of social support during quit attempts. Patients who inform their friends, family and co-workers of their intentions, and engage them in a quit attempt, do better. Physicians, nurses, medical assistants, pharmacists, respiratory therapists and other healthcare workers can provide considerable support for patients attempting to quit, simply by expressing encouragement and congratulations.

Treatment

A. COUNSELING

Counseling can be provided in many formats. Brief physician counseling (as little as 3 minutes) delivered in the context of a well visit, acute care visit, or chronic care visit is effective (Figure 7–2). Group, in-person,

and telephone counseling are all effective when delivered with multiple contacts over time by a trained counselor. Generally, there is a dose-response relationship between the extent and duration of contact.

One easily applied approach developed and tested in a series of randomized clinical trials is called the "5 A" approach:

Ask—Identify tobacco status at all visits

Advise—Encourage all tobacco users to quit

Assess—Collect information including interest in quitting

Assist—Provide help developing a plan for quitting, providing practical counseling and skills training, arranging for pharmacotherapy and referral for counseling

Arrange—Follow-up

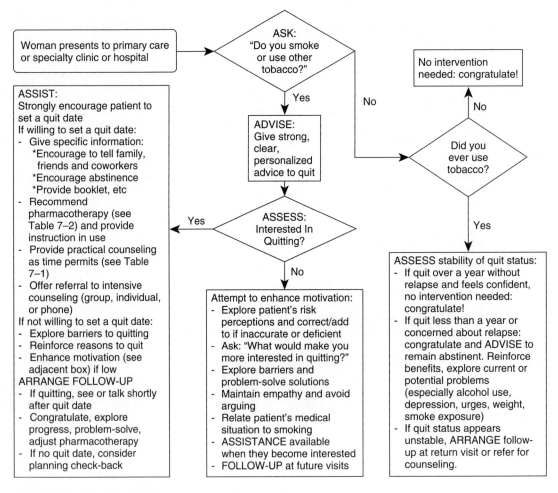

Figure 7–2. "5A" Method of tobacco cessation counseling.

Table 7–1 also lists techniques for counseling patients to quit smoking.

1. Counseling parents and adolescents—Young children exposed to tobacco smoke are at increased risk for respiratory illnesses, including initiation of asthma and chronic otitis media. The "5 A" model can be applied to parents, with special attention to firm advice about the effects of second-hand smoke on children. The primary recommendation should be for parents who smoke to quit. If a parent is unwilling to quit, recommend that they only smoke outside the house, wearing a separate jacket to keep smoke from permeating clothing that children come in contact with.

All preadolescent and adolescent girls are at high risk for experimenting with tobacco and progressing to dependency. Anticipatory guidance can be given at school physicals and well visits, beginning at age 11 or younger and continued regularly. Girls who have already experimented; have friends, siblings, or parents who smoke; who would accept a cigarette from a friend if offered; or who are doing poorly in school are at higher risk. Young girls profoundly underestimate the addictive nature of nicotine. Dependence can develop rapidly, and health care providers should emphasize that even experimentation is very risky. Young girls also overestimate the prevalence of smoking among their peers. As with women, 70% of adolescent daily smokers wish they had never started smoking. Unfortunately, there is very little known about what might work to help an adolescent quit smoking.

2. Counseling about weight gain—Weight gain of from 5 to 10 pounds (2–4 kg) is common when quitting. Women tend to gain more weight than men and be more concerned about it. Weight gain is usually caused both by metabolic changes and by increased caloric intake. However, excessive attention to weight control while quitting can undermine a quit attempt.

Physicians may emphasize the following points in counseling their patients to quit smoking:

- Weight gain from quitting smoking for most women is much less of a health concern than continued smoking.
- Weight gain may be lessened by increasing exercise such as walking, eating more fruits and vegetables, and avoiding an increase in fatty food intake.
- It is best not to focus too much on weight control until the patient is firmly established as a nonsmoker. It is generally not a good idea to attempt to lose weight while quitting smoking.
- Nicotine gum and sustained-release bupropion are associated with less initial weight gain, but there is no evidence for a sustained effect over time.

Table 7–1. Brief counseling techniques and examples for smokers planning a quit attempt.

Technique	Examples
Provision of cessation information	• Abstinence is required for success due to addictive nature of nicotine • Urges usually last just a few minutes; withdrawal usually decreases after 1–3 weeks. • Body begins to heal immediately after quitting (blood pressure and pulse decrease within hours)
Specific advice around quit date	• Get rid of all tobacco paraphernalia from house and car before quit date • Choose a date that gives enough time to prepare (1–4 weeks) but not so far out that there is no motivation to prepare • Review medication plans
Elicit past experiences	• Think of quit attempts that end in relapse as partial successes rather than failures • Review past quit attempts and relapses, and problem-solve for future attempt • Ask about current concerns
Anticipate high-risk situations	**Most common causes of relapse are:** • Substance abuse, including alcohol • Social situations with smokers, including household members who smoke • Depression, stress, and anxiety • Uncontrolled withdrawal symptoms • Weight gain • Higher level of dependence (ie, more than 1 pack per day) **Anticipate possibility of relapse:** • Best to avoid any smoking, even a puff • If slip, immediately return to non-smoking • If smoke more than 1 cigarette or recurrent slips, contact office or counselor
Provide and arrange for support	• Provide repeated encouragement and caring from practitioner and office staff • Acknowledge the difficulty of quitting • Elicit feelings about smoking and quitting • Encourage obtaining additional social support from friends, family, and coworkers

3. Counseling and pregnancy—Pregnant women should receive special attention regarding tobacco use because of the very serious potential for fetal harm. The major role of tobacco use in negative obstetric outcomes should be explained to all women of child-bearing age, since the best time to quit is before becoming pregnant. Initial obstetric visit forms and history taking should include meticulous inquiry into both current and former tobacco use, as well as exposure to second-hand smoke.

Almost half of women who smoke prior to becoming pregnant will have quit or cut down dramatically before their first obstetric visit. However, they are at significant risk for relapse. Unlike most other adult smokers, pregnant women may underreport smoking.

There is considerable controversy and uncertainty regarding the potential role for screening urine for cotinine in pregnant women. Any pregnant patient who either continues to smoke or has quit in the year previous to becoming pregnant should have her smoking status tracked as a pregnancy-related "vital sign" along with weight, blood pressure, and fundal height. In addition to brief office support and counseling, she should be strongly encouraged to receive intensive counseling from a trained cessation counselor. She should also receive counseling postpartum from both her obstetric and pediatric care providers about the importance of continued abstinence for her own health and the health of her baby. The well-proven impact of maternal smoking on sudden infant death syndrome, asthma, respiratory infections and otitis media can be emphasized. Without clinical reinforcement, well over half of women who quit during pregnancy will relapse to smoking within the first 6 months postpartum.

B. PHARMACOTHERAPY

There are 5 pharmaceutical products approved by the US Food and Drug Administration (FDA) for treating tobacco dependence (Table 7–2). An additional nicotine replacement product in lozenge form is also being approved by the FDA. Four of them are different delivery systems for nicotine replacement (patch, gum, inhaler, and spray). The fifth product is sustained-release bupropion, an oral medication that acts on the central nervous system (also used as an antidepressant). These agents have all been compared with placebo in large randomized clinical trials. However, there have been very few comparative trials between agents. Almost all trials have included substantial counseling with frequent follow-up in addition to medication. The absolute benefit from the medications increases markedly as the "dose" of counseling and instruction is increased.

Clonidine and nortriptyline have not been approved by the FDA for smoking cessation but efficacy has been shown in randomized trials. However, the evidence base is not as strong, they are more complex to prescribe, and are associated with more side effects than bupropion and the nicotine replacement therapies. Therefore, clonidine and nortriptyline should be reserved for patients in whom the FDA-approved medications are contraindicated.

Because of lack of comparative trials, choice of pharmacotherapy may be guided by patient preference, previous experiences (both positive and negative), cost, specific contraindications, and clinician familiarity. In general, the nicotine patch and sustained-release bupropion are the easiest and least expensive agents to use. Although less well-studied, there is some evidence that combination nicotine replacement therapy may increase long-term abstinence (patch with either gum or nasal spray).

The nicotine patch has not been studied in patients who have unstable angina or who have had a myocardial infarction in the last month. The patch has been shown to be safe but not necessarily effective in adolescents.

No cessation medication has been approved for use during pregnancy. Nicotine itself is associated with fetal risk, including neurotoxicity. Sustained-release bupropion has not been studied specifically in pregnant women, although it is classified as category B. When pregnant women are unsuccessful quitting smoking with counseling alone, clinicians can reasonably consider pharmacotherapy. If nicotine replacement is used, consider dosing at the lower end and using an intermittent delivery form such as nicotine gum (there have been concerns raised around the continuous levels of nicotine provided by the patch). If sustained-release bupropion is used, consider dosing at 150 mg once daily rather than twice daily.

C. COMPLEMENTARY THERAPY

The US Public Health Service guideline group conducted a meta-analysis on 5 randomized trials of acupuncture as a cessation technique. No evidence for effectiveness was found. A similar review of hypnosis found insufficient evidence to support its use as a treatment for smoking cessation. A number of herbal and homeopathic remedies are available, but none have been tested in randomized controlled trials.

Aversive smoking, in which a patient smokes intensively to the point of physical discomfort including nausea, has been shown to be effective. However, it involves some increased health risk, requires careful clinical oversight, and has not proved popular with smokers.

When to Refer to a Specialist

Primary care clinicians can appropriately treat most women who use tobacco. All the medications that have

Table 7–2. FDA-approved pharmacotherapy for smoking cessation.[a]

Medication	Usual dose/duration	Precautions	Side Effects	Pros and Cons
Nicotine patch	• 21 mg patch for 4 weeks • 14 mg patch for 2 weeks • 7 mg patch for 2 weeks OR • 15 mg/16 hr for 8 weeks (consider lower initial dose if smoke fewer than 11 cigarettes per day)	History of allergic reaction to adhesives	Local skin reactions, insomnia	**Pros:** Easiest nicotine replacement therapy product to use Available over the counter Lower abuse potential **Con:** Fixed daily dose
Nicotine polacrilex gum	• 2 mg and 4 mg dose • May use up to 24 pieces per day—aim for at least 9 pieces per day initially • Often patients do not use enough	Peptic ulcer disease, full dentures, TMJ	Throat and mouth irritation, dyspepsia	**Pros:** Available over the counter unobtrusive to use Can use on schedule and ad lib for individual cravings **Cons:** Requires more instruction in proper use (briefly chew to activate then park, avoid acidic beverages before use) Expensive if used extensively
Nasal spray	• 1–2 doses/h up to 3–6 months	Severe reactive airway disease	Severe nasal irritation, tearing, sneezing, cough	**Pro:** Pharmacokinetics most similar to smoking—fast delivery **Cons:** Smaller number of RCT participants Highest abuse potential Cost Most annoying side effects
Nicotine inhaler	• 6–16 cartridges per day for up to 6 months	Severe bronchospastic disease	Cough, throat and mouth irritation	**Pros:** User controls dosing Provides similar hand/mouth stimulation to cigarettes **Cons:** Expensive Use is obvious
Sustained-release bupropion	• 150 mg/d for 3 days, then 150 mg twice daily for 8 weeks—begin 10 days before discontinuing smoking (150 mg daily continued dosing also effective	History of seizure or predisposition to seizures (anorexia/ bulimia, meds, family history, stroke etc)	Dry mouth, insomnia, agitation	**Pro:** Easy to use oral medication No nicotine **Con:** Increases seizure risk in unscreened population (1 in 1000)

[a]Instruct all users to abstain from smoking while using the above agents. Pregnancy, lactation, and recent myocardial infarction or unstable angina are relative contraindications. All nicotine replacement therapies can result in symptoms of nicotine overdose if more nicotine than baseline smoking is delivered.

been shown to be effective can be prescribed or recommended by primary care physicians. Brief counseling by physicians has been shown to increase quit success. However, patients making a quit attempt can further increase their likelihood of success by receiving additional counseling support by a trained cessation specialist.

Unfortunately, the availability of intensive tobacco treatment counseling support varies widely in different areas of the country. In addition, many insurance plans still do not provide coverage for these well-proven services, and most smokers are simply not willing to attend group programs.

In many states, there are now toll-free phone lines where women who want help quitting can receive in-depth evidence-based counseling sessions over the phone, as well as learn about local resources. In some states, nicotine patches may be available through these phone lines for uninsured smokers. A number of web sites are also available that provide information about local treatment resources; chat rooms and discussion groups on the Internet help provide social support to smokers.

Most smoking cessation medications can be prescribed to women without difficulty. Caution should be exercised when prescribing either sustained-release bupropion or nicotine replacement for a pregnant woman. Consultation may be useful if the clinician is unfamiliar with the risk-benefit profile during pregnancy. If a woman is at significantly increased risk for seizure due either to medications or to past history, and the use of bupropion is strongly desired, consultation with a psychiatrist or a physician with specialized tobacco treatment experience may be considered.

For women who have attempted to quit multiple times using medication and intensive counseling, referral to an intensive multidisciplinary tobacco treatment clinic may be useful. However, these do not exist in many areas.

Prognosis

A woman who continues to smoke faces a 40% chance of dying prematurely of a tobacco-related disease. Absolute risk of dying is low until she reaches her 50s. A woman who quits adds about 3–7 years to her life expectancy depending on her smoking history and time of quit. It is very important to emphasize to patients that switching to a "light" cigarette is not an effective means of decreasing risk.

The odds of success for any given quit attempt vary dramatically depending on the amount of assistance that a smoker uses. For an unassisted "cold turkey" quit attempt, the odds of being a nonsmoker 1 year later are around 5–10% at best. With pharmacotherapy and

counseling, this can be increased to 20–35%. Prognosis is improved in patients who smoke fewer cigarettes, are highly motivated, and believe they will be successful.

A clinical practice guideline for treating tobacco use and dependence: A US Public Health Service report. The Tobacco Use and Dependence Clinical Practice Guideline Panel, Staff, and Consortium Representatives. JAMA 2000;283:3244. [PMID: 10866874] http://jama.ama-assn.org/issues/v283n24/abs/jst00005.html

Rigotti NA: Clinical practice. Treatment of tobacco use and dependence. N Engl J Med 2002;346:506. [PMID: 11844853]

NUTRITION

General Considerations

Good nutrition is not just about eating healthy foods; it is about eating the right amount and having enough variety to supply the body with needed nutrients. Nutrition advice for women can be simple: eat a diet that is low in fat (particularly saturated fat); high in fruits and vegetables (5 servings per day); and has adequate calcium, vitamin D, and folate intake. People given a brief motivational message by physicians along with self-help pamphlets on nutrition continued to have a low fat, high fiber diet after 1 year.

Nutrition Recommendations

A. FATS

Fat intake and its relationship to cardiovascular disease is of particular importance since women have only a slightly lower risk than men of dying of cardiovascular disease. The evidence that shows eating a high-fat diet (particularly foods high in saturated fats) increases the risk of coronary heart disease (CHD), stroke, peripheral vascular disease, and overall mortality is strong.

Medications that lower serum lipids increase blood insulin levels. Diets low in fat decrease insulin levels; when lipid-lowering medications are combined with a low-fat diet, the effects on lowering cholesterol and LDL are additive and independent. Women at high risk for or who have cardiovascular disease need to be reminded that it is optimal to combine medications with a low fat diet. High fat diets have also been linked to colon cancer. The relationship of fat intake to breast cancer is less clear. Fats are also calorie dense with 9 calories per gram of weight, while carbohydrates and proteins only have 4 calories per gram of weight.

The US Preventive Services Task Force (USPSTF), USDA "Dietary Guidelines for Americans" (1995), Surgeon General, and American Cancer Society all recommend a low-fat diet (particularly one low in saturated fats and cholesterol). The American Heart Association (1993), National Research Council (1989),

National Cancer Institute (1986), and National Cholesterol Education Program (1993) all recommend limiting dietary fat to 30% or less of total calories, saturated fat to 8–10% or less of total calories, and cholesterol to 300 mg or less per day.

B. Fruits, Vegetables, and Fiber

Less than one fourth of American women eat 5 servings of fruits or vegetables a day. Eating 5 or more servings of fruits or vegetables, with some whole grains, helps people get the recommended intake of 20–35 grams of fiber per day. Fruits and vegetables also supply vitamins and other nutrients that appear to be health-protective.

People who have higher intakes of fruits and vegetables have decreased risk for some cancers, CHD, and some chronic diseases including strokes and advanced age-related macular degeneration. High fiber intake decreases serum cholesterol and LDL, decreases risk of myocardial infarction and deaths from CHD, improves glycemic control in diabetics, helps with weight control, and improves gastrointestinal function. The relationship between colon cancer and fiber intake has been recently challenged, however.

The USPSTF recommends that "Adults and children age 2 years and over should be encouraged to eat a variety of foods with an emphasis on the consumption of whole grains, cereals, legumes, vegetables, and fruits." The USDA "Dietary Guidelines for Americans" (1995): The Food Guide Pyramid recommends 3–5 servings per day of vegetables; 2–4 servings per day of fruits; and 6–10 servings per day of bread, cereal, rice, and pasta. The American Dietetic Association and the National Cancer Institute recommend eating 20–35 grams of fiber every day.

C. Calcium and Vitamin D

According to the National Institutes of Health, 70% of women have a daily calcium intake below the recommended level. In the Framingham population, vitamin D deficiency was found in 14% of women and it increased with age. Adequate calcium and vitamin D intake is needed to achieve optimal peak bone mass, and in later years modifies the rate of bone loss associated with aging (Table 7–3). Women who have higher milk intake in childhood and adolescence attain greater peak bone mass. Women with greater peak bone mass are at lower risk for osteoporosis.

Adequate levels of calcium intake can be achieved by eating calcium rich foods (dairy products), calcium-fortified foods or taking calcium supplements. Calcium absorption and retention are negatively affected by inadequate vitamin D, certain medications (eg, glucocorticoids), achlorhydria of the stomach, and foods that contain high amounts of oxalic acid (spinach and beans) or phytic acid (whole grains, nuts, and seeds).

Table 7–3. Optimal Daily Calcium and Vitamin D Intake

Calcium Intake	Vitamin D Intake
1300 mg for adolescent girls	200 IU for females ages 1–49 years
1000 mg for women aged 19–50 years	400 IU for women aged 50 years
1200 mg for women older than 50 years	600–800 IU for women over age 65 years
1300 mg for pregnant or nursing women	200 IU for pregnant or nursing women

Recommendations of the Standing Committee on the Scientific Evaluation of Dietary Reference Intakes (Institute of Medicine).

Solar radiation results in the cutaneous synthesis of vitamin D. Fifteen to 30 minutes of sun exposure daily is usually sufficient to maintain adequate vitamin D production. Vitamin D synthesis, however, depends on the intensity of the sun and the amount of skin exposed. Cutaneous production of vitamin D may be deficient in northern latitudes. Age-related skin changes also result in decreased production of vitamin D. Milk is vitamin D fortified with 100 IU per 8 ounces. Other dairy products generally have no vitamin D. A multivitamin or vitamin D supplements should be considered for older women and for women with less sun exposure.

Supplemental vitamin D reduces the risk of bone fracture in older women. Adequate calcium intake may reduce bone loss, particularly in women with below average calcium intake (< 400 mg daily). There is no evidence that shows giving adequate calcium alone decreases fractures.

The USPSTF recommends that women consume adequate amounts of calcium and vitamin D. The NIH Consensus Development Conference on Optimal Calcium Intake states that adequate vitamin D is essential for optimal calcium absorption. The preferred source of calcium is calcium-rich foods, such as dairy products. Eating calcium-fortified foods and taking calcium supplements are other means by which optimal calcium intake can be reached.

D. Folate

Each year in the United States about 2500 infants are born with neural tube defects (NTDs), spina bifida, and anencephaly. There is direct evidence that the consumption of folic acid (folate) or multivitamins containing folate before and during early pregnancy can reduce the incidence of NTDs. It is estimated that 75% of American women of reproductive age do not consume enough folate to reduce the risk of NTDs.

All women who may become pregnant (even if using birth control), should take 0.4 mg of folate daily. To ensure adequate folate during the first 28 days of pregnancy, women should begin taking adequate doses of folate at least 1 month before conception and continue throughout the first trimester of pregnancy. For women who have had at least 1 infant affected with an NTD, supplementation with a higher dose of folate—4 mg of folate daily—is recommended.

Folate deficiency is also thought to be a factor in cardiovascular disease; people with lower folate blood levels tend to have higher homocysteine levels. Higher homocysteine levels have been associated with cardiovascular disease, and folate supplementation decreases homocysteine levels. Patients with cardiac disease who took supplemental vitamin B (1 mg/d of folate, 400 μg/d of B_{12}, and 10 mg/d of pyridoxine) decreased their risk for new cardiac events by 32%.

Foods rich in folate include legumes, leafy green vegetables, yeast, liver, and oranges. Fortified cereals generally have 0.1 mg per serving. Breads and flours are fortified with folate as well, but the amounts may not be enough to ensure adequate intake. Most multivitamins (including prenatal vitamins) contain 0.4–0.8 mg of folate. Women need to start taking folate 1–3 months before pregnancy. Since many pregnancies are unplanned, it is recommended that all women who may become pregnant ensure adequate folate through the diet or supplements.

The USPSTF recommends that all women of childbearing age take a daily multivitamin or supplement containing 0.4–0.8 mg of folic acid. The US Department of Health and Human Services recommends that all women capable of becoming pregnant should consume 0.4 mg of folic acid per day for the purpose of reducing their risk of having a pregnancy affected with spina bifida or other NTDs.

E. VITAMINS A, C, AND E

Vitamins, minerals, and other food supplements are concentrated forms of nutrients and need to be treated with the same respect as prescription medications.

For **vitamin A,** doses above the recommended daily allowance (RDA) of 5000 IU are not recommended. Vitamin A deficiency leads to xerophthalmia, a common cause of blindness in undeveloped countries. Vitamin A deficiency is rare in the United States because foods are fortified with vitamin A. Vitamin A and beta-carotene are not recommended for primary or secondary prevention of CHD or cancer. Excess intake of vitamin A has been associated with birth defects (as little as 10,000 IU/day). High intake of vitamin A has also been associated with osteoporotic fractures. A randomized controlled trial (the CARET study) of beta-carotene found that persons given supplements had an increased risk of cancer.

The RDA for **vitamin C** is 60 mg. There is only weak evidence that vitamin C (1000 mg/d) decreases the severity of the common cold. There is insufficient evidence to recommend vitamin C supplementation for the primary or secondary prevention of CHD or cancer. Vitamin C is safe even at very high doses consumed over long periods of time. High doses may, however, cause dyspepsia and diarrhea in some people. High doses of vitamin C may interfere with tests for occult blood in the stool and urine, leading to false-negative results. There is controversy as to whether vitamin C supplementation contributes to excess iron absorption in hereditary hemochromatosis.

The RDA for **vitamin E** is 15 IU. Higher doses of vitamin E (400–800 IU) have antioxidant effects and remove free radicals that may be responsible for vascular changes in cardiovascular disease and possibly cancer. There is good direct evidence from a randomized controlled trial (the HOPE trial) that vitamin E does not decrease the risk of cardiovascular events or death in men and women with known cardiovascular disease. There is insufficient evidence to recommend it for the primary prevention of cancer. Vitamin E is generally safe in high doses over long periods of time. However, it may induce a vitamin K–related coagulopathy and bleeding in patients taking warfarin, so prothrombin times may need to be monitored more closely.

Body Weight

There is common agreement with the principle that all people, including women, should match their intake of calories to their overall energy needs and that they should maintain a level of physical activity that matches their energy intake. Despite the wisdom of this statement, in the year 2000 more than 56% of the U.S. adult population was overweight (36% are overweight and 20% are obese), compared with 45% in 1991 (32% were overweight and 13% obese). The definition of overweight is a body mass index (BMI) > 25 and > 30 for obesity (Table 7–4). The equation to calculate BMI follows:

$$BMI = \text{weight in kg} \div \text{height in m}^2$$

Related to the increasing epidemic of obesity, the incidence of diabetes has almost doubled in the last 10 years with the incidence increasing from 4.9% to 7.3%. Men are slightly more likely than women to be obese (20.2% versus 19.4%, respectively). However, diabetes

Table 7–4. Body mass index chart.

Height (in)	Body mass index																
	19	20	21	22	23	24	25	26	27	28	29	30	31	32	33	34	35
	Body Weight (lbs)																
58	91	96	100	105	110	115	119	124	129	134	138	143	148	153	158	162	167
59	94	99	104	109	114	119	124	128	133	138	143	148	153	158	163	168	173
60	97	102	107	112	118	123	128	133	138	143	148	153	158	163	168	174	179
61	100	106	111	116	122	127	132	137	143	148	153	158	164	169	174	180	185
62	104	109	115	120	126	131	136	142	147	153	158	164	169	175	180	186	191
63	107	113	118	124	130	135	141	146	152	158	163	169	175	180	186	191	197
64	110	116	122	128	134	140	145	151	157	163	169	174	180	186	192	197	204
65	114	120	126	132	138	144	150	156	162	168	174	180	186	192	198	204	210
66	118	124	130	136	142	148	155	161	167	173	179	186	192	198	204	210	216
67	121	127	134	140	146	153	159	166	172	178	185	191	198	204	211	217	223
68	125	131	138	144	151	158	164	171	177	184	190	197	203	210	216	223	230
69	128	135	142	149	155	162	169	176	182	189	196	203	209	216	223	230	236
70	132	139	146	153	160	167	174	181	188	195	202	209	216	222	229	236	243
71	136	143	150	157	165	172	179	186	193	200	208	215	222	229	236	243	250
72	140	147	154	162	169	177	184	191	199	206	213	221	228	235	242	250	258
73	144	151	159	166	174	182	189	197	204	212	219	227	235	242	250	257	265
74	148	155	163	171	179	186	194	202	210	218	225	233	241	249	256	264	272
75	152	160	168	176	184	192	200	208	216	224	232	240	248	256	264	272	279
76	156	164	172	180	189	197	205	213	221	230	238	246	254	263	271	279	287

is diagnosed in more women (8.2%) than men. Childhood obesity and the weight gain associated with pregnancy are risk factors for adult obesity. Obesity is also associated with a variety of other conditions including hypertension, cardiovascular disease, degenerative arthritis, gallbladder disease, sleep apnea, and some cancers including breast and pancreatic cancer, and overall mortality risk.

Obesity or overweight is a very complex problem, with components that are both societal and genetic. Over the last 30 years lifestyles have become increasingly more sedentary, fast food more prevalent, and portions larger. Despite our easier access to fresh fruit and vegetables and low calorie food options, this epidemic continues. From a health promotion point a view, little is known about what providers can do to help patients. A recent Cochrane Review analyzing the effectiveness of health professionals' management of overweight patients found few studies that tested interventions to improve physicians' skills or the provision of institutional support to improve weight control. They recommended that physicians use "good clinical judgment" until more studies are done. However, people that participate in weight loss programs that include behavioral approaches, as well as dietary and exercise counseling do generally lose 5% of their body weight or more. While this might not result in a person's returning to their ideal body weight, small weight losses can have great health benefits, including prevention of or improved control of diabetes and hypertension, and improvements in sleep apnea and degenerative arthritis symptoms and overall sense of well being.

General principles of behavior change and support may be useful for helping women who are overweight. Setting small goals—such as improving nutrition, increasing physical activity, and losing 5–10% of current body weight—may be more attainable, result in immediate improvements in health, and improve health outcomes. If a woman lacks self-confidence because of weight issues, cognitive therapy skills may be useful. See Chapter 16 for more information on obesity and its treatment.

Nutrition During Pregnancy

Pregnant women can follow the same general principles already outlined, including ensuring adequate intake of folate. Alcohol should be avoided in all trimesters, because of its known association with Fetal Alcohol Syndrome. Iron deficiency is common during pregnancy and is associated with prematurity and low birth weight infants. However, there is no evidence that replacing iron in pregnancy improves outcomes.

Report of the US Preventive Services Task Force. Guide to Clinical Preventive Services, 2nd ed. International Medical Publishing, Inc, 1996.

Schatzkin A et al: Lack of effect of a low-fat, high-fiber diet on the recurrence of colorectal adenomas. Polyp Prevention Trial Study Group. N Engl J Med 2000;342:1149. [PMID: 10770979]

PHYSICAL ACTVITY

General Considerations

The value of regular physical activity for reducing the risk of cardiovascular disease, type 2 diabetes, some cancers (including breast and colon cancer), and osteoporosis is well established. Physical activity also decreases stress and is as effective as medications in treating depression.

Despite the benefits of exercise, only 24% of adults report participating in regular, sustained physical activity (5 or more times per week for 30minutes or longer), and 27% of Americans participated in no leisure time physical activity at all. Physicians are in a unique position to influence patients; however, in a recent survey, only 28% of patients reported receiving advice to increase their physical activity level. Identifying strategies to increase physical activity is a major public health challenge.

The Role of Physical Activity Over a Lifetime

Young women establish habits for physical activity that will last a lifetime. Physical activity can help women cope with PMS (premenstrual syndrome) and the stress of work or a young family. Physical activity helps women make strong bones; however, if they are elite athletes, special attention needs to be given to calcium intake and hormonal status. Women who become amenorrheic with exercise may need estrogen replacement to prevent bone loss. Similarly, women who exercise too much, especially if they have menstrual changes, may need to be evaluated for anorexia nervosa.

A. PREGNANCY

Being physically active before, during, and after pregnancy has several benefits: an improved sense of well being and decreased discomforts, a shorter second stage of labor, faster recovery after labor, and decreased weight gain after pregnancy. There is no evidence that a moderate exercise program is harmful to the fetus. Women can continue the activities they did prior to pregnancy or start a moderate exercise program. Starting a new vigorous exercise program during pregnancy is not advised because of (1) concerns about overheating, particularly in early pregnancy, as this has been identified as a risk to the fetus and (2) concerns about the possibility of ketosis or hypoxia and their potential for harmful effects to the fetus.

The hormone relaxin peaks in the third trimester, preparing the pelvis to widen and become more malleable for delivery. Relaxin increases the laxity of all joints and the woman's center of gravity also shifts as the uterus expands. These 2 changes increase the risk of falls, which are more common during pregnancy. Sports that require balance or coordination may be more difficult, and women should avoid these or be advised to use great caution if they choose to hike, horseback ride, or ski during later pregnancy. Because of pressure on the vena cava and the resulting increase in maternal blood pressure, women should avoid exercises in the supine position in the third trimester. Scuba diving is also not recommended at any time during pregnancy.

The American College of Obstetricians and Gynecologists have the following recommendations about exercise during pregnancy:

- Exercise at an intensity, duration, and frequency that does not cause pain, shortness of breath, or excessive fatigue.
- Avoid exercises in the supine position in the third trimester.
- Avoid exercise that requires exceptional balance or extreme range of motion in the third trimester.

B. MENOPAUSE

Physical activity helps counteract the decrease in basal metabolic rate that occurs as women age and after menopause. Women who maintain a normal weight and are fit have lower estrogen levels and decreased risk for breast cancer and uterine cancer. A lower baseline level of estrogen in exercising women also helps lessen the wide fluctuations of estrogen that occur during menopause. Physical activity decreases the risk and improves the control of cardiovascular risk factors including hypertension, diabetes, and hypercholesterolemia. Flexibility and strength helps prevent common muscular conditions such as rotator cuff syndrome and can help prevent or improve back problems. Weight bearing exercise helps maintain bone mass in the hips and low back.

C. OLDER WOMEN

Women who are moderately or very physically active in later life have better health status, lower health care utilization, improved quality of life, less disability, less cardiovascular disease, and lower overall mortality rates. Women who start or increase their levels of physical activity derive the same benefits. Flexibility and strengthening become increasingly important in helping women to prevent the normal muscle loss that begins to occur in older people and to maintain better control of balance. Osteoporosis occurs in over 50% of women who are age 80 or older. Only half of the women with osteoporosis suffer an osteoporotic fracture. Fitness interventions that have included exercises to improve balance, including Tai Chi, decrease the risk of falling and trips to the emergency department, but did not decrease osteoporotic fractures.

Physical activity decreases the symptoms of osteoarthritis and can help to delay a joint replacement. Staying active is important in maintaining function and independence in old age. Many people feel that they should do less if they have a chronic disease. Paradoxically, this is the group that benefits most from physical activity.

Integrating Exercise Counseling into Clinical Practice

The USPSTF recommends that clinicians counsel patients to incorporate regular physical activity into their daily routines to prevent CHD, hypertension, obesity, and diabetes. The Centers for Disease Control and Prevention recommends 30 minutes of moderate to vigorous activity on most days. To maintain energy balance and an ideal weight, many women will need to accumulate at more than 30 minutes of exercise. The Institute of Medicine recommends accumulating 60 minutes of moderate activity on most days. The American College of Sports Medicine advises that before starting a new program of vigorous exercise (ie, running a 10-minute mile) patients who are at moderate risk for cardiovascular disease undergo a diagnostic exercise tolerance test (ETT). Moderate risk is defined as being 55 or older, and having two or more risk factors (diabetes, hypertension, family history of premature cardiovascular disease, obesity (BMI > 30), tobacco use, or hyperc-

holesterolemia/low high-density lipoprotein levels). Patients at high risk for cardiovascular disease (ie, existing symptoms or signs) are advised to undergo testing before beginning moderate exercise.

Questions to ask in obtaining a physical activity history follow:

- How many times per week do you exercise?
  ☐ none ☐ 1–2 ☐ 3–4 ☐ 5+
- How many minutes does your exercise usually last?
  ☐ 1–14 ☐ 15–29 ☐ 30
- Is your exercise moderate to vigorous?
  ☐ yes ☐ no

Examples of moderate to vigorous exercise include brisk walking, active gardening, jogging, swimming, or bicycling (Table 7–5). If a woman answers 5 or more times per week, 30 minutes per session, and yes to moderate to vigorous, then they are active. If not, ask if she is considering increasing her physical activity in the next 6 months and how confident she is that she can do this.

Physician advice, including the use of exercise prescriptions and motivational counseling, has been shown to help patients initiate physical activity. However, advice alone does not lead to sustained increases in activity over time. Providing additional support, such as vouchers to exercise clubs or motivational and tailored counseling by health educators, has had some success in helping people to maintain these gains. To avoid injuries, advise the patient to (1) increase activity levels gradually, (2) listen to her body (if something begins to hurt, do not work through it, rest), (3) use protective equipment (such as helmets for bicycling, skating, and snowboarding; elbow, wrist, and knee protectors for in-line skating; and goggles for handball and racquetball), and (4) make sure equipment and shoes are in good shape. Writing an exercise prescription may be helpful. Have the patient choose the activity, agree on the frequency and duration of the activity, and write it on a prescription pad!

Discuss the importance of physical activity as often as possible. Remind people who have chronic diseases and disability, that exercise is essential for their well-being. Provide information for patients on how to increase and maintain exercise levels. Learn about the resources provided by health care organizations. Many health plans offer discounts or coverage for fitness programs or the use of exercise facilities. Some health plans have health educators that can help support behavior change. Learn about resources in your community. The USPSTF in the Guide to Community Preventive Services found that multicomponent community interventions such as signs to use the stairs, creation of walking trails, self-help groups and social support, school pro-

Table 7–5. Exercise intensity guide.

Light activity (4 or less calories burned per min; 100 calories in ½ hour)	Moderate activity (5–7 calories burned per minute; 150–200 calories in ½ hour)	Strenuous activity (7 calories burned per min; 250–300 calories in ½ hour)
Walking slowly	Walking briskly	Running
Light housekeeping	Mopping, sweeping	Hiking uphill or backpacking
Weeding	Washing windows, washing car	Building a fence
Carpentry	Mowing (push mower), raking	Moving furniture
Stretching	Calisthenics, low impact aerobics	Strenuous aerobics, stairmaster
Baseball	Rowing, canoeing	Soccer, football, basketball
Fishing	Swimming with moderate effort	Fast swimming
Bowling	Cycling at a moderate pace	Fast cycling
Table tennis	Tennis (doubles)	Tennis, racquetball
Golf with a power cart	Golf carrying clubs	Skiing

grams, and media campaigns are effective in increasing physical activity levels.

Report of the US Preventive Services Task Force. Guide to Clinical Preventive Services, 2nd ed. International Medical Publishing, Inc, 1996. http://odphp.osophs.dhhs.gov/pubs/guidecps

Relevant Web Sites

[The American College of Sports Medicine]
http://www.acsm.org
[American Dietetic Association]
http://www.eatright.org
[Sites for smokers who want to quit]
www.quitnet.org www.trytostop.org

[USPHS guidelines and consumer and practitioner guides and tools]
www.surgeongeneral.gov/tobacco
[The US Department of Agriculture (USDA) Dietary Guidelines]
http://www.health.gov/dietaryguidelines/dga2000/document/front cover.htm
[Interactive tool from the USDA to help calculate caloric and nutrient intake]
http://147.208.9.133/Default.asp
[A tool to calculate BMI from National Institute of Health and obesity guidelines]
http://www.nhlbisupport.com/bmi/   http://www.nhlbi.nih.gov/guidelines/obesity/ob_home.htm
[The National Cancer Institute]
http://www.cancer.gov/

SECTION III

Psychiatric & Behavioral Disorders

Eating Disorders

Deborah S. Cowley, MD

Eating disorders are common and potentially serious illnesses characterized by disturbed eating behavior, such as restriction of intake or binge eating, combined with excessive concerns about body weight or shape. These conditions may take the form of anorexia nervosa, bulimia nervosa, or binge eating disorder.

ANOREXIA NERVOSA

Anorexia nervosa is characterized by purposeful behavior designed to produce marked weight loss, a morbid fear of becoming fat, and amenorrhea. This disorder is most common in young women, and has its onset in adolescence or early adulthood. Ninety percent of cases of anorexia nervosa occur in girls or women, with the lifetime prevalence of the disorder among women being approximately 0.5–1%. Anorexia nervosa is more prevalent in industrialized societies, in which there is an abundance of food and in which the ideal of feminine beauty includes being very thin. The disorder is most common among Caucasian women and is rare in non-Western developing countries. With exposure to Western standards of beauty, rates of anorexia nervosa among non-Western women increase significantly. Although earlier studies suggested that anorexia nervosa was more common among middle- to upper-income groups, this finding has not been borne out by studies done between the 1980s and the present.

 ESSENTIALS OF DIAGNOSIS

- *Refusal to maintain minimal normal weight for age and height (weight less than 85% of recommended level).*
- *Intense fear of gaining weight or becoming fat, even though underweight.*
- *Disturbance of body image or denial of seriousness of low body weight.*
- *Amenorrhea (ie, absence of menstrual periods) for at least 3 consecutive cycles.*

General Considerations

Anorexia nervosa is often difficult to diagnose. Eating disorders in general go undetected in clinical settings in up to 50% of cases. Patients with anorexia nervosa usually are unconcerned about their weight loss and may present instead with vague and nonspecific symptoms, such as weakness, fatigue, or dizziness. Often, family members bring the patient to the physician because they are concerned about significant weight loss or amenorrhea. Even with diagnosis of the disorder, patients may deny the seriousness of their condition, refuse to accept the diagnosis, and be very difficult to engage in treatment.

Two subtypes of anorexia nervosa have been described. Patients with the restricting subtype lose weight by dieting, fasting, or excessive exercise. Patients with the binge eating/purging subtype binge eat and then purge by inducing vomiting or misusing laxatives, diuretics, or enemas. Some patients do not binge eat, but purge after eating small amounts of food. Of note, recent studies suggest that the majority of women with the restricting subtype of anorexia nervosa go on to develop the binge eating/purging subtype and that only 12% of women with anorexia nervosa report never having had regular binge/purge behaviors.

Pathogenesis

No single cause for anorexia nervosa has been identified. Instead, the disorder appears to result from a combination of sociocultural, psychological, and physiologic factors. These factors lead to dieting behavior, which seems to be the most common trigger for the development of a serious eating disorder in vulnerable persons. Starvation effects and psychological changes resulting from severe restriction of food intake then reinforce maladaptive eating behavior and help sustain the eating disorder.

Sociocultural factors include pressure for women in Western societies to be physically attractive and thin. Over the past few decades, as average weights of fashion models have decreased, the prevalence of eating disorders has risen. Misguided attempts to achieve an unrealistic weight through dieting can contribute to the development of eating disorders, both by direct physiologic effects (caloric deprivation producing a physiologic predisposition to binge) and by psychological issues (an erosion of self-esteem related to the inability to measure up to an unrealistic ideal). Gymnasts, ballet dancers, jockeys, and other athletes in fields valuing thinness or low weight, may also diet and are at increased risk for the development of eating disorders. In fact, in 1992 the American College of Sports Medicine coined the term "the female athlete triad" to describe the triad of disordered eating, amenorrhea, and osteoporosis seen in some female athletes.

Psychological factors thought to be important in the etiology of anorexia nervosa have included individual personality traits, as well as family factors. Patients with anorexia nervosa often display perfectionism, rigid and obsessional thinking, restricted affect, and introversion. Whether these traits predate and contribute to the development of the disorder or are a result of the illness remains unclear. Although family psychopathology has been examined as a cause of the development of anorexia nervosa, there is no reliable evidence of this as the sole cause. Family dynamics may be disturbed prior to the diagnosis but may also become dysfunctional as family members try to deal with the illness. Disturbances in the family that may contribute to or exacerbate eating disorders include enmeshment or overinvolvement among family members, particularly the patient and her parents; physical or sexual abuse; low tolerance for expression of negative emotions, such as anger; poor communication in general; and lack of empathy by the parents for the children's emotional experience. In enmeshed families, disturbed eating behavior may represent the child's attempt to separate from her parents, express independence, and exert some control over her life.

Ambivalence about adult roles, including sexual ones, also may play a part, as evidenced by the fact that extreme weight loss results in a body shape resembling that of a prepubertal girl and in loss of reproductive functioning.

Although cross-cultural variability in rates of anorexia nervosa suggests a large effect of sociocultural factors in the etiology of the disorder, there is also strong evidence that vulnerability to the development of this condition is familial and probably genetically transmitted. Female first-degree relatives of patients with anorexia nervosa have increased rates of both anorexia and bulimia, while concordance rates in monozygotic twins of patients with anorexia nervosa are higher than those in dizygotic twins (50% vs 14%). These findings point to underlying heritable and biologic risk factors for anorexia nervosa.

Of note, many of the symptoms of eating disorders are similar to those resulting from starvation. These include preoccupation with food, hoarding food, binge eating when food is available, depression, and abnormal taste preferences. Thus, these symptoms and behaviors may be the outcome of physiologic effects of food restriction rather than the cause of the disorder. Interestingly, leptin levels in anorexia nervosa appear to be inappropriately high, when adjusted for body weight as a percent of ideal body weight. This may contribute to a blunted physiologic response to being underweight.

Clinical Findings

A. SYMPTOMS AND SIGNS

Symptoms of anorexia nervosa include an intense preoccupation with the need to lose weight, and the principal indicator of the disorder is refusal to maintain a minimally normal body weight. Girls and women with anorexia nervosa are intensely fearful of weight gain and body fat and typically do not feel reassured even by ongoing weight loss. Instead, they generally deny that they have a problem and continue to insist that they are too fat even when emaciated. This disturbance of body image often reaches delusional proportions. There may be ritualization of eating behavior, including hoarding of food and compulsions about weighing, measuring, and counting (eg, counting the number of Cheerios eaten for breakfast).

Most patients are intensely preoccupied with food. Despite the fact that the word **anorexia** means absence of appetite, these patients are hungry most of the time. Other associated symptoms may include concerns about eating in public, a strong need to control one's environment, rigid thinking, perfectionism, and lack of spontaneity and emotional expressiveness. Many patients display symptoms of depression, including depressed mood, social withdrawal, irritability, insomnia, and anhedonia. Patients with anorexia nervosa may also have comorbid obsessive-compulsive disorder, with obsessions and rituals both related and unrelated to food, or comorbid substance abuse or dependence.

The cardinal physical sign of anorexia nervosa is excessive thinness and low body weight. Other findings on physical examination may include hypotension, bradycardia, hypothermia, dry skin, hypercarotenemia, lanugo (fine, downy body hair), acrocyanosis, and atrophy of the breasts. Intestinal dilatation from chronic constipation and decreased intestinal motility from laxative abuse may occur.

The amenorrhea of anorexia nervosa is a consequence of the low estrogen levels (due, in turn, to decreased pituitary secretion of follicle-stimulating hormone [FSH] and luteinizing hormone [LH]) and typically follows weight loss but may precede it in some individuals. Menarche can be delayed if anorexia nervosa is already present.

B. LABORATORY FINDINGS

Laboratory tests are often unremarkable, but may show abnormalities including leukopenia, mild anemia, rare thrombocytopenia, hyponatremia, or hypoglycemia. Hypokalemia with an increase in serum bicarbonate may indicate frequent self-induced vomiting or use of diuretics, while a non–anion gap acidosis is characteristic of laxative abuse. Hypercortisolemia may be present, and thyroid function tests often reflect the euthyroid sick syndrome with decreased thyroxine and triiodothyronine levels but normal or decreased thyroid stimulating hormone levels. Women with anorexia nervosa have low estrogen levels and prepubertal patterns of FSH and LH secretion.

Differential Diagnosis

The differential diagnosis of anorexia nervosa includes other causes of significant weight loss, including diabetes mellitus, inflammatory bowel disease, malignancies, hyperthyroidism, and AIDS as well as causes of amenorrhea, including hypothalamic dysfunction, polycystic ovary syndrome, pituitary prolactinomas, and ovarian failure. However, these conditions are not associated with distorted body image, the desire for further weight loss, or the conviction that one is fat despite being underweight. Severe weight loss may accompany major depression, psychotic disorders may be associated with bizarre eating behaviors, and obsessive-compulsive behavior is characterized by obsessions and rituals. However, again, none of these conditions is associated with the disturbed body image and fear of weight gain pathognomonic of anorexia nervosa. Patients with bulimia nervosa binge-eat and perform compensatory behaviors, such as purging, to avoid weight gain; however, these patients are able to maintain a minimally normal body weight.

Complications

Complications of anorexia nervosa include electrolyte imbalance (metabolic alkalosis and hypokalemia), cardiovascular disturbances (bradycardia, tachycardia, hypotension, congestive heart failure, ECG changes, ventricular arrhythmias, and sudden death), renal abnormalities (decreased glomerular filtration rate, increased blood urea nitrogen, and pitting edema), hematologic problems (pancytopenia and reduced serum complement levels), skeletal abnormalities (osteoporosis and associated pathologic fractures), endocrine abnormalities (amenorrhea and hypogonadism), metabolic abnormalities (low basal metabolic rate, hypercholesterolemia, altered glucose metabolism, impaired temperature regulation), and dermatologic abnormalities (lanugo, scaly skin, and hypercarotenemia). When self-induced vomiting is present, the gastrointestinal and dental complications of bulimia nervosa (see following section, Bulimia Nervosa) may occur also. Anorectic women may have great difficulty conceiving because of prolonged anovulation. Low prepregnancy weight and poor nutritional status during pregnancy both are associated with low birth weight. If a pregnant anorectic patient purges through vomiting or diuretic/laxative abuse, electrolyte imbalance may put the fetus in further jeopardy. Anorexia nervosa is associated with increased rates of stillbirth, preterm birth, delivery by cesarean section, and postpartum depression.

Treatment

The first goal of treatment is to engage the patient and to build a relationship with the patient and her family. The patient's denial of the seriousness of her illness often makes it challenging to motivate her to pursue treatment. Finding and focusing on a symptom that is distressing to the patient (eg, depression, insomnia, amenorrhea, dizziness) may help in building a treatment alliance. The highest priority in the treatment of anorexia nervosa is restoration of normal body weight, followed by the establishment of healthy eating patterns.

A. HOSPITALIZATION

Hospitalization is indicated when weight has dropped below 75% of ideal body weight, if weight loss is rapid, or when the patient is medically unstable (eg, marked hypokalemia, arrhythmias, heart rate less than 35–40 beats per minute, symptomatic hypotension). The inpatient treatment team determines a target weight (generally a range rather than a single figure) that will support normal menstrual cycles and reverse bone demineralization. There is a trend toward using body mass index, which is calculated by weight (kg)/[height (m)]^2, rather than weight alone, and toward taking into account the patient's age. Initial goals of inpatient programs include weight gain of up to 2–3 pounds per week and caloric intake that usually starts at about 1000–1600 kcal/d, increasing as needed up to as much as 70–100 kcal/kg/d.

Typically, a behavior modification program is designed in which the patient's adherence to daily weight and behavior goals leads to previously agreed-on results, including positive reinforcers (eg, increased privileges) and negative reinforcers (eg, withholding of privileges). Discussions about food generally are held only with the dietician to avoid engaging the whole team in struggles about food. Patients are encouraged to gain weight only at the recommended rate and not any faster, to avoid medical complications of refeeding (eg, hypophosphatemia, cardiac arrest, delirium). Forced feeding via nasogastric tube is a last resort reserved for life-threatening situations. The goal is for the patient to assume responsibility for a rational pattern of eating rather than for the staff to impose its program on the patient.

B. Psychotherapy

1. Individual therapy—Forms of individual psychotherapy for anorexia nervosa include cognitive restructuring (especially with respect to beliefs about food and attractiveness), interpersonal therapy, and psychodynamic approaches that emphasize an understanding of the psychological conflicts underlying the problem behavior.

2. Family therapy—Patients with anorexia nervosa tend to be younger than patients with other eating disorders. The younger the patient, the more likely she is to benefit from therapy that addresses issues within the family, on whom she is still emotionally dependent. Education of the patient and the family, and helping the family to improve communication and conflict management patterns, are important parts of family therapy. For the older adolescent, family therapy may focus on allowing the patient to achieve greater independence.

3. Group therapy—Group therapy for patients with anorexia nervosa may be most useful in nonacute stages of treatment to provide ongoing support over a period of years and to help the patient maintain therapeutic gains made earlier in a more intensive treatment setting. At any stage of treatment, group therapy offers one distinct advantage over other forms of treatment: the opportunity for group members to confront each other about the ways in which they try to fool themselves and their clinicians as well as the problematic ways in which they interact with peers.

C. Medication

There are few data concerning the usefulness of psychotropic medications in treating anorexia nervosa. If major depression is present, indications for antidepressant medication are the usual ones (severe and pervasive mood disturbance accompanied by vegetative symptoms such as insomnia and fatigue). Patients with anorexia nervosa may be more susceptible to orthostatic hypotension as a side effect of some antidepressants. Because cardiac arrhythmias are a complication of anorexia nervosa, the least cardiotoxic antidepressants should be prescribed. Fluoxetine has been shown to be effective in preventing relapse of anorexia nervosa, even in the absence of depression, and in facilitating maintenance of normal body weight. However, fluoxetine has not been shown to be effective in the initial restoration of normal weight in patients with anorexia nervosa and low body weight.

A recent open study suggests that the atypical antipsychotic olanzapine may cause clinically significant weight gain in outpatients with anorexia nervosa. Atypical antipsychotics such as olanzapine also may be helpful in treating obsessive-compulsive symptoms and ideas about food and weight loss that approach delusional proportions. Randomized, double-blind controlled trials indicate that zinc supplementation enhances weight gain and decreases anxiety and depression in patients with anorexia nervosa. Finally, although estrogen may lead to increases in bone density in very low weight women with anorexia nervosa, it appears that estrogen or other treatments used for postmenopausal osteoporosis do not generally reverse osteoporosis or osteopenia. The most effective treatment for decreased bone density appears to be weight gain and resumption of normal menses.

When to Refer to a Specialist

Because of the possibility of grave complications, every patient with anorexia nervosa should be referred to a specialist in eating disorders. The best treatment for these patients is care by a multidisciplinary team, including a psychiatrist or psychologist with expertise in eating disorders, a dietician, and the primary care physician. The primary care physician's role is to assess and monitor the patient's physical health status and body weight in regular visits (eg, every 3–4 weeks at first, and less often as the patient improves). The primary care physician should set a weight loss limit beyond which more intensive and structured treatment will be necessary, and assess the need for hospitalization.

Prognosis

In studies of hospitalized or tertiary referral populations followed for at least 4 years after onset of illness, approximately 44% of the patients had their weight restored to within 15% of the recommended level and attained regular menstruation, about 24% did not come within 15% of the recommended level and continued with absent or sporadic menstruation, and about 28% had an intermediate outcome. In a recent 21-year follow-up study, 51% of patients were fully recovered, 21% were partially recovered, and 10% continued to meet diagnostic criteria for anorexia nervosa. Sixteen percent were deceased, due to causes related to anorexia nervosa, primarily suicide and cardiac arrest. Predictors of poor outcomes include longer duration of illness, psychiatric comorbidity, self-induced vomiting, previous treatment failures, greater severity of social and psychological problems, being married, and lower initial weight.

Becker AE et al: Eating disorders. N Engl J Med 1999;340:1092. [PMID: 10194240]

Eddy KT et al: Longitudinal comparison of anorexia nervosa subtypes. Int J Eat Disord 2002;31:191. [PMID: 11920980]

Franko DL et al: Pregnancy complications and neonatal outcomes in women with eating disorders. Am J Psychiatry 2001;158:1461. [PMID: 11532732]

Kaye WH et al: Double-blind placebo-controlled administration of fluoxetine in restricting and restricting-purging-type anorexia nervosa. Biol Psychiatry 2001;49:644. [PMID: 11297722]

Klump KL, Kaye WH, Strober M: The evolving genetic foundations of eating disorders. Psychiatr Clin North Am 2001;24:215. [PMID: 11416922]

Lowe B et al: Long-term outcome of anorexia nervosa in a prospective 21-year follow-up study. Psychol Med 2001;31:881. [PMID: 11449385]

Mehler PS: Diagnosis and care of patients with anorexia nervosa in primary care settings. Ann Intern Med 2001;134:1048. [PMID: 11388818]

Miller MN, Pumariega AJ: Culture and eating disorders: a historical and cross-cultural review. Psychiatry 2001;64:93. [PMID: 11495364]

West RV: The female athlete. The triad of disordered eating, amenorrhoea, and osteoporosis. Sports Med 1998;26:63. [PMID: 9777680]

Nielsen S: Epidemiology and mortality of eating disorders. Psychiatr Clin North Am 2001;24:201. [PMID: 11416921]

Powers PS, Santana CA, Bannon YS: Olanzapine in the treatment of anorexia nervosa: An open label trial. Int J Eat Disord 2002;32:146. [PMID: 12210656]

Practice guideline for the treatment of patients with eating disorders (revision). American Psychiatric Association Work Group on Eating Disorders. Am J Psychiatry 2000;157 (1 Suppl):1. [PMID: 10642782]

Su JC, Birmingham CL: Zinc supplementation in the treatment of anorexia nervosa. Eat Weight Disord 2002;7:20. [PMID: 11930982]

BULIMIA NERVOSA

Bulimia nervosa is characterized by frequent episodes of binge eating, followed by compensatory behaviors designed to prevent weight gain from bingeing. Like other eating disorders, bulimia nervosa is most common in young women. Ninety to 95% of patients with bulimia are women, and the disorder affects between 1.1% and 4.2% of women in the United States.

The onset of symptoms tends to be later in bulimia nervosa than in anorexia nervosa. The mean age of onset of binge eating is approximately 18 years, with self-induced vomiting beginning about 1 year later.

 ESSENTIALS OF DIAGNOSIS

- *Recurrent, uncontrolled episodes of binge eating.*
- *Recurrent inappropriate compensatory behavior to prevent weight gain, such as self-induced vomiting, misuse of laxatives or diuretics, strict dieting or fasting, or excessive exercise.*
- *Binge eating and compensatory behaviors both occur, on average, at least twice a week for 3 months.*
- *Overconcern with weight and body shape.*

General Considerations

Binges involve eating a larger amount of food than most people would in similar circumstances in a similar period of time (2 hours or less). The food consumed during binges varies according to the individual's tastes and what is available, but sweet, high calorie foods are generally favored as well as foods that require little or no preparation (eg, chips or cookies that can be eaten from the bag.)

Bulimia is divided into two subtypes, according to the types of compensatory behaviors used to control weight in the face of binge eating. In the purging subtype, the patient regularly uses self-induced vomiting, laxatives, diuretics, or enemas to lose weight. In the nonpurging subtype, the patient instead uses other compensatory behaviors, such as fasting or excessive exercise.

Pathogenesis

The onset of symptoms in bulimia nervosa usually occurs during or following a period of dieting. Stringent dieting and caloric restriction produce a physiologically based predisposition to binge-eat when the self-imposed restriction is lifted. Overconsumption of food through binge eating may also follow periods of stress, tension, or other negative emotions, such as anxiety, anger, and depression. Because the normal consequence of overconsumption is weight gain, the patient may try to control weight gain by additional stringent dieting. This behavior sets up a cycle of alternating fasting (or near-fasting) and binge eating. Often, girls first learn about vomiting as a means of controlling caloric intake from a friend. They may copy the behavior initially on a trial basis but later become reliant on the practice to avoid weight gain and the feelings of guilt and shame that follow binge eating.

Recent family and twin studies suggest that over 50% of the variance in bulimia nervosa can be accounted for by genetic factors. Moreover, there appears to be a significant heritable component not only for diagnosed eating disorders, such as bulimia and anorexia nervosa, but also for related attitudes and behaviors, such as body dissatisfaction, binge eating, self-induced vomiting, and dietary restraint. Family members of patients with bulimia nervosa also have been found to have higher rates of mood disorders, substance abuse and dependence (particularly alcoholism), and obesity.

Clinical Findings

A. SYMPTOMS AND SIGNS

Symptoms of bulimia nervosa include frequent binge eating and the compensatory behaviors noted above. Binges are often precipitated by negative feelings, life stress, or extreme hunger produced by dieting. The person usually conducts the binge in private, consuming the food rapidly, and continuing even after uncomfortably full. Most persons with bulimia nervosa induce vomiting after binge eating. Feelings of shame and disgust often follow the binge, with or without the self-induced vomiting. Comorbid psychiatric disorders may include major depression, dysthymia, anxiety disorders, substance abuse, and personality disorders.

There are usually few (if any) outward signs to alert the clinician. Body weight is usually normal, although premorbid obesity is common. Erosion of dental enamel from stomach acid is common. A few bulimic women have visible calluses on the dorsal aspects of their hands (Russell's sign, caused by teeth abrading the skin), as well as fresh abrasions and scarring. Some patients have obvious parotid hypertrophy.

B. LABORATORY FINDINGS

Laboratory findings are generally nonspecific, although the serum amylase level may be elevated and hypokalemia with increased serum bicarbonate may be present as a result of frequent self-induced vomiting. However, laboratory tests are often normal and the diagnosis is made most commonly through history. This is extremely difficult because most bulimic patients are secretive about their bingeing out of a sense of shame. Questioning about abnormal eating and weight-control practices should be matter-of-fact and nonjudgmental and should persist as long as the physician suspects an eating disorder. For example, a physician might say, "Some young women are extremely concerned about their appearance and weight and do things like throwing up after eating to try to avoid the calories. Is that something that you ever do?" A patient may deny the problem initially but later acknowledge it and accept help.

Differential Diagnosis

Binge-eating and purging often occur in patients with anorexia nervosa who, unlike those with bulimia, are unable to maintain a normal body weight. Disturbed eating behavior may accompany Kleine-Levin syndrome, Klüver-Bucy syndrome, major depression, and the impulsive behavior seen in borderline personality disorder. However, the diagnosis of bulimia nervosa is not given unless the patient exhibits overconcern with body shape and weight and indulges in inappropriate compensatory behaviors, such as purging, misuse of diuretics or laxatives, or excessive exercise.

Complications

Complications include electrolyte imbalance (metabolic alkalosis and hypokalemia), gastrointestinal problems (constipation, esophagitis, gastritis, and perforations of the esophagus or stomach [Mallory-Weiss tears]), cardiovascular disturbances (orthostatic hypotension and potentially lethal arrhythmias), dental problems (increased caries and upper incisor erosions), and endocrine disturbances leading to irregular menses or amenorrhea. As in anorexia nervosa, menstrual disturbances may interfere with the ability to conceive. Purging is potentially dangerous to the fetus because of the severe electrolyte imbalance that can occur. Pregnant women with active bulimia during pregnancy have been reported to have higher rates of cesarean section and postpartum depression. Low birth rate and low 5-minute Apgar scores also have been reported in association with bulimia nervosa.

Treatment

A. HOSPITALIZATION

Bulimia nervosa usually does not require inpatient treatment. Hospitalization should be considered when the binge eating and purging occupy so much of a patient's time that normal work and socialization are impossible. Although hospitalization is required to treat suicidality and life-threatening electrolyte imbalance, treatment is directed at stabilizing the patient in the face of these complications rather than at the underlying eating disorder.

B. PSYCHOTHERAPY

1. Individual psychotherapy—In contrast to patients with anorexia nervosa, individuals with bulimia nervosa usually are quite distressed by their symptoms and readily engage in treatment. Of the psychotherapies, cognitive-behavioral therapy has received the most systematic study and appears to bring about in most patients substantial change in eating and weight-control practices and in the attitudes that contribute to the disordered behaviors. This approach includes (1) modification of attitudes with respect to body shape and its relation to self-worth, (2) education in nutrition and rational weight regulation (eg, many bulimic patients do not know that severe caloric restriction predisposes to binge eating), (3) identification of precipitants of binge eating (primarily through record-keeping), (4) increasing "damage-control" skills (getting back on track after a binge), (5) increasing the repertoire of maneuvers for dealing with intensely unpleasant affective states (which often act as precipitants of binge eating), (6) increasing problem-solving skills in general (for some patients, binge eating becomes an all-purpose approach for dealing with problem situations), (7) increasing social contacts.

One especially promising behavioral approach known as exposure with response prevention combines having the patient consume food in the treatment setting with preventing the usual pathologic response (vomiting). For some patients, the binge eating occurs only when vomiting can be guaranteed, so learning to resist the urge to vomit translates into stopping binge eating.

Individual interpersonal or psychodynamic psychotherapy can help address underlying issues that precipitate and maintain symptoms. Treatment often includes work on interpersonal issues and relationships, self-esteem, alternative ways to manage emotions, and gender-role expectations.

2. Group therapy—In group therapy for bulimia nervosa, psychoeducational approaches plus the cognitive-behavioral methods described previously are the most widely used techniques. In the group format, there is also the opportunity to observe and modify disturbed interpersonal interactions in a setting that approximates interactions with friends and family more closely than does individual therapy.

3. Family therapy—It is unusual for bulimic patients to undergo family therapy except for adolescents still living with their families of origin. Family therapy also may have some usefulness in younger adult patients with ongoing conflicts with their parents. Patients with bulimia frequently have intimate relationships and, in some cases, may benefit from couples therapy.

4. Self-help—Controlled trials have shown that self-help treatments are effective in the treatment of bulimia nervosa. For example, self-help materials given with 4 face-to-face guidance sessions over 4 months was superior to a waitlist control condition in one controlled trial. In another study, both fluoxetine and a self-help manual reduced the frequency of self-induced vomiting and these two treatments had additive effects.

C. MEDICATION

Tricyclic antidepressants, monoamine oxidase inhibitors, and fluoxetine have been shown in double-blind, placebo-controlled studies to reduce bulimic symptoms significantly more than placebo. Depressed and nondepressed bulimic patients appear to respond equally well to the "antibinge" effects of antidepressants. This finding suggests that the drugs may exert direct central effects on the neurotransmitter systems that regulate appetite and eating behavior. Although 50–75% reductions in binge-eating and vomiting are seen in most trials, only about 20% of patients achieve full remission. Serotonin reuptake inhibitors, such as fluoxetine, are the most commonly used antidepressants because of their lower rates of side effects, greater safety, and effectiveness for ruminations and obsessive thinking often seen in bulimic patients. Doses of serotonin reuptake inhibitors are usually higher than those used for treatment of depression. For example, the effective dose of fluoxetine for bulimia nervosa is 60 mg/d, or 3 times the usual antidepressant dosage. Monoamine oxidase inhibitors are effective in producing short-term reduction of bulimic symptoms, but the decision to prescribe a medication that requires stringent dietary restrictions must be considered carefully in patients who have serious problems with impulse control concerning oral intake. Use of bupropion is not recommended in eating disorder patients because of an observed increase in the risk of seizures.

Although antidepressants appear to be effective in bringing about short-term behavior change in many patients, relapses are common following cessation of medication. A 52-week, controlled trial of maintenance treatment with fluoxetine versus placebo after successful acute fluoxetine treatment showed significantly lower relapse rates in patients who took the medication continuously.

Some recent studies suggest that the combination of cognitive-behavioral therapy and antidepressant medication is superior to either treatment alone.

When to Refer to a Specialist

Most bulimic women benefit from referral to a skilled therapist who is experienced in treating eating disorders. Suicidal ideation mandates referral to a psychiatrist or psychologist or for psychiatric hospitalization. Patients with comorbid mood disorders, anxiety disorders, substance abuse, or personality disorders are more difficult to treat and should be referred to a psychiatrist or psychologist.

Prognosis

With adequate treatment, the prognosis is good for bringing the problem behavior under control. Approximately 70% of patients completing treatment programs consisting of psychotherapy, medication, or both report considerable improvement. A meta-analysis of outcome studies found that 30% of women with bulimia nervosa relapsed within the 5 to 10 years following treatment. Poorer outcomes are associated with more severe initial symptoms requiring hospitalization, longer duration of illness, delayed treatment, greater frequency of self-induced vomiting, high levels of impulsivity, premorbid history of obesity, and substance abuse.

Bacaltchuk J, Hay P: Antidepressants versus placebo for people with bulimia nervosa. Cochrane Database Syst Rev 2001;(4): CD003391. [PMID: 11687198]

Hay PJ, Bacaltchuk J: Psychotherapy for bulimia nervosa and binging. Cochrane Database Syst Rev 2001;(3):CD000562. [PMID: 11686968]

Mitchell JE et al: The relative efficacy of fluoxetine and manual-based self-help in the treatment of outpatients with bulimia nervosa. J Clin Psychopharmacol 2001;21:298. [PMID: 11386493]

Romano SJ et al: A placebo-controlled study of fluoxetine in continued treatment of bulimia nervosa after successful acute fluoxetine treatment. Am J Psychiatry 2002;159:96. [PMID: 11772696]

Walsh BT et al: Medication and psychotherapy in the treatment of bulimia nervosa. Am J Psychiatry 1997;154:523. [PMID: 9090340]

Wilson GT et al: Cognitive-behavioral therapy for bulimia nervosa: time course and mechanisms of change. J Consult Clin Psychol 2002;70:267. [PMID: 11952185]

BINGE EATING DISORDER

Binge eating disorder is characterized by recurrent episodes of binge eating, a feeling of loss of control over and distress about overeating, and the lack of compensatory behaviors, such as self-induced vomiting, fasting, excessive exercise, or overuse of laxatives or diuretics. As with other eating disorders, binge eating disorder is most common in women, although up to 35% of individuals with this condition are male.

 ESSENTIALS OF DIAGNOSIS

- *Recurrent episodes of uncontrolled binge eating, occurring on average at least 2 days a week for 6 months.*

- *Binge eating episodes are associated with 3 of the following: eating rapidly; eating until uncomfortably full; eating large amounts when not hungry; eating alone because embarrassed by how much one is eating; or feeling disgusted with oneself, depressed, or guilty after overeating.*
- *Distress regarding overeating.*
- *No associated compensatory behaviors (eg, purging, fasting).*
- *Does not occur only during the course of anorexia or bulimia nervosa.*

General Considerations

Binge eating disorder is not an established diagnosis in *The Diagnostic and Statistical Manual of Mental Disorders,* 4th ed—Text Revision but instead is included as a condition requiring further study. Binge eating disorder occurs in 2–5% of the general population, in 30% of participants in weight loss programs, and in up to 70% of persons attending Overeaters Anonymous. Women with binge eating disorder are older than those with bulimia nervosa, are less likely to have a history of anorexia nervosa, are less likely to have been treated for an eating disorder, and are more commonly obese. These women report high rates of childhood abuse and have levels of psychopathology, such as depression and personality disorders, intermediate between those of patients with bulimia nervosa and obese women.

Pathogenesis

The onset of binge eating usually is in late adolescence or the early 20s, often after significant weight loss from dieting. Binge eating may be a response to caloric restriction and often is triggered by dysphoric moods, such as depression, anxiety, and tension. Thus, factors important in the onset and maintenance of this condition are similar to those seen in bulimia nervosa. However, these patients do not develop compensatory behaviors.

Clinical Findings

Symptoms of binge eating disorder, in addition to episodes of binge eating, include self-loathing and disgust after overeating, low self-esteem, interpersonal sensitivity, depression, anxiety, dieting and significant weight fluctuations, and functional impairment at work and in social settings. The patient may be overweight or obese but usually has no other abnormal findings on physical examination or laboratory testing.

Differential Diagnosis

Binge eating disorder is distinguished from bulimia nervosa by the lack of compensatory behaviors. Overeating may accompany depression or anxiety disorders, but in these cases does not include binges or associated symptoms such as eating more rapidly than usual, eating until uncomfortably full or when not hungry, eating alone, or feelings of self-disgust or guilt with overeating.

Complications

The major complications of binge eating disorder are obesity, depression, substance abuse, anxiety, and functional impairment.

Treatment

Cognitive-behavior therapy and interpersonal therapy, provided either as individual or group psychotherapies, are both effective in the treatment of binge eating disorder, with binge eating recovery rates of 70–80% after acute treatment and about 50–60% at 1-year follow-up. One study of dialectical behavior therapy produced similar rates of improvement in binge eating. Serotonin reuptake inhibitor antidepressants appear to have some efficacy in decreasing binge eating, although they are less effective than psychotherapy.

When to Refer to a Specialist

Patients with binge eating disorder may be difficult to identify in primary care settings, given the lack of characteristic clinical findings, unless the clinician asks specifically about binge eating behaviors. Since the specific psychotherapies discussed above are the treatments of choice for this condition, women with binge eating disorder should be referred, when possible, to a therapist skilled in one of these treatment modalities.

Prognosis

The long-term prognosis of binge eating disorder is unknown. The treatment studies discussed above suggest that at least 50–60% of women with this condition maintain significant reductions in binge eating 1 year after treatment. However, weight loss with these treatments usually is modest and, even in patients who maintain improvements in eating behaviors, the weight lost often is regained at 1-year follow-up.

EATING DISORDER NOT OTHERWISE SPECIFIED

Eating disorder not otherwise specified is a common eating disorder diagnosis, given to about 50% of patients presenting to specialty eating disorders centers. The diagnosis appears to be most common in adolescents. These patients have subsyndromal forms of eating disorders, for example meeting criteria for anorexia nervosa but not having 3 months of amenorrhea, or binge eating and purging less frequently than needed to meet full criteria for bulimia nervosa. Treatment depends on the individual clinical situation but is similar to that outlined above for women meeting full criteria for the particular eating disorder.

de Zwaan M: Binge eating disorder and obesity. Int J Obes Relat Metab Disord 2001;25(Suppl 1):S51. [PMID: 11466589]

Dingemans AE, Bruna MJ, van Furth EF: Binge eating disorder: a review. Int J Obes Relat Metab Disord 2002;26:299. [PMID: 11896484]

Striegel-Moore RH et al: Comparison of binge eating disorder and bulimia nervosa in a community sample. Int J Eat Disord 2001;29:157. [PMID: 11429978]

Telch CF, Agras WS, Linehan MM: Dialectical behavior therapy for binge-eating disorder. J Consult Clin Psychol 2001;69:1061. [PMID: 11777110]

Wilfley DE et al: A randomized comparison of group cognitive-behavioral therapy and group interpersonal psychotherapy for the treatment of overweight individuals with binge-eating disorder. Arch Gen Psychiatry 2002;59:713. [PMID: 12150647]

Relevant Web Sites

[National Institute of Mental Health]
www.nimh.nih.gov
[National Eating Disorders Association]
www.nationaleatingdisorders.org
[Anorexia Nervosa and Related Eating Disorders, Inc.]
www. anred.com
[Academy for Eating Disorders]
www.aedweb.org

Chemical Dependency

9

Joyce A. Tinsley, MD, & Steven M. Juergens, MD

General Considerations

Synonymous terms for chemical dependency include addiction, psychoactive substance dependence, and substance use disorder. Chemical dependency is a chronic, progressive disease characterized by continuous or periodic impaired control of—and preoccupation with—the psychoactive substance. The addicted person continues to use substances despite suffering social, physical, emotional, and legal consequences.

An integral part of the disease is denial. Denial is a defense mechanism that includes a range of psychological maneuvers designed to reduce awareness of the fact that alcohol and/or drugs is a cause of the person's problems. Dealing with denial can be especially frustrating for clinicians who mistake it for conscious deception.

A. EPIDEMIOLOGY

Lifetime prevalence rates among women are 8.2% for alcohol dependence, 5.9% for drug dependence (not including nicotine), and 18% for the combination of alcohol and drug dependence. Women have about half the prevalence rate of men. Addiction problems have apparently increased in recent cohorts; the highest prevalence rate in both women and men is between the ages of 25 and 34. Recent data have shown that the ratio of male to female teenagers dependent on alcohol is 1:1.

B. PRESENTATION IN WOMEN

The identification of substance abuse in women is more difficult than in men because there is more stigma associated with substance abuse for women, and they tend to hide it because of shame. However, there are no gender differences in the criteria used to make the diagnosis.

Women tend to drink less than men, and alcoholic women drink less than alcoholic men. Women are more likely to date the onset of their drinking problems to stressful events. For all age groups, more women than men abstain. Females are less likely to drink daily, to drink continuously, or to engage in binges; however, women drink alone more frequently. Although alcohol abuse begins at later ages in women, they seek treatment at about the same age as men. This is indicative of a "telescoping" in the course of addiction in women, in

that most have had fewer drinking years prior to treatment than their male counterparts. Women abuse prescription drugs more than men, often mixed with alcohol. They use illicit drugs to a lesser extent, except for stimulants, which may be related to weight loss issues.

Women are often motivated to seek treatment when health and family problems arise, while men tend to enter treatment in the face of job or legal problems. Women are more likely to stay with an alcoholic partner but when women enter treatment for chemical dependency, they are more likely to be divorced. Compared with men, women report lower self-esteem, greater symptom severity, and more psychiatric symptoms once in treatment. They are more likely than men to seek care for alcoholism in nonspecialized settings, such as mental health agencies, emergency services, and primary care. These are settings in which depression and anxiety are often addressed while addictions are ignored.

Role deprivation—which occurs when there is a lack or loss of being a wife, mother, or worker—appears to increase the use of alcohol by women. This may be due to reduced feelings of self-worth or reduced contact with role partners that could provide feedback about the excessive drinking. However, divorce or separation among women who are problem drinkers actually leads to fewer problems with alcohol, perhaps because the marriage was dysfunctional (ie, an "alcoholic marriage").

There is a higher incidence of anxiety, depression, eating disorders, and sexual abuse in substance abusing women than in substance abusing men. Personality disorders are common in both genders. Women are more likely than men to have borderline personality disorder characterized by interpersonal instability, and men are more likely to have antisocial personality disorder characterized by legal problems.

Genetic factors seem to play a role in alcoholism for both women and men. It is estimated that at least half the liability to alcoholism is a result of genetic factors, which is higher than the genetic liability for coronary artery disease, stroke, peptic ulcer disease, or major depression.

Kessler RC et al: Lifetime and 12-month prevalence of DSM-III-R psychiatric disorders in the United States: Results from the National Comorbidity Study. Arch Gen Psychiatry 1994;51: 8. [PMID: 8279933]

Substance Abuse and Mental Health Services Administration. *Substance use among women in the United States* (Analytic Series A-3). Department of Health and Human Services, 1997.

Substance Abuse and Mental Health Services Administration. *Summary of findings from the National Household Survey on Drug Abuse.* Department of Health and Human Services, 2000.

Clinical Findings

A. SYMPTOMS AND SIGNS

The Diagnostic and Statistical Manual of Mental Disorders, 4th ed—Text Revised (DSM-IV-TR) lists diagnostic criteria for psychoactive substance abuse (Table 9–1). Tolerance and withdrawal are frequent symptoms; although neither is necessary for the diagnosis of substance dependence to be made. There are 10 classes of psychoactive substances: alcohol, amphetamines or similar acting sympathomimetics, cannabis, cocaine, hallucinogens, nicotine, inhalants, opioids, phencyclidine (PCP), and sedative-hypnotics. The symptoms of addiction are the same across all categories; however, some symptoms are more or less salient depending on the class of substance.

B. SCREENING TOOLS

Physicians often have a low index of suspicion for substance abuse in their female patients. Systematic screening for substance abuse can help physicians to identify addiction in their patients. Questions that are routine and nonjudgmental work best, although the physician may still encounter evasiveness and defensiveness to questions about substance use. Over 100 addiction screening questionnaires are available. While most of them were developed for men, in practice they are useful in both genders. Two of the most frequently used are the Short Michigan Alcoholism Screening Test

Table 9–1. DSM-IV-TR criteria for substance abuse and dependence.

Abuse
A. A maladaptive pattern of substance use leading to clinically significant impairment or distress, as manifested by one (or more) of the following, occurring at any time during the same 12-month period:
1. Recurrent substance use resulting in a failure to fulfill major role obligations at work, school, or home (eg, repeated absences or poor work performance related to substance use; substance-related absences, suspensions, or expulsions from school; neglect of children or household).
2. Recurrent substance use in situations in which it is physically hazardous (eg, driving an automobile or operating a machine when impaired by substance use).
3. Recurrent substance-related legal problems (eg, arrests for substance-related disorderly conduct).
4. Recurrent substance use despite having persistent or recurrent social or interpersonal problems caused or exacerbated by the effects of the substance (eg, arguments with spouse about consequences of intoxication, physical fights).
B. The symptoms have never met the criteria for substance dependence for this class of substance.
Dependence
A maladaptive pattern of substance use, leading to clinically significant impairment or distress, as manifested by 3 (or more) of the following occurring at any time in the same 12-month period:
1. Tolerance.
2. Withdrawal.
3. The substance is often taken in larger amounts or over a longer period than was intended.
4. There is a persistent desire or unsuccessful efforts to cut down on or control substance use.
5. A great deal of time is spent in activities necessary to obtain the substance (eg, visiting multiple doctors or driving long distances), use the substance (eg, chain-smoking), or recover from its effects.
6. Important social, occupational, or recreational activities are given up or reduced because of substance use.
7. The substance use is continued despite knowledge of having had a persistent or recurrent physical or psychologic problem that is likely to have been caused or exacerbated by the substance (eg, current cocaine use despite recognition of cocaine-induced depression, or continued drinking despite recognition that an ulcer was made worse by alcohol consumption).
Specify if:
With physiologic dependence: evidence of tolerance or withdrawal.
Without physiologic dependence: no evidence of tolerance or withdrawal.

Reproduced, with permission, from American Psychiatric Association: *Diagnostic and Statistical Manual of Mental Disorders,* 4th ed, Text Revision. American Psychiatric Association, 2000.

(Table 9–2) and the CAGE Questionnaire (Table 9–3). Two positive responses to the CAGE indicate an alcohol use disorder. However, 1 positive response from a woman signals a problem.

Even briefer screening tools are being sought. In one study, a positive response to the question "Have you ever had a drinking problem?" correctly identified 70% of alcoholics, with equal benefit for men and women. If the patient was also asked "When was your last drink?" and the response indicated that it was less than 24 hours ago, the accurate identification of alcoholism rose to more than 90%.

The Two-item Conjoint Screen (TICS), another questionnaire, identified current alcohol and other drug problems in nearly 80% of young and middle-aged patients by asking 2 questions. A positive response to either question was interpreted as a positive screen for current substance abuse: (1) In the last year, have you ever drunk or used drugs more than you meant to? and

Table 9–2. Short Michigan Alcoholism Screening Test (SMAST).

---

1. Do you feel you are a normal drinker? *(No)*[1]
2. Does your spouse, a parent, or other close relative ever worry or complain about your drinking? *(Yes)*
3. Do you ever feel guilty about your drinking? *(Yes)*
4. Do friends or relatives think you are a normal drinker? *(No)*
5. Are you able to stop drinking when you want to? *(No)*
6. Have you ever attended a meeting of Alcoholics Anonymous? *(Yes)*
7. Has drinking ever created problems between you and your spouse, a parent, or other close relative? *(Yes)*
8. Have you ever gotten into trouble at work because of your drinking? *(Yes)*
9. Have you ever neglected your obligations, your family, or your work for 2 or more days in a row because you were drinking? *(Yes)*
10. Have you ever gone to anyone for help about your drinking? *(Yes)*
11. Have you ever been in a hospital because of drinking? *(Yes)*
12. Have you ever been arrested for drunken driving, driving while intoxicated, or driving under the influence of alcoholic beverages? *(Yes)*
13. Have you ever been arrested, even for a few hours, because of other drunken behavior? *(Yes)*

---

[1]Answers suggestive of alcoholism are shown in parentheses after each question. Three or more indicate a diagnosis of alcoholism; two indicate the possibility of alcoholism; one or less indicates that alcoholism is unlikely.
Reproduced, with permission, from Selzer ML, Vinokur A, van Rooijen L: A self-administered Short Michigan Alcoholism Screening Test (SMAST). J Stud Alcohol 1975; 36:117.

Table 9–3. CAGE Screening Test for Alcoholism.

Have you ever felt the need to	**C**ut down on drinking?
Have you ever felt	**A**nnoyed by criticism of your drinking?
Have you ever felt	**G**uilty about your drinking?
Have you ever taken a morning	**E**ye opener?

INTERPRETATION: Two "yes" answers are considered a positive screen. One "yes" answer should raise a suspicion of alcohol abuse.

Modified and reproduced, with permission, from Mayfield D et al: The CAGE questionnaire: Validation of a new alcoholism screening instrument. Am J Psychiatry 1974; 131:1121.

(2) Have you felt you wanted or needed to cut down on your drinking or drug use in the last year? Questions can easily be added to a routine interview. Positive responses should be followed up with inquiry into past or present use of other drugs.

C. LABORATORY FINDINGS

Laboratory tests are not as reliable as screening tools for identifying addiction. For alcohol, unexplained laboratory abnormalities may lead to suspicion of abuse. Data that suggest further inquiry are elevations in the following: mean corpuscular volume (MCV);†liver function tests, such as serum gamma-glutamyltransferase (SGGT; a particularly sensitive test), aspartate aminotransferase (AST), and alanine aminotransferase (ALT); uric acid; high-density lipoprotein (HDL) cholesterol; triglycerides; and amylase. The measurement of carbohydrate-deficient transferrin (CDT) is an expensive test being studied as a marker for heavy drinking and relapse. In women, SGGT and CDT have been shown to have moderate sensitivity in screening for alcohol problems. Combining these tests substantially enhances sensitivity.

Other substances induce fewer laboratory changes. In injecting drug users, in particular, test results may be positive for hepatitis infection and HIV, as well as other sexually transmitted diseases. Urine and blood tests remain valuable tools in screening and monitoring. Studies are assessing the advantages of saliva and hair analyses for use in some circumstances, although these tests are unlikely to be used for routine screening.

Allen JP et al: Carbohydrate-deficient transferrin, gamma-glutamyltransferase, and macrocytic volume as biomarkers of alcohol problems in women. Alcohol Clin Exp Res 2000;24:492. [PMID: 10798585]

American Psychiatric Association: *Diagnostic and Statistical Manual of Mental Disorders*, 4th ed, Text Revision. American Psychiatric Association, 2000.

Brown RL et al: A two-item conjoint screen for alcohol and other drug problems. J Am Board Fam Pract 2001;14:95. [PMID: 11314930]

Cyr MG, Wartman SA: The effectiveness of routine screening questions in the detection of alcoholism. JAMA 1988;259:51. [PMID: 3334771]

Complications

There are health consequences of addiction that are specific to women. Women show an increased susceptibility to alcoholic liver disease and require less alcohol use over a shorter period of time to cause damage. Based on the risk of developing alcoholic liver disease, heavy drinking for women is defined as daily consumption of 1½ or more drinks containing 1.5 oz liquor, 12 oz of beer, or 5 oz of wine. This compares to 4 or more drinks per day for men.

There is an association between alcohol consumption and breast cancer as well as between alcohol and osteoporosis. Neuropsychological impairment develops more rapidly in women than in men, and there is a greater magnitude of differences in brain volumes between alcoholic and nonalcoholic women than between alcoholic and nonalcoholic men, suggesting a greater sensitivity to alcohol neurotoxicity among women. Hypertension develops more rapidly in women than men, and women require a lower total lifetime dose of ethanol than men to develop alcoholic cardiomyopathy.

HDL cholesterol is elevated in both men and women and may have a protective effect against cardiovascular disease. Even so, consuming 1 or 2 drinks per day places women at risk for other health problems and should not be encouraged.

The way in which women metabolize alcohol may contribute to its harmful effects on their health. Women become more intoxicated when given the same amount of alcohol as men, even when weight is taken into consideration. This may be because women have less body water than men leading to a smaller volume of distribution and a higher blood alcohol concentration. Another contributing factor may be that women show less activity of alcohol dehydrogenase in the stomach. Alcohol may increase the permeability of endotoxin, which triggers liver damage in women. This may be another reason that women have a higher rate than men of alcoholic liver disease.

There is relatively little literature about gender-related health problems resulting from illicit drug use. Certainly, intoxicated women risk exposure to sexually transmitted diseases because of impaired judgment and relationships with men who have addictions. Heterosexual women are contracting HIV at an increasing rate. All injecting drug users risk infection with hepatitis B and C viruses, HIV, and bacteremias, with the attendant complications of these infections.

The consequences of nicotine dependence have become a medical nightmare for women who smoke. It is speculated that cigarette smoking creates an antiestrogen effect that accelerates osteoporosis, development of cataracts, and wrinkling of the skin. Like men, women are at increased risk for cardiovascular disease, cancer, and respiratory disease.

Lung cancer is the leading cause of cancer in women. In 1959, 26 per 100,000 women died of lung disease caused by smoking; and in 1986 the number of deaths increased to 155 per 100,000. Men continue to smoke in greater numbers than women. Quit rates for men and women are similar; however, there may be gender differences in the obstacles to smoking cessation. Women may be more susceptible to depression, low levels of social support, and weight gain upon discontinuation of nicotine.

Day CP: Who gets alcoholic liver disease: nature of nurture? J R Coll Physicians of London 2000;24:557.

Hommer D et al: Evidence for a gender-related effect of alcoholism on brain volumes. Am J Psychiatry 2001;158:198. [PMID: 11156801]

Okuyemi KS, Ahluwalia JS, Harris KJ: Pharmacotherapy of smoking cessation. Arch Fam Med 2000;9:270. [PMID: 10728115]

Pregnancy & the Newborn

There is strong interest in identifying pregnant women who abuse substances. One study found the 1 characteristic that best differentiates pregnant drug or alcohol users from those who abstain during pregnancy is past use of alcohol, especially in the month preceding pregnancy. Other risk factors for substance use during pregnancy include moderate to severe depression, living alone or with small children, and living with someone who uses drugs. Screening tests for the obstetric population have largely been adapted from those in general use, such as the CAGE and SMAST. The most sensitive screening tests in obstetric patients appear to be those that ask about tolerance, the diminished effect of alcohol with continued use. Such a tool is the T-ACE, which uses 3 questions from the CAGE questionnaire. The rationale for using questions about tolerance is that they seem to elicit less defensiveness. The tolerance question in the T-ACE is: "How many drinks does it take to make you high" or "How many drinks can you hold?" A response that it takes more than 2 drinks indicates the presence of tolerance.

Children of chemically dependent women may be profoundly affected by maternal substance use. Addiction affects a mother's ability to parent effectively. Abandonment, abuse, physical and cognitive deficits, decreased interpersonal skills, and emotional difficulty and lability occur more frequently in children who have parents with an addiction. Evidence that substance abuse causes harm to the fetus is most convincing for alcohol. Fetal alcohol syndrome (FAS) and fetal alcoholic effects (FAE) are among the leading causes of mental retardation in the Western world, with an incidence of 1–3 per 1000 births, and perhaps as high as 25 per 1000 births in women who drink heavily. It is believed that fetal vulnerabilities such as malnutrition exacerbate the toxicity of alcohol. An estimated 9–11% of women have used an illicit drug during pregnancy. The fetal health effects of illicit substances are not as clear as they are for alcohol. It is apparent that FAS is a leading cause of mental retardation and that it is entirely preventable.

The minimal criteria for FAS include growth retardation below the 10th percentile; signs of neurologic abnormality, developmental delay, or intellectual involvement; and characteristic facial dysmorphology with at least 2 of the distinguishing features. These features are microencephaly, microphthalmos and/or short palpebral fissures, and a poorly developed philtrum, with a thin upper lip or flattening of the maxillary area. Children born with less than the full constellation comprise those with FAE. There appears to be a continuum of effects from subtle cognitive-behavioral dysfunction to severe morphologic effects.

There is no safe amount of alcohol a woman can consume during pregnancy. However, even a reduction in heavy drinking is associated with improved neonatal outcomes compared with women who continue to drink heavily. Over time the craniofacial abnormalities of FAS diminish and weight normalizes, but microencephaly and short stature remain. Mental retardation, poor judgment, and distractibility cause lifelong psychosocial problems.

The harm of using cocaine during pregnancy has been widely advertised. However, there are conflicting views about whether or not maternal cocaine use causes irreversible fetal damage. A recent systematic review found that among children aged 6 years or younger, there is no convincing evidence of developmental toxic effects attributable solely to maternal cocaine use. There is evidence that high-dose cocaine use during pregnancy leads to a disproportionately small head circumference, a finding that was not present if the mother used cocaine at low or moderate doses. Long-term studies are needed to better define the teratogenic effects of cocaine and other illicit drugs as well.

Smoking cigarettes during pregnancy causes low birth weight, spontaneous abortion, and prematurity. In 1995, low birth weight attributable to maternal smoking cost $263 million in excess direct medical costs for neonatal care. Even quitting as late as the 30th week of gestation improves neonatal outcome. Behavioral approaches to smoking cessation should be tried during pregnancy before pharmacologic approaches are

used. Then, the risks versus benefits of adding medication for smoking cessation must be considered for each individual patient.

Bateman DA, Chiriboga CA: Dose-response effect of cocaine on newborn head circumference. Pediatrics 2000;106:E33. [PMID: 10969117]

Chasnoff IJ et al: Screening for substance use in pregnancy: a practical approach for the primary care physician. Am J Obstet Gynecol 2001;184:752. [PMID: 11262483]

Effects of alcohol on fetal and postnatal development. In: *Secretary of Health and Human Services: Alcohol and Health Ninth Special Report to the US Congress.* Department of Health and Human Services, 1997:193.

Lightwood JM, Phibbs CS, Glantz SA: Short-term health and economic benefits of smoking cessation: low birth weight. Pediatrics 1999;104:1312. [PMID: 10585982]

Treatment

When the diagnosis of a substance use disorder is made or suspected, the physician needs to further explore the problem. For instance, the clinician may begin by better understanding the patient's reasons to pursue sobriety and readiness to do so. Whenever possible the physician presents facts from the patient's history and results from the physical and laboratory examinations that provide evidence of harm caused by the substance abuse. In the discussion, the clinician should emphasize that addiction is a treatable disease and the individual is not at fault for having it. However, without treatment, it is a disease that affects not only the addicted person but also others.

A. MANAGING DENIAL

The patient may deny that drugs or alcohol are a problem. Close friends and family are usually effective in helping the patient accept the need for treatment. A strategy that may clarify the presence or severity of a problem is to make an agreement with the patient to reduce use markedly for a period of time to determine how long limited alcohol intake is possible. The clinician may recommend Alcoholics Anonymous (AA) and discuss the patient's response to this or ask the patient to see a chemical dependency professional for a second opinion. Follow-up is essential when addiction is suspected. If denial predominates initially, continued discussion and concern are appropriate and may encourage treatment acceptance later. If the person has been treated, continued monitoring for abstinence from alcohol and addicting drugs is valuable since relapse is common. It is concerning when patients return to "controlled" use of alcohol or drugs because usually "once an addict, always an addict" holds true. The physician should evaluate the extent of the relapse and discuss the realities that women who continue to drink develop serious long-term health problems much more frequently than those who abstain.

An important concept for the clinician to appreciate is cross addiction. For example, if a patient who has a history of dependence on alcohol begins to use another drug, such as an opiate for chronic pain, there is risk of relapse back to using the original drug of choice or becoming addicted to the new drug. Abstinence from all addicting substances is advisable. If medically necessary, a time-limited use is recommended.

Few primary care physicians do the actual addiction treatment, so being comfortable and familiar with referral options to addiction professionals, outpatient and inpatient chemical dependency programs, and mutual help programs is important. Going to an open AA meeting, visiting a reputable treatment center, and getting to know a good addiction professional are simple ways to become more knowledgeable.

B. Treatment Principles

For tobacco addiction, the combination of behavioral therapy and nicotine replacement can lead to a quit rate of approximately 30%. Strategies to help patients quit smoking include the following: (1) establish a therapeutic alliance; (2) advise the patient to quit; (3) assess motivation to quit, identifying specific incentives and barriers to quitting; (4) work with the patient to set a "stop date"; (5) assist through nicotine replacement therapy, bupropion, and/or behavioral strategies; (6) follow up in 2–3 days, then weekly thereafter.

The general principles of intensive treatment for alcohol dependence and dependence on other drugs are identical. The patient is initially detoxified and abstinence from addicting drugs is emphasized. Most programs are group-oriented with individual counseling and family meetings as needed. There are educational sessions regarding various aspects of addiction. Therapy sessions often focus on "here and now" issues such as adjustment to life without chemicals, breakdown of denial, and stresses on family, friends and job. Patients are introduced to AA and other self-help programs, such as Women for Sobriety.

Treatment programs may be outpatient or inpatient; the length of stay can be fixed or variable. Most addiction treatment is provided on an outpatient basis. Inpatient treatment is more comprehensive, eliminates drug access, and may offer more medical and psychiatric services. However, it is more disruptive, expensive, stigmatized, and may be artificially safe, postponing critical learning tasks. There have not been adequate studies to assess whether or not there is an advantage for women to be treated in same-sex versus mixed programs, although women may have a personal preference that

should be honored if possible. Specialized recovery services for women may include assertiveness training, additional therapies for victims of sexual and physical abuse, issues of parenting, self-esteem, and childcare. Positive female role models in recovery can be especially beneficial in navigating life without substances.

C. Common Pharmacologic Agents in Treatment of Addiction

Withdrawal syndromes caused by cessation of alcohol, sedatives, opiates, stimulants, and nicotine each have characteristic features. Only withdrawal from alcohol and sedatives produce life-threatening syndromes, unless the patient is medically compromised. Opiate withdrawal can be extremely uncomfortable and consequently contributes to a cycle of use that is difficult to overcome.

1. Alcohol withdrawal—Alcohol is the substance that most frequently requires detoxification. The distinctive symptoms of alcohol withdrawal can range from mild (eg, sweating, anxiety, insomnia, tachycardia, and mild hypertension) to severe (eg, severe hypertension, delirium tremens, and convulsions). Most detoxification can be accomplished on an outpatient basis unless there are significant medical (ie, past history of delirium tremens, withdrawal seizures, or significant cardiac disease), psychiatric (ie, suicidality), or social (ie, lack of an environment that would allow detoxification) complications.

Benzodiazepines are the most common agents used for alcohol withdrawal. Chlordiazepoxide (25–50 mg), lorazepam (1–2 mg), or diazepam (5–10 mg) 4 times per day for 1 or 2 days and then orally tapering by 20% per day can be used in outpatient therapy; taper with daily visits to assess symptoms. The patient should have another person with them to monitor her status, and the patient should not drive. Higher doses and closer monitoring may be needed with more severe withdrawal symptoms, in which case inpatient detoxification is best. Lorazepam is the treatment of choice in the elderly and in those with significant liver disease. Its advantages include renal excretion, a relatively short half-life, and no metabolites. It can be given orally, intramuscularly or intravenously. Thiamine 100 mg twice a day and multivitamins should be given as well.

2. Disulfiram and naltrexone—Drugs most useful in helping the patient abstain from alcohol include disulfiram and naltrexone. Disulfiram inhibits aldehydedehydrogenase, which leads to increased levels of acetaldehyde in the metabolism of alcohol. This causes the toxic reaction of nausea, vomiting, tachycardia, flushing, dyspnea and headache if alcohol is ingested. The usual dose is 250 mg per day and if an aversive agent is appropriate, it can be started 48–72 hours after cessation of alcohol. It is most effective when it is used as part of a comprehensive recovery plan, is dispensed by a professional, and includes a consequence for discontinuing treatment.

Naltrexone is an opioid antagonist used after detoxification as some patients find it very helpful in reducing craving. It is usually prescribed 50–100 mg daily or 100–150 mg 3 times weekly. Side effects are minimal; however it is expensive. It is most effective when used in the context of a recovery plan. Naltrexone can also be used in the treatment of opiate addicts in highly motivated individuals.

3. Benzodiazepine and barbiturate withdrawal— Benzodiazepine and barbiturate withdrawal should be done pharmacologically. Even withdrawal from a low dose of sedative taken for a few months goes more smoothly if it is gradual. Such conservative detoxification is done over weeks (eg, 10% every 3–7 days). With shorter-acting benzodiazepines, such as lorazepam, it may be advantageous to switch to a longer-acting agent such as clonazepam for withdrawal. Inpatient detoxification by an experienced staff is recommended if there is significant difficulty with the detoxification, high doses are being abused, social support is inadequate, or there are medical or psychiatric complications. Carbamazepine and valproic acid are also effective treatments for sedative withdrawal.

4. Opiate withdrawal and maintenance—Conventional detoxification of opiates is accomplished by gradual reduction in opiate dose over several days or weeks. Breakthrough withdrawal symptoms can be managed by slowing the rate of medication reduction. Adding clonidine, an α_2-agonist that suppresses autonomic symptoms of withdrawal, can accelerate the process. Methadone maintenance is indicated for the heroin addict who injects the drug. It is an attempt to interrupt an addict's lifestyle, decrease criminality, promote stability and employment, and reduce injecting drug abuse with its risk of HIV infection. Methadone maintenance is a tightly regulated, although valuable and underused treatment.

Buprenorphine is a partial opioid agonist that is effective for use in facilitating opiate withdrawal and as a maintenance drug. It is anticipated that the Food and Drug Administration will approve it for use outside of a regulated treatment program because it is considered to have less abuse potential than methadone. This will give opiate-addicted patients greater choice in selecting a treatment, and physicians will be allowed to prescribe it from their offices. Training sessions on the use of buprenorphine are underway.

Prognosis

The prognosis for recovery among women in treatment for chemical dependency appears to be the same as for men. Higher socioeconomic stability, low antisocial personality traits, a lack of psychiatric and medical problems and contact with treatment and mutual help groups such as AA are associated with better outcome.

Relevant Web Sites

[National Institute on Alcohol Abuse and Alcoholism]
www.niaaa. nih.gov
[National Institute of Drug Abuse]
www.nida.nih.gov
[American Society of Addiction Medicine]
www.asam.org
[American Academy of Addiction Psychiatry]
www.aaap.org
[Tobacco Cessation Guidelines]
www.surgeongeneral.gov/tobacco
[Alcoholics Anonymous]
www.alcoholics-anonymous.org
[Women for Sobriety]
www.womenforsobriety.org
[Narcotics Anonymous]
www.na.org
[Cocaine Anonymous]
www.ca.org
[Marijuana Anonymous]
www.marijuana-anonymous.org

Anxiety & Panic Disorder

Deborah S. Cowley, MD

10

ESSENTIALS OF DIAGNOSIS

- *Severe anxiety symptoms, including 1 or more of the following:*
  - *Sudden, unexpected attacks of fear or panic*
  - *Excessive, unrealistic worry*
  - *Obsessive thoughts and repetitive, compulsive behaviors*
  - *Reexperiencing of the event, avoidance, and increased arousal following a traumatic event*
  - *Fear or phobias.*
- *The anxiety and/or phobia leads to significant functional impairment or distress.*
- *The fear or avoidance is not due to a substance (eg, drug, medication), general medical condition, or another psychiatric disorder.*

Anxiety is a common experience that serves as an adaptive response to danger or threat. In anxiety disorders, however, anxiety occurs without clear cause or out of proportion to the magnitude of external events. Such "pathologic" anxiety is distressing and debilitating and interferes with normal functioning.

Many patients with anxiety disorders are seen and treated in primary care rather than in psychiatric settings. Thus, primary care providers must be able to recognize and manage anxiety disorders.

General Considerations

A. EPIDEMIOLOGY

Anxiety disorders affect at least 5–10% of the general population. Lifetime prevalence rates in the general population are as follows: 1.5–3.5% for panic disorder, with or without agoraphobia; 5% for generalized anxiety disorder (GAD); and 2% for social anxiety disorder. Rates of posttraumatic stress disorder (PTSD) vary considerably (1–14% lifetime) depending on the population samples. Specific phobias occur in approximately 10% of the general population. Approximately 5–10% of patients presenting to both primary care and subspe-

cialty medical clinics have clinically significant anxiety disorders.

B. PRESENTATION IN WOMEN

Panic disorder, particularly panic with agoraphobia, is 2–3 times more likely to develop in women than in men. Women are twice as likely to have GAD, 2–3 times as likely to suffer from specific phobias, and more likely to report significant social anxiety. Obsessive-compulsive disorder (OCD) occurs at about the same rate in men and women.

The reasons for the greater prevalence of anxiety disorders among women are unclear but may include hormonal factors, sexual differences in the structure and neurochemistry of the regions of the brain that mediate anxiety, the types of life stressors and feelings of powerlessness experienced by women, and their higher rate of sexual abuse.

C. GENETICS

Panic disorder appears to have a heritable component; the risk of developing the disorder increases to 17% in first-degree relatives of affected people. Precipitants of initial panic attacks include life stress and exposure to marijuana and stimulant drugs, such as cocaine, amphetamines, and caffeine. OCD has a genetic component and has been linked to altered serotonin function in the brain. Social anxiety disorder is transmitted in families and may be inherited.

Clinical Findings

Most patients with anxiety disorders seek medical care from their primary care providers and are often preoccupied with the physical symptoms of the disorder. This focus on somatic symptoms can divert attention from the underlying anxiety disorder and result in unnecessary, costly, and invasive medical work-ups.

Several distinct anxiety disorders, each differing in clinical presentation, cause, and treatment, have been described over the past 20 years. Most patients complaining of anxiety symptoms have situational anxiety or an adjustment disorder with anxious mood, in which clinically significant anxiety occurs in the context of ongoing life stress. More chronic anxiety disorders include panic disorder, GAD, OCD, PTSD, phobic disorders (eg, agoraphobia, specific phobias), and social anxiety disorder. The American Psychiatric Association's *Diagnostic and Statistical Manual of Mental Disorders,* 4e, Text Revision (DSM-IV-TR) lists diagnostic criteria for these disorders.

A. SYMPTOMS AND SIGNS

1. Panic disorder—The peak age of onset of panic disorder is between the late teens and mid-30s. Panic disorder is characterized by recurrent, unexpected attacks of intense fear associated with 4 of the following 13 symptoms:

1. Palpitations/accelerated heart rate
2. Sweating
3. Trembling or shaking
4. Shortness of breath
5. Choking
6. Chest pain
7. Nausea or abdominal distress
8. Dizziness
9. Feelings of unreality (derealization) or detachment from oneself (depersonalization)
10. Fear of losing control or going crazy
11. Fear of dying
12. Numbness or tingling
13. Chills or hot flushes.

At least 1 panic attack must lead to a month or more of worry about having another attack (anticipatory anxiety), anxiety about the possible consequences or meaning of the attack, or a significant change in behavior as a result of the attack. Panic disorder usually is accompanied by fear of having another panic attack (anticipatory anxiety) and often leads to phobic avoidance or agoraphobia.

2. Generalized anxiety disorder—GAD usually begins in childhood or adolescence and is characterized by chronic, excessive worry lasting 6 months or longer that is difficult to control, causes significant functional impairment, and is accompanied by 3 of the following 6 symptoms:

1. Restlessness or the feeling of being "on edge"
2. Fatigability
3. Trouble concentrating or feeling as though one's mind "goes blank"
4. Irritability
5. Muscle tension
6. Sleep disturbance.

3. Obsessive-compulsive disorder—The peak age of onset in women is in their 20s. OCD is characterized by persistent, irrational thoughts or images (obsessions) and repetitive behaviors that the patient feels driven to perform to reduce anxiety (compulsions) and that significantly interfere with her life. Examples of compulsive rituals include handwashing, checking, counting, or arranging objects in a rigid order.

Obsessions, compulsions, and other neuropsychiatric symptoms have been described in children following streptococcal infections (PANDAS, or pediatric autoimmune neuropsychiatric disorders associated with group B α-hemolytic streptococcal infections).

OCD may result from disturbances in a neural circuit involving the frontal cortex, thalamus, and basal ganglia. Symptoms of OCD may develop in patients with disorders of the basal ganglia such as Sydenham's chorea, Tourette's syndrome, and other movement and tic disorders.

4. Posttraumatic stress disorder—PTSD follows a traumatic, life-threatening event and is characterized by the following: reexperiencing the trauma in dreams, intrusive memories, or flashbacks; avoiding situations associated with the trauma; emotional numbing; and increased arousal in the form of an exaggerated startle response, temper outbursts, and insomnia. PTSD has been described and studied primarily in male combat veterans. In women, PTSD may follow rape or sexual abuse, other traumatic events, and accidents.

The risk of developing PTSD depends on the intensity and duration of exposure to an unusual and extreme stressor. The risk increases with greater intensity and duration of exposure to the stressor and is higher in people with fewer social supports and in those who have preexisting psychiatric disorders.

5. Phobic disorders—For persons suffering from these disorders, particular situations or objects are feared and avoided. Specific phobias are common and include fear of heights, spiders, the dark, and so on. **Agoraphobia** refers to numerous fears of situations or settings in which escape would be difficult without embarrassment (eg, crowds, tunnels, bridges, movie theaters, checkout lines at grocery stores). Agoraphobia often accompanies panic disorder, but it may occur alone.

6. Social anxiety disorder—The onset of this disorder is typically seen in childhood or adolescence, often following a history of marked shyness (behavioral inhibition) or a specific humiliating experience. The patient fears and avoids being judged; being the center of attention; or standing out in a situation, such as public speaking, meeting new people, or eating or writing in front of other people.

B. Screening Methods

The diagnosis of an anxiety disorder is made based on the patient's history, since there are no pathognomonic physical findings or laboratory tests. There are several rating forms available to assess anxiety symptoms. These include the Hamilton Rating Scale for Anxiety and the Yale-Brown Obsessive-Compulsive Scale. Although these rating forms can be helpful in evaluating treatment, a few diagnostic questions are more helpful in diagnosing an anxiety disorder.

For example, for panic disorder, the patient can be asked, "Have you ever had an attack when you suddenly felt frightened or anxious?" If the answer is yes, the patient should be asked whether this ever has happened for no apparent reason, or "out of the blue." Some people may not admit to feeling frightened but report instead sudden attacks of racing heart, shortness of breath, or dizziness.

For OCD, screening might include questions such as, "Is there anything that you have to do over and over again and you cannot resist doing it, like washing your hands again and again or checking something several times to make sure you have done it right?" Patients can be asked a general question about phobias such as, "Is there anything you fear so much that you always avoid it, like animals, heights, crowds, closed spaces, driving, public speaking, or being the center of attention?"

To screen for PTSD, the patient can be asked whether she has experienced a traumatic or life-threatening event that still affects her. In screening for anxiety disorders, it is important to assess how much the symptoms impair the patient's function and interfere with her life.

American Psychiatric Association: *Diagnostic and Statistical Manual of Mental Disorders,* 4th ed., Text Revision, American Psychiatric Association, 2000.

Bottas A, Richter MA: Pediatric autoimmune neuropsychiatric disorders associated with streptococcal infections (PANDAS). Pediatr Infect Dis J 2002;21:67.

Foa EB, Street GP: Women and traumatic events. J Clin Psychiatry 2001;62(Suppl 17):29. [PMID: 11495093]

Goodman WK et al: The Yale-Brown Obsessive-Compulsive Scale (Y-BOCS). Part I. Development, use, and reliability. Arch Gen Psychiatry 1989;46:1006. [PMID: 2684084]

Gorman JM: Generalized anxiety disorder. Clin Cornerstone 2001;3:37. [PMID: 11351785]

Hamilton M: The assessment of anxiety states by rating. Br J Med Psychol 1959;32:50.

Hidalgo RB, Barnett SD, Davidson JR: Social anxiety disorder in review: two decades of progress. Int J Neuropsychopharmacol 2001;4:279. [PMID: 11602035]

Jenike MA: An update on obsessive-compulsive disorder. Bull Menninger Clin 2001;65:4. [PMID: 11280957]

Yehuda R: Post-traumatic stress disorder. N Engl J Med 2002; 346:108. [PMID: 11784878]

Differential Diagnosis

The psychiatric differential diagnosis of anxiety disorders includes agitated depression, mania, and psychotic disorders. Anxiety symptoms also may result from medical illnesses or substance abuse or withdrawal. Table 10–1 lists some of the conditions to include in the medical differential diagnosis; however, most of them are uncommon causes of significant anxiety symptoms. In the presence of a clear-cut, typical history of an anxiety disorder in a young and apparently healthy woman, the medical work-up need not be exhaustive; it should be designed to rule out only the conditions strongly suggested by the patient's history and physical examination. In older patients and those not responding to initial treatment of the anxiety disorder, a more extensive medical work-up is indicated.

Table 10–1. Medical differential diagnosis of anxiety.

System or Agent	Disorder or Drug
Cardiac	Arrhythmias
	Coronary artery disease
	Congestive heart failure
Respiratory	Hyperventilation
	Asthma
	Pulmonary embolus
	Chronic obstructive pulmonary disease
Endocrine	Cushing's syndrome
	Hyperparathyroidism
	Hyper- or hypothyroidism
	Hypoglycemia
	Menopausal symptoms
	Pheochromocytoma
	Carcinoid
	Insulinoma
Neurologic	Temporal lobe epilepsy
	True vertigo
	Tic disorders (obsessive-compulsive disorder)
	Tumor
	Akathisia
Medication or drugs	Alcohol withdrawal
	Caffeinism
	Sedative withdrawal
	Cocaine
	Amphetamines
	Marijuana
	Steroids
	Sympathomimetics
	Theophylline
Other	Electrolyte disturbance
	Collagen vascular disease

Several medical conditions warrant special mention. Mitral valve prolapse often occurs together with panic attacks, especially in women. This usually benign medical condition most often requires no specific treatment and does not change the approach to diagnosis or treatment of panic attacks. Irritable bowel syndrome also commonly coexists with anxiety disorders and may respond well to treatment of anxiety, especially with tricyclic antidepressants. Chest pain can be a symptom of panic attacks and may lead to invasive, expensive cardiac work-ups.

The most common and most frequently overlooked conditions causing anxiety symptoms are substance abuse and depression. Alcohol or sedative withdrawal, caffeine, marijuana, and stimulants (such as cocaine and amphetamines) often provoke anxiety or panic symptoms, but the patient may not spontaneously report drug or alcohol use. Many depressed people complain primarily of anxiety, and their depressive symptoms may be missed. Because major depression frequently coexists with anxiety, all anxious patients should be asked about symptoms of depression. Screening for substance abuse and for depression is described in Chapters 9 and 11, respectively.

Complications

Two thirds of patients with panic disorder have a lifetime history of depression, and one third have coexisting depression and panic disorder. The latter group has been shown to have lower treatment response rates than patients with panic disorder alone. Panic disorder also has been linked with an increased rate of suicide attempts.

Depression commonly coexists with OCD, PTSD, and social phobia. Most anxiety disorders are associated with an increased rate of alcohol and sedative abuse and dependence. Abuse of these drugs may alleviate anxiety symptoms temporarily and represent a form of "self-medication"; however, repeated use and withdrawal may provoke more anxiety.

Treatment

A. GENERAL MEASURES

Patients with anxiety disorders usually are quite relieved to be assured that they have a treatable condition. Many of these patients believe they are "going crazy" or are suffering from a life-threatening disorder. Providing information about their anxiety disorder is extremely helpful. A small number of patients continue to insist that they have a "medical" disorder or that there is something wrong with them that the doctors have been unable to diagnose. Such patients may benefit from an empathic approach in which the provider does not attempt to argue or convince them otherwise but instead sympathizes with the difficulty of their position, discusses anxiety disorders using a medical model (eg, emphasizing the increased adrenalin), and explains that psychological factors such as life stressors can exacerbate any condition, including theirs, and thus deserve attention.

In addition to education, general measures helpful for people with anxiety disorders include avoidance of caffeine, alcohol, and illicit drugs; adequate sleep; exercise; and when possible, avoidance of life stressors such as moving to a new home or major changes in routine. In initiating treatment, the provider needs to be reassuring, optimistic, and available to answer questions and take telephone calls.

B. PHARMACOTHERAPY

Effective medication is available for panic disorder, OCD, GAD, and social anxiety disorder. Medications provide useful adjuncts in the treatment of PTSD. Specific phobias, on the other hand, should be treated with psychotherapy (see the following section) and do not respond to pharmacotherapy.

1. Antidepressants—Most antidepressants, including selective serotonin reuptake inhibitors (SSRIs), tricyclic antidepressants, monoamine oxidase (MAO) inhibitors, and newer agents such as venlafaxine, are effective in treating panic disorder. An exception is bupropion, which may exacerbate panic symptoms. The SSRIs (fluoxetine, sertraline, paroxetine, citalopram, escitalopram, and fluvoxamine) and venlafaxine are now the medications of choice for panic disorder, primarily because they have fewer side effects than the older antidepressants. There are several important points to keep in mind when prescribing antidepressants for panic and anxiety disorders. First, many anxious patients are sensitive to and fearful of medication side effects. Thus, these drugs should be started at very low doses, (eg, 5–10 mg of paroxetine, 12.5 mg of sertraline, or 2 mg of fluoxetine syrup daily). Second, anxious patients often experience increased anxiety or "overstimulation" in the first week or two of antidepressant treatment. They should be warned that this effect might occur and be reassured that it will pass. If necessary, benzodiazepines can be prescribed initially to help reduce anxiety. Although small doses of antidepressants are necessary at first, patients with panic disorder usually require full antidepressant doses for therapeutic efficacy and thus need to have their doses steadily increased, as rapidly as they can tolerate, to the usual therapeutic level. Finally, antidepressants may take up to 10–12 weeks to reach their full effect in anxiety disorders, compared with 4–6 weeks in depression. In general, success rates for antidepressant treatment of panic disorder are approximately 70–80%, with a placebo response rate of about 30%. The optimal duration of antidepressant treatment for panic disorder is unclear. In patients being treated with imipramine for panic disorder, the dose can be cut in half after 6 months but discontinuation of medication at this point in therapy results in high relapse rates. (See Chapter 11 for a full list and discussion of antidepressants and their side effects.)

Specific types of antidepressant medications are helpful in other anxiety disorders. The treatment of choice for social anxiety disorder is an SSRI. MAO inhibitors are also effective, while tricyclics are not. β-Blockers such as atenolol, 50–100 mg/d, may be helpful when prescribed regularly or as needed in circumscribed social anxiety, such as fears of performance or public speaking. β-Blockers do not appear superior to placebo in the treatment of more generalized or severe social anxiety disorder. Antidepressants such as venlafaxine, SSRIs, and imipramine have been shown to be beneficial in managing GAD.

The treatment of choice for OCD is 1 of the serotonergic antidepressants: clomipramine, 150–300 mg/d; fluoxetine, 20–80 mg/d; sertraline, 50–200 mg/d; paroxetine, 20–50 mg/d; citalopram, 20–80 mg/d; escitalopram 10–20 mg/day or fluvoxamine, 150–300 mg/d. A moderate to marked therapeutic response occurs in 40–60% of patients given 1 of these medications; the response can take up to 12 weeks and is uncommon with placebo. If one of these agents is ineffective, another may work for the patient. Although all of these agents are effective, clomipramine has more anticholinergic and other side effects, so it may be less well tolerated.

In patients with PTSD, antidepressants are helpful in treating depression, panic attacks, and intrusive symptoms. SSRIs are effective in alleviating emotional numbing and avoidance. Hyperarousal symptoms may respond to β-blockers or clonidine. Insomnia has been treated symptomatically with trazodone, and mood instability and anger outbursts may improve with a mood stabilizer such as valproic acid. Of note, prazosin, an α-adrenergic antagonist long used as an antihypertensive, has been shown to be very effective in treating the traumatic nightmares associated with PTSD as well as other PTSD symptoms.

2. Anxiolytics—Traditionally, people presenting with anxiety symptoms have been treated with anxiolytics, primarily benzodiazepines. Benzodiazepines are indeed quite effective for GAD and situational anxiety symptoms. Alprazolam (Xanax), 2–6 mg/d; clonazepam (Klonopin), 1–3 mg/d; lorazepam (Ativan), 3–8 mg/d; and diazepam (Valium), 20–60 mg/d all have been shown to be effective in panic disorder, with alprazolam being comparable in efficacy to antidepressants but with a much more rapid onset of action. The starting dosage of alprazolam for panic disorder is 0.25–0.5 mg (or an equivalent dosage of another benzodiazepine) 3 times daily (Table 10–2).

Benzodiazepines are also useful as treatment adjuncts in OCD and social anxiety disorder, although the high rate of alcohol abuse and dependence in patients with social anxiety disorder dictates caution in prescribing these medications in this group. Patients with other anxiety disorders usually require lower doses

Table 10–2. Pharmacokinetics of benzodiazepines commonly prescribed for anxiety disorders.

Generic Name (Trade Name)	Dosage Equivalent (mg)	Onset of Action	Elimination Half-Life (hours)[1]	Hepatic Metabolism
Alprazolam (Xanax)	1.0	Intermediate	6–20	Oxidation
Chlordiazepoxide (Librium)	20.0–25.0	Intermediate	5–100	Oxidation
Clonazepam (Klonopin)	0.5	Intermediate	18–50	Oxidation, nitroreduction
Clorazepate (Tranxene)	15.0	Fast	30–100	Oxidation
Diazepam (Valium)	10.0	Fast	30–100	Oxidation
Lorazepam (Ativan)	1.5–2.0	Intermediate	10–20	Conjugation
Oxazepam (Serax)	30.0	Slow	5–21	Conjugation

[1]Elimination half-lives include those of all active metabolites.

of benzodiazepines than do patients with panic disorder.

The advantages of benzodiazepines include a rapid onset of action, efficacy when used as needed, and a low rate of adverse effects. The greatest disadvantages are the development of tolerance (need for a higher dose to achieve a therapeutic effect or loss of anxiolytic effects altogether) and dependence. Anxious patients without a history of substance abuse are unlikely to abuse benzodiazepines; however, they may develop tolerance and withdrawal symptoms with attempted discontinuation, especially with higher doses and longer duration of treatment. Other side effects of benzodiazepines include memory loss for recently acquired information (anterograde amnesia), sedation, impaired driving ability, and incoordination. The patient should be advised not to drive if she feels sleepy while taking the medication.

The primary indications for use of benzodiazepines in anxiety disorders are (1) disabling symptoms, with significantly impaired function and (2) inability to tolerate other medication or to benefit from psychotherapeutic treatments. Benzodiazepines should be avoided in people with a history of alcohol or substance abuse themselves or a family history of alcoholism in a first-degree relative.

The pharmacokinetic properties of the benzodiazepines commonly used for anxiety disorders are given in Table 10–2. Compounds with a more rapid onset of action are more suitable for use "as needed." Elimination half-lives increase with a patient's age and in patients with liver disease. The risk of side effects of benzodiazepines increases with age; hip fractures are significantly more common in elderly people taking benzodiazepines with a long half-life than in those taking a benzodiazepine with a short half-life. This is a particularly important consideration in elderly women with osteoporosis. Benzodiazepines that are metabolized by conjugation, have no active metabolites, and have relatively short half-lives (such as oxazepam, temazepam, and lorazepam) are preferable in elderly or medically ill patients.

Buspirone (BuSpar), a non–habit-forming and nonsedating medication, is available for treatment of generalized anxiety. Buspirone takes 2–3 weeks at doses of 30–60 mg/d for full effect. Its most common side effects include dizziness, gastrointestinal upset, and headaches. No tolerance or withdrawal symptoms have been reported with this medication. Its benign side effect profile makes buspirone an attractive treatment for GAD.

Gabapentin, initially developed as an anticonvulsant, has proven to be an effective, non–habit-forming anxiolytic treatment for patients with panic disorder and social anxiety disorder. Doses range from 100–3600 mg daily in 3 divided doses, and side effects can include dizziness, incoordination, and sedation. Some patients find gabapentin to be effective and well tolerated when used as needed for anxiety symptoms. In addition, its efficacy for chronic neuropathic pain makes it a useful anxiolytic in patients with comorbid anxiety and chronic pain.

C. PSYCHOTHERAPY

The mainstay of treatment for phobic disorders (agoraphobia, specific phobias) is behavior therapy, in which the patient confronts the feared situation either in her imagination, with the therapist, or on her own (exposure therapy), often using relaxation or other techniques to become less and less fearful of it (desensitization). Behavior therapy is also quite effective in OCD, for which it consists of a combination of exposure and response prevention, (eg, preventing the patient from washing her hands if she fears dirt and contamination).

Specific forms of cognitive-behavioral therapy have been developed for panic disorder and GAD. In this therapy, the patient identifies and confronts distorted thoughts (eg, "If I have a panic attack, I will have a heart attack and die") and learns specific techniques to deal with and tolerate anxiety symptoms. Cognitive-behavioral therapy has a high success rate (80–90%), takes about 12–20 sessions, and gives the patient a valuable feeling of mastery of her disorder. Although this therapy usually is done best with the help of a trained therapist, patient manuals (such as one by Barlow and Craske) are available. Both individual and group cognitive-behavioral treatments have been developed for social anxiety disorder.

PTSD usually requires more intensive psychotherapeutic approaches, including both group and individual treatment. Specific forms of psychotherapy for PTSD include desensitization, flooding, and stress inoculation therapy. The general goal is to allow the patient to confront or recall the trauma and integrate the event into their life while reducing intrusive memories, flashbacks, and hyperarousal. Patients can be gradually desensitized to stimuli or situations that remind them of the traumatic event, either in their imagination, by talking about the event, or by confronting real-life situations that arouse painful memories or flashbacks. Sudden, overwhelming exposure to feared situations (or flooding) can be a very effective treatment but may exacerbate comorbid depression, substance abuse, panic attacks, or suicidal ideation and so should be used with caution. Stress inoculation therapy emphasizes identifying stress reactions, rehearsing coping skills, and applying these skill in feared situations. All of these approaches are best carried out by a therapist with expertise in treating PTSD.

The optimal treatment for most anxiety disorders usually is a combination of medication and psychotherapy. Some people prefer to avoid medication or cannot tolerate side effects and so may choose psychotherapy alone, whereas others prefer a medical model and do not wish to spend the time required for psychotherapy. The success of treatment can be monitored using rating scales and diaries; many of the treatments for anxiety disorders take weeks to work, and identifying small gains in the first few weeks of treatment can be encouraging.

D. COMPLEMENTARY THERAPY

The major anxiolytic herbal agent has been kava kava, which derives from the plant *Piper methysticum.* Kava kava has been used in Polynesia for centuries during ceremonial occasions and has been shown in several double-blind trials to be effective for generalized anxiety. However, recent reports of hepatitis associated with kava kava treatment have limited its use.

Ballenger JC: Current treatments of the anxiety disorders in adults. Biol Psychiatry 1999;46:1579. [PMID: 10599485]

Barlow DH: *Anxiety and Its Disorders: Second Edition.* Guilford Press, 2001.

Barlow DH, Craske MG: *Mastery of Your Anxiety and Panic II.* Graywind Publications, 1994.

Mavissakalian M, Perel JM: Clinical experiments in maintenance and discontinuation of imipramine therapy in panic disorder with agoraphobia. Arch Gen Psychiatry 1992;49:318. [PMID: 1558466]

Pande AC et al: Treatment of social phobia with gabapentin: a placebo-controlled trial. J Clin Psychopharmacol 1999;19:341. [PMID: 10440462]

Taylor F, Raskind MA: The alpha-1-adrenergic antagonist prazosin improves sleep and nightmares in civilian trauma posttraumatic stress disorder. J Clin Psychopharmacol 2002;22:82. [PMID: 11799347]

Issues of Pregnancy, Lactation, & Menstruation

Many forms of anxiety, particularly panic disorder and agoraphobia, are significantly more prevalent in women than in men. Although anxiety disorders can begin at any stage of life, they are most likely to develop in childhood, adolescence, or young adulthood. Because they occur during the childbearing years, important questions arise regarding their course and management during pregnancy and lactation.

Many women with anxiety disorders note that their symptoms worsen premenstrually, even in the absence of premenstrual syndrome. The course of these disorders during pregnancy is quite variable. Symptoms of OCD often begin or worsen during pregnancy, whereas panic attacks may subside or continue unchanged. It is clearly preferable to plan a pregnancy during an asymptomatic period, discontinue medication, and use psychotherapeutic approaches as needed during the pregnancy. It is important to taper benzodiazepines slowly to avoid uncomfortable withdrawal symptoms or seizures. In the case of an unplanned pregnancy or severe symptoms, it may be necessary to make difficult choices concerning treatment, taking into account both the safety of the fetus and the mental health of the mother. These decisions should be made, when possible, with the full, informed collaboration of the woman and, if appropriate, with the participation of her partner.

Medications should be avoided whenever possible during pregnancy but especially in the first trimester. The use of antidepressants during pregnancy and lactation is reviewed in Chapter 12. First- and second-trimester exposure to benzodiazepines has been associated with an increased risk of cleft lip and palate and cardiocirculatory defects, although these findings have not been replicated in more recent, large studies and may be attributable, at least in part, to concurrent heavy smoking. Both tricyclic antidepressants and benzodiazepines given close to term may provoke a neonatal withdrawal syndrome. Benzodiazepines are contraindicated during lactation because they may cause lethargy, jaundice, and poor feeding in the infant. Concerns about medication use in pregnancy must be weighed against evidence that maternal anxiety can affect the fetus adversely. In primates, anxiety leads to placental vasoconstriction and fetal hypoxia; in humans, there has been one case report of a spontaneous abortion during a panic attack. Given the paucity of knowledge and lack of clear clinical guidelines, it may be helpful to obtain psychiatric consultation, gather information from the company manufacturing the drug to be prescribed and a local teratogen information service, and keep in close contact with the patient's obstetrician.

When to Refer to a Specialist

Anxiety disorders can often be treated successfully in the primary care setting with a combination of reassurance, education, medication, problem-solving to assist in dealing with life stressors, and encouragement of the patient to confront feared situations. Referral to a psychiatrist, psychologist, or other mental health provider is indicated in the following situations:

(1) Diagnostic uncertainty: If the presenting complaints are confusing, complicated, or atypical, a psychiatric evaluation may be helpful in clarifying the diagnosis and the appropriate approach to treatment.

(2) Treatment failure: When the first-line treatments outlined in this chapter do not help, other diagnoses should be reconsidered. Evaluation by a specialist is helpful to obtain suggestions of alternative treatments or to initiate a specific psychotherapeutic or medication treatment program.

(3) **Comorbidity, severe illness, or suicidality:** Patients with comorbid depression, substance abuse, or personality disorders or persons who are very ill or are suicidal are more difficult to treat and should be referred to a specialist. Acutely suicidal patients should be referred for emergent consultation or hospitalization.

Of note, a recent study showed that panic disorder can be treated within primary care settings very effectively using a collaborative care model, in which a psychiatrist sees the patient for 2 or 3 visits in collaboration with the primary care provider. This enhanced treatment model was more effective and more cost-effective than treatment as usual within primary care.

Roy-Byrne PP, Katon W, Cowley DS, Russo J: A randomized effectiveness trial of collaborative care for patients with panic disorder in primary care. Arch Gen Psychiatry 2001, 58:869-876. [PMID: 11545671]

Prognosis

Surprisingly, little is known about the long-term prognosis of anxiety disorders. In general, they tend to have a chronic, fluctuating, waxing and waning course with exacerbations during periods of life stress. Naturalistic studies of patients with panic disorder treated in anxiety clinics show improvement in about 40–50%, worsening or continued symptoms in 15–30%, and discontinuation of symptoms in approximately 30%. The prognosis for anxiety disorders is worse in those with comorbid depression, substance abuse, or personality disorders.

Roy-Byrne PP, Cowley DS: Course and outcome in panic disorder: a review of recent follow-up studies. Anxiety 1994-95;1:151. [PMID: 9160567]

Relevant Web Sites

[Anxiety Disorders Association of America]
www.adaa.org
[Obsessive-Compulsive Foundation]
www.ocfoundation.org

Mood Disorders

11

Jennifer D. Bolen, MD, Patricia L. Paddison, MD, Edward K. Rynearson, MD & Fanny Correa, MSW, CT

ESSENTIALS OF DIAGNOSIS

- *Depressed mood.*
- *Loss of interest or pleasure.*
- *Sleep and/or appetite changes.*
- *Decreased concentration.*
- *Psychomotor agitation or retardation.*
- *Fatigue.*
- *Suicidal thoughts.*
- *Negative thinking or excessive guilt.*

General Considerations

A. EPIDEMIOLOGY

Mood disorders are common and disabling illnesses seen frequently in the primary care setting. Approximately 17 million Americans each year are affected with a mood disorder; rates among women are twice that of men. The estimated annual cost of depression in the United States is $43.7 billion. Epidemiologic studies demonstrate repeatedly that 13–20% of people in any community sample exhibit depressive symptoms. Other studies show 1-year prevalence rates for major depression in the range of 2.6–6.2%. Lifetime prevalence for male and female patients combined is 14% (9–26% in women and 5–12% in men), and the female-to-male ratio is 2–3:1. The highest rates of major depression occur in patients who are between 18- and 44-years-old, with the highest occurrence between 25 and 34 years.

Thirty percent of depressions in women start in association with a reproductive event such as menarche, menses, pregnancy, childbirth, infertility, menopause, or oral contraceptive exposure. In addition, women predominate with respect to unipolar depression, seasonal depression, and rapid-cycling mood disorders.

Currently, a biopsychosocial model is used to attempt to understand the causes of mood disorders. Biologic factors include heredity, age, physical illness, circadian cycles, and endocrine physiology. Psychological factors include personality features that may predispose to mood disturbance. Some personality traits found more often in women are correlated with vulnerability to depression; these include passive, avoidant, dependent, and learned helplessness features. Social factors particularly prevalent in the lives of women include poverty, abuse, gender discrimination, caretaking burdens, and low socioeconomic status. Factors such as culture and ethnicity impact differently on men and women. All of the above influences are hypothesized to affect people on a biochemical level, causing dysregulation of basic neurophysiology at the cellular level of the brain, leading to mood disturbance.

Serotonin, norepinephrine, dopamine, and the endorphins are 4 of the neurotransmitter systems believed to be important in mood regulation. Additional neuroreceptors are being studied. Both estrogen and progesterone have effects on these receptor systems and are hypothesized to be significant in female-specific disturbances such as premenstrual syndrome (PMS), postpartum mood disorders, and perimenopausal complaints (see Chapter 12 for details). The additional dysfunction in the hypothalamic-pituitary-adrenal axis seen in depression currently is being studied. Mood disorders also may be associated with thyroid dysfunction, particularly hypothyroidism.

B. PRESENTATION IN WOMEN

Numerous population and cross-cultural studies have shown that depression, mood disturbances, mood cycling, and bereavement have a higher prevalence in women than in men. This gender difference begins to emerge in early adolescence.

Continuing research into mood disorders highlights the fact that these disturbances are complex and have multifactorial causes. There are unique biopsychosocial factors that predispose women to these reactions, such as hormonal changes, reproductive losses, poverty, cultural influences, and abuse. A clinician, determining treatment for a woman suffering from disordered mood must rely on an integrated model that includes all the factors that may influence the patient's mood status.

American Psychiatric Association: *Diagnostic and Statistical Manual of Mental Disorders*, 4th ed, Text Revision. American Psychiatric Association, 2000.

Angold A, Worthman CW: Puberty onset of gender differences in rates of depression: a developmental, epidemiologic and neuroendocrine perspective. J Affect Disord 1993;29:145. [PMID: 8300975]

Established Populations for the Epidemiologic Studies of the Elderly. Arch Intern Med 1998;158:2341. [PMID: 9827785]

Narrow WE et al: Use of services by persons with mental and addictive disorders: Findings from the National Institute of Mental Health Epidemiological Catchment Area Program. Arch Gen Psychiatry 1993;50:95. [PMID: 8381266]

Weissman MM et al: Sex differences in rates of depression: cross-national perspectives. J Affect Disord 1993;29:77. [PMID: 8300980]

Risk Factors

Risk factors for depression include prior episodes, family history, prior suicide attempts, female gender, recent childbirth, medical comorbidity, alcohol or substance abuse, and recent separation or bereavement. Other risk factors include hormonal fluctuations, genetic factors, sleep disturbance, predisposing psychiatric and medical illnesses, history of depression, medications, psychological factors, and social factors.

A. Hormonal Fluctuations

Hormonal fluctuations are known to interact with neurotransmitters, the neuroendocrine axis, and circadian systems. Girls begin to outnumber boys in rates of depression at the time of menarche.

Infertility and reproductive losses have a negative impact on mood in many women. Reproductive hormonal manipulation to enhance fertility or treat perimenopausal irregular bleeding sometimes disrupts mood homeostasis (see Chapter 12 for details).

B. Genetic Factors

The effects of genetic factors on mood are well documented. A study conducted on female twin pairs showed an influence from genetics on the liability for major depression. Another study showed greater heritability for major depression in women than in men.

C. Sleep Disturbance

A sleep disturbance may contribute to the risk of major depression. Sleep studies show that female patients have higher total sleep requirements than male patients and yet often are relatively sleep deprived. Insomnia often precedes the onset of depression; perimenopausal women, in particular, may have disrupted sleep because of vasomotor symptoms at night; or postpartum women may have disrupted sleep related to infant feeding.

D. Predisposing Psychiatric and Medical Illnesses

Examples of the many illnesses associated with mood disorders include anxiety disorders, substance abuse, eating disorders, posttraumatic stress disorder, sleep disorders, hypothyroidism, and hyperthyroidism. Autoimmune illness is more prevalent in women than in men, and the resultant pain symptoms and steroid exposure are added risk factors for depression and mood instability. Also, stroke and dementia often are accompanied by depression.

E. History of Depression

Depression is frequently a recurrent illness with 30% of patients becoming chronically depressed and 20% exhibiting a recurrent course. The chance of another episode of depression developing is 50% after 1 episode, 80% after 2 episodes, and 90% after 3 episodes.

F. Medications

A careful evaluation of any patient's mood should include a review of current and recent medication exposure. There are well known medications commonly used in primary care that may predispose a patient to mood changes such as narcotics, benzodiazepines, and glucocorticoids. Other agents may cause fatigue or symptoms that may be confused with depression. Consultation with a pharmacist is often helpful in particular cases.

G. Psychological Factors

Cognitive and personality styles, as discussed previously, may affect mood. Family and culture-bound traditions regarding female roles emphasize responsibility toward family over self, dependency, compliance, self-sacrifice, and physical beauty, rather than assertiveness, self-direction, physical expression in work and play, and independent creativity.

H. Social Factors

Women's economic status often places them at risk for living in or on the margin of poverty. They are frequently burdened with numerous responsibilities caring for children, elderly family members, working outside the home and doing the "second shift" after returning home from their jobs. Although marriage decreases the risk of depression in men, married women are more likely to be depressed than their single counterparts. An unhappy marriage is a major risk factor for depression in women. The number of children in the home has a positive correlation with rates of depression. Domestic violence and history of prior or current victimization also afflict women more commonly than men and are major risk factors for depression. Dysfunctional work environments, in which low status, poor pay, and sexual harassment are factors, contribute toward an increased risk for dysphoric and depressed mood. Bereavement in women triggered by reproductive losses, death of a child, divorce, or widowhood can precipitate a depressive episode.

Brandis M: A feminist analysis of the theories of etiology of depression in women. Nurs Leadersh Forum 1998;3:18. [PMID: 10458848]

Dixit AR, Crum RM: Prospective study of depression and the risk of heavy alcohol use in women. Am J Psychiatry 2000;157:751. [PMID: 10784468]

Frank JB et al: Women's mental health in primary care. Depression, anxiety, somatization, eating disorders, and substance abuse. Med Clin North Am 1998;82:359. [PMID: 9531930]

Kendler KS et al: Genetic risk factors for major depression in men and women: similar or different heritabilities and same or partly distinct genes? Psychol Med 2001;31:605. [PMID: 11352363]

Kendler KS, Prescott CA: A population-based twin study of lifetime major depression in men and women. Arch Gen Psychiatry 1999;56:39. [PMID: 9892254]

Prevention

Prevention efforts related to mood disorders must become a priority in our society given the frequency of these illnesses and the attendant morbidity, suffering, and risk of suicide in affected individuals. The impact on children growing up with an affected mother has been well documented. The cost in actual dollars and loss of function is substantial. Targets for prevention efforts would include societal, cultural, and public health changes that reduce the risk factors reviewed earlier in this chapter.

Clinical Findings

A. SYMPTOMS

Common symptoms of depression include anger, sadness, feelings of loss and emptiness, and lowered frustration tolerance or coping. Symptoms must not be caused by substance use or an organic condition.

B. DIAGNOSTIC CRITERIA

1. Major depressive episode—The Diagnostic and Statistical Manual of Mental Disorders, 4e, Text Revision (DSM-IV-TR) criteria for a major depressive disorder require that "5 (or more) of the following symptoms have been present during the same 2-week period and represent a change from previous functioning; at least 1 of the symptoms is either (1) depressed mood or (2) loss of interest or pleasure."

The additional symptoms referred to in the criteria established by the American Psychiatric Association (APA) include (3) weight loss or gain, (4) insomnia or hypersomnia, (5) psychomotor agitation or retardation, (6) fatigue or low energy, (7) feelings of worthlessness or excessive guilt, (8) diminished ability to think or concentrate, and (9) recurrent thoughts of death, suicidal ideation, or suicide attempt. Beck Depression Inventory scores are usually in the range of the upper teens to greater than 20 on a scale of 0–63. (The Beck Depression Inventory, a self-administered multiple-choice questionnaire that takes minutes to complete, is a well-established and easily understood clinical tool that indicates both presence of depression and degree of severity.)

2. Adjustment disorder with depressed mood—This condition is defined as the development of symptoms, either emotional or behavioral, in response to an identifiable stressor (or stressors) that has occurred in the preceding 3 months; and the patient experiences a drop in mood and other symptoms common to depression but does not fulfill criteria for major depression. The reaction causes impairment in social or occupational functioning and distress in excess of what would be expected from exposure to the stressor and is of a significant level and has not lasted longer than 6 months. Once the stressor has been eliminated, the symptoms do not last for longer than another 6 months.

3. Dysthymic disorder—A patient who is chronically depressed for at least 2 years and has at least 2 of the following symptoms is diagnosed as having dysthymic disorder: (1) changes in appetite, (2) insomnia or hypersomnia, (3) low energy or fatigue, (4) diminished self-esteem, (5) poor concentration or difficulty with decision-making, and (6) feelings of hopelessness. Scores on the Beck Depression Inventory usually are elevated but not in the range seen for major depression. During the 2-year period, the person has never been free from the symptoms for more than 2 months at a time. No major depressive episode has been present during the first 2 years of the disturbance. The symptoms cause clinical distress or impairment in social or occupational functioning.

4. Seasonal depression—Known also as seasonal affective disorder (SAD), seasonal depression requires identification of a regular temporal relationship between the onset of mood episodes and a particular time of the year, eg, regular occurrence of a depressive episode in the fall or winter. The change from depression to euthymia or hypomania also occurs at a characteristic time of the year, eg, depression disappears in the spring. In the previous 2 years, 2 depressive episodes must have occurred following the same seasonal pattern, and no nonseasonal depressions may have occurred outside the pattern. Seasonal depressive episodes must outnumber the nonseasonal episodes that have occurred over the patient's lifetime. This disorder is more common in female than male patients and often presents with striking hypersomnia, lethargy, weight gain, and dysthymia.

5. Rapid-cycling bipolar disorder—This disorder is a disturbance of mood meeting criteria for major depression at times and for mania or hypomania at other times. These cycles must occur at least 4 times annually, and the episodes must meet the criteria for a major depressive, manic, mixed, or hypomanic episode. This disorder is much more common in female than male patients.

6. Bipolar disorder—Bipolar disorder has several separate criteria sets depending on the subtype as defined in DSM-IV-TR. This disorder refers to an individual suffering from a mood disturbance that includes cycles of elevated mood states. **Mania** is defined as a period of elevated mood with at least 3 of the following symptoms present: (1) sense of grandiosity, (2) decrease in the need for sleep, (3) increase in talkativeness, (4) thought racing, (5) distracted or agitated easily, (6) buying sprees, (7) sexual indiscretion.

7. Cyclothymia disorder—Criteria for this disorder include at least a 2-year history of cyclic mood disturbance with elevation of mood and depression of mood. Neither of these mood states fulfills criteria for major depression or mania. The person has not been without symptoms for more than 2 months during the 2-year period.

8. Postpartum depression—See Chapter 12.

9. Premenstrual dysphoric disorder—See Chapter 12.

Beck AT et al: An inventory for measuring depression. Arch Gen Psychiatry 1961;4:561.

Evaluation

Up to 75% of patients with identified depressions are treated in the primary care setting, although many cases go unrecognized and untreated. Depression can be missed easily if other presenting complaints such as somatic symptoms are emphasized, if the depression is masked, or if the patient is not asked specific questions about depressive symptoms. Unfortunately, inquiry into the patient's mental health in the medical setting can be perceived as a lack of validation on the part of the provider of the patient's presenting complaints. Providers need to attend to the patient's presenting problems seriously, as well as to offer educational information regarding the importance of additional inquiry concerning mental health. If depression is identified coincident with the patient's presenting illness or routine well care, timely evaluation of the mood problem is indicated assuming the patient is willing. If additional evaluation by a mental health specialist is indicated, further education may be necessary for the reluctant patient.

Brochures that define depression and mood disturbance are available for placement in waiting areas. These materials inform patients of the contemporary understandings of depressive illness (ie, that it is not a weakness, that often it does not abate without treatment, that lack of treatment has ramifications in terms of quality of life and risks of suicide and substance abuse, and that treatment is successful when well-established clinical guidelines are followed).

Women who have depression often seek medical attention for such complaints as fatigue, pain, or headache. If depression is suspected, a screening tool such as the Beck Depression Inventory can be used during the visit. The inventory also can direct a clinician to critical problem areas such as suicidality, sleep disturbance, and weight change, although it cannot substitute for the provider's careful history.

In brief visits there may not be time to attend to more than the primary presenting problem; if a mood disorder is suspected, the patient should be asked to come back as soon as possible for additional evaluation and history.

A thorough past and current medical and mental health history, including psychosocial aspects, is the standard for evaluation. Included also are a history of recent stressors, medication exposure, substance use, prior treatment efforts, past or current abuse, and psychiatric illness or suicide in other family members. Most important are the patient's mind-set concerning her mental health and the provider's impression of her psychological status.

The history must include attention to hormonal status, cyclic mood changes, pregnancy or prepregnancy status, any physical condition that can aggravate or cause depression, medication (over the counter and prescribed), herbal remedies, and substance exposure. Inquiries are made concerning job and family satisfaction, recent loss or trauma, and recent major stressors. Evaluation of suicidal or homicidal ideation, self-harm impulses, and parenting safety are priorities in history gathering.

Studies show that the strongest predictors for major depression are recent stressful life events, a positive family history, a prior episode, and the presence of other psychiatric disorders. A positive history in these areas warrants further evaluation of depression and predepression symptoms. The discovery of predepression symptoms such as sleep disturbance, mild anhedonia, changes in function at work or home, and beginning loss of motivation might prompt preventive measures to attempt to circumvent the development of a more chronic and refractory depression subtype. The recommendation of increased exercise, stress reduction and relaxation training might prevent a major depressive episode. If the person has a positive history, early intervention with medications and/or therapy is important. Certainly, monitoring a patient under these circumstances is warranted.

Additional evaluation of a patient with a mood disorder generally includes a physical examination, a test of thyroid function, additional laboratory studies if indicated, and an electrocardiogram (ECG) if the patient is elderly or has a history of cardiac disturbance.

Psychological testing is not routine in the work-up of patients with mood disorder; however, it is indicated if the differential includes the possibility of dementia or unusual memory and cognitive problems beyond those typical of depressed patients. Many perimenopausal and geriatric patients complain of memory difficulties, and the extent of the evaluation depends on the provider's clinical intuition regarding the presence of organic factors.

Depression Guideline Panel: *Depression in Primary Care.* Vol 1. *Diagnosis and Detection.* (Clinical Practice Guideline No. 5, AHCPR Publication No. 93-0550.) US Department of Health and Human Services, Public Health Service, Agency for Health Care Policy and Research, 1993.

Differential Diagnosis

The most common depression diagnoses in primary care settings are major depressive episode, adjustment disorder with depressed mood, and dysthymic disorder. However, busy primary care providers are not in a position to go through the DSM-IV-TR with each patient presenting with a mood disturbance. In general, keep an index of suspicion for medical and/or psychiatric comorbidities in the evaluation of a depressed patient. (See the section of When to Refer to a Specialist for more input.)

Treatment

Dysfunction in terms of parenting, work, interpersonal relationships, marriage, and general quality of life is high for depressed people. Suicide rates of depressed people range from 10% to 15%. Susceptibility to other illnesses may be increased. Research is currently looking at cardiovascular risks and altered immune function with depression in both men and women. Poor self-care and high-risk health behaviors such as smoking, overeating, lack of exercise, and alcohol abuse are additional problems associated with depression. It is hoped that identifying depressed patients and initiating treatment will minimize the morbidity of untreated depression.

The current standard for treatment is to increase detection and treatment in primary care, to strive for complete remission, to enhance compliance, to ameliorate long-term side effects, and to refer more refractory patients to psychiatry for more aggressive treatment.

Excellent studies have been done proving the efficacy of treatment for mood disorders; rates of response to treatment are reported to be in the range of 60–80%. Studies of mild to moderate depression have shown equal effectiveness of antidepressant pharmacotherapy and cognitive/behavioral or interpersonal psychotherapy. Antidepressant medications are indicated strongly for severe depressions. A combination of antidepressants and weekly psychotherapy is often the initial treatment of choice. Chronic forms of major depression are often difficult to treat. A recent 12-week study of patients with chronic depression demonstrated 85% recovery responses to a combination of antidepressants and a subtype of cognitive therapy.

Patients who have been in psychotherapy in the past and are presenting with an acute or chronic depression may opt for pharmacotherapy only. Patients in whom depression is refractory or recurrent often benefit from supportive psychotherapy because medications may take longer to be effective in subsequent episodes, and the interim suffering is often great. Feelings of hopelessness and the possibility of suicide must be monitored in more refractory and treatment-resistant patients. At times, the type of treatment initiated is influenced by a patient's resources, prior treatment experiences, access and belief system. Clinicians need to weigh these factors in their treatment recommendations and review with the patient the risks of not selecting a modality that is known to be beneficial.

In addition to initiating one of the treatments outlined in the following sections, it is helpful for the clinician to provide educational material for the patient. Resources for patients regarding treatment can be found on web sites (see following section, Relevant Web Sites).

A. PSYCHOTHERAPY

Psychotherapy alone may be recommended in adolescents with depression, patients with mild and situational mood disturbances, and women who are strongly opposed to taking medication. Pregnant patients and those planning a pregnancy are good candidates for psychotherapy alone. The initial response to psychotherapy may be somewhat slower than to medication, a fact best explained to the patient when weighing the pros and cons of the options for treatment.

Psychotherapy is practiced by a diverse group of providers with a variety of academic degrees and training; the most common practitioners are therapists with a masters degree, psychologists with a PhD degree, and psychiatrists with an MD degree. Referrals should be made to known therapists with excellent reputations, good training, and a track record of reasonable outcomes. Attempting to provide a good match between therapist and patient is beneficial. Most states have licensing boards for mental health practitioners and have on record any disciplinary actions related to licensed professionals. Boundary violations such as sexual abuse are not uncommon in the therapy profession and can be highly damaging to patients. Referrals should be made with caution and the patients told to trust their instincts regarding therapists. It is helpful to inform patients that they have several options and to encourage them to recontact the primary provider if an initial referral does not work well.

"Side effects" of psychotherapy need to be considered. In some instances, increased insight may precipitate life changes, with subsequent increase in stressors (eg, a patient who leaves a miserable marriage and undergoes a change in financial status, a major relocation, or a reduction in contact with her children). Therapy also may be the setting in which child abuse experiences that have been dormant for years are brought into conscious awareness, with the attendant psychological pain.

B. PHARMACOTHERAPY

1. Antidepressants—Pharmacotherapy is indicated in cases of severe depression, of milder but chronic depression that has not responded to an adequate trial of psychotherapy, and of depression with anxiety and multiple vegetative symptoms. At times medications are tried because a depressed patient is unwilling or unable to seek psychotherapy. Numerous other factors may contribute to the decision to prescribe antidepressants, such as a history of severe pain, fibromyalgia, longstanding fatigue, or severe PMS.

When a provider decides to recommend a medication trial to a patient, the first action is inform the patient of pros, cons, and alternative options of pharmacotherapy. In cases of severe mood disturbance, the risks need to be explained to the patient should she decide not to take the medication. It is helpful to stress that the initial prescription is a trial of medication and that if the benefits outweigh the side effects, the trial will become longer term treatment.

Choosing an initial agent depends on the provider and the patient. Providers should prescribe agents with which they are familiar and that they use frequently; patients often can participate in the selection when given adequate information about the side-effect profiles common to these agents.

It is important to inform patients that all antidepressants studied demonstrate equal efficacy in the treatment of depression; greater than 70% of depressed patients respond with mood improvement. Antidepressant effects are not immediate and often take from 10 days to 8 weeks to appear. Twelve weeks may be a more typical trial length in a patient with a history of chronic or more resistant depression.

Studies and experience show that side effects of all antidepressants are most common in the initial and early phases of treatment. One study of patients taking antidepressants found minimal complaints of side effects at the 6-month point.

Patients should be warned that antidepressants can augment the effects of alcohol. In general, taking antidepressants is a contraindication to alcohol use because of the negative interactions between alcohol and antidepressants, such as the depressive effects of alcohol on the central nervous system and the negative effects of alcohol on sleep quality.

Discontinuation/withdrawal type syndromes coming off antidepressants or with missed dosages need to be reviewed with patients. They are especially common with the shorter half-life agents such as venlafaxine and paroxetine. Symptoms include lightheadedness, dizziness, visual lag, vertigo, and other flu-like symptoms such as myalgia, nausea, insomnia and sensory disturbances. They may be short lived or in some cases persist over weeks.

The selective serotonin reuptake inhibitors (SSRIs) include fluoxetine, sertraline, paroxetine, fluvoxamine, citalopram, and escitalopram. SSRIs are first-line agents for the treatment of most depressions seen in primary care. Compared with tricyclic antidepressants (TCAs), SSRIs have an improved side-effect profile. Table 11–1 compares the advantages and side effects of TCAs with those of SSRIs.

Gastrointestinal symptoms, nervousness, insomnia, and headaches are common complaints of patients taking SSRIs and tend to be early-phase side effects. Sexual dysfunction (decreased libido and/or delayed or absent orgasm) with SSRIs tends to be a longer term adverse side effect. Treatment of this side effect has been tried with the addition of various agents, such as bupropion, buspirone, stimulants, sildenafil, and *Gingko biloba* as well as lowering dose and drug skip days. Most of these interventions have had variable results. At times, the wish to avoid sexual side effects on the part of the patient may simplify the selection of an initial antidepressant agent or result in a complete switch to an agent during the treatment of a given episode. SSRIs are much safer in overdose than TCAs. The greater expense of these agents is offset by better compliance and lower utilization. In addition, generic forms are now entering the market.

TCAs still in common use include amitriptyline, nortriptyline, desipramine, imipramine, and protriptyline. The TCAs have stood the test of time (up to 5 decades) and are often a good choice for patients with pain syndromes or headaches. They are second- or third-line agents for depression treatment after trials of SSRIs or venlafaxine have failed. They are generally inexpensive and provide latitude in terms of flexibility of dosage. Data on long-term exposure to these older agents are abundant. The downside of these drugs is their side-effect profile (Table 11–2) and high lethality

Table 11–1. Comparison of tricyclic antidepressants (TCAs) with selective serotonin reuptake inhibitors (SSRIs).

		TCAs	SSRIs
Advantages		Effective	Effective
		Dosage flexibility	Single daily dose
		Variety of types available	Six types available
		Long-term data available	Newer than TCAs
		Inexpensive	Expensive, generic available for fluoxetine and others coming out
		Better with pain conditions	Better with obsessive-compulsive disorder
Disadvantages		Dry mouth	
		Constipation	Occasional loose stools, flatulence
		Heart block, prolonged QT	Can trigger premature ventricular contractions in some patients
		Tachycardia	Rare reports of bradycardia
		Postural hypotension	
		Weight gain	Weight loss early, some reports of weight gain over time
		Sedation in some types of depression	Lightens sleep cycle
		Anorgasmia	Anorgasmia, decreased libido
		Lethal in overdose	Much safer than TCAs in overdose
		Cognitive side effects	Gastrointestinal side effects
			Jitteriness
			Akathisia
			Asthenia
			Headache
			Psychomotor agitation
			Extrapyramidal reactions

in overdose. Weight gain, constipation, dry mouth, and postural hypotension can be adverse effects.

Bupropion, neither a TCA nor an SSRI, has the following advantages: no sexual side effects, efficacy in SAD, a tendency toward activation rather than sedation, and no weight gain. Its drawbacks include the necessity to take it 2 times daily, lowering of seizure threshhold, minimal anxiolytic effects, and lightening of the sleep cycle (bedtime dosage should be avoided). Avoid use in patients with a history of bulimia, prior seizures, or head injury patients. It has also been marketed for smoking cessation.

Trazodone is an antidepressant that usually causes sedation; its use as a primary antidepressant is limited, therefore, because of difficulty achieving a therapeutic dose. It also can cause heart block and priapism on rare occasions and has less of an antipanic effect than other agents. It is an inexpensive agent useful at bedtime to help with sleep. It is often prescribed with more activating agents, such as SSRIs and bupropion, when insomnia is an early side effect.

Venlafaxine is an antidepressant with both SSRI and norepinephrine reuptake inhibition activity. It is frequently selected for patients in whom 2 SSRI trials have failed. The common side effects of this agent are similar to those seen with the SSRIs (see Table 11–2).

This agent may elevate blood pressure gradually and blood pressure monitoring in the office and at home is recommended. Avoid using in patients who are hypertensive.

Nefazodone is an antidepressant that targets several serotonergic receptors. Sexual side effects are generally not a problem with this agent, and it is marketed as especially effective in an anxious, depressed patient with sleep disruption. Drawbacks include twice daily dosing, tiredness as a common side effect at higher dosages, and a black box warning for hepatotoxicity. Avoid use in patients with known liver disease or elevated liver function tests. Monitoring guidelines are unclear at this time but a baseline set of liver function tests would seem reasonable pretreatment with repeats after drug initiation.

Mirtazapine, a broad-spectrum antidepressant, has a niche with the elderly depressed patient who is losing weight and cannot sleep. At low dose, sedation and weight gain are common side effects. At higher dosages, the side-effect profile changes, and this agent seems more similar to an SSRI. It is often a second- or third-line choice. Sexual side effects are not common with this agent.

One agent soon to be released is duloxetine, a dual agent similar to venlafaxine.

Table 11–2. Side-effect profiles of antidepressant medications.

Drug	Anticholinergic[1]	Central Nervous System		Cardiovascular		Other	
		Drowsiness	Insomnia/ Agitation	Orthostatic- Hypotension	Cardiac Arrhythmia	Gastrointestinal Distress	Weight Gain (Over 6 kg)
Amitriptyline	4	4	1/2	4	3	1/2	4
Desipramine	1	1	1	2	3	1/2	1
Doxepin	3	4	1/2	3	2	1/2	3
Imipramine	3	3	1	4	3	1	3
Nortriptyline	1	2	1/2	1	2	1/2	2
Protriptyline	2	1	1	2	2	0	0
Trazodone	0	4	0	1	1	1	1
Bupropion	0	1/2	2	0	1/2	1	0
Fluoxetine	0	0	2	0	0	3	0
Paroxetine	1/2	1/2	1	0	1/2	3	0
Sertraline	0	1/2	1	0	1/2	3	0
Monoamine Oxidase Inhibitors (MAOIs)	1	1	2	2	0	1	2
Venlafaxine	1/2	1/2	2	0	1/2	3	0
Nefazodone	1/2	1/2	0	2	1/2	2	1/2
Mirtazepine	2	3	0	1	—	0	2
Citalopram	1	0	0	0	—	2	1

Sources: Data from the Depression Guideline Panel 1993; Pies 1998, Whooley and Simon 2000. Ratings may vary depending on dose, age of patient, length of treatment, and individual variation.
0 = absent or rare
1 = modest
2 = significant
3 = moderately high
4 = high
[1]Dry mouth, blurred vision, urinary hesitancy, constipation.

Monoamine oxidase inhibitors (MAOIs) can be used in patients who have a history of a positive response to these agents or in whom standard trials of the other antidepressant groups have failed to help. Refer the patient to a psychiatrist if these agents seem indicated. The significant drawbacks of MAOIs include hypertensive crisis if combined with tyramine-containing foods or sympathomimetic drugs, dietary restrictions, weight gain, drug interactions, postural hypotension, and the necessity for a washout period of approximately 2 weeks between stopping one of these drugs and beginning another type of antidepressant. The serotonin syndrome is a risk factor for patients exposed to SSRIs and MAOIs in a close temporal relationship. This syndrome of autonomic instability can be life-threatening.

2. Mood stabilizers—Mood stabilizers are prescribed for patients with bipolar disorder, rapid cycling, and refractory and recurrent unipolar depression. Medications in this category include lithium, carbamazepine, and valproic acid. They all require close monitoring of the patient and laboratory screening of drug levels and specific blood tests (such as complete blood cell count, liver function tests, or thyroid-stimulating hormone [TSH] measurement) depending on the agent during treatment. Because lithium can cause hypothyroidism and renal disease, levels of TSH and creatinine should be monitored during exposure. Often combinations of 2 of these 3 agents are prescribed in patients with rapid-cycling bipolar or unipolar disorders or patients with refractory mania. Other anticonvulsants are being used off label for mood stabilizing effects and treatment of depression. These include lamotrigine, gabapentin, and topiramate to name a few.

3. Augmentation—The term augmentation applies to the addition of a second agent to a patient's regimen when the primary agent has provided a partial response, or when a mild relapse has occurred and the clinician does not want to increase the dosage of the primary agent. The augmenting agent boosts the positive treatment effect of the primary agent. Common augmentation agents include lithium in low dosage (300–900 mg/d), sodium liothyronine (Cytomel) (25–50 mcg (micrograms)/day), buspirone, bupropion, trazodone, TCAs, and SSRIs. Before starting augmentation strategies, review accurate diagnoses (rule out bipolar, character disorder, substance abuse). Refer to a psychiatrist for more complex regimens such as the addition of an atypical antipsychotic or the use of lamotrigine due to the risk of Stevens-Johnson syndrome.

4. Dosage guidelines—Table 11–3 presents the standard dosage ranges for antidepressants. In patients with high anxiety or panic, SSRIs should be started at low dosages (2–5 mg of fluoxetine, 12.5–25 mg of sertraline, 5–10 mg of paroxetine, 5–10 mg of citalopram, and 5 mg of escitalopram); short-acting benzodiazepines should be prescribed as needed in the early phase to treat adrenergic side effects, which generally clear in 2–3 weeks. If the patient's sleep pattern is a significant presenting problem or deteriorates, trazodone or an alternative agent may be added at bedtime. The bedtime agent can be discontinued after a few weeks to months, although some patients continue to need it for the duration of treatment.

Elderly patients should be started on antidepressant therapy with low dosages, eg, 10 mg of citalopram. Given that elderly patients often take a number of other prescription medications, select an antidepressant that has a lower likelihood of P-450 drug interactions. All patients must be monitored carefully for side effects and drug interactions. The likelihood of antidepressants causing P-450 interactions is more common with fluoxetine, fluvoxamine, nefazodone, and paroxetine and less common with citalopram, mirtazapine and venlafaxine. Sertraline and bupropion fall in the middle of the above 2 groups.

5. Trial and treatment time guidelines—An adequate trial of an antidepressant is at least 6 weeks for TCAs or 8–12 weeks for SSRIs. The time frame is usually started after a patient titrates up to a therapeutic dose, which may take 1–2 weeks on an outpatient basis. For patients who respond initially and relapse partially during their treatment, one can increase the dosage within the drug's therapeutic range. The side effect profile and recommended dosage guidelines often dictate the drug's upper dosage limit. Blood levels of the drugs are called for infrequently because of lack of availability or reliability; it is best to leave it to a psychiatric consultant to order these tests.

Medications are started at low dosages and increased during the first 1–2 weeks depending on tolerance. It is best to see patients again within 7–14 days of initiating medication to evaluate mood, anxiety, sleep, functional status, side effects, and suicidal ideation. If a patient is feeling better and having minimal side effects, the dosage can be adjusted at this first return visit and the patient can be seen again in 2–6 weeks. If the patient is doing well and a therapeutic dosage has been determined with reasonable certainty, subsequent visits can be scheduled for every 2–4 months. Frequency of visits in the first 3 months of antidepressant therapy depend in part on side effects, clinical response, and confidence in the dosage adjustment. Remember that the goal of treatment for depression is to strive for complete remission of symptoms. Patients should be told to call or schedule an appointment if their mood falters and cycles down over a period of several days or if associated symptoms of depression reemerge, such as sleep disturbance or panic. At the 9-month point for patients with first-onset, single-episode depression, one can begin to educate the patient about tapering off medications. Tapering may start after 9–12 months of therapy and is best done over a period of several weeks with monitoring. If symptoms of depression return, medication can be restarted or increased to the level that was most effective or brought full remission.

C. RESISTANT AND RECURRENT ILLNESS

Treatment resistance is most common in patients with complex psychiatric conditions, significant comorbidities, or personality disorder. Patients who responded in the past but relapsed after drug discontinuation and failed to respond again after retreatment are another example of resistant patients. Patients with resistant illness are best referred for psychiatric consultation because they may require multiple medications, electroconvulsive therapy (ECT), or mood stabilizers. These patients also need increased support for living with a chronic illness.

Even in the best of circumstances, mood disorders are often similar to other medical illnesses (ie, chronic, recurrent, and lifelong). Longer periods of medication maintenance are recommended for patients with recurrent depression, and the guidelines for duration of treatment are 2–5 years of therapy to lifelong. Undertreatment of depression puts patients at higher risk for recurrence.

D. ADDITIONAL THERAPIES

ECT is helpful in some conditions such as rapid cycling mixed mania and dysphoria, psychotic depression, and resistant depression. The side effects include short-term memory impairment, stigma, and often, rapid relapse after treatment stops even when medications have been restarted. Outpatient maintenance ECT has become more common in responders.

Phototherapy is indicated if a patient has SAD alone or in combination with major depression, dysthymic disorder, or both, and requires sitting near the light

Table 11–3. Pharmacology of antidepressant medications.

Drug	Therapeutic Dosage Range (mg/d)	Average (Range) of Elimination Half-Lives (h)[1]	Potentially Fatal Drug Interactions
Tricyclics			
Amitriptyline (Elavil, Endep)	75–300	24 (16–46)	Antiarrhythmics, monoamine oxidase inhibitors (MAOIs)
Clomipramine (Anafranil)	75–300	24 (20–40)	Antiarrhythmics, MAOIs
Desipramine (Norpramin, Pertofrane)	75–300	18 (12–50)	Antiarrhythmics, MAOIs
Doxepin (Adapin, Sinequan)	75–300	17 (10–47)	Antiarrhythmics, MAOIs
Imipramine (Janimine, Tofranil)	75–300	22 (12–34)	Antiarrhythmics, MAOIs
Nortriptyline (Aventyl, Pamelor)	40–200	26 (18–88)	Antiarrhythmics, MAOIs
Protriptyline (Vivactil)	20–60	76 (54–124)	Antiarrhythmics, MAOIs
Trimipramine (Surmontil)	75–300	12 (8–30)	Antiarrhythmics, MAOIs
Heterocyclics			
Amoxapine (Asendin)	100–600	10 (8–14)	MAOIs
Bupropion (Wellbutrin)	225–450	14 (8–24)	MAOIs (possibly)
Maprotiline (Ludiomil)	100–225	43 (27–58)	MAOIs
Trazodone (Desyrel)	150–600	8 (4–14)	—
Selective Serotonin Reuptake Inhibitors (SSRIs)			
Fluoxetine (Prozac)	10–40	168 (72–360)[2]	MAOIs
Paroxetine (Paxil)	20–50	24 (3–65)	MAOIs[3]
Sertraline (Zoloft)	50–150	24 (10–30)	MAOIs[3]
Monoamine Oxidase Inhibitors (MAOIs)[4]			For all three MAOIs: Vasoconstrictors,[5] decongestants,[5] meperidine, and possibly other narcotics
Isocarboxazid (Marplan)	30–50	Unknown	
Phenelzine (Nardil)	45–90	2 (1.5–4.0)	
Tranylcypromine (Parnate)	20–60	2 (1.5–3.0)	
Newer antidepressants			
Venlafaxine (Effexor)	75–300	5–11	MAOIs
Mirtazepine (Remeron)	15–45	20–40	MAOIs
Nefazodone (Serzone)	300–600	3	MAOIs
Fluvoxamine (Luvox)	50–250	15	MAOIs
Citalopram (Celexa)	20–60	35	MAOIs
Escitalopram (Lexapro)	10–20	27–32	MAOIs

Reproduced from *Depression Guideline Panel: Depression in Primary Care: Detection, Diagnosis and Treatment. Quick Reference Guide for Clinicians.* (Clinical Practice Guideline No. 5, AHCPR Publication No. 93-0552.) Department of Health and Human Services, Agency for Health Care Policy and Research, 1993. Pies 1998, Whooley and Simon 2000.

[1]Half-lives are affected by age, sex, race, concurrent medications, and length of drug exposure.
[2]Includes both fluoxetine and norfluoxetine.
[3]By extrapolation from fluoxetine data.
[4]MAO inhibition lasts longer (7 days) than drug half-life.
[5]Including pseudoephedrine, phenylephrine, phenylpropanolamine, epinephrine, norepinephrine, and others.

panel daily for 30–60 minutes of morning exposure. Headache is a possible side effect. A family history of retinal eye disease is an indication for ophthalmologic consultation before panel exposure. Outdoor midday exposure to natural light for 1 hour also has been shown to have benefit and can be combined with exercise or other outdoor activities.

Other therapies include support groups, group psychotherapy, day treatment, exercise, movement therapies, and acupuncture, but their effectiveness is variable. Sleep deprivation is another intervention that has demonstrated some effectiveness. Newer therapies being studied include transcranial magnetic stimulation, vagus nerve stimulation, and even neurosurgery.

E. COMPLEMENTARY THERAPIES

St. John's Wort has been a prescription antidepressant in Europe for some time in the treatment of mild depression. In the United States, it is a popular over-the-counter agent. Evidence-based studies are ongoing. Studies have shown both efficacy and lack of efficacy. All studies seem to show that the *Hypericum* extracts are well tolerated. Recent reports have shown it to have some deleterious drug interactions with cyclosporine, digoxin, warfarin, protease inhibitors, theophylline, carbamazepine, and in one instance oral contraceptives.

Altshuler LL et al: The Expert Consensus Guideline Series. Treatment of depression in women. Postgrad Med 2001;(Spec No):1. [PMID: 11500997]

Cott JM: Herb-drug interactions: focus on pharmacokinetics. CNS Spectrums 2001;6:827.

Depression Guideline Panel: *Depression in Primary Care.* Vol 2. *Treatment of Major Depression.* (Clinical Practice Guideline No. 5, AHCPR Publication No. 93-0551.) US Department of Health and Human Services, Public Health Service, Agency for Health Care Policy and Research, 1993.

Depression Guideline Panel: Depression in Primary Care: Detection, Diagnosis and Treatment. *Quick Reference Guide for Clinicians.* (Clinical Practice Guideline No. 5, AHCPR Publication No. 93-0552.) Department of Health and Human Services, Public Health Service, Agency for Health Care Policy and Research, 1993.

Desai HD, Jann MW: Major depression in women: a review of the literature. J Am Pharm Assoc (Wash) 2000;40:525. [PMID: 10932463]

Fava M: Augmentation and combination strategies in treatment-resistant depression. J Clin Psychiatry 2001;62:4. [PMID: 11575733]

Frank E et al: Interpersonal psychotherapy and antidepressant medication: evaluation of a sequential treatment strategy in women with recurrent major depression. J Clin Psychiatry 2000;61:51. [PMID: 10695647]

Keller MB et al: A comparison of nefazodone, the cognitive behavioral-analysis system of psychotherapy, and their combination for the treatment of chronic depression. N Engl J Med 2001;345:232. [PMID: 10816183]

Kornstein SG: The evaluation and management of depression in women across the life span. J Clin Psychiatry 2001;62:11. [PMID: 11676428]

Kornstein SG, McEnany G: Enhancing pharmacologic effects in the treatment of depression in women. J Clin Psychiatry 2000;61:18. [PMID: 10926051]

Meltzer-Brody SE: St. John's Wort: clinical status in psychiatry. CNS Spectrums 2001;6:835.

Mendes de Leon CF et al: Depression and risk of coronary heart disease in elderly men and women: New Haven EPESE, 1982–1991.

Pies RW: Handbook of Essential Psychopharmacology. American Psychiatric Press, Inc., 1998.

Practice guidelines for major depressive disorder in adults. American Psychiatric Association. Am J Psychiatry 1993;150:1. [PMID: 8465906]

Richelson E: Pharmacology of antidepressants. Mayo Clin Proc 2001;76:511. [PMID: 11357798]

Stotland NL, Stotland NE: Depression in women. Obstet Gynecol Surv 1999;54:519. [PMID: 10434272]

Walsh BT: *Child Psychopharmacology.* American Psychiatric Press, Inc., 1998.

Whooley MA, Simon GE: Primary care: managing depression in medical outpatients. N Engl J Med 2000;343:1942. [PMID: 11136266]

Age-Related Aspects of Depression

A. ADOLESCENCE

Adolescents often experience moodiness that seems related to their stage of development. For severely distressed patients, referral to psychotherapy is often advisable in lieu of medication treatment because adolescents have many psychosocial issues to be unraveled and appreciated, which may require a considerable amount of time. The effectiveness of medication is less well studied and demonstrated in this age group, and these patients are often sensitive to side effects. Adolescents also present challenges in the areas of compliance and impulsivity.

For adolescents who continue to be depressed after a course of psychotherapy, a trial of medication is indicated. SSRIs are much safer than other antidepressants if taken in overdose, and they are better tolerated than older agents. Because antidepressants are rapidly metabolized in adolescents and children, they require the same weight-adjusted doses used for adults. Split-dose regimens in the short half-life agents sometimes sustain a more even blood level in adolescents, related to the more rapid biodegradation of these agents in this age group.

B. MID-LIFE

For women in their 20s, 30s, and 40s, pregnancy and prepregnancy issues must be assessed in terms of treatment options. These women are in the age group most commonly treated for depression and often experience a number of the reproductive factors believed to be important in depression onset eg, delivery, hormonal changes associated with birth and lactation, miscarriage, oral contraceptive exposure, perimenopausal changes, and PMS (see Chapter 12 for details). Additional factors to be considered include death of aging parents, caretaking burdens, work stress, divorce, financial stressors, and at times, the onset of conditions related to aging such as breast cancer or autoimmune illnesses. This age group is better informed than older generations in terms of treatment for depression and is an optimal group for both psychotherapy and pharmacotherapy.

C. LATER LIFE

Older women with depression are a particularly challenging group to treat. They are often medically complex and may be taking many medications. Some older women are recently widowed, and bereavement symptoms may confuse their diagnosis. Members of this generation have been less open about mental health, and may feel more stigmatized than younger people do today if a psychiatric diagnosis is applied to themselves or a family member. In this age group, compromised physical health, memory impairment, high-risk for falling, drug interaction risk, and sensitivity to the side effects of antidepressants are important aspects of clinical treatment. Supportive psychotherapy, social services, and personal support are important treatment interventions.

When to Refer to a Specialist

Referral of the patient to a psychiatrist depends on the clinician's level of comfort with differential diagnosis of mood disorders, ability to distinguish affective illness from primary anxiety disorders, and confidence in working with the pharmacotherapy of mood disorders; another factor is the patient's willingness to see a consultant.

Patients with the following characteristics should be referred: (1) those considered at high risk for suicide, homicide, or self-abusive behavior; (2) patients with a history of past or current psychosis, dissociation, rapid cycling, resistant symptoms, mania, eating disorder, severe personality disorder, or active substance abuse; (3) noncompliant patients; (4) those highly sensitive to side effects of medication; (5) patients with partial or no response to 2 adequate medication trials; (6) those who relapse or experience breakthrough during treatment; and (7) those with complex medical conditions.

Referral for psychotherapy is common in the primary care setting. Phototherapy, ECT, day treatment, inpatient treatment, and psychological testing are less frequent referral requests. When a psychiatrist is consulted, he or she may take over the treatment of the patient, initiate treatment and refer the patient back to the primary care provider for continuation, or make recommendations to the primary provider, who initiates or tailors the treatment.

Prognosis

Outcomes for the management of mood disorders depend on numerous factors. Uncomplicated, single episode depression has an excellent prognosis with state of the art intervention. Depressions that are resistant to treatment occur in up to 30% of those treated. Newer strategies for treatment will improve prognosis. Emphasis on more complete remission with current treatments may prevent relapse and improve prognosis.

Relevant Web Sites

[The National Women's Health Information Center (US Department of Health and Human Services)]

www.4women.gov

[American Psychiatric Association]

www.psych.org/public_info

[The Journal of the American Medical Association; patient page on depression, 09/27/2000 issue]

www.jama.com

■ BEREAVEMENT

Edward K. Rynearson, MD & Fanny Correa, MSW, CT

The presumption that pathologic responses to death occur in coherent form, duration, and incidence is based on early reports of cases in treatment rather than reliable measurement and comparison. Freud's brilliant speculation that mourning (normal bereavement) and melancholia (pathologic grief) were separate but related was transformed into an a priori principle by subsequent theoreticians. This fruitful model was so compelling that clinical facts were strained to make them fit. The belief in the model led to a number of clinical axioms:

- Mourning is inevitable and necessary and resolves in months.
- Mourning follows a sequence of discrete stages.
- Grief is a denial or aberrant fixation of mourning.
- Catharsis and active mourning promise recovery.

These clinical suppositions of the nature of grief were excessively simple; they were misleading, not because they were wrong, but because they were not entirely right. Several authors have reviewed the empiric work available to verify these presumptions about grief, and in all cases, the data cannot support them. The danger of such empiric refutation, however, is that the concepts, which have usefulness and relevance, will be discarded entirely.

To study so subjective and diverse a referent as pathologic grief requires, first, a tentative approach that is tolerant of multiple hypotheses, and second, a softening of the demand of empiric validation until the development of precise and specific measurement tools. Until then, it is advisable to remain skeptical when presented with certainties about the nature of pathologic grief and its treatment.

Gender as a Risk Factor

A review of clinical studies of grief demonstrates that a disproportionate number of women present for psychotherapy (3–4 times the frequency of men). The increased risk in women to develop unrecovered grief is consistent with epidemiologic surveys that demonstrate the high risk among women in the general population for affective disorders, anxiety disorders, and somatization disorders.

The explanation for the apparent vulnerability of women remains obscure. To overemphasize the biologic and neuropsychological uniqueness of women denies the uniqueness of their emotional attachments, of their primary role as caregivers, and of their economic calamity and role dysjunction when their spouse dies—all of which alone or in combination might be overwhelming. It would be misleading to deny the significance of any of the biopsychosocial variables that differentiate women's responses to grief from men's. Perhaps seeking help for intense grief responses is a more adaptive response than the prototypical male behavior of persistent stoicism and resistance of support. Clarification of these possibly gender-related responses to loss must await further, controlled research.

Psychotherapy

There are few controlled studies on treating unrecovered grief with psychotherapy. Studies limited to support groups and short-term (15–20 sessions) individual psychotherapy demonstrate a measurable effectiveness during the first year of treatment. Patients undergoing treatment show a significant increase in their rate of recovery, but untreated patients show the same frequency of recovery after 2 years. Both treated and untreated patients demonstrate the same frequency of nonrecovery (15–30%).

Researchers are now focusing on the timing of intervention and whether participants were recruited or pursued treatment. Early interventions may interfere with family and social support systems and prevent individuals from finding resolution through their own coping mechanisms.

Comorbidity & Medications

Affective and anxiety disorders include many of the signs and symptoms of pathologic grief. Nearly half of patients with uncomplicated bereavement meet diagnostic criteria for depressive disorder during the first year of bereavement, and one third meet criteria for an anxiety disorder as well. Those affective and anxiety re-

sponses begin to subside after 4–6 months of bereavement without treatment, but a sizable minority of persons (20%) remain depressed or anxious for many years. The presence of the following symptoms is not characteristic of "normal" grief and may be helpful in differentiating bereavement from a major depressive episode:

1. Excessive or inappropriate guilt (EXCEPT about actions taken or not taken by the survivor around the time of the death).
2. Suicidal thoughts (EXCEPT feelings that the survivor should have died with or instead of the deceased).
3. Preoccupation with feelings of worthlessness.
4. Marked psychomotor retardation.
5. Prolonged and marked functional impairment.
6. Hallucinations (other than thinking that he or she hears the voice of, or transiently sees, the deceased person).

Withholding medication from patients in whom refractory affective and anxiety disorders present would border on clinical negligence, yet few studies have examined the use of psychotropic medication in patients with bereavement-related depression or anxiety. One controlled trial and 2 open pilot studies using antidepressants (nortriptyline, paroxetine, and bupropion) have shown robust effects in decreasing depressive symptoms in patients meeting criteria for major depression in the context of bereavement. In 1 of these trials, symptoms of both grief and depression were assessed. Although, in the past, bereavement has been considered not to be responsive to treatment with antidepressants, in this open trial of bupropion, improvement in depressive symptoms was associated with decreases in the intensity of grief. The judicious use of medication in combination with psychotherapy seems a reasonable alternative, particularly in cases of refractory or intense and dysfunctional affective and anxiety disorders, for which there is abundant evidence of their effectiveness. Knowing that the patient and members of the extended family have a history of effective use of pharmacotherapy may alert the clinician to the inclusion of medication during the early phase of treatment.

When to Refer to a Specialist

Referral to a psychiatrist should not be delayed by the promise of spontaneous recovery. Recent studies have documented that patients who show a particularly intense and dysfunctional response within the first 3–6 months of grieving are at high risk for nonrecovery. Patients who are unable to function at home or at work because of their despondency or who become preoccupied with suicide at any point during their recovery should be referred for psychiatric consultation.

Nonrecovery

Careful studies of patients treated for pathologic grief invariably report that 15–30% are nonresponders. Grief-stricken patients should not be demoralized further by the offer of a therapy that promises short-term recovery or a narrow model that insists on one of several underlying causes. Because failed recovery is common to every prospective outcome study of pathologic grief, clinicians must be prepared to recognize and acknowledge therapeutic limitations rather than anticipate short-term recovery.

There is no known strategy or combination of strategies that ensures recovery, and patients should be reassured that failed recovery is not tantamount to personal failure. For purposes of ongoing support, clinicians need to maintain an optimism about the future, including an image of self-stability, that does not require "recovery" of what has been lost. Accommodating to this distressing subjective state requires steadfast courage and commitment. Perhaps all that can be offered is an empathic reassurance that both the clinician and the patient are doing their best.

Allumbaugh DL, Hoyt WT: Effectiveness of grief therapy: a meta-analysis. J Couns Psychol 1999;46:370.

Bergen L: *Death and Dying: Theory, Research, Practice.* William C. Brown, 1979.

Freud S: Mourning and melancholia. In: *Complete Psychological Works of Sigmund Freud* (standard edition). Vol 14. Hogarth Press, 1957.

Horowitz MJ et al: Pathological grief and the activation of latent self-image. Am J Psychiatry 1980;137:1157. [PMID: 7416259]

Jacobs SC: Attachment theory and multiple dimensions of grief. Omega 1987–1988;18:41.

Jacobs S: *Pathologic Grief: Maladaption to Loss.* American Psychiatric Press, 1993.

Kato PM, Mann T: A synthesis of psychological interventions for the bereaved. Clin Psychol Rev 1999;19:275. [PMID: 10097872]

Kessler RC et al: Lifetime and 12-month prevalence of DSM-III-R psychiatric disorders in the United States: Results from the National Comorbidity Survey. Arch Gen Psychiatry 1994; 51:8. [PMID: 8279933]

Parkes CM, Weiss RS: *Recovery from Bereavement.* Basic Books, 1983.

Prigerson HG et al: Consensus criteria for traumatic grief: A preliminary empirical test. Br J Psychiatry 1999;174:67. [PMID: 10211154]

Raphael B: *The Anatomy of Bereavement.* Basic Books, 1983.

Reynolds CF 3rd et al: Treatment of bereavement-related major depressive episodes in later life: a controlled study of acute and continuation treatment with nortriptyline and interpersonal psychotherapy. Am J Psychiatry 1999;156:202. [PMID: 9989555]

Rynearson EK: *Retelling Violent Death.* Brunner-Routledge, 2001.

Shut H et al: The efficacy of bereavement interventions: Determining who benefits. Handbook of Bereavement Research: Consequences, Coping and Care 2001:705.

Zisook S et al: Bupropion sustained release for bereavement: results of an open trial. J Clin Psychiatry 2001;62:227. [PMID: 11379835]

Zygmont M et al: A post hoc comparison of paroxetine and nortriptyline for symptoms of traumatic grief. J Clin Psychiatry 1998;59:241. [PMID: 9632035]

Hormonally Related Psychiatric Mood Disorders: PMS & Depression During Pregnancy, Postpartum, & Perimenopause

12

Patricia L. Paddison, MD

The peak onset of psychiatric disorders is during the childbearing years, with the greatest risk of psychiatric hospitalization occurring in the postpartum period. Estrogen appears to interact with multiple neurotransmitters, and there are specific estrogen receptors in the brain. Animal research suggests that estrogen acts as a serotonin agonist, an acetylcholine agonist, a norepinephrine agonist, and also down-regulates dopamine-2 receptors. The clinical implications of this are uncertain, but it appears likely that estrogen could be an augmentation strategy for a more robust response to antidepressants and antipsychotic medications as well as a primary treatment. Studies are looking at the therapeutic uses of estrogen for mood disorders. The most promising data are coming from studies examining treatment of depression during the postpartum period and during perimenopause. This chapter reviews the diagnosis and treatment of premenstrual syndrome (PMS) as well as depression occurring during pregnancy, the postpartum, and in the perimenopausal period.

PREMENSTRUAL SYNDROME

 ESSENTIALS OF DIAGNOSIS

- *Depression/hopelessness.*
- *Anxiety/tension.*
- *Mood swings/affective lability.*
- *Anger/irritability.*
- *Decreased interest in activities.*
- *Changes in sleep and/or appetite.*
- *Decreased concentration.*

- *Feeling out of control or overwhelmed.*
- *Bloating, breast tenderness.*

General Considerations

Premenstrual syndrome has long been recognized clinically as a constellation of physical and mood symptoms occurring in the week prior to menses. In recent years, the diagnosis of premenstrual dysphoric disorder (PDD) has been developed to describe disabling mood symptoms that occur exclusively during the premenstrual period.

Clinical Findings

The diagnostic criteria for PDD, as listed in the *Diagnostic Statistical Manual of Mental Disorders,* 4th edition, Text Revised (DSM-IV-TR) include at least 5 of the following 10 symptoms:

1. Depression/hopelessness
2. Anxiety/tension
3. Mood swings/affective lability
4. Anger/irritability
5. Decreased interest in activities
6. Changes in sleep
7. Changes in appetite
8. Decreased concentration
9. Feeling out of control/overwhelmed
10. Bloating or breast tenderness.

One of the 5 must be a mood symptom (as listed 1 through 4).

Premenstrual symptoms must occur during the week before menses, remit within a few days after the onset of menses, and interfere with occupational or social functioning. All criteria should be confirmed for at least 2 consecutive menstrual cycles, using a rating scale.

Differential Diagnosis

Many women report premenstrual symptoms but only 5–10% meet criteria for PDD. Many women have a few symptoms but do not meet all the criteria for the disorder. Women who present to clinics complaining of PMS may have other medical and psychiatric disorders. Although they recall symptoms as occurring premenstrually, they may actually have more persistent depression lasting throughout the menstrual cycle. Cohen and Bailey found that 38.8% of women presenting with symptoms of PMS had major depression and/or anxiety disorders. It is important to have patients chart symptoms on a daily rating scale to prospectively confirm the diagnosis. Women in whom PDD has been diagnosed may be at risk for major depression developing in their lifetime.

Treatment

A. ANTIDEPRESSANTS

Fluoxetine (Prozac) and sertraline (Zoloft) are the only antidepressants approved by the US Food and Drug Administration for the treatment of PDD. Fluoxetine has proved effective at both 20 mg/d and 40 mg/d with continual dosing throughout the menstrual cycle. Sertraline has proved effective at 50 mg/d. Many antidepressants have been studied and shown effective for PDD including paroxetine (Paxil), citalopram (Celexa), venlafaxine (Effexor), clomipramine (Anafranil), and fluvoxamine (Luvox). Selective serotonin reuptake inhibitors (SSRIs) seem to be more efficacious than noradrenergic antidepressants, such as bupropion (Wellbutrin), desipramine (Norpramin), and maprotiline (Ludiomil).

Luteal phase dosing (using an SSRI during days 14–28 of the menstrual cycle) has been shown to be effective for fluoxetine, sertraline, and citalopram. Advantages of luteal phase dosing include fewer long-term side effects and less expense. The major disadvantage is adjusting to the short-term side effects and then discontinuing the medication, only to reexperience the short-term side effects when restarting the medication 2 weeks later. Currently, the US Food and Drug Administration has only approved sertraline for luteal phase dosing.

Long-term use of fluoxetine in PDD has been well tolerated, and efficacy has persisted when it has been used longer than 6 months. Many women relapse when they stop treatment, as early as 1 to 2 cycles off of medication.

B. ANTIANXIETY MEDICATIONS

Studies have been mixed regarding the efficacy of buspirone and alprazolam in the treatment of PDD. The National Institute of Mental Health (NIMH) found alprazolam to be no better than placebo in a double-blind crossover study. In a patient who may be fighting for the control of irritability or anger, it seems best to avoid agents that may disinhibit behavior and instead use an SSRI, which helps impulsive behavior. Other concerns of using alprazolam would be causing tolerance, dependence, and withdrawal symptoms, which are a greater concern in women with a history of substance abuse.

C. OVULATION SUPPRESSORS

Gonadotropin-releasing hormone agonists (GnRHa) have been tried as an alternative to surgical oophorectomy to abolish the menstrual cycle and premenstrual symptoms. Double-blind randomized studies have shown reductions in physical symptoms, although the onset of action is up to 2 to 3 months. Women with moderate to severe premenstrual depressive symptoms do not seem to respond to GnRHa treatment. In addition, these agents have no efficacy in the treatment of major depression; the diagnosis of major depression can be missed if the differential diagnosis is not carefully done. Add-back therapy with estrogen and progesterone during GnRHa treatment can cause depression.

Adverse effects include hypoestrogen symptoms such as osteoporosis after only several months of use as well as a possible increased cardiovascular risk, which limits the duration of GnRHa treatment to about 6 months. GnRHa is not currently indicated by the US Food and Drug Administration for treatment of premenstrual symptoms or PDD.

D. ORAL CONTRACEPTIVES AND HORMONES

There is no convincing evidence that progesterone in any form helps PDD, and it may exacerbate the depressive symptoms. The American College of Obstetrics and Gynecology (ACOG) does not recommend oral contraceptives for treatment of PDD.

E. DIURETICS

Diuretics have not been well studied in PMS. The only double-blind placebo-controlled study used spironolactone 100 mg/d in a small group of patients.

F. COMPLEMENTARY THERAPIES

Lifestyle changes that seem the most helpful include exercise and abstaining from caffeine and alcohol throughout the month. An alternative medicine approach that seems most helpful is the use of calcium carbonate (600 mg twice daily), which may not help until after the second or third cycle; use with caution in patients with a history of kidney stones.

Other alternative approaches that have been reported to be helpful include the following: vitamin B_6, no more than 100 mg/d to avoid the risk of peripheral neuropathy; magnesium, 250–1000 mg/d (use with caution in patients with a history of kidney stones); vitamin E, 400 IU/d (may be helpful, but studies are mixed); evening primrose oil, 2–4 g/d standardized to 8% gamma-linolenic acid; chaste berry, 20–40 g/d (which is recommended by the German Commission E and helpful only for cyclic mastalgia); and black cohosh, 20 mg twice daily (which is recommended by the German Commission E, but it may cause abnormal bleeding).

When to Refer to a Specialist

A patient should be referred to a specialist when the diagnosis is in question; if the patient is suicidal; if her anger or irritability is threatening to herself, her family, or coworkers; if there are complicating comorbid disorders, such as substance abuse or personality disorders; if the patient requires hospitalization; or if initial attempts at treatment are unsuccessful. If the patient displays significant impulsivity or irritability, or the diagnosis is uncertain, she should be evaluated by a psychiatrist to rule out bipolar disorder, which may be exacerbated by the use of SSRIs.

ACOG Practice Bulletin; Clinical management guidelines for obstetrician-gynecologists: Premenstrual Syndrome. Obstetrics & Gynecology 2000. Number 15 April.

Chavez ML, Spitzer MF: Herbal and other dietary supplements for premenstrual syndrome and menopause. Psychiatric Annals 2002;32:61.

Bailey JW, Cohen LS: Prevalence of mood and anxiety disorders in women who seek treatment for premenstrual syndrome. J Womens Health Gend Based Med 1999;8:1181. [PMID: 10595331]

Pearlstein TJ, Stone AB: Long-term fluoxetine treatment of late luteal phase dysphoric disorder. J Clin Psychiatry 1994;55: 332. [PMID: 8071300]

Schmidt PJ et al: Alprazolam in the treatment of premenstrual syndrome: a double-blind placebo-controlled trial. Arch Gen Psychiatry 1993;50(6):467. [PMID: 8498881]

Steiner M, Born L: Diagnosis and treatment of premenstrual dysphoric disorder: an update. Int Clin Psychopharmacol 2000; 15(Suppl 3):S5. [PMID: 11195269]

Wang M et al: Treatment of premenstrual syndrome by spironolactone: a double-blind, placebo-controlled study. Acta Obstetricia et Gynecologica Scandinavica 1995;74:803. [PMID: 8533564]

DEPRESSION DURING PREGNANCY

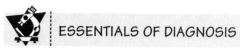 ESSENTIALS OF DIAGNOSIS

- *Depressed mood.*
- *Sleep and appetite changes.*
- *Lack of pleasure in usual activities.*
- *Hopelessness or suicidal thoughts.*
- *Low birth weight infants.*

General Considerations

Despite the commonly held belief that pregnancy is associated with a heightened sense of well-being and improvement in psychiatric symptoms, the chance of becoming depressed during pregnancy is the same as that for nonpregnant women (around 10–15%). A recent study of 9000 women in England who were monitored for depression during pregnancy and postpartum found higher rates of depression at 32 weeks of pregnancy (13%) than at 8 weeks postpartum (9%). Women who are taking antidepressants at the time of conception and stop their medications may relapse into depression.

Clinical Findings

The symptoms of depression in pregnancy are the same as depression at any other time. These symptoms include loss of interest in activities that give pleasure, depressed mood, sleep and appetite changes, hopelessness and suicidal thoughts. Women who are depressed during pregnancy are likely to have low birth weight infants. Whether this is a result of not eating well or a biochemical effect of depression on the fetus is unclear.

Treatment

The same treatment modalities are effective in depression in pregnant and nonpregnant women. However, the choice of treatments during pregnancy is difficult because of concerns about risks to the fetus. Ideally, medication should be avoided whenever possible during the first trimester, and preconception folic acid should be administered. Special consideration should be given to the pros and cons of treating depressed women with medications versus psychotherapy. There are few studies on treating depression during pregnancy, and these must be examined carefully to determine whether researchers controlled for depression in women who stopped their medications because there are profound effects of untreated depression on fetuses and infants. Many studies lump together any in utero exposure, making it difficult to understand differences in exposure by trimester compared with treatment in pregnancy in general. There have been no studies examining the differences in specific trimester exposure (first versus second versus third). Further examination is required to determine the effects of untreated depression versus antidepressant therapy on a fetus.

The most widely studied antidepressant during pregnancy has been fluoxetine. Thousands of women have been monitored during pregnancy while taking fluoxetine and the consensus is that there is no increased incidence of major congenital malformations in their children. A study in 1996 of women calling a teratogen hotline in San Diego, California found no increase in major malformations with exposure to fluoxetine. This study (which was not controlled for effects of depression) found higher rates of premature delivery, poorer neonatal outcomes, and lower birth weights in infants exposed to fluoxetine. However, treated women had a higher maternal age and the results have not been replicated in other studies. A review of available studies concluded that exposure to antidepressants in utero did not significantly increase the rate of major congenital malformations, did not affect the perinatal condition, and did not cause delays in neurodevelopmental milestones.

A 1998 study examined pregnancy outcomes in women who had taken antidepressants at some point during pregnancy (most of whom discontinued their medications when they discovered that they were pregnant). This controlled study only looked at sertraline, paroxetine, and fluvoxamine and was prospectively controlled for depression. It found no increases in spontaneous abortion and no differences in birth weights. The rate of malformations was not significantly different from that in women who did not take antidepressants during pregnancy (4.1% vs 3.8%). A study of citalopram found no increases in malformations. This study controlled for year of birth, maternal age, parity, and smoking habits and found that antidepressant use in pregnancy did not increase the risk of infant mortality or low birth weights.

A recent multicenter, prospectively controlled study of venlafaxine use in pregnancy did not find any differences in rates of malformations. However, there are some concerns regarding use of venlafaxine in pregnancy due to possible elevations in blood pressure. Another concern is the drug is not highly protein bound and as a result fetuses may have higher serum levels than maternal serum levels. This study compared venlafaxine exposure with SSRI exposure with nonteratogenic exposure to medications such as loperamide, Echinacea, sumatriptan, and dextromethorphan, using a meta-analysis of the available literature. The rates of spontaneous abortion were 12% in the venlafaxine group, 12% in the SSRI group, and 7% in the nonteratogenic medication

group. These results raise the question of whether there may be a possible association between first trimester exposure to antidepressants and higher rates of spontaneous abortion and indicate a need for further study.

Complications

A. IN UTERO EXPOSURE TO ANTIDEPRESSANTS

The best study to date is the controlled follow-up report of children exposed to fluoxetine or tricyclic antidepressants in utero up to 7 years postexposure. The conclusion was that there was no significant difference between the groups in measures of IQ, distractibility, arousability, activity level, temperament, mood, or behavior problems.

B. EFFECTS OF UNTREATED DEPRESSION

Lower birth weight is a consistent outcome of untreated depression in pregnancy. One study found lower levels of corticotropin-releasing hormone in depressed pregnant adolescents. Presumed alterations in cortisol functioning and/or genetic factors may predispose offspring of depressed parents to an earlier onset of depression and a more chronic course. One study of pregnant women with elevated Center for Epidemiologic Studies-depression (CES-D) scores (who were presumably more depressed than other pregnant women) found infants with lower birth weights, excessive crying, and infant inconsolability. Pediatricians who were not aware of survey scores were able to distinguish infants of the more depressed mothers from those of mothers who were not depressed. The decision to use medications in pregnancy is a difficult one. Most women discontinue antidepressant therapy hoping to avoid medication effects on their infants. Clinicians must consider the outcomes of untreated depression on the patient, the fetus, other children, and the spouse in presenting to the patient a balanced view of the risks and benefits of using medication during pregnancy.

Higher dose requirements for antidepressants are common in the second trimester of pregnancy due to the physiologic effects of pregnancy, which include increased cardiac output, lowered serum albumin levels, decreased gut motility, increased hepatic function, and changes in metabolic enzymes. The net effect is a higher dose requirement for many medications. A recent study found that women taking antidepressants during pregnancy required an increased dose of their antidepressant to achieve a stable mood in the second trimester.

When to Refer to a Specialist

When treating a pregnant woman with a history of depression, it is wise to refer to a psychiatrist well versed in the treatment studies and to establish a relationship in the event that the patient's depression worsens. Sometimes psychotherapy is effective in women who are afraid to use antidepressants in pregnancy. Any thoughts of harming oneself or the baby should mandate immediate referral to a specialist.

Chambers CD et al: Birth outcomes in pregnant women taking fluoxetine. N Engl J Med 1996;335:1010. [PMID: 8793924]

Einarson A et al: Pregnancy outcome following gestational exposure to venlafaxine: a multicenter prospective controlled study. Am J Psychiatry 2001;158:1728. [PMID: 11579012]

Ericson A et al: Delivery outcome after the use of antidepressants in early pregnancy. N Engl J Med 1996;55:503.

Ericson A et al: Delivery outcome after the use of antidepressants in early pregnancy. Eur J Clin Pharmacol 1999;55:503. [PMID: 10501819]

Evans J et al: Cohort study of depressed mood during pregnancy and after childbirth. BMJ 2001;323:257. [PMID: 11485953]

Hostetter A: Dose of selective serotonin uptake inhibitors across pregnancy: clinical implications. Depression and Anxiety 2000;11:51. [PMID: 10812529]

Jacobsen T: Effects of postpartum disorders on parenting and on offspring. In: Miller LJ (editor): *Postpartum Mood Disorders.* American Psychiatric Press, 1999:119.

Kulin NA et al: Pregnancy outcome following maternal use of the new selective serotonin reuptake inhibitors: a prospective controlled multicenter study. J Am Med Assoc 1998;279:609. [PMID: 9486756]

Marcus SM et al: Treatment guidelines for depression in pregnancy. Int J Gynecol Obstet 2001;72:61. [PMID: 11146079]

Nulman I et al: Neurodevelopment of children exposed in utero to antidepressant drugs. N Engl J Med 1997;336:258. [PMID: 8995088]

Robert E: Treatment of depression in pregnancy. N Engl J Med 1996;335:1056. [PMID: 8793933]

Schmeelk K et al: Maternal depression and risk for postpartum complications: role of prenatal corticotropin-releasing hormone and interleukin-1 receptor antagonist. Behav Med 1999;25:88. [PMID: 10401538]

Weissman MM et al: Offspring of depressed parents. 10 years later. Comment in: Arch Gen Psychiatry 1998;55:949.

Wisner KL et al: Risk-benefit decision making for treatment of depression during pregnancy. Am J Psychiatry 2000;157:1933. [PMID: 11097953]

Zuckerman BS et al: Maternal depressive symptoms during pregnancy and newborn irritability. J Dev Behav Pediatr 1990;11:190. [PMID: 2212032]

POSTPARTUM

 ESSENTIALS OF DIAGNOSIS

- *Sluggishness.*
- *Fatigue/exhaustion.*
- *Hopelessness or depression.*
- *Disturbances in sleep and appetite.*
- *Confusion.*
- *Uncontrollable crying.*
- *Lack of interest in baby.*
- *Fear of harming baby or oneself.*
- *Mood swings.*

General Considerations

The rates of depression in the postpartum period are the same as for nonpregnant women (around 10–15%). If a woman has a previous history of depression, the rate of postpartum depression increases to 25%. With a previous history of postpartum depression, the woman has a 50% chance of recurrence. It is important to ask a woman whether her depression was present in pregnancy before it was recognized in the postpartum.

Postpartum mood episodes with psychotic features occur in 1 of 500 to 1 in a 1000 deliveries. Postpartum psychosis can present as mania or an acute psychotic episode with hallucinations and delusions. Psychotic episodes during the postpartum period are often associated with greater confusion and emotional lability than non-puerperal psychoses. Women with a history of bipolar disorder or prior postpartum psychosis are at higher risk (up to 70–90%) for exacerbation in the postpartum period. Untreated postpartum psychosis is a psychiatric emergency and carries with it a 4% risk of infanticide. The risk of infanticide is much higher when psychosis or delusions are present, such as command hallucinations to kill the infant or delusions that the infant might be possessed.

Clinical Findings

Symptoms of depression include sluggishness, fatigue, exhaustion, feelings of hopelessness or depression, disturbances of appetite and/or sleep, confusion, uncontrollable crying, lack of interest in the baby, fears of harming the baby or oneself, and mood swings.

Differential Diagnosis

It is very important to rule out thyroid disease in any depressed patient, but especially in the postpartum depressed patient in whom fatigue and sleeplessness often are attributed to taking care of an infant rather than a disease process. A thyroid-stimulating hormone should be measured on any women appearing depressed and should probably be routinely done at the 6 week postpartum visit to the gynecologist. Postpartum depression must be differentiated from postpartum blues. This transient syndrome occurs several days after delivery in the majority of women; is characterized by unexplained crying, feeling overwhelmed, and mood lability; and remits spontaneously without specific treatment. Warning a pregnant patient that this may occur is important and prevents her from feeling that these symptoms indicate that she is a bad mother. In evaluating more severe postpartum depression and psychotic episodes, substance abuse and other primary psychiatric disorders such as bipolar disorder or schizophrenia must be ruled out.

Treatment

A. ANTIDEPRESSANTS

All antidepressants are excreted in breast milk. Currently, the American Psychiatric Association recommends using sertraline for women who are depressed and breast-feeding their infant. A recent study looking at platelet serotonin levels in breast-feeding women on sertraline found no changes in the infants, thus pointing to no demonstrable serotonin effect in the infants. Paroxetine as well as sertraline have been shown to produce minimal serum blood levels in infants who are being breast-fed.

There have been isolated case reports of jitteriness, decreased appetite, and difficulty sleeping in breast-fed infants whose mothers were taking fluoxetine. These effects were associated with high serum levels in the infants and went away when the mother stopped taking fluoxetine. The symptoms resumed when she restarted the medication.

It is more difficult to assess the effects of medications on a newborn infant than it is in a 3- or 4-month-old infant. The mother will not be able to assess changes in sleeping, feeding, and behavior patterns easily.

B. ANTIPSYCHOTICS

Any delusions or psychotic behavior must be treated with antipsychotic medications (such as haloperidol, olanzapine, and risperidone), and these patients should be referred to a psychiatrist.

C. HORMONAL TREATMENT

There have been a few studies describing successful treatment with the use of hormones for both postpartum depression and psychosis. One study in women with histories of puerperal psychoses or puerperal depression used high dose Premarin that was dropped to 0.625 mg in 2 weeks. Heparin was administered at the same time to reduce embolic phenomena. Most women did well. It is important to note the use of heparin because the immediate use of hormones in the postpartum period may predispose women to embolic phenomena. Two subsequent studies looked at the use of sublingual estrogen 1 mg every 4–6 hours based on serum levels (average dose 4 mg/d) for 8 weeks; one treated postpartum depression while the other treated postpartum psychosis. All of these studies noted a rapid onset of action, which is remarkable because psychotic depression normally may take months to improve with traditional treatment.

A recent, double-blind, placebo-controlled study using mifepristone (RU-486) in patients with psychotic major depression showed rapid relief in symptoms after a 4-day course of 600 mg mifepristone. The presumed mechanism of action was of central glucocorticoid antagonism even though it is also a progesterone-receptor antagonist. These are noteworthy studies for clinicians looking for rapid onset of action in patients who are at high risk for infanticide.

Complications

The impact of untreated postpartum depression on children is profound. One study found that children of depressed mothers had lower vocabulary scores and higher levels of behavior problems. There was a relationship between severity and chronicity of maternal depressive symptoms and lower vocabulary scores and more behavior problems. Another study compared postpartum depressed mothers with controls and found no differences in babies aged 0–6 months but found differences at age 1. The infants of the depressed mothers had lower scores on intellectual measures. Depressed mothers were more irritable and did not attach to their infants as well as the nondepressed mothers. As early as 1951, Bowlby described the potential adverse impact of maternal separation history (emotional or physical) on the infant. The failure to attach well to a caregiver is predictive of long-term relationship problems for the infant as well as conduct disorders and behavioral problems. Animal studies dating back to 1962 by Harlow document this adverse effect.

When to Refer to a Specialist

If any thoughts or fears of harm coming to the baby exist, a referral to a specialist should be facilitated as quickly as possible and hospitalization should be considered. Weekly therapy in addition to medication is indicated in any woman with a postpartum mood disorder. Many women will have thoughts or fears of harm coming to the baby without wanting to directly harm the baby. This is part of an obsessional thought process of depression, which is different from a command hallucination or delusional process. The mother is very disturbed by the thoughts and does not want to harm her baby. Nevertheless, all such patients should be referred to a specialist.

Brennan P et al: Chronicity, severity, and timing of maternal depressive symptoms: relationships with child outcomes at age 5. Dev Psychol 2000;36:759. [PMID: 11081699]

Miller LJ: Postpartum depression. JAMA 2002;287:762. [PMID: 11851544]

Murray L: The impact of postnatal depression on infant development. J Child Psychol Psychiatry 1992;33:543. [PMID: 1577898]

Weinberg MK, Tronick EZ: The impact of maternal psychiatric illness on infant development. J Clin Psychiatry 1998;59 (Suppl 2):53. [PMID: 9559760]

Ahokas A et al: Positive treatment effect of estradiol in postpartum psychosis: a pilot study. J Clin Psychiatry 2000;61:166. [PMID: 10817099]

Ahokas A et al: Estrogen deficiency in severe postpartum depression: successful treatment with sublingual physiologic 17β-estradiol: a preliminary study. J Clin Psychiatry 2001;62:332. [PMID: 11411813]

Altschuler LL et al: The expert consensus guideline series. Treatment of depression in women. Postgrad Med 2001;(SpecNo): 1. [PMID: 11500997]

Belanoff JK et al: Rapid reversal of psychotic depression using mifepristone. J Clin Psychopharmacol 2001;21:516. [PMID: 11593077]

Epperson N et al: Maternal sertraline treatment and serotonin transport in breast-feeding mother-infant pairs. Am J Psychiatry 2001;158:1631. [PMID: 11578995]

Sichel DA et al: Prophylactic estrogen in recurrent postpartum affective disorder. Biol Psychiatry 1995;38:814. [PMID: 8750040]

PERIMENOPAUSE

 ESSENTIALS OF DIAGNOSIS

- Irritability.
- Tearfulness/depressed mood.
- Sleep disruption.
- Lack of motivation/energy.
- Poor concentration.
- Anxiety.

General Considerations

The rates of depression decrease after menopause. If a woman is going to get depressed after the childbearing years, it is during perimenopause (approximately 45–55 years old) according to the National Comorbidity Survey. Criteria for diagnosing depression during perimenopause are identical to diagnostic criteria used at any other stage of life.

Differential Diagnosis

It is important to distinguish depression from perimenopausal symptoms such as irritability, night sweats, hot flashes, and disrupted sleep. Follicle-stimulating hormone has been shown to be an inconsistent measure in perimenopausal women and is not useful diagnostically until the patient has missed at least 6 months of menstrual cycles. Whether to use hormones or antidepressants is a clinical decision that must be determined by both the patient and the clinician. Currently, the approved treatment for depression is antidepressants.

Treatment

A. Antidepressant Versus Hormone Therapy

Currently, the usual regimen of antidepressant therapy is the standard for perimenopause/menopause depression. There have been suggestions that postmenopausal women receiving hormone replacement therapy (HRT) have a more robust response to SSRIs than women not receiving HRT. However, Kornstein found similar response rates in postmenopausal women to sertraline and imipramine.

Transdermal estradiol has been studied in perimenopausal depressed women. Women were given 100 μg of unopposed transdermal estradiol twice a week for 12 weeks. Remission was achieved in 68% of the group.

B. Complementary Therapy

The use of St. John's Wort has been helpful for mild depression but has not been helpful in more severe depression. Typical dosages are 300 mg 3 times daily. St. John's Wort has significant interactions with medications such as oral contraceptives, coumadin, virus protease inhibitors, cyclosporine, digoxin, theophylline, and carbamazepine. Use of alternative medicines for the treatment of perimenopausal symptoms are reviewed in Chapter 18, Menopause and Hormone Replacement Therapy.

Kessler RC: Sex and depression in the National Comorbidity Survey I: Lifetime prevalence, chronicity and recurrence. J Affect Disord 1993;29:85. [PMID: 8300981]

Kornstein SG: The evaluation and management of depression in women across the life span. J Clin Psychiatry 2001;62(suppl 24):11. [PMID: 11676428]

de Novaes Soares C et al: Efficacy of estradiol for the treatment of depressive disorders in perimenopausal women: a double-blind, randomized, placebo-controlled trial. Arch Gen Psychiatry 2001;58:529. [PMID: 11386980]

Relevant Web Sites

[The National Women's Health Information Center (US Department of Health and Human Services)]
www.4woman.gov

[American Psychiatric Association]
www.psych.org
[Depression After Delivery, Inc]
www.depressionafterdelivery.com
[Depression Awareness, recognition, and treatment program of the National Institute of Mental Health]
www.nimh.nih.gov/ publicat/index.cfm

[Postpartum education for parents]
www.sbpep.org
[American College of Obstetricians and Gynecologists]
www.acog. com/
[JAMA patient pages]
www.jama.com

Domestic Violence

13

Nancy Sugg, MD, MPH

Throughout any woman's life span, she will be at risk for violence from partners and family members. Domestic violence may take the form of financial control, loss of autonomy in daily activities, social isolation, verbal or psychological abuse, physical abuse, sexual coercion, or rape. Medical providers are in a unique position to recognize and begin to intervene in the violence. For many patients, the medical provider is the first person to whom they confide their abuse.

 ESSENTIALS OF DIAGNOSIS

- *Controlling behavior by partner resulting in loss of personal autonomy.*
- *Verbal or psychological abuse; threats of harm.*
- *Intentional physical injury or forced sexual contact.*

General Considerations

A. Adolescent Women

Adolescence is a time of separating from a dependent relationship with family and forming new relationships with intimate partners. For many young women, it is also a time of experiencing physical violence at the hands of family members, intimate partners, or both.

A survey of Massachusetts teenagers found that 18–20% of female students had experienced physical and/or sexual abuse from a dating partner. The health consequences of abuse for adolescents often take the form of risky behaviors, such as an increase in substance use, unhealthy weight control, promiscuity, pregnancy, and suicide attempts.

The prevalence of date rape among female adolescents is as high as 20–68%. Many adolescents do not recognize sexual assault by a dating partner as rape. More disturbingly, both males and females perceive that sexual coercion and the use of force are acceptable in certain situations, especially if the woman sexually excites the man.

B. Adult Women

Because of the multiple definitions of intimate partner violence (IPV) and the lack of reports, reliable statistics on the annual incidence of domestic violence are limited. However, available data show alarming rates of domestic violence. Among a nationally representative sample of women, 34.6% had experienced IPV at some point in their lifetime; two thirds of the victims classified the assaults as serious and recurrent.

Although the rate of homicides resulting from IPV has steadily declined from 1981 to 1998, 1 of 3 female homicides are committed by intimate partners, compared with only 1 of 20 male homicides. Firearms are the weapon of choice for most of the female homicides resulting from IPV.

C. Pregnant Women

For many women, pregnancy is a time of increased physical violence and fear. Physical violence affects not only the health of the mother but also the health and safety of the unborn child.

The prevalence of IPV during pregnancy ranges from 0.9% to 20%. IPV may be more common than other pregnancy-related complications, such as preeclampsia, gestational diabetes, and placenta previa.

Pregnant teenagers are already considered at high-risk for a poor outcome and battering only adds to that likelihood. The rate of physical and/or sexual violence among pregnant teenagers is high (29%); ex-boyfriends, ex-husbands, parents, and stepparents are common perpetrators. Pregnant teenagers who experience violence are more likely to use illicit drugs, smoke cigarettes, and drink alcohol than pregnant teenagers who do not experience violence.

D. Elderly Women

Elder abuse evokes the vision of a frail elderly person victimized by their adult child. However, spouses are the common perpetrators of elder abuse. The estimated national incidence ranges from 51,000 to 186,000 annually. The definition of elder abuse includes physical and psychological injury; sexual abuse; and withholding of food, clothing, and medical care. Other definitions have included financial exploitation, isolation, and neglect.

[No authors listed] Elder abuse and neglect. Council on Scientific Affairs. JAMA 1987;257:966. [PMID: 3806880]

Abbott J et al: Domestic violence against women. Incidence and prevalence in an emergency department population. JAMA 1995;273:1763. [PMID: 7769770]

Alpert EJ, Cohen S, Sege RD: Family violence: an overview. Acad Med 1997;72(1 Suppl):S3. [PMID: 9008581]

Alpert EJ: Violence in intimate relationships and the practicing internist: new "disease" or new agenda? Ann Intern Med 1995; 123:774. [PMID: 7574196]

Dearwater SR et al: Prevalence of intimate partner abuse in women treated at community hospital emergency departments. JAMA 1998;280:433. [PMID: 9701078]

Gazmararian JA et al: Prevalence of violence against pregnant women. JAMA 1996;275:1915. [PMID: 8648873]

Martin SL et al: Physical abuse of women before, during, and after pregnancy. JAMA 2001;285:1581. [PMID: 11268265]

Martin SL et al: Violence in the lives of pregnant teenage women: associations with multiple substance use. Am J Drug Alcohol Abuse 1999;25:425. [PMID: 10473006]

McCauley J et al: Relation of low-severity violence to women"s health. J Gen Intern Med 1998;13:687. [PMID: 9798816]

Paulozzi LJ et al: Surveillance for homicide among intimate partners–United States, 1981-1998. Mor Mortal Wkly Rep CDC Surveill Summ 2001;50:1. [PMID: 11678352]

Pillemer K, Finkelhor D: The prevalence of elder abuse: a random sample survey. Gerontologist 1988;28:51. [PMID: 3342992]

Plichta SB, Falik M: Prevalence of violence and its implications for women"s health. Women"s Health Issues 2001;11:244. [PMID: 11336864]

Rickert VI, Wiemann CM: Date rape among adolescents and young adults. J Pediatr Adolesc Gynecol 1998;11:167. [PMID: 9806126]

Silverman JG et al: Dating violence against adolescent girls and associated substance use, unhealthy weight control, sexual risk behavior, pregnancy, and suicidality. JAMA 2001;286:572. [PMID: 11476659]

Weinbaum Z et al: Female victims of intimate partner physical domestic violence (IPP-DV), California 1998. Am J Prev Med 2001;21:313. [PMID: 11701303]

Clinical Findings

Any woman, regardless of socioeconomic class, level of education, professional status, ethnic or religious group, age, or race, has the potential to be a battered woman. There is no "classic" battered woman; therefore, screening for abuse in all patients is essential. However, there are symptoms and signs that should compel the medical provider to ask direct questions regarding violence.

A. SYMPTOMS AND SIGNS

1. Chronic pain—Headache, abdominal pain, or pelvic pain are examples of chronic pain and may be a signal of ongoing abuse. Thirty-six percent of women who were referred to a gastroenterologic practice for work-up of abdominal pain admitted to experiencing physical or sexual abuse as an adult. Patients with functional bowel disorder had a higher risk of physical abuse than those who had organic bowel disorders, with an

odds ratio of 11:39. Similarly, a significant percentage of women with chronic pelvic pain without pelvic pathology had a history of experiencing physical abuse as an adult. Clearly, patients with chronic pain must be evaluated for a history of both physical and sexual abuse.

2. Somatic complaints—Many women in abusive relationships seek medical attention not for traumatic injury but for somatic complaints. Physical symptoms, such as headache, loss of appetite, chest pain, and fainting, tend to increase as the level of violence from an intimate partner escalates. Patients with 6 or more symptoms were 5 times more likely to report abuse compared with patients with 0 to 2 symptoms. Diarrhea and vaginal discharge are two of the most strongly associated symptoms of abuse. The stress of battering may cause patients to present with vague symptoms for which an organic source cannot be found even after an exhaustive work-up. The patients may be labeled as hypochondriacal or hysterical, thereby obscuring the underlying problem of abuse.

In an emergency department study, some symptoms associated with abuse (urinary tract infections, neck pain, vaginitis, foot wound, suicide attempts, and finger fracture) lacked sensitivity and positive predictive value. The use of these symptoms alone would only identify 20% of the women in physically abusive relationships. Therefore, all patients should be asked routinely.

3. Injury—Multiple injuries, especially involving the head and face, should raise a strong suspicion of IPV. The most common injuries involving the head, face, arms, hands, and legs are contusions and abrasions. Twenty-seven percent of injuries were inflicted with weapons, and blunt instruments (pipes, bottles, and broomsticks) are the most common. Eighty-one percent of IPV injuries involve the maxillofacial area, usually the middle third of the face. One third of patients had facial fractures, most commonly nasal. Other types of injuries suspicious for intentional injury are old injuries and bruises in various stages of healing, burns in unusual places, lacerations or abrasions in the genital area, ruptured tympanic membranes, and human bites. Any injuries that do not match the explanation given by the patient certainly need further investigation.

Marital rape is a common form of physical violence in abusive relationships. Forced vaginal intercourse accounts for the majority of marital rape incidents, but anal intercourse; being hit, kicked, or burned during sex; and insertion of objects into the anus and vagina are also described frequently by abused women. Women associate these acts with urinary tract infections, vaginal and anal bleeding, urinary incontinence, unwanted pregnancies, and sexually transmitted diseases. Because rape may not result in obvious injuries and because women may be embarrassed to describe marital rape, it often is not revealed unless the medical provider asks direct questions about abuse.

4. Adverse pregnancy outcomes—Despite the lack of consensus in the literature, there are many potential mechanisms for IPV to result in poor pregnancy outcomes. Trauma, especially to the abdomen, can lead to placental abruption or direct fetal injury. The emotional stress associated with battering may indirectly lead to delay in seeking prenatal care, poor nutrition, and substance abuse.

5. Alcohol abuse—Battered women are at higher risk than others for alcohol abuse. Patients currently in abusive relationships admit to having a problem alcohol problem significantly more often than nonabused patients, and they have higher scores on the CAGE questionnaire. For many women, the use of alcohol may be a means of calming the anxiety and numbing the pain of abuse. Among women attending an alcohol treatment program, 61% had experienced physical and/or sexual abuse at some point in their lives. It is clear that alcoholic women need to be screened for violence and that battered women need to be screened for alcoholism. Both issues need to be addressed to provide optimal treatment.

6. Psychiatric Illness—Repeated emotional and physical violence has a major effect on women's mental health. Many women report more pain and lasting damage being inflicted by the emotional and verbal abuse than by physical injury. Perpetrators frequently demean and belittle their partners in order to erode self-esteem and increase emotional vulnerability. Medical providers and mental health professionals seldom screen all patients for physical abuse and very rarely screen for emotional abuse.

Depression is an extremely common sequela of domestic violence. Over 55% of depressed women have experienced physical abuse during their adult life and 14% are currently being abused. Women who are depressed and abused have more severe depression and more comorbid psychiatric problems. Despite the severity of the depression, these women are less likely to be receiving mental health care and only 28% report the abuse to a health or mental health provider.

Women living with physical assaults often experience higher levels of depression, anxiety, and posttraumatic stress disorder. More than half of women who suffer IPV have a psychiatric diagnosis and when compared with nonvictims have significantly higher rates of mood and eating disorders. Two thirds of women who are victims of severe violence (eg, kicked, bitten, hit with a fist or an object, beat up, choked, strangled, or threatened with a knife or gun) have a psychiatric diagnosis and have significantly higher rates of mood disor-

der, eating disorder, substance dependence, antisocial personality disorder, and schizophrenia compared with nonvictims.

B. Screening Instruments

1. Patient interview—One of the first steps in asking about abuse is to provide an environment that encourages women to talk about the abuse. Hanging posters on the subject of domestic violence in the waiting room or having brochures available in the women's bathroom conveys a willingness to attend to the issue. If health history forms are available, a question about physical violence or threat of violence is important; abused women will know that the health provider is concerned about the issue, and nonabused women will understand that it is a standard question asked of all women. Although health surveys are useful in collecting information, verbal inquiry yields higher positive response rates than self-administered questionnaires.

Creating a safe environment for the discussion of abuse is also critical. At some point in the interview, the patient must be spoken with alone. A partner, adult child, or caregiver refusing to leave should raise suspicion of abuse. Sometimes compelling an overly protective partner to leave the room can be difficult. Asking the partner to fill out forms or sending the patient to the bathroom for a urine sample accompanied by a female nurse or physician are techniques that can create the needed privacy. It is also important to make sure that children are in a safe place. Ideally, the children could be invited to play in a supervised playroom. If this is not available, a social worker, nurse, or staff member could entertain the children in an area separate from the waiting room. Fear that the partner may take the children will constrain the patient from revealing abuse.

The patient must be reassured that all information will be kept confidential. The issue of confidentiality is especially important if the practitioner or physician also provides health care to the abuser. However, confidentiality cannot be maintained if a child or elderly person is at risk for—or is currently—being abused. If a report to the appropriate state protective department needs to be filed, it is essential that the patient be made aware of the pending report and that issues of safety be discussed.

When asking about physical violence, the best approach is a direct question aimed at specific behavior. Initially, it is reasonable to ask open-ended questions about how things are going at home and how the couple resolves conflicts; but at some point, a direct question about abuse needs to be asked.

The physician should avoid using phrases such as "abused," "battered woman," or "domestic violence" because these terms may mean different things to different women. It is often helpful to begin by stating that all women are screened for IVP, describing the health risks of violence, and/or conveying that many women find themselves in violent relationships. These openings should lead into direct questions about being hit, hurt, or threatened at home.

McFarlane and colleagues developed the Abuse Assessment Screen (AAS) for evaluating abuse during pregnancy. Modifications of the screening tool have been used for research purposes and also adapted to different clinical settings. Below are 4 questions from the AAS that are useful in a variety of clinical settings:

1. Within the past year, have you been hit, slapped, kicked, or otherwise physically hurt by someone?

2. Since you have been pregnant, have you been hit, slapped, kicked, or otherwise physically hurt by someone?

3. Within the past year, has anyone forced you to have sexual activity?

4. Are you afraid of your partner?

It is imperative that all pregnant women be screened for physical violence during prenatal visits throughout the pregnancy. Furthermore, any pregnant woman who presents with an injury needs to be asked if the injury was inflicted intentionally. Women should be asked about abuse in each trimester of pregnancy.

2. Assessing the elderly—The physical examination is of paramount importance in looking for evidence of physical abuse and neglect in elderly women. The skin is often the most revealing organ because it can provide information on hydration, hygiene, nutrition, and physical abuse. Evidence of restraints around the wrist or waist should be noted.

Decubiti or other skin irritation (eg, burns from prolonged exposure to urine or feces) may be signs of neglect. The genital and rectal areas need to be examined for signs of sexually transmitted diseases and trauma.

Because many forms of abuse of elderly women cannot be identified by a physical examination, the medical provider needs to ask questions of both the patient and the caregiver to discover potential abuse. Patients need to be assessed concerning their daily activities such as cooking, eating, bathing, dressing, and walking, as well as regarding issues such as incontinence and ability to use a bathroom. This assessment gives the provider an idea of the types of stress a caregiver encounters and a sense of whether basic needs are being met appropriately. It is important to obtain information regarding who lives in the home, whether drugs or alcohol are abused by household members, what financial arrangement exists, and whether the elderly patient has social support other than that of the caregiver.

Many elderly patients do not provide information about abuse because of fear of retaliation or fear of being forced to move into a nursing home if the caregiver leaves. However, some elderly patients do not provide the information because they do not recognize neglect or financial exploitation as abuse.

Campbell JC, Alford P: The dark consequences of marital rape. Am J Nurs 1989;89:946. [PMID: 2619795]

Danielson KK et al: Comorbidity between abuse of an adult and DSM-III-R mental disorders: evidence from an epidemiological study. Am J Psychiatry 1998;155:131. [PMID: 9433353]

Drossman DA et al: Sexual and physical abuse in women with functional or organic gastrointestinal disorders. Ann Intern Med 1990;113:828. [PMID: 2240898]

Kyriacou DN et al: Risk factors for injury to women from domestic violence against women. N Engl J Med 1999;341:1892. [PMID: 10601509]

Le BT et al: Maxillofacial injuries associated with domestic violence. J Oral Maxillofac Surg 2001;59:1277. [PMID: 11688025]

McCauley J et al: The "battering syndrome": prevalence and clinical characteristics of domestic violence in primary care internal medicine practices. Ann Intern Med 1995;123:737. [PMID: 7574191]

McFarlane J et al: Assessing for abuse during pregnancy. Severity and frequency of injuries and associated entry into prenatal care. JAMA 1992;267:3176. [PMID: 1593739]

Petersen R et al: Violence and adverse pregnancy outcomes: a review of the literature and directions for future research. Am J Prev Med 1997;13:366. [PMID: 9315269]

Muelleman RL, Lenaghan PA, Pakieser RA: Nonbattering presentations to the ED of women in physically abusive relationships. Am J Emerg Med 1998;16:128. [PMID: 9517685]

Rapkin AJ et al: History of physical and sexual abuse in women with chronic pelvic pain. Obstet Gynecol 1990;76:92. [PMID: 2359571]

Rice C et al: Self-reports of physical, sexual and emotional abuse in an alcoholism treatment sample. J Stud Alcohol 2001;62:114. [PMID: 11271959]

Scholle SH, Rost KM, Golding JM: Physical abuse among depressed women. J Gen Intern Med 1998;13:607. [PMID: 9754516]

Treatment & Follow-Up

Once a patient reveals abuse, it is important for the provider to communicate that he or she is concerned about the issue and that the problem is serious. There are multiple ways of approaching the problem: (1) assure the patient that she does not deserve to be beaten, (2) address the fact that assault is a criminal act and that the patient has the right to be safe in her own home, or (3) focus on the health consequences of ongoing abuse. One of the most devastating responses a health care provider can make is no response. If the provider does not address the issue, the woman's sense of hopelessness and isolation is intensified.

Assessing safety is the next critical step. The primary issue is whether it is safe for the patient to return home that day; the provider should ask her that question directly. If the patient wishes to return home, she needs to begin making a safety plan in case the violence starts again. A detailed plan does not need to be completed in the office or clinic, but the patient needs to be encouraged to think about safety. The patient should plan escape routes from each room in the house. She should think about how she will access money and transportation if she needs to leave suddenly. She should think about where she could go in an emergency, such as the home of a friend or relative, and possibly leave clothing there for future needs. She should have important documents (such as children's birth certificates and health insurance cards), bank books, and credit cards, and her prescription medication easily accessible.

If the patient does not feel it is safe to return home, a safe place must be located (eg, home of friends or relatives or a shelter—the location of which is confidential). The safety plan does not stop here, however, because the period of separation and divorce can be one of the most dangerous for an abused woman. She may need a protection order or a restraining order, and it is important to find out whether she knows how to obtain these documents.

It is crucial to be aware of factors that may increase the risk of a lethal outcome, but it is not always possible to ask about each danger sign. The following situations were found to be associated with risk of homicide:

1. Increase in frequency or severity of violence in the last year.
2. Presence of firearms in the home.
3. Sexual abuse.
4. Abuse of drugs or alcohol by the batterer.
5. Violent episodes outside the home perpetrated by the abuser.
6. Abuser threatens to kill the woman (or she believes he is capable of killing).
7. Attempts by the abuser to control all aspects of the woman's life.
8. Violent jealousy expressed by the abuser.
9. Battering during pregnancy.

Ending a battering relationship is a process. Some women are capable of leaving very quickly; others may not be able to leave. There are a variety of reasons that women remain in an abusive situation. One of the most compelling is the real threat of death if she leaves. It is important for the provider to respect the serious dilemmas that many women face in leaving an abusive relationship, including fear, economic insecurity, religious convictions, fear of police involvement, and family or cultural pressures.

Health care providers need to monitor the course of a battering relationship as they would follow any health problem. Domestic violence should be listed on the problem list and the situation reassessed at subsequent visits. Continued support for the woman is crucial.

When to Refer to a Specialist

It is important for health care providers to investigate the resources available in their community. Keeping an up-to-date list of resources saves time and prevents frustration.

Before an abused woman leaves the office, she should know how to contact the police and the local shelter in an emergency. Some areas have city or statewide hotlines that can give the patient the telephone numbers she needs for her area. Brochures are handy, but they may be dangerous if they are found by the batterer. It may be prudent to have the woman memorize the most important numbers or hide them in a safe place.

Teenage women are at a disadvantage when it comes to accessing social services. Because most teenagers are under the age of majority, representatives of social service organizations are not as likely to get involved without parental consent. Child protective services are geared to respond to abuse of young children and often do not expend great effort in protecting adolescents from abuse. Because of their age, female adolescents often are denied access to shelters for battered women; legally, they cannot file assault charges unless they are emancipated adults. This state of affairs often leaves abused adolescent women without advocacy or resources. Caught in limbo between childhood and adulthood, adolescent women are at risk for battering from multiple sources and lack appropriate avenues for help. Helping the adolescent find someone to confide in, such as a school guidance counselor, teacher, minister, or counselor at a local teen center, may be the most valuable action that can be taken. However, for some teenagers, the health care provider may be the safest advocate, and subsequent visits will need to be scheduled to talk about issues such as safety, defining limits in relationships, and building self-esteem.

Elderly women may have difficulty finding shelters that can address their specific needs, especially if they are physically disabled or mentally impaired. Many women may remain in abusive situations or relationships because they fear that nursing home placement is the only alternative.

Campbell JC: Nursing assessment for risk of homicide with battered women. ANS Adv Nurs Sci 1986;8:36. [PMID: 3089133]

Medicolegal Issues

A. DOCUMENTATION

Proper documentation in the medical chart is crucial for any criminal or civil proceedings that may follow for the patient. It is also important as a means of verifying that the medical provider has acted responsibly in intervening in a situation of domestic violence.

For an acute assault, the date, time, and place of the incident need to be recorded. The most important aspect to record, however, is the name of the alleged assailant and the relationship to the patient. Terms such as "boyfriend" and "cousin" are not specific enough. Recording the relationship is necessary also because violence by an intimate partner or caretaker has a higher probability of being repeated than violence inflicted by a stranger. The mechanism of injury should be described and all visible signs of injury should be documented. Any evidence of old injuries should be documented also. Finally, clinicians should document that safety was assessed and information on appropriate resources was given.

B. LEGAL MANDATES

Medical providers must know the legal statutes regarding reporting child abuse, elder abuse, and IPV. Almost all states have mandatory reporting for child abuse and elder abuse. Many states or local governments require reporting of all injuries involving a knife or gun or injuries inflicted on a vulnerable adult (ie, developmentally delayed or severely physically or mentally impaired). Still others mandate reporting felonious injuries such as broken bones or injuries requiring hospitalization. Recently, a few states enacted legislation making domestic violence—regardless of age, vulnerable status, or type of injury—a mandatory police report with criminal penalties for noncompliance.

Relevant Web Sites

[American College of Obstetrics and Gynecologists (ACOG)]
www.acog.com
[American Medical Association]
www.ama-assn.org
[Family Violence Prevention Fund]
www.fvpf.org

Sexual Abuse

14

Jennifer D. Bolen, MD & Naomi F. Sugar, MD

Sexual abuse can be defined as sexual contact with a child who does not or cannot consent by virtue of immaturity or social status. The perpetrator may be an adult or a person who has authority over the child, such as a baby-sitter, older relative, or family friend. Girls are victimized by family members in 30–50% of cases.

Severe sexual abuse involves oral, anal, or vaginal penetration. **Less severe** sexual abuse involves fondling over clothing or exhibitionism. Severe sexual abuse is more damaging than less severe abuse and causes more numerous and profound sequelae.

General Considerations

In 1999, reported rates of child sexual abuse ranged from 15% to 32%. A study of 2003 women between the ages of 18 and 22 showed there were no differences in the rates of sexual abuse among ethnic groups. Another study showed no differences in sexual abuse rates among women of different economic status. Broad-based population studies of the prevalence of childhood sexual abuse indicate that between 12% and 40% of adult women have experienced sexual abuse before the age of 17. Although this chapter addresses the concerns of women, it should be noted that 16% of men have been sexually abused in childhood.

Finkelhor D et al: Sexual abuse in a national survey of adult men and women: prevalence, characteristics, and risk factors. Child Abuse Negl 1990;14:19. [PMID: 3210970]

Kendler KS et al: Childhood sexual abuse and adult psychiatric and substance use disorders in women: an epidemiological and cotwin control analysis. Arch Gen Psychiatry 2000;57:953. [PMID: 11015813]

Roosa MW, Reinholtz C, Angelini PJ: The relation of child sexual abuse and depression in young women: comparisons across four ethnic groups. J Abnorm Child Psychol 1999;27:65. [PMID: 10197407]

Vogeltanz ND et al: Prevalence and risk factors for childhood sexual abuse in women: national survey findings. Child Abuse Negl 1999;23:579. [PMID: 103391515]

Wyatt GE, Peters SD: Methodologic considerations in research on the prevalence of child sexual abuse. Child Abuse Negl 1986;10:241. [PMID: 3486702]

Prevention

Preventing sexual abuse of children is a goal for all societies. The factors that put children at risk are complex and challenging for any culture to eradicate. A number of studies have documented specific risk factors that increase risk of abuse: parental inadequacy, unavailability, and poor parent-child relationship. Girls who live away from a biologic parent for extended periods of time and those who reside with a stepfather are at higher risk. Parental drug or alcohol abuse and marital conflict are also risk factors for child sexual abuse. However, many children who are sexually abused have none of these risk factors. Changes that may improve prevention are slow in coming. Studies have shown that children seldom report the abuse. One study found that children had difficulty remembering or they belittled or denied the experience even when the abuse was videotaped by the perpetrator.

Finkelhor D: Current information on the scope and nature of child sexual abuse, in the future of children. 1994;4(2). Available at: http://www.futureofchildren.org/information2827/information_show.htm?doc_id=74220. Accessed November 3, 2002.

Sjoberg RL, Lindblad F: Limited disclosure of sexual abuse in children whose experiences were documented by videotape. Am J Psychiatry 2002;159:312. [PMID: 11823279]

Clinical Findings

All patients should be asked about a history of sexual abuse because many patients fail to disclose the information spontaneously. In a random review of medical charts at a psychiatric emergency department, only 6% of the charts noted a history of childhood sexual abuse. However, when physicians were asked to query their next 50 patients verbally about abuse, 70% of patients reported sexual contact before the age of 17 initiated by someone 5 or more years older. A study in a primary care setting noted that while women with a history of child sexual abuse suffered more physical and psychosocial symptoms, their symptoms were not reflected in their medical charts.

To screen for a history of sexual abuse, clinicians should routinely ask all patients about adverse sexual experiences during the initial interview. How and when to obtain these histories are matters of clinical judgment. Generally, an appropriate time to ask about abuse is when taking the past medical history after inquiring about menses and pregnancy. The clinician may ask questions such as: "Has anyone ever touched you against your will? Have you had any adverse sexual experiences?" If a patient says yes, the clinician should ask, "How old were you when it started? Who was the abuser, and how old was that person? What made it stop? What happened physically to you during the abuse?"

Framing the initial questions using the words **against your will** and **adverse experiences** allows the patient to define the abuse in her own way. Specifically naming the types of abuse is an attempt to take away any shame patients may feel in describing the acts. Knowing the duration of abuse and whether the perpetrator lived in the home helps the clinician evaluate the severity of the abuse. Inquiring about what made the abuse stop gives the clinician information about what the patient experienced and the degree of family dysfunction. Poor outcomes are associated with longer duration of abuse and more physically intrusive abuse.

Clinicians should be aware that abuse survivors may be particularly anxious regarding medical visits. This anxiety may be manifested by appearing disorganized and/or forgetful or behaving in a guarded and/or overly controlling manner. The pelvic examination can be difficult for these patients. It may help to delay the pelvic examination until the next visit if the patient is particularly anxious. These patients may call back for instruction on medications or procedures that were discussed during the office visit; anxiety often causes them to "space out" or dissociate through part of the interview or examination. Therefore, written instructions can be helpful.

Although clinicians may fear that raising the subject of abuse may cause decompensation on the part of the patient, ignoring the subject only contributes to continued isolation and possible development of psychopathology. The patient needs to understand the value of determining the effects of sexual abuse, namely, the complex relationship between childhood experiences and adult health and body experiences. The clinician can express concern that retraumatization during the examination be minimized and problem-solve with the patient to reduce that risk, eg, by talking and keeping eye contact. It is appropriate at this time to ask the patient if she feels she has worked through the effects of the abuse. If the abuse appears to be unresolved, consider referring her to a mental health professional experienced in abuse (see following section, When to Refer to a Specialist).

The clinical presentation is often complicated further by other potentially damaging experiences such as physical and psychological abuse, parental psychopathology, parental neglect, alcoholism, and severe family dysfunction. The long-term effects of the abuse are influenced by these factors.

Briere J, Zaida LY: Sexual abuse histories and sequelae in female psychiatric emergency room patients. Am J Psychiatry 1989;146:1602. [PMID: 2589554]

Hulme PA: Symptomatology and health care utilization of women primary care patients who experienced childhood sexual abuse. Child Abuse Negl 2000;24:1471. [PMID: 11128178]

Complications

A. MEDICAL

Medical complications that may be associated with sexual abuse include chronic pelvic pain, premenstrual syndrome (PMS), somatization disorder, pain syndromes, pseudoseizures, headaches, asthma, and gastrointestinal complaints (Table 14–1). Chronic pelvic pain with normal laparoscopic findings has been associated with a history of sexual abuse. Very high rates of sexual abuse have been noted in women who complain of severe PMS. A Canadian study concluded that women with a history of childhood sexual abuse reported a greater number of painful body areas than women with no history of abuse; in addition, sexually abused women tended to use health services more often, had more surgeries, and had fibromyalgia more often than nonabused women. Other studies have shown that patients with a history of childhood sexual abuse visit emergency departments more often than those with no history of abuse. Clinicians have noted that pain management may be more difficult in cancer patients with a history of sexual abuse. Patients referred to a gastroenterology clinic who had a history of abuse (sexual and physical) reported more medical symptoms and were more frequent users of health care services than nonabused patients.

B. PSYCHIATRIC

Psychiatric complications that may be associated with sexual abuse include substance abuse, depression or suicide, eating disorders, sexual disorders, borderline personality disorder, and anxiety disorders (eg, posttraumatic stress disorder [PTSD]), and dissociative disorders) (Table 14–2).

Table 14–1. Medical complications of sexual abuse.

Chronic pelvic pain
Premenstrual syndrome
Somatization disorder
Hypochondriases
Pseudoseizures
Headaches
Asthma
Gastrointestinal complaints

Table 14–2. Psychiatric complications of sexual abuse.

Substance abuse
Depression
Suicide
Sexual disorders
Eating disorders
Borderline personality disorder
Anxiety disorders (eg, PTSD)
Dissociative disorders (eg, MPD)

PTSD, posttraumatic stress disorder; MPD, multiple personality disorder.

Many women in the early stages of recovery from sexual abuse engage in self-destructive behaviors, including substance abuse, involvement in abusive relationships, promiscuity, and self-cutting; self-cutting is considered self-mutilation rather than a suicide attempt. High rates of sexual abuse are seen among women in substance abuse treatment programs.

One model of the way that childhood trauma predisposes persons to numerous medical and psychiatric complications uses the concept of inescapable stress. This concept involves inescapable shock, and the effects of exposure include (1) deficits in learning to escape novel adverse situations, (2) decreased motivation for learning new contingencies, (3) chronic subjective distress, and (4) increased tumor genesis and immunosuppression. The "learned helplessness syndrome" that follows is caused by lack of control. This syndrome is related to depression and PTSD. Some authors have postulated HPA (hypothalamic-pituitary axis) dysregulation is part of the physical impact of childhood abuse trauma putting survivors at risk for health events.

When victims are faced with repeated trauma, they commonly use the defense mechanisms of dissociation, repression, and denial. Each mechanism is an appropriate way to cope with present trauma when no other modes of coping are available. However, continuing to use these defense mechanisms in adulthood, long after the original trauma has occurred, may be maladaptive.

Women with a history of childhood abuse tend to have a number of interpersonal dysfunctions including problems with intimate partner relations, disturbed sexual functioning, and difficulties in the parental role. Many trauma survivors use dissociation; they may say, "It's happening to someone else," or describe being "in the wallpaper" while the abuse was taking place.

Dissociation as a defense enables the victim to escape overwhelming stimuli. Repression involves pushing the memories into the unconscious mind. In denial, the victim claims the experiences are unimportant.

Using these defense mechanisms in adulthood may predispose the woman to manage current stress by somatizing anxiety. Thus, a woman may complain of nonspecific somatic complaints, such as PMS, abdominal pain, or headaches, when the real issue is marital discord or work problems.

Clinicians may better understand their patients' underlying psychopathology and ultimately be more helpful by evaluating them in the context of the inescapable stress concept and the defense mechanisms of dissociation, repression, and denial (see following section, Treatment).

Arnow BA et al: Childhood sexual abuse, psychological distress, and medical use among women. Psychosom Med 1999;61: 762. [PMID: 10593627]

Arnow BA et al: Severity of child maltreatment, pain complaints and medical utilization among women. J Psychiatr Res 2000; 34:413. [PMID: 11165309]

Deep AL et al: Sexual abuse in eating disorder subtypes and control women: the role of comorbid substance dependence in bulimia nervosa. Int J Eat Disord 1999;25:1. [PMID: 9924647]

DeLillo D: Interpersonal functioning among women reporting a history of childhood sexual abuse: empirical findings and methodological issues. Clin Psychol Rev 2001;21:553. [PMID: 11413867]

Drossman DA et al: Sexual and physical abuse in women with functional or organic gastrointestinal disorders. Ann Intern Med 1990;113:828. [PMID: 2240898]

Finestone HM et al: Chronic pain and health care utilization in women with a history of childhood sexual abuse. Child Abuse Negl 2000;24:547. [PMID: 10798843]

Fleming J et al: The long-term impact of childhood sexual abuse in Australian women. Child Abuse Negl 1999;23:145. [PMID: 10075184]

Golding JM et al: Prevalence of sexual abuse history in a sample of women seeking treatment for premenstrual syndrome. J Psychosom Obstet Gynaecol 2000;21:69. [PMID: 10994179]

Green CR et al: Do physical and sexual abuse differentially affect chronic pain states in women? J Pain Symptom Manage 1999;18:420. [PMID: 10641468]

Heim C et al: Abuse-related posttraumatic stress disorder and alterations of the hypothalamic-pituitary-adrenal axis in women with chronic pelvic pain. Psychosom Med 1998;60:309. [PMID: 9625218]

Liebschutz JM et al: Physical and sexual abuse in women infected with the human immunodeficiency virus: increased illness and health care utilization. Arch Intern Med 2000;12:1659. [PMID: 10847259]

Longstreth GF et al: Group psychotherapy for women molested in childhood: psychological and somatic symptoms and medical visits. Int J Group Psychother 1998;48:533. [PMID: 9766093]

Thakkar RR, McCanne TR: The effects of daily stressors on physical health in women with and without a childhood history of sexual abuse. Child Abuse Negl 2000;24:209. [PMID: 10695516]

van der Kolk BA: *Psychological Trauma.* American Psychiatric Press, 1987.

van der Kolk BA: The body keeps the score: memory and the evolving psychobiology of posttraumatic stress. Harv Rev Psychiatry 1994;1:253.[PMID: 9384857]

Weiss EL, Longhurst JG, Mazure CM: Childhood sexual abuse as a risk factor for depression in women: psychosocial and neurobiological correlates. Am J Psychiatry 1999;156:816. [PMID: 10360118]

Treatment

Often a combination of individual psychotherapy, pharmacotherapy, and possibly, group therapy is advised in treating abuse survivors. Antidepressant medication is often helpful because these drugs target mood, panic, and the "positive" symptoms of PTSD (eg, autonomic hyperarousal, hypervigilance, nightmares, and flashbacks). The selective serotonin reuptake inhibitors (SSRIs) such as paroxetine (Paxil), sertraline (Zoloft), citalopram (Celexa), and fluoxetine (Prozac) have an improved side effect and safety profile. Sertraline (Zoloft) has been approved by the US Food and Drug Administration for the treatment of PTSD. Clinically, all the SSRIs seem to be equally effective. Prazosin has been beneficial in the treatment of PTSD-related nightmares. Tricyclic antidepressants (TCAs), monoamine oxidase (MAO) inhibitors, and some of the newer antidepressant medications such as venlafaxine (Effexor) or nefazodone (Serzone) also appear effective. Sometimes the addition of low-dose trazodone (Desyrel) in the 25–50 mg range helps with the nightmares and sleep disturbances. TCAs are sometimes added at night or as primary agents when chronic pain is a central complaint. Prescribing habit-forming agents such as the benzodiazepines should be avoided, although they are helpful in treating the acute reactivation of memories on a short-term basis (less than 3 weeks). These drugs may be helpful for someone whose symptoms have caused extreme impairment. Neuroleptics should be avoided.

The patient should be an active participant in treatment planning, although there are situations in which the survivor is so disabled that participation in the planning of the initial phase of treatment is minimal. At other times, patients may have their own, fixed agenda for treatment. These agendas are sometimes helpful and always illuminating, and they should be listened to before decisions are made; however, the clinician needs to stay within his or her domain of ethical, sensible, and well-founded treatment.

Treatment and recovery, when possible, enable the patient to go from feeling like a victim to feeling like a survivor and ideally to becoming someone who thrives in life. The health care provider plays an integral part in the development of a new relationship between the survivor and her body and between the survivor and her support network.

An important issue in the treatment of abuse survivors has to do with the relationship between the survivor and her health care provider. The patient may distort the relationship due to her experiences with authority figures in the past; the distortion may be toward either a heightened positive or an increased negative perception. Clinicians should be cautious and maintain professional boundaries to avoid these distortions.

When to Refer to a Specialist

Refer a patient to a mental health provider if she is experiencing severe symptoms (eg, suicidal ideation, posttraumatic sequelae, severe panic attacks, sleep disturbance, depression, self-mutilation, or involvement in abusive relationships). The difficult-to-manage patient who is noncompliant with the treatment of serious medical problems also should be referred. An in-depth mental health evaluation can help determine treatment recommendations.

Every primary care clinician should have the names of at least 2 experienced clinicians who work in the area of sexual abuse so that a referral may be made when needed. Physical therapy involving pelvic floor exercises, biofeedback, or other types of movement therapy for chronic pelvic pain that has no underlying pathology also are quite helpful. Here, too, the referral should be made to someone experienced in the area of sexual abuse.

Relevant Web Sites

[American Academy of Child and Adolescent Psychiatry]
http://www.aacap.org/publications/factsfam
[American Psychological Association]
http://www.apa.org/releases/sexabuse/
[American Professional Society on the Abuse of Children]
http://www.apsac.org/public.html

Evaluating Sexual Dysfunctions

15

Julia R. Heiman, PhD

Sexual dysfunctions are disorders that impair or prevent participation in sexual activity. Many women experience sexual dysfunction but either do not choose to view it as a problem or are unwilling to volunteer the information to a primary care physician. The reasons for the latter usually include some combination of the woman's discomfort, her perception of discomfort in her health care provider, or the physician does not ask adequate questions. This stalemate has continued for many generations, assisted by broader cultural resistance to the idea that sex can be a problem or to the acknowledgment that women's sexuality is important. Women's sexuality has been seen as incidental in comparison to diseases and conditions that are life-threatening or severely compromising of general functioning. In significant contrast, male erectile problems have been the subject of extensive research.

The prevalence of sexual dysfunction is not known precisely, and epidemiologic studies that include sexual dysfunction are rare, especially in women. Based on a random probability sample of US adults between 18 and 59 years old, recent estimates showed that 43% of women reported experiencing 1 or more sexual problems for several months or more during the past year, compared with 31% of men. The most common problem was lack of sexual interest reported by nearly one third of the female sample. More clinic-based data suggest that sexual dysfunctions are even more common. In a study of 329 women between the ages of 18 and 79 years, orgasm difficulties were reported by 58% and painful intercourse by 29%.

Sexual problems can be a source of distress, can cause pain and discomfort, can result from a disease such as diabetes, and can have a ripple effect on other areas of a woman's life. Examples of effects in other areas of life are the avoidance of forming enduring relationships, the avoidance of having children although they are desired, ongoing relationship distress or dissolution, or discontinuance of a sexuality impairing medication prescribed for a serious medical condition. A woman may feel that a sexual complaint is not only embarrassing but insignificant. It is the responsibility of the health care provider to include sexual disorders in the realm of health care. Unfortunately, little attention is given in medical and professional training programs concerning how to appropriately ask about sexual complaints, the treatment of sexual complaints, and the connections between sexual complaints and other areas of a woman's life.

Laumann EO, Paik A, Rosen RC: Sexual dysfunction in the United States: prevalence and predictors. JAMA 1999;281:537. [PMID: 10022110]

Rosen RC et al: Prevalence of sexual dysfunction in women: Results of a survey study of 329 women in an outpatient gynecological clinic. J Sex Marital Ther 1993;19:171. [PMID: 8246273]

SCREENING

Office screening formats usually include some combination of symptom checklists and interviews. Brief questions about sexual functioning can be included in the general screening. (Research suggests that patients are more likely to answer questions than to initiate sexual information.) Two possible questions are as follows:

1. Are you currently experiencing any sexual concerns or problems? (If an interview format is used, the clinician may consider probing for information about problems of desire, arousal, orgasm, or pain.)

2. (If the patient has answered yes to the previous question.) Does the problem bother you enough that you want to do something about it?

The first question allows the person to raise a wide variety of issues, including contraception, sexual abuse, and safe sex. In fact, separate questions about these issues can be asked in the same period of the assessment. The second question helps the clinician evaluate whether the person expresses enough distress to want to pursue help. If she does not, the information is useful in determining whether the symptoms are related to another problem such as depression, genital injury or sensitivity, endocrine problems, or medication-related disorders, or whether they fit into a broader disease pattern such as that of diabetes or a neurologic disorder.

It is important for the clinician not to assume that a patient is heterosexual until this fact has been made clear by the patient. Some sexual complaints, such as vaginismus, are clearly less common in lesbian women; others are just as common. For example, lack of lubrication can be a bothersome issue regardless of sexual orientation.

Table 15–1. Female sexual dysfunctions.[1]

Sexual desire disorders

Hypoactive sexual desire disorder: Persistent absence or deficiency of sexual feelings and desire for sexual activity. Take into account factors that affect sexual functioning such as age, sex, life context. Rule out other psychiatric disorders such as major depression.

Sexual aversion disorder: Persistent or recurrent aversion to and avoidance of genital contact with a sexual partner. Rule out other psychiatric disorders such as major depression or obsessive-compulsive disorder.

Sexual arousal disorder

1. Partial or total lack of physical response as indicated by lack of lubrication and vasocongestion of genitals, or
2. Persistent lack of a subjective sense of sexual excitement and pleasure during sex. (This criterion is omitted from *DSM-IV*, but it is important for clarification.)

Inhibited female orgasm

Persistent delay or absence of orgasm. Lack of coital orgasm is usually considered a normal variation of female sexual response if the woman is able to experience orgasm with a partner using other, noncoital methods.

Sexual pain disorders

Dyspareunia: Recurrent genital pain before, during, or after intercourse. Rule out vaginismus and lack of lubrication.

Vaginismus: Recurrent involuntary spasm of the outer third of the vagina interfering with or preventing coitus. Rule out physical disorder or other psychiatric disorder (rare).

Sexual dysfunctions not otherwise specified

Examples:(1) Anesthesia with arousal and orgasm, (2) too rapid orgasm, (3) genital pain during noncoital activities, (4) lack of pleasure during sex.

Sexual satisfaction

A woman may be satisfied despite the preceding symptoms, but the partner may be dissatisfied. The problem may be a difference in desire rather than hypoactivity of one partner.

---

[1]Using modified *DSM-IV-TR* classification with expansion (Basson et al., 2000). For all diagnoses, specify psychogenic, biogenic, or both; lifelong or acquired; generalized or situational.

DIFFERENTIAL DIAGNOSIS

Diagnosing sexual dysfunctions in women requires knowledge of the basic disorders and their modifiers. Table 15–1 shows the categories of the American Psychiatric Association's *Diagnostic and Statistical Manual of Mental Disorders,* 4th ed—Text Revision (DSM-IV-TR) used as a guide for clinical assessment. There are 6 major categories that, when modified by the variables lifelong/acquired and generalized/situational, provide a thorough description of the extent of the sexual problem. It is important to ask about each basic category, even if the patient states only one, and to identify which dysfunction occurred first. For example, a pain disorder preceded by an arousal disorder (lack of lubrication) suggests a different treatment from a pain disorder that preceded an arousal disorder. In addition, the symptoms must be accompanied by marked distress or interpersonal difficulty to qualify as a disorder in the DSM-IV-TR. Diagnoses of dysfunctions in women are currently under reconsideration. The results of a consensus conference proposed several modifications that the participant researchers and practitioners agreed were important. Additions included subjective as well as genital sexual arousal signs and both organic and psychogenic etiologies.

1. Desire Disorders

Hypoactive Sexual Desire Disorder

A. DIAGNOSIS

When a woman reports a desire disorder, it is important to clarify whether she is simply uninterested in sex but able to respond sexually or she is aversive to sex. Hypoactive sexual desire disorder is a common complaint; 30–50% of patients (mostly women) in sex therapy clinics report the condition, and 27–32% of women in the study by Laumann et al reported lack of sexual interest as a problem in the past year.

There are 2 major problems with this diagnosis: (1) there are no norms for sexual desire across age cohorts and (2) the reasons for the development and maintenance of the complaint are variable and imprecise, suggesting it is a heterogeneous diagnosis. There is also increasing evidence of overlap between hypoactive sexual desire disorder and sexual arousal disorder. Certainly, physical factors can play a role (Table 15–2); in particular, general health, depression, hormonal status, and use of recreational drugs and medications should be reviewed. It should be kept in mind that taking exogenous estrogens, whether through oral contraceptive or hormone replacement therapy will result in increased sex hormone binding globulin (SHBG) and related decreased free testosterone. Psychological and interpersonal factors are as likely if not more likely to play a role. Sudden events (such as job loss or family trauma), cumulative factors (such as the psychological response to aging, an especially sensitive issue in women because of the stricter cultural norms for women's attractiveness), and life milestones (such as childbirth, children leaving home, or ongoing relationship distress) commonly have an impact on sexual desire.

Table 15–2. Summary of factors and treatment approaches for female sexual dysfunction.[1]

Physical Factors[2]	Treatment Action
1. Illness/disease	
Diabetes, neurologic disorder, pelvic inflammatory disease, endometriosis	Treat illness; inform of its sexual effects; refer if adjustment to illness remains a problem.
Depression, anxiety, panic	Refer for consultation concerning medication or psychotherapy, or both.
2. Endocrine status	
Menstrual disorders including anovulatory cycles, thyroid conditions, elevated prolactin	Endocrine work-up; consider nonhormonal treatment; with hormonal and other medication, consider sexual side effects and inform patient.
Menopausal	Discuss alteration of hormonal status; consider topical lubricants. For patient information, have list of reference books on menopause available; discuss sexual consequences.
3. Medications	
Antidepressants, neuroleptics, diuretics, hormones, other vasoactive substances	Change medication or reduce dosage if appropriate. Note drug interactions (eg, antidepressants and hormones).
4. Recreational drugs	
Alcohol, nicotine, cocaine, cannabis	If heavy use, refer to treatment; if moderate use, ask if patient can stop for 3 months or dramatically reduce. If not able to do latter, refer for substance abuse treatment or more extensive evaluation.
5. Surgeries	
Abdominal repairs, hysterectomy	Careful physical examination and review of records. If over 1 year since surgery and no physical signs of problems, refer for consultation.
6. Genitourinary pain	
Interstitial cystitis	Alleviate symptoms of recurrent pain. If no improvement, refer for specialized or psychological treatment of pain.
Psychological Factors	**Treatment Action**
1. Acute or chronic stress	
Symptoms of fatigue, poor motivation, sleep disturbance, distractibility, poor coping style	Rule out depression; acknowledge degree of stress; refer for evaluation.
2. Gender identity	Refer for consultation.
3. Sex role satisfaction	Give information and book list; refer for counseling.
4. Sexual knowledge	Give information; refer.
5. Sexual attitudes and values (including religious)	Give information; refer for psychological or religious counseling.
6. Negative body image	Give book list; refer for therapy.
Negative history, aging, illness, surgery, trauma, body weight	
Interactional Factors	**Treatment Action**
1. History of physical, sexual, or emotional abuse (as a child or adult)	Consider books; refer for therapy.
2. Prior relationships	Consider broader interpersonal issues that may benefit from treatment.
Patterns of attachment (chaotic, stressed, clinging) and sex (always poor, decreasing, stopped suddenly)	
3. Current relationship	Give information about impact of relationship on sex; offer to speak with partner; refer.
Partner's health, satisfaction, commitment	
4. Sexual preferences	Recommend discussion with partner; if refused or no effect, refer.
One partner focused on sexual position or pattern	

[1]The examples given here are not inclusive. See text for more details.
[2]Although listed separately, physical, psychological, and interactional factors overlap and interact with each other.

B. TREATMENT

Appropriate treatment depends on the outcome of the assessment of the patient's health and psychosocial issues. Generalized and lifelong low sexual desire suggests the need for a screening for endocrine disorders, illness, and long-term medication use. Depression is a possible diagnosis in women with low sexual desire. The use of testosterone has been shown to increase desire but is viewed cautiously as a long-term intervention because of its potential cardiovascular side effects. Preliminary trials that are searching for a safe and effective means of delivering testosterone show that there may be some benefit to "replacing" the testosterone decreases that occur with aging/menopause or oophorectomy. Shifren et al tested a transdermal testosterone patch in women who had undergone an oophorectomy and hysterectomy and found that the 300 µg dose of testosterone significantly improved sexual activity frequency, pleasure-orgasm, depression and positive well-being, but only nonsignificant increases occurred in sexual thoughts-desire. This dose also produced total testosterone levels well above the norms available for premenopausal women, although no changes in lipid or liver functioning were found. Recently, a female androgen insufficiency syndrome has been proposed; it attempts to specify the consequences of decreased androgens in terms of sexuality, mood, and well-being. Other chemical treatments such as yohimbine, antidepressants, and dopamine agonists all appear to carry more of a placebo than a true effect on low desire, although there may be a subgroup that is as yet undescribed for whom these interventions are effective. It is also true that some of the pharmaceutical agents being tested on women's sexual arousal may secondarily help desire, in part because desire and arousal have been found to overlap in women's experience of sexual response.

The patient also may benefit from information conveyed by the physician. For example, a woman can be informed that there are no current norms for sexual desire at different ages. On the other hand, sexual desire is not expected to go from 2–3 times per week to zero times per week between the ages of 20 and 40 unless something is wrong. Desire and behavioral frequencies (the latter more dependent on the availability of a partner) remain quite stable in women, decreasing generally with age or in the context of a long-term relationship in most couples, regardless of sexual orientation. There are no data on the percentage of couples who stop having sex while maintaining a good relationship; this occurrence may be more common in lesbian couples.

If there is no medical disorder, or if the medical disorder has been addressed with no desire change, individual or couples therapy can be recommended. Controlled treatment studies are rare. Trudel et al found that cognitive behavior therapy could be helpful for women with hypoactive sexual desire disorder. The clinical literature can provide an estimate of the effectiveness of treatments. Hypoactive sexual desire is one of the more difficult sexual disorders to treat with psychotherapy. One study showed a success rate below 50%. Treatment duration varies but is often 15–45 sessions. Better treatment outcomes are associated with the absence of a global and lifelong desire disorder.

Sexual Aversion Disorder

A. DIAGNOSIS

Sexual aversion disorder is a much rarer desire disorder than hypoactive sexual desire disorder and is usually accompanied by low sexual desire and occasionally by vaginismus or dyspareunia. Women with this disorder may have a history of sexual or physical abuse or may have extensive negative, unexpressed feelings about their relationships. Physical factors rarely are involved, although there may be concomitant significant anxiety, a phobic response to sexual stimuli or obsessive-compulsive symptoms that may respond to specific treatment.

B. TREATMENT

Psychological intervention, combining individual and couples therapy, can be useful. Therapy typically includes cognitive-behavioral techniques, desensitization, and working through of past issues of abuse. Couples work often focuses on conflict areas, emotional differences, and issues of control. Specific aversions of phobic dimensions, such as aversion to semen, can be difficult to remove and may need to be diminished somewhat and then worked around (eg, avoiding manual stimulation to orgasm). In occasional cases, a significant level of anxiety augments rather modest aversion symptoms, and a course of anxiolytics can be helpful. However, it is probably wise to have a clinician experienced in sexual and anxiety disorders give a second opinion before trying an antianxiety medication. Although no outcome statistics are available for these disorders, the duration and success of therapy are estimated to be similar to those of hypoactive sexual desire.

Sexual Arousal Disorder

A. DIAGNOSIS

This disorder is relatively uncommon in women unless there are concomitant menopausal, dyspareunia, or anorgasmic symptoms. Women who report lack of lubrication are somewhat more likely to be menopausal or perimenopausal; however, data from the study by Laumann et al demonstrate that 18–19% of women between the ages of 18 and 39 reported trouble lubricating. It should be noted that physical and subjective sexual arousal are not necessarily correlated in women; however, a continual lack of lubrication may lead to discomfort in sex, which will then impair subjective arousal. Also, women's partners sometimes interpret lack of lubrication to mean lack of interest, which can result in a distressed sexual relationship.

B. TREATMENT

Reviewing possible physical causes for this complaint is the first step. The recommendation of topical lubricants such as K-Y Jelly, Astroglide or estrogenic compounds depends on the woman's physical condition and her risk factors for estrogen therapy. If the woman has another, concurrent sexual dysfunction that preceded her sexual arousal problem, such as genital pain, lack of orgasm or desire, that condition should be addressed first and the woman referred for therapy. There is increasing evidence that desire and arousal domains overlap significantly in women. The effectiveness of treatment for sexual arousal disorder is essentially unknown because the condition is so rarely treated in the absence of pain or orgasmic dysfunction. Since the availability of sildenafil (Viagra) for men, there has been interest in differentiating sexual arousal disorder and treating it in women. Thus far, only 1 controlled, double-blind study has shown sildenafil to be effective, and in that case, it was in women younger than 30 years not using hormonal contraceptives. Other systemic and local vasocongestive agents are being tested currently.

Orgasmic Disorders

A. DIAGNOSIS

These disorders are common sexual complaints, with approximately 10% of women reporting global, lifelong lack of orgasm and at least 50% reporting situational and intermittent orgasmic problems. Until recently, it has been rare for an orgasmic problem to have a physical basis, although it is important to review surgeries, use of recreational drugs and alcohol, and medications carefully. With the advent and frequent prescription of selective serotonin reuptake inhibitor (SSRI) antidepressants, reports of medication-induced anorgasmia have become more frequent. Orgasm delay also can occur with other medications, including the monoamine oxidase (MAO) inhibitor antidepressants.

Psychological and interpersonal factors frequently contribute to lack of orgasm, including early family history messages about sex as shameful, a view of the parents as untrustworthy or abandoning, unpleasant earlier sexual experiences, and ineffective current sexual techniques of both partners. Male partners of nonorgasmic women often are quite distressed by and feel responsible for the woman's orgasm problem. Although the partner can be helpful by providing physical and emotional attention, taking primary responsibility for a woman's orgasm is counterproductive and can contribute to a continuing lack of orgasm, because the female partner is likely to feel pressured to perform. The woman often feels inhibited and embarrassed about this problem, which makes her less likely to disclose it to a primary care provider than if she had a sexual pain problem.

B. TREATMENT

It is rare that primary (lifelong, generalized) orgasmic disorder has a physical basis. There is evidence that it can be treated effectively by masturbation or traditional sex therapy techniques or both. Individual, group, and couples therapy have been shown to be effective. Books are available dealing with body image, relaxation, self-observation, tolerance of sexual arousal tension, acceptance of sexual feelings, and sensual touching that may be used alone or with a partner. Lack of progress using any of the techniques described in the books should be evaluated by a brief counseling consultation. Therapy is usually effective in about 88–90% of cases for becoming orgasmic during masturbation and in about 75% for experiencing orgasm in partner activities. Therapy usually takes 15–20 sessions, unless there are issues in the woman's history such as sexual assault or other interpersonal trauma or serious conflicts. Situational or intermittent problems with orgasm are more likely to be related to relationship problems and require additional therapy.

In the case of SSRI-induced anorgasmia, reducing the drug dosage, changing the antidepressant, augmenting with a second antidepressant (eg, bupropion) or other medication (eg, buspirone) has been found to work idiosyncratically.

Sexual Pain Disorders

1. Dyspareunia

A. DIAGNOSIS

Of the sexual pain disorders, dyspareunia—recurrent genital pain before, during, or after intercourse—is the most variable in presentation. Its diagnosis requires a careful physical examination to identify the type of pain and possibly its physical basis, which may be injury, endometriosis, scarring, or unusual skin sensitivity. Differential diagnosis is essential. A common diagnosis that requires a physical examination is vulvar vestibulitis, and recent advances have been made in the medical treatment of this disorder. Pain of a diffuse and long-term nature is difficult to treat, and the clinician should keep in mind the possibility of referral during the assessment to evaluate potential psychological factors that could be addressed simultaneously. Psychological factors include development issues, such as guilt and shame surrounding sex; traumatic sexual events, such as rape or even painful sex from consensual experiences; and relationship distress, such as unresolved conflicts and anger.

B. TREATMENT

Dyspareunia may be related to organic factors, not all of which can be treated. For example, pain sensitivity may remain after scar tissue is removed. Nevertheless, referral to a psychotherapist could help because behavioral patterns and emotions (eg, fear or tension) may be maintaining the pain. Physical therapy involving perineal or vaginal biofeedback may be particularly helpful for women with ongoing dyspareunia. Letting the patient know when no more can be done about the pain on a physical level is important. In addition, it is useful for the patient to discuss with her partner the need to rely on noncoital sexual expression. Low doses of antidepressants may provide temporary help for dyspareunia but are best considered reluctantly, only after consultation with a specialist in sexual disorders, because of the likelihood of the medications affecting desire or orgasmic response. Referral to a specialist also may help in managing the pain by finding ways for the patient to control her focus and relax.

2. Vaginismus

A. DIAGNOSIS

Vaginismus is defined as the recurrent involuntary spasm of the outer third of the vagina interfering with intercourse; it is often accompanied by much embarrassment on the part of the patient and frustration for the couple. Vaginismus is less common than dyspareunia, but both are infrequent and together account for about 10% of sexual complaints. A primary care provider is likely to see patients with this disorder when symptoms have existed for some time and either relationship distress or desire for pregnancy is prominent. Again, a careful physical examination is important, as is questioning about the initial conditions under which symptoms appeared. Once established, the vaginismus response is enduring and usually requires both a mechanical and a psychological approach to treatment. Psychological factors typically include past and present strong sexual inhibition; less common factors include sexual trauma (rape or incest). Frequently, unexpressed negative feelings toward a sexual partner or other important male figures are involved. Phobia about sexual response or intercourse also may be part of the clinical picture. Finally, in vaginismus, as in dyspareunia, a repeated experience with pain can establish a pain-tension-pain cycle that maintains itself independently of overt psychological factors.

B. TREATMENT

The usual recommendation is a dilation procedure, using a series of graduated dilators coupled with relaxation, although increasingly referral to a physical therapist for genital biofeedback is helpful. Gradual involvement of the partner includes his use of dilators or fingers, gradual insertion of his penis, and reliance on the woman's guidance to control the pace and duration of the sexual activity. For severely phobic women, additional techniques and systematic desensitization may be necessary. Although clinicians 20 years ago reported rapid and easy success with vaginismus (10–14 sessions), more recently they report more demanding problems; perhaps patients with milder problems are being treated through self-help methods.

Other Sexual Complaints

Lack of sensation in the genital area may be an issue for women who have experienced neurologic disease or injury; the potential for recovery from the underlying illness determines whether the problem can improve or the patient needs to accommodate to the problem. Surgeries in the pelvic area may have an effect on the sensation of orgasm, a possibility with some women following hysterectomy. The factor of autonomic nerve damage has been underresearched but is suggested by the outcomes of some patients. Lack of feeling without physical findings suggests the need for a referral for evaluation to help identify and manage psychological factors. A patient with noncoital genital pain, like those with other pain disorders, needs careful evaluation for possible physical sensitivity or injury. Early psychological referral is recommended unless symptoms remit quickly, given the propensity for pain to result in behavioral patterns that may maintain it. When sexual dissatisfaction is based on different levels of sexual desire between the patient and her partner, but both are within the limits of typical variation (eg, 2–3 times a week; 1 time a month), it may be helpful to let the patient know the usual variations in desire. If differences in desire are well outside the usual range (several times a day; less than once in 6 months), referral for therapy may be offered.

American Psychiatric Association: *Diagnostic and Statistical Manual of Mental Disorders,* 4th ed—Text Revision. American Psychiatric Association, 2000.

Bachman G et al: Female androgen insufficiency: the princeton consensus statement on definition, classification, and assessment. Fertil Steril 2002;77:660. [PMID: 1193711]

Basson R et al: Report of the international consensus development conference on female sexual dysfunction: definitions and classifications. J Urol 2000;163:888. [PMID: 10688001]

Bergeron S et al: Vulvar vestibulitis syndrome: a critical review. Clin J Pain 1997;13:27. [PMID: 9084950]

Burman B, Margolin G: Analysis of the association between marital relationships and health problems: an interactional perspective. Psychol Bull 1992;112:39. [PMID: 1529039]

Caruso S et al: Premenopausal women affected by sexual arousal disorder treated with sildenafil: a double-blind, cross-over, placebo-controlled study. BJOG 2001;108:623. [PMID: 11426898]

Heiman J, LoPiccolo J: *Becoming Orgasmic: A Sexual and Personal Growth Program for Women,* 2nd ed. Prentice Hall, 1988.

Heiman JR, Meston CM: Empirically validated treatment for sexual dysfunction. Annu Rev Sex Res 1997;8:148. [PMID: 10051893]

Laumann EO, Paik A, Rosen RC: Sexual dysfunction in the United States: prevalence and predictors. JAMA 1999;281:537. [PMID: 10022110]

Leiblum SR, Rosen RC (editors): *Sexual Desire Disorders.* Guilford, 1988.

Leiblum SR, Rosen RC (editors): *Principles and Practices of Sex Therapy,* 3rd ed. Guilford, 2000.

Shifren et al: Transdermal testosterone treatment in women with impaired sexual function after oophorectomy. N Engl J Med 2000;343:682. [PMID: 10974131]

Trudel G et al: The effect of a cognitive-behavioral group treatment program on hypoactive sexual desire in women. Sex Relationship Ther 2001;16:145.

Valins L: *When a Woman's Body Says No to Sex: Understanding and Overcoming Vaginismus.* Penguin, 1992.

When to Refer to A Specialist

Primary care practitioners cannot be expected to provide all the treatment options available for sexual disorders. In some cases, even the diagnostic work-up may benefit from a specialist's consultation to avoid inefficient referral or unnecessary treatment. Conditions under which a referral should be considered include the following:

1. The physician is uncertain of the diagnosis. If the problem appears to be long-term yet situational, and possibly contributed to by a myriad of physical, psychological, and interpersonal factors, an early referral may prevent dissatisfaction and save both money and time for the patient.

2. The factors surrounding the sexual problem appear to be in an area in which the primary care provider has limited expertise. Common areas include psychological and interpersonal factors as well as the nonphysical consequences of illness or normal physiologic processes. For example, some women have a mixture of psychological reactions to menopause and the events surrounding it, as do their partners. The psychological

reactions can be even more extensive in response to a disease like multiple sclerosis; the complaint of loss of sexual functioning may be a patient's "flag" for fears of a number of interpersonal losses. Lack of specialized training and knowledge in the area of sexuality may be an issue, particularly regarding the factors that determine a good sex life, predictors of relationship endurance and happiness, and sexual values and attitudes. Well-intentioned advice to "have a glass of wine to relax before sex" or "take a vacation" has been offered in the past by primary care providers. For an ongoing sexual problem, the patient may benefit more from a brief consultation with a therapist.

3. The symptoms are intense or severe. A 35-year-old woman who has never been able to have intercourse because of vaginismus is best referred to a specialist in sexual problems after a careful history and physical examination. Similarly, a patient who reports extensive distress or serious relationship problems associated with a sexual dysfunction may benefit most by rapid referral to a specialist in sexuality or relationships.

Whether referring for a second opinion, an evaluation, or treatment, several factors can increase the likelihood of success. It is useful to keep a short list of names of specialists in the areas of sexuality, psychiatry, psychology, relationship distress, gynecology, urology, and endocrinology. One should ask for verbal or written feedback from the referral agent; written reports take longer and bear a cost to patients. It is possible, however, that the patient may refuse to give permission for information exchange, especially in the case of a referral for psychotherapy or management of psychiatric medication. Also important are the manner and message used in presenting the referral to the patient. One should explain briefly the reason for the referral; if referring to a nonmedical specialist, one might state that both normal and problematic functioning are established to be result from an interaction of the mind and the body. If referring to a psychiatrist, psychologist, social worker, or nurse, one should specify the referral agent's area of expertise, eg, sexuality, pain disorders, diagnosis, medication interactions. The recommendation of a therapist for recovery from rape, sexual abuse, or physical abuse might be accompanied by the statement that some people find that therapy speeds the recovery process. In the case of a referral to a marital or relationship therapist, it may be worthwhile to mention that distressed relationships take a toll on individual family members' health (increased clinic visits have been reported), work efficiency, and general functioning. Perhaps the most important message the patient needs to hear is that a referral will increase the likelihood that the problem will be dealt with quickly and thoroughly, with less cost to health and quality of life.

Relevant Web Sites

These sites can change rapidly in terms of their emphasis and their longevity is not guaranteed. If they are not to your taste, continue to search, as there are many for women and men on sexual health.

[Official web site of the American Society of Sex Educators, Counselors and Therapists]

www.sexuality.org

[Women's sexual health, one of several sites]

www.womenssexualhealth.com

SECTION IV

Metabolic & Endocrine Disorders

Obesity

16

Paul Mystkowski, MD

Determination of the ideal body weight is an imperfect science. However, in most populations, the body mass index (BMI), defined as BMI = weight in kg ÷ height in m^2, is probably the most clinically practical measure of body weight associated morbidity. While less applicable to certain populations (eg, lean athletes with relatively high BMI values due to large muscle mass, but clearly at low cardiovascular risk), BMI is easily determined in the office setting and, in general, an excellent predictor of obesity-related complications.

 ESSENTIALS OF DIAGNOSIS

- *Overweight persons have a BMI from 25 to 30.*
- *Obese persons have a BMI greater than 30.*

General Considerations

A. EPIDEMIOLOGY

The prevalence of overweight and obesity in the United States continues to increase despite its identification by the United States government and World Health Organization as a priority public health issue. A primary goal of the Public Health Service's National Health Promotion and Disease Prevention Objectives is to "reduce overweight to a prevalence of no more than 20% among people aged 20 years and older and no more than 15% among adolescents aged 12–19." Unfortunately, this goal has been difficult to achieve. As of the year 2000, 65% of American adults were either overweight or obese, while the prevalence of obesity in children has more than doubled from the 1970s until 1999. Thus, despite national efforts to address the growing epidemic of obesity, the prevalence of obesity continues to increase in both children and adults.

The high prevalence of obesity also has a substantial economic impact. Direct and indirect costs of obesity are approximately $117 billion per year in 2000 and represents ~7% of all health care dollars in the United States. Moreover, this negative economic impact may also occur on a more individual level, particularly in women. The University of Michigan Health and Retirement Study found that obese women accumulated a net worth ~60% less than that of normal weight peers, whereas body weight had no effect on the net worth of men.

B. PRESENTATION IN WOMEN

Overweight and obesity can present with several features unique to women, particularly with respect to fertility, pregnancy, menopause, and cancer risk.

1. Fertility—Several studies have demonstrated that overweight and obese women have about a 2-fold increased risk of anovulation relative to women with BMI values between 20 and 25 kg/m^2, although these findings have not been universally demonstrated. Clearly, however, maintaining a normal body weight prepregnancy has beneficial effects on maternal and fetal well-being.

Obesity is a significant risk factor, although not a requirement, for developing polycystic ovary syndrome (PCOS), a syndrome clinically defined as the presence of hyperandrogenism and ovulatory dysfunction with no other identifiable cause (see Chapter 20). The prevalence of obesity in women in PCOS is dependent on the population studied and can range from 38% in a population of English women to 87.5% in a population of Pennsylvanian women. Exercise and weight loss is particularly effective in treating PCOS in an obese woman.

2. Pregnancy—Excess maternal body weight significantly increases morbidity during and after pregnancy for both the mother and the fetus. Overweight and obese women have a 6.5- and 20-fold increased risk of gestational diabetes, respectively, compared with women with normal BMIs. In addition, the risk of developing hypertension and preeclampsia are increased 20-fold and 10-fold, respectively, in obese women. The risk of thromboembolic disease and urinary tract infections are also increased in obese women.

3. Menopause—Menopause is classically associated with weight gain ranging from 1 to 5 kg, primarily in the form of intra-abdominal fat (rather than subcutaneous fat, which confers less metabolic risk), and most likely occurs secondary to the associated estrogen deficiency. The Postmenopausal Estrogen Progesterone Interventions Trial (PEPI) was probably the first large-scale prospective trial demonstrating that this weight gain and body fat redistribution can be prevented with the use of hormone replacement therapy (HRT). While HRT is not indicated for weight reduction, its potential benefit in attenuating menopausal weight gain might be a consideration for its use in obese women with other indications for its use, such as osteoporosis or menopausal symptoms.

4. Cancer risk—Cancer risk increases with BMI for several types of cancer specific to women. While obesity reduces the risk of developing breast cancer in premenopausal women, increasing BMI correlates with increased breast cancer risk in the postmenopausal woman. In addition, the risk of ovarian, endometrial, colon, and gallbladder cancer is increased in obese women. Thus, minimizing weight gain in women may have important implications for minimizing cancer risk, particularly in those with other risk factors for these types of cancer.

Bongain A, Isnard V, Gillet JY: Obesity in obstetrics and gynaecology. Eur J Obstet Gynecol Reprod Biol 1998;77:217. [PMID: 9578282]

de Groot LC: High maternal body weight and pregnancy outcome. Nutr Rev 1999;57:62. [PMID: 10079705]

Espeland MA et al: Effect of postmenopausal hormone therapy on body weight and waist and hip girths. Postmenopausal Estrogen-Progestin Interventions Study Investigators. J Clin Endocrinol Metab 1997;82:1549. [PMID: 9141548]

Flegal KM et al: Prevalence and trends in obesity among US adults, 1999–2000. JAMA 2002;288:1723. [PMID: 12365955]

Galtier-Dereure F, Boegner C, Bringer J: Obesity and pregnancy: complications and cost. Am J Clin Nutr 2000;71 (5 Suppl):1242S. [PMID: 10799397]

Lu GC et al: The effect of the increasing prevalence of maternal obesity on perinatal morbidity. Am J Obstet Gynecol 2001;185:845. [PMID: 11641663]

Prevalence of overweight among children and adolescents: United States 1999. Washington, DC: National Center for Health Statistics: 2001.

Strauss RS, Pollack HA: Epidemic increase in childhood overweight, 1986–1998. JAMA 2001;286:2845. [PMID: 11735760]

Pathogenesis

A. Leptin

The basic equation governing body weight seems straightforward: Caloric flux = caloric consumption − caloric expenditure. Caloric consumption and expenditure have long been considered factors predominantly influenced by psychosocial elements of human society, but the discovery of leptin in 1995 revolutionized the understanding of body weight regulation. Zhang et al discovered that the ob/ob mouse, an inbred strain of mouse commonly used as a model of obesity and diabetes, failed to produce a novel, adipocyte-derived hormone, ultimately called leptin (from the Greek leptos, meaning thin). Leptin administration to these mice induced fat-specific weight loss, reduced food intake, restored fertility, and ameliorated their diabetes, suggesting that leptin plays a critical role in mammalian metabolism and body weight regulation. Leptin administration even reduced food intake and fat mass in otherwise normal mice. Thus, the discovery of leptin represented one of the first modern steps toward considering obesity as a disorder of body weight regulation at a physiologic and molecular level, rather than purely a psychological and motivational disease.

B. Current Models of Energy Homeostasis

1. Peripheral signals of fuel stores—Current models of energy homeostasis propose that some peripheral signal, either hormonal or neural, acts upon the hypothalamus to exert effects that regulate body weight in a fashion as tightly regulated as blood pressure or blood glucose (Figure 16–1). Some of the hormonal signals contributing to this process include leptin, insulin, and estradiol. As might be expected with hormones that exert classic negative feedback to control body weight, these hormones circulate in proportion to fat mass and their administration into the central nervous system (CNS) reduces food intake and can increase energy expenditure. Moreover, deficiency of these hormones is associated with increased food intake, while impaired signaling of these hormones within the CNS, particularly the hypothalamus, is associated with weight gain. Rising levels of these hormones (as might result from increased fat mass) engage hypothalamic neuronal systems that concomitantly (1) activate catabolic neurons (which reduce food intake and increase energy expenditure) and (2) inhibit anabolic neurons (which increase food intake and reduce energy expenditure). Conversely, declining levels of these hormones (as might occur with fasting or ovariectomy) inhibits catabolic

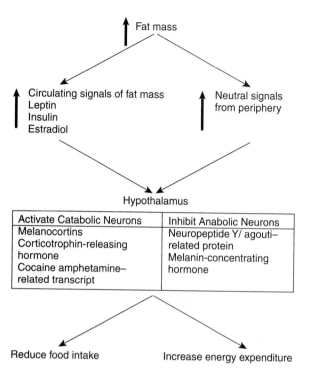

Figure 16–1. Proposed model for the regulation of energy balance. In this model, increasing fat mass leads to the production of hormonal and neural signals that act upon neuronal populations in the hypothalamus to maintain energy homeostasis. These neurons induce behaviors and physiology (reduced food intake and increased energy expenditure) that ultimately attenuate weight gain.

hypothalamic neuronal populations and activates anabolic neuronal populations. In this way, fasting or weight loss engage pathways that serve to preserve energy stores, contributing to the challenge of sustained weight loss.

2. Central effectors of peripheral signals—One example of these catabolic neuronal populations is the hypothalamic melanocortin system. Increased circulating leptin levels (such as might occur from weight gain due to high fat feeding or leptin administration to obese leptin-deficient mice) are proposed to induce behavior resulting in weight loss (or attenuating weight gain) by activation of these melanocortin neurons in the hypothalamus. In contrast, fasting is associated with reductions in leptin levels and hypothalamic melanocortin signaling, favoring behavior that increases food intake and reduction of energy expenditure. The role of the melanocortin system on body weight regulation is largely derived from characterization of genetic models with melanocortin signaling defects. Rodents and humans with defective melanocortin signaling are obese, while rodents that are genetically manipulated to overproduce melanocortins are lean. In fact, up to 10% of all morbidly obese humans may have defective melanocortin receptors, suggesting that melanocortin-agonist might represent a future therapy for obesity in humans.

A prototype anabolic neuronal population is the melanin concentrating hormone (MCH) system of the lateral hypothalamus. MCH administration into the brain of rodents increases food intake, while rodents lacking MCH are hypophagic and lean. No humans with defective MCH signaling have yet been identified, but from a theoretic perspective, development of an MCH antagonist might represent another mechanism by which to treat obesity. Other examples of anabolic signals include neuropeptide Y (produced by the hypothalamus) and ghrelin (a hormone of the stomach). Characterization of these anabolic signals may ultimately prove useful in treating wasting syndromes, such as seen with cancer.

Keeping this physiology in mind, it is probable that a combination of environmental and genetic elements affects these hormonal and hypothalamic signaling pathways in ways that contribute to human obesity. As an example, in certain strains of rodents, high-fat diets seem to impair hypothalamic leptin signaling, thereby reducing leptin's catabolic effects and potentially mediating the greater weight gain observed in these rodents, compared with rodents fed normal-fat diets. While many of these findings have yet to be clearly demonstrated in humans, initial insights into the body weight regulation of rodents have already contributed to the understanding of human obesity and a reasonable conclusion from these insights is that, while a poor diet and sedentary lifestyle contribute to obesity, the effect of these lifestyle choices on an individual's genetic capacity to regulate body weight may further compound the problem.

3. Estradiol as a catabolic signal—Interestingly, circulating leptin levels are higher in women than in men, even when comparing populations with similar fat mass. The significance of this effect, as well as the underlying mechanism by which it occurs, is not clear, but may reflect a contribution of gonadal steroids to energy balance. Estradiol, in particular, has characteristics of a classic hormonal negative-feedback signal of energy balance. In humans and rodents, fasting reduces estradiol levels, while weight gain increases estradiol levels. In rodents, estradiol administration potently induces hypophagia, loss of body fat, and increased lean mass, while estradiol deficiency results in fat-specific weight gain. The contribution of estradiol to body weight regulation in humans, however, is less substantial. In menstruating women, food intake is inversely related to estradiol levels and estrogen deficiency resulting from oophorectomy or menopause leads to ~2 kg weight gain. Estrogen's role in regulating the body weight of humans can also be assessed by examining the effects of estrogen deficiency and excess in men. While the body weight effects have not been well characterized, men with genetic aromatase deficiency (thereby inducing estrogen deficiency) are insulin resistant, a feature classically associated with accumulation of intra-abdominal fat. Male patients with gender dysphoria treated with high-dose estradiol represent a human model of estrogen excess, but it appears that estradiol has little effect on body weight and body composition in these patients. Thus, the contribution of estradiol to human energy homeostasis is probably small, but delineating the mechanism by which estrogens exert their catabolic effects in rodents may ultimately contribute to understanding human obesity.

Mystkowski P, Schwartz MW: Gonadal steroids and energy homeostasis in the leptin era. Nutrition 2000;16:937. [PMID: 11054599]

Schwartz MW et al: Central nervous system control of food intake. Nature 2000;404:661. [PMID: 10766253]

Zhang Y et al: Positional cloning of the mouse obese gene and its human homologue. Nature 1994;372:425. [PMID: 7984236]

Prevention

Primary prevention of obesity represents the ideal method of treating obesity and its comorbidities. Interestingly, however, few studies have prospectively evaluated methods for obesity prevention in populations. One of the strongest predictors of adult obesity is BMI during adolescence. Thus, interventions focused on achieving healthy body weight during this period may represent a particularly potent method of preventing obesity in adulthood.

A. IN UTERO CORRELATES TO ADULT BODY WEIGHT

The correlation between birth weight and adult BMI appears to be J-shaped, ie, extremes of birth weight increase the risk for developing adulthood obesity, although the specific mechanisms underlying these effects remain numerous and speculative.

Gestational diabetes that requires insulin treatment increases the risk of adulthood obesity for the offspring. In contrast, mild gestational diabetes (ie, well controlled with diet and exercise) does not appear to significantly increase the risk of adulthood obesity. Thus, aggressive prevention, detection, and management of gestational diabetes may confer some benefit to the offspring with respect to preventing obesity.

B. BREAST-FEEDING AND BODY WEIGHT

Several observational studies have suggested that increased duration of breast-feeding during infancy correlates with a protective effect against adulthood obesity in the offspring. While this intervention has not been prospectively evaluated, the possible beneficial effect of breast-feeding on the adult body weight of the offspring represents another potential benefit of breast-feeding.

C. POPULATION-BASED INTERVENTIONS WITH DEMONSTRATED EFFICACY

Few intervention trials have been performed that demonstrate efficacy in the prevention of fat gain during childhood and adolescence. In a 1999 study, children who watched less television and played fewer video games had a lower BMI than their sedentary counterparts. Until more data accumulates, it is difficult to make an evidence-based, comprehensive listing of formal recommendations to prevent the development of obesity in children, but some reasonable suggestions can be made (Table 16–1).

Dietz WH, Gortmaker SL: Preventing obesity in children and adolescents. Annu Rev Public Health 2001;22:337. [PMID: 11274525]

Gillman MW et al: Risk of overweight among adolescents who were breastfed as infants. JAMA 2001;285:2461. [PMID: 11368698]

Gortmaker SL et al: Reducing obesity via a school-based interdisciplinary intervention among youth: Planet Health. Arch Pediatr Adolesc Med 1999;153:409. [PMID: 10201726]

Robinson TN: Reducing children's television viewing to prevent obesity: a randomized controlled trial. JAMA 1999;282:1561. [PMID: 10546696]

Whitaker RC et al: Gestational diabetes and the risk of offspring obesity. Pediatrics 1998;101:E9. [PMID: 9445519]

Table 16–1. Suggestions for primary prevention of obesity in children.

Maternal interventions—particularly in high-risk mothers
Strive for healthy body weight before conception
Avoid excessive weight gain during pregnancy
Aggressively screen for and treat gestational diabetes in at-risk populations
Consider the potential beneficial effects of breast-feeding on the risk of obesity in the offspring

Family-based interventions
Consume a balanced diet with < 30% of calories from fat and high in fruits and vegetables
Minimize exposure to high-fat foods (i.e., rather than restricting access in the house, do not purchase these foods)
Limit time spent watching television or playing video games to < 2 hours per day or less
Create a climate in which physical activity is an attractive option for children rather than a mandate

School-based interventions
Reverse the decline in time spent during physical education
Make tasty, low-fat diets easily recognizable and available in cafeterias
Promote the value of healthy lifestyle choices (reduced television viewing, balanced low-fat diets, increased moderate to vigorous exercise)
Convey the promotion of these healthy lifestyles to parents

Whitaker RC, Dietz WH: Role of the prenatal environment in the development of obesity. J Pediatr 1998;132:768. [PMID: 9602184]

Clinical Findings

From the physician's perspective, one approach to the management of obesity is to focus the history and physical examination on 3 specific elements.

1. Identify barriers to weight loss

Several practical concerns can impair successful, sustained weight loss for a given patient. For example, specific dietary suggestions for a patient who cannot cook and eats out for most of their meals are different than for someone whose spouse cooks for them at home. Cultural factors can also have a significant impact on food choice.

Since many exercise programs require being outside, bad weather can impair the opportunity to exercise. In addition, obesity is more prevalent in poor, higher crime, urban areas, with a higher potential for more physical risk upon leaving the home. This problem can be circumvented by exercising in the home or in enclosed public areas (eg,

shopping malls, community centers, or church gyms) or by taking advantage of the increasing availability of work-related fitness centers.

Financial considerations can also impact on successful weight loss. Many patients cannot afford to join a club or purchase equipment that allows them to exercise at home. Low-fat foods, such as fruits and vegetables, tend to be more expensive than high-fat foods and many insurance companies do not cover obesity medication and surgical intervention. While pharmaceutical companies often have financial assistance programs, financing bariatric surgery is still a challenge. Some larger institutions have charity programs that assist with the financing of significant surgery. In addition, there is increasing pressure for legislation that might compel insurance companies to cover bariatric surgery in the future, particularly in patients with multiple obesity-related comorbidities.

Many of these practical barriers to successful weight loss can be addressed by formally enlisting the services of a social worker (who may be aware of community programs), a physical therapist (who can suggest activities a patient can easily access in their area), and a dietician who can assist with practical food choices.

2. Identify obesity-related comorbidities

Table 16–2 outlines suggested screening interventions for every patient with a BMI > 25 kg/m^2.

3. Evaluate for possible secondary causes of obesity

Using the analogy to hypertension, most obesity is "essential," but certain medical conditions and medications can contribute to weight gain and every patient should be evaluated, at least clinically, for the secondary causes of weight gain outlined in the following Differential Diagnosis section.

Differential Diagnosis

A. THYROID DISEASE

Thyroid hormone deficiency is commonly implicated as a cause of weight gain in the general population. However, several studies have demonstrated that the treatment of hypothyroidism does not typically lead to significant weight loss. Nonetheless, it seems reasonable to screen all overweight patients with a plasma thyroid-stimulating hormone, especially since hypothyroidism is an easily reversible disease with its own host of comorbidities, independent of its relatively small contribution to body weight. While classically associated with weight loss, hyperthyroidism may actually be associated with weight gain, likely as a result of increased appetite. Weight gain in this setting typically resolves when the patient is rendered euthyroid. Conversely, patients with

Table 16–2. Suggestions for screening for obesity-related comorbidities.

Obesity-related Comorbidity	Suggested Screening Mechanism
Diabetes	Yearly fasting glucose

Dyslipidemia
  Hypercholesterolemia
  Hypertriglyceridemia
  Low HDL syndrome
	Yearly fasting lipid panel, unless stable

Hypertension	Yearly blood pressure check

Cardiac disease
  Coronary artery disease
  Left ventricular hypertrophy
  Congestive heart failure
	Clinical history and document electrocardiogram in high-risk patients

Stroke and peripheral vascular disease	Evaluate if symptoms
Menstrual disturbances/infertility	Clinical history and examination
Degenerative joint disease	Clinical history and examination
Sleep apnea	Clinical history and examination
Restrictive and obstructive lung disease	Clinical history and examination
Gallstones	Evaluate if symptoms
Gastro-esophageal reflux disease (GERD)	Evaluate if symptoms
Hypogonadism	Evaluate if symptoms
Skin infections	Clinical history and examination
Colon cancer	Assess family history Consider flexible colonoscopy every 5 years after age 50
Endometrial cancer	Clinical history and examination
Breast cancer	Physical examination, and mammogram as indicated
Psychiatric disturbances	Clinical history and examination

hyperthyroidism who present with weight loss can be expected to gain roughly 3–5 kg once they are rendered euthyroid, irrespective of how this is achieved. Minimizing the degree to which a patient is hypothyroid after treatment for hyperthyroidism seems to attenuate this weight gain.

B. CORTISOL EXCESS

Endogenous and exogenous cortisol excess can lead to dramatic increases in body weight. Rapid weight gain (> 10% per year) is one of the most sensitive, albeit nonspecific, symptoms of endogenous cortisol excess. Other markers for cortisol excess include mood disturbance, hypertension, diabetes, and classic physical findings and symptoms (eg, buffalo hump, easy bruising, supraclavicular fat pad prominence, gluteal atrophy, and acanthosis nigricans). However, none of these findings are particularly specific to the syndrome.

The use of exogenous glucocorticoid therapy can typically be determined by the patient's medical history, and the best approach to minimizing weight gain in this setting is to minimize the dose administered. Patients with rapid weight gain and at least 2 other hallmark findings of Cushing's syndrome are reasonable candidates for screening for endogenous cortisol excess. The tests of choice for screening are either the overnight dexamethasone suppression test (1 mg of oral dexamethasone at 11 PM with a serum cortisol drawn at 8 AM the next day) or a 24-hour urine-free cortisol. Patients with cortisol excess will typically have morning cortisol values > 5 (after 1 mg of dexamethasone the night prior) or 24-hour urine cortisol values > 200. If cortisol excess is confirmed, further evaluation should probably be performed in consultation with an endocrinologist.

C. MEDICATIONS

Several classes of medication have been associated with weight gain, although typically the risk of weight gain is outweighed by the benefits of treatment with these medications. The mechanism by which weight gain occurs with these agents is not well known, but may reflect drug-induced impairment of CNS pathways that otherwise regulate body weight very tightly.

1. Drugs for diabetes—Ironically, intensive medical treatment of diabetes, a common morbidity of obesity, with insulin, sulfonylureas, or thiazolidinediones (TZDs) may contribute to further weight gain. In the Diabetes Control and Complications Trial, intensive insulin therapy of patients with type 1 diabetes was associated with a 4.75 kg weight gain, compared with less intensively treated controls. Interestingly, this increase in weight represented an increase in both lean and fat mass. In the United Kingdom Prospective Diabetes Study (UKPDS), intensive therapy with either insulin or sulfonylureas for patients with type 2 diabetes was associated with a 3.5 kg weight gain, compared with less intensively treated controls. The weight increase was more pronounced in patients treated with insulin (4 kg) than in patients treated with the sulfonylurea glibenclamide (1.7 kg) and did not correlate with improved glycemic control. Monotherapy with pioglitazone or rosiglitazone (TZDs) has been associated with ~3–4 kg increases in body weight, most of which is adipose tissue. Acarbose treatment in the UKPDS was weight neutral but had a higher dropout rate relative to other agents and was less potent (a 0.5% reduction in A1C over the 3-year treatment period).

Thus, the drug of choice for the obese patient with diabetes is probably metformin (see following section on Indirect Medical Therapy). Failing this, addition of sulfonylureas, TZDs, or insulin to metformin, rather than substitution, is likely to attenuate the weight gain side effect of intensive control. In addition, bedtime NPH (neutral protamine Hagedorn) seems to have less of an association with weight gain than daytime insulin administration.

2. Psychotropic medications—Older antipsychotics (eg, haloperidol and fluphenazine) seem to be associated with less weight gain (~ 0.5 kg) than some of the newer antipsychotics. Clozapine and olanzapine have been associated with ~4 kg weight gain during 10 weeks of treatment, while risperidone seems to be associated with ~2 kg weight gain. Treatment with molindone, an older antipsychotic, is actually associated with slight weight loss. Lithium therapy has also been associated with weight gain (sometimes dramatic), although alternative agents for bipolar illness (such as carbamazepine and valproic acid) are also associated with weight gain.

Broad generalizations can be made regarding the risk of weight gain associated with the use of antidepressant medications. Tricyclic antidepressants (TCAs) are classically associated with weight gain (up to 1.4 kg/month of therapy) and amitriptyline, compared with nortriptyline and imipramine, seems to be the agent with the highest risk. Selective serotonin reuptake inhibitors (SSRIs) can also have significant effects on body weight. Both sertraline and paroxetine have been associated with weight gain, with increases ranging from 7–26% in patients treated with paroxetine. Fluoxetine, in contrast, is associated with an initial temporary weight loss. Bupropion has been classically associated with a ~1 kg weight loss versus placebo, nefazodone seems to be weight neutral, and mirtazapine is implicated with significant weight gain.

Thus, if weight gain effects have a significant influence on the choice of antidepressant medication, it seems prudent to consider the newer SSRIs, bupropion, and nefazodone as first-line agents, while using other agents, particularly the TCAs, as second-line therapy.

3. Antiseizure medications—In addition to their antiseizure indications, these agents are increasingly being used to treat various pain syndromes, particularly painful diabetic neuropathies. While therapeutic efficacy is of the utmost importance in choosing one of these drugs, considering their effects on body weight may be useful for patients whose treatment options are less restrictive. Carbamazepine, valproic acid, vigabatrin, and gabapentin are all implicated in weight gain to various degrees. The degree of weight gain appears to be dose-dependent with valproic acid and gabapentin. Phenytoin and phenobarbital appear to be weight neutral.

4. Other medications—Hormonal methods of birth control have also been implicated in weight gain, but when formally studied, the effect appears to be small in most populations, on the order of 0.3 kg. Minimizing the amount of progesterone (or the relative androgenicity) in oral contraceptive formulations and avoiding depot-medroxyprogesterone may reduce the risk of weight gain associated with these methods of birth control.

Some of the central-acting antihypertensive agents (eg, clonidine and methyldopa) have also been associated with weight gain, although the degree to which they contribute is not clear. The use of weight neutral agents, including angiotensin-converting enzyme (ACE) inhibitors, β-blockers other than propranolol, and calcium-channel blockers other than nisoldipine, may minimize the effects of hypertension therapy on body weight.

Allison DB, Casey DE: Antipsychotic-induced weight gain: a review of the literature. J Clin Psychiatry 2001;62(Suppl 7):22. [PMID: 11346192]

Fava M: Weight gain and antidepressants. J Clin Psychiatry 2000;61(Suppl 11):37. [PMID: 10926053]

Gupta S: Weight gain on the combined pill—is it real? Hum Reprod Update 2000;6:427. [PMID: 11045873]

Holman RR, Cull CA, Turner RC: A randomized double-blind trial of acarbose in type 2 diabetes shows improved glycemic control over 3 years (U.K. Prospective Diabetes Study 44) Diabetes Care 1999;22:960. [PMID: 10372249]

Intensive blood-glucose control with sulfonylureas or insulin compared with conventional treatment and risk of complications in patients with type 2 diabetes (UKPDS 33). UK Prospective Diabetes Study (UKPDS) Group. Lancet 1998;352:837. [PMID: 9742976]

Jallon P, Picard F: Bodyweight gain and anticonvulsants: a comparative review. Drug Saf 2001;24:969. [PMID: 11735653]

Miyazaki Y et al: Improved glycemic control and enhanced insulin sensitivity in type 2 diabetic subjects treated with pioglitazone. Diabetes Care 2001;24:710. [PMID: 11315836]

Complications

A. MEDICAL

The medical complications associated with obesity are summarized in Table 16–2. In general, the risk of developing these conditions correlates with increasing BMI, and weight loss has been demonstrated to improve the management of these disorders. Moreover, for patients with BMI values over 30 kg/m^2, mortality risk is also directly correlated to increasing BMI. Few studies have prospectively assessed the potential mortality benefit in patients with intentional weight loss, although Williamson found that in obese patients with diabetes, intentional weight loss was associated with a 25% reduction in mortality over a 12-year period.

B. PSYCHOSOCIAL

Obesity is associated with work discrimination, depression, suicide, binge-eating disorder, sexual abuse, body image distortion, and relatively reduced quality of life. Many have argued that some of these psychosocial disturbances are causative factors in weight gain, suggesting that weight loss would not result in the improvement of these morbidities. This notion, however, is not clearly supported by the literature.

Depression and anxiety scores improve in the first year after bariatric surgery (see following Treatment section). While this is encouraging, the Swedish Obesity Study (which prospectively compared the effects of bariatric surgery on obese patients with patients treated with behavioral intervention) demonstrates that these improvements may not be fully sustained at 2 years postoperatively, suggesting that while depression and obesity may be closely linked comorbidities, one does not appear to cause the other. Nonetheless, given the relatively increased prevalence of psychiatric illness in the obese population, it seems prudent to address the issue and consider formal psychological intervention to optimize the well-being of the obese patient.

Quality of life is another factor significantly influenced by body weight. While patients in the Swedish Obesity Study took more sick leave in the first year postoperatively, the number of sick leave days per year gradually declined to below that of controls in a weight-loss dependent fashion over 4 years. Patients in the surgical group also reported significant improvements in health-related quality of life, compared with controls. Similarly, the Nurses Health Study demonstrated that weight gain was associated with impairments in quality of life scores that seemed to improve with weight loss. Thus, improved quality of life should be another consideration when counseling a patient about the benefits of weight loss.

Fine JT et al: A prospective study of weight change and health-related quality of life in women. JAMA 1999;282:2136. [PMID: 10591335]

Wadden TA et al: Psychosocial aspects of obesity and obesity surgery. Surg Clin North Am 2001;81:1001. [PMID: 11589242]

Williamson DF et al: Intentional weight loss and mortality among overweight individuals with diabetes. Diabetes Care 2000;23:1499. [PMID: 11023143]

Treatment

A. INDICATIONS FOR THERAPY

Patients with a BMI > 25 kg/m^2 are candidates for diet and exercise intervention. Patients with a BMI > 30 kg/m^2 or > 28 kg/m^2 with two or more obesity related comorbidities are candidates for medical therapy in conjunction with diet and exercise intervention (see below). Patients should be considered for surgical therapy of obesity (bariatric surgery) if they (1) have a BMI > 40 kg/m^2 or > 35 kg/m^2 and 2 or more obesity related co-morbidities, (2) have failed diet, exercise, and medical intervention, and (3) are otherwise psychosocially fit for surgery.

B. TREATMENT GOALS

One of the keys to achieving successful lifestyle change is to set reasonable goals. For example, most population-based studies would suggest it is highly unlikely for a 300-pound patient to achieve a weight loss of 100 lbs in 1 year due to lifestyle intervention and sustain this lifelong. This degree of weight loss entails a commitment to lifestyle change that most patients are not willing or able to achieve. Thus, while this degree of weight loss should be commended if it occurs, it is statistically unreasonable to expect it.

Reasonable goals for the physician are (1) to identify and treat obesity related co-morbidities, (2) assess patients for secondary causes of obesity, (3) encourage LIFELONG diet and exercise intervention, and (4) provide treatment options, recognizing their limitations.

Reasonable goals for most patients are to (1) comply with the suggested treatment regimen, (2) recognize that these changes must occur lifelong to maintain efficacy, and (3) aim for ~10% weight loss or even attenuation of weight gain. A goal rate of change should be ~1–2 pounds per week.

C. DIET

Lifestyle modification including sustainable changes in diet and increased exercise is probably the safest form of therapy for obesity available. However, the finding that ~90% of patients who lose weight regain that weight by 5 years suggests that lifestyle modification is difficult for most patients to maintain. Nonetheless, several recommendations regarding the goals of diet and exercise can be made based on their effects on metabolic risk from obesity as well as their association with sustained weight loss.

Since much of the metabolic risk from obesity is related to adverse affects on the cardiovascular system, it seems prudent to follow guidelines that minimize this risk. The American Heart Association (AHA) dietary guidelines represent current best evidence and opinion on dietary interventions that optimize lipid profile and blood pressure for a general population and are summarized in the Box. Dietary guidelines to achieve weight loss and weight maintenance are more controversial. At any given moment, there are a host of books on the New York Times Bestseller list advocating a particular diet over another. In fact, many of these diets promote variations of the same themes Table 16–3. Clearly, a reduction in caloric intake is required to achieve sustained weight loss, yet the degree to which this should occur, as well as the best mechanism for achieving this is still not clear.

Some insight into effective dietary strategies for weight loss and maintenance can be gleaned from data from the National Weight Control Registry (NWCR), a database of patients who have successfully, intentionally, and persistently reduced their weight by 30 pounds for > 1 year. Patients in this cohort reported an average weight loss of 30 kg, a mean reduction in BMI of 10 kg/m^2, and duration of weight loss maintenance of 5.5 years. These body weight effects were associated with a mean caloric consumption of 1381 kcal/day, with 24% of these calories derived from fat. Astrup et al recently evaluated the efficacy of low-fat, but freely feeding, intervention trials on weight loss and concluded that a 10.2 % reduction in fat calories was associated with ~3.2 kg weight loss maintenance. Thus, the association of consumption of a low-fat diet with sustained weight loss, in concert with the diet's beneficial effects on cardiovascular risk, suggest that a diet with < 30% of calo-

Table 16–3. Categorization of some popular diet programs.

Moderate Fat, High Carbohydrate, Moderate Protein	High Fat, Low Carbohydrate	Low Fat, Very High Carbohydrate, Moderate Protein
DASH diet	Dr. Atkins diet revolution	Ornish Diet
USDA food pyramid guide	Protein Power	Eat More, Weigh Less
Weight Watchers	The Carbohydrate Addict's Diet	The New Pritikin Program
ADA diet	Dr. Bernstein's Diabetes Solution	
	Life Without Bread	

USDA, United States Department of Agriculture; ADA, America Diabetes Association.

ries from fat is probably the best recommendation for most overweight and obese patients, a diet consistent with the AHA guidelines. The National Heart, Lung, and Blood Institute suggests that a woman reduce her caloric intake by 500-1000 kcal/day, or strive for a goal of 1000-1200 kcal/d. Very low calorie diets (VLCD, < 800 kcal/d) are not recommended for prolonged weight loss maintenance due to their associated risk of nutritional deficiencies and their lack of benefit, relative to conventional low calorie diets (LCD, < 1800 kcal/day), on weight loss at one year. The importance of formal consultation with a nutritionist to achieve these nutritional goals cannot be overemphasized.

AMERICAN HEART ASSOCIATION DIETARY GUIDELINES 2000

Consume a variety of fruits and vegetables (5 or more servings per day) and a variety of grain products (6 or more servings per day)

Limit intake of

- Saturated fat to < 10% of daily caloric intake, < 7% if low-density lipoprotein (LDL) cholesterol level is elevated

- Trans-fatty acid (found in foods containing partially hydrogenated vegetable oils) to < 10% of daily caloric intake

- Cholesterol to < 300 mg/d, < 200 mg/d if LDL cholesterol level is elevated

- Sodium < 2.4 g/d

- Alcohol to ≤ 1 glass per day for women and ≤ 2 glasses per day for men

D. EXERCISE

Exercise intervention alone (without reductions in caloric intake) is typically only associated with modest reductions (~1 to 2.5 kg) in body weight relative to non-exercising controls. However, exercise intervention can improve cardiovascular fitness (as measured by oxygen consumption) by up to 16%, independent of its effects on body weight. Moreover, patients in the NWCR reported that their weight loss was associated with the equivalent of 1 hour of moderate physical activity per day. Only 9% of this cohort reported that their weight loss occurred without substantial increases in physical activity. These findings support the notion that increased physical activity has beneficial effects on inducing and maintaining weight loss, while improving cardiovascular fitness independent of weight loss, a point that should be emphasized with patients. It is a common experience that many patients embark upon an exercise regimen, only to stop if they do not observe a weight loss benefit. It is imperative, however, that physicians encourage their patients to exercise independent of the weight loss effects, since the cardiovascular benefits are substantial.

Another challenge has been making evidence based recommendations regarding the type and duration of exercise. Initial recommendations are dependent upon the functional status of an individual but, since most patients are able to engage in walking as physical activity, initial goals of walking 30 minutes per day 3 times per week are reasonable. Within limits, the more frequently that an activity be engaged and sustained, the greater the potential benefit. Special precautions should be observed in patients at risk for coronary artery disease and these patients should probably undergo formal treadmill testing to assess functional status and cardiovascular risk. In patients who have difficulty walking, eg, due to musculoskeletal problems, then non–weight bearing exercises, such as cycling and swimming, may be a useful option. Consultation with a physical therapist for the determination of exercises that an individual patient can perform is often useful.

One of the most critical roles of the physician in engaging dietary and exercise interventions for our patients is to emphasize that these interventions need to represent lifestyle changes, not just short-term whims. We must educate patients that regression to previous habits will lead to regression to previous weight, while also assisting them with achieving changes that can be sustained lifelong.

E. INDIRECT MEDICAL THERAPY

1. Metformin—In the UKPDS, the 2–5 kg weight gain related to intensive diabetes treatment with sulfonylureas or insulin did not occur in patients treated with metformin. While the specific mechanism for this effect is unknown, metformin is generally well tolerated, reduces the risk of cardiovascular complications in patients treated for diabetes, and does not lead to weight gain, thereby suggesting that metformin should probably represent the first-line agent in treating the overweight or obese patient with diabetes.

Metformin has been studied as a primary weight loss agent in obese patients without diabetes (initial mean BMI = ~32 kg/m^2) and is associated with about 1 kg weight loss over 1 year compared with placebo-treated controls.

2. Estrogen replacement—While there is no clear evidence that pharmacologic estrogen treatment of humans, unlike rodents, induces weight loss, the PEPI trial suggests that HRT may attenuate the weight gain associated with menopause. Thus, it seems reasonable to consider this beneficial effect when presenting the option of HRT to women for other indications, such as symptomatic hot flashes or osteoporosis. Certainly,

however, HRT would not be indicated for weight loss alone.

F. DIRECT MEDICAL THERAPY

There are currently only 3 weight control agents approved by the US Food and Drug Administration (FDA): phentermine, sibutramine, and orlistat. Given the redundant physiology regulating body weight, these agents probably must be continued indefinitely to maintain weight loss, although the efficacy or safety of these agents with use longer than 1 year has not been clearly established. In addition, insurance companies have been reluctant to pay for these agents, making their lifelong use not only potentially risky but also potentially expensive. Nonetheless, these agents may positively contribute to the psychological aspects of "jump-starting" weight loss programs and can be used to break the cycle of elements contributing to excess body weight. As an example, overweight or obese patients with joint pain that limits exercise may have less pain as a result of weight loss induced by these agents, thereby allowing more exercise to occur.

Medical therapy for obesity is indicated for patients with a BMI > 30 kg/m^2 or a BMI > 28 kg/m^2 with 2 or more obesity-related comorbidities. While monotherapy is generally the first choice, phentermine or sibutramine can also be used in conjunction with orlistat, although there is little published evidence documenting synergistic effects.

1. Phentermine—This drug induces anorexia by increasing noradrenergic signaling in the CNS. It has gained some notoriety as half of the fenfluramine/phentermine ("fen/phen") combination that was associated with cardiac abnormalities, which ultimately led to the FDA withdrawing fenfluramine from the market. In general, it is fairly well tolerated but should not be used in patients with uncontrolled hypertension or those at risk for cardiac dysrhythmias. In addition, it is a schedule IV drug and should be used cautiously in patients with a history of stimulant drug abuse. The longest available prospective trials evaluating the effect of phentermine on body weight demonstrated an 8.1% weight loss over 9 months compared with placebo. Phentermine is relatively inexpensive and in 2002 cost approximately $23 per month.

2. Sibutramine—This medication also acts centrally to block uptake of norepinephrine and serotonin, resulting in anorexia and possibly an increase of energy expenditure. It is also a schedule IV drug and its contraindications and side effect profile are similar to that of phentermine with a comparable weight loss effect. In a 2001 study, sibutramine responders sustained a 4% weight loss versus placebo after 44 weeks. In 2002, sibutramine cost roughly $100 per month.

3. Orlistat—This agent is not absorbed systemically and inhibits the action of pancreatic lipase, thereby blocking absorption of 30% of fat calories. Fatty diarrhea, which can often be unpredictable if the patient is noncompliant with a low-fat diet, is its major side effect and can significantly impair compliance. Another potential side effect is the malabsorption of fat-soluble vitamins. Thus, orlistat must be prescribed with fat-soluble vitamin supplementation. In a 1999 study, 120 mg/d of orlistat for 104 weeks resulted in a 4% weight loss, compared with placebo. The cost of 1 month of treatment with orlistat in 2002 (120 mg three times daily) was about $110.

G. Surgery

Surgical treatment of obesity probably represents the most effective method currently available for achieving significant long-term weight loss. In general, surgery is indicated for patients who have been unable to achieve weight loss after 1 year of standard dietary, exercise, and medical intervention and who have a BMI > 40 kg/m^2 or a BMI > 35 kg/m^2 plus 2 obesity-related comorbidities.

Bariatric surgery induces weight loss by restricting the amount of food ingested and inducing malabsorption. Several different surgeries have been proposed over the years, but the currently recommended procedures of choice are the Roux-en-Y gastric bypass procedure (GBP) and the vertical-banded gastroplasty (VBG), both of which are restrictive procedures endorsed by a National Institute of Health (NIH) consensus conference in 1991. However, based on prospective studies performed subsequent to the development of these guidelines, GBP is probably the superior procedure with respect to efficacy and safety.

In GBP, a 10–30 mL portion of the stomach cardia is transected from the remainder of the stomach. The jejunum is then split and the proximal end of the distal part of the jejunum is anastomosed to the cardia via a gastrojejunostomy, forming the Roux-en-Y portion of the procedure. Thus, food travels through the cardia into the distal half of the jejunum and ileum, "bypassing" the majority of the stomach and the duodenum and proximal jejunum. The distal end of the proximal jejunum (which drains the bypassed portion of the stomach and duodenum) is then anastomosed to the distal second part of the jejunum via a jejunojejunostomy, allowing acid and digestive enzymes of the stomach, liver, and pancreas to digest food that ultimately reaches the distal jejunum and ileum via the cardia and Roux-en-Y portion of the jejunum (Figure 16–2).

The small cardiac pouch and the reduced exposure to digestive products of the foregut induce a restrictive physiology as well as a "dumping syndrome," if dietary indiscretions occur. In this dumping syndrome, high

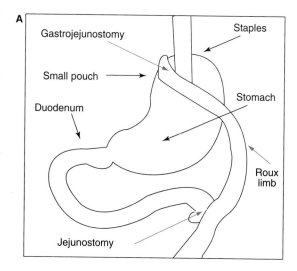

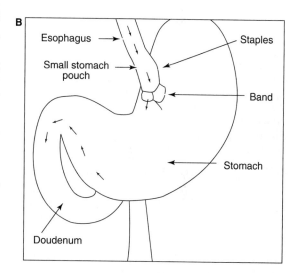

Figure 16–2. Two Common Surgical Procedures for Inducing Weight Loss (Bariatric Surgery) **A:** Roux-en-Y Gastric Bypass (GBP) In this procedure, formation of a 10-30 cc gastric pouch pouch induces restrictive physiology. The jejunostomy drains gastric and pancreaticobiliary secretions into the alimentary stream and reduces the risk of bile reflux esophagitis. The standard GBP (short-limb) calls for a 50 cm roux limb. Increasing the length of the roux limb to 100 cm (long-limb GBP) may improve weight loss but also increases malabsorption and risk of nutritional sequelae (eg, osteopenia). **B:** Vertical Banded Gastroplasty (VBG) In this procedure, weight loss is primarily induced by restrictive physiology, without malabsorption. The procedure is easier to perform than GBP but is less efficacious and can lead to troublesome vomiting and gastroesophageal reflux. Few centers are currently performing this procedure.

carbohydrate liquid meals pass through the proximal gut too quickly to be adequately digested, resulting in nausea, diarrhea, diaphoresis, and light-headedness. These symptoms function as potent negative conditioning responses that further facilitate the efficacy of the surgery, particularly during the first year after surgery.

Several studies have demonstrated the long-term efficacy and safety of bariatric procedures, but few have done so in a prospective fashion. Perhaps the largest study to prospectively evaluate the effects of bariatric surgery versus usual care is the Swedish Obesity Study (SOS). Started in 1987, this study used 18 criteria to match patients treated with behavioral intervention to patients treated with surgery. The 3 surgeries performed were gastric banding (where a band is used to constrict the proximal stomach to induce restrictive physiology), VBG, or GBP. The overall complication rate in the 251 patients who underwent surgery was ~13%; 2.2% of all patients required another operation, and there was a perioperative mortality rate of 0.2%.

The initial BMI in both groups was 41 kg/m². Eight years after enrollment, patients who had surgical intervention showed a 16% weight loss (with the most pronounced effects in the GBP group), a 5-fold risk reduction for the development of diabetes, and significant improvements in quality of life and missed days from work, compared with control patients treated with behavioral intervention. Interestingly, there was no difference in blood pressure between groups at the 8-year follow-up period, but the mechanism for this effect is not clear. More data are required to fully assess whether these interventions improve mortality.

Thus, while medical therapy plays a role in the treatment of morbid obesity, surgical intervention remains the most effective long-term method of sustained weight loss and probably represents the treatment of choice for patients with multiple obesity-related comorbidities. Unfortunately, access to a surgeon experienced with these procedures can be limited.

H. COMPLEMENTARY THERAPY

Allison et al recently reviewed a host of alternative medicine approaches to weight loss. A treatment was considered "alternative" if it was *not* categorized as the following: (1) FDA-approved for weight loss, (2) an agent under development by a pharmaceutical company, (3) surgery, (4) cognitive-behavioral techniques to promote weight-reducing changes in diet and exercise behavior. While many of the trials testing the efficacy of these techniques demonstrated benefit in uncontrolled case series, few alternative interventions have been rigorously tested in randomized, controlled trials. Therefore, firm conclusions regarding the efficacy of specific interventions may be hard to clearly justify because of the absence of well-designed prospective trials. In addition,

health care providers are reminded that "natural" and safe can be mutually exclusive, as evidenced by the use of ma huang, a plant-derived ephedrine. The FDA is currently evaluating limitations on the amounts of ma huang available in over-the-counter preparations, since it has been associated with heart attack, seizure, dysrhythmias, high blood pressure, and even death. Another consideration in the use of alternative medical treatments is that the FDA does not directly regulate most of these agents; therefore, potency and purity for a given product may be highly variable. Nonetheless, a summary of the effects of some popular interventions is shown in Table 16–4.

[No authors listed] Effect of intensive blood-glucose control with metformin on complications in overweight patients with type 2 diabetes (UKPDS 34). UK Prospective Diabetes Study (UKPDS) Group. Lancet 1998;352:854. [PMID: 9742977]

[No authors listed] NIH conference. Gastrointestinal surgery for severe obesity. Consensus Development Conference Panel. Ann Intern Med 1991;115:956. [PMID: 1952493]

Allison DB et al: Alternative treatments for weight loss: a critical review. Crit Rev Food Sci Nutr 2001;41:1; discussion 39. [PMID: 11152041]

Astrup A et al: The role of low-fat diets in body weight control: a meta-analysis of ad libitum dietary intervention studies. Int J Obes Relat Metab Disord 2000;24:1545. [PMID: 11126204]

Balsiger BM et al: Bariatric surgery. Surgery for weight control in patients with morbid obesity. Med Clin North Am 2000; 84:477. [PMID: 10793653]

Charles MA et al: Effect of weight change and metformin on fibrinolysis and the von Willebrand factor in obese nondiabetic subjects: the BIGPRO1 Study. Biguanides and the Prevention of the Risk of Obesity. Diabetes Care 1998;21:1967. [PMID: 9802752]

Freedman MR, King J, Kennedy E: Popular diets: a scientific review. Obes Res 2001;9(Suppl 1):1S. [PMID: 11374180]

Krauss RM et al: AHA Dietary Guidelines: revision 2000: A statement for healthcare professionals from the Nutrition Com-

Table 16–4. Summary of some alternative methods of weight control.

Intervention	Effect on Obesity
Acupuncture	Few randomized trials, no clear benefit
Acupressure	Few randomized trials, no clear benefit
Hypnosis	Possible modest benefit, possible adverse psychological effects in adolescents
St. John's wort	Few randomized trials, no benefit
DHEA	May improve body composition, toxicity of long-term use not known

DHEA, dihydroepiandrostenedione.

mittee of the American Heart Association. Circulation 2000;102:2284. [PMID: 11056107]

Torgerson JS, Sjostrom L: The Swedish Obese Subjects (SOS) study–rationale and results. Int J Obes Relat Metab Disord 2001;25(Suppl 1):S2. [PMID: 11466577]

Wirth A, Krause J: Long-term weight loss with sibutramine: a randomized controlled trial. JAMA 2001;286:1331. [PMID: 11560538]

Yanovski SZ, Yanovski JA: Pharmacotherapy for obesity. N Engl J Med 2002;346:591. [PMID: 11856799]

When to Refer to a Specialist

Endocrinology referral should be considered for patients who have failed to achieve attenuation of weight gain or a 10% weight loss after a formal 1-year trial of diet and exercise intervention. The primary goals of this assessment would be to reevaluate treatment goals, obesity-related comorbidities, and medical and surgical treatment options. In addition, endocrinology consultation should be considered in patients with documented thyroid dysfunction, evidence of cortisol excess, or refractory hypercholesterolemia.

Relevant Web Sites

[The National Heart, Lung, and Blood Institute (NHLBI) Clinical Guidelines on the Identification, Evaluation, and Treatment of Overweight and Obesity in Adults is an evidence based, comprehensive review of the management of the overweight and obese patient. This is an excellent and complete reference for healthcare providers.]
http://www.nhlbi.nih.gov/guidelines/obesity/ob_home.htm

[The CDC maintains a web site tracking body weight and diabetes trends in the United States] http://
www.cdc.gov/nccdphp /dnpa/obesity/trend/index.htm

[The NIH maintains an information site for patients on obesity surgery]
http://www.niddk.nih.gov/health/nutrit/pubs/gasturg.htm

[The US Surgeon General has renewed the promotion of overweight and obesity as a public health risk]
http://www.surgeongeneral.gov/topics/obesity/default.htm

[Healthfinder is a government sponsored web site with links to various useful sites]
http://www.healthfinder.gov/scripts/SearchContext.asp?topic=592

[Aim for a Healthy Weight is an NHLBI site intended for patients and healthcare providers and maintains links and information on a broad array of obesity-related topics. It also contains some useful Palm programs for BMI assessment and dietary planning.]
http://www.nhlbi.nih.gov/health/public/heart/obesity/lose_wt/index.htm

[The National Weight Control Registry maintains a web site that updates their most recent findings and also allows for patient recruitment into the study. This has many other useful links for both patients and providers.]
http://www.lifespan.org/services/bmed/wt_loss/nwcr/

Thyroid Disorders

17

James W. Benson, Jr, MD

Thyroid disorders are more common in women than men. Graves' disease favors women by a ratio of 10:1, and thyroid nodules are 3 times more common in women than men. Postpartum autoimmune thyroiditis and struma ovarii are of course unique to female patients.

Because 1.4% of women older than 50 years may have unsuspected, overt hypothyroidism or hyperthyroidism, the American College of Physicians has recommended that women over the age of 50 be screened with a thyroid-stimulating hormone (TSH) measurement. If the TSH is undetectable or 10 mIU/L or more, a free T4 should be done.

GENERAL CONSIDERATIONS

To appreciate the changes in circulating thyroid hormone concentrations in thyroidal and nonthyroidal disease, it is necessary to understand normal thyroid physiology, including synthesis, protein binding, and peripheral metabolism.

Inorganic iodide is transported actively into the thyroid gland for use in synthesis of thyroid hormone, which involves 3 steps (Figure 17–1): (1) organification occurs when iodide is bound to tyrosine residues attached to the large intrathyroidal protein thyroglobulin, (2) iodotyrosines are coupled to form triiodothyronine (T3) and thyroxine (T4), and (3) proteolysis frees T4 and T3 from thyroglobulin for release into the circulation. Both iodide uptake and thyroid hormone synthesis are stimulated by thyrotropin, or TSH, secreted by the pituitary gland. Circulating thyroid hormones exert negative feedback on TSH, which is under the control of hypothalamic thyrotropin-releasing hormone (TRH) (Figure 17–2).

More than 99% of thyroid hormone in the bloodstream is bound to thyroxine-binding globulin (TBG), albumin, and prealbumin. Only unbound, "free" T4 and T3 are biologically active. Processes that increase TBG transiently decrease the levels of free T4 and T3, because hormone attaches to open binding sites. Rapid equilibration occurs, however, as the low level of free thyroid hormone decreases its own disposal rate by autoregulation, reaching a new steady state with normal levels of free T4 and T3.

The peripheral metabolism of T4 is critical for hormone action and is affected significantly by nonthy-roidal factors, especially during acute illness. Thyroxine is degraded by removal of iodine (deiodination) (Figure 17–3). Removal of an iodine from the outer ring by 5'-deiodinase to form T3 accounts for 50% of the metabolic fate of T4. Of circulating T3, 80% is produced by deiodination of T4 and 20% by direct thyroidal secretion. Biologic activity of T3 is at least twice that of T4, although the plasma concentration is only 1/50 that of T4. Because T4 is converted intracellularly to T3, it is unclear whether T4 is just a prehormone for T3 or has independent biologic potency. The other 50% of T4 is deiodinated at the inner ring by 5-deiodinase to form reverse T3 (rT3), which is biologically inactive.

HYPERTHYROXINEMIA (INCREASED T4)

An elevated T4 is not uncommon, and the differential diagnosis for it is large. Table 17–1 outlines the possible causes of this condition. It may occur with thyrotoxicosis or euthyroidism.

THYROTOXICOSIS

ESSENTIALS OF DIAGNOSIS

- *Tachycardia.*
- *Tremor.*
- *Hyperkinesis.*
- *Weight loss.*
- *Nervousness.*

Clinical Findings

A. SYMPTOMS AND SIGNS

The first step in evaluating the patient is to identify clinical thyrotoxicosis. Thyrotoxic patients under the age of 60 years usually manifest all the signs and symptoms of hyperthyroidism. In the elderly, only weight loss, tachycardia (especially atrial fibrillation), or failure to thrive may be present. Detection during pregnancy may be particularly difficult because findings of hypermetabolism (except for weight loss) are consistent with pregnancy itself. The signs of thyrotoxicosis are as fol-

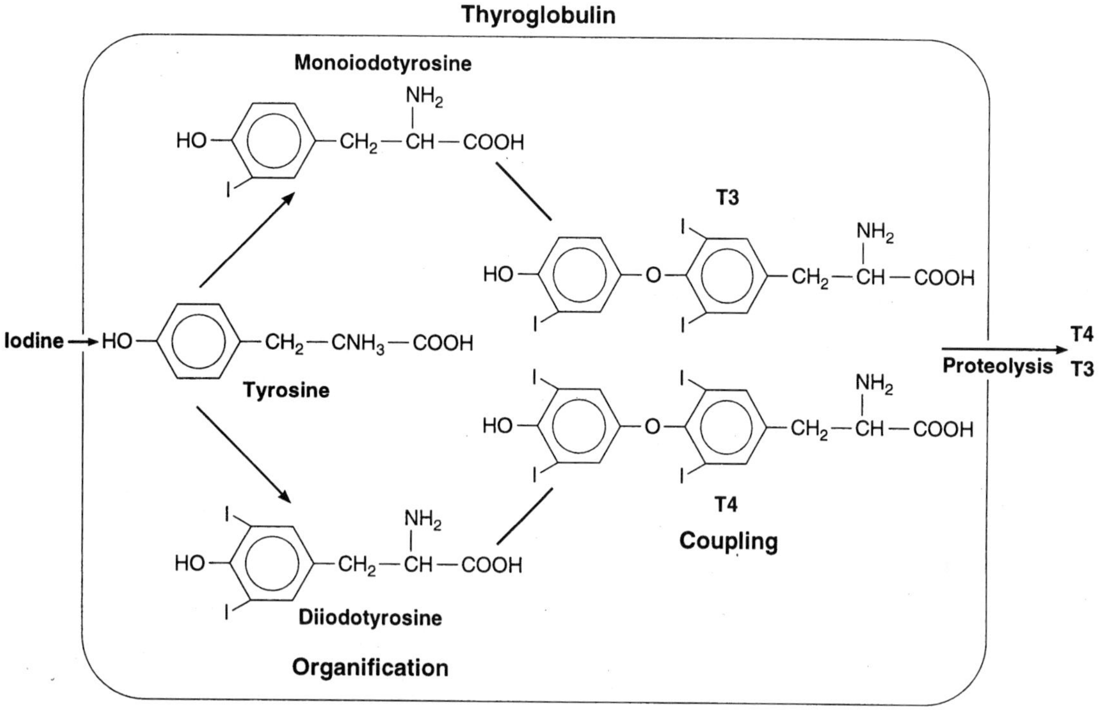

Thyroglobulin

Figure 17–1. Thyroid hormone synthesis.

lows: (1) tachycardia, (2) tremor, (3) skin changes, (4) hyperkinesis, (5) lid lag, (6) muscle weakness, and (7) systolic hypertension (wide pulse pressure).

Patients may present with a variety of possible symptoms: weight loss, palpitations, heat intolerance, shakiness, hyperdefecation, insomnia, nervousness, polydipsia, oligomenorrhea or amenorrhea, or easy fatigability.

Graves' disease, the most common cause of thyrotoxicosis, is an autoimmune disorder mediated by thyroid-stimulating immunoglobulin (TSI) usually presenting in patients between 20 and 50 years of age. Graves' orbitopathy can be detected in most patients using sensitive testing, but clinically significant disease characterized by exophthalmos, congestive findings of conjunctival injection and chemosis, periorbital edema, and paresis of extraocular muscles occurs in only 50% of patients. In most patients in whom eye disease develops, clinical findings occur within 6 months before or after the onset of thyrotoxicosis. The severity of orbitopathy is unrelated to the level of thyroid hormone and probably is mediated by a related but different immune phenomenon. Lid lag alone is not an indicator of Graves' orbitopathy because it is mediated by sympathomimetic activity, which is increased in all forms of thyrotoxicosis. Decreased visual acuity from optic nerve compression is a rare complication. Patients with clini-

cally apparent orbitopathy should be referred to an ophthalmologist for baseline measurement of exophthalmos and visual acuity. Any patient complaining of progressive exophthalmos, decreased visual acuity, or diplopia should be reassessed by an ophthalmologist.

The cause of toxic nodule and toxic multinodular goiter is unknown, but these conditions do not appear to be autoimmune in nature and are not associated with eye disease or other autoimmune diseases.

Hydatidiform mole and choriocarcinoma both can produce human chorionic gonadotropin (HCG), which is homologous to TSH. Occasionally, enough HCG is produced to cause clinical thyrotoxicosis. This unusual cause of hyperthyroidism should be considered if there is anything to suggest retained products of conception.

Subacute thyroiditis is virally mediated, with biopsy showing polymorphonuclear leukocytes (PMNs) and giant cells. A prodrome of fever, myalgia, headache, and occasionally upper respiratory tract infection is followed by exquisite tenderness of the diffusely enlarged thyroid gland, signs and symptoms of thyrotoxicosis, and an elevated erythrocyte sedimentation rate (ESR). Spontaneous resolution occurs uniformly within 4–6 weeks, usually with a transient period of hypothyroidism. Permanent thyroid dysfunction or recurrence is rare.

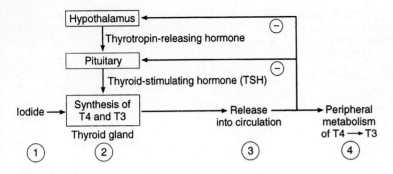

Figure 17–2. Normal thyroid physiology.

Autoimmune (painless) thyroiditis is an indolent disorder; biopsy shows lymphocytic infiltration. The thyroid gland is diffusely enlarged and nontender. The ESR is normal, and antithyroid antibodies are detected in 50% of patients.

The mechanism by which thyrotoxicosis occurs in both forms of thyroiditis is leakage of stored hormone from the inflamed gland. Although autoimmune thyroiditis may occur in anyone, the most common setting is within 6 months postpartum. In fact, this condition develops in about 5% of women after delivery, with spontaneous remission occurring within 3 to 6 months. Spontaneous remission usually includes a period of transient hypothyroidism; however, permanent hypothyroidism may develop in 20% of patients. Women

with postpartum depression should be screened for painless thyroiditis, particularly the hypothyroid phase. Because there is also an increased incidence of Graves' disease during the postpartum period, diagnostic separation of these two entities is important and may be difficult in a woman who is breast-feeding. RAIU is contraindicated because radioactive iodine is excreted in breast milk for up to 1 week after oral administration to the mother. If the patient is symptomatic, breast-feeding should be terminated to permit RAIU and definitive treatment.

Struma ovarii (benign or malignant ovarian dermoid containing thyroid tissue) is a rare cause of thyrotoxicosis. Suspicion is raised if RAIU is suppressed, no thyroid tissue is palpable, and spontaneous resolution does

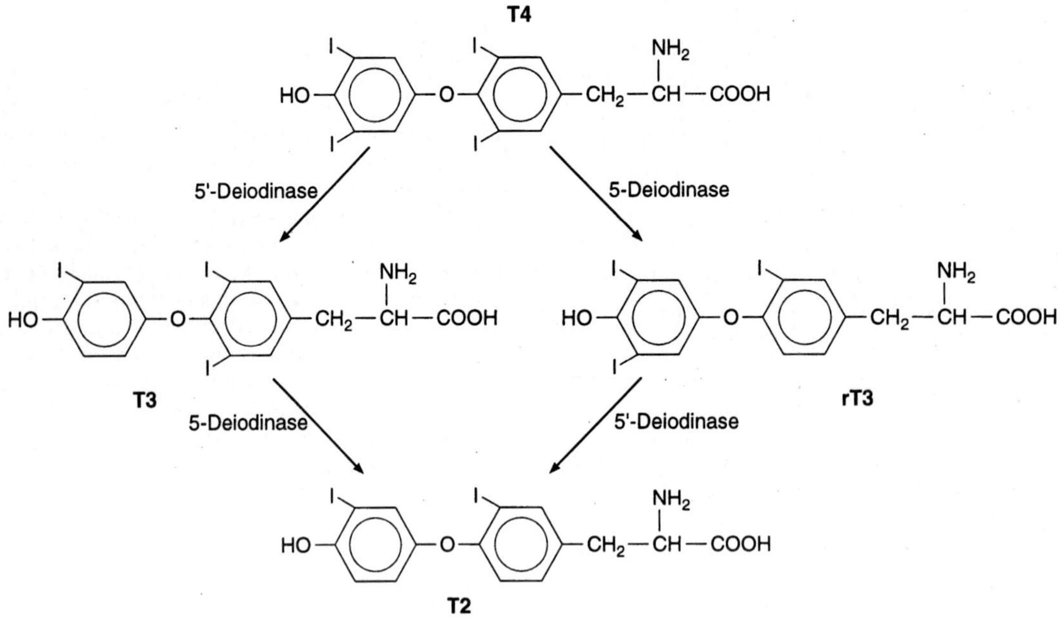

Figure 17–3. Peripheral metabolism of T4.

Table 17–1. Causes of hyperthyroxinemia.

Suppressed RAIU	I. Clinical thyrotoxicosis with suppressed TSH
	  A. Increased release from damaged thyroid gland
	    1. Subacute thyroiditis
	    2. Autoimmune thyroiditis
	  B. Amiodarone and iodides, (eg, SSKI)
	  C. Factitious
	  D. Struma ovarii

Increased RAIU	E. Overproduction by thyroid gland
	    1. Graves' disease
	    2. Toxic nodule
	    3. Toxic multinodular goiter
	II. Clinical thyrotoxicosis (with pathologic increase in TSH)
	  A. Hydatidaform mole and choriocarcinoma
	  B. Thyrotropin-producing pituitary tumor

III. Clinical euthyroidism
  A. Normal TSH
    1. Increased TBG (increased total T4, but normal free T4)
      a. Pregnancy
      b. Hereditary TBG excess
      c. Acute intermittent porphyria
      d. Hepatitis and primary biliary cirrhosis
      e. Drugs
        i. Estrogens and oral contraceptives
        ii. Methadone
        iii. Heparin
        iv. Perphenazine
        v. 5-Fluorouracil
    2. Peripheral conversion defect
  B. Low TSH: first trimester of pregnancy
  C. High TSH
    1. Acute psychiatric illness
    2. Thyroid-resistance syndrome

TSH, thyroid-stimulating hormone; SSKI, saturated solution of potassium iodide; TBG, thyroxine-binding globulin.

not occur, or if a pelvic mass is palpable. Factitious thyrotoxicosis must be considered if RAIU is suppressed, particularly among medical personnel. Iatrogenic exogenous thyroid hormone excess historically has been a frequent cause of elevated free T4, but with titration of dose using sensitive assays for TSH, this cause is becoming less common. Finally, a unique form of thyrotoxicosis in which overproduction of thyroid hormone occurs but RAIU is decreased because of dilution by nonradioactive iodine can be precipitated by iodine-rich medications such as amiodarone and saturated solution of potassium iodide (SSKI).

B. SPECIAL TESTS

The mechanism of thyrotoxicosis can be classified as either thyroid overproduction or "other." The critical test in differentiating between these 2 categories is the 4-hour radioactive iodine uptake (RAIU), which is nearly always high (occasionally normal) in patients with overproduction and suppressed in those with all other causes of thyrotoxicosis. Although the RAIU is mandatory, a thyroid scan is unnecessary except in defining a single toxic nodule or struma ovarii (which would require pelvic scanning).

Diagnosis

Almost all patients with thyrotoxicosis have elevated free T4 levels. Confirmation requires a suppressed level of TSH (except in the rare conditions of TSH overproduction). In most cases, the TSH is less than 0.1 mIU/L. A normal TSH rules out the diagnosis. If the free T4 is normal but clinical suspicion is high, a free T3 level should be obtained; "T3 toxicosis" may occur, particularly in toxic nodules, or recurrent Graves' disease after radioactive iodine therapy. Other laboratory abnormalities may include mild hypercalcemia, elevated aspartate aminotransferase (AST) and alkaline phosphatase, low cholesterol, and mild neutropenia.

Treatment

Because thyroiditis (whether painful or silent) resolves spontaneously, treatment is warranted only for symptomatic patients (ie, β-blockers for heart rate in excess of 100 beats per minute or severe tremor). The usual starting dose of atenolol is 25–50 mg daily, with increases as needed to keep the heart rate below 100 beats per minute. Because iodine uptake is impaired and synthetic processes damaged, treatment with either radioactive iodine or thionamides would be unsuccessful. β-Blockers are relatively contraindicated during breastfeeding because they are concentrated in breast milk, which may lead to bradycardia in the infant.

Analgesic treatment initially should consist of acetaminophen, nonsteroidal anti-inflammatory agents, or salicylates. Although salicylates are probably the most effective medication, there is some risk of displacing thyroid hormone from TBG, thereby worsening the thyrotoxic state. Salicylates should be avoided in severely thyrotoxic patients. High-dose steroids (prednisone, 30–40 mg/d) should be reserved for patients with severe pain unresponsive to the previously mentioned measures because the recurrence rate may be as high as 20% following cessation of therapy.

For treatment of Graves' disease, there are 3 standard options in addition to use of β-blockers. In the United States, ablation with I-131 is the most frequently recommended method. Treatment with a single oral dose of 6–12 mCi has a 95% cure rate at 6 months. The major side effect is permanent hypothyroidism, which develops in 60% of patients by 1 year and 90% by 10 years. There is no evidence of an increased incidence of cancer or abnormalities of reproduction. Radioactive iodine is contraindicated in pregnancy and breast-feeding. It is not used commonly in children or adolescents, although there are few data to suggest toxicity in this age group. In elderly or severely thyrotoxic patients, pretreatment with a thionamide may be appropriate for 6–8 weeks to reduce the risk of radiation thyroiditis causing an unacceptable rise in circulating thyroid hormone levels.

The second option is treatment with thionamides (propylthiouracil, 100 mg orally 3 times daily, or methimazole, 10–30 mg orally daily), which interfere with thyroid hormone synthesis. Thionamides can modulate cellular immunity in vitro, although a similar effect in clinical disease is unclear. Propylthiouracil also decreases peripheral conversion of T4 to T3. A euthyroid state is reached in about 4–12 weeks, after which titration of the dosage downward is necessary at a rate of 30% every 2–4 months. Treatment is continued for 12–18 months. After discontinuation of treatment, remission persists in only 40% of patients by 5 years. Most recurrences appear within the first 6 months after therapy is stopped. Remission is not present if TSH or free T3 is abnormal while the patient is still receiving therapy. Although standard practice is to treat with ablative therapy (I-131 or surgery) if thyrotoxicosis recurs after 1 year of thionamide treatment, there is some evidence, particularly in children, that the remission rate continues to increase with longer duration of therapy; the rate may be as high as 70% after 5 years of treatment.

Radioactive iodine is preferred over medical treatment for Graves' disease because of predictability of rapid cure and lack of side effects. Rash or arthralgias occur in about 1–5% of patients who take thionamides, and 0.3% suffer transient life-threatening agranulocytosis (usually within the first 3 months of therapy). A white blood cell count (WBC) with differential should be obtained if a fever or sore throat develops. Periodic WBC counts are not recommended because both thyrotoxicosis and treatment with thionamides can cause mild neutropenia.

The third treatment option, thyroidectomy, is reserved for patients in the second trimester of pregnancy who are unable to tolerate propylthiouracil (methimazole is contraindicated because of scalp defects in the fetus) and patients in whom treatment with the other 2 approaches has failed.

In symptomatic hyperthyroidism with elevated free T4 and free T3 with suppressed TSH, the decision to treat is straightforward. However, approximately 2% of the population has "subclinical hyperthyroidism" defined as a TSH below 0.1 mIU/L with normal free T3 and free T4. The natural history of this condition has not been well established. In at least 50% of such patients, TSH returns to normal within 1 year. On the other hand, overt thyrotoxicosis will develop at a rate of 5% per year in a subset of such patients with multinodular goiters. Patients with subclinical hyperthyroidism have lower bone densities and in the elderly there is a 3-fold increased risk of atrial fibrillation. In the elderly (60 yrs or older), patients with symptoms, or those with goiters, treatment with I-131 (preferable) or thionamides is reasonable. In other patients, it is acceptable simply to follow thyroid function tests 2–3 times per year.

Thyrotoxicosis during pregnancy constitutes a high-risk pregnancy; treatment should be managed by an endocrinologist or perinatologist. Fetal demise is increased in patients with untreated hyperthyroidism or hypothyroidism. Because thionamides cross the placenta easily but thyroid hormones do not, a maternal plasma concentration of free T4 must be maintained in the high-normal range. The baby is at risk for neonatal goiter, which may compromise delivery, and transient neonatal thyrotoxicosis, because TSI crosses the placenta. Both complications may occur even if the mother is euthyroid if the presence of TSI persists. Both the pediatrician and the obstetrician must be aware of the diagnosis. Patients should not become pregnant until their thyrotoxicosis has remitted or been treated definitively. Postpartum, propylthiouracil is the treatment of choice if the mother does not wish to terminate breast-feeding to receive radioactive iodine, although hypothyroidism and goiter may occur in the infant.

Except as a temporizing measure, thionamides are not appropriate for treatment of toxic uninodular or multinodular goiters because remission is unlikely. Definitive therapy with radioactive iodine is recommended. Surgery is an acceptable option, but pretreatment with thionamides to achieve euthyroidism is recommended to decrease the risk of thyroid storm precipitated by surgical manipulation of the toxic gland.

Complications

The acute, life-threatening worsening of thyrotoxicosis called thyroid storm is fortunately rare. Manifestations include fever, tachycardia, vomiting, diarrhea, abnormal liver function tests, and altered mental status (usually agitation but occasionally apathy or coma). High-output congestive heart failure (CHF) and tachyarrhythmias may require treatment.

The mechanism of thyroid storm—a medical emergency—is unclear. In some cases, direct injury to the thyroid gland, from either surgical manipulation or I-131 therapy may release stored thyroid hormone. However, most cases are associated with acute nonthyroidal conditions, such as infection, other surgery, or trauma. Circulating total T4 and T3 do not correlate with the severity of disease and in fact are no higher in thyroid storm than in typical thyrotoxicosis. Free thyroid hormone levels are higher in thyroid storm, perhaps because an inhibitor of binding to TBG is released during acute illness, thus displacing thyroid hormone into the unbound, biologically active state.

Immediate treatment of thyroid storm must be initiated in the hospital. Because there are no definitive tests to confirm thyrotoxic crisis, clinicians should treat as such if the diagnosis is suspected. Treatment includes inhibition of thyroidal hormone synthesis and release, blockade of peripheral conversion and action, and supportive measures (Table 17–2). All therapies should be initiated simultaneously except that propylthiouracil must be given before iodide to prevent enrichment of intrathyroidal iodine stores and continued production of thyroid hormone. For temperature control, salicylates should be avoided because they inhibit binding to TBG and thus may increase free hormone levels. Steroids traditionally have been used because patients may have unsuspected autoimmune adrenal insuffi-

ciency. If CHF is present, β-blockade may be highly effective in decreasing the high-output state, but it should be administered in an intensive care unit with hemodynamic monitoring because sympathetic blockade may worsen CHF, particularly in patients with underlying cardiac disease. Treatment of the underlying illness is critical to survival.

When to Refer to a Specialist

Thyrotropin-producing pituitary tumors causing thyroxicosis are rare, and patients in whom such a tumor is suspected should be referred to an endocrinologist.

EUTHYROIDISM

Particularly in the inpatient setting, elevation of total T4 without clinical thyrotoxicosis is common, usually caused by increased TBG levels or decreased conversion to T3. In contrast to the situation in thyrotoxicosis, TSH is not suppressed. Although the conditions and medications are associated with increased TBG and consequent high total T4 levels, the measured free T4 remains normal. It is recommended that *only* free T4 measurements be used.

As described previously, T4 is metabolized peripherally by deiodination. In various conditions, 5'-deiodinase is inactivated, causing circulating T3 to fall, frequently below normal, with a reciprocal increase in rT3 (Figure 17–4). Inhibition of 5'-deiodinase may be caused by acute illness, starvation, and medications such as amiodarone, propylthiouracil, steroids, and β-blockers. In 10% of patients, free T4 increases to above the normal level because of both decreased peripheral metabolism and increased TSH responding to low T3 levels. Confirmation of this condition is made by demonstrating a normal or minimally elevated TSH level. The level of free T3 is low, although it is not always measured. No treatment is required. A low free T3 during acute illness is meaningless, unless free T4 is

Table 17–2. Treatment of thyroid storm.

Medication	Inhibitory Site
Propylthiouracil, 300 mg PO q6h (give before iodide or ipodate)	Synthesis and deiodination
SSKI, 10 drops in water po tid or sodium iodide 1 g IV over 24 h	Release
Atenolol 50 mg PO q6h prn or propanolol 1 mg IV prn	Sympathomimetic and deiodinase
Supportive measures: IV hydration Acetaminophen/cooling blanket Hydrocortisone, 100 mg IV q8h Digoxin for congestive heart failure	

SSKI, saturated solution of potassium iodide.

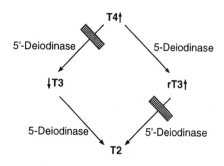

Figure 17–4. Peripheral thyroid hormone metabolism in acute illness.

also low and TSH is elevated. Amiodarone and oral cholecystographic agents are structurally similar to T4 and compete for 5'-deiodinase. Although the mechanism is uncertain in acute illness, free fatty acids released during acute physiologic stress may inhibit this reaction.

As many as 20% of acutely hospitalized patients with a spectrum of psychiatric illnesses are hyperthyroxinemic. Because the free T3 level is normal and the TSH level is normal or mildly elevated, central pituitary stimulation is the presumed mechanism. Such patients are not clinically thyrotoxic, and laboratory test results return to normal within 1–3 weeks.

Peripheral thyroid hormone resistance is a rare condition, probably caused by an intracellular defect in pituitary and peripheral tissues. Despite high levels of free T4 and free T3, patients are clinically normal or mildly hypothyroid with increased TSH. A pituitary tumor must be ruled out. No treatment is available or necessary.

HYPOTHYROXINEMIA

Hypothyroxinemia may be the result of primary thyroid dysfunction, pituitary disease leading to underproduction of TSH, or abnormalities of thyroid hormone metabolism or binding. The most common etiologies of primary hypothyroxinemia are autoimmune (eg, Hashimoto's thyroiditis) and amiodarone (Table 17–3). Pituitary hypofunction is an uncommon cause of profound hypothyroxinemia, although mild depression of TSH and free T4 is frequently seen in the intensive care unit secondary to dopamine and endogenous and exogenous steroids. If TSH and free T4 are both low, a pituitary magnetic resonance imaging scan must be done to rule out pituitary tumor. Decreased binding to TBG is easily identified by low T4 and normal free T4.

HYPOTHYROIDISM

The signs and symptoms of hypothyroidism can be nonspecific and subtle. Common signs include (1) bradycardia, (2) hypothermia, (3) hypokinesis, (4) skin changes (skin may be doughy, dry, and cold), (5) hoarseness, (6) pericardial effusion, (7) delayed relaxation phase of deep tendon reflexes, and (8) diastolic hypertension. A variety of symptoms may manifest: fatigue, cold intolerance, failure to lose weight or modest weight gain, constipation, muscle cramps, weakness, or menorrhagia.

The signs and symptoms—including hypertension—are reversible with thyroid hormone replacement therapy. The laboratory abnormalities, which include combined hyperlipidemia (increased triglycerides and

Table 17–3. Causes of hypothyroxinemia.

I. Hypothyroidism
  A. Primary (thyroidal failure)—increased TSH
    1. Post-ablative (I-131 or surgery)
    2. Thyroiditis
      a. Transient (recovery phase in subacute or autoimmune thyroiditis)
      b. Permanent (autoimmune including Hashimoto's)
    3. External radiation
    4. Congenital dyshormonogenesis
    5. Medications
      a. Amiodarone
      b. Lithium
      c. Iodides (eg, SSKI)
      d. Thionamides (propylthiouracil and methimazole)
  B. Secondary (pituitary or hypothalamic failure)—low TSH
    1. Tumor (primary or metastatic)
    2. Infiltrative (sarcoidosis, hemochromatosis, histiocytosis, lymphoma)
    3. Inflammation (hypophysitis)
    4. Ablation (surgery or radiation therapy)
    5. Medications
      a. Dopamine
      b. Steroids
II. Euthyroidism—normal TSH
  A. Decreased binding to TBG (low total T4, but normal free T4)
    1. "Euthyroid sick" syndrome
    2. Hereditary decreased TBG
    3. Nephrotic syndrome
    4. Chronic renal failure
    5. Cirrhosis
    6. Medications
      a. Androgens
      b. Steroids
      c. Salicylates
      d. L-asparaginase
  B. Altered intracellular metabolism
    1. Phenytoin
    2. Carbamazapine

TSH, thyroid-stimulating hormone; SSKI, saturated solution of potassium iodide; TBG, thyroxine-binding globulin.

low-density lipoprotein cholesterol), macrocytic anemia, elevated liver function levels, high creatine phosphokinase (CPK), and hyponatremia, also resolve with correction of thyroid hormone deficiency. The possibility of hypothyroidism should be considered in any patient with hyperlipidemia. Measurement of TSH is mandatory to confirm primary hypothyroidism. If free T4 is unequivocally low and there is no other reason for an inappropriately low TSH (eg, euthyroid sick syndrome), evaluation for pituitary disease is indicated. When total T4 is low because of decreased binding to

TBG, free T4 will still be normal. It is recommended that *only* free T4 measurements be obtained.

EUTHYROID SICK SYNDROME (LOW T4, LOW T3)

As many as 70% of critically ill patients have total T4 levels below normal; often the levels are undetectable. On the basis of their normal TSH and return of total T4 to normal with resolution of the intercurrent illness, these patients are euthyroid. The low total T4 level is caused by interference with binding to TBG. The inhibitor remains speculative, but the same fatty acid purported to inactivate 5'-deiodinase during acute stress has been implicated, as have immunoglobulins. Measurement of free T4 shows a normal or minimally depressed result, confirming euthyroidism. Thyroid hormone replacement is unnecessary because the patient is euthyroid.

The euthyroid sick syndrome has prognostic implications: the lower the total T4, the higher the mortality rate, probably as a reflection of the severity of the underlying illness. The total T4 will improve concurrently with improvement in the acute illness. Mild secondary hypothyroidism also may be present in acute illness because TSH is normal or mildly decreased despite a free T4 level slightly lower than normal. The response of TSH to TRH is blunted in the presence of high-dose steroids (either exogenous or endogenous) and dopamine infusion. From a teleologic perspective, this response may be appropriate (as is the shift to biologically inactive reverse T3,) because the body is already in a catabolic state. Only if TSH is undetectable or there is other reason to suspect pituitary insufficiency should an additional work-up be initiated. A transient increase in TSH to above normal usually is seen during the recovery phase either because of transient decrease in free T4 caused by increased binding to TBG as the inhibitor is removed or because of recovery from mild secondary hypothyroidism. In both acute and recovery phases, serial measurements of free T4 and TSH every 5–7 days are appropriate.

Treatment

In symptomatic hypothyroidism with low free T4 and high TSH, the decision to treat is straightforward. In patients with "subclinical hypothyroidism," however, with normal free T4 and a mild elevation of TSH (usually between 5 and 10 mIU/L), the decision is more difficult. There is disagreement about whether these patients are normal, recovering from painless thyroiditis, or in the process of developing frank hypothyroidism. Studies have shown that frank hypothyroidism develops

at a rate of 5% per year in patients with antithyroid antibodies and not at all in patients without antibodies. In patients with TSH levels above 10 mIU/L, treatment with thyroid hormone may lead to mild improvement in lipids, some cardiac function tests, and subjective symptoms. Benefits are equivocal in patients with TSH between 5 and 10 mIU/L. This condition is recognized in about 8% of men and 15% of women over the age of 60. Replacement therapy should be started if one of the following exists:

1. Positive antimicrosomal or antithyroglobulin antibodies
2. Goiter
3. TSH above 10 mIU/L
4. Development of low free T4
5. Strong clinical suspicion of symptomatic hypothyroidism (bradycardia, delayed deep tendon reflexes, unexplained fatigue, or weight gain)

In the absence of these indications, observation with repeat TSH every 6 months is adequate.

Standard replacement of thyroid hormone is with synthetic L-thyroxine, which has a plasma half-life of 7 days; this treatment avoids the swings in plasma concentration encountered with T3 (sodium liothyronine [Cytomel]) or with desiccated thyroid, which contains T3 in the amount of 15%.

If the patient is allowed nothing by mouth for more than 1 week, L-thyroxine may be given parenterally (intravenously is preferable) at 80% of the oral dose. Oral absorption may be impaired by malabsorption syndrome or by simultaneous ingestion of ferrous sulfate, cholestyramine, sucralfate, calcium or aluminum hydroxide. Food interferes with absorption, so L-thyroxine should be taken on an empty stomach.

The level of TSH should be maintained within the normal range, which requires approximately 1.6 μg/kg/d once daily. Patients without coronary artery disease may be started immediately on full replacement dosage. Adjustment of the dosage to normalize TSH should be made no sooner than 8 weeks after initiation of therapy. Once TSH is in the normal range, a change in dosage is rarely needed, and periodic measurement of TSH is not necessary. Increases in circulating thyroid hormone levels increase myocardial oxygen demand, thereby increasing risk of angina pectoris or myocardial infarction in patients with coronary artery disease. In such patients, treatment should be started with 25–50 μg/d and increased by 25–50 μg every 4 to 8 weeks if tolerated. Antianginal medications may need to be initiated or increased.

If patients complain of depression or decreased cognition on adequate L-thyroxine replacement, the combination of L-thyroxine and T3 (Cytomel) may be helpful. In combination therapy, 10–12.5 µg of T3 is substituted for 50 µg of L-thyroxine (eg, a person taking 150 µg of L-thyroxine would be converted to 100 µg of L-thyroxine and 10 to 12.5 µg of T3.

For patients requiring surgery, preoperative treatment of hypothyroidism is preferable but not mandatory. Increased sensitivity to anesthetics and narcotics, decreased ability to excrete a water load with consequent risk of hyponatremia, and decreased inotropic and chronotropic myocardial function are reasons to delay elective surgery such as laminectomy or cholecystectomy. Fortunately, however, there are good data showing that most patients with undiagnosed hypothyroidism undergoing major nonelective surgery such as coronary artery bypass grafting do well, with minimally increased morbidity and no increased mortality. Emergent and semiemergent surgery should proceed without rapid replacement therapy but with careful perioperative monitoring.

Complications

Profound hypothyroidism, usually in the setting of intercurrent illness such as sepsis, CHF, or cerebrovascular accident, may lead to the complication myxedema coma. The clinical findings can include hypercapnea caused by decreased ventilatory drive, hypothermia, bradycardia, CHF, and hyponatremia. Supportive measures include adequate ventilation, body warming, water restriction, treatment of CHF, and administration of steroids in case autoimmune adrenal disease coexists. Adequate thyroid hormone replacement should be administered immediately, although the dosage is controversial. Because T3 is not available commercially for intravenous administration, L-thyroxine, 500 µg intravenously, is recommended, followed by 100 µg daily thereafter.

Because in acute illness there is almost always inhibition of 5′-deiodinase, it is reasonable (but unproved) to provide T3 orally also, if possible, at a rate of about 10 µg every 8 hours. There is an increased risk of acute myocardial infarction or arrhythmia during rapid replacement therapy.

THYROID NODULE

About 5% of the population over the age of 40 years have a palpable thyroid nodule; however, at autopsy half the population has at least 1 nodule. Exposure to face or neck irradiation in childhood increases the risk of palpable abnormality to 30%, with peak incidence at age 30. Most nodules, even those appearing after exposure to irradiation, are benign; only 5% of nodules are malignant. In irradiated patients, 30% are malignant. The benign lesions include cysts, colloid nodules, and cellular follicular adenomas.

Screening

Patients with a history of face or neck irradiation in childhood for thymus enlargement, tonsil and adenoid hypertrophy, acne, or cancer should have annual neck palpation for at least 30 years after exposure. A patient with a family history of medullary carcinoma of the thyroid requires annual examination; members of families with multiple endocrine neoplasia syndrome II (hyperparathyroidism, pheochromocytoma, and medullary carcinoma of the thyroid) should be screened annually with a provocative test of calcitonin secretion such as calcium infusion or tested for the same mutation in the RET proto-oncogene as the proband. Ultrasonography is not an appropriate screening method because of the high incidence of abnormality (50%) with no discrimination between benign and malignant lesions.

Clinical Findings

Thyroid nodules are usually palpable if they are larger than 1 cm in diameter. They are usually round, smooth, and nontender. Physical examination and history rarely can distinguish between benign and malignant lesions. Even rock-hard nodules may represent benign thyroiditis. Sudden onset of a painful, tender nodule usually represents hemorrhage into a preexisting solid or cystic nodule. Rapid growth, particularly in an irregular, hard nodule, suggests anaplastic carcinoma. Presence of cervical nodes must raise concern about malignant disease. Size is not a good discriminator.

Diagnosis

First, euthyroidism should be confirmed by determining the level of TSH. If hypothyroidism or hyperthyroidism is detected, attention should be directed to diagnosis and treatment of the metabolic abnormality. Differentiation of benign from malignant lesions has been enhanced and simplified by fine-needle aspiration biopsy, which is safe and inexpensive. Adequacy of specimen and accuracy of cytologic interpretation depend on experience; patients should be referred to a center specializing in this procedure—one at which at least 30 biopsies are performed yearly. About 70% of biopsies are read as benign; the false-negative rate is 1–5%. A malignant cytologic classification is the result in 5% of biopsies, with a false-positive rate of 0–5%. A suspicious classification is given in 10–15% of biopsies, of which 25% are cancer. Approximately 10–15% of biopsies are indeterminate because of an inadequate number of cells, usually in the setting of hemorrhage.

Fine-needle aspiration biopsy should be the first step in diagnosis. Ultrasonography cannot discriminate between benign and malignant nodules. Because most nodules are "cold" (do not take up radionuclide), radionuclide scanning is not helpful as an initial procedure. Cancer can be expected in about 30% of patients undergoing surgery if the diagnostic approach shown in Figure 17–5 is used.

Treatment

Malignant lesions and suspicious lesions should be removed by an experienced surgeon. Near-total thyroidectomy is indicated for clearly malignant nodules, most of which are papillary carcinoma. The extent of surgery for suspicious nodules remains controversial. The differential diagnosis between follicular carcinoma and adenoma may be equally difficult to confirm at frozen section. If there is considerable doubt, at least a subtotal thyroidectomy should be undertaken.

If cancer is confirmed, referral to an endocrinologist is appropriate. Papillary carcinoma, which represents 70% of malignant lesions, has an excellent prognosis, with no decrease in life expectancy if (1) the patient is under 40 years of age, (2) the lesion is less than 3 cm in diameter, and (3) there is no vascular or capsular invasion. Lymph-node invasion is common and unrelated to mortality rate. Follicular carcinoma accounts for 20% of malignant lesions and is more aggressive, with a 10-year mortality rate of 30%; most of the mortality is the result of local recurrence. Treatment in both types of differentiated carcinomas includes adequate surgical removal, suppressive doses of L-thyroxine (enough to suppress TSH to below normal), and usually, ablation of residual normal and malignant thyroid tissue with I-131. Anaplastic carcinoma is unresponsive to any treatment and uniformly fatal. Medullary carcinoma and lymphoma are intermediate in responsiveness to therapy.

Treatment of benign nodules remains controversial. Although suppression with L-thyroxine is standard procedure in some centers, many institutions do not recommend it routinely for 3 reasons: (1) controlled studies of up to 3 years show no difference in likelihood of shrinkage or enlargement between patients who undergo thyroid suppression and those who do not; (2) administration of suppressive doses of L-thyroxine may have adverse consequences, including atrial fibrillation and decreased bone mineral density; and (3) there is no evidence that suppression prevents malignancy. Suppression of remaining thyroid tissue following removal of benign nodule is equally uncertain; however, in patients who were exposed previously to face or neck irradiation, the incidence of recurrent nodule decreases from 30% to 7% with suppression. Annual palpation of the benign nodule or remaining gland after surgery is recommended; if progressive enlargement or recurrence is found, biopsy should be repeated.

THYROID FUNCTION DURING PREGNANCY

Early Pregnancy

Thyroid function changes in a predictable manner during the first trimester of pregnancy. Coincident with rising HCG levels, free T4 and free T3 increase and TSH decreases, consistent with the thyroid-stimulating activity of HCG. These alterations peak at 6 to 12 weeks and return to normal by 20 weeks. Even when free T4 or TSH is out of the normal range, clinical thyrotoxicosis is not observed. Treatment is not necessary for this normal physiologic phenomenon. In fact, understanding of this condition is critical for prevention of unnecessary intervention. Close follow-up is equally important, however, because Graves' disease can present during pregnancy and must be aggressively man-

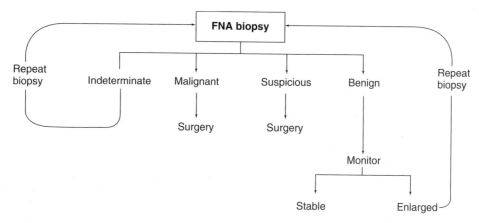

Figure 17–5. Evaluation of thyroid nodule. (FNA, fine-needle aspiration.)

aged. If the patient is symptomatic or thyroid function fails to normalize by 20 weeks, treatment with propylthiouracil should be considered.

The relationship of this physiologic phenomenon to hyperemesis gravidarum remains controversial. Although up to 50% of women with hyperemesis gravidarum have an elevated free T4, they are not clinically thyrotoxic, and conversely, most pregnant patients with high free T4 do not have hyperemesis gravidarum. Because free T4 elevation is self-limited, treatment with propylthiouracil should be avoided if possible.

Late Pregnancy

Throughout pregnancy, TBG levels increase progressively under the influence of increasing circulating estrogen levels. Consequently, total T4 levels increase progressively to above normal limits by the third trimester. However, there is actually a slight decrease in free T4 and increase in TSH, both within normal limits. In 75% of patients receiving thyroid replacement therapy for hypothyroidism who are unable to respond to TSH stimulation, frankly elevated TSH can be documented. Therefore, a TSH level should be obtained in each trimester of pregnancy in patients on replacement therapy. The dosage of thyroid replacement should be increased, frequently as much as 40%, to normalize TSH, although the significance of these mild abnor-malities late in pregnancy is unclear. Finally, the thyroid gland enlarges by about 20% as detected by ultrasonography during pregnancy. In the iodine-sufficient United States, however, there is no increase in incidence of clinical goiter during pregnancy.

MEDICATIONS THAT ALTER THYROID FUNCTION TESTS

Many commonly prescribed medications have an effect on thyroid function tests either by altering binding to proteins or by changing thyroid metabolism. These medications are classified here according to mechanism of action and in Table 17–4 by changes in thyroid function tests.

A. Increased TBG
  1. Estrogens (including oral contraceptives)
  2. Methadone
  3. Heparin
  4. Perphenazine
  5. 5-Fluorouracil (5-FU)
B. Decreased TBG or binding to TBG
  1. Androgens
  2. Steroids
  3. Salicylates
  4. L-asparaginase

Table 17–4. Medications affecting thyroid function.

Medication	Total T4	Free T4	Free T3	TSH	Mechanism
Dopamine	D	D	D	D	Pituitary suppression
Steroids	D,N,I	D,N,I	D,N	D,N,I	Pituitary suppresion; deiodinase block
Methimazole	D	D	D	I	Decreased synthesis
Propylthiouracil	D	D	D	I	Decreased synthesis, deiodinase block
Inorganic iodides and amiodarone	D	D	D	I	Synthetic defect
					Block release
	I	I	I	D	Iodine repletion
Amiodarone	N,I	N,I	D	N,I	Deiodinase block
β-Blockers	N,I	N,I	D	N,I	Deiodinase block
Lithium	D	D	D	I	Block release
Estrogens					
Methadone					
Heparin	I	N	N	N	Increased thyroxine-binding globulin
5-Fluorouracil					
Perphenazine					
Androgens					
Steroids					
L-asparaginase	D	N	N	N	Decreased thyroxine-binding globulin
Salicylates					
Phenytoin	D	D	N	N	Decreased intracellular metabolism
Carbamazepine					

D, decreased; N, normal; I, increased.

C. Increased synthesis of thyroid hormone
 1. Amiodarone
 2. Inorganic iodide (eg, SSKI)
D. Decreased synthesis of thyroid hormone
 1. Thionamides (propylthiouracil and methimazole)
 2. Inorganic iodides (eg, SSKI) in patients with intrinsic defect in thyroid hormone synthesis such as Hashimoto's thyroiditis
 3. Amiodarone (same mechanism as SSKI)
E. Decreased release of stored thyroid hormone
 1. Inorganic iodide (eg, SSKI)
 2. Amiodarone
 3. Lithium carbonate
F. Decreased peripheral conversion of T4 to T3
 1. Propylthiouracil (not methimazole)
 2. Steroids
 3. Amiodarone
 4. β-Blockers
G. Altered intracellular metabolism of thyroid hormone
 1. Phenytoin
 2. Carbamazepine
H. Decreased TSH secretion
 1. Steroids
 2. Dopamine

A few medications require special comment. Inorganic iodides act at multiple steps in thyroid hormone physiology. They uniformly interfere with diagnostic radioactive iodine uptake by competing for uptake into the thyroid gland. They may precipitate reversible myxedema in patients with damaged synthetic processes but paradoxically may cause thyrotoxicosis in iodine-deficient patients with autoimmune thyroid disease. Finally, they inhibit release of thyroid hormone from the gland, leading to hypothyroidism and goiter. The class III antiarrhythmic agent amiodarone, because of structural similarity to the thyronines and its iodine content, has many often clinically important effects on thyroid hormone synthesis and action. Depending on the baseline status of the thyroid gland, amiodarone may cause either hypothyroidism or hyperthyroidism, both of which are reversible. In addition, amiodarone is a potent inhibitor of 5′-deiodinase.

The mechanism of action of antiseizure medications on thyroid hormone metabolism is obscure, but it appears to involve increased intracellular disposal ac-

counting for decreased circulating hormone levels but normal TSH and euthyroid clinical status. A low free T4 may occur as often as 20% of the time. No treatment is indicated, but if there is any other reason to suspect pituitary dysfunction, further evaluation should be undertaken.

GLOSSARY OF THYROID FUNCTION TESTS

T4—total thyroxine concentration, of which 99.9% is inactive, bound to plasma proteins.

RT3U—resin-T3-uptake, which is an indirect reciprocal measurement of T4 binding to TBG; ie, if TBG increases, RT3U decreases. (This test is no longer necessary since free T4 and free T3 can now be accurately measured.)

Free T4—biologically active thyroxine unbound to protein and not influenced by changes in thyroxine-binding globulin (TBG). In all cases this determination is preferred over the total T4. **Total T3**—total triiodothyronine, of which 99% is bound to protein.

Free T3—biologically active triiodothyronine unbound to protein and not influenced by changes in TBG. Preferred measurement.

TSH—thyrotropin (thyroid-stimulating hormone), which is secreted by the pituitary gland and controls thyroid function. Most laboratories now use sensitive TSH assays capable of measuring 0.1 mIU/L (second generation) or 0.01 mIU/L (third generation). Discussion in this chapter refers to the second-generation assays.

RAIU—radioactive iodine uptake, which is the percentage of an oral dose of I-123 or I-131 taken up by the thyroid gland in 4 or 24 hours.

Thyroid scan—nuclear imaging with I-123 or ^{99}Tc to show functional anatomy of the thyroid gland.

Burrow GN: Thyroid function and hyperfunction during gestation. Endocr Rev 1993;14:194.[PMID: 8325252]

Gharib H: Fine-needle aspiration biopsy of the thyroid: an appraisal. Ann Intern Med 1993;118:282. [PMID: 8420446]

Ingbar SH, Braverman LE (editors): *Werner's The Thyroid.* Lippincott, 1986.

Roti E et al: The use and misuse of thyroid hormone. Endocr Rev 1993;14:401. [PMID: 8223339]

Menopause

18

Julie Pattison, MD & Dawn P. Lemcke, MD

Menopause is the last stage of a biologic process in which a woman's ovaries cease follicular activity and gradually produce decreasing levels of sex hormones, associated initially with vasomotor symptoms and genitourinary atrophy and eventually with increasing risk of coronary heart disease and osteoporosis. Women today are living one third of their lives in menopause. Accumulating evidence of risks and benefits of hormone replacement therapy (HRT) indicate that the emphasis should be placed on its use for treatment of the initial symptoms in the lowest effective dose for the shortest duration, at least for combined estrogen/progestin therapy. Increasingly, solutions other than traditional oral hormone replacement for treatment of menopausal symptoms and associated disorders are being advised.

ESSENTIALS OF DIAGNOSIS

- *Amenorrhea for 6 to 12 months.*
- *Vasomotor symptoms.*
- *Elevated follicle-stimulating hormone (FSH).*

General Considerations

Menopause is defined as the cessation of menstrual periods. Women typically become menopausal between the ages of 45 and 55, with the average age of menopause being 51. A clinical diagnosis of menopause is made when a woman of typical age has been amenorrheic for up to 6 months and has typical symptoms of hot flushes or night sweats. A menopausal range FSH in this situation is pathognomonic. The actual serum FSH concentration that is diagnostic varies depending on the assay used, but it will always be above the upper limit of normal for a premenopausal woman, except for the midcycle menstrual surge. An FSH level of 10–25 mIU on day 3 of the menstrual cycle suggests that the ability to conceive is no longer likely. A high FSH concentration after 6 days off a low-dose oral contraceptive (ie, just prior to starting a new pill package) is also indicative of menopause. Women with prior hysterectomy with intact ovaries may have no vasomotor symptoms, and therefore sometimes diagnosis of menopause may only be made clinically with signs of estrogen deficiency on examination or by significantly or persistently elevated FSH levels. Serum estradiol levels are not sufficiently sensitive for use in diagnosis of menopause.

Perimenopause is the menopausal transition that occurs 2 to 8 years before menopause and the year following the last menstrual cycle. Ovaries produce decreasing quantities of estrogen, progesterone, and androgens. During this time, anovulatory (estrogen only) cycles of varying length are interspersed with normal ovulatory cycles. This results in menstrual irregularity, with variable cycle length and amount or duration of flow, sometimes with light spotting or heavy breakthrough bleeding. Irregularity increases and then missed menses occur. Some women note hot flushes, night sweats, and vaginal dryness more typical of the postmenopausal period.

During perimenopause, ovarian function varies considerably, with extended periods of estrogen deficiency associated with increased FSH secretion followed by occasional ovulation with estradiol production and normal FSH secretion. Because serum FSH levels may rise to the postmenopausal range during some cycles, elevated levels of FSH should not be used to diagnose menopause in menstruating women.

Endometrial hyperplasia may occur in this transition period, secondary to anovulation with associated prolonged estrogen stimulation and progesterone deficiency. Endometrial evaluation should occur if a woman has heavy or prolonged vaginal bleeding or persistent intermenstrual bleeding. Women should be made aware of the risk of unintended pregnancy during perimenopause.

Menopause occurs as ovarian follicle activity stops. Menses cease, ovarian hormone production declines further, and the gonadotropins luteinizing hormone (LH) and FSH rise indefinitely. Estrogen levels drop to about one tenth of the level before menopause and progesterone production becomes almost absent. Ovarian androgen production falls only 30%, because high LH levels stimulate ongoing production and adrenal glands continue to produce androgens as well. Aromatization of the ovarian and adrenal androgen androstenedione by some peripheral tissues, especially adipose cells, produces the weak estrogen estrone, which is the major circulating estrogen in the postmenopausal period. Therefore, obese women tend to have higher post-menopausal endogenous estrogen levels and may have fewer estrogen deficiency symptoms.

Menopause occurs 2 years earlier on average in women who smoke, and also occurs earlier in women who are nulliparous, have had prior hysterectomy, or have had more regular menstrual cycles. A family history of early menopause or personal history of type 1 diabetes mellitus may also be associated with earlier menopause.

Clinical Findings

A. EARLIER EFFECTS OF ESTROGEN DEFICIENCY

1. Vasomotor symptoms—The most common acute menopausal symptoms are the vasomotor symptoms, including hot flushes (flashes), night sweats, and day sweats. Hot flushes occur in 75% of women; 50–75% have cessation of vasomotor symptoms by 5 years and most are significantly improved by 2 years after menopause onset. Hot flushes are centrally mediated, temporally related to pulses of LH secretion. They may occur from once daily up to several times daily. Hot flushes are associated with inappropriate peripheral vasodilation with increased skin blood flow and perspiration resulting in rapid heat loss, decrease in core body temperature below normal, and resultant shivering. Vasomotor symptoms are usually more intense in women who have abrupt menopause, such as that related to a surgical menopause or chemotherapy.

2. Sleep disturbance and irritability—One of the most bothersome symptoms of menopause is sleep disruption. This occurs in mid-life when insomnia is already prevalent. Hot flushes may occur as often as every hour and are frequently associated with arousal from sleep. In some women, this causes chronic sleep disturbance with symptoms of fatigue, difficulty concentrating, forgetfulness, irritability, and other psychological symptoms sometimes associated with menopause. Several studies have attempted to sort out the contribution of menopause to mood disorders that are common in mid-life. Most long-term studies have not found an association between menopause and depression. It appears that more important than estrogen deficiency are a woman's stresses (eg, physical limitations and chronic illnesses, children leaving home, marital discord, career and financial stresses, aging parents), emotional make-up, cultural background, and changing role in her family.

3. Urogenital atrophy—The vagina and urethra are estrogen sensitive tissues. Atrophy of these tissues develops in many women within the first 2 to 3 years of menopause onset. This may be associated with decreased vaginal lubrication, decreased vaginal wall elas-ticity, and narrowing and shortening of the vagina. This may result in dyspareunia and may eventually cause diminished libido. Continuing sexual activity may prevent some of the vaginal wall changes, even without estrogen treatment.

Diminished production of androgens has been thought to be a potential cause of decreased libido. Studies of androgen treatment for sexual dysfunction have had conflicting results. More commonly, decreased libido appears to be secondary to dyspareunia or to mood disorder.

Atrophy of the urethra and bladder trigone may cause urinary frequency with stress or urge incontinence as well as increased frequency of urinary tract infections.

4. Other disorders—The collagen content of the skin is reduced by estrogen deficiency, leading to wrinkling and other aging changes. Fluctuating estrogen levels may trigger migraines and may be the first noticed symptom of perimenopause.

B. LATER EFFECTS OF ESTROGEN DEFICIENCY

1. Osteoporosis—Accelerated bone loss occurs in the perimenopausal years and in the first years after menopause, during which skeletal mass may decline 1–5% per year. Depending on a woman's baseline bone mass and her propensity toward more rapid rate of bone loss, osteoporosis with fractures and chronic bone pain may occur in as little as 10 years. Of all of the consequences of osteoporosis, hip fractures cause the majority of morbidity and mortality. Twenty to thirty percent of women die within 6 months of a hip fracture and many who survive are never able to live independently again. Vertebral compression fractures cause about 50% of all fractures and are associated with loss of height, kyphosis, as well as acute and chronic back pain (see Chapter 19, Osteoporosis).

2. Cardiovascular disease (CVD)—Cardiovascular disease, primarily coronary heart disease and stroke, are the main cause of mortality in women. Before menopause, women have relative protection from coronary heart disease. After menopause, the incidence of myocardial infarction increases rapidly, such that as women age, the incidence becomes similar to that in men.

Treatment

A. HORMONE REPLACEMENT THERAPY

1. Earlier menopausal conditions—Estrogen is very effective for treating early menopausal symptoms. It is the most effective therapy for hot flushes and sweats, with significant improvement noted within days to 1 month. Estrogen replacement therapy (ERT) is also effective in treating menopause-related sleeplessness and associated transient cognitive symptoms. Doses of estrogen necessary to control vasomotor symptoms vary greatly among women. Because it now seems prudent to start with the lowest dose possible of estrogen, examples of starting doses are 0.3 mg/d of oral conjugated equine estrogen (CEE), 0.5 mg/d of oral estradiol or .05 mg weekly of transdermal estradiol. If these doses are ineffective at 1 month, then an increase is reasonable. Vasomotor symptom response to estrogen usually occurs as quickly as 14 days after beginning therapy, so it is easy to titrate quickly to ease a woman's discomfort from these symptoms. ERT, in general is not effective for the treatment of depression. The Heart and Estrogen/progestin Replacement Study (HERS) showed that women who were affected by vasomotor symptoms before starting HRT did seem to have improved emotional measures when compared with the placebo group. In contrast, the women who were without vasomotor symptoms did not appear to have benefit on emotional measures and actually had a decline in physical measures related to quality of life.

Progestins are the next most effective treatment for vasomotor symptoms but may have an adverse impact on mood as well as weight. Recommended beginning doses for progestins would be 10 mg/d of medroxyprogesterone, 20–80 mg/d of megestrol acetate (Megace), or 10 mg/d of norethindrone acetate. Micronized progesterone (100–200 mg/d) may be less likely to aggravate mood disturbance and could be used for those women who cannot tolerate other progestin preparations. Studies of progestins for effectiveness of decreasing vasomotor symptoms have not to date been head-to-head trials with ERT. The randomized, placebo-controlled trials that have been done have shown an 85% decrease in symptoms in women treated with megestrol and norethindrone acetate.

Systemic or local estrogen reverses vaginal atrophy and increases vaginal secretions. Increases in local estrogen therapy dosage for genitourinary atrophy symptoms is more effective and potentially less harmful than increases in systemic estrogen dose. Treatment of vaginal atrophy with estrogen may eliminate dyspareunia and improve libido. The effect of testosterone therapy on libido is questionable, but the addition of testosterone may be helpful for those women whose vasomotor symptoms are refractory to ERT. This seems to be the case in young women who have a sudden surgical menopause; they may benefit from the addition only after large doses of estrogen have failed. The most common testosterone preparations in the United States are in combination with estradiol with either 1.25 or 2.5 mg of methyltestosterone. Because of the potential side effects (eg, adverse impact on lipid profile and risk of CVD), the lowest dose of testosterone should be used;

it should be continued only if it clearly alleviates symptoms. Vaginal estrogen has been shown to reduce the incidence of urinary tract infections. Studies of the effect of estrogen on urinary incontinence are conflicting, but it is reasonable to try this estrogen therapy in a symptomatic patient.

Skin changes, such as skin dryness and decreased thickness, related to estrogen deficiency are reversible with estrogen.

Continuous estrogen is an effective therapy in some women whose migraines worsen in intensity or occur more frequently during perimenopause, but it may also aggravate migraine in others and therefore may be contraindicated in women with complicated migraine.

2. Later menopausal conditions—In the past 5 years, the notion that HRT decreases CVD has been shattered by the first randomized, placebo-controlled studies to evaluate this issue. Previously, the evidence seemed to strongly favor HRT for decreasing the risk of CVD by approximately 50%.

The original HERS trial was a randomized, placebo-controlled trial of 2763 postmenopausal women with documented coronary artery disease (CAD). This was a secondary prevention trial comparing CEE 0.625 mg and medroxyprogesterone 2.5 mg with placebo; the primary endpoints of the trial were nonfatal myocardial infarction or death from coronary heart disease (CHD) death. In addition, secondary outcome measures of coronary revascularization, unstable angina, congestive heart failure, resuscitated cardiac arrest, cardiovascular accidents (CVAs) or transient ischemic attacks (TIAs), and peripheral vascular disease were measured along with all cause mortality. The results were published after 4.1 years of follow-up.

In the HERS II trial, the treatment groups were unblinded, and women were offered the choice of remaining on HRT or continuing without it. Many women, with input from their primary care providers decided to remain within their randomized groups; this afforded an opportunity for continued follow-up. This group numbered 2321, which was 93% of the women surviving the original HERS trial. The planned follow-up was 4 years, but the study was terminated after 2.7 years because the investigators believed there was no benefit to continuing. The primary outcomes for HERS II were the same as in HERS.

Finally, in July 2002, the Women's Health Initiative (WHI) reported the initial data on the estrogen and progestin arm, which was terminated after only 5.2 years because of an increase in health risks. The planned length of the study was 8 years. The WHI is a multicenter trial that enrolled 161,809 postmenopausal women between 1993 and 1998 into a set of trials involving lifestyle issues and 2 arms of HRT. One arm was estrogen and progestins for women who had an intact uterus and an estrogen only arm for those women who had undergone hysterectomy. The majority of these women did not have CHD, so it was largely a primary prevention trial. Primary outcomes were CHD and invasive breast cancer and secondary outcomes were hip fracture; endometrial, colorectal, and other cancers; CVA, and pulmonary embolism. The following paragraphs present the primary and secondary outcome measures of the HERS, HERS II, and WHI trials:

CHD: Because CHD is the major cause of mortality in postmenopausal women, this outcome was an important revelation to the medical community. The HERS trial revealed that there was no difference in the CHD endpoints between the 2 groups at a follow-up of 4.1 years. This lack of effect occurred despite an overall decrease in low-density lipoprotein cholesterol and an increase in high-density lipoprotein cholesterol. In addition, there was a time trend that showed more CHD events during the first year in the group treated with HRT and fewer events in the fourth and fifth year compared with the placebo group. There was speculation that there was an increase in prothrombotic factors when HRT was first started that then decreased with time. The HERS trial was continued to assess whether longer use of HRT might prove beneficial. At 6.8 years of follow-up, the results again revealed no statistically significant difference in any of the CHD endpoints in either group, so the decrease seen in the final years of the HERS trial did not continue. Finally, the WHI also reported early data in July 2002 that revealed no statistically significant differences in CHD endpoints between the estrogen plus progestin group and placebo group. The majority of these women did not have CHD upon entry into the study, and therefore, this primary prevention study arrived at the same conclusions as the secondary prevention trials from HERS and HERS II. The WHI also found the same increase in the incidence of CHD in the first year that declined in the following years of HRT. There also have been a number of smaller randomized, placebo-controlled trials that have come to the same conclusions as the above-mentioned large studies for both primary and secondary prevention of CHD.

CVA: This endpoint was evaluated in all studies. The only trial to find a significant increase in CVA and TIA was the WHI; the hazard ratio was 1.41 for this outcome. Interestingly, there was no increase in these events in the first year as there were for CHD events, but rather CVAs and TIAs occurred in the second year and persisted. When adjusting for other confounding variables of age and blood pressure, this increased risk still prevailed.

Venous thromboembolic disease: This entity has been a well-known complication of estrogen therapy in any form and its risk was reconfirmed in all 3 of the aforementioned trials. In HERS, the relative hazard ratio was 2.89; in HERS II, the adjusted harzard ration was 3.08; and in the WHI, the hazard ratio was 2.13 for pulmonary embolism. These studies emphasize and make clear the increased risk of venous thromboembolic disease whether in a relatively healthy population (such as in the WHI) or a population with already existing comorbidities (such as in the HERS trials).

Hip fracture: Estrogen has been used for the treatment and prevention of osteoporosis. While estrogen's effectiveness for this indication has been well accepted, these trials were some of the first randomized trials that have been done to assess the true effect. In the initial HERS trial, hip fracture was a secondary endpoint, but because of the follow-up interval and statistical power of the study, there was no benefit noted. In the HERS II trial, with longer follow-up, there again was no benefit found. Despite those findings, the WHI found a hazard ratio of .76 for all osteoporotic fractures and .66 for hip fractures. Despite these numbers, the study investigators commented that overall rate for fractures was low, and these numbers—while statistically significant—were nominally so.

Breast cancer: Many epidemiologic studies found an increased risk of breast cancer associated with HRT use, while there were some that did not find an increased risk. When increased risk was found, it was generally seen after therapy for 5 years or longer. In HERS and HERS II, there was no statistically significant increased risk of breast cancer noted in the 6.8 years of follow-up. The WHI reported the increased risk of breast cancer in July 2002, and this was the reason that the trial was terminated early. This applies only to the estrogen plus progestin arm as the estrogen only group continues. The hazard ratio was 1.26, which reached nominal statistical significance only for invasive breast cancer and not carcinoma in situ. Also, like many of the epidemiologic studies, the risk seemed to occur at year 5 and beyond. This has important implications for women who may wish to use HRT for symptom relief for short periods of time, since they may be reassured that they are not increasing their risk of breast cancer.

Other cancers: Data on other cancers was collected from these studies. An interesting finding in all 3 of the trials was a statistically significant decrease in colorectal cancer (hazard ratio of .65). A clear reason for this has not been given. Other cancers including lung and endometrial did not appear to be affected by HRT.

Endometrial cancer is increased in women using unopposed estrogen, with a 2- to 6-fold risk compared with nonusers, increasing to an 8-fold risk for 10–20 years of use. Risk increases after 3 years use and persists longer than 10 years after discontinuation of estrogen. Risk also increases with increasing estrogen dose. The risk for death is probably not as significant, as endometrial cancer is largely curable. The addition of a progestin in sufficient dose and for sufficient duration (eg, medroxyprogesterone 5 mg for 12 days monthly added to conjugated estrogen 0.625 mg/d) appears adequate to eliminate almost all of this risk. Cyclic use of unopposed estrogen (eg, 25 days monthly) does not reduce the risk for development of endometrial cancer. Absolute risk, if any, of unopposed vaginal estrogen use is not well studied. Prevention of the increased risk of uterine cancer associated with unopposed ERT is the only reason for adding a progestin to ERT.

Risk of ovarian cancer related to hormone replacement has also been evaluated. The results of a retrospective observational study that reviewed 44,241 postmenopausal women in the Breast Cancer Detection Demonstration Project revealed an increased risk, especially for more than 10 years of hormone use. Overall, unopposed estrogen users had a 60% increased risk (relative risk 1.6) of ovarian cancer compared with never users. Risk increased with duration of use, such that those who used ERT for 10–19 years had a relative risk of 1.8 and those with 20 or more years had a relative risk of 3.2. Women who used combined estrogen and progestin did not have an increased risk, but the number of women using this combination was small. The results of this study are consistent with a large prospective study that monitored 46,260 former and current ERT users for 14 years. It showed increased risk of ovarian cancer mortality with estrogen, with risk limited to women who used estrogens for 10 or more years and which lasted for up to 29 years after cessation. A Swedish study found that estrogen use alone and combined HRT may be associated with increased ovarian cancer risk. More data is needed to determine whether estrogen-progestin use is associated with increased risk.

The above studies have helped clarify 2 very important issues: (1) HRT should not be started or continued with the intent of either primary or secondary prevention of CHD in postmenopausal women, and (2) the overall risk-benefit ratio may not be favorable to hormone use because there are clear increases in venous thromboembolism, CVA, biliary disease, and CHD. If all of these factors are placed in a global index perspective, there would be an excess risk of 19 events per 10,000 person years of HRT use (Table 18–1). If a patient's major need is for symptom relief, HRT still is a good short-term option. If, on the other hand, she has an increased risk of invasive breast cancer and no other

Table 18–1. Risk of adverse events associated with hormone replacement therapy.

Adverse Event	Number of Cases	Estimated Hazard Ratio (95% CIs)
Coronary heart disease	286	1.29 (1.02–1.63)
Breast cancer	290	1.26 (1.00–1.59)
Stroke	212	1.41 (1.07–1.85)
Pulmonary embolism	101	2.13 (1.39–3.25)
Colorectal cancer	112	0.63 (0.43–0.92)
Endometrial cancer	47	0.83 (0.47–1.47)
Hip fracture	106	0.66 (0.45–0.98)
Death due to other causes	331	0.92 (0.74–1.14)

Results from JAMA 2002;288:321.
CI, confidence interval.
Absolute excess risks per 10,000 woman-years attributable to estrogen plus progestin were 7 more CHD events, 8 more strokes, 8 more pulmonary embolisms, and 8 more invasive breast cancers. Absolute risk reductions per 10,000 woman-years were 6 fewer colorectal cancers and 5 fewer hip fractures. The absolute excess risk of events included in a global index to summarize the balance of risks and benefits was 19 per 10,000 woman-years.

needs, HRT is probably not appropriate. In women who have been taking the combination of estrogen and progestin for CHD protection, it would be wise to discontinue the regimen but remember the risk of osteoporosis.

3. Side effects of HRT or ERT—There is a 2- to 3-fold increased risk of gallstones or cholecystectomy in women using ERT. In HERS, the risk of gallbladder disease was 38% higher among women who were receiving combination HRT than in those receiving placebo. Estrogen can significantly increase triglycerides, which can cause increased risk of pancreatitis in women with preexisting severe hypertriglyceridemia. ERT can exacerbate preexisting liver disease. In the Nurses' Health Study, there was an increased risk of systemic lupus erythematosus developing in estrogen users. In the same study, new-onset asthma appeared to be associated with estrogen use. Data are conflicting on whether or not ERT worsens airway function in women with established asthma. Unopposed ERT may increase the risk for Raynaud's phenomenon. A large observational study showed an increased risk of dry eye syndrome in postmenopausal women. One small study of asymptomatic uterine leiomyomas did not show growth in 1 year on standard doses of HRT.

Other side effects of ERT include bloating, headache, and breast tenderness in a small percentage of women. These adverse effects are usually mild and often improve within a few months of therapy. Unopposed ERT in women with a uterus is associated with unpredictable uterine bleeding in 35–40% of women per year. Side effects of progestins can include bloating, weight gain, irritability, and depression. In most women, these are mild and dose related. Micronized progesterone may have fewer side effects than progestins.

Absolute contraindications to the use of HRT are breast cancer, endometrial cancer, ovarian cancer, undiagnosed breast mass or vaginal bleeding, and active vascular thrombosis (eg, myocardial infarction, stroke, and deep venous thrombosis). Relative contraindications are CHD, cerebrovascular disease or other vascular occlusive disease, previous thromboembolic disease, chronic liver disease, severe hypertriglyceridemia, gallbladder disease, and endometriosis. A few small studies of use of hormones in women with a history of endometrial cancer have found no adverse effect on recurrence or survival of the disease, and an ongoing study sponsored by the National Cancer Institute is designed to determine whether women with a history of early stage uterine cancer can safely take ERT.

4. Common therapeutic regimens—The most common hormone regimens consist of oral continuous estrogen with or without progestin. Low dose oral contraceptives are an attractive early menopausal/perimenopausal alternative for eligible women (eg, nonsmoking, no CVD, etc.) who have vasomotor symptoms but who are still having fairly frequent menstrual bleeding, especially if they also need contraception. The main risk is the slight increase in cardiovascular and thromboembolic risk. For the majority of women who are not actively menstruating, HRT is a more preferable option secondary to its lower cardiovascular and thrombotic risk. Oral estrogen is typically prescribed in the form of CEE 0.3 mg–0.625 mg/d or micronized estradiol 0.5 mg–1 mg/d. Daily use of estrogen is preferable to cyclic use to decrease vasomotor symptoms, which can occur if there are days off estrogen. Transdermal estradiol preparations avoid the first-pass liver effect, which may be beneficial in reducing coagulation risk. Vaginal preparations are increasingly popular, given the risks associated with prolonged oral HRT use, and are especially effective for symptoms of genitourinary atrophy. Creams such as conjugated estrogen 0.5–2 g or micronized estradiol 2–4 g are typically prescribed daily for 1 to 2 weeks, then reduced to 50% or less of the initial daily dose once or twice weekly. For genitourinary symptoms, vaginal estrogen can be discontinued entirely in some women after 6 months or continued as infrequently as 2 to 4 times monthly. An estrogen vaginal ring containing 2 mg of micronized estradiol is available and lasts for up to 90 days. Estrogen-only regimens are appropriate for women who have undergone hysterectomy. Progestins such as medroxyprogesterone 2.5 mg/d or 5 mg for 12 days monthly should be added to the oral and transdermal estrogen preparations in women with a uterus. Oral micronized progesterone (200 mg/d for 12 days) reduces risk for endometrial hyperplasia similar to continuous or cyclic (12 day) medroxyprogesterone. Combination oral and patch formulations are available. Continuous HRT regimens are the most widely accepted, as the cyclic regimens are associated with cyclic menstrual type bleeding. Vaginal bleeding may occur during the first 6 to 8 months of continuous regimens, but amenorrhea is usually achieved by 1 year, especially on the lower doses of estrogen. If progestins are not tolerated, women with an intact uterus taking unopposed estrogen should undergo annual endometrial surveillance. In light of the risks associated with long-term HRT use, if a woman wishes to use hormones and has no contraindications, it seems most prudent to use the formulation, dosage, frequency and duration of hormone(s) that causes the least systemic exposure possible to accomplish the goals of treatment.

B. Selective Estrogen Receptor Modulators (SERMs)

SERMs are estrogen-like therapies that have tissue-selective estrogen agonist and antagonist properties. Results of the effectiveness of SERMs, such as raloxifene and tamoxifen, in reducing breast cancer risk, improving bone density, and preventing osteoporotic fractures are accumulating. Tamoxifen has been proved to reduce breast cancer risk. It increases bone density, but substantially less so than with ERT and bisphosphonates, and bone loss has been reported in some women taking it. Side effects include hot flushes and increased risk for thromboembolism and endometrial cancer. Raloxifene may be more beneficial for menopausal women because, unlike HRT and tamoxifen, it appears to have no effect on endometrial proliferation in early studies. It appears to reduce risk for breast cancer in early studies. However, it does have an increased risk of thromboembolism and hot flushes. Cardiac benefits are currently being studied (Raloxifene Use for the Heart, RUTH study). Raloxifene is less effective than bisphosphonates for treatment of osteoporosis (see Chapter 19, Osteoporosis).

C. Nonhormonal Therapies

Nonhormonal therapies have become increasingly important to postmenopausal women, particularly with increasing evidence of their benefits and of the risks of long-term HRT. Even in women who elect short-term HRT use, nonhormonal therapy benefits are additive.

1. Lifestyle approaches—Lifestyle approaches include eating a healthy diet, exercising regularly, quitting smoking, decreasing alcohol intake, and reducing stress.

a. Diet—A diet high in fiber and low in fat decreases CHD risk. Decreasing caloric intake and associated weight loss in overweight women reduces CHD risk (see Chapter 7). Increased intake of soy products may decrease hot flushes and other menopausal symptoms.

b. Exercise—Regular aerobic exercise reduces CHD risk (see Chapter 7). Weight-bearing exercise and strengthening decreases osteoporosis risk, decreases risk of falls, may improve mood, helps prevent weight gain and may help sleep.

c. Tobacco cessation—Smoking accelerates menopause and associated long-term risks by 2 years on average. Smoking cessation greatly reduces risk for CHD and should be a priority for all women (see Chapter 7). It also reduces risk for osteoporosis.

d. Alcohol intake decrease—Moderation of alcohol intake may decrease hot flushes and osteoporosis/fall risk.

e. Stress reduction and relaxation—Stress is associated with increased CHD risk as well as worsened mood. In addition to aerobic exercise, a menopausal woman may benefit from focusing efforts on reducing stress and relaxation.

2. Bisphosphonates—There is increasing evidence of the effectiveness of alendronate and risedronate for prevention of osteoporotic fracture, even more so than with ERT and SERMs. Another advantage of these agents is that unlike ERT, there is no increased thromboembolic risk and no effect on breast or endometrial tissue (see Chapter 19, Osteoporosis).

3. Individual conditions—Associated with menopause and treatment of those conditions with nonpharmacologic therapies can be very effective.

a. Vasomotor symptoms—Nonpharmacologic interventions include dressing in layers and identifying and avoiding triggers (eg, hot rooms, spicy foods, caffeine, alcohol). Antidepressants such as fluoxetine, paroxetine, and venlafaxine have been shown to be superior to placebo for treatment of hot flushes. Belladonna alkaloids are effective but potentially habituating, so should be used for only short periods of time. Clonidine is much less effective and has limiting side effects of dry mouth, sedation, and hypotension, even in patch form. Gabapentin may be effective, but there

is little data. Herbal preparations are reviewed in the following section, Complementary Therapy.

b. Genitourinary atrophy—Vaginal lubricants and moisturizers can be very effective for vaginal dryness and dyspareunia. Regular sexual stimulation can prevent decreasing vaginal size. Vaginal estrogen is effective (see above).

c. Cardiovascular disease—Menopausal women should have their risk factors for CVD assessed and be counseled regarding risk factor reduction, which may include optimal control of elevated blood pressure, diabetes, and hyperlipidemia (eg, statins) as well as tobacco cessation and other lifestyle modifications (see Chapter 29, Risk Factors for Coronary Artery Disease and Their Treatment). The clinician should also ensure that each women ingests adequate folic acid (400 IU/d in typical woman).

d. Osteoporosis—Risks for osteoporosis should be assessed and modified as possible, which may include tobacco cessation, optimization of calcium and vitamin D intake, alcohol intake reduction, improvement of vision, fall prevention strategies and increased physical activity. Bone density screening should be obtained if indicated.

e. Breast cancer—In addition to routine breast cancer screening with clinical breast examination and mammography as indicated, modifying lifestyle to reduce risks, such as eating a low-fat diet and incorporating exercise into a woman's daily routine to prevent obesity may be helpful. Clinicians should discuss use of tamoxifen for prevention in women at high-risk.

f. Colon cancer—Colon cancer screening should begin at age 50, or age 40 if patient is at high risk. In addition, a low-fat, high-fiber diet may have a protective effect. Aspirin and other nonsteroidal anti-inflammatory drugs have also been associated with some reduction in colon cancer risk, but side effects may make prophylactic risks outweigh benefits and therefore they are not currently recommended. Calcium has shown similar efficacy.

D. COMPLEMENTARY THERAPY

Given the increased concern regarding HRT, there has been increased interest in alternatives to treat symptoms and disorders associated with menopause. Although concerns regarding safety and effectiveness remain, some research is available to guide the choices of women and their providers; in addition, several studies are underway.

Several alternative preparations have been evaluated for treatment of vasomotor symptoms. Progesterone cream has been studied in a randomized trial for treatment of hot flushes; doses of ¼ teaspoon per day was superior to placebo. In 1 double-blind, placebo-controlled study, hot flushes were reduced by 45% in women who took 60 g of soy protein isolate daily compared with 30% in the placebo group. In another study, women who took 400 mg of soy extract and 50 mg of isoflavone daily significantly reduced their hot flushes after 6 weeks. In 1 small double-blind, placebo-controlled German study, 8 mg/d of black cohosh was compared with 0.625 mg/d of conjugated estrogen and placebo. Women using black cohosh had fewer vasomotor and vaginal symptoms then women receiving estrogen, but there was an unlikely failure to show a difference between estrogen and placebo groups. In another randomized, placebo-controlled trial in women with a history of breast cancer, there was no difference in hot flushes between the treatment and placebo groups.

Dong quai, evening primrose oil, St. John's wort, ginseng, ginkgo, valerian root and other herbals have not been shown to be effective treatments for menopausal symptoms. More extensive review of complementary approaches is available in Chapter 58, Integrative Approaches to Women's Health: Herbals.

Effects of estrogen or estrogen/progestin regimens on heart disease risk factors in postmenopausal women. The Postmenopausal Estrogen/Progestin Interventions (PEPI) Trial. JAMA 1995; 273:199. [PMID: 7807658]

Grady D et al: Cardiovascular disease outcomes during 6.8 years of hormone therapy. Heart and Estrogen/progestin Replacement Study follow-up (HERS II). JAMA 2002;288:49. [PMID: 12090862]

Grodstein F et al: A prospective, observational study of postmenopausal hormone therapy and primary prevention of cardiovascular disease. Ann Intern Med 2000;133:933. [PMID: 11119394]

Herrington DM et al: Effects of estrogen replacement on the progression of coronary-artery atherosclerosis. N Engl J Med 2000;343:522. [PMID: 10954759]

Hulley S et al: Noncardiovascular disease outcomes during 6.8 years of hormone therapy. Heart and Estrogen/progestin Replacement Study follow-up (HERS II). JAMA 2002;288:58. [PMID: 12090863]

Lacey JV et al: Menopausal hormone replacement therapy and risk of ovarian cancer. JAMA 2002;288:334. [PMID: 12117398]

Risks and benefits of estrogen plus progestin in healthy postmenopausal women: principal results From the Women's Health Initiative randomized controlled trial. JAMA 2002; 288:321. [PMID: 12117397]

Rodriguez C et al: Estrogen replacement therapy and ovarian cancer mortality in a large prospective study of US women. JAMA 2001;285:1460. [PMID: 11255422]

Perimenopausal & Postmenopausal Bleeding

Atypical endometrial hyperplasia and cancer must be ruled out in women with abnormal perimenopausal bleeding. In addition, evaluation of the etiology of bleeding, especially in women on hormones, may further direct changes in therapy. Controversy remains regarding the appropriate method for endometrial surveillance, but common methods used are endometrial biopsy by pipelle and transvaginal ultrasound (TVUS). Other diagnostic tests such as dilatation and curettage or assessment of the uterine cavity with ultrasonography or hysteroscopy should be performed if abnormal bleeding continues after initial evaluation by endometrial biopsy or TVUS or if office endometrial sampling is indicated but unsuccessful.

Endometrial surveillance is indicated in any perimenopausal woman with a history of abnormal acyclic bleeding, including spotting or heavy vaginal bleeding, as well as in any woman who has uterine bleeding after a period of amenorrhea (eg, for 1 year or more), whether or not she is on HRT.

In women receiving unopposed ERT with an intact uterus, a biopsy should be performed before starting ERT and then yearly, whether or not there is uterine bleeding. TVUS usually cannot be substituted because of the thick endometrial lining in these women. Likewise, in women taking ERT and innovative progestin regimens that are not well studied, such as cyclic progestins every 2 to 3 months, a biopsy or TVUS should be performed yearly.

In women receiving combination HRT, regular monitoring for bleeding should be performed while on therapy. In these women, the likelihood of bleeding is related to the number of years since menopause, with less frequent bleeding occurring the further a woman is from menopause when she starts HRT.

Continuous combined HRT (eg, conjugated estrogen 0.625 mg/d or its equivalent and medroxyprogesterone 2.5 mg to 5 mg/d) is associated with a low risk of endometrial hyperplasia and induces amenorrhea within 60–75% of women by 6 months of use. Endometrial surveillance by biopsy or TVUS should be performed if bleeding is unusually heavy and persistent in the start-up months or if bleeding continues for more than 6 months after starting continuous combination HRT.

In women taking cyclic combined HRT, a biopsy should be performed when bleeding is acyclic or lasts for 10 days or longer. If bleeding is cyclic but begins before the tenth day of progestin administration, the clinician may increase the dosage or duration of progestin or both before performing a biopsy. If bleeding remains early or late (ie, before the eighth day or after the seventeenth day) in the 12-day course of progestin in spite of these manipulations, a biopsy should be performed.

Women taking tamoxifen or raloxifene should undergo referral to a gynecologist for any episode of vaginal bleeding. TVUS cannot be substituted because of the thickness of the endometrial lining.

Some controversy remains regarding the role of TVUS compared with endometrial sampling. In the Postmenopausal Estrogen/Progestin Interventions (PEPI) trial, an endometrial double layer thickness of 4 mm or less by TVUS was sufficient to rule out endometrial cancer in women taking continuous combined HRT for 4 years, although 50% had a thicker endometrium and required biopsy. In women not taking hormones, the same cutoff of 4 mm or less would yield a false-negative rate for endometrial cancer of 0.25–0.5%, which compares favorably with endometrial biopsy. Women with persistent bleeding who have an endometrial thickness of 4 mm or less by TVUS should undergo further evaluation, especially if there is any increased risk of developing endometrial cancer (eg, obesity; chronic anovulation; tamoxifen use; or family history of uterine, ovarian, breast, or colon cancer).

Relevant Web Sites

[The American College of Obstetricians and Gynecologists]
www.acog.org
[NCI Web site for patients]
www.cancer.gov
[North American Menopause Society]
www.menopause.org
[National Osteoporosis Foundation]
www.nof.org

Osteoporosis

Dawn P. Lemcke, MD

Osteoporosis is a major cause of morbidity and mortality, particularly in postmenopausal women. It is defined as bone mass 2.5 standard deviations (SDs) below the mean of a young, healthy person. A decline of bone mass by 1 SD is by definition **osteopenia,** which increases the relative risk of fracture by 50–100%. At present, prevention is clearly the most effective way to decrease this morbidity and mortality. The current mainstays of prevention are discontinuation of smoking, calcium and vitamin D supplementation, appropriate exercise, and antiresorptive agents. Treatments for established osteoporosis continue to be in a state of flux as new agents are evaluated.

 ESSENTIALS OF DIAGNOSIS

- *Low bone mass.*
- *Microarchitectural deterioration of bone tissue.*
- *Bone fragility.*
- *Presence of fractures.*
- *Increase in fracture risk.*

General Considerations

A. Epidemiology

Osteoporosis represents a major public health problem in the United States, affecting 15–20 million persons per year, most of whom are postmenopausal women. The disease accounts for 1.3 million fractures per year. The major manifestations of osteoporosis are proximal hip fractures accounting for 250,000 fractures per year, distal forearm and Colles' fractures representing another 250,000 fractures per year, and vertebral fractures in the amount of 500,000 fractures per year. By the year 2020, using conservative estimates taking into account the aging of the population and increase in incidence of osteoporotic fractures, the cost of such fractures may be approximately $62 billion. It is estimated that 15% of white women will fracture a hip in their lifetime, with a mortality rate between 5% and 20% in the year following the fracture related to complications. For many women, a fracture means the loss of independent living

and a marked change in the quality of life, factors that add to the impact of the disease. A recent study revealed that in a population of women over age 50, 40% had osteopenia and 7% had frank osteoporosis.

B. Risk Factors

Although there are known risk factors for osteoporosis, risk factor assessment in individual patients may miss up to 30% of women who are at highest risk for fracture. Although risk factor assessment is important, it should not be the sole method by which preventive measures or treatments are offered to patients.

Definitive risk factors for osteoporosis are shown in Table 19–1. In the National Osteoporosis Risk Assessment (NORA) study, the factors that were associated with an increased risk of fracture were advanced age, low body weight, frailty, cigarette smoking, lack of exercise, personal or family history of fracture, and corticosteroid therapy. Many of these risk factors have to do with increased risk of falls rather than with metabolic causes of low bone mass. Therefore, an important part of prevention is to decrease risk of falls.

Recommendations for calcium intake have been somewhat controversial, but it is clear that failure to achieve peak bone mass in adolescence can be related directly to calcium intake (Figure 19–1). The attainment of peak bone mass helps prevent osteoporosis later. After menopause, appropriate calcium and vitamin D intake along with other measures also can help in the prevention of osteoporosis.

Physical inactivity markedly reduces bone mass secondary to the loss of mechanical loading on bone, which acts to increase bone mass. Athletes have somewhat greater bone mass, unless they are suffering from the female athlete triad; this triad consists of the interrelated medical disorders of disordered eating, amenorrhea, and osteoporosis (see Chapter 8).

Alcohol intake in women also may increase risk of osteoporosis because alcohol impairs bone remodeling. Despite this, studies have conflicting results regarding whether or not alcohol intake truly increases the risk of fracture.

Smoking represents a significant risk factor for decreased bone mass and thus a preventable cause of osteoporosis. A study comparing female twins who were discordant for smoking revealed that those who smoked

Table 19–1. Risk factors for osteoporosis.

Nonmodifiable
Female sex
Age over 65 years
Slight build
Family history of osteoporosis
White, Hispanic, or Asian race
Premature menopause
Surgical menopause
History of atraumatic fracture
Loss of 1 in or more in height
Above average height
Dementia
Modifiable
Estrogen deficiency
    Particularly early menopause (younger than 45-years-old)
    Premenopausal amennorhea lasting longer than 1 year
Sedentary lifestyle
Low calcium intake
Failure to achieve peak bone mass
Weight below normal
Cigarette smoking
Impaired eye sight
Fall risk

1 pack of cigarettes a day throughout their adult life had an average decrease in bone density of 5–10% compared with their nonsmoking twins. This decrease is in the range that effectively increases the risk of fracture. Female patients of all ages who smoke should be urged to quit; physicians should be attentive to opportunities for early intervention concerning possible osteoporosis in these patients.

Amenorrhea, usually caused by a decreased level of estrogen, is a clear risk factor for osteoporosis. Important causes of amenorrhea are natural or surgical menopause, anorexia nervosa, and prolactinoma. Other important types include hypothalamic amenorrhea and exercise-induced amenorrhea. Drugs, including luteinizing hormone-releasing hormone (LH-RH) agonists and antiestrogens, also provoke anovulation. A careful history including menstrual and exercise history should help the physician to decide which women need further testing. Early intervention in amenorrheic women is important, although a study reported that anorectic women who achieved 80% of recommended weight and took estrogen and calcium supplementation did not fare any better in bone mass preservation than those who had no intervention. There are factors that appear to protect women from osteoporosis (Table 19–2).

Pathogenesis

Bone mass in women peaks shortly after puberty at the end of the growth period (approximately age 17); however, small gains in bone mass may be achieved up to age 30. This period is followed by progressive loss of bone mass. The pattern of bone loss is different in women than in men. Women not only have a slow, protracted phase, which is also present in men, but they also have an accelerated phase that occurs in the postmenopausal period. It is this accelerated phase in menopause that is believed to account for up to 40% of loss of bone mass. The accelerated phase may last for 5–10 years and generally ceases by age 70 when it returns to the normal bone loss of aging (Figure 19–2).

The slow phase of bone loss is due to decreased bone formation. There is continued activity of osteoclasts, but osteoblasts fail to recreate bone leading to a decrease in bone mass. In the accelerated phase of osteoporosis, there is a marked increase in osteoclastic activity with continued osteoblastic activity, which cannot maintain the same rate of activity as osteoclasts. A major contributor to the accelerated phase of bone loss

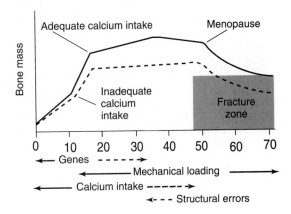

Figure 19–1. Major determinants of bone mass at various ages. (Reproduced, with permission, from Heaney R: Nutritional factors in bone health. In: Riggs BL, Melton L J III (editors): *Osteoporosis: Etiology, Diagnosis, and Management.* Raven Press, 1988.)

Table 19–2. Protective factors against osteoporosis.

Increased BMI
African-American race
Estrogen therapy
Diuretics
Exercise

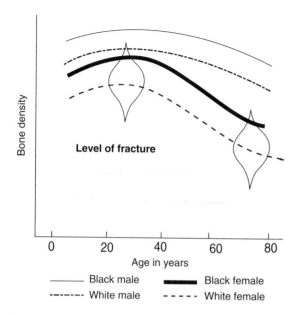

Black male ———   Black female ━━━
White male - - - - -   White female - - - -

Figure 19–2. Effect of sex and race on peak bone mass. Individual values about regression lines (for white women this is given by a top-shaped figure). This figure illustrates the rapid perimenopausal bone loss, but also that low bone density at young ages predisposes to fractures in later life. (Reproduced, with permission, from Riggs BL: Osteoporosis. In: DeGroot LJ et al (editors): *Textbook of Endocrinology,* 2nd ed. WB Saunders and Company, 1989. Reproduced, with permission, from Riggs BL, Melton LJ: The prevention and treatment of osteoporosis. N Engl J Med 1992;327:620.)

in menopausal women is the loss of intrinsic estrogen. The primary effect of estrogen on bone is to decrease bone turnover by decreasing osteoclastic activity. Other factors that contribute to osteoporosis are decreased absorption of calcium from the gastrointestinal tract, which occurs with aging; elevated parathyroid hormone (PTH) levels caused by decreased serum calcium levels; and decreased vitamin D levels, which occur with aging. The risk of fracture, particularly in the elderly, is affected by the type of fall and use of protective devices.

Screening

A. GUIDELINES

To date, none of the major health organizations (eg, American College of Physicians, American College Obstetrics and Gynecology, Canadian Task Force, and United States Preventive Services Task Force) recommend routine screening for bone density, and there are

no clear guidelines regarding intervals of screening and subsequent treatment. If a mass screening strategy were used, the percentage of women receiving estrogen therapy would increase and lifetime risk of hip fracture would decrease. The cost-effectiveness of such a strategy has not been determined. At present, most authorities recommend a selective screening approach to osteoporosis. The criteria for bone mass measurement as recommended by the National Osteoporosis Foundation (NOF) are as follows:

1. All women should be counseled regarding risk factors for osteoporosis and encouraged to discontinue smoking, increase exercise, and have adequate intake of calcium and vitamin D.
2. Bone mineral density (BMD) should be measured in women younger than age 65 with 1 or more risk factors (in addition to menopause) (Table 19–1). All women without risk factors should have BMD measured at age 65.
3. Postmenopausal women who seek medical attention for a fracture (to confirm the diagnosis and determine severity.)
4. Women who are considering therapy for osteoporosis, in whom BMD would facilitate the decision.
5. Women who have been on hormone therapy for prolonged periods of time.

Figure 19–3 is the NOF's guidelines about how to approach screening for osteoporosis.

Besides the recommendations for who should be screened, there are also recommendations for who should not be screened. If the decision to treat or alter treatment will not be affected by the results of bone density testing, it is not appropriate to measure bone mass. For example, some menopausal women plan to undergo hormone replacement therapy regardless of the results of bone mass screening.

The NOF has made helpful recommendations regarding the decision to treat after screening (Figure 19–3). Therapy should be initiated to decrease the risk of fracture in women with BMD below −2 SD (who have no risk factors) and in women with T scores −1.5 SD (with risk factors). In addition, women over the age of 70 who have multiple risk factors, especially prior fracture, are at high enough risk for the disease to begin therapy without having their BMD measured.

B. METHODS FOR MEASURING BONE MASS

Bone mass can be measured accurately in a number of ways, including single-photon absorptiometry, dual-photon absorptiometry, dual-energy x-ray absorptiometry, quatitative computed tomography (QCT), ultrasonography, and biochemical markers. It is clear from

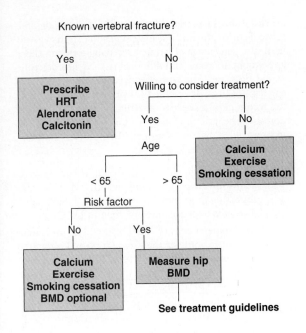

Figure 19–3. A suggested algorithm for evaluation and management of osteoporotic fractures. (Reprinted with permission from Johnston CC Jr: Physician's Guide to Prevention: Treatment of Osteoporosis, 1998, National Osteoporosis Foundation, Washington DC 2003.)

many studies that the bone mass measure is correlated with risk for subsequent fracture at all sites.

1. Single-photon absorptiometry—This method is limited to peripheral sites and cannot be used to measure spine and hip density. It is well tolerated by patients, with short scan times of 10–20 minutes and a cost of $35–125. It is relatively accurate and precise and may be most helpful in hyperparathyroidism, in which peripheral cortical bone is reduced more than trabecular bone.

2. Dual-photon absorptiometry—This method measures spine and hip density. From a patient standpoint, it is more cumbersome than single-photon absorptiometry, with scan times of up to 60 minutes. It is slightly more costly than single-photon absorptiometry.

3. Dual-energy x-ray absorptiometry (DEXA)—This method largely has replaced the other types of absorptiometry and currently represents the best method of determining bone density. It is rapid, with scan times of 10 minutes, costs approximately $100, and is precise. An excellent test for monitoring patients over time, it can measure density at any site; most commonly, the hip and spine are evaluated.

4. Quantitative computed tomography (QCT)—An accurate method of determining bone density, its use is limited because of its cost ($100–400) and radiation exposure, which makes it unsuitable for monitoring patients.

5. Ultrasonography—Ultrasound of the calcaneus is a relatively new technique for measuring BMD and predicting risk of fracture. There have now been 2 large studies, including the recent NORA trial that have demonstrated the ability of ultrasound to predict future fracture risk. Ultrasound appears to be an equal to DEXA in this regard. Using ultrasound to screen patients for osteoporosis is very attractive due to its portability and lower cost when compared with other methods. Both studies conclude that it should not be considered the gold standard in diagnosing osteoporosis. Its place is to screen large groups of women and refer those who appear to have low BMD for further testing.

6. Biochemical markers—There are various urinary chemical markers that can be used to assess bone turnover. For many reasons, these markers are not appropriate tests for screening patients for osteoporosis and should not be used for that purpose. Their proposed value is in monitoring women who are receiving therapy to assess effectiveness earlier than radiographic methods would allow. For example, if a women has undergone a DEXA and is found to be in the osteoporotic range, therapy is begun. Various studies have shown that a decline in the urinary markers correlates with increased BMD and therefore decreased fracture risk. If the markers remained elevated, a change in therapy (either adding a second agent or dose adjustment of the original agent) might be recommended. Using this approach, ongoing bone loss could be assessed before the 2 years that are recommended for most radiographic tests.

C. INDICATIONS FOR MEASURING BONE DENSITY

Besides the possibility of a mass screening that includes menopausal women, potential indications for bone density measurement include the following:

(1) Therapy for osteoporosis—Bone mass would be monitored to assess therapeutic efficacy. DEXA scanning is the most appropriate for this indication because of its precision. Unfortunately, there are no protocols for monitoring therapy in this way.

(2) To identify "fast losers" of bone—Such patients would benefit from aggressive therapy.

(3) Patients at high risk for osteoporosis—Evaluation would be done for patients undergoing anticonvulsant therapy and thyroid replacement therapy and those with amenorrhea, anorexia nervosa, alcoholism, multiple atraumatic fractures, or breast cancer.

Clinical Findings & Diagnosis

Most often osteoporosis is a silent disease without signs and symptoms until fractures occur. Some of the manifestations of the disease are loss of height; spinal deformity, especially kyphosis; and fractures, which may lead to pain. Although osteomalacia may present with diffuse bone pain, osteoporosis does not, unless the patient has suffered a fracture. If a patient with known osteoporosis without fractures experiences back pain, the pain is usually caused by other factors such as nerve compression, facet joint arthropathy, degenerative disk disease, or muscle dysfunction.

In a patient who has documented osteoporosis, a careful history and physical examination and several laboratory tests should be performed to rule out secondary causes of osteoporosis (Table 19–3). These factors may be identified in 20% of women with vertebral fractures. The most common causes of secondary osteoporosis are endocrinopathies. Other causes that should be considered are malignant tumors, (particularly multiple myeloma), renal insufficiency, liver disease, collagen vascular diseases (such as systemic lupus erythematosus and rheumatoid arthritis), and drugs.

In searching for secondary causes, the history should include a drug and alcohol history and a menstrual history. Standard laboratory tests should include a chemistry battery, complete blood cell count, creatinine level, and urinary calcium test. Additional laboratory tests that may be performed if indicated are tests for PTH, thyroid-stimulating hormone (TSH), serum protein electrophoresis (SPEP), urine protein electrophoresis (UPEP), 25-OH-vitamin D, prolactin, and urinary calcium. The level of urinary calcium excretion in a woman with documented osteoporosis may help in determining not only the cause of the osteoporosis but

Table 19–3. Secondary causes of osteoporosis.

Endocrinopathies
Hypogonadism
Hyperthyroidism
Hyperparathyroidism
Cushing's syndrome
Hyperprolactinemia
Acromegaly
Diabetes mellitus
Gastrointestinal diseases
Malabsorption syndromes
Chronic obstructive jaundice
Primary biliary cirrhosis
Subtotal gastrectomy
Inflammatory bowel disease
Drugs
Anticonvulsants
Chronic use of heparin
Overreplacement with thyroid hormone
Glucocorticoids
Anxiolytics
Cytotoxic drugs
Vitamin A and retinoids
Lithium
GnRH agonists

GnRH, gonadotropin-releasing hormone.

also the effective therapy. Normal urinary calcium excretion in women is 100–250 mg/d. Factors that increase calcium excretion include high calcium intake, renal calcium leak, high level of bone resorption, and furosemide therapy. Decreased levels of calcium excretion may be secondary to vitamin D deficiency, small-bowel disease, low calcium intake, and thiazide therapy.

Medications as secondary causes for osteoporosis deserve special mention. Glucocorticoid therapy represents a significant risk for osteoporosis. Although the true incidence of glucocorticoid-induced osteoporosis is not known, current data suggest the incidence to be 30–50%. Doses of prednisone of 7.5 mg or greater appear to cause significant loss of trabecular bone in most patients. Lesser doses do not appear to have a significant effect in premenopausal women, but postmenopausal women lose bone when taking lower doses. The mechanism of glucocorticoid-induced osteoporosis is both systemic and skeletal. The systemic effects include a decrease in calcium absorption and increase in renal excretion of calcium, decrease in gonadal hormone secretion, and muscle wasting. The skeletal effects of glucocorticoids that lead to osteoporosis are an inhibition of osteoblastic activity, increased sensitivity to PTH and 1,25-[OH]2D3, and possibly, stimulation of osteoclasts.

Thyroid hormone replacement, used commonly by many women, may present a risk for osteoporosis if the patient is "overreplaced," thus suppressing the TSH level. It is recommended, therefore, that the supersensitive TSH measurements be used to monitor women undergoing thyroid replacement to maintain their hormone levels in the normal range to prevent bone loss.

Prolonged use of heparin may accelerate bone loss in women and increase the risk for osteoporosis. Heparin is used as an alternative to warfarin during pregnancy. While the use of heparin is brief, a study of 184 women revealed that there was a mean decline in hip density by 5%, and 2.2% of the women suffered osteoporotic vertebral fractures. While the heparin is discontinued after delivery and bone density increases, it is unclear if BMD recovery is complete. Low-molecular-weight heparin appears to have a lesser risk of BMD loss but current studies are small.

High doses of medroxyprogesterone (such as those used for contraception and endometrial pathology) has been shown to increase bone resorption as well as reduce BMD. There has not been an increase in fractures noted and BMD appears to recover completely when the agent is discontinued. Therefore depot medroxyprogesterone should still be considered as an appropriate choice of contraception for young women.

Other drugs that have been shown to interfere with normal bone remodeling and therefore increase risk of osteoporosis are anticonvulsants, cyclosporine, vitamin A, and retinoids.

Although it may not be possible to avoid using these medications, special attention should be given to other interventions that may offset the effects of the medications. These interventions might include ensuring appropriate calcium and vitamin D intake, recommending exercise, and treating estrogen deficiency or documented osteoporosis at an early stage. In addition, screening for osteoporosis while on these therapies should not be forgotten.

There are medications that have been shown to be protective of bone and increase BMD. Hydrochlorothiazide has been shown to increase calcium absorption in the gastrointestinal tract and increase BMD. This effect is believed to be modest at best. Hydrochlorothiazide should not be the only treatment for a women with osteoporosis, but it may be additive to other conventional therapies. The effects of statins on BMD and fracture risk have been studied with conflicting results. Again, statins may increase BMD, but they should not be considered as preventive or sole treatment of osteoporosis.

Diagnosis of osteoporosis is made on the basis of a finding of decreased bone density by one of the methods described in the preceding Screening section.

Prevention & Treatment

There are several options available for both the prevention and the treatment of osteoporosis. Table 19–4 summarizes the current treatment options and their mechanisms of action. The drugs for treatment and prevention of osteoporosis fall into two general categories: those that inhibit bone resorption and those that stimulate bone formation. Most of the drugs available fall into the antiresorptive category.

A. ESTROGEN

In the past decade, estrogen was considered the first-line therapy for both prevention as well as treatment of osteoporosis. With the recent release of the Women's Health Initiative Study (WHI) and the Heart and Estrogen/progestin Replacement Study (HERS) II trial, this approach will likely change in the next decade. These studies show an increased risk of breast cancer and no benefit in secondary prevention of cardiovascular disease in women on a regimen of daily estrogen and progestin (see Chapter 18 for more detail). Because there are now other agents, specifically bisphosphonates, that do not affect breast cancer risk and are very effective for prevention and treatment of osteoporosis, these may be more appropriate as first-line agents. The mechanism of estrogen's effect on bone has not been elucidated fully, but the drug most likely works by increasing osteoblastic activity and thus decreasing bone resorption. Postmenopausal estrogen therapy should be started soon after menopause, because there is accelerated bone loss at that time. Beginning therapy within 3–5 years of natural menopause and within 6–12 months of surgical menopause should prevent bone loss. It is known that in premenopausal women who suddenly become estrogen deficient rapid bone loss en-

Table 19–4. Drug therapy for osteoporosis.

Antiresorptive Drugs
Estrogen
Biphosphonates
Calcium
Calcitonin
Vitamin D
1, 25-[OH]2D3
Selective estrogen receptor modulators (SERMs)
Drugs that Stimulate Bone Formation
Sodium fluoride
Low intermittent doses of parathyroid hormone
Phosphate and calcitonin
Growth hormone
AFDR (coherence therapy)

sues, resulting in the loss of up to 8% of their BMD per year, compared with 1–2% in normal menopause. This occurs in patients who have undergone surgical menopause or chemotherapy and in those patients who have radiation-induced amenorrhea or who have received therapy with GnRH agonists. Estrogen given postmenopausally rapidly normalizes bone resorption and formation, thus reestablishing bone balance. The effective doses of estrogen necessary to prevent bone loss are 0.625 mg/d of conjugated estrogen, 1 mg/d of 17-β-estradiol, or 50–100 mg/d of transdermal estrogen. Although there have been no definitive studies, it is believed that serum estradiol levels of 60 pg/mL represent the protective level for bone. Lower doses of estrogen are being used to decrease side effect profiles and perhaps risk of breast cancer but without clear data on their effectiveness on protecting against fractures. There is preliminary data that BMD is increased with conjugated equine estrogen doses of 0.3 mg/d; however, without fracture risk as the end point, it is hard to recommend this therapy over other more proven therapy.

The effect of estrogen on the maintenance of bone mass continues for as long as therapy is continued, and a positive effect has been shown up to age 75. After age 75, even long-term therapy may not be protective against fracture. Any time that estrogen is discontinued, bone loss proceeds at a rate similar to that of the early menopausal period. Studies have shown that 7 years of estrogen therapy is the minimal requirement for the effective maintenance of bone mass. Many studies have shown a 50% reduction in hip and wrist fractures and a 90% decrease in vertebral fractures with use of estrogen therapy.

In women with established osteoporosis, estrogen therapy increases vertebral bone mass by 5% and reduces risk of vertebral fractures by 50%. Thus, although estrogen is an effective therapy when speaking about osteoporosis, a discussion of risks and benefits in each patient should be undertaken as well as alternative treatments. The place for estrogen therapy may be in women who are perimenopausal with estrogen deficiency symptoms. In this scenario, estrogen could be used for a brief time for symptom relief as well as osteoporosis prevention, and long-term therapy could be reassessed at another time.

B. BISPHOSPHONATES

There are now many bisphosphonates for both prevention and treatment of osteoporosis. Those available are etidronate, alendronate, risedronate, pamidronate, and zoledronate. Of those available, only alendronate and risedronate are approved by the US Food and Drug Administration (FDA) for osteoporosis treatment and prevention. The bisphosphonates act as antiresorptives by inhibiting osteoclastic activity. Well-done, randomized, placebo-controlled trials of cyclic etidronate, alendronate and risedronate have shown that they all increase BMD in somewhat of a dose-dependent fashion, and decrease risk of vertebral and nonvertebral fractures by 30–50%.

Etidronate was the first bisphosphonate studied for use in osteoporosis. The trials revealed an increase in BMD and a decrease in vertebral fractures. Because of some question about long-term effect on bone mineralization (similar to the fluoride studies), etidronate was never approved by the FDA for use in osteoporosis. The newer bisphosphonates do not have these concerns, and their use has superceded the use of etidronate.

Alendronate in a dose of 10 mg/d or 70 mg/wk has shown consistent increase in BMD by 7–10% and a decrease in vertebral and nonvertebral fractures by approximately 50%. These studies were largely conducted in women with low BMD and evidence of osteoporotic fractures. When alendronate's use in women with low BMD without fracture was evaluated, no statistically significant decrease in fracture was found. Subset analysis did reveal that there was a decreased risk of fracture that was statistically significant in women with the lowest BMD (greater than −2.5 SD). Therefore, alendronate's value in this particular setting is uncertain.

Risedronate in a dose of 5 mg/d or 30 mg/wk is also an effective therapy for osteoporosis in women who have evidence of other osteoporotic fractures.

Combination therapy with various pharmacologic agents has been explored with the thought that the effect may be additive and thus more beneficial. Estrogen and bisphosphonates have been evaluated and have shown that the effect of the 2 agents is indeed more efficacious in increasing BMD than either alone. There is no data on whether this translates into a decreased risk of fracture and therefore this approach should be used only in special populations. This approach might be recommended for women who continue to lose bone on monotherapy, have very rapid loss of bone, or those who have had several osteoporotic fractures. Other combinations of agents have also shown promise for additive effect.

Pamidronate and zoledronate are intravenous bisphosphonates that may be considered as alternatives for women with osteoporosis. These agents may be appropriate for women who cannot tolerate the oral bisphosphonates or have contraindications to them. These agents require infusion 1–4 times per year; zoledronate is the easier of the 2 agents to infuse and has the most data in regards to BMD.

Patients must be carefully instructed how to use oral bisphosphonates properly so that absorption is maximized and the incidence of pill-induced esophagitis is decreased. Because the oral bisphosphonates are poorly absorbed, they must be taken on an empty stomach with nothing to eat for 30–60 minutes after taking the dose. In addition, the patient needs to take the medication with adequate fluid and remain upright after taking the medication to prevent esophagitis and esophageal ulcers. If these precautions are followed, the incidence of gastrointestinal side effects is no different than that of placebo. Risedronate is reported to have a lower overall incidence of gastrointestinal side effects when compared with alendronate.

Bisphosphonates have also been shown to prevent osteoporosis in lower doses than those needed for already established disease. The doses recommended are 5 mg/d or 35 mg/wk of alendronate or 5 mg/d or 35 mg/wk of risendronate.

Due to the recent questions regarding estrogen use, bisphosphonates may supercede estrogen as first-line therapy for both prevention and treatment of osteoporosis. Other candidates for bisphosphonate therapy are patients receiving either short- or long-term glucocorticoid therapy, premenopausal women undergoing chemotherapy likely to induce premature ovarian failure and rapid bone loss, and those with other chronic medical conditions known to cause bone loss. Many providers have now begun the practice of beginning bisphosphonate therapy at the start of glucocorticoid therapy that is anticipated to be longer than 2 months.

C. CALCITONIN

The action of calcitonin is to inhibit osteoclastic activity on bone. While studies have shown an increase in BMD associated with intranasal use of calcitonin, there are no good studies that show a decrease in fracture risk at any site. Because of this, calcitonin should be considered perhaps as a last alternative to other more effective therapies. Some clinicians will continue to use calcitonin in the setting of acute fractures because there is some data that it helps with pain relief by increasing endogenous endorphin release.

D. SELECTIVE ESTROGEN RECEPTOR MODULATORS (SERMs)

SERMs are a relative new class of drugs that holds great promise for not only osteoporosis treatment but also breast cancer treatment and prevention. The two drugs available in this class are tamoxifen and raloxifene. Tamoxifen, a drug used commonly in the treatment of breast cancer, appears to have both antiestrogenic and proestrogenic properties depending on the body site. It appears to act as an estrogen agonist on lipids, sex-binding hormones, and (as recently discovered), the skeleton. In a recent small study, 140 postmenopausal women with breast cancer received placebo or 10 mg twice daily of tamoxifen. In the follow-up examination

after 1 year, researchers found a 61% increase in bone density at the spine of women who received tamoxifen. Although this study did not document a decrease in fractures, it was encouraging that women with breast cancer may be protected from osteoporosis despite their inability to take estrogen. Further studies that document decreases in fractures with the increase in bone density will help clarify the role of tamoxifen in treating osteoporosis. At the present time, candidates for this therapy should probably be limited to women with breast cancer who are not candidates for estrogen therapy. Raloxifene is another SERM that has shown not only an increase in BMD but also a decrease in vertebral fractures of approximately 35%. The Multiple Outcomes of Raloxifene Evaluation (MORE) trial also appeared to show a substantial decrease in the risk of developing breast cancer in those women taking raloxifene. This finding has prompted the Study of Tamoxifen and Raloxifene (STAR trial) as a head-to-head comparison of tamoxifen and raloxifene in the prevention of breast cancer in women at higher risk. Women with an increased risk of breast cancer who want to prevent or treat osteoporosis are candidates for SERM therapy. However, until the results of the STAR trial are available, whether raloxifene therapy actually prevents breast cancer is unclear.

E. PARATHYROID HORMONE

Intermittent subcutaneous administration of PTH has recently been shown to increase BMD and decrease vertebral and nonvertebral fractures. The mechanism of action appears to be more bone formation than breakdown. The study was done in a population of women with prior fracture and low BMD. The beneficial effects were seen fairly quickly, in a period of 21 months compared with other therapies that may not show benefit for 3–5 years. This fact may help establish the drug's place in the treatment regimen of osteoporosis. PTH therapy is very costly, and therefore, there will be a very small number of patients in whom its use can be justified. Patients who are candidates are those who are rapidly losing bone and need a more immediate effect to prevent ongoing fracture.

F. PHYTOESTROGEN/ISOFLAVONES

There has been much public interest in natural approaches to treatment and prevention of menopause-related conditions including osteoporosis. Plant estrogens, because of their weak estrogenic activity have been advocated as a reasonable therapy for osteoporosis as well as estrogen-deficiency symptoms. Despite animal data that appeared to show increased BMD, human studies have not shown this to be true nor have they shown a decreased risk of fracture. Therefore, if women wish to take phytoestrogens, they should not be considered to be on effective therapy for osteoporosis prevention or treatment.

G. CALCIUM

In numerous studies throughout the last decade, the effectiveness of calcium supplementation in the prevention and treatment of osteoporosis has been found. It is also clear that adequate calcium and vitamin D intake is integral to bone health and full effectiveness of other therapies that may be used for prevention or treatment. Adequate calcium intake is essential to bone health in all age groups of women. It is important that adolescent women have adequate calcium intake so that they may achieve peak bone mass. A recent, randomized, double-blind, placebo-controlled study of 94 adolescent white girls showed that increasing calcium intake from 960 mg/d (80% of recommended daily allowance) to approximately 1300 mg/d (110% of recommended daily allowance) resulted in increases in total bone density. The form of calcium used in this study was calcium citrate malate. This increase in bone density may serve as protection later against osteoporotic fractures.

In an important recent study of women who had been menopausal for more than 5 years with baseline calcium intakes of less than 400 mg/d, benefit was seen from calcium supplementation of 500 mg/d. These women, compared with a group treated with placebo, had no statistically significant bone loss at the spine, hip, and radius. The positive effect was not seen in women in the first 5 years of menopause, when bone loss is quite rapid. Two forms of calcium were used in

the study, calcium carbonate and calcium citrate malate. Of the two forms, calcium citrate malate had more of a stabilizing influence on bone density than calcium carbonate, possibly because of variations in absorption.

In another confirmatory, placebo-controlled study, postmenopausal women with average calcium intakes of 750 mg/d showed slowing of bone loss by 43% over a 2-year period with calcium supplementation of 1000 mg/d. The form of calcium used in this study was calcium lactate-gluconate.

From the studies described in the preceding paragraphs of women of varying ages, the following conclusions can be drawn:

1. Appropriate calcium intake is important for women of all ages for maintenance of bone health.
2. The amounts of calcium necessary for bone health may vary by age, menopausal status, and pregnancy status.
3. Different forms of calcium may have different bioavailabilities.
4. Dietary calcium is preferable to supplements when possible.

Figure 19–4 shows the recommendations for calcium intake for women of various ages. An assessment of the dietary intake of calcium is an easy task during the history; use the guideline that each serving of dairy

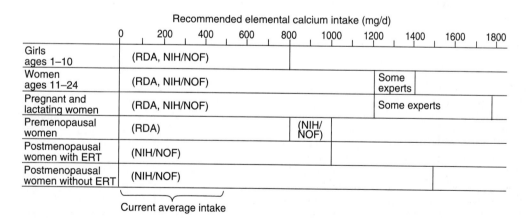

Figure 19–4. Recommended and current average calcium intakes in women of different ages. Although recommendations regarding intake vary, it is certain that the current average intake of 550 mg/d among adults in the United States falls well below recommended levels. RDA, recommended daily allowance; NIH, National Institutes of Health; NOF, National Osteoporosis Foundation. (Reproduced, with permission, from Utian WH et al: Calcium supplementation for the prevention and treatment of osteoporosis: A consensus opinion. Menopause Management Supplement, May/June 1994.)

food contains approximately 300 mg of calcium. For women who do not have adequate calcium in their diet, supplemental calcium is an option. To ensure bioavailability of calcium supplements, it is recommended that they be taken with food, that chewable forms be used when possible for higher availability, and that amounts larger than 500 mg be taken in 2 doses. It may be appropriate to recommend the citrate form of calcium for patients who take H_2-blockers, elderly women who may have achlorhydria, and those with a history of nephrolithiasis. Although there has been mention of the risk of nephrolithiasis with increasing levels of calcium supplementation, the available data do not support this concern as a factor that should limit recommendations to women. All women should be counseled about adequate calcium intake either in their diet or with supplementation.

H. Vitamin D

With the aging process, serum levels of vitamin D decline. The levels appear to be low enough to affect fracture thresholds in women over the age of 60. This decrease is secondary to decreased gastrointestinal absorption, decreased vitamin D synthesis by the skin, and renal deficiencies in the production of 1, 25-[OH] 2D3. It was the previous belief that only homebound, nursing home patients or those with chronic medical illnesses were at risk for vitamin D deficiency. Newer research has shown that up to 40% of healthy women with osteoporosis may be vitamin D deficient. Given this knowledge it would be reasonable to recommend that all postmenopausal women take vitamin D supplements. While the exact effective dose is not clear, 400–1000 IU/d is a reasonable recommendation without likelihood of harm. The dosage that has shown efficacy in women in nursing homes is 800 U/d of vitamin D or 150,000–300,000 units of intramuscular calciferol.

Another study of vitamin D revealed that in Boston at 42 degrees north latitude, perimenopausal women may lose bone mass in the winter months. Bone mass increased gradually during the summer months, but yearlong bone mass showed a slight decline. This decrease was presumed to be secondary to decreased sunlight, and therefore decreased vitamin D synthesis in the winter months. With supplementation of 400 U/d of vitamin D, the wintertime loss of bone density was slowed when compared with placebo. With vitamin D supplementation, there was a small but significant increase in bone density through the years; however, no correlation with decreased fractures was reported. This information may help physicians in recommending vitamin D supplementation to perimenopausal women in a similar geographic area, although it may not apply to all women.

I. Sodium Fluoride

Because fluoride increases osteoblastic activity, it has been considered a possible therapeutic agent for osteoporosis. Studies have shown that fluoride increases bone density in the spine but not at other sites containing trabecular bone. The increase in bone density depends also on adequate calcium intake of 1500 mg/d. Despite the increase in bone density, most studies have shown an increase in nonvertebral fractures associated with fluoride use and no significant decrease in vertebral fractures. This increase in fractures is caused by the formation of abnormal bone that may be poorly mineralized and mechanically defective. In addition, fluoride has side effects of gastrointestinal upset and lower extremity pain.

Fluoride may be more beneficial in decreasing fractures if given in a cyclic fashion or in a slow-release preparation. The previous studies were done with preparations that were not sustained release. A randomized, controlled trial of slow-release fluoride given in a cyclic fashion to women with documented osteoporosis showed encouraging results. When compared with placebo, the fluoride-treated group had an increase in bone mass of 4–6% and a decrease in fractures. Side effects for the two groups were similar.

Because of the concerns about safety and effectiveness and the questions about type of preparation and regimen, fluoride should not be considered effective treatment for osteoporosis.

J. Exercise

It is known that exercise is necessary for bone health: a sedentary lifestyle can increase the risk for osteoporosis. This fact has led to speculation that exercise might be viewed as a preventive measure for osteoporosis. From studies of exercise for prevention of osteoporosis, however, it is clear that exercise alone in the perimenopausal period does not maintain bone density. In postmenopausal women, the decreased risk of fracture that is found in the group that exercised, was largely due to increased muscle strength and improved balance that prevented falls, as opposed to true changes in BMD. A regimen of aerobic exercise 3–5 days a week for cardiovascular fitness and for attainment of peak bone mass and prevention of falls is recommended for all women.

L. Fall Prevention

One of the major reasons that fractures occur is falling. One of the biggest preventive measures that can be taken to decrease fractures is to prevent these falls. Attention to issues such as failing eye sight, obstacles in the home, and urinary incontinence have shown to decrease risk of fall and subsequent fracture.

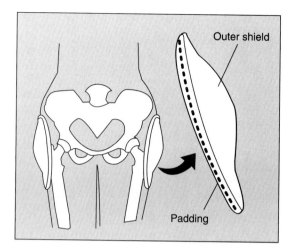

Figure 19–5. The hip protector. The two padded protectors are worn inside pockets on a stretchy undergarment. (From Kannus P et al: Prevention of hip fracture in elderly people with the use of a hip protector. N Engl J Med 2000;343:1506.)

M. HIP PROTECTORS

Hip protectors are a very simple measure that has proved effective. This device was evaluated in a nursing home population of frail, ambulatory patients at risk for fracture; it is designed to protect the greater trochanter should a sideways fall occur. A diagram of the simple device is shown in Figure 19–5. An impressive 60% decrease in both hip and pelvic fractures was found, despite many falls. Hip protectors should be considered for patients similar to the population in this study; it is a simple, nonpharmacologic way to prevent fractures. When the number needed to treat was evaluated, only 41 patients needed to use the device for 1 year to prevent 1 fracture. While there are now many hip protectors on the market, the device discussed here is the only 1 that has been studied to ascertain risk reduction for fractures.

Table 19–5 gives comparative costs of some of the more common treatments mentioned in the discussion.

When to Refer to a Specialist

The primary care provider should ensure appropriate calcium and vitamin D intake and take menstrual histories in women of all age groups to assess the potential for osteoporosis. If there is a concern for osteoporosis, the primary care provider should begin the assessment and evaluation, provided he or she is able to do so. The specialists most commonly recognized as experts in metabolic bone disease and osteoporosis are endocrinologists and rheumatologists. The following groups of patients may benefit from the input of a specialist:

1. Patients with documented osteoporosis who may not be candidates for estrogen therapy or oral bisphosphonate therapy because of personal preference or other diseases (eg, breast cancer). The specialist will discuss other options for treatment.

2. Women with documented osteoporosis who continue to have osteoporotic fractures despite treatment

Table 19–5. Cost of major drugs used in the treatment of osteoporosis.[1]

Drug	Daily dose	Cost per month
Conjugated estrogen (Premarin)	0.625 mg	$19.28
Medroxyprogesterone acetate	2.5 mg	$8.95
Conjugated estrogen plus medroxyprogesterone (PremPro)	3.125 mg	$28.68
Alendronate (Fosamax)	10 mg	$63.50
Risedronate (Actonel)	5 mg	$58.64
Calcitonin nasal spray (Miacalcin)	200 IU	$58.99
Calcium carbonate		
Tums	200 mg 2 tablets BID	$3.43
Tums Ultra	400 mg 1 tablet BID	$4.41
Oscal + D	500 mg 1 tablet BID	$6.67
Calcium citrate		
Citracal	200 mg 2 tablets BID	$8.24
Citracal + D	315 mg 1 tablet BID	$8.78
Citracal liquitabs	500 mg 1 tablet BID	$8.26

[1]Prices represent the cost to the pharmacist for 30 days' treatment according to average wholesale price listings. Data from Red Book Update, June 2001.

with appropriate agents. The specialist can help ensure that secondary causes have been ruled out and discuss treatment options, such as intravenous therapies or PTH therapy.

3. Women undergoing treatment for osteoporosis who have a considerable amount of related disability. These patients might benefit from a multidisciplinary osteoporosis clinic to address rehabilitation, nutrition, exercise, and the psychosocial aspects of osteoporosis.

Cundy T et al: Bone density in women receiving depot medroxyprogesterone acetate for contraception. BMJ 1991;303:13. [PMID: 1830502]

Cummings SR et al: The effect of raloxifene on risk of breast cancer in postmenopausal women: results from the MORE randomized trial. Multiple Outcomes of Raloxifene Evaluation. JAMA 1999; 281:2189. [PMID: 10376571]

Cummings SR et al: Effect of alendronate on risk of fracture in women with low bone density but without vertebral fractures; results from the Fracture Intervention Trial. JAMA 1998; 280:2077. [PMID: 9875874]

Dawson-Hughes B et al: A controlled trial of the effect of calcium supplementation on bone density in postmenopausal women. N Engl J Med 1990;323:878. [PMID: 2203964]

Dawson-Hughes B et al: Effect of vitamin D supplementation on wintertime and overall bone loss in healthy postmenopausal women. Ann Intern Med 1991;115:505. [PMID: 1883119]

Ettinger B et al: Reduction of vertebral fracture risk in postmenopausal women with osteoporosis treated with raloxifene: results from a 3-year randomized clinical trial. Multiple Outcomes of Raloxifene Evaluation (MORE) Investigators. JAMA 1999;282:637. [PMID: 10517716]

Felson DT et al: The effect of postmenopausal estrogen therapy on bone density in elderly women. N Engl J Med 1993;329: 1141. [PMID: 8377776]

Hopper JL, Seeman E: The bone density of female twins discordant for tobacco use. N Engl J Med 1994;330:387. [PMID: 8284003]

Kannus P et al: Prevention of hip fracture in elderly people with use of a hip protector. N Engl J Med 2000;343:1506. [PMID: 11087879]

Lindsay R et al: Effect of lower doses of conjugated equine estrogen with and without medroxyprogesterone acetate on bone in early postmenopausal women. JAMA 2002;287:2668. [PMID: 12020302]

Lloyd T et al: Calcium supplementation and bone mineral density in adolescent girls. JAMA 1993;270:841. [PMID: 8340983]

Love RR et al: Effects of tamoxifen on bone mineral density in postmenopausal women with breast cancer. N Engl J Med 1992;326:852. [PMID: 1542321]

Lufkin EG et al: Treatment of established postmenopausal osteoporosis with raloxifene: a randomized trial. J Bone Miner Res 1998;13:1747. [PMID: 9797484]

McClung MR et al: Effect of risendronate on the risk of hip fracture in elderly women. Hip Intervention Program Study Group. N Engl J Med 2001;344:333. [PMID: 11172164]

Melton LJ 3rd, Eddy DM, Johnston CC Jr: Screening for osteoporosis. Ann Intern Med 1990;112:516. [PMID: 2180356]

Mezquita-Raya P et al: Relation between vitamin D insufficiency, bone density, and bone metabolism in healthy postmenopausal women. J Bone Mineral Res 2001;16:1408. [PMID: 11499863]

Neer RM et al: Effect of parathyroid hormone (1-34) on fractures and bone mineral density in postmenopausal women with osteoporosis. N Engl J Med 2001;344:1434. [PMID: 11346808]

Osteoporosis prevention, diagnosis and therapy. JAMA 2001;285: 785. [PMID: 11176917]

NOF Physicians Guide 2001.

Pak C et al: Slow-release sodium fluoride in the management of postmenopausal osteoporosis. A randomized controlled trial. Ann Intern Med 1994;120:625. [PMID: 8135445]

Reid IR, et al: Intravenous zoledronic acid in postmenopausal women with low bone mineral density. N Engl J Med 2002; 346:653. [PMID: 11870242]

Schneider DL, Barrett-Connor EL, Morton DJ: Thyroid hormone use and bone mineral density in elderly women. Effects of estrogen. JAMA 1994;271:1245. [PMID: 7848399]

Siris E et al: Identification and fracture outcomes of undiagnosed low bone mineral density in postmenopausal women: results from the National Osteoporosis Risk Assessment. JAMA 2001;286:2815. [PMID: 11735756]

Utian WH et al: Calcium supplementation for the prevention and treatment of osteoporosis: A consensus opinion. Menopause Management Supplement, May/June 1994.

Watts NB et al: Intermittent cyclical etidronate treatment of postmenopausal osteoporosis. N Engl J Med 1990;323:73. [PMID: 2113611]

Relevant Web Sites

[National Osteoporosis Foundation. An excellent site for professionals and patients alike. Includes the latest consensus on diagnosis, treatment, and screening of osteoporosis.]
www. nof.org

Polycystic Ovary Syndrome

Lorna A. Marshall, MD

ESSENTIALS OF DIAGNOSIS

- *Oligomenorrhea with cycle lengths greater than 35 days or fewer than 8 menstrual cycles per year.*
- *Clinical or laboratory evidence of androgen excess.*
- *Exclusion of related disorders.*

General Considerations

Polycystic ovary syndrome (PCOS) is common, although its estimated prevalence depends on the criterion used for diagnosis. It may affect 6–10% of women in the reproductive age group. At least 90% of women who present with hirsutism and irregular menses have PCOS. Stein and Leventhal first described women with a triad of obesity, hirsutism, and anovulation in 1935. This triad is now known to be associated with a wide spectrum of hormonal, cardiovascular, and neoplastic changes and is more broadly classified as polycystic ovary syndrome. Importantly, neither obesity nor hirsutism is felt to be essential for the diagnosis of PCOS. In fact, about 10–30% of women with PCOS are considered lean. In general, any woman with anovulation and evidence of androgen excess is considered to have PCOS as long as related disorders have been excluded.

Pathogenesis

Although the pathogenesis of PCOS continues to be a subject of considerable debate, most investigators now believe that insulin resistance plays a critical role. Contemporary theories suggest that multiple factors, including insulin resistance and a cross-reactivity of insulin with ovarian insulin-like growth factor receptors (Figure 20–1), contribute to the development of PCOS. Because of the extreme sensitivity of the ovary to insulin, even small increases in insulin can cause the ovary to produce increasing amounts of androgens. The final result is noncyclic gonadotropin and androgen production, chronic anovulation, and a broad range of metabolic changes and associated increased morbidity and mortality.

The "polycystic ovary" develops when a state of anovulation persists for any length of time. The presence of the polycystic ovary is neither pathognomonic for PCOS nor is it essential to make the diagnosis. It is characterized by double the surface area, a thicker tunica, and 4 times more ovarian hilus cell nests than the normal ovary. Twenty to 100 small cystic follicles are present in the periphery of the ovary, and represent both growing and atretic follicles. When there are large patches of luteinized theca-like cells, the term "hyperthecosis" has been applied. The process is the same as in PCOS, but serum androgen levels are usually higher, amenorrhea is likely, hyperinsulinemia is more prominent, and acanthosis nigricans is likely.

Prevention

PCOS is thought to be a genetic disorder, possibly with autosomal or X-linked dominant transmission in some families. However, early diagnosis soon after puberty may allow the patient and provider to institute dietary and exercise modifications, as well as to initiate oral contraception. Suppression of ovarian androgens by oral contraceptive pills (OCPs) decreases the severity of hirsutism and insulin resistance associated with PCOS. It is not yet known whether the use of insulin-sensitizing agents in adolescence may play a similar role in preventing the severe manifestations of PCOS.

Franks S: Polycystic ovarian syndrome. New Engl J Med 1995;333:853. [PMID: 7651477]

Franks S et al: The genetic basis of polycystic ovarian syndrome. Hum Reprod 1997;12:2641 [PMID: 9455828]

Govind A, Obhral MS, Clayton RN: Polycystic ovaries are inherited as an autosomal dominant trait: analysis of 29 polycystic ovary syndrome and 10 control families. J Clin Endocrinol Metab 1999;84:38. [PMID: 9920059]

Stein IF, Leventhal ML: Amenorrhea associated with bilateral polycystic ovaries. Am J Obstet Gynecol 1935;29:181.

Clinical Findings

A. SYMPTOMS AND SIGNS

The diagnosis of PCOS can usually be established by history and physical examination. Most women have been overweight or have had difficulty losing weight since puberty. However, normal weight should not exclude the diagnosis of PCOS, since 10–30% of patients

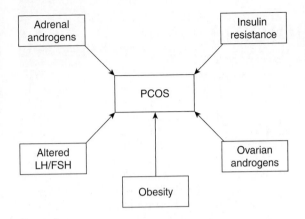

Figure 20–1. Etiologies of polycystic ovary syndrome (PCOS). LH, luteinizing hormone; FSH, follicle-stimulating hormone.

with PCOS are considered to have the "lean" variant of the disorder.

A menstrual history should be taken. Anovulation presents as primary or secondary amenorrhea in 50% of women with PCOS and as irregular, heavy bleeding in 30%. Women with adult-onset congenital adrenal hyperplasia or idiopathic hirsutism usually have regular menses. The high androgen levels present in patients with adrenal or ovarian tumors usually result in amenorrhea. A history of medications and dietary supplements should exclude androgen-containing preparations.

In both the history and physical examination, the provider should search for clinical evidence of androgen excess, including acne, hirsutism, and signs of virilization.

Close to one third of normal women between the ages of 15 and 44 have hair growth on the upper lip, lower abdomen, or breasts. In addition, 6% to 9% have hair growth on the chin and sides of the face. Hirsutism is excess body hair in women that follows an androgenic growth pattern. It is central in distribution, following the midline of the body. Coarse, terminal hairs suggest androgen excess, whereas finer, less pigmented, and slower growing vellus hairs do not. In contrast, hypertrichosis is a generalized increase in hair throughout the body, is present in both men and women, and does not warrant an investigation. Any methods that were used to control hirsutism and the frequency of their use should be documented. Assessing the severity of hirsutism from examination alone may be difficult if the patient has used mechanical methods frequently to control the hair growth. Correlation between history of hair growth and examination results should be ascertained carefully. Careful documentation

is made of hair growth on the upper lip, chin, breast and midsternal area, midline upper abdomen, lower abdomen and escutcheon, upper arm, inner thigh, upper back, and lower back. Several scoring systems are available for quantifying the severity of hirsutism, with the system of Ferriman and Gallwey being most commonly used.

For women with PCOS, hirsutism begins at the time of menarche and worsens gradually with age. Weight gain may worsen signs of hyperandrogenism in polycystic ovary syndrome. Use of oral contraceptives may delay the onset or arrest the progression of hirsutism. A woman may first complain of hirsutism in her mid-30s after she has stopped taking oral contraceptives. Rapidly progressive hirsutism or hirsutism that is noted first before menarche raises the possibility of an androgen-dependent tumor or Cushing's syndrome.

Ethnicity and race may be important to note. Since the concentration of hair follicles per unit area is greater in Caucasians than Asians, Asian women may have very elevated androgen levels with mild or no hirsutism. Adult-onset adrenal hyperplasia has a higher incidence in Ashkenazi Jews, Hispanics, and those of central European ancestry, whereas idiopathic hirsutism is common in women of Mediterranean ancestry.

Significant scalp hair loss, deepening of the voice, increased muscle mass, and clitoromegaly are signs of virilization. They usually are associated with higher androgen levels, although some scalp hair loss and slight changes in pitch can be seen with milder androgen excess. Before signs of virilization appear in a woman with an androgen-producing tumor, decrease in breast size and change in body contour to a more masculine habitus often are noted. Sometimes previous pictures of the patient are useful for comparison.

Acanthosis nigricans refers to velvety, verrucous, hyperpigmented skin changes, usually at the nape of the neck, at the axilla, in the groin area, and underneath the breasts. Its presence suggests the severe androgen excess and insulin resistance associated with hyperthecosis, but it can also be present in normal women.

A pelvic examination should be performed. Varying degrees of clitoral enlargement are seen in hirsute women. In general, the glans should be less than 7–8 mm in diameter. A glans size greater than 1 cm in diameter suggests virilization. Most androgen-producing ovarian tumors are too small to be palpated on examination. However, some larger nonsecreting ovarian tumors are associated with hyperplasia of the surrounding stroma and subsequent hirsutism.

Central obesity, hypertension, pigmented striae, proximal muscle weakness, facial plethora, and increased dorsocervical and supraclavicular fat suggest Cushing's syndrome.

Some women with PCOS may feel stigmatized and less feminine than other women. One study showed that a woman with body hair was rated by college students as more aggressive, unsociable, nonconformist, and independent and significantly less friendly, moral, and relaxed than the same woman without body hair.

A patient's reaction to hirsutism depends on her racial and cultural background, her perception of body image, and the severity of her symptoms. Most women in whom the onset of hirsutism occurs after puberty do not show any changes in gender identification. Compared with nonhirsute women, hirsute women tend to have greater body weight, more mood disturbances, fewer sexual partners, more body image problems, and more somatic complaints.

The effect of excessive androgens on behavior in women is not known; studies on this topic have been contradictory. Some studies have shown that high androgen levels correlate with greater sexual interest, especially with regard to masturbation. Antiandrogens given for the treatment of hirsutism may diminish this effect. This potentially undesirable side effect should be considered when counseling women with PCOS about treatment options for hirsutism.

B. LABORATORY FINDINGS

PCOS is generally believed to be a clinical diagnosis. Laboratory evaluation has in the past been reserved to exclude related disorders. Some argue that a hormonal evaluation is not necessary if hirsutism is mild or moderate and has been slowly progressive since puberty. Currently, additional evaluation is usually recommended to define the degree of insulin resistance and exclude glucose intolerance in women with PCOS.

If hirsutism is severe, recent in onset, or rapidly progressive, an evaluation should be initiated. The 2 key tests for exclusion of androgen-producing tumors are measures of testosterone and dehydroepiandrosterone sulfate (DHAS). Testosterone is the best marker for ovarian androgen secretion. If the testosterone level is greater than 200 ng/dL, an androgen-producing tumor, usually ovarian, is likely to be present and a referral should be initiated. Some women with hyperthecosis but no ovarian tumors have testosterone levels that are close to 200 ng/dL. On the other hand, some postmenopausal women with testosterone-producing tumors may have testosterone levels slightly less than 200 ng/dL. If the testosterone level is greater than 100 ng/dL and a tumor is strongly suspected in a woman of this age group, the evaluation to locate a tumor should continue.

DHAS is almost exclusively an adrenal product. Although it is not an androgenic steroid, it is a marker of androgenic steroid production by the adrenal gland. When DHAS levels are greater than 700 mg/dL, an adrenal tumor should be suspected. DHAS measurement is not a suitable tool to exclude adult-onset adrenal hyperplasia. Mild elevations of DHAS are consistent with PCOS.

If Cushing's syndrome is suspected from the history and clinical findings, testing for cortisol excess (eg the overnight dexamethasone suppression test) should be done. One milligram of dexamethasone is given at bedtime; the 8:00 AM cortisol level should be less than 6 mg/dL to exclude Cushing's syndrome.

Selective use of 17-hydroxyprogesterone (17OH-P) is appropriate to exclude the most common type of adult-onset congenital adrenal hyperplasia, 21-hydroxylase deficiency. Its use should be considered in patients who are members of ethnic groups that are at high risk for this disorder. However, women with PCOS often have elevated baseline levels of 17OH-P. If an early morning 17OH-P level is less than 200 ng/dL, 21-hydroxylase deficiency is unlikely. If it is greater than 800 ng/dL, the diagnosis is likely and a referral to a medical or reproductive endocrinologist should be initiated. If the level is between 300 and 800 ng/dL, an adrenocorticotropin hormone (ACTH)-stimulation test should be performed. The response of 17OH-P to intravenous administration of 0.25 mg of ACTH is believed to differentiate women with attenuated adrenal hyperplasia from those who have a slightly elevated baseline 17OH-P caused by another process, such as PCOS. The interpretation of this test is sometimes difficult, and referral to a medical or reproductive endocrinologist to determine the protocol and interpret the results is useful.

Free testosterone, sex-hormone-binding globulin, and androstenedione levels generally are not useful in the differential diagnosis of PCOS, only adding expense to the evaluation.

Prolactin, thyroid-stimulating hormone (TSH), and gonadotropin levels should be measured as part of an evaluation for oligomenorrhea or amenorrhea. Altered gonadotropin secretion in PCOS results in a preponderance of luteinizing hormone (LH) secretion and elevated serum levels of LH. In normal patients, LH measurements should be very similar to follicle-stimulating hormone (FSH). An elevated LH value (LH/FSH > 2) is consistent with PCOS, but 20–40% of women with PCOS do not have high LH levels.

All women in whom PCOS is diagnosed should be screened for hyperinsulinemia and glucose intolerance. There is no completely satisfactory method to determine insulin resistance in a clinical practice setting. A fasting glucose-to-insulin ratio has been shown to correlate with insulin sensitivity as measured by the insulin-glucose clamp test for insulin resistance. A ratio of less than 4.5 is consistent with insulin resistance. However, this test is not necessarily predictive of a response to insulin-sensitizing drugs. In fact, some investigators believe that all women with PCOS are insulin resistant and are therefore candidates for insulin-sensitizing agents. A useful strategy in the evaluation of the PCOS patient would be to obtain a fasting insulin and glucose, and a 2-hour glucose following ingestion of 75 g of glucola. The diagnosis of glucose intolerance can be made as follows:

- Fasting glucose: > 126 mg/dL indicates type 2 diabetes; 116–125 mg/dL indicates impaired glucose tolerance
- 2 hours after 75 g glucola: > 200 mg/dL indicates type 2 diabetes; 140–199 mg/dL indicates impaired glucose tolerance

Screening for lipoprotein abnormalities should be part of the evaluation of a PCOS patient, since hyperinsulinemia is associated with a higher risk of hypertension, hypertriglyceridemia, and decreased high-density lipoproteins.

Laboratory findings in PCOS are summarized in Table 20–1.

C. Imaging Studies

The diagnosis of PCOS does not depend on the ultrasonographic appearance of the ovaries, although a wide spectrum of sonographic appearances of the ovary in PCOS has been described. The "polycystic ovary" becomes apparent whenever anovulation persists for any length of time. Follicular growth is stimulated, but not to the point of full maturation and ovulation, resulting in enlarged ovaries with multiple tiny follicular cysts. This occurs whether or not androgens levels are elevated. In addition, as many as 25% of normal young women will demonstrate sonographic findings typical of polycystic ovaries. Therefore, the ultrasonographic finding of "polycystic ovaries" should be interpreted as "consistent with but not diagnostic of PCOS."

When the testosterone level is greater than 200 ng/dL, ultrasonography, preferably transvaginal, is recommended to exclude a tumor. These tumors are small, often 1–2 cm in size, and sometimes cannot be detected clearly with any imaging technique. For the adrenal gland, computed tomography and magnetic resonance imaging (MRI) are the best tests to localize a tumor.

D. Special Tests

An endometrial biopsy should be performed when anovulation has been long-standing. Endometrial cancer is more common as age increases, but even women younger than 30 years old with PCOS have been diagnosed with endometrial hyperplasia and cancer.

Laparoscopy should not be done solely to make the diagnosis of PCOS. The classic appearance of the PCOS ovary is with a smooth, thick, pearly white capsule.

Table 20–1. Laboratory findings in polycystic ovary syndrome (PCOS).

Test	Value	Comments
Luteinizing hormone (LH)	Normal or high	LH/FSH level > 2 strongly suggests PCOS
Follicle-stimulating hormone (FSH)	Low-normal or low	
Thyroid-stimulating hormone (TSH)	Normal	
Prolactin	Normal or slightly increased	
Testosterone	Usually > 50 ng/dL	Normal levels do not exclude PCOS if clinical evidence of androgen excess is present
Dehydroepiandrosterone sulfate (DHAS)	Normal or slightly increased	Rarely in range of adrenal tumor
17-OH progesterone	Normal or slightly increased	Should be measured in early morning. Levels over 200 ng/dL prompt ACTH
Estradiol	Normal for early follicular phase	
Estrone	Slightly high in obese PCOS patients	Generally not clinically useful to measure
Sex hormone binding globulin (SHBG)	Low	Generally not clinically useful to measure
Free testosterone	Normal or increased	Generally not clinically useful to measure
Fasting glucose/insulin ratio	Ratio < 4.5 suggests insulin resistance	May not identify all women who would benefit from insulin-sensitizing agents

When an ovarian or adrenal tumor cannot be detected but suspicion remains high, selective catheterization of the ovarian and adrenal vessels can be useful in localizing the tumor. Adrenal tumors occasionally produce testosterone, so that both ovarian and adrenal veins need to be catheterized when testosterone levels are elevated.

Consensus Development Conference on Insulin Resistance. November 5–6, 1997. American Diabetes Assoc. Diabetes Care 1998;21:310. [PMID: 9540000]

Ferriman D, Gallwey JD: Clinical assessment of body hair growth in women. J Clin Endocrinol Metab 1961;21:1440.

Kitzinger C, Willmott J: 'The thief of womanhood': women's experience of polycystic ovarian syndrome. Social Science & Medicine. 2002;54:349. [PMID: 11824912]

Legro RS, Finegood D, Dunaif A: A fasting glucose to insulin ratio is a useful measure of insulin sensitivity in women with polycystic ovary syndrome. J Clin Endocrinol Metab 1998;83:2694. [PMID: 9709933]

Differential Diagnosis

Several disorders result in oligomenorrhea or amenorrhea, usually without evidence of androgen excess. Prolactin levels are rarely above 50 ng/mL in PCOS; higher levels should prompt an MRI to exclude a pituitary tumor. Hypothyroidism can result in oligomenorrhea and sometimes an increase in vellus, but not terminal hair. Women with ovarian failure as a cause of amenorrhea have elevated FSH levels. Women may have oligomenorrhea or amenorrhea from hypothalamic dysfunction. Similarly, some women may have chronic anovulation without androgen excess, and without the typical profile of a woman with hypothalamic dysfunction. These women usually have no evidence of androgen excess, but may have "PCOS-like" ovaries on ultrasound. Currently, the most practical approach is to require either laboratory or clinical evidence of androgen excess to assign the diagnosis of PCOS and to avoid using ultrasound findings to make the diagnosis.

When hirsutism is severe, ovarian and adrenal tumors can usually be excluded by testosterone and DHAS measurements. Adult-onset congenital adrenal hyperplasia is usually associated with normal menses, as is idiopathic hirsutism. The term "idiopathic hirsutism" is often applied to women with normal ovulatory function and no evidence of ovarian or adrenal androgen overproduction, although the existence of this diagnosis is currently controversial. These women are thought to have increased skin 5-alpha reductase activity as a primary problem. Currently, most clinicians believe that irregular menses are necessary to assign the diagnosis of PCOS. Cushing's syndrome and acromegaly are rare causes of hirsutism but should be considered if the onset is later in life. Rapid progression of hirsutism or the appearance of virilization should prompt exclusion of other disorders even when the diagnosis of PCOS has been made previously.

Complications

When women with PCOS conceive, those pregnancies are associated with a higher risk of complications, including early pregnancy loss, gestational diabetes, and pregnancy-induced hypertension. In addition, the ovulation induction medications that are often necessary for pregnancy to occur result in a greater chance of multiple gestations and their associated risks. The risk of pregnancy loss in women with PCOS may be as high as 30–50%, or 3-fold that of the normal population. The cause for this is unclear, but may be related to elevated LH levels, hyperinsulinemia, or obesity.

Women with PCOS have a 3-fold increased risk for endometrial cancer. The increased estrone levels from conversion of androgens to estrogen as well as absent progesterone production contribute to excessive estrogenic stimulation of the endometrium in PCOS. Thirty percent of young women with endometrial cancer have PCOS.

It is now clear that the consequences of PCOS extend beyond the confines of reproduction. Impaired glucose intolerance or type 2 diabetes develops in about 40–50% of obese women with PCOS and 10% of nonobese women with PCOS. Hyperinsulinemia is thought to be an independent risk factor for coronary artery disease, as are the hyperlipidemia and increased levels of hypofibrinolytic PAI-1 observed in PCOS.

Legro RS et al: Prevalence and predictors of risk for type 2 diabetes mellitus and impaired glucose tolerance in polycystic ovary syndrome: a prospective, controlled study in 254 affected women. J Clin Endocrinol Metab 1999;84:165. [PMID: 9920077]

Wild S et al: Cardiovascular disease in women with polycystic ovary syndrome at long-term follow-up: a retrospective cohort study. Clin Endocrinol 2000;52:595. [PMID: 10792339]

Treatment

Treatment of the patient with PCOS depends on the specific manifestations, whether they be hirsutism, anovulatory infertility, irregular menses, or glucose intolerance. No single treatment can correct all of the manifestations of PCOS.

A. LIFESTYLE MODIFICATIONS

Weight loss is an excellent treatment for PCOS in the obese woman and has been shown to reduce insulin resistance, increase the frequency of ovulation and menses, and improve fertility. Strategies to promote weight loss should be part of any treatment plan for the obese woman with PCOS. However, many women do not wish to delay conception waiting to see if lifestyle modifications will result in ovulation and pregnancy. In addition, the provider should be careful not to withhold ovulation induction medications.

Lifestyle modifications are probably less useful for lean women with PCOS.

B. Oral Contraceptive Pills

OCPs are an excellent long-term treatment option for women with PCOS. Unless pregnancy is desired and ovulation induction is planned, OCPs or cyclic progestins should be administered to prevent endometrial hyperplasia or neoplasia (see Chapter 47). Medroxyprogesterone acetate can be prescribed 5–10 mg daily for 10–12 days of every 1 to 2 months to ensure complete, synchronous withdrawal bleeding. However, OCPs are generally a better option, since the estrogen in OCPs opposes the effect of androgen on the hair follicle, resulting in a reduced rate of hair growth and finer, less pigmented hair, while its progestin protects the endometrium from hyperplasia. In addition, OCPs suppress pituitary secretion of LH, which drives ovarian testosterone production. Most monophasic OCPs are appropriate for the treatment of PCOS. Preparations with ethynodiol diacetate have not been shown to be more effective than those with ethinyl estradiol. No more than 30–35 mg of ethinyl estradiol is necessary. The 19-nortestosterone derivatives such as levonorgestrel should be avoided because of their greater androgenic activity. The best progestins to prescribe are norethindrone and the newer, less androgenic progestins (desogestrel, norgestimate, and gestodene). There are some data that OCPs are less successful in the management of PCOS symptoms in the patients with the highest BMI (body mass index).

The new combination pill drospirenone-ethinyl estradiol is a spironolactone analogue with antiandrogenic properties. This new pill may prove to be an excellent treatment option for women with PCOS.

C. Insulin-sensitizing Agents

There has been increasing interest in insulin-sensitizing agents such as metformin or the thiazolidinediones in the management of PCOS. The role of these medications derives from the role of insulin and insulin resistance in the evolution of PCOS. Their most successful role has been as a sole agent or adjunctive agent in ovulation induction for PCOS. Although they are being used in the management of androgen-associated symptoms of PCOS, their role in the long-term management of PCOS in hopes of reducing cardiovascular morbidity and mortality is unclear. In addition, they have not yet been shown to be effective treatments for hirsutism.

Metformin is the most evaluated insulin-sensitizing agent. Doses of 1500 mg/d may increase menstrual cyclicity, improve ovulation, and improve fertility. About half of women with PCOS can expect a sustained positive response. Women who are morbidly obese (> 42 kg/m^2) may not respond well to this dose, and may need 2000–2500 mg/d to see a response. The most common side effect of metformin is nausea and diarrhea, and many women tolerate this medication better if the dose is increased gradually to the recommended one. The most serious side effect is lactic acidosis. Women who are prescribed metformin should have creatinine < 1.4 mg/dL, normal hepatic function, and no cardiac or respiratory disease that reduces peripheral perfusion.

Thiazolidinediones such as rosiglitazone or pioglitazone are probably also effective in women with PCOS, but fewer studies have been performed and the ideal dosing has not been determined. D-chiro-inositol is in clinical development and may eventually increase options available to women with PCOS.

The mechanism of action of insulin-sensitizing agents in women with PCOS is still unclear. They may act by decreasing insulin resistance and reducing hyperinsulinemia and therefore ovarian androgens or they may act directly on the production of ovarian androgens.

How to choose patients that may benefit from insulin-sensitizing agents is also unclear. Some endocrinologists use the fasting glucose-insulin ratio to choose candidates for treatment. A ratio less than 4.5 has been shown to correlate well with the glucose-insulin clamp test for insulin resistance. Others believe that all patients with PCOS are insulin-resistant whatever their test results, and therefore should be offered treatment. At this time, there are not enough data in adolescents to justify the use of these agents outside of study protocols.

D. Specific Treatments for Hirsutism

Mechanical treatments are effective by themselves for mild hirsutism and can be used in conjunction with medical therapy for more severe hirsutism. Bleaching is most successful with vellus hair growth but frequent use can result in skin irritation. Plucking is painful but can be useful for mild hirsutism in localized areas. Plucking has not been shown to decrease or increase the rate of hair growth. For larger areas, shaving commonly is used, but it carries a stigma when stubble is apparent. Depilatories and waxing also are used for larger areas but can cause significant skin irritation. Electrolysis is not really permanent, although it is often advertised to be. It can be expensive and time-consuming and may eventually cause skin thickening. Intense pulsed light systems and lasers have been developed specifically to target hair follicles. However, the development of these techniques has often been commercially driven and few controlled studies are available for evaluation.

Several antiandrogens are available for clinical use. The efficacy and safety of spironolactone have been established clearly. Spironolactone competitively inhibits the androgen receptor, and may also inhibit biosynthesis of ovarian and adrenal androgens. Spironolactone is most effective when given in doses of 100–200 mg/d; the dose may be lowered to 50 mg/d to maintain an effect. Because hyperkalemia is a theoretic risk of treatment, potassium levels should be monitored at follow-up visits. An undesirable side effect of spironolactone is abnormal bleeding; the addition of OCPs corrects the abnormal bleeding and augments the treatment of hirsutism. Spironolactone alone treats only the hirsutism associated with PCOS and does not alter the hormonal or metabolic manifestations of the syndrome. Currently the combination of OCPs and spironolactone is the most practical and effective therapy in most circumstances and has the added benefit of providing contraception. Cyproterone acetate is used widely in Europe but not available in the United States. Flutamide is being studied currently as a treatment for hirsutism. Enthusiasm for flutamide has been limited by reports of idiosyncratic severe acute hepatitis. An initial dose of 250 mg/d can be lowered to 125 mg for maintenance. Even lower doses such as 62.5 mg have been shown to be effective and may have an improved safety profile. Liver function tests should be monitored during treatment. Finasteride (5 mg/d), a 5-alpha reductase inhibitor, and ketoconazole (400 mg/d) have also been studied as treatments for hirsutism. One clinical trial showed that spironolactone, flutamide, and finasteride were equally effective after 6 months of treatment.

All medical therapies for hirsutism should be considered to be long-term. When the effectiveness is to be monitored, the 3-month growth cycle of hair should be considered. Any interruption in androgen-mediated growth cannot be seen until the next cycle of growth. The patient should be advised that 3–6 months of treatment might be required before any improvement in hirsutism is seen. It is also important to advise the patient that excess hair will not fall out and needs to be removed by mechanical means after about 6 months of medical therapy. The goal of therapy is to arrest or attenuate the growth of new hair.

Eflornithine HCl 13.9% is a new topical treatment for hirsutism that inhibits ornithine decarboxylase, which is essential for the rapidly growing cells of the hair follicle. It is a promising, convenient therapy that results in some burning or stinging on application but less than 1% is absorbed, so no systemic side effects should be expected.

E. Induction of Ovulation

PCOS is associated with oligomenorrhea or amenorrhea. These patients usually require ovulation induction to conceive. In women with high levels of androgens, ovulation induction is often difficult, requiring high doses of clomiphene or gonadotropins.

Reduction in insulin levels through weight loss and the use of insulin-sensitizing agents have emerged as important tools to assist ovulation in women with PCOS. Metformin has been shown to increase both spontaneous and clomiphene-induced ovulation rates. It is less clear whether insulin-sensitizing agents are effective adjuvants to gonadotropin therapy or to in vitro fertilization. Metformin in a dose of 500 mg 3 times a day may be prescribed in addition to clomiphene for women who do not ovulate on 100 mg/d. Nestler has proposed an algorithm for managing ovulation induction in women with PCOS (Figure 20–2). Probably, the most compelling argument for use of insulin-sensitizing agents is to avoid multiple gestations associated with gonadotropin use.

Women with PCOS are also at higher risk for complications of ovulation induction, including ovarian hyperstimulation and multiple pregnancies. Increased rates of spontaneous pregnancy loss have been associated with elevated LH levels, such as those seen in PCOS.

Metformin is a pregnancy category B medication. The current recommendation is to stop the medication when pregnancy occurs, but at least 1 study suggests that metformin may reduce the incidence of pregnancy loss and is safe to take in the first trimester.

F. Other Treatments for PCOS

Surgical treatment of PCOS has a long history. Laparotomy with ovarian wedge resection was first described in by Stein and Leventhal in 1935. All 7 patients in their initial series resumed regular menses after removal of one half to three quarters of each ovary, and 2 became pregnant. This procedure is no longer performed because of the risk of severe periadnexal adhesions. Laparoscopy with ovarian "drilling" using a laser or cautery has replaced the wedge resection and continues to have a place in the management of PCOS. In some cases, electrocautery of the ovarian cortex reduces androgens and facilitates the success of ovulation-inducing agents.

Gonadotropin-releasing hormone agonists plus estrogens and progestins, OCPs, or flutamide are also useful but are much more expensive and should be used only in selected cases with high testosterone levels.

G. Complementary Therapies

Patients may seek complementary medicine approaches for the management of some symptoms of PCOS. In Chinese medicine, normal menstrual periods are essential for maintaining a balance in the body, and many herbal treatments are directed toward the restoration of

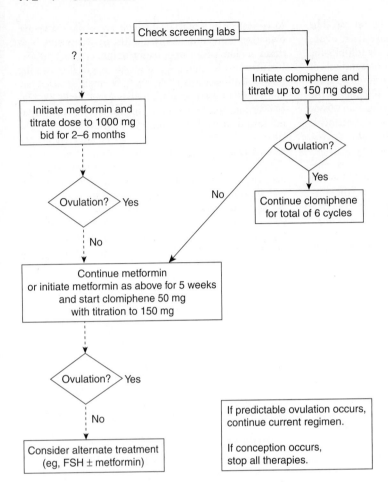

Figure 20–2. Algorithm for the use of metformin in the induction of ovulation in women with polycystic ovary syndrome. FSH, follicle-stimulating hormone. (Reproduced with permission from Nestler JE et al. Fertil Steril 2002;77:209.)

normal menstruation. The herb licorice is offered specifically to restore menses in women with elevated testosterone levels, such as those with PCOS. Many herbs probably have estrogenic, anti-estrogenic, or progestogenic activity. Knowledge of any herbal medicines or dietary supplements used by the patient is essential as a hormonal treatment plan is formulated.

A large variety of nutritional supplements and herbs are available for the management of obesity associated with PCOS, including pyruvate, 5-hydroxytryptophan, guarana, and ma huang. Ma huang (ephedra sinica) is a central nervous system stimulant with many adverse side effects.

Farquhar C, Vandekerckhove P, Lilford R: Laparoscopic "drilling" by diathermy or laser for ovulation induction in anovulatory polycystic ovary syndrome. Cochrane Database Syst Rev 2002;(4):CD001122. [PMID: 11687100]

Jakubowicz DJ et al: Effects of metformin on early pregnancy loss in the polycystic ovary syndrome. J Clin Endocrinol Metab 2002;87:524. [PMID: 11836280]

Moghetti P et al: Metformin effects on clinical features, endocrine and metabolic profiles, and insulin sensitivity in polycystic ovary syndrome: a randomized, double-blind, placebo-controlled 6-month trial, followed by open, long-term clinical evaluation. J Clin Endocrinol Metab 2000;85:89. [PMID: 10634370]

Moghetti P et al: Comparison of spironolactone, flutamide, and finasteride efficacy in the treatment of hirsutism: a randomized, double blind, placebo-controlled trial. J Clin Endocrinol Metab 2000;85:89. [PMID: 10634370]

Nestler JE et al: Strategies for the use of insulin-sensitizing drugs to treat infertility in women with polycystic ovary syndrome. Fertil Steril 2002;77:209 [PMID: 11821072]

Velazquez E, Acosta A, Mendoza SG: Menstrual cyclicity after metformin therapy in polycystic ovary syndrome. Obstet Gynecol 1997;90:392. [PMID: 9277650]

When to Refer to a Specialist

If the diagnosis of PCOS is unclear, a medical endocrinologist, a reproductive endocrinologist, or sometimes a pediatric endocrinologist can help clarify the diagnosis and recommend a treatment plan. When a patient with PCOS desires conception and does not ovulate while taking 100 mg of clomiphene, she should be referred to a reproductive endocrinologist or to a gynecologist who has experience with complicated ovulation induction.

Prognosis

PCOS is a genetic disorder, with lifelong effects on reproductive and general health. Women who respond well to oral contraceptives can use them for the duration of their reproductive years, and this can be a quite satisfactory long-term treatment option. In addition, weight loss in the obese patient with PCOS has been shown to improve the hormonal profile and may decrease the risk of long-term sequelae of PCOS such as diabetes, endometrial cancer, and hypertension. Moderate or severe hirsutism is usually a long-standing problem that may improve somewhat with medical and mechanical therapies but usually never goes away completely.

Women with PCOS should have periodic monitoring for glucose intolerance, hypertension and lipid abnormalities. If they are not taking OCPs, monitoring of the endometrium is also recommended.

Relevant Web Sites

[Polycystic Ovarian Syndrome Society] A national organization operated by women with PCOS

www.pcosupport.org

[American Society for Reproductive Medicine] Patient information and professional guidelines available to all users

www.asrm.org

SECTION V

Breast Disease

Evaluation of Breast Masses

21

Debra G. Wechter, MD

ESSENTIALS OF DIAGNOSIS

- *Verify that a true breast mass is present.*
- *Use appropriate imaging studies and special tests to help determine whether a mass is suspicious for malignancy.*

General Considerations

Whenever a woman or her provider finds a breast abnormality, the primary concern is the possibility of cancer. Therefore, the focus of the evaluation must be on proving whether a mass is benign or malignant. Fortunately, most abnormalities found by women and their providers are benign. Most palpable abnormalities are cysts, fibroadenomas, or even just benign asymmetric breast tissue.

Clinical Findings

A. SYMPTOMS AND SIGNS

Most breast masses are asymptomatic and are found by a provider on clinical breast examination or by a woman performing self examination. Occasionally, a woman will have breast pain that will lead her to self examination. She may then feel an area of breast tissue that she thinks is abnormal and accounts for her pain. More often than not, this will be a benign area of normal or asymmetric breast tissue. However, a cyst, fibroadenoma, or fat necrosis can certainly cause pain. Cancer is less likely to be associated with pain as its initial symptoms. There may be associated nipple discharge, but this is not as likely if the mass is benign.

The following information about a woman's history helps determine the appropriate level of suspicion necessary in evaluating a breast mass:

Length of time the mass has been present

Variation with the menstrual cycle

Change in size, shape, or texture

How the mass was discovered

Associated pain, nipple discharge, skin change

Age at menarche, regularity of menses, time of last menstrual cycle

Age at menopause

Number of pregnancies and births

Age at first live birth

History of breast-feeding

Family or personal history of breast or ovarian cancer

Age at which affected first-degree relative was diagnosed with breast or ovarian cancer

Previous breast operations and results of pathology tests

Exogenous hormone usage

Many of these facts help assess a woman's personal risk for breast cancer. However, this is of little consequence compared with the data obtained from imaging studies and tissue diagnosis, since more than 75% of women with breast cancer have no identifiable risk factors. Whether the risk seems high or low, further evaluation should be the same.

Physical examination should focus on characterizing the mass and comparing findings in both breasts. The key is to determine whether a mass is normal for a particular woman based on her age and hormonal status. As with the woman's history, the examination is important, but it merely changes the level of suspicion and does not give information as specific as imaging and tissue diagnosis. Breast examination continues to be important, however, since it can detect up to 50% of breast cancers not detected by mammography alone.

It is important to examine a woman in both the sitting and supine positions. When the patient is sitting with her arms raised above her head, look for asymmetry, puckering, or dimpling and then have her tense the pectoralis major muscle by having her press both hands on her hips. When the patient is supine, the arm on the side to be examined should again be raised above the head to flatten the breast as much as possible. Any skin changes such as erythema or peau d'orange (thickened skin with more visible pores) should be noted, as should any nipple retraction or eczematous type change of the areola. Associated nipple discharge should be characterized as unilateral or bilateral, single duct or multiple ducts, and by color. Discharge that is clear, serosanguineous, bloody, or dark like old blood is a matter for concern, whereas gray, green, yellow, or beige discharge is likely benign. Lymph nodes in the cervical, supraclavicular, and axillary regions should be evaluated as well.

A mass should be described by bidimensional size, location by distance from the areolar margin or nipple, and by position on a clock. It should be characterized further by assessing its borders (smooth, vague, irregular), texture (firm, soft, rubbery), mobility, whether fixed to overlying skin or underlying chest wall, and whether it is dominant or nondominant. A dominant mass persists throughout the menstrual cycle and is distinctly different from other normal areas of nodularity in either breast, whereas a nondominant mass is one that seems similar to other areas of normal breast tissue. Careful documentation of findings on clinical breast examination is crucial.

There are certain pitfalls in evaluating a breast mass. A prominent rib or costochondral junction may be mistaken for a mass, especially in slender women. A prominent axillary tail can masquerade as a breast mass. Most women have increased fibroglandular tissue density and nodularity in the upper outer quadrants of the breast that may be mistaken for a true breast mass. Another area that can be tricky is along the inframammary crease. This area is often more nodular than other areas in the breast, so clinicians can be fooled into thinking a normal area of nodularity is of concern; conversely, a malignant mass can be hard to distinguish in this area too. The areolar margin is a similarly difficult area that may feel nodular especially when compared with the paucity of tissue directly beneath the nipple-areolar complex. Even trickier to examine are women who have breast implants, are pregnant or lactating, or have had previous breast surgery.

In pregnancy or lactation, the breast tissue can be very spongy in texture and more nodular than usual.

With previous breast surgery, sometimes there can be a paucity of breast tissue at the surgical site, making the immediately adjacent surrounding breast tissue more prominent and suggestive of a mass. Women who have had breast cancer treated with previous partial mastectomy and radiation can be difficult to examine as well because of the postoperative and radiation-induced changes in the breast. A sebaceous cyst may occur in the skin of the breast, but it can be diagnosed because of its superficial location and overlying punctum in the skin.

B. Imaging Studies

The most common imaging studies used to evaluate abnormal breast examination findings are mammography and ultrasound. Imaging studies are complementary to examination, and it is important to remember that if a mass is clinically suspicious, normal mammographic and ultrasound results do not rule out the possibility of cancer.

1. Mammography and ultrasonography—Five to 15% of palpable cancers are not identified on mammography. There are no strict guidelines as to when to order either mammography or ultrasonography. In general, however, any woman 30 years of age or older should have mammography for evaluating a palpable mass that is dominant or concerning. It is important to order this as a diagnostic rather than a screening mammogram, since the radiologist will approach the study differently. First of all, a marker of some sort will be placed on the skin overlying the mass so that this area will be viewed more carefully. Secondly, additional mammographic views such as coned-down, compression, or spot magnification views may be done as well. A radiologist will correlate clinical symptoms and signs with imaging findings. It is critical to give information to the radiologist about the location of the mass unless the patient can clearly point it out. Marking the skin overlying the mass or drawing a picture of the mass on a breast diagram are other methods of communicating this information. Bilateral mammography is useful to perform for several reasons. First, it may demonstrate multicentric ipsilateral breast cancer, confirm the presence of a cancer evident on examination, and may show nonpalpable contralateral breast carcinoma. Second, it may document the presence of a lesion that is benign and does not require any further evaluation, such as a lipoma, galactocele, or oil cyst. If tissue diagnosis is planned with fine-needle aspiration (FNA) or core biopsy, mammography should be performed first since a hematoma at the biopsy site could obscure the lesion and give a false-positive reading.

Ultrasound has become a very useful tool over the past several years. Previously, the best ultrasound could do was to distinguish a solid mass from a cyst. With improvements in ultrasound technology, this modality can distinguish simple from complex cysts, with cyst complexity ranging from a single septation or minimal debris to wall nodularity. Solid lesions can be more completely characterized by examination of the borders, relationship of height to width, and type of sonographic shadowing to determine whether a mass looks malignant. Ultrasound is usually the test of choice in younger women whose breasts are often dense on mammography making detection of abnormalities more difficult. There is no exact age cutoff below which mammography should not be done, but it is probably reasonable to perform ultrasound first in women younger than 30 years, and add bilateral mammography if there is a suspicious lesion that might be cancerous. Between the ages of 30 and 40 is a gray zone, but at 40 years and older, mammography and ultrasound are complementary and should both be performed in most patients.

2. Magnetic resonance imaging—Magnetic resonance imaging (MRI) is another tool that is still finding its place in the breast imaging armamentarium. A clear-cut indication is suspected rupture in a patient with implants. It is not a good screening test for breast disease, although it is being evaluated for this purpose in clinical trials studying certain high-risk groups of patients. It does have its uses in patients with known or suspected breast cancer, but its clinical applicability is continuing to evolve.

C. SPECIAL TESTS

There are 3 primary diagnostic methods used for tissue evaluation of breast masses—FNA, core needle biopsy, and excisional biopsy. There are advantages and disadvantages to each approach.

FNA is simple to perform in the office. The skin overlying the mass is aseptically prepared and then locally anesthetized. A needle attached to a syringe is inserted into the mass, fixing the mass in place with one hand while the other is used to insert the needle. Once in the mass, suction is applied to the syringe, making several passes into the mass. Then, the needle is removed from the breast, releasing the suction just before pulling out of the skin so that the cells obtained stay in the needle rather than getting aspirated into the syringe. The cells obtained are then expelled onto a slide, sprayed with fixative, and then examined by a pathologist. This technique can be performed in the office with little equipment, takes little time, and yields results quickly. However, this does not always give a histologic diagnosis such as fibroadenoma or cancer, but merely gives a cytologic diagnosis. This can be read as benign, atypical, suspicious, malignant, or indeterminate. If malignant, the difference between invasive and in situ disease cannot always be detected, thus not giving enough useful information to plan a single stage opera-

tion to treat the breast as well as stage the axillary nodes. Atypical findings are troublesome, often requiring further diagnostic tests such as excisional biopsy to make a definitive diagnosis. For instance, a fibroadenoma is a very cellular proliferative lesion, so FNA may yield atypia on cytologic examination, requiring surgical removal of a benign lesion. Given the other options available for tissue diagnosis, FNA has less applicability than it had previously. FNA should not be confused with cyst aspiration, which has as its goal removal of fluid from a cyst without necessarily involving cytologic examination.

FNA has variable sensitivity and specificity reported in the literature with false-negative rates ranging from 1% to 35%, and false-positive rates that are as low as 0%. Its accuracy depends on technique and cytopathology expertise. One method of trying to improve the usefulness of FNA is the triple test—an evaluation of the concordance of FNA, mammography, and physical examination—initially described for palpable masses in women 40 years of age and older. It has been shown to be 100% accurate if all 3 components are concordantly either benign or malignant. As initially described, however, 40% of masses had nonconcordant results leading to open biopsy. A modification using the triple test score assigns 1, 2, or 3 points for a benign, suspicious, or malignant result for each component. One study categorized masses scoring 6 points or higher as malignant and masses scoring 4 points or less as benign. Only 8% of patients with a score of 5 required open biopsy.

Core biopsy has been touted as a superior diagnostic technique when compared with FNA. In a study by Clarke et al, core biopsy was added to the triple test, creating a quadruple test. In patients in whom breast cancer was suspected because of clinical examination or radiographic findings, FNA had a sensitivity of only 60% compared with 96% for core biopsy. When mammographic findings were not suspicious but clinical examination indicated malignancy, the sensitivity of FNA was low at 53% while the sensitivity of core biopsy remained high at 95%.

The core biopsy technique, in addition to having greater sensitivity, has better specimen quality and a higher sampling success rate. One study showed that 74% of women who had core biopsy needed no further tissue sampling.

Core biopsy, like FNA, can be performed in the office if there is an easily palpable mass. If the mass is small, deep, mobile, or vaguely palpable, core biopsy can be performed under ultrasound guidance or by stereotaxic biopsy, depending on how the lesion is best visualized on imaging. When done in the office, usually by a specialist, a local anesthetic is used for the skin and subcutaneous tissue. A small incision is made to allow easy passage of the needle, and several cores of tissue are removed using a core biopsy instrument, usually spring loaded, with a large bore needle. These cores are then placed in formalin and sent for pathologic examination. By obtaining enough tissue for histologic diagnosis, the lesion can be characterized more accurately and completely. It is possible to distinguish in situ from invasive disease, and tumor studies such as estrogen and progesterone receptors can be obtained.

It is important to correlate the pathologic diagnosis with the examination to be sure that it fits with the clinical impression. If the mass is suspicious by examination or imaging, and the core biopsy result is benign or indeterminate, then further evaluation is necessary. One of the advantages of core biopsy is the ability to obtain a histologic diagnosis, and, if malignant, to allow planning for a single definitive operation to treat the breast cancer and stage the axillary nodes, if clinically indicated.

Excisional biopsy has been the gold standard for diagnosis in the past, but with the advent of FNA and core biopsy, this is no longer the initial diagnostic procedure of choice for most palpable masses. It has the advantage of removing a mass entirely, thus obviating the need for follow-up, but involves an operation done by a specialist with an incision and need for some type of anesthetic. There is very little risk (such as infection or bleeding) with excisional biopsy, but the incision can thicken or widen with healing, or pucker or indent depending on the amount of breast tissue removed. When removing a benign lesion such as a fibroadenoma, very little surrounding breast tissue is taken, while excisional biopsy of a suspicious mass entails removal of a rim of normal breast tissue to create a clear margin in case the mass proves to be malignant. This procedure may be done in the office or operating room with anesthesia ranging from local anesthetic alone to general anesthesia depending on the size of the mass, the available facilities and the preference of the patient and provider.

This procedure is not to be confused with an incisional biopsy, which now is rarely performed and removes only part of a mass. This is usually done when there is a large mass suspicious for cancer that cannot be diagnosed in a less invasive manner.

Evaluation of Breast Masses During Pregnancy & Lactation

Pregnancy and lactation create special circumstances that make evaluation and treatment of a breast mass more difficult. It is important to pursue evaluation despite these difficulties to rule out the possibility of cancer, which occurs in about 1 in 3000 pregnant women. Seven to 14% of breast cancers in women under the age of 40 and 0.2 to 3.8% of all breast cancers occur during pregnancy.

It is important to remember that the approach to the pregnant or lactating patient should be the same as for other women with certain exceptions. The same history should be taken. Examination is more difficult as the breasts become larger, more nodular, and different in texture.

Mammography should be avoided even though the dose of radiation to the fetus is very low. Ultrasound is the best first step because it is safe and accurate. If ultrasound shows a cyst, galactocele, or benign lymph node, then no further evaluation is necessary. Other benign fat-containing lesions such as lipoma, hamartoma, or lipid cyst are usually nonpalpable but are still within the differential diagnosis. If ultrasound shows a solid mass, then tissue diagnosis is the next step. Note that FNA is not as accurate in these patients because the increased cellularity of the breast tissue can lead to a false-positive result. Core biopsy is the best choice. Excisional biopsy is technically more difficult because the breast tissue is more vascular. If biopsy is done during lactation, there is a higher risk of infection and milk fistula.

The most common solid masses are lactating adenomas and fibroadenomas. Lactating adenoma is unique to pregnancy and usually regresses after lactation. A fibroadenoma can increase in size during this time because of hormonal influences but then may involute. If cancer is found on core biopsy, bilateral mammography should be performed. Although the density of breast tissue is believed to hamper the usefulness of mammography in these patients, 78% of pregnancy associated breast cancers are identified on mammography.

Differential Diagnosis

The list of possible diagnoses for a palpable breast mass is long, but the most common abnormality is a cyst or fibroadenoma. Other likely considerations include breast cancer, fat necrosis, lipoma, sebaceous cyst, phyllodes tumor, or intramammary lymph node. Less common entities include lymphoma, sarcoma, or metastasis.

The history given by a woman with a breast mass will often make one of these diagnoses seem more likely than another. Physical examination is useful, but cannot always distinguish benign from malignant lesions. Imaging and diagnostic tests are most helpful.

Cysts arise from dilatation or obstruction of collecting ducts in the breast. They are more common in premenopausal women older than 40 years of age. Less than 10% of masses in women under 40 years old are cysts. Cysts may fluctuate with the menstrual cycle or other hormonal changes. On examination, a cyst may feel firm, smooth, round or oval, mobile and well demarcated from surrounding breast tissue. If it is tense with fluid, a cyst may be very hard or tender.

A fibroadenoma results from periductal fibrous tissue proliferation within the breast lobules. The median age for discovery of a fibroadenoma is 30 years. It may be difficult to distinguish a fibroadenoma from a cyst on clinical examination, although a fibroadenoma may feel firmer. These masses are more common in the upper outer quadrant of the breast.

A phyllodes tumor is an uncommon mass that is usually clinically indistinguishable by examination and imaging from fibroadenoma. Tissue diagnosis is key.

A lipoma in the breast feels similar to a lipoma elsewhere in the body but again can be difficult to diagnose without the very characteristic appearance seen on imaging.

Fat necrosis may feel firm, vaguely bordered and perhaps have overlying skin change, mimicking cancer. A history of trauma or previous surgery helps make a diagnosis, but again imaging and tissue diagnosis are key.

Breast cancer is suspected when there is a hard, irregular or vaguely bordered mass, which may have associated abnormalities such as bloody or clear nipple discharge, nipple retraction, peau d'orange, fixation to skin or chest wall, or adenopathy in the axilla, neck or supraclavicular area.

Treatment

The goal in evaluating any palpable breast mass is to determine if it is benign or malignant. It is best to try to make a diagnosis with imaging and either FNA or core biopsy, leaving excisional biopsy as a last resort in most cases. FNA has been claimed to be the initial evaluation of choice, but it has its drawbacks. If aspiration yields cyst fluid, and the cyst resolves, a 4- to 6-week follow-up ensues. If the cyst recurs, it is still unknown whether the cyst is malignant or benign. If ultrasound is performed at this point, the cyst may look complex if there is any hemorrhage with the aspiration. This may lead to further unnecessary imaging or even operation. If aspiration yields no fluid, the lesion may be a solid mass or a cyst with very viscous fluid, requiring further imaging to evaluate. All breast abnormalities should be imaged first with mammography, ultrasound, or both before doing any invasive diagnostic tests, realizing that these modalities are not readily available to everyone. An algorithm is presented in Figure 21–1 as a guide to evaluation, realizing that choices may be altered depending on the availability of resources and the preferences of patient and provider. (See Chapter 35 for the treatment of breast cancer.)

A. CYSTS

The advent of breast ultrasound has changed the management of breast cysts. Previously, if examination suggested a cyst, and mammography corroborated this, or showed no abnormality, diagnostic aspiration was performed. If benign appearing cyst fluid was obtained, and the cyst resolved, follow-up would ensue, with either repeat aspiration or excisional biopsy if the mass recurred since there was no other way of ruling out the possibility of malignancy. If bloody fluid was obtained, or if cytologic examination suggested atypia or malignancy, then excisional biopsy was performed. This algorithm is still practiced especially when ultrasound is not readily available, but ultrasound examination may obviate the need for additional invasive diagnostic procedures in some cases.

Cysts can be characterized by ultrasound as simple or complex. Only 0.3% of complex cysts prove to be malignant. Simple cysts are merely fluid-filled without septations, debris, or intramural nodules. If ultrasound is performed and a simple cyst is seen, it may be left alone. If the patient is symptomatic or anxious, then aspiration is reasonable. The fluid should be discarded and only sent for cytologic examination if it is bloody. Sending cyst fluid for examination may not uncommonly result in findings of atypia, which would indicate the need for biopsy. This may be a problem in patients in whom the cyst has subsequently resolved by examination and imaging studies. A complex cyst may have findings ranging from a single septation to an intramural nodule. Cysts with debris or single septations may be aspirated, again sending the fluid for cytologic examination only if suspicious in appearance, or followed with examination and repeat ultrasound. Cysts that are more complex but without intramural nodules should be aspirated and followed up in 4 to 6 weeks with an examination and a repeat ultrasound if the fluid is not suspicious. If the fluid is suspicious, it should be sent for cytologic examination. If a definitive diagnosis is made, appropriate treatment should be initiated, and if not, excisional biopsy should be performed. Lesions with intramural nodules are most suspicious. Core biopsy of the nodule under ultrasound guidance or excisional biopsy should be performed.

B. FIBROADENOMAS

A fibroadenoma may be suspected based on the patient's age, history, physical examination, and imaging studies. The options for evaluation include follow-up examination and imaging studies, FNA, core biopsy, or excisional biopsy. If the clinical scenario supports a diagnosis of fibroadenoma, follow-up is not unreasonable as long as there is the understanding that malignancy cannot be ruled out entirely. In a young woman with an obvious fibroadenoma, proceeding straight to excisional biopsy is appropriate especially if the mass is growing or otherwise bothersome. Given that malig-

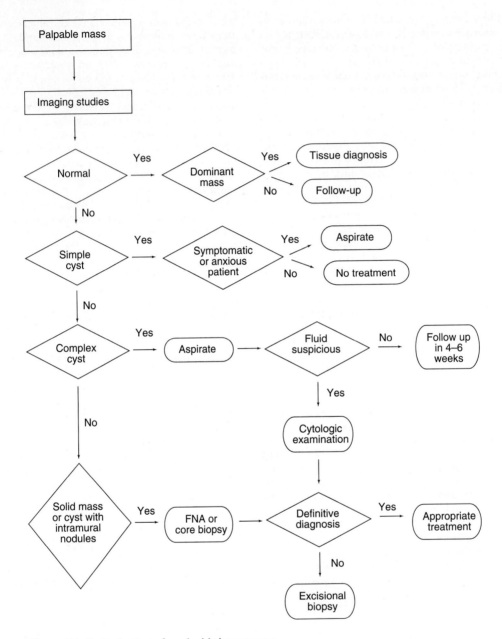

Figure 21–1. Evaluation of a palpable breast mass.

nancy is unlikely in this case, core biopsy may be an unnecessary first step since it will not contribute to surgical planning. If a woman is concerned about the diagnosis, but not anxious to have the mass removed, then core biopsy is a better first choice, still leaving the option of excisional biopsy open.

C. Other Dominant or Nondominant Masses

With respect to other solid dominant breast masses, obtaining as much information as possible from imaging and then assessing whether tissue diagnosis is required using core biopsy (performing excisional biopsy as a last option) is the best approach. If follow-up is elected, then the mass should be reevaluated at least every 3 to 4 months for 1 year. For nondominant breast masses, if imaging studies show no abnormality, then follow-up and reassurance are reasonable options.

When to Refer to a Specialist

Any breast mass that cannot be proven to be benign to the satisfaction of both the provider and patient should be referred to a specialist. Simple cysts that do not require aspiration do not require referral. If a cyst is proven to be simple by ultrasound, and aspiration is elected, this may be performed by the primary care provider if he or she is familiar with the procedure. Otherwise a specialist should evaluate any cyst requiring aspiration, whether simple or complex, or any solid mass warranting further evaluation. Depending on local expertise, the evaluating specialist may be a surgeon or a radiologist.

Beitler AL, Hurd TC, Edge SB: The evaluation of palpable breast masses: common pitfalls and management guidelines. Surg Oncol 1997;6:227. [PMID: 9775409]

Clarke D, Sudhakaran N, Gateley CA: Replace fine needle aspiration cytology with automated core biopsy in the triple assess-ment of breast cancer. Ann R Coll Surg Engl 2001;83:110. [PMID: 11320918]

Hansen N, Morrow M: Breast disease. Med Clin North Am 1998;82:203. [PMID: 9531923]

Hogge JP et al: Imaging and management of breast masses during pregnancy and lactation. Breast J 1999;5:272. [PMID: 11348301]

Liberman L et al: Palpable breast masses: is there a role for percutaneous imaging-guided biopsy? AJR Am J Roentgenol 2000; 175:779. [PMID: 10954467]

Morris A et al: Accurate evaluation of palpable breast masses by the triple test score. Arch Surg 1998;133:930. [PMID: 9749842]

Morris KT et al: Usefulness of the triple test score for palpable breast masses. Arch Surg 2001;136:1008. [PMID: 11529822]

Morrow M: The evaluation of common breast problems. Am Fam Physician 2000;61:2371. [PMID: 10794579]

Pruthi S: Detection and evaluation of a palpable breast mass. Mayo Clin Proc 2001;76:641. [PMID: 11393504]

The Steering Committee on Clinical Practice Guidelines for the Care and Treatment of Cancer. 1. The palpable breast lump: information and recommendations to assist decision-making when a breast lump is detected. Can Med Assoc J 1998;158:S3.

Venta LA et al: Management of complex breast cysts. AJR Am J Roentgenol 1999;173:1331. [PMID: 10541113]

Benign Breast Disorders

Joan E. Miller, MD

Breast symptoms, such as pain, tenderness, nipple discharge, and lumps, are common reasons for a visit to a health care provider. Because breast cancer and benign breast disorders may present with the same symptoms, it is critical to rule out a malignant condition as the cause for the presenting symptom.

MASTODYNIA (MASTALGIA)

 ESSENTIALS OF DIAGNOSIS

- Pain in the breast. Can be intermittent, cyclic, or constant.
- Often there is no identifiable cause.

General Considerations

Mastodynia is common. Most women experience some breast tenderness during the luteal phase of their menstrual cycle. It is more common in premenopausal women although estrogen replacement therapy in postmenopausal women can cause breast tenderness. Women often worry that mastodynia is a sign of breast cancer, but it rarely is a presenting symptom of cancer.

Mastodynia often causes anxiety in the patient, who fears that an underlying cancer is the cause of the pain. Some women experience pain that is sufficient enough to have an impact on their lifestyle and activities. They may avoid exercise, sexual activity or intimate contact because of breast pain. The health care provider should acknowledge the patient's fears and concerns. An open discussion of these issues leads to a better patient-provider relationship and improved patient satisfaction.

Clinical Findings

Breast pain may occur alone or with other signs and symptoms such as nodularity, masses, or breast swelling. Mastodynia is usually cyclical and often worsens during the luteal phase of the menstrual cycle. When it is persistent and noncyclic, it requires evaluation to rule out an underlying breast cancer or other cause.

The history should include the location and character of the pain, exacerbating or alleviating factors, the timing and relationship to the menstrual cycle, medications, risk factors for breast cancer (family history, age at menarche, pregnancy history, past history of breast disease), past medical history (including injuries to the chest and breast), and impact of the pain on lifestyle.

Physical examination should include evaluation of the heart, lungs, chest wall, breasts, and associated lymph nodes. Pregnancy should be ruled out when appropriate. A thorough breast examination must be performed to identify any dominant masses or other abnormalities. Screening mammography should be performed if age appropriate. Diagnostic mammography and/or ultrasonography should be used to evaluate any masses or palpable abnormalities. Ultrasonography can be used to distinguish cysts from solid lesions. Hormonal evaluation is usually not indicated.

Differential Diagnosis

Pain in the breast can be due to mammary sources (such as normal luteal phase hormonal changes, pregnancy, cysts, fibroadenomas, mastitis, or breast cancer) or nonmammary sources (including costochondritis, muscle strains, or angina).

Treatment

Most women with mastodynia require no treatment other than reassurance that they do not have a serious problem such as cancer. A pain chart or calendar may be helpful in evaluating women who experience severe or persistent pain. Treatments for mastodynia have ranged from dietary therapy to hormonal manipulation. Physical factors such as wearing a properly fitted brassiere are important. Often analgesics such as nonprescription nonsteroidal anti-inflammatory drugs (NSAIDs) or acetaminophen are helpful. Postmenopausal women taking hormone replacement therapy may respond to lowering the dose of estrogen.

Advocates for dietary therapy recommend a low-fat, high-fiber diet. A randomized, controlled trial of 21 patients who had cyclic mastodynia for at least 5 years found that patients who followed a low fat (less than 15% of calories), high complex carbohydrate diet for

6 months had a significant reduction in premenstrual breast swelling and tenderness. Vitamin E supplementation has gained popularity although there are no good studies to support its use. Avoidance of caffeine has been advocated; however, several studies have failed to find a relationship between caffeine intake and mastalgia.

Low sodium diet and diuretics have been used, but no studies have been done to evaluate their effects. A study comparing women with mastodynia to symptom-free age-matched controls showed no difference in premenstrual total body water:weight ratio, suggesting that diuretics should not be beneficial.

Evening primrose oil, a natural product with a high content of gamma linolenic acid (an essential fatty acid that is thought to act via prostaglandin mediators), has been recommended at doses of 1000 mg 3 times daily or 1500 mg twice daily. It may take up to 4 months to get a beneficial response. It is said to have few side effects.

Bromocriptine is a long-acting dopaminergic drug that suppresses prolactin. A European multicenter study of bromocriptine at 2.5 mg orally twice daily found improvement in breast pain and tenderness. However, side effects of headache, nausea, and vomiting resulted in a 26% dropout rate.

Danazol, a synthetic steroid which suppresses the pituitary-ovarian axis, has been shown to be effective in 2 controlled trials, but side effects such as bloating, weight gain, menstrual irregularities, leg cramps, and decreased libido may make it unacceptable. Thromboembolic disease and pseudotumor cerebri have been reported with the use of danazol. Total daily doses of 100–400 mg orally given (2nd one) in 2 divided doses have been used. Tapering the dose to 100 mg on alternate days or 100 mg per day during the luteal phase (days 14–28) only has been tried. Danazol is potentially teratogenic and an effective nonhormonal method of contraception is required when danazol is prescribed.

Tamoxifen, a partial estrogen antagonist, has been shown to be beneficial in treating cyclic mastodynia but has many side effects including hot flushes, menstrual irregularity, nausea, headaches, depression, and increased thromboembolic risk. Daily doses of 10–20 mg given orally for 3 months have been studied.

Nafarelin, an octapeptide analogue of gonadotropin-releasing hormone (GnRH) used as a nasal spray, was not found to be significantly different from placebo and had side effects of vasomotor symptoms, menstrual irregularities, headaches, and nausea. Long-term use may cause osteoporosis.

Micronized progesterone (100 mg) as a vaginal cream at bedtime on days 10–25 of the menstrual cycle for 6 months was effective in a placebo-controlled trial. No major side effects were reported.

When to Refer to a Specialist

Women who have an abnormal breast examination or imaging study should be referred to a breast surgeon for evaluation and possible biopsy. A palpable abnormality on breast examination, even if not seen on mammogram, needs further evaluation. Women whose pain is not relieved by more conservative measures should probably see a specialist prior to initiating a hormonal treatment such as bromocriptine, danazol, or tamoxifen.

Ader DN, Browne MW: Prevalence and impact of cyclic mastalgia in a United States clinic-based sample. Am J Obstet Gynecol 1997;177:126. [PMID: 9240595]

Boyd NF et al: Effect of a low-fat high-carbohydrate diet on symptoms of cyclic mastopathy. Lancet 1988;2:128. [PMID: 2899188]

Dogliotti L, Mansel RE: Bromocriptine treatment of cyclical mastalgia/fibrocystic breast disease: update on the European trial. Br J Clin Pract Suppl 1989;43:26. [PMID: 2488563]

Faiz O, Fentiman IS: Management of breast pain. Int J Clin Pract 2000;54:228. [PMID: 10912311]

Fentiman IS et al: Studies of tamoxifen in women with mastalgia. Br J Clin Pract Suppl 1989;68:34. [PMID: 2488564]

Maddox PR, Harrison BJ, Mansel RE: Low-dose danazol for mastalgia. Br J Clin Pract Suppl 1989;68:43. [PMID: 2488565]

Nappi C et al: Double-blind controlled trial of progesterone vaginal cream treatment for cyclical mastodynia in women with benign breast disease. J Endocrinol Invest 1992;15:801. [PMID: 1291593]

Preece PE et al: Mastalgia and total body water. BMJ 1975;4:498. [PMID: 1238148]

Steinbrunn BS, Zera RT, Rodriguez JL: Mastalgia: Tailoring treatment to type of breast pain. Postgrad Med 1997;102(5):183. [PMID: 9385340]

MASTITIS

 ESSENTIALS OF DIAGNOSIS

- *Tender, erythematous wedge-shaped area in breast.*
- *Staphylococcus aureus and Streptococcus are most common causes.*
- *Nonlactating women require evaluation to rule out malignant disease.*

General Considerations

Puerperal mastitis is thought to be a retrograde infection that results from disruption of the epithelium of the nipple-areola complex. Risk factors include nipple fissuring, milk stasis, skipped breast feedings, change in feeding patterns, and mechanical obstruction (eg, because of a tight brassiere strap). *Staphylococcus aureus* and *Streptococcus* species are the most common bacteria associated with mastitis.

Mastitis in nonlactating women is uncommon. Duct ectasia, a benign condition affecting the major breast ducts, may be associated with periductal mastitis, periareolar abscess, and mammary fistula. The cause is unclear but anaerobic infection may play a role. Chronic infectious disorders, such as tuberculosis, and inflammatory disorders, such as vasculitis, may present as mastitis. Inflammatory breast cancer can be confused with mastitis. Breast cysts occasionally present with an inflamed area of skin overlying the cyst.

Prevention

To help prevent puerperal mastitis, breast-feeding should be done regularly and the breast should be emptied of milk. Proper positioning of the infant is important to allow the child to take the whole nipple and latch on. This helps prevent sore nipples. If dried milk secretions build up in a duct, these should be loosened using moist, warm compresses. Milk should be expressed until the duct opening is clear. Tight-fitting clothing should be avoided. Some clinicians advocate avoiding underwire bras. Not wearing a brassiere has been recommended by some.

Clinical Findings

A. SYMPTOMS AND SIGNS

Puerperal mastitis presents as a tender, warm, swollen, wedge-shaped area of the breast. Fever, chills, flu-like aching, and other systemic signs may be seen. Purulent material may be expressed from the nipple. Streptococcal infections often cause a diffuse cellulitis with no localization, whereas staphylococcal infections tend to be more localized and deeply invasive with possible abscess formation. A fluctuant mass with point tenderness and erythema suggests an abscess.

Signs of periductal mastitis or duct ectasia include noncyclic mastalgia, periareola breast mass, periareola breast abscess, nipple discharge, nipple retraction, and mammary fistula. Inflammatory carcinoma can present with inflamed, indurated skin and tenderness.

B. LABORATORY AND IMAGING STUDIES

Breast milk or purulent discharge can be expressed and sent for Gram's stain and culture. This is not routinely needed.

Women who do not respond to antibiotics or who have a questionable diagnosis should have a thorough breast examination followed by ultrasonography and, if appropriate, mammography.

Differential Diagnosis

The differential diagnosis for puerperal mastitis includes engorgement, plugged duct, and all the causes for an inflammatory breast mass in nonlactating women. Engorgement occurs early in the postpartum period and involves both breasts in a generalized fashion. Fever and signs of systemic illness are absent. A plugged milk duct is usually unilateral and noticed after nursing when a small discrete mass remains.

The differential diagnosis of mastitis in a nonlactating woman includes inflammatory carcinoma, periductal mastitis/duct ectasia, inflammatory cyst, tuberculosis, sarcoidosis, oleogranulomatous mastitis (mammoplasty in Hong Kong has been done with injections of paraffin or beeswax), parasitic infections (hydatid disease, filariasis), actinomycosis, blastomycosis, sporotrichosis, giant cell arteritis, and idiopathic.

Complications

Mastitis, if not treated adequately, can lead to abscess or sepsis.

Treatment

Puerperal mastitis should be treated with antibiotics that are active against *Staphylococcus aureus* and *Streptococcus* and also safe for the nursing infant. Drainage of milk from the breast by nursing or breast pumping should be done. Some recommend oxytocin nasal spray to enhance milk letdown. Warm compresses or warm baths may be used. If an abscess is present, drainage is needed.

Periductal mastitis/duct ectasia usually requires surgical treatment, although some recommend treatment with metronidazole and a first-generation cephalosporin antibiotic. A mixture of anaerobic and aerobic bacteria can be involved.

Percutaneous drainage of inflammatory cysts should be curative. If not, further evaluation needs to be performed.

When to Refer to a Specialist

A woman with mastitis that results in an abscess or does not resolve with typical treatment should be referred to a breast surgeon. Inflammatory breast lesions in nonlactating women that do not resolve with antibiotics or have worrisome findings on imaging studies should be evaluated by a specialist to rule out carcinoma.

Lawrence RA: The puerperium, breastfeeding, and breast milk. Curr Opin Obstet Gynecol 1990;2:23. [PMID: 2102300]

NIPPLE DISCHARGE

 ESSENTIALS OF DIAGNOSIS

- *Spontaneous, unilateral, single duct discharge that is clear or bloody may signify cancer.*
- *Spontaneous bilateral milky discharge is galactorrhea and suggests that hyperprolactinemia may be present.*
- *Nonspontaneous, multiductular, bilateral discharge is usually benign.*

General Considerations

Nipple discharge is more common in benign than in malignant conditions. In one study, 9% of 6266 women who had breast surgery for benign lesions and 3.4% of 2437 women who had surgery for malignant conditions had nipple discharge as their chief complaint.

Nipple discharge can be physiologic, pathologic, or galactorrhea. Galactorrhea is the spontaneous discharge of milk-like fluid due to elevated prolactin levels. Hyperprolactinemia can be due to normal postpartum lactation, thyroid disease, medications, excessive nipple stimulation and pituitary adenoma.

In postmenopausal women, the most common cause of nipple discharge is duct ectasia, which is a benign condition affecting the major breast ducts. The second and third most common causes are intraductal papilloma and carcinoma, respectively.

Clinical Findings

Nipple discharge can be spontaneous or nonspontaneous (expressed by manipulating the breast and nipple), unilateral or bilateral, and from a single duct or multiple ducts. Discharge may be green, gray, black, milky, serous, serosanguineous, sanguineous, or watery. With a single-duct discharge, a trigger point may be found; pressure at that point produces maximal discharge.

A woman seeking medical attention for nipple discharge should be asked about her age, menstrual history, pregnancy status, past history with attention to endocrine disorders and chest trauma, medications, and characteristics of the discharge. The patient should also be asked whether she has any associated symptoms such as breast mass, pain, headache, or visual changes.

Physical examination with a thorough breast examination should be performed. Patients with galactorrhea unrelated to pregnancy should also have thyroid and neurologic examinations, including visual field testing. Age appropriate screening mammography should be performed. If a palpable abnormality is found on breast examination, the work-up should be done as it would for any breast mass. Ultrasonography may be useful in identifying intraductal abnormalities.

The characteristics (eg, unilateral, bilateral, single duct or multiple ducts, and color) of the nipple discharge should be noted at the time of examination. Discharge can be tested for occult blood using a urine dipstick or a stool occult blood card. Cytologic analysis of the discharge is rarely useful.

Patients with galactorrhea should have thyroid-stimulating hormone (TSH) and prolactin levels measured. Patients with hyperprolactinemia need evaluation for a possible pituitary adenoma. In the absence of secondary causes of hyperprolactinemia, such as medications, nipple stimulation, pregnancy or hypothyroidism, patients with an elevated prolactin level should undergo pituitary gland imaging by computed tomography (CT) or magnetic resonance imaging (MRI). Prolactin elevations secondary to medications are generally less than 100 ng/mL.

Patients with unilateral discharge, especially single duct discharge, need evaluation for underlying malignant disease or intraductal papilloma. Mammography should be performed. Galactography or ductography may be obtained by injecting a radiopaque dye into the discharging duct; however, this test may be supplanted by ultrasonography in certain centers. Surgical biopsy may be needed for definitive diagnosis.

Differential Diagnosis

Galactorrhea due to hyperprolactinemia can be due to excessive nipple stimulation (sexual activity or exercise related), hypothyroidism, medications, pituitary adenoma, chest trauma, chronic renal failure, or tumors such as bronchogenic carcinoma and hypernephroma. Some of the medications that may cause hyperprolactinemia include estrogen-containing oral contraceptives, phenothiazines, reserpine, opiates, H_2-receptor blockers, calcium channel blockers, tricyclic antidepressants, alpha-methyldopa, marijuana, and isoniazid.

Bloody discharge can be seen with carcinoma, intraductal papilloma, and near-term pregnancy. The bloody discharge in a prepartum woman is attributed to vascular engorgement and should clear within a few weeks. If it persists, further evaluation is required. Patients with periductal mastitis/duct ectasia may have unilateral or bilateral discharge, which can vary in color.

Discharge that is nonspontaneous, bilateral, and nonbloody (usually green, gray, black) can be seen in healthy women.

Treatment

Treatment depends on the cause of the nipple discharge. Galactorrhea due to a pituitary tumor secreting prolactin can be treated medically or surgically. Pituitary microadenomas (< 1 cm) can be treated with bromocriptine or cabergoline. Macroadenomas are usually treated surgically. Hypothyroidism is treated with thyroid replacement therapy to normalize the TSH and prolactin level. If medications are the cause, then the health care provider and patient must decide whether the benefits of the medication justify the side effects of high prolactin levels.

Cancers and intraductal papillomas require surgery. Duct ectasia usually requires duct excision.

When to Refer to a Specialist

Patients with a mass, unilateral spontaneous discharge, single duct discharge, bloody or watery discharge or an abnormal mammogram should be referred to a breast surgeon. Patients with hyperprolactinemia due to a pituitary tumor or unidentified cause should be referred to an endocrinologist.

Prognosis

One study showed that the likelihood of cancer increases if the nipple discharge is, in order of increasing frequency, serous (6%), serosanguineous (13%), sanguineous (28%), or watery (33%). There is also a high risk of cancer when the following factors are present: a mass, unilateral discharge, single duct discharge, abnormal mammographic findings, and the patient is older than 50 years.

Leis HP Jr: Management of nipple discharge. World J Surg 1989; 13:736. [PMID: 2696228]

Morrison C: The significance of nipple discharge: Diagnosis and treatment regimes. Lippincotts Prim Care Pract 1998;2:129. [PMID: 9727109]

FIBROCYSTIC BREAST CHANGE

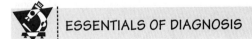

ESSENTIALS OF DIAGNOSIS

- *Includes various histologic diagnoses: cysts, hyperplasia, atypical hyperplasia, fibrosis, sclerosing adenosis, duct ectasia, fibroadenoma, papilloma.*

General Considerations

Fibrocystic breast change is a common term that is used to describe lumpy breasts that may be painful; it is not clinically useful. Synonyms for fibrocystic breast change include mammary dysplasia, chronic cystic mastitis, fibrocystic disease, cystic hyperplasia, mastopathia. Clinicians have labeled women with breast lumps that are not malignant as having fibrocystic change. Histologically, cysts, hyperplasia, atypical hyperplasia, sclerosing adenosis, duct ectasia, fibrosis and fibroadenoma can be seen. These pathologic diagnoses are all benign, but the risk of developing breast cancer varies depending on whether the lesion if proliferative or nonproliferative. Some clinicians support using the proliferative versus nonproliferative categorization of benign lesions rather than lumping them as fibrocystic change.

Some health care providers advocate that the benign histopathologic and clinical changes that fall into the category of fibrocystic change be viewed as minor aberrations of normal processes. The concept of aberrations of normal development and involution (ANDI) provides a framework for understanding some of the benign lesions that have been lumped under fibrocystic change. Normal development and involution of breast tissue is divided into 3 stages: (1) early reproductive period, (2) mature reproductive period, and (3) involution. Abnormalities or aberrations may occur during these stages resulting in different clinical and pathologic conditions. Table 22–1 summarizes the ANDI concept.

Palpable nodularity is present in at least 50% of women. Autopsy studies determined that 58% of women had histologic changes that have been called fibrocystic change. Clinical studies estimate that 7–10% of women have breast cysts.

Prevention

There are no data to show a consistent association between benign breast lesions and diet, smoking status, caffeine, or methylxanthine ingestion. Oral contraceptive use may decrease the risk of benign breast conditions. There may be an increased risk with long-term use of estrogen replacement therapy.

Clinical Findings

Women in whom fibrocystic change has been diagnosed may complain of mastodynia, nodularity, breast mass, inflammatory lesion, or nipple discharge. Abnormal changes such as architectural distortion and microcalcifications may be seen on mammography, and these can be similar to changes seen with malignancy. Biopsy may be needed to differentiate.

Table 22–1. Aberrations of normal development and involution.

Stage (Peak Age in Years)	Normal Process	Aberration		Disease State
		Underlying Condition	Clinical Presentation	
Early reproductive period (15–25)	Lobule development	Fibroadenoma	Discrete lump	Giant fibroadenoma; multiple fibroadenoma
Mature reproductive period (25–40)	Stroma formation Cyclic hormonal effects on glandular tissue and stroma	Juvenile hypertrophy Exaggerated cyclic effects	Cyclic mastalgia and nodularity— generalized or discrete	
Involution (35–55)	Lobular involution (including microcysts, apocrine change, fibrosis, adenosis)	Macrocysts Sclerosing lesions	Discrete lumps Radiographic abnormalities	
	Ductal involution (including periductal round-cell infiltrates)	Duct dilatation	Nipple discharge	Periductal bacterial infection and abscess formation
	Epithelial turnover	Periductal fibrosis Mild epithelial hyperplasia	Nipple retraction Histologic report	Epithelial hyperplasia with atypia

(Reproduced with permission from Hughes LE: Benign breast disorders: The clinician's view. Cancer Detect Prev 1992;16:1.)

Differential Diagnosis

Breast lesions can present as masses or be seen as abnormalities on imaging studies. The diagnoses that have been lumped under the term fibrocystic change include cysts, hyperplasia, atypical hyperplasia, fibrosis, sclerosing adenosis, duct ectasia, fibroadenoma, and papilloma.

Treatment

Once an underlying malignant condition is ruled out, most benign breast disorders need no further treatment. Women with atypical hyperplasia need close follow-up. Clinical examinations twice a year and annual mammograms are recommended. Tamoxifen prophylaxis could be considered.

Cysts may be aspirated or monitored (see Chapter 21, Evaluation of Breast Masses for more detail).

When to Refer to a Specialist

Patients should be referred to a specialist if they have a solid mass needing biopsy, recent nipple retraction, bloody nipple discharge, bloody fluid aspirated from a cyst, recurrent breast cyst after aspiration, or for any condition that is not clearly benign.

Prognosis

The risk of breast cancer developing depends on the pathologic diagnosis. Dupont and Page showed the relative risk for developing breast cancer is as follows: proliferative disease without atypia (hyperplasia) 1.9, atypical hyperplasia 4.4, atypical hyperplasia with a positive family history of breast cancer 4.8–20, cysts 1.2–1.9, and cysts with a positive family history of breast cancer 1.9–4.5. Other studies have confirmed that women with atypical hyperplasia have about a 4-fold increased risk of breast cancer compared with women without proliferative changes. There is a synergistic effect of atypical hyperplasia and family history of breast cancer. Women with both these risk factors have a relative risk up to 20 times that of women without proliferative changes or a positive family history.

In 1986, a consensus statement was released concerning the pathologic diagnosis and risk of breast cancer. It is believed that nonproliferative breast lesions (such as apocrine metaplasia, sclerosing adenosis, cysts, duct ectasia, fibroadenoma, fibrosis, mild hyperplasia, and mastitis) do not increase a woman's risk of subsequently developing breast cancer. Proliferative lesions do increase the risk. There is a slight increased risk (1.5–2.0 ×) with moderate or severe hyperplasia. Atypical hyperplasia (ductal or lobular) increase the risk 4 to 5 times.

Studies of breast cysts and the relative risk of developing breast cancer have shown variable results. A consensus statement published in 1986 indicated no increased risk, but other studies have found an increased relative risk varying between 1.7 and 7.5 for women with palpable breast cysts. Some researchers have looked at the concentration of sodium and potassium in the cyst fluid to try to identify which cysts are more high risk, but no difference between cyst types was found. Cancer rarely develops in cysts, but cysts may be a marker of a generalized increase in epithelial activity within the breast.

More recent data on the long-term risk of breast cancer in women with fibroadenoma contradicts the 1986 consensus statement. The histologic features of the fibroadenoma influence the breast cancer risk. Fibroadenomas that contain cysts greater than 3 mm in diameter, sclerosing adenosis, epithelial calcifications, or papillary apocrine changes are classified as complex. The relative risk of developing invasive breast cancer in women with complex fibroadenomas ranges from 2.24 to 3.10 (varying control groups). Having a positive family history of breast cancer or proliferative changes (with or without atypia) increases risk. In addition, the increased risk of breast cancer persists for longer than 20 years after the diagnosis of complex fibroadenoma.

A recent study evaluated the risk of breast cancer in women with biopsy-confirmed benign breast disease and the postmenopausal use of exogenous female hormones. Women with proliferative changes without atypia had a relative risk of breast cancer of 1.8 and women with atypical hyperplasia had a relative risk of 3.6 compared with women who had had biopsies with nonproliferative benign histology. There was no increased risk beyond the risk associated with their histo-logic diagnosis for women who were currently receiving hormone replacement therapy or for women who had been taking hormone replacement therapy for 5 or more years.

Byrne C et al: Biopsy confirmed benign breast disease, postmenopausal use of exogenous female hormones, and breast carcinoma risk. Cancer 2000;89:2046. [PMID: 11066044]

Cady B et al: Evaluation of common breast problems: guidance for primary care providers. CA Cancer J Clin 1998;48:190. [PMID: 9449933]

Charreau I et al: Oral contraceptive use and risk of benign breast disease in a French case-control study of young women. Eur J Cancer Prev 1993;2:147. [PMID: 8461865]

Dixon JM et al: Risk of breast cancer in women with palpable breast cysts: a prospective study. Edinburgh Breast Group. Lancet 1999;353:1742. [PMID: 10347986]

Dupont WD et al: Long-term risk of breast cancer in women with fibroadenoma. N Engl J Med 1994;331:10. [PMID: 8202095]

Dupont WD, Page DL: Risk factors for breast cancer in women with proliferative breast disease. N Engl J Med 1985;312:146. [PMID: 3965932]

Goehring C, Marabia A: Epidemiology of benign breast disease, with special attention to histologic types. Epidemiol Rev 1997;19:310. [PMID: 9494790]

Hansen N, Morrow M: Breast disease. Med Clin North Am 1998;82:203. [PMID: 9531923]

Hughes LE: Benign breast disorders: The clinician's view. Cancer Detect Prev 1992;16:1. [PMID: 1551132]

Is "fibrocystic disease" of the breast precancerous? Arch Pathol Lab Med 1986:110:171. [PMID: 3606334]

Levinson W, Dunn PM: Nonassociation of caffeine and fibrocystic breast disease. Arch Intern Med 1986;146:1773. [PMID: 3530165]

Lubin F et al: A case-control study of caffeine and methylxanthines in benign breast disease. JAMA 1985;253:2388. [PMID: 3981766]

Ory H et al: Oral contraceptives and reduced risk of benign breast diseases. N Engl J Med 1976;294:419. [PMID: 12334129]

Breast Augmentation & Disorders of the Augmented Breast

23

Kian J. Samimi, MD

Breast augmentation using silicone implants was first introduced in the early 1960s. Before the introduction of silicone implants, various techniques for breast reconstruction and augmentation dating back to the 19th century had yielded unpredictable results. Initial reports associating silicone implants with rheumatic disorders were published in the 1980s. In response to these reports and media publicity, the Food and Drug Administration in 1992 mandated a moratorium on the use of silicone implants. Since then, numerous studies have failed to establish a link between connective tissue disorders and silicone implants. This prompted the American College of Rheumatology to issue the following statement in 1995: "These studies provide compelling evidence that silicone implants expose patients to no demonstrable additional risk for connective tissue or rheumatic disease."

Breast implants consist of an outer shell and a filler substance. Different materials have been used for the shell in the past, but essentially all implants used in the United States over the last 10 years have silicone shells. The filler material determines the implant type. The US Food and Drug Administration (FDA) presently approves only saline implants, which have a well-documented safety record, for cosmetic augmentation. Silicone implants may be used for breast reconstruction as part of a study and are pending approval by the FDA. Other implant types (such as using organic oils as filler substance) are being evaluated but are not FDA approved.

Wolfe P: "Silicone breast implants and the risk of fibromyalgia and rheumatoid arthritis." Presented at the American College of Rheumatology, 59th National Science Meeting, San Francisco, CA, October 21-26, 1995, Arthritis and Rheumatism, 1995;38:S265.

General Considerations

Approximately 1–2 million females in the United States, 1% of the adult female population, have breast implants. The vast majority has been placed for cosmetic reasons. Surveys have shown that 90–95% of women are satisfied with the outcome.

Indications for breast implant placement include congenital causes such as Poland's syndrome (congenital absence of pectoralis major muscle and breast); acquired absence of the breast following mastectomy; and cosmetic correction of hypomastia, involution, and ptosis.

Breast implants can be placed using a variety of techniques: inframammary, periareolar, and axillary incisions are most common (Figure 23–1). Endoscopic transumbilical augmentation is less commonly used. Periareolar incisions have a slightly higher incidence of hypoesthesia of the nipple. The implants are placed subglandular (under the breast parenchyma) or submuscular (under the pectoralis muscle). While the subglandular placement was the most common with silicone implants, saline implants are most often placed in a submuscular position. The submuscular position provides an additional layer of soft tissue covering and camouflages the normal wrinkling of the implant wall, which occurs with saline implants. It also has been shown to reduce the incidence of capsular contracture (see following section on Disorders). The anesthesia ranges from local to general. Early complications including implant infection, seroma formation, and hypoesthesia or hyperesthesia at the surgical sites are rare.

Women with breast implants may have decreased milk production. A recent study suggested women who have had breast augmentation have higher incidence (64% vs 7%) of inadequate milk production than women who have not had the procedure. This was seen mostly in women with periareolar incisions. A periareolar approach may transect milk ducts and therefore is avoided by many plastic surgeons. Further, many of these women may have had augmentations for breast hypoplasia and had decreased lactation potential initially. Breast milk from women who have silicone implants does not contain increased levels of silicone.

Examining the Augmented Breast

Typically, patients are in their 30s, successful, self-confident and well informed. When examining the breast, a horizontal incision above the inframammary fold, a round incision in the outer margin of the areola, or a straight scar within the axilla can be seen. These scars

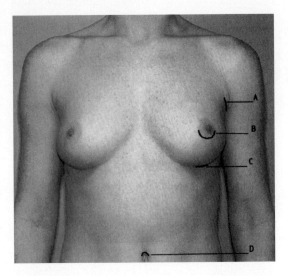

Figure 23–1. Axillary, periareolar, inframammary, and umbilical incisions for breast augmentation are marked.

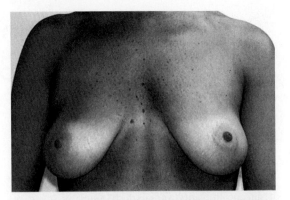

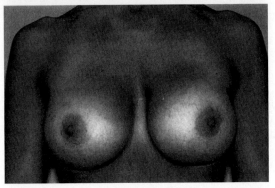

Figure 23–2. Preoperative and postoperative saline breast implant augmentation for treatment of glandular ptosis.

tend to fade and may be barely noticeable after several years. Palpation of the augmented breast will reveal whether a silicone or saline implant has been used. A silicone implant feels very similar to breast tissue, and the presence of the implant may be noticed only on firmer palpation. Saline implants do not feel as soft as a silicone. Also, the wall of the implant may be felt along the medial and inferior border of the breast. Rippling (wrinkling) of the implant may be noted in these areas. This is a normal finding with saline implants (Figure 23–2).

Women who have breast implants should follow the same routine schedule for mammography as women who do not have implants. Mammography of the augmented breast requires special techniques and therefore should only be performed at facilities accredited by the American College of Radiologists. Only about two thirds of the breast parenchyma can be visualized using standard techniques. The Eklund displacement technique involves manually pushing the implant towards the chest wall and selectively compressing the breast. This improves the amount of breast parenchyma visualized from 56% to 64% for subglandular implants and from 75% to 85% for submuscular implants. There have been reports of implant deflation with standard mammography techniques; the risk of this should be lower with the Eklund technique.

Baker JL Jr: Classification of spherical contractures. Presented at the Aesthetic Breast Symposium, Scottsdale, Arizona, 1975.

Brinton LA et al: Characteristics of a population of women with breast implants compared with women seeking other types of plastic surgery. Plast Reconstr Surg 2000;105:919. [PMID: 10724251]

Cunningham BL, Lokeh A, Gutowski KA: Saline-filled breast implant safety and efficacy: a multicenter retrospective review. Plast Reconstr Surg 2000;105:2143. [PMID: 10839417]

Eklund GW et al: Improve imaging of the augmented breast. AJR Am J Roentgenol 1988;151:469. [PMID: 3261503]

Hurst NM: Lactation after augmentation mammoplasty. Obstet Gynecol 1996;87:30. [PMID: 8532261]

Silverstein MJ, Handel N, Gamagami P: The effect of silicone gelfilled implants on mammography. Cancer 1991;68 (5 Suppl):1159. [PMID: 1913498]

DISORDERS

Capsular Contracture

 ESSENTIALS OF DIAGNOSIS

- *Increasing firmness and deformity of the augmented breast.*

General Considerations

The incidence varies according to the different implant types and placement techniques. Any implanted foreign body will induce an inflammatory reaction, which results in a fibrous capsule or scar. The degree of capsule formation is variable and unpredictable. The newer saline implants with a textured surface have a drastically lower incidence of capsular contracture than silicone implants. The incidence according to the implant manufacturer is between 5% and 20%. The Saline Prospective Study found a 9% incidence of Baker grade III or IV contractures (see following Diagnosis section) at 3 years.

Clinical Findings

On examination, firmness of the implant is noted. There may be a palpable capsule surrounding the implant. The breast has an unnatural appearance, frequently with upward displacement of the implant and descent of the breast parenchyma over the implant (Figure 23–3). Firmness of the underlying implant differentiates this from the natural ptosis of the breast tissue, which occurs with age. The patient complains of increasing firmness, implant displacement and, in the later stages, breast pain. Implants in place for more than 10 years may have palpable calcifications in the capsule. These are also seen on mammogram.

Diagnosis

The Baker classification is used to grade the degree of firmness:

Grade I: No palpable capsule
Grade II: Minimal firmness
Grade III: Moderate firmness
Grade IV: Severe contracture

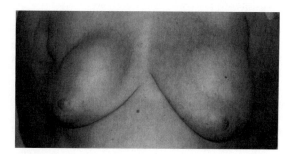

Figure 23–3. Capsular contracture is evident in the right breast.

In essence, grades I and II are considered normal and acceptable results. The examining physician notices a grade III capsular contracture with a palpable capsule surrounding the implant more often than the patient. Because the hardening occurs slowly, the patient may not be aware of an existing grade II or grade III contracture. Implant malpositioning or deformity and increasing pain are signs of a grade IV contracture. The amount of breast tissue visualized on mammography decreases with increasing capsular contracture.

Treatment

Intervention is indicated for grade III or IV contractures. Closed capsulectomy by forcefully manipulating the breast and capsule has been largely abandoned because of possible implant rupture. Surgically incising or completely excising the capsule is the treatment of choice. Because implants with a textured surface seem to reduce the risk of capsular contracture, smooth-walled implants should be replaced with textured implants. The patient may still develop a significant capsular contracture and ultimately require removal of the implants. At present, there are no medical treatments for the prevention or treatment of capsular contracture. Massage and displacement exercises of the augmented breast help prevent the development of capsular contracture. In these exercises the implant is pushed forcibly around the pocket to prevent formation of a tight capsule. These need to be performed daily for years after augmentation because the onset of contractures may be late.

Baker JL Jr: Classification of spherical contractures. Presented at the Aesthetic Breast Symposium, Scottsdale, Arizona, 1975.

Handel N et al: Factors affecting mammographic visualization of the breast after augmentation mammaplasty. JAMA 1992; 268:1913. [PMID: 1404718]

Implant Leak

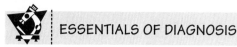 ESSENTIALS OF DIAGNOSIS

- *Sudden or gradual volume loss of implant.*
- *Evidence of leak by ultrasonography or magnetic resonance imaging (MRI).*

Clinical Findings

Risk factors for an implant leak include implant older than 10 years, attempts at manipulation of capsule (closed capsulotomy), and iatrogenic (such as biopsy, needle localization, aspiration, mammogram).

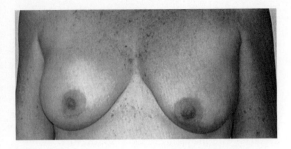

Figure 23–4. Deflated saline implant is easily recognized in the left breast.

A. Symptoms and Signs

Patients will notice a loss of breast volume. The rate of deflation can be very slow; ultimately, breast asymmetry will develop (Figure 23–4). Frequently, the initial complaint will be a misfitting bra or clothing. A burning sensation may be reported.

B. Imaging Studies

Routine screening mammograms may suggest a rupture if disruption of the implant wall is seen. Calcifications are not a sign of rupture. Mammograms alone are inadequate to work-up a suspected leak or smaller rupture. Sensitivity is low, especially with the more common intracapsular rupture. Ultrasonography is the most practical tool in the work-up of a suspected implant rupture. A sensitivity of 70% and specificity of 85% have been reported. These results are highly operator dependent. The most accurate tool is MRI with specificity reaching 100%. The accuracy can be improved by the use of breast surface coils. The high cost of MRI limits its use. The algorithm in Figure 23–5 can help the clinician work-up a suspected leak or rupture.

Diagnosis

A fully deflated implant is easily recognized, while a slow leak may be difficult to detect initially. Leaking saline implants will usually lose most of their volume within a few weeks. A small tear may stop leaking when the implant loses some saline and the pressure within decreases. The patient almost always notices the volume loss, so she is aware of the leak when she seeks medical attention. No diagnostic tests beyond a physical examination are necessary. Breast asymmetry and marked wrinkling of the implant wall are noted (Figure 23–4). There are no systemic or local adverse reactions associated with a saline leak.

Silicone implants have a very slow rate of deflation. All silicone implants allow for diffusion of silicone oil and this process is called **"bleed."** Bleed is normal and

should not cause a noticeable change in implant volume. A **leak** results from a small hole in the implant wall and a thin coating of silicone is deposited around the implant. Again, examination will be normal. A major tear is considered a **rupture.** A significant portion of the gel is outside of the implant. The silicone is not absorbed. It is contained in the capsule and therefore does not cause a loss of breast volume. Physical examination may reveal an area of induration or an irregular capsule, although the examination is frequently normal. Even when **extrusion** of silicone occurs into the adjacent soft tissues through a tear in the capsule, the examination may be normal. Extracapsular extrusion of silicone is the only instance in which adverse reactions may occur. An inflammatory reaction to the extruded silicone may manifest as an induration, erythema, or necrosis of the overlying skin. There are reports of silicone migration into the axilla and subsequent neurologic symptoms. Enlarged axillary nodes have been biopsied and found to contain silicone. These are isolated, rare reports and seem to be associated with the use of a certain type of low viscosity silicone in the late 1970s. No association between silicone implant rupture and rheumatologic disorders has been established.

The only common findings on examination associated with silicone implant rupture are breast asymmetry and capsular contracture.

Treatment

Surgical removal of the ruptured or leaking implant is the appropriate therapy for both saline and silicone implants. Any deflated saline implant should be removed. If the patient wishes to have the implant replaced, this should not be delayed beyond 4 weeks because the skin envelope may contract. Older saline implants do not have to be routinely exchanged as a leak is easily diagnosed and causes no adverse reactions.

Any silicone implant, which has signs of a leak or rupture, should be removed. As the incidence of implant failure increases significantly with age, silicone implants older than 10 years with a suspected leak should also be removed. Ultrasonography may be used in the work-up. Although MRI is more accurate, its use should be reserved for patients who are reluctant to have an older implant removed. The patient has to decide whether she wants to have the implants replaced during the same surgery. Frequently, patients (especially older women) do not want to have the implants replaced. It is important for the physician to inform the woman that she will not regain the preimplant shape of her breast. Atrophy of the breast parenchyma occurs naturally with age and seems to be accelerated with breast implants. Marked ptosis following removal of

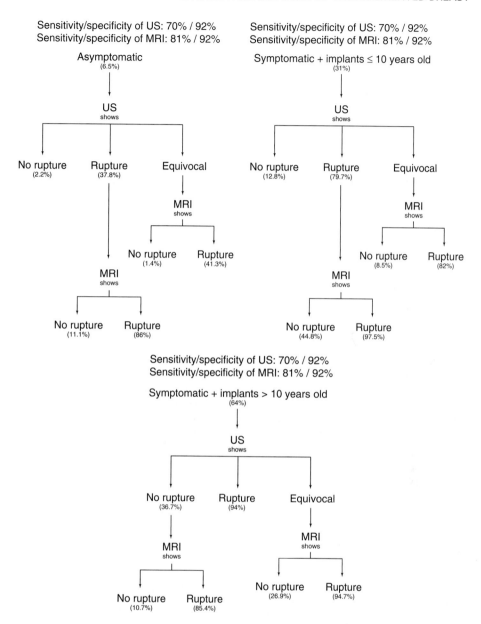

Sensitivity/specificity of US: 70% / 92%
Sensitivity/specificity of MRI: 81% / 92%

Asymptomatic
(6.5%)

US
shows

No rupture (2.2%)   Rupture (37.8%)   Equivocal

MRI
shows

No rupture (1.4%)   Rupture (41.3%)

MRI
shows

No rupture (11.1%)   Rupture (86%)

Sensitivity/specificity of US: 70% / 92%
Sensitivity/specificity of MRI: 81% / 92%

Symptomatic + implants ≤ 10 years old
(31%)

US
shows

No rupture (12.8%)   Rupture (79.7%)   Equivocal

MRI
shows

No rupture (8.5%)   Rupture (82%)

MRI
shows

No rupture (44.8%)   Rupture (97.5%)

Sensitivity/specificity of US: 70% / 92%
Sensitivity/specificity of MRI: 81% / 92%

Symptomatic + implants > 10 years old
(64%)

US
shows

No rupture (36.7%)   Rupture (94%)   Equivocal

MRI
shows

No rupture (10.7%)   Rupture (85.4%)

MRI
shows

No rupture (26.9%)   Rupture (94.7%)

US, ultrasonography;
MRI, magnetic resonance imaging

Figure 23–5. Algorithm illustrating the work-up of silicone implant rupture. (Data from Chung KC, Greenfield ML, Walters M: Decision-analysis methodology in the work-up of women with suspected silicone breast implant rupture. Plast Reconstr Surg 1998;102:689.)

breast implants will develop in most women; this requires a breast lift (mastopexy) to correct. Replacement should be with a saline implant until other implants are FDA approved.

Collis N, Sharpe DT: Silicone gel-filled breast implant integrity: a retrospective review of 478 consecutively explanted implants. Plast Reconstr Surg 2000;105:1979. [PMID: 10839395]

Holmich LR et al: Prevalence of silicone breast implant rupture among Danish women. Plast Reconstr Surg 2001;108:848. [PMID: 11547138]

Rheumatologic Disorders

 ESSENTIALS OF DIAGNOSIS

- *Presence of silicone breast implants.*
- *Symptoms of connective tissue disease, such as malaise, weight loss, joint swelling, pain, and stiffness.*

General Considerations

The term "human adjuvant disease" was first used in the Japanese literature to describe symptoms of connective tissue disease arising in women injected with paraffin for breast augmentation. Other publications from Japan showed an association between injection of various substances and connective tissue diseases. This was followed by reports associating breast implants with autoimmune diseases. The association between silicone breast implants and autoimmune diseases has been examined in more than 30 epidemiologic studies involving over 500,000 women. No statistical connection between silicone breast implants and autoimmune diseases has ever been shown. The syndrome "silicone associated disorders" has also been used to describe a fibromyalgia-like condition in women with silicone breast implants. There have been no epidemiologic studies to support this association.

As mentioned above, all silicone gel implants "bleed" and a small amount of silicone is deposited outside of the implant. This results in elevated blood and tissue silicone levels. This may induce an immune response. There have been no laboratory or epidemiologic data linking this immune response to an immune disease.

Carcinogenesis

No study has credibly found an association of breast implants and breast cancer. Recent epidemiologic studies have not demonstrated any delay in diagnosis or poorer survival among women with breast implants who have breast cancer. Despite this, several issues may affect the diagnosis and treatment of breast cancer in women with breast implants.

In the presence of an implant, less breast tissue is visualized on mammography and special techniques have to be used. The incidence of false-negative mammograms is increased. However, this does not seem to delay diagnosis.

The presence of an implant may require an open biopsy instead of a needle aspiration or core needle biopsy for the diagnosis of a suspected lesion. This is because of distortion on mammography and potential perforation of the implant. The threshold for an open biopsy depends on the practitioner's experience and location of the lesion. Needle localizations and stereotactic biopsies may also be limited. Due to the prevalence of breast implants, most general surgeons are comfortable performing open biopsies, but occasionally, the plastic surgeon will be asked to perform the open biopsy.

Treatment of diagnosed breast cancer also has to be modified. Lumpectomy and radiation yields poor results in women with breast implants. The oncologic surgeon may not be able to achieve negative margins on lumpectomy in patients with subglandular implants. Radiation will induce formation of a thick capsule. For these reasons, mastectomy with immediate reconstruction is more often recommended for women with breast implants.

Birdsell DC, Jenkins H, Berkel H: Breast cancer diagnosis and survival in women with and without breast implants. Plast Reconstr Surg 1993;92:795. [PMID: 8415960]

Bondurant S, Ernster V, Herdman R, (editors): Safety of Silicone Breast Implants (Report of the Committee on the Safety of Silicone Breast Implants, Division of Public Health Promotion and Disease Prevention, Institute of Medicine). National Academy Press, 1999.

Deapen D et al: Breast cancer stage at diagnosis and survival among patients with prior breast implants. Plast Reconstr Surg 2000; 105:535. [PMID: 10697158]

Douglas KP et al: Roentgenographic evaluation of the augmented breast. South Med J 1991;84:49. [PMID: 1846050]

Handel N et al: Breast conservation therapy after augmentation mammaplasty: is it appropriate? Plast Reconstr Surg 1996;98: 1216. [PMID: 8942907]

Hoshaw SJ et al: Breast implants and cancer: causation, delayed detection, and survival. Plast Reconstr Surg 2001;107:1393. [PMID: 11335807]

Leibman AJ, Kruse BD: Imaging of breast cancer after augmentation mammoplasty. Ann Plast Surg 1993;30:111. [PMID: 8387738]

Silverstein MJ et al: Breast cancer diagnosis and prognosis in women following augmentation with silicone gelfilled prostheses. Eur J Cancer 1992;28:635. [PMID: 1591087]

SECTION VI

Urologic Disorders

Lower Urinary Tract Pain

24

Kathleen C. Kobashi, MD, Ali Sarram, MD, & Fred Govier, MD

 ESSENTIALS OF DIAGNOSIS

- *Dysuria is a symptom complex with many causes.*
- *Dysuria and pyuria may indicate bacterial cystitis.*
- *Dysuria without pyuria should not be diagnosed as an infection.*
- *Hematuria without infection needs to be evaluated with intravenous pyelography or similar studies and cystoscopy.*

General Considerations

Normal functioning of the lower urinary tract (LUT) represents a delicate balance between the bladder and outlet and between the voluntary and involuntary control mechanisms through the autonomic and somatic nerve supply. Although the neurologic control of the LUT is incompletely understood, it generally is agreed that sympathetic innervation is responsible for urine storage and parasympathetic innervation for evacuation of urine. Somatic innervation is through the pudendal nerve to the pelvic floor muscles and the periurethral striated muscle. The bladder acts as a passive storage reservoir during filling and actively contracts during urination. During storage, the bladder outlet must maintain a pressure that exceeds bladder pressure. The role of the bladder neck smooth muscle is to maintain a constant tone or pressure during bladder filling (storage phase). With bladder muscle contraction during the emptying phase, the bladder neck muscle relaxes, which decreases the outlet resistance and promotes emptying.

Appreciating the delicate balance between bladder storage and emptying is crucial to understanding the symptoms associated with lower urinary tract pain (LUTP) and how seemingly innocuous occurrences external to the urinary tract can contribute to its dysfunction.

Pathogenesis

Pain is a noxious sensation carried by nerve fibers from the site of tissue injury to the brain. Acute pain is beneficial when it alerts the person to the site of injury. Once injury is recognized, treated, and healed, persistent pain becomes chronic and is no longer beneficial. Chronic pain can severely affect quality of life by decreasing motivation, limiting physical activities, and disrupting sleep patterns.

There are 3 types of pain: somatic, visceral, and neuropathic. Somatic pain arises from skin, muscles, and bones. Rapid transmission by fibers to the cerebral cortex allows the source of pain to be localized quickly, yielding a fast response. Descriptions of somatic pain include "sharp," "stabbing," and "throbbing." Visceral pain arises from the internal organs and is carried on slower fibers through the limbic system (emotional center). The source of pain is poorly localized and often described in emotional terms such as "awful" or "agonizing." Neuropathic pain is generated in damaged nerve fibers. Its messages also are carried through the limbic system and often are described as "electrical," "shock-like," or a "painful numbness." These descriptions can be helpful in identifying the type of pain, especially in the pelvis where all 3 types can coexist. The role of the limbic system explains why visceral and neuropathic pain (with afferent transmission through the limbic system) present with significant emotional overlay, which is not seen in somatic pain (in which the limbic system is bypassed).

The concept of "triggers" and "amplifiers" can be used to understand the pathogenesis of LUTP. In this model, factors such as infection, anatomic abnormalities, or trauma can trigger LUTP. Potential symptom amplifiers can then enhance these symptoms. Figure 24–1 contains a depiction of this model.

Patients with LUT symptoms often complain of a mixture of somatic, visceral, and neuropathic pain. This is often associated with urinary frequency and urgency. Normal bladder capacity ranges from 400 to 600 mL. An initial sense of bladder awareness occurs when the volume is approximately 250–300 mL, with gradually increasing awareness of fullness and the urge to urinate with progressive filling. When the volume in the bladder is less than 200–300 mL, the bladder may have difficulty generating and sustaining a contraction. Without a

detrusor contraction, the outlet has difficulty maintaining relaxation. When there is a source of irritation in or around the LUT, the urge to urinate may occur at very low volumes (30–100 mL). At this low volume, coordinated detrusor contraction and outlet relaxation may not occur, and urination may be hesitant, slow, and interrupted, with a sense of incomplete emptying. This condition can become exacerbated when the sense of urge is intense or painful at low volumes. Chronic straining to initiate or sustain urination against "tight" pelvic muscles can contribute further to the voiding dysfunction. In summary, increased bladder sensitivity can become associated quickly with a voiding dysfunction. Irrespective of what may have caused the irritation initially, the voiding dysfunction can be responsible for chronically maintaining the symptoms.

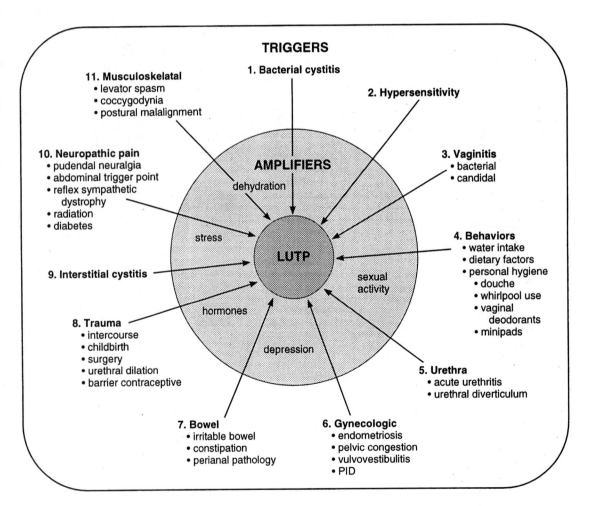

Figure 24–1. Factors triggering lower urinary tract pain (LUTP) with potential symptom amplifiers.

Clinical Findings

A. SYMPTOMS AND SIGNS

Symptoms of pain or discomfort in the bladder, ure-thra, or both are a common complaint. The causes of these symptoms range from acute bacterial cystitis to pelvic floor myalgia. Sensations arising from the pelvic organs and supporting musculoskeletal tissue are poorly localized and travel via common pathways to the central nervous system. Consequently, impulses originating in the internal abdominal or pelvic organs or the bones, muscles, and nerves of the pelvis can generate impulses that are perceived as originating in the bladder or ure-thra. These sensations may be described as sharp, heavy, stabbing, aching, burning, cramping, a severe sense of urgency, or an unrelenting awareness of the bladder. The factors contributing to symptoms of LUTP are often multiple and additive and can be influenced by factors seemingly unrelated to the LUT.

Most women with LUTP note increased frequency of urination compared with their previous habits. Although urinating every 3 hours is not excessive, it may be bothersome for someone who used to urinate every 4–6 hours. The key is to determine what bladder volumes signal the urge to urinate and what happens if the signals are ignored. A record of voiding times and volume of urination over several days and nights is invaluable. A bladder that can hold 600 mL at night but holds only 100–300 mL during the day suggests hyper-sensitivity of the LUT. A woman who gets out of bed while awake to urinate several times with very small volumes but is able to hold her urine all night once she falls asleep has a different problem than someone who wakes up every 2 hours to urinate 100 mL.

Hematuria is the abnormal presence of erythrocytes in the urine and must be distinguished from myoglo-binuria and hemoglobinuria. This distinction can be made by confirming the presence of red blood cells on microscopic analysis after a urine dipstick is found to be positive for blood. Hematuria, either macroscopic or microscopic, is frequently the first symptom of a signif-icant urologic disease and warrants evaluation to deter-mine its cause. In female patients, hematuria must be either localized to the urinary tract or established to have a gynecologic source. This distinction may be made by obtaining a catheterized urine specimen.

B. LABORATORY FINDINGS

A voided urinalysis should always be done. A voided specimen is collected mid-stream as the patient urinates into a sterile specimen container. Microscopic examina-tion of a spun specimen allows for immediate assess-ment of hematuria and pyuria (infection) and contami-nation. If the specimen appears contaminated with squamous epithelial cells or contains red blood cells, obtaining an immediate catheterized specimen can eliminate confusion about whether culture results accu-rately represent the status of the bladder. Routine cul-ture of a urine specimen that is chemically negative for leukocyte esterase, nitrates, and blood is not indicated unless the patient needs the additional reassurance that there is no bacterial infection requiring antibiotics.

A urine specimen collected with a small-caliber (12F or 14F) catheter also provides an accurate determina-tion of the postvoid residual (PVR), which is important in patients who have frequency and a sensation of in-complete emptying. Alternatively, an ultrasonographic estimation of the PVR can be done. A voided urine sample can be sent for cytologic study as an initial screen to rule out carcinoma in situ of the bladder, which can be present with symptoms of LUT irritation. This assessment is especially important in women with a present or past history of smoking. When significant hematuria is found, an upper tract evaluation should be done before cystoscopy.

Evaluation

A. HISTORY

A complete history is the most important aspect of the initial evaluation of a patient with LUTP. Specific questions include:

1. What are your current symptoms?
2. Can you describe your pain?
3. Are the symptoms the same all the time?
4. What were your bladder habits before this prob-lem started?
5. Did you have infections, frequency, or daytime or nighttime incontinence as a child? If so, were any procedures performed such as a meatotomy, ure-throtomy, or urethral dilation?
6. Do symptoms vary with your menstrual cycle?
7. Do any of the following exacerbate your symp-toms?

   –Dehydration (increased physical activity and sweating or decreased fluid intake)

   –Dietary factors (coffee, carbonation, acidic foods, juices, spicy foods, sugar, aspartame)

   –Physical factors (sitting or standing for pro-longed periods, car rides, lifting)

   –Emotional factors (stress, anxiety, depression, fa-tigue)
8. What relieves your symptoms?
9. What is your normal daily fluid intake of the fol-lowing: coffee (include decaffeinated), tea, car-

bonated beverages (seltzer, sparkling water), fruit juices (especially citrus and cranberry), alcohol, water, milk?

10. What was going on in your life at the time of the onset of symptoms?

   –Becoming sexually active

   –Being with a new sexual partner

   –Using a new form of birth control

   –Experiencing hot weather

   –Injuring lower back or tail bone

   –Undergoing a pelvic operation or a minor gynecologic procedure

   –Suffering from a pelvic organ infection

   –Suffering from a perianal process, such as fissure or hemorrhoid

11. What is your biggest fear concerning these symptoms?

12. Do you have a history of physical, sexual, or emotional abuse that may have some significance for your current symptom complex?

B. Physical Examination

Ensure the patient has voided shortly before the examination. It is important to explain the examination to the patient as it progresses. Having the woman positioned and draped in a manner allowing observation of facial expressions can be helpful in permitting her to feel like a participant in the process. First, the external genitalia are inspected visually for signs of irritation, discharge, and atrophic changes.

Next, a finger is introduced gently through the introitus, with pressure kept against the posterior vaginal wall. Ask the patient to identify when she is having discomfort or pain and if the discomfort is the same as or different from her symptomatic episodes. Initially, the introitus is palpated circumferentially; the finger is introduced gently to the level of the cervix or vaginal cuff, with the pressure kept posteriorly. The levator muscles are palpated gradually following the arc of pubic bone, pushing up on the genitourinary diaphragm lateral to the bladder and urethra. This should be done on both sides, with the physician observing for symptom reproduction. The lateral pelvic sidewalls also are palpated, as is the anterior vaginal wall. The clinician begins with the urethra just proximal to the meatus and gently palpates toward the bladder neck. The urethra should feel like a midline spongy tube with a "gutter" on either side. These gutters may be obscured by a previous anterior colporrhaphy, anterior vaginal wall mass (cyst or infected glands), or urethral diverticulum.

Moving superiorly, the physician gently palpates the base of the bladder. A sense of urge is normal, but a sense of pain, burning, cramping, or aching is not. A bimanual examination is begun by gently putting downward pressure in the suprapubic area while pushing upward on the base of the bladder in the midline with the vaginal finger. Next, the clinician moves the vaginal finger lateral to the bladder and pushes up on the pelvic floor support immediately adjacent to the pubic bone. Pain in this area is consistent with myofascial pain. Bimanual examination of the uterus and ovaries is performed, again with careful assessment for pain reproduction. When pain is reproduced, the same spot should be assessed with abdominal and vaginal pressure independently to determine whether the pain is generated by abdominal or vaginal trigger points or the tissue in between. A speculum examination is performed to look for signs of vaginitis or cervicitis.

The final part of the examination is an assessment of the patient's ability to contract and relax the pelvic floor muscles. This muscle group should be supple and nontender at rest. There should be circumferential tightening of muscles around the vagina without lifting of the buttocks and immediate relaxation on command. It may be difficult to feel contraction if muscles are tight and in spasm. Verbal encouragement to relax or not to hold back often initiates relaxation. Once the muscles are relaxed, any tender areas are palpated again. Often, the pain decreases, which provides immediate feedback to the patient, indicating that at least part of the pain is related to tension in the pelvic muscles and can be lessened by muscle relaxation.

Differential Diagnosis

A. Infection

Health care providers should be careful not to diagnose a urinary tract infection based on the symptoms alone. To diagnose a urinary tract infection with certainty, a clean catch or catheterized urine specimen must be examined microscopically, and a urine culture must be obtained. Classic diagnostic criterion requires a urine culture showing greater than 100,000 colony-forming units (CFU) per milliliter of urine. It has become increasingly apparent, however, that 20–40% of women with symptomatic urinary tract infections present with bacteria counts of less than 10^5 CFU/mL of urine. Thus, in dysuric women, an appropriate threshold value for defining significant bacteriuria is greater than 10^2 CFU/mL of a known pathogen when the urine specimen is collected appropriately.

B. Lower Urinary Tract Hypersensitivity

This term has replaced others such as urethral syndrome, chronic trigonitis, chronic urethritis, and chronic nonbacterial cystitis. It refers to an overly sensitive bladder, which can contribute to the cascade of events leading to uncoordinated low-volume urination;

voiding dysfunction; and eventually, pain before, during, or after urination. Usually, the pain is worse before or after urination, and patients often report that the pain feels different from that of a bacterial bladder infection. Identifying all the potential triggers and eliminating as many of them as possible, while increasing water intake, modifying the diet, and working with pelvic muscle relaxation, can alleviate symptoms and minimize the number of symptomatic episodes.

C. INTERSTITIAL CYSTITIS

Women who have interstitial cystitis (IC) typically report frequency and urgency of urination as well as suprapubic, perineal, vulvar, or vaginal discomfort before, during, or after urination. Pain during or after sexual intercourse also is reported commonly. The diagnosis of IC is made based on symptoms, functional bladder data (cystometrogram), and cystoscopic criteria. There are no specific blood, urine, or bladder biopsy criteria to confirm the diagnosis. The exact incidence of IC is not known. An epidemiologic study showed the median age of onset of symptoms was 40 years, with 25% of the patients younger than 30 years. The social, economic, and psychological costs of this syndrome are significant, and often difficult to appreciate. The cause is unknown, and there is no known cure. Etiologic concepts currently being considered include infection, vascular or lymphatic obstruction, psychological factors, glycosaminoglycan alterations, reflex sympathetic dystrophy, toxic urinary agents, and immunologic factors. With the wide variety of potential causative factors, it is not surprising that no single intervention is uniformly successful and that often a combination of interventions is required to control symptoms.

IC is thought to be associated with poorer quality of life and higher levels of depressive symptoms. Rothrock and colleagues found that patients in whom IC was diagnosed reported compromised quality of life across various domains, including physical functioning and ability to function in one's normal role, and vitality. Patients also suffered from more severe depressive symptoms, which was associated with greater compromise in physical and social functioning. To the astute clinician, this underscores the importance of recognizing and treating possible associated psychological factors in a patient with LUTP.

D. NEUROPATHIC PAIN

The diagnosis of neuropathic pain rarely is considered in women who present with LUTP, but it should be considered first in women who describe their pain as "burning" or "electric shock-like" sensation. The mechanism of nerve injury may never be known; the injury can be perpetuated by local trauma, pelvic floor spasm, or repeated injury to the peripheral nerves. Trauma to the pudendal nerve has been attributed to events and activities such as vaginal childbirth, horseback riding, and prolonged cycling. Reflex sympathetic dystrophy has been reported in women with chronic bladder pain. Exposure of the pelvic organs to radiation can damage the blood supply and the nerves, leading to symptoms of LUTP.

E. MUSCULOSKELETAL PAIN

Musculoskeletal pain is probably the most frequently missed diagnosis in patients who present with pain in the pelvis and an altered voiding pattern. Typically, this pain is poorly localized, dull, and aching. Health care providers are not accustomed to thinking of the pelvic musculoskeletal system as a source of pain when patients attribute their discomfort to their internal organs. Timely recognition of such contributing disorders allows healthcare workers to appropriately diagnose and treat these patients with standard techniques of physiotherapy, such as applications of heat and cold, massage, and muscle stretching, strengthening, and relaxation. The value of these techniques has been demonstrated in patients with extremely refractory chronic pain, and they now are employed early in the management of patients with LUTP.

F. MALIGNANCY

Dysuria with persistent hematuria should initiate a work-up directed at detecting urologic malignancy. Transitional cell carcinoma and carcinoma in situ of the bladder often present with persistent dysuria and hematuria despite attempts at symptomatic relief with antibiotics and analgesics. When a patient presents with gross hematuria, whether painless or associated with abdominal or flank pain, a thorough investigation is imperative, even if only a single episode of bloody urine is reported. Evaluation should begin with a urine culture. If the urine culture is positive and hematuria resolves with treatment, further evaluation usually is not indicated unless a repeat urinalysis shows persistent hematuria. In patients with culture-negative urine, further urologic evaluation is necessary. Evaluation typically includes cytologic study of the urine, intravenous pyelography or similar studies, and cystoscopy.

Although the presence of a small number of red blood cells in the urine is normal and does not require extensive urologic evaluation, there is controversy concerning the degree of microscopic hematuria that requires evaluation. A widely accepted upper limit of normal is 5 red blood cells/high-powered field. Often hematuria is detected on dipstick only, and the patient is referred to a urologist before true hematuria is documented. Because dipstick tests generally are based on the peroxidase-like activities of red blood cells and hemoglobin, there may be false-positive results. Therefore, all patients who have dipstick-positive urine should have a microscopic evaluation of the urine sediment. A standard urologic evaluation is prompted by the findings of microscopic hematuria in 2 of 3 clean-catch uncatheterized specimens. An issue of concern is how to manage hematuria in patients undergoing anticoagulant therapy. Studies have shown that approximately 20% of these patients have significant disease that will show up if appropriate studies are performed.

G. OTHER

Urinary tract pain in women with vulvovaginal inflammation generally occurs during the act of urination, but it typically is felt as the urine contacts the external tissues rather than while it passes through the urethra. Chemical irritation of the external genitalia from soaps, douches, perfumes, and contraceptive preparations also is felt as pain on the external tissues. Urethral diverticula should be considered in women with recurrent LUT infections, pain during urination, painful coitus, and postvoid dribbling. On physical examination, there is usually a sense of fullness to palpation in the anterior vaginal wall. Endometriosis, pelvic inflammatory disease, pelvic congestion, and vulvar vestibulitis (vulvodynia) are disorders that can present with symptoms primarily localized to the LUT and need to be considered in the differential diagnosis of LUTP of uncertain cause.

Held P et al: Epidemiology of interstitial cystitis. In: Hanno P (editor): *Interstitial Cystitis.* Springer-Verlag, 1990.

Rothrock et al: Depressive symptoms and quality of life in patients with interstitial cystitis. J Urol 2002;167:1763. [PMID: 11912405]

Treatment

Once malignancy and infection have been excluded, treatment begins with reassurance and education concerning the structure and function of the LUT and its interrelationship with the gynecologic, gastrointestinal, and musculoskeletal systems. Use of anatomic diagrams can be helpful in assisting the patient to understand the concepts being discussed. A working partnership between physician and patient needs to be established with the goal of obtaining symptom control and allowing the patient to get on with life. If the goal is to "cure" the disease, the patient is at risk for continual disappointment as one treatment after another fails to bring permanent symptom relief. Terms such as "dysfunctions" and "symptomatic episodes" or "flare-ups" are most accurate and do not lead to the expectation that antibiotics will help. It is crucial to ensure that the office personnel who patients communicate with (in person or on the phone) understand the importance of terminology. Getting mixed messages from different persons fuels fear, frustration, and anxiety.

A. BEHAVIORAL STRATEGIES

Common sense is important in using behavioral recommendations. Using a diary to record time and volume of urination can be important in demonstrating objective improvement to the patient. Increasing the water intake to dilute the urine and flush out the LUT is important. The optimal volume varies. A general guideline is to drink enough water to keep the color of urine pale yellow. Avoiding particular foods or fluids also can relieve the discomfort, although the rationale for this intervention is not known. Foods typically reported to exacerbate symptoms are coffee; tea (even decaffeinated); and substances that are carbonated, acidic, or spicy.

It is important to recognize the potential of voluntary or involuntary pelvic muscle contraction in symptom generation, perpetuation, or exacerbation. Voluntary pelvic floor relaxation can ease symptoms. Many times patients need instruction in pelvic muscle localization and contraction before they can understand how to relax this muscle group. Anything that promotes generalized relaxation and stress management (eg, aerobic exercise or distraction) should be used when possible. The provider must present these behavioral strategies as valid treatments so that the patient will accept them.

B. PHARMACOLOGIC MANAGEMENT

A variety of medications can be used to treat LUTP syndromes. Often, a combination of drugs is needed. Table 24–1 lists the medications most commonly used and the symptoms that indicate various treatment plans. In particular, the use of α-blockers (eg, prazosin) can be helpful in patients with obstructive voiding symptoms. The list of medications should be regarded as a general guideline and, in refractory conditions, a trial of 1 more agent or 1 more combination may be the key in breaking the pain cycle. Realistic expectations for treatment outcome are necessary.

C. PHYSIOTHERAPY

A comprehensive physiotherapy evaluation and treatment regimen is invaluable to women with LUTP. Patients with refractory symptoms who see physical therapists with a special interest in pelvic floor dysfunction can have surprising success. Weiss et al evaluated the effectiveness of manual physical therapy in patients with IC and LUTP. With a mean follow-up of 1.5 years, the investigators noted that 70% of patients with IC had moderate to marked improvement of their symptoms.

Table 24–1. Medications for treatment of lower urinary tract pain.

Medication	Dosage	Symptom	Sign
Antidepressants			
Amitriptyline	10–75 mg qhs[1]	Sleep disruption; sharp, burning, shock-like pain; bladder/urethral burning or constant awareness	Increased pelvic muscle tone; tender bladder
Doxepin	10–75 mg qhs[1]		
Trazodone	50 mg qhs[1]		
Fluoxetine	20 mg qd		
Imipramine	10–25 mg tid[1]		
α-Blockers			
Terazosin	1–10 mg qhs[2]	Hesitancy; slow stream, sense of incomplete emptying	Abnormal uroflow; ± tender pelvic muscles
Prazosin	0.5–2.0 mg tid[1]		
Phenoxybenzamine	10–20 mg bid[2]	Postvoiding pain/spasm	
Antispasmodics			
Oxybutynin	5 mg tid[1]	Frequency; discomfort with full bladder; severe urgency	Involuntary detrusor contraction on cysto-metrogram
Hyoscyamine	1–2 tablet tid		
Flavoxate	1 tablet tid		
Skeletal muscle relaxants			
Carisoprodol	350 mg tid	Postvoiding pain; dyspareunia	Increased tone of pelvic muscles; pain reproduction with palpation
Cyclobenzaprine	10 mg qd–tid[1]		
Methocarbamol	100 mg bid		
Anesthetics			
Phenazopyridine	100–200 mg tid	Hypersensitivity; pain during urination; pain localized to meatal area during urination or intercourse	Tender introital area or perimeatal area
Lidocaine jelly 2%	Apply intra-vesically prn		
Lidocaine ointment 5%			
Anticonvulsants			
Carbamazepine	100–200 mg bid,[1] gradually increase to qid prn	Neuropathic pain	Sensory deficits-perineum/lower extremity; dysesthesia

[1]Start with lowest dosage and gradually increase as necessary for symptom control.
[2]May divide into tid if sedation not a problem.

Most patients can be referred for physiotherapy assessment after their first or second visit. Patients almost universally report that they gain some improvement if not total symptom relief.

D. TREATMENTS SPECIFIC TO INTERSTITIAL CYSTITIS

Even patients with a confirmed diagnosis of IC may respond well to some of the simple behavioral strategies. It is best to start by reviewing what the patient knows about IC, what she knows about self-help strategies, and how well she has tried to incorporate these strategies into her life. Patients and their families can be reas-sured that most women arrive at a treatment strategy by combining behavioral, pharmacologic, and physiotherapeutic techniques, which allows them to have a reasonably pain-free, functional life. Current treatment for IC is aimed at symptomatic relief through a variety of means including dietary modification; intravesical instillations of various pharmacologic agents including dimethyl sulfoxide (DMSO), hydrocortisone, sodium bicarbonate, heparin, and oxychlorosene; and use of oral agents such as amitriptyline, hydroxyzine, nifedipine, and sodium pentosan polysulfate. Other methods used to treat IC include transcutaneous nerve stimulation, neuromodulation (sacral nerve root stimulator), surgical enlargement of the bladder (augmentation cystoplasty), substitution cystoplasty, and cystectomy with urinary diversion.

E. Sacroneuromodulation

It has become increasingly apparent that urinary symptoms of urgency, frequency, and LUTP may have a neurologic component. Consequently, the effects of neuromodulation for the treatment of such symptoms has been the focus of much research over the past 2 decades. This treatment involves placement of leads that stimulate the sacral nerves responsible for bladder sensory and motor function. After favorable response to a temporary test stimulator is assured, a permanent device is implanted. As the clinical experience with this device has expanded, the Interstim (Medtronic, Minneapolis, MN) has been found to be successful not only in the treatment of patients with urinary frequency and urgency, but also in those with idiopathic urinary retention or refractory LUTP. In a series from Melbourne, Australia, Maher and colleagues reported a statistically significant improvement in the mean voided volume and daytime frequency and nocturia episodes in patients with intractable IC in response to percutaneous sacral nerve root neuromodulation. They also reported a decrease in mean bladder pain from 8.9 to 2.4 points on a scale of 0 to 10.

Maher CF et al: Percutaneous sacral nerve root neuromodulation for intractable interstitial cystitis. J Urol 2001;165:884. [PMID: 11176493]

Weiss JM: Pelvic floor myofascial trigger points: manual therapy for interstitial cystitis and the urgency-frequency syndrome. J Urol 2001;166(6):2226. [PMID: 11696740]

When to Refer to a Specialist

Patients with symptoms refractory to conventional therapy should be referred to a specialist for further work-up and therapy. Moreover, patients with persistent microscopically confirmed hematuria or gross hematuria in absence of a urinary tract infection should be referred to a urologist for a hematuria work-up.

Baker P: Musculoskeletal origins of chronic pelvic pain: diagnosis and treatment. Obstet Gynecol Clin North Am 1993;20:719. [PMID: 8115087]

Bavendam T: A common sense approach to lower urinary tract hypersensitivity in women. Contemp Urol 1992;4:25.

Bemelmans BL, Mundy AR, Craggs MD: Neuromodulation by implant for treating lower urinary tract symptoms and dysfunction. Eur Urol 1999;36:81. [PMID: 10420026]

Brockoff D: Understanding pain and pain medications. Interstitial Cystitis Association, 1990.

Early experience with physical therapy in the management of pelvic pain in female urologic patients: 1992. In: Annual Meeting of American Urological Society, Western Section. Maui, Hawaii.

Fleischmann J et al: Clinical and immunological response to nifedipine for the treatment of interstitial cystitis. J Urol 1991;146:1235. [PMID: 1942269]

Galloway NT, Gabale DR, Irwin PP: Interstitial cystitis or reflex sympathetic dystrophy of the bladder? Semin Urol 1991; 9:148. [PMID: 1853012]

Hanno P et al: *Interstitial Cystitis.* Springer-Verlag, 1990.

Hanno PM, Buehler J, Wein AJ: Use of amitriptyline in the treatment of interstitial cystitis. J Urol 1989;141:846. [PMID: 2926877]

Koziol JA: Epidemiology of interstitial cystitis. Urol Clin North Am 1994;21:7. [PMID: 8284848]

Krieger JN: Urinary tract infections in women: causes, classification, and differential diagnosis. Urology 1990;35:4. [PMID: 2404372]

Leach GF, Bavendam TG: Female urethral diverticula. Urology 1987;30:407. [PMID: 3118546]

Moldwin RM, Sant GR: Interstitial cystitis: a pathophysiology and treatment update. Clin Obstet Gynecol 2002;45:259. [PMID: 11862078]

Mulholland SG et al: Pentosan polysulfate sodium for therapy of interstitial cystitis: A double-blind placebo-controlled clinical study. Urology 1990;35:552. [PMID: 1693797]

Oravisto KJ: Epidemiology of interstitial cystitis. Ann Chir Gynaecol Fenn 1975;64:75. [PMID: 1137336]

Parsons CL, Koprowski PF: Interstitial cystitis: Successful management by increasing voiding intervals. Urology 1991;37:207. [PMID: 2000675]

Perez-Marrero R et al: Prolongation of response to DMSO by heparin maintenance. Urology 1993;41(Suppl):64. [PMID: 8420097]

Petersen T, Husted S: Prazosin treatment of neurological patients with lower urinary tract dysfunction. Int Urogynecol J 1993; 4:106.

Phillips HC, Fenster HN, Samsom D: An effective treatment for functional urinary incoordination. J Behav Med 1992;15:45. [PMID: 1583673]

Rapkin AJ, Mayer EA: Gastroenterologic causes of chronic pelvic pain. Obstet Gynecol Clin North Am 1993;20:663. [PMID: 8115083]

Ratliff TL, Klutke CG, McDougall EM: The etiology of interstitial cystitis. Urol Clin North Am 1994;21:21. [PMID: 8284842]

Schuster GA, Lewis GA: Clinical significance of hematuria in patients on anticoagulant therapy. J Urol 1987;137:923. [PMID: 3573184]

Seigel SW et al: Long-term results of a multicenter study on sacral nerve stimulation for treatment of urinary urge incontinence, urgency-frequency, and retention. Urology 2000;56(6 Suppl 1):87. [PMID: 11114569]

Tanagho EA, Schmidt RA: Electrical stimulation in the management of the neurogenic bladder. J Urol 1988;140:1331. [PMID: 3057221]

Theoharides TC: Hydroxyzine in the treatment of interstitial cystitis. Urol Clin North Am 1994;21:113. [PMID: 8284834]

Turner ML, Marinoff SC: Pudendal neuralgia. Am J Obstet Gynecol 1991;165:1233. [PMID: 1951579]

Wishard W, Nourse M, Mertz J: Use of chlorpactin WCS 90 for relief of symptoms due to interstitial cystitis. J Urol 1957; 77:420.

Relevant Web Sites

http://www.ichelp.com/
http://www.niddk.nih.gov/health/urolog/pubs/cystitis/cystitis.htm
http://www.nlm.nih.gov/medlineplus/interstitialcystitis.html

Acknowledgment:

The editors wish to acknowledge the contribution of Tamara G. Bavendam, MD, who wrote this chapter in the previous edition of this book.

Urinary Incontinence

25

Kathleen C. Kobashi, MD & Fred E. Govier, MD

The International Continence Society (ICS) defines urinary incontinence as the "involuntary loss of urine that represents a hygienic or social problem to the individual and which is objectively demonstrable." The estimates of the prevalence of urinary incontinence vary with the profiles of the groups considered. Urinary incontinence is estimated to affect 13 million Americans. The estimated annual cost of treating urinary incontinence in patients older than 65 years is $26.3 billion, or $3565 per patient. Approximately 10–20% of women aged 15–64 years, 40% of women older than 60 years, and more than 50% of institutionalized patients (including both sexes) are affected. Wolin found that 50% of 4211 nulliparous women 18–25 years of age reported involuntary loss of urine with some type of activity, 16% on a daily basis.

Women may delay reporting urinary incontinence because of embarrassment or because they are unaware that successful treatment options are available. Primary care providers may not routinely ask about bladder control problems for similar reasons or because they are not comfortable with the initial evaluation and treatment options. Although it is rapidly changing, education concerning urinary incontinence is lacking at all levels of medical education. Clinicians must have the basic information necessary to perform initial incontinence evaluations, institute treatment, and refer appropriate patients to specialists.

 ESSENTIALS OF DIAGNOSIS

- Urge urinary incontinence is a sudden insuppressible sensation to void, resulting in variable leakage of urine.
- Stress urinary incontinence is characterized by symptoms of leakage of urine with coughing, sneezing, laughing, lifting, or other physically strenuous activities.

General Considerations

Incontinence is categorized based on the circumstances precipitating the involuntary loss of urine and symptoms associated with the incontinence. Table 25–1 shows the various causes of urinary incontinence. A patient often has more than one type of incontinence and more than one causative factor.

Stress urinary incontinence (SUI) is defined as urine leakage with a sudden increased intra-abdominal pressure, such as that seen with laughing, coughing, lifting, walking, or changing position, *without* concomitant rise in detrusor (bladder-generated) pressure. The proposed mechanism of SUI is that increase in intra-abdominal pressure resulting from various activities is transmitted to the bladder, causing the intravesical (within the bladder, but not due to the bladder) pressure to rise above the urethral pressure. Under normal circumstances, the urethral pressure rises approximately 250 msec prior to any increase in the detrusor pressure, and this rise is sufficient to prevent urinary leakage from occurring.

Patients with **urge urinary incontinence (UUI)** describe a sudden insuppressible sensation to void, resulting in variable leakage of urine. Urgency can occur secondary to a sensory or a motor dysfunction. With sensory urgency, the desire to urinate is so intense the person "lets go" of the urine to relieve the severe urgency. Motor urgency occurs with a bladder or detrusor contraction that cannot be suppressed voluntarily.

Mixed incontinence includes components of both SUI and UUI.

Overflow incontinence may occur in cases in which the bladder is full to capacity such that any further urine production results in frequent low-volume loss of urine (ie, "overflow"). The clinician should be aware that patients who actually suffer from overflow incontinence may describe symptoms of urgency or stress incontinence. A patient's ability to empty the bladder must be evaluated to ensure that overflow incontinence is not being overlooked.

Total incontinence can be due to severe intrinsic sphincter deficiency or the rare condition of vesicovaginal or ureterovaginal fistula. An often overlooked type of incontinence is **functional incontinence,** which is the loss of urine due to entities extrinsic to the urinary tract. Factors that limit patient mobility such as stroke or neurologic disease may result in incontinence. Other barriers may include heavy doors to toilets or poor wheelchair access that could prevent a patient from

Table 25–1. Etiologies of various types of urinary incontinence.

Stress urinary incontinence	Urge urinary incontinence	Overflow incontinence
Trauma	**Neurologic**	**Trauma**
Childbirth	Spinal cord injury	Myogenic detrusor damage (2° to overdistension)
Pelvic surgery	Back surgery	**Neurologic**
Physiologic	Multiple sclerosis	Diabetes mellitus (70% decreased sensation; 15%
Atrophic vaginitis (hormonal)	Cerebrovascular accident	acontractile)
Pelvic prolapse	Parkinson's disease	**Obstruction**
Medication side effects	Aging	Previous anti-incontinence surgery
α-blockers (hypertension)	**Obstruction**	Malignancy
β-antagonists	Uncommon in females without prior	**Medication side effects**
Benzodiazepines (muscle relaxants)	pelvic surgery	Drugs with anticholinergic side effects
Iatrogenic	Cystocele, vault prolapse	Sympathomimetic drugs
Postoperative (eg, rectal surgery,	Previous pelvic surgery	
back surgery)	Malignancy	
	Fibrosis	
	Aging	
	Atrophic vaginitis	
	Iatrogenic	
	(Long-term indwelling catheter)	
	Other	
	Infection	
	Tumor/carcinoma in situ	
	Stones	
	Interstitial	

reaching the toilet facilities in time. Finally, medications such as diuretics can contribute to incontinence by causing precipitous filling of the bladder over a short period of time.

The importance of urinary incontinence is determined by the impact of the incontinence episodes on a person's quality of life. Quality-of-life issues are different for every individual. Activity restriction, fluid restriction, and staying near bathrooms may eliminate accidents, making extra protection unnecessary; yet cause negative changes in an individual's quality of life. Questions that can help the patient and her provider understand the significance of the problem are "What have you done to minimize your episodes of urine leakage?" and "What impact have these changes had on your quality of life?"

Constantinou CE: Resting and stress urethral pressures as a clinical guide to the mechanism of continence in the female patient. Urol Clin North Am 1985;12:247. [PMID: 4039486]

Payne CK: Epidemiology, pathophysiology and evaluation of urinary incontinence and overactive bladder. Urology 1998; 51(2A Suppl):3. [PMID: 9495728]

Wagner TH, Hu TW: Economic costs of urinary incontinence in 1995. Urology 1998;51:355. [PMID: 9510336]

Wolin LH: Stress incontinence in young, healthy nulliparous female subjects. J Urol 1969;101:545. [PMID: 5776039]

Pathogenesis

The lower urinary tract has 2 main functions: storage and expulsion of urine, each of which can be evaluated with regard to the bladder or the bladder outlet. Consideration of incontinence in terms of the functional abnormalities responsible simplifies treatment, and therefore it is important to first understand the contribution of the bladder and bladder outlet to the storage and expulsion of urine.

A. Physiology

Proper balance between the bladder and the bladder outlet is required to maintain urinary continence. The mechanism of female continence involves normal bladder function, an intact urethral sphincter, a well-supported urethra, and intact autonomic (pelvic and hypogastric) and somatic (pudendal) innervation. Incontinence occurs when the bladder pressure exceeds the pressure of the bladder outlet. In women, the bladder outlet mechanism consists of the smooth muscle of the bladder neck and urethra, the skeletal muscle of the urinary sphincter and pelvic floor, and the urethral mucosa. The bladder serves as a low-pressure storage receptacle for urine.

The urethra has an important role in preserving continence (intrinsic urethral factors) independent of its anatomic position. Normal urethral mucosa is moist and supple, supplied by a rich vascular network. The mucosa has abundant folds that facilitate complete coaptation of the tissue to create a "mucosal seal" effect that contributes to sustaining continence. Normal estrogen levels are important for maintaining the folds of the mucosa and the ample vascular supply. Smooth muscle in the wall of the urethra also provides compressive forces that maintain urethral closure.

Normally, the bladder and proximal urethra occupy an intra-abdominal position above the level of the pelvic floor muscles. With strong myofascial support, the intra-abdominal position is maintained even during activities that increase intra-abdominal pressure. This results in equal pressure transmission to the bladder and proximal urethra, and there is no loss of urine (Figure 25–1). In patients with SUI, weakened anatomic support allows the proximal urethra and bladder neck to rest at or below the level of the pelvic muscles. Consequently, pressure increases are transmitted to the bladder but not to the proximal urethra. At times of increased intra-abdominal pressure, bladder pressure exceeds outlet pressure and leakage occurs (Figure 25–2).

The innervation of the bladder and outlet involves an intricate system that coordinates relaxation of the detrusor muscle and contraction of the pelvic floor and sphincter during filling of the bladder and contraction of the detrusor and relaxation of the pelvic floor and

sphincter during voiding. During increases in intra-abdominal pressure, reflex skeletal muscle contraction increases the tone of the pelvic floor and urethra. Voluntary contraction is an important adjunct to the reflex contraction and is dependent on a woman's awareness of how and when to use this muscle group effectively.

B. PATHOPHYSIOLOGY

Urinary incontinence can result from a failure to properly store the urine or failure to properly empty the bladder. In women, urinary incontinence is typically due to a storage abnormality secondary to increased bladder pressure, decreased outlet resistance, or a combination of the two.

1. Failure to store because of the bladder—Increased bladder pressures can result from uninhibited detrusor contractions or from decreased compliance ("stretchability") of the bladder, resulting in the inability of the detrusor muscle to fill and store urine at low pressures. When detrusor instability or decreased compliance is suspected, it is important to determine whether there is an underlying neurologic abnormality.

2. Failure to store because of the bladder outlet—Impaired function of the female bladder outlet can result from the following: (1) prolapse or herniation of the bladder and urethra into the vaginal space, commonly referred to as a cystourethrocele; (2) incompetence of the involuntary smooth muscle at the bladder

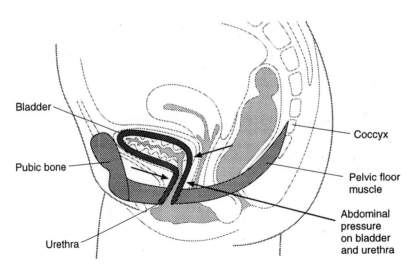

Figure 25–1. With normal support, the bladder neck and proximal urethra are maintained in an intra-abdominal position. During stressful maneuvers, the bladder and proximal urethra receive equal pressure transmission (arrows), and continence is maintained. (Reproduced, with permission, from Bavendam TG: J Enterostomal Therapy 1990;17:58.)

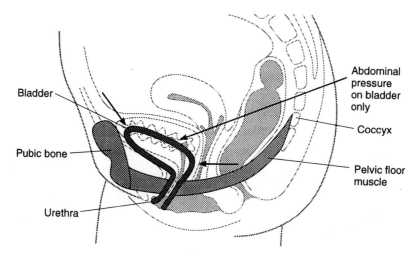

Figure 25–2. With weakened anatomic support, the bladder base sags (relaxes) into the vaginal space. Increased intra-abdominal pressure (arrows) is transmitted to the bladder but not to the proximal urethra. When the bladder pressure exceeds the outlet pressure, urinary leakage occurs. (Reproduced, with permission, from Bavendam TG: J Enterostomal Therapy 1990;17:59.)

neck; (3) weakness of the skeletal muscle of the external sphincteric mechanism; or (4) intrinsic urethral sphincter deficiency. The cystourethrocele can be corrected by surgery, but if there are other contributing factors to the incontinence, surgery alone may not result in perfect bladder control and normal voiding function.

Loss or decreased strength of voluntary contraction of the skeletal muscles of the pelvic floor or nerve injury resulting in the impairment of the reflex contraction of the pelvic floor and urethra at times of increased intra-abdominal pressure can result in urinary incontinence. The pelvic floor muscles are supplied by the pudendal nerve, which can be damaged by uncomplicated vaginal deliveries. This damage may not be apparent or relevant until the woman becomes older and begins to experience menopause or the generalized nerve and muscle deterioration that occurs with aging.

3. Failure to empty because of the bladder outlet—The most common cause of failure to empty the bladder in women is previous anti-incontinence surgery resulting in outlet obstruction. Impaired detrusor contraction can also result in inability to empty the bladder. Possible etiologies are detrusor injury secondary to a lifetime of infrequent voiding, diabetic sensory neuropathy, lower back injury, or surgical damage of the sensory or motor nerves to the bladder. The female urethra is short, and many women, despite impaired detrusor contractility, can void by pelvic floor relaxation and Valsalva or Crede maneuvers. The Valsalva maneuver involves voluntary "bearing-down," and the Crede maneuver requires manual compression of the abdomen or suprapubic region to induce an increase in intra-abdominal pressure that results in expulsion of urine.

4. Failure to empty because of the bladder—Although urinary incontinence is *not* a normal part of the aging process, there are multiple changes that occur with aging that make the development of incontinence more likely. Gradual decrease in bladder elasticity may result in smaller bladder capacity. Deterioration in the sensory nerves to the bladder may impair the sensation of bladder filling. Consequently, the first sensation a person experiences may be a strong urge to void that can be accompanied by loss of urine. The detrusor muscle becomes less able to generate a voluntary contraction and to sustain the contraction until the bladder is empty, resulting in incomplete bladder emptying. The nerves supplying the lower urinary tract undergo the same gradual deterioration as the rest of the body. Mobility decreases, making it more difficult to get to the bathroom quickly. Nighttime production of urine increases. Estrogen levels decrease, impairing the health of the lower urinary tract tissues and compromising continence.

Prevention

Prevention of some of the changes that occur with aging is clearly not feasible in all cases. However, there is literature to support the concept that women who undergo vaginal delivery are at higher risk for developing SUI compared with women who undergo cesarean sections. With regard to UUI, simple behavioral modifications, such as avoidance of caffeine or alcohol and limitation of fluid intake can be helpful in minimizing these symptoms. Postmenopausal women may benefit from the use of local hormone replacement therapy with vaginal estrogen cream, which theoretically increases adrenergic receptor density and sensitivity at the bladder neck and proximal urethra, increases blood flow to the urethral mucosa thereby facilitating the mucosal seal effect, and increases the sensory threshold of the bladder thereby decreasing urgency.

Clinical Findings

Proper and thorough evaluation of patients is imperative in order to provide effective treatment of urinary incontinence. Clearly, much of this can be done at the primary care level, and a brief description of an appropriate evaluation is described below. Patients with complicated urologic, neurologic, or medical histories that may affect voiding function, and patients with refractory urinary incontinence should be referred to a specialist (see When to Refer to a Specialist).

A. SYMPTOMS AND SIGNS

A careful voiding history can provide the clinician with very valuable information. Important issues on which to concentrate include the nature of the leakage, the timing of the leakage, the circumstances under which leakage occurs, urinary frequency during the daytime and nighttime, and patient-perceived emptying ability. It is also important to assess whether a patient experiences urinary tract infections or irritative voiding complaints (symptoms that may mimic the symptoms of infection).

SUI is characterized by symptoms of leakage of urine with coughing, sneezing, laughing, lifting, or other physically strenuous activities. Patients with UUI describe a sensation of a sudden uncontrollable urge to void that may result in urinary loss. Urgency may occur without any physical activity and can often result in large volumes of urinary leakage.

Up to 65% of patients are estimated to have mixed incontinence. Patients with overflow incontinence may also describe symptoms of SUI or UUI, and physicians must be cognizant that symptoms in overflow incontinence may mimic these conditions. In any case in which incomplete bladder emptying may be a possibility, postvoid residual volume should be assessed by bladder ultrasound or in and out catheterization.

Sporadic incontinence may be related to dietary factors. For reasons that are not clear, spicy or acidic foods and caffeinated, alcoholic, or carbonated beverages can be irritating to the bladder and thereby contribute to incontinence. Common offenders are coffee and tea (even decaffeinated types), alcoholic beverages, citrus fruits, tomatoes, and cranberries.

Pregnancy and delivery carry a risk of initiating persistent stress incontinence. A number of women experience incontinence for the first time during pregnancy. Most of these women regain continence during the first 3 months of the postpartum period; however, continence may continue to return for up to 12 months after delivery. There is evidence that suggests that vaginal delivery can contribute to the development of SUI via various mechanisms such as nerve compression and exaggeration of laxity of the supporting structures of the pelvic organs. As the baby's head travels through the birthing canal, compression of the nerves between the head and the mother's pelvis can cause neural damage that can result in sphincteric laxity and relaxation of the pelvic floor as well as detrusor dysfunction.

The importance of obstetric factors such as episiotomy, length of labor, and type of anesthetic in the causation of incontinence remains controversial.

Some women find incontinence exacerbated premenstrually and nonexistent during the early part of their menstrual cycle. Many women report changes in their bladder function as one of their first symptoms of the perimenopausal period. Local hormone replacement therapy and some of the theories behind the mechanism by which estrogen therapy may help continence is presented in the treatment section below.

Changes in vesicourethral function can occur after simple or radical hysterectomy. Historically, internal urethrotomy or repeated urethral dilations were performed for a variety of complaints in women and young girls. Although there may be no immediate effect on the continence mechanism, as the woman ages, the damage may become clinically significant. The urethra tends to scar as it heals. Scarring leads to a stiff, noncompliant urethra that can contribute to either SUI if it scars open or bladder outlet obstruction if it scars shut.

Diabetes, congestive heart failure, and venous insufficiency can increase urinary output, particularly at night when the patient is in a recumbent position. Nighttime incontinence is often associated with a large volume of urine produced by the kidneys at night. Urine production during sleep increases with aging secondary to decreasing ability to concentrate the urine. It is important to recognize that this problem is not one of lower urinary tract function. Any individual who produces 2 L of urine at night would need to get up during the night to void.

Neurologic diseases or injuries, back or brain surgeries, closed head injuries, and strokes all need to be recognized and optimally managed before definitive management of urinary incontinence. When there is a history of incontinence or voiding difficulties concomitant with neurologic symptoms such as visual disturbances, numbness, tingling, or lack of coordination, neurologic consultation should be sought. Even if intermittent, multiple sclerosis must be considered in the face of this constellation of symptoms.

Pelvic radiation therapy can cause a decrease in bladder compliance and damage to the urethra and the nerves that supply the lower urinary tract. These effects can manifest years after the treatment is administered.

Previous back, brain, rectal, or pelvic or retroperitoneal surgery can result in neurologic changes that may affect bladder control. Patients who have undergone previous anti-incontinence or pelvic prolapse repair surgeries can present with voiding complaints that vary from stress incontinence to urgency with or without incontinence, and incomplete bladder emptying. This group of patients is best served by a referral to a specialist.

Incontinence associated with a morning diuretic may be improved by changing to a lower dosage to be taken in both the morning and evening. α-Blockers (prazosin, terazosin, and phenoxybenzamine) can precipitate incontinence by relaxing the bladder neck and decreasing outlet resistance. Sedatives and hypnotics can decrease perception of the bladder signals and impair mobility, causing a delay in getting to the bathroom. Some antidepressant medications may contribute to incontinence because of impaired bladder emptying secondary to the anticholinergic side effects. Diuretics may exacerbate incontinence by increasing urine production.

Smoking can contribute to lung disease and chronic cough that may exacerbate SUI.

Pain, discomfort, or loss of urine associated with intercourse or climax may limit the frequency or pleasure associated with sexual activity. Hilton found that 24% of 324 sexually active women experienced urinary incontinence with intercourse. Loss of urine at climax is secondary either to a triggered detrusor contraction or to outlet relaxation. If the volume of urine lost is small or intermittent and the patient does not have urinary incontinence at any other time, the likelihood of finding a solution or "cure" is low. The physician can provide an explanation to the patient such as the following: "Intercourse and orgasm provide a complex stimulation to the nerves of the pelvic organs. At times, the messages traveling to and from the brain and organs get confused or cross over to different organs, resulting in urinary incontinence. It is impossible to block the parts of the signals that trigger the urinary incontinence." It is important to reassure the woman that the condition is fairly common and will not necessarily get worse or begin to affect her during other activities.

B. Physical Examination

The physical examination includes an abdominal examination, a pelvic examination in the lithotomy position, a rectal examination, and a screening neurologic examination.

Two separated posterior blades of a Grave's vaginal speculum are used to examine the vagina. One blade is placed posteriorly against the rectum with gentle downward pressure. The anterior vaginal wall and urethra are then examined in the resting and straining positions. Attention is paid to the urethral and bladder positions, the degree of estrogenization of the vaginal epithelium, and the presence of urinary leakage with straining. Normal vaginal tissues are moist and contain folds of vaginal epithelium. Atrophic tissues are dry, thin, and friable. The urethral meatus often looks erythematous and prominent in the hypoestrogenic state. If the urethral mucosa has a fungating or friable appearance, the patient should be referred to a urologist for evaluation.

With normal anatomic support, the bladder base is "tucked up" behind the pubic bone and not readily visible when the posterior blade is placed. A small degree of bladder descent with restoration of the normal position upon cessation of a Valsalva maneuver is considered normal. Movement or rotational descent half-way into the vaginal cavity is considered mild, and movement down to the level of the introitus is moderate. Prolapse of the bladder into the vagina at rest or through the introitus with stress is considered severe.

The blade is then placed to retract the anterior vaginal wall anteriorly, and the posterior wall of the vagina is examined at rest and during strain. Rectal examination can facilitate demonstration of the degree of laxity of the posterior wall (rectovaginal septum) and the integrity of the perineal body. The second blade retracts the posterior wall while the anterior wall is retracted, and the apex of the vagina is evaluated. Apical descensus can involve the uterus or the cuff of the vagina. An enterocele is considered in cases in which only the top of the vagina descends without any identifiable foreshortening of the posterior vaginal wall. With concomitant shortening of the posterior wall, vaginal vault prolapse is suspected.

Rectal examination is an important part of the anatomic and neurologic examination. Attention should be paid specifically to (1) anal sphincter tone (lax sphincter is highly suggestive of neurologic impairment or damage to the external anal sphincter from birth trauma or rectal/anal surgery); (2) the degree of rectocele and integrity of the perineum; (3) the ability to localize and contract the sphincteric mechanism; and (4) the bulbocavernosus reflex (BCR), which is an indication of intact pudendal afferent and efferent nerve supply. The BCR is elicited by squeezing firmly but gently over the clitoris and observing or feeling for contraction of the anal sphincter, upward movement of the urethral meatus, and/or contraction of the bulbocavernosus muscle around the vaginal introitus. The remainder of the neurologic examination includes sensory evaluation of the perineum, perianal region, and lower extremities, and evaluation of lower extremity reflexes. A patient with any obvious asymmetry or markedly diminished sensation should be referred for neurologic evaluation.

C. LABORATORY TESTS

Urinalysis is obtained in all patients with irritative voiding symptoms (frequency, urgency, urge incontinence, nocturia, dysuria) or sudden onset of urinary incontinence. Any urinalysis suggestive of infection (white cells, bacteria, nitrate or leukocyte esterase positivity) is sent for culture and sensitivity. Treatment of a positive urine culture with an appropriate antibiotic, prescribed according to the sensitivities, should span 3–5 days.

In the face of hematuria without evidence of infection, complete evaluation should be initiated. This work-up should include a cystourethroscopy to evaluate the lower urinary tract and upper tract evaluation with radiographic imaging (intravenous pyelogram or CT-IVP). Cytology of the first urine specimen obtained in the morning should also be considered, particularly in those patients with a history of smoking.

D. EVALUATION OF BLADDER FUNCTION

Assessment of bladder function can be as simple as observing for urinary leakage as a patient coughs or strains in a supine or erect position. Other simple evaluation tools include measurement of postvoid residual volume (by in and out catheterization or bladder ultrasound) and voiding diaries (to establish a patient's voiding and leakage patterns), both of which can be performed by the primary care team to obtain initial valuable information.

A thorough functional bladder evaluation may include the more complex formal multichannel urodynamics, which are performed by most urologists and select gynecologists. Urodynamics are helpful in identifying significant urethral and detrusor dysfunction. Addition of video imaging during the urodynamics study ("Video Urodynamics") provides a very sophisticated examination that correlates real-time bladder and urethral position and function, and is performed only by subspecialists in the field of voiding dysfunction.

"Eyeball urodynamics" can be performed in the primary care office to provide a simple means of evaluating bladder function. A Foley catheter is placed and a catheter-tip syringe is placed into the catheter and held straight up perpendicular to the patient's body. The bladder is filled with sterile fluid via gravity drainage, keeping track of the volume instilled. Normal bladder capacity is 300–600 mL. The patient is asked to inform the examiner of their first sensation of "something filling the bladder," their first urge to void, and strong urge to urinate. The column of fluid within the catheter barrel is observed for any rise that may indicate uninhibited contractions of the bladder or stiffness (decreased compliance) of the bladder. When the patient feels full, the catheter is removed and the patient is asked to strain in both the lithotomy and standing positions to examine for SUI. She is then asked to void, and postvoid residual urine is measured. Normal postvoid residual is generally considered to be less than 100 mL.

E. CYSTOSCOPIC EXAMINATION

Cystoscopy is performed by the urologist and is necessary to rule out any intravesical pathology in patients with hematuria or irritative voiding symptoms. If there is any question regarding whether or not a patient needs cystoscopy, consultation with a specialist should be obtained.

Fantl JA et al: Diuretics and urinary incontinence in community-dwelling women. Neurourol Urodynam 1990;9:25.

Hilton P: Urinary incontinence during sexual intercourse: a common, but rarely volunteered symptom. Br J Obstet Gynaecol 1988;95:377. [PMID: 3382610]

Khan Z, Bhola A, Starer P: Urinary incontinence during orgasm. Urology 1988;31:279. [PMID: 3347980]

Viktrup L et al: The symptoms of stress incontinence caused by pregnancy or delivery in primiparas. Obstet Gynecol 1992; 79:945. [PMID: 1579319]

Differential Diagnosis

The differential diagnosis for urinary incontinence depends on the clinical findings. The primary determination that must be made is whether the patient is experiencing SUI, UUI, mixed incontinence, or overflow incontinence. Patients may certainly experience a combination of any of the above and/or total urinary incontinence that may make it difficult to discern the etiology of the incontinence. Table 25–1 lists multiple factors that may contribute to the development of urinary incontinence.

Treatment

Treatment of urinary incontinence begins after an accurate assessment of all factors contributing to the incontinence and after all contributing medical problems, environmental factors, and behavioral changes have been addressed. Knowing the options and understanding the risk-benefit ratios are the keys to a successful surgical outcome.

In considering the treatment options, it may be helpful to categorize the ailment into issues of *failure of urine storage* or *problems with bladder emptying*. On occasion, simultaneous treatment for ineffective bladder storage and bladder emptying may need to be instituted (eg, concomitant anticholinergic medication and clean intermittent catheterization). Multiple interventions are often necessary, particularly in the older patient population, and frequent changes in the treatment plan are common because of the balance that must exist between bladder storage and emptying (Figure 25–3).

Vaginal estrogen replacement is important for the treatment of urinary incontinence of any cause and should be recommended for all postmenopausal women with significant urinary tract complaints (infection, irritative voiding symptoms, or incontinence) who do not have significant contraindications to hormone replacement therapy.

The exact mechanism of action of estrogen on the continence mechanism is speculative. Theoretically, estrogen enhances the effects of α-agonists, perhaps by increasing the density of α-receptors. Estrogen also promotes mucosal proliferation and increases submucosal blood flow, thereby enhancing the "mucosal seal" effect. Healthy urethral mucosa is moist and this moisture facilitates the sealing effect of the mucosa as it adheres to itself. In the presence of a hypoestrogenic effect, the mucosa may be dry and atrophic and consequently, the mucosal seal does not occur effectively. Estrogen is indicated in patients noted to have atrophic changes in the vagina. Intravaginal use at a dose of ⅛ applicator 3 times a week amplifies the local effect of the estrogen greater than the effect of oral estrogen on the urethral and vaginal epithelium. Estrogen is usually used in combination with other medications, pelvic floor exercises, and behavioral modification to get maximal benefit.

Oral estrogen supplementation has been implicated in increasing the risk of endometrial cancer when unopposed by progestins, and an association between estrogens and breast cancer has been shown with long-term use (longer than 5 to 10 years). However, this effect has not been definitively demonstrated with the use of vaginal hormone creams. Numerous studies have examined the effect of vaginally administered estrogens on the endometrium and have shown minimal or no proliferation with varying doses. Vaginal administration of estrogens avoids the first-pass effect through the liver seen with oral dosage, and therefore, the risks of alteration in clotting factors and plasma renin substrate are less likely to occur. Some recent studies have indicated that consideration of local hormone replacement therapy even in those patients who have had a remote history of breast cancer is reasonable. Consider consulting with the oncologist before starting any hormone replacement in patients with a history of breast cancer.

A. STRESS URINARY INCONTINENCE

1. Nonsurgical options—When counseling patients about treatment alternatives for SUI, all options must be considered. Many patients wish to try noninvasive therapy before surgery. Regardless of treatment choice, the goal is to improve continence and maximize the patient's quality of life.

a. Medications—α-Agonists stimulate the α-receptors of the bladder neck and proximal urethra, resulting in smooth muscle stimulation and increased bladder outlet resistance. Table 25–2 lists the available α-agonists. α-Stimulators are useful in the treatment of mild to moderate SUI but are usually not sufficient to treat severe SUI. For maximal results, α-agonists should be used in conjunction with pelvic floor exercises and estrogens.

α-Stimulants should be used with caution in elderly patients, particularly those patients with cardiac disease, hypertension, or hyperthyroidism, as α-agonists can

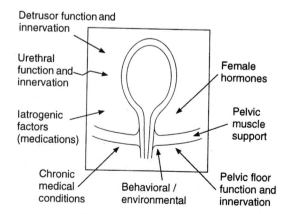

Figure 25–3. Pictorial representation of the multiple factors contributing to the urinary continence mechanism.

Table 25–2. Agonists for stress urinary incontinence.

Medication	Dosage
Ephedrine sulfate	25–50 mg orally qid
Pseudoephedrine (Sudafed, Actifed)	30–60 mg orally tid
Chlorpheniramine maleate (Ornade)	1 tablet orally bid
Guaifenesin (Entex LA)	50 mg orally qd or bid

cause drowsiness, anxiety, weakness, insomnia, headache, tremor, palpitations, cardiac arrhythmias, and respiratory difficulty. Tachyphylaxis may be seen. Ephedrine and pseudoephedrine, the active agents in many decongestants and antihistamines, are stereoisomers of each other and stimulate both α- and β-receptors in addition to inducing the release of norepinephrine.

Tricyclic antidepressants (TCAs) increase bladder outlet resistance via inhibition of peripheral reuptake of norepinephrine. This, in turn, increases stimulation of the α-receptors in the smooth muscle of the bladder neck and proximal urethra. The TCAs also have anticholinergic and musculotrophic effects in addition to a strong direct inhibitory effect on the detrusor that is neither anticholinergic nor antiadrenergic. These effects make TCAs ideal for treatment of mild SUI, UUI, and mixed incontinence. The primary agent in this category is imipramine, which is administered at a dosage of 10–25 mg 2 or 3 times daily. Dosage may be increased up to a total 150 mg/d; higher doses are often used in the treatment of depression.

Adverse effects of TCAs can be divided into α-adrenergic and anticholinergic effects. The medication is generally well-tolerated, but it is contraindicated in patients with cardiac arrhythmia or heart block. Adrenergic side effects include tachycardia, restlessness, blood pressure elevation, and exacerbation of heart block. Anticholinergic effects include orthostatic hypotension, dry mouth, ataxia, tachycardia, restlessness, hallucinations, and mental status changes. The latter effects are typically seen only at the higher doses used to treat depression.

b. Behavioral therapy—All patients deemed to be mentally and physically fit for active participation are candidates for behavioral modification. However, the candidates who appear to benefit the most are those who suffer from only mild SUI. Patients must also be dedicated to compliance with the program in order to benefit maximally. Patients are encouraged to limit fluid intake to 40–50 ounces per day (unless there is a medical contraindication to fluid restriction) and to avoid consumption of caffeinated or alcoholic beverages.

Weighted vaginal cones have been used in Europe and are currently available in the United States. Women learn to isolate and properly contract their pelvic muscles by holding these tampon-like weights in the vagina. The use of Kegel exercises and vaginal weights have had variable success in the literature. In a study of women with SUI who were treated with weighted vaginal cones, 19 of 27 (70%) of patients had complete cure or a greater than 50% improvement.

Conversely, only 7 of 50 (14%) of patients with severe SUI had similar success. Wilson and Borland studied 34 women with genuine SUI treated with vaginal weight training for 6 weeks. Subjective improvement was reported in 23 (47%). At a mean follow-up of 15.8 months (range 12–24), 14 (41%) still reported continued improvement.

Cammu et al showed that the cure/improved rates in 2 groups of 30 women who underwent either pelvic floor exercises with weighted vaginal cones or pelvic floor exercises alone were similar. However, patients in the cone group either dropped out of the study or discontinued cone therapy upon completion of the 12-week study. Use of the vaginal cones can decrease the number of visits to the physical therapist without affecting therapeutic outcome. Pelvic muscle exercises can be effective in increasing the resting tone of the striated muscles of the urethral and pelvic floor.

The main limiting factors for pelvic muscle exercises are the woman's ability to localize and contract the pelvic floor muscles and her motivation to learn the exercise regimen. Women who are successful with pelvic muscle exercises find the treatment regimen to be compatible with their lifestyle on a long-term basis.

Methods to improve pelvic muscle localization, which leads to more effective exercises, include verbal feedback from the examiner, biofeedback, and use of weighted vaginal cones. Verbal feedback is accomplished by inserting 1 or 2 fingers in the vagina or 1 finger in the anus while instructing the woman to squeeze on the finger or fingers, lift or pull in on the vaginal muscles, use the muscles she would use to stop the flow of urine, or hold back on rectal gas. Many women find it easier at first to localize the anal muscle than the vaginal muscles. At the time of muscle contraction, the physician observes for contraction of the abdominal, thigh, and buttock muscles. When inappropriate muscles are contracted, the woman is given verbal feedback and asked to repeat the contraction while relaxing the muscle she does not need to use. The only muscles that should be contracted are the pubococcygeus muscles around the examining fingers. Follow-up visits are important to ensure continued exercise of the proper muscles and provide reinforcement and motivation.

c. Biofeedback—Biofeedback (BFB) is an excellent treatment option for those patients who would benefit from a nonsurgical approach to their incontinence based on either individual preference or clinical situation. It is helpful for women who are unable to localize the proper muscle groups for pelvic floor strengthening on their own. It is also a method in which the patient takes an active role in the management of her health care issues. BFB employs monitoring equipment to facilitate the development of conscious control of various body functions of which the patient is unaware. A vaginal probe is inserted to measure the activity of the levator ani musculature, and surface electrodes detect contractions of the abdominal or gluteal muscles that might otherwise be mistaken by the patient as contraction of the pelvic floor musculature. Patients are taught to tighten the sphincter muscle without increasing abdominal pressure, and the BFB equipment relays auditory or visual feedback to patients regarding measurements of the physiologic activity.

Moderate success was noted in a study in which 5 of 14 (36%) patients had significant decrease in SUI symptoms following 6 BFB sessions over a 3-week period. The response was durable over the period of follow-up, although the length of follow-up was not specified. It is important for the clinician to understand and relay to the patients that long-term success with pelvic floor exercises is only possible if the patient continues with the exercises following completion of their course of BFB. Biofeedback can be accomplished using surface electromyography or a pneumatic compression device. Biofeedback training can be delivered by physicians, biofeedback therapists, nurses, social workers, psychologists, or physical therapists who have received training in pelvic muscle neuromuscular education. Treatment success can be achieved by reviewing the patient's progress, providing positive reinforcement and encouragement, and possibly changing therapeutic approaches.

There have been many attempts to use electrical stimulation to strengthen the pelvic muscles passively. This form of therapy has been used for several years in Europe and is gradually gaining support in the United States. Specialists who offer a broad spectrum of treatment options may recommend transvaginal electrical stimulation for some women; it can be effective for both SUI and UUI.

2. Surgical options—

a. Urethral bulking injection therapy—Over the past couple of decades, a variety of periurethrally and transurethrally injected bulking agents have been developed and studied for treatment of SUI. The goal is to increase periurethral compressive forces by injecting a material beneath the mucosa that facilitates mucosal coaptation at the bladder neck and proximal urethra (Figure 25–4 and Figure 25–5). The only agents currently available for use in the United States are glutaraldehyde cross-linked collagen (Contigen) and pyrolytic carbon-coated zirconium beads (Durasphere). Autologous fat, which does not require approval by the US Food and Drug Administration (FDA), has also been explored as a urethral bulking agent.

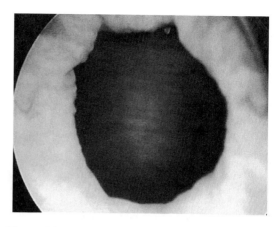

Figure 25–4. Cystoscopic view of urethra prior to urethral bulking injection.

Patients with symptoms of pure SUI are candidates for consideration of urethral bulking injection. Injection therapy can be offered to those patients who are not surgical candidates, those who wish to undergo conservative management, those who prefer to avoid the 6-week activity limitation required following surgical anti-incontinence procedures, those who are of child-bearing age, and those who have not had complete resolution of their SUI following surgical repair. Contraindications to injection therapy include active urinary tract infection, uncontrolled urinary urgency or detrusor instability, or hypersensitivity to the bulking agent. Patients planning to undergo collagen injection receive an intradermal skin test approximately 4 weeks before the injection to ensure absence of hypersensitivity to the agent.

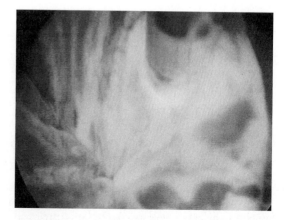

Figure 25–5. Coapted urethral mucosa following transurethral injection of Durasphere.

Urethral bulking agents can be injected in the office or "surgicenter" setting with or without light intravenous sedation. Technically, injection can be performed transurethrally or periurethrally under local anesthesia with minimal patient discomfort.

Glutaraldehyde cross-linked collagen is a purified bovine dermal collagen that is cross-linked to glutaraldehyde to decrease antigenicity and increase the stability of the material. It is suspended in a solution of lidocaine and saline, and other than the cross-linking, is identical to the collagen used for cosmetic applications.

In 1989, Shortliffe et al described urethral bulking by injection of glutaraldehyde cross-linked bovine collagen for the treatment of SUI. The series was small, including 16 men and 1 woman. Herschorn subsequently reported the first long-term follow-up of 187 patients who underwent collagen injection. Herschorn's series illustrated diminishing success with longer follow-up; at 6 months 90.3% were cured or improved, but at a mean follow-up of 22 months (range 4 to 69), only 75% were cured or improved (23% and 52%, respectively) and 25% failed. It is well established that multiple injections are warranted in most patients who undergo collagen injection.

An advantage of pyrolytic carbon-coated zirconium beads over collagen is that no skin-testing is necessary, and, in theory, the synthetic nature of the material would make it more likely to be durable over biodegradable agents.

In the original clinical trial examining pyrolytic carbon-coated zirconium beads, 115 of 178 (65%) patients were available for follow-up at 12 months. Patients underwent a mean of 1.7 injections, with 43% undergoing a single treatment, 40% undergoing 2 treatments, and 13% undergoing 3 treatments. Mean total volume injected per patient was 7.6 mL. Thirty-six of 115 (31%) reported being completely dry, and 66% were improved.

Urethral bulking with injectables theoretically offers patients treatment for SUI with minimal discomfort and essentially no recovery time. Unfortunately, the materials that have been studied to date offer variable success rates that leave significant room for improvement. The ideal injectable agent would be a cost-effective, nonimmunogenic permanent material with no potential for migration and properties that allow technically easy injection. The search for this material continues, but urethral bulking continues to be a viable, conservative option for the treatment of SUI.

b. Needle suspensions—Because of poor long-term results, needle suspensions such as the Raz, Stamey, and Pereyra have fallen by the wayside.

c. Retropubic suspensions—Retropubic bladder neck suspensions, such as the Burch procedure, have stood the test of time. In a meta-analysis of the literature regarding anti-incontinence procedures, the retropubic suspensions demonstrated an overall success rate of 83% at 48 months follow-up. Retropubic suspensions involve restoring the normal anatomic position of the bladder neck by securing the periurethral tissue to the pubic bone. This is only successful in patients with urethral hypermobility and is not useful for those with an intrinsic weakness of the urethral sphincter.

d. Pubovaginal slings—The pubovaginal sling procedure is considered the gold standard for the treatment of SUI in women. Originally described for the treatment of intrinsic sphincter deficiency, pubovaginal slings have been used to treat other types of SUI. There have been many modifications of the technique over the years but the principles behind the pubovaginal sling still hold today. The sling is placed beneath the proximal urethra and bladder neck to provide support and compression and to prevent proximal urethral descent during increased intra-abdominal pressure. Numerous materials—such as autologous tissues, cadaveric (allograft) tissues, and synthetics—have been used over the years to construct the sling, and newer materials continue to be introduced in an attempt to decrease morbidity and improve durability of the procedure and patient satisfaction. The choice of sling material is ultimately made by patient and surgeon preference. Each material has its own advantages, disadvantages and inherent complications.

Autologous fascia has been the gold standard material for the pubovaginal sling. Use of autologous fascia, whether it is rectus fascia or fascia lata, has been associated with success rates of 82–84% at 48 months. Complications related to the sling material are extremely rare with most complications consisting of de novo detrusor instability or urinary retention.

Advantages of using fascia include that it is a strong, natural tissue that does not pose a risk of rejection or infectious transmission. Also, degeneration of autologous fascia over time appears to be limited. Disadvantages of fascia are dependent on the type of fascia used and include limitation in the maximum length of fascia attainable, patient morbidity secondary to pain at the incision site, potential for abdominal wall hernia or leg muscle herniation, and a theoretical concern of compromised tissue quality if there has been prior lower abdominal surgery or radiation therapy to the area.

Allografts are tissues harvested from human donors. The risk of HIV transmission from soft tissue allografts is 1 in 1.7 million to 1 in 8 million, which is lower than the risk of HIV infection from a blood transfusion. In fact, there have been no reports of HIV transmission due to transplantation of fascia. Since 1985, all donors have been screened for HIV and other viruses, and more than 60,000 organ transplants and 1 million tissue transplants have been performed without an increase in disease transmission.

Another potential risk of cadaveric fascia transplantation is the transmission of prions. Prions are proteinacious particles that are the causative agents of spongiform encephalopathy, of which the most common is Creutzfeldt-Jakob disease. Prions are very resistant to treatments that target nucleic acids such as radiation. However, prions may be destroyed by denaturing agents. A treatment process has been designed that addresses the risk of prion disease without affecting the tensile strength of the graft. The patented processing technique involves solvent-dehydration followed by freeze-drying. Despite the theoretic risk and heightened worldwide awareness of prion-transmitted diseases, there are no cases of a transmissible spongiform encephalopathy associated with cadaveric fascia lata.

The FDA regulates licensed tissue banks that process cadaveric fascia. The tissue banks are required to perform an extensive process of donor selection, donor testing, and a multi-step tissue processing in order to remove tissue antigenicity and the risk of disease transmission. Prior to harvesting, donors are screened for a history of carrying hepatitis and other viruses. Serologic tests for HIV, hepatitis B virus, hepatitis C virus, human T-cell lymphotropic virus type I (HTLV-I), and syphilis are then performed. The tissue is processed by one of several techniques: freeze-drying alone, freeze-drying with gamma-irradiation, or solvent dehydration.

Allograft fascia lata is an attractive alternative to autologous fascia lata because the morbidity associated with graft harvesting is avoided. Early reports have demonstrated that operative time, hospital stay, and postoperative time may be decreased with the use of allograft fascia. With respect to the effectiveness, early results with cadaveric fascia lata have been promising. Cure rates of 85–87% have been reported, but the follow-up is still short (less than 48 months). However, although cadaveric fascia lata is approved by the FDA, there are no regulations as to the quality or thickness of the fascia that is harvested, a fact that may be reflected in the variable results from one center to another. There have been reports of failure rates as high as 40%, but the tissue processing technique used in these 2 opposing groups was different (the former, solvent-dehydrated and the latter, freeze-dried). The differences in success posed by varying processing techniques is being studied in more detail as is the use of cadaveric dermis, which also appears to show great promise.

In recent years there has been interest in using synthetic materials as an alternative to autologous fascia in the pubovaginal sling procedure in order to decrease operative time, postoperative pain, and need for hospi-

talization as well as to improve the durability of the results. In theory, the ideal sling material should last the lifetime of a patient and should not be at risk for degradation. It is debated that the biomechanical properties of synthetic material may be superior to those of autologous tissue.

SUI cure rates using synthetic slings in general have been reported to be 77–90% at a mean follow-up of 4–8 years. The concept of a permanent mesh is appealing as a sling material because it does not have the added morbidity of harvesting the graft; the material is permanent and therefore the results of the procedure should be durable; and there is also no risk of transmittable diseases. Despite apparent long-term durability, synthetic slings are more prone to infection and erosion. However, complication rates with synthetics appear to vary with the type of material used, and various newer more loosely woven materials have shown excellent early and intermediate results.

One of the new and promising synthetics used today is the tension-free vaginal tape (TVT) procedure. The procedure involves the implantation of a polypropylene (prolene) mesh tape beneath the mid-urethra without tension. Early results have revealed a cure rate of 80–87% with another 9.6–11% of patients significantly improved and approximately 3.3% who did not respond.

e. Artificial urinary sphincter—In the United States, the artificial urinary sphincter (AUS) is used predominantly in men, although it is used extensively in women in Europe. The AUS consists of an inflatable fluid-filled cuff that is placed around the urethra. The cuff is attached to a pump that is placed in the labia and a reservoir that is placed adjacent to the bladder. When the patient wishes to void, the fluid in the cuff is "pumped" out of the cuff into the reservoir, allowing the urine to flow from the bladder. The cuff automatically refills over the ensuing few minutes. The disadvantages of using the AUS in women is that the shorter urethra in women allows only a short length on which to place the device. If there are problems with atrophy or erosion of the urethral tissue beneath the cuff, alternatives are limited. Other risks include infection, malfunction, and erosion of the cuff through the bladder neck tissue.

f. Concomitant pelvic prolapse repair—The main indication for repair of pelvic prolapse is patient discomfort from the prolapsing organ. Cystoceles can be associated with voiding difficulties, incomplete bladder emptying, urinary incontinence, or recurrent urinary tract infections, or conversely, there may be no symptoms. Very large cystoceles can be associated with hydronephrosis from elongating and "kinking" of the distal ureters, and renal ultrasonography or intravenous pyelography is indicated before the decision is made to monitor a large cystocele conservatively. Pessaries are a good option for many women who are not interested in surgery. Women can be instructed to insert and remove the pessaries themselves.

B. URGE URINARY INCONTINENCE

The true incidence of bladder overactivity in the general population has been estimated to be 10%. In the absence of other pathology such as urinary tract infection, bladder tumors, or bladder stones, symptoms of urgency and urge incontinence may be caused by bladder overactivity. The term "detrusor instability" is used to describe the urodynamic findings of detrusor overactivity in patients with no neuropathology. Any rise in bladder pressure as the patient attempts to inhibit micturition falls into this definition. In those patients with neurologic disease, the same urodynamic findings are termed "detrusor hyperreflexia." In other words, the terminology describes the same condition but indicates whether or not the patient has a neurologic cause for the unstable bladder.

Treatment of detrusor instability or hyperreflexia is optimally nonsurgical, with surgical therapy used only as a last resort.

1. Nonsurgical options—

a. Medications—Agents that inhibit bladder contractility can thereby increase bladder capacity and may also decrease intravesical pressures. Also, sustained elevation of intravesical pressures above 40 cm H_2O, seen especially in those patients with myelodysplasia, put the patient at risk for upper tract damage. Patients who fall into this group should be evaluated with renal ultrasound to rule out the presence of hydronephrosis.

Anticholinergic medications competitively inhibit acetylcholine at the postganglionic autonomic (muscarinic) receptors. Musculotropics act directly on smooth muscle contractility by a papavarine-like action and also have varying anesthetic properties. Medications and their respective dosages are listed in Table 25–3. Probantheline is more selective than atropine for the lower urinary tract.

Adverse effects of this group of medications vary with the systemic absorption and tend to be the most pronounced with oxybutynin (Ditropan). Effects include dry mouth, constipation, blurred vision, tachycardia, drowsiness, precipitation of urinary retention, and confusion. Narrow-angle glaucoma is an absolute contraindication to the use of this group of medications. The adverse effects often result in poor compliance on the part of the patients. The hepatic metabolites of oxybutynin are responsible for the severity of its side effects. Patients who are unable to tolerate the adverse effects of oral oxybutynin, have not responded to other oral therapies, and who are willing to undergo catheterization are candidates for intravesical oxybutynin. Intravesical instillation of oxybutynin bypasses the liver, and therefore the tolerance of this route of administration is better.

Table 25–3. Medications used to treat "overactive bladder."

Medication	Tradename	Dosage
Anticholinergics		
Probantheline bromide	(Probanthine)	15–30 mg orally qid
Hyoscyamine sulfate	(Levsin, Levsinex, Cystospaz, Anaspaz)	1 mg orally bid (available in capsule, slow-release, elixir)
Musculotropics		
Oxybutynin	(Ditropan)	2.5–5.0 mg orally qd to tid May try intravesical instillation
Oxybutynin—extended-release	(Ditropan XL)	5–30 orally qd
Tolterodine	(Detrol)	2 mg orally bid
Tolterodine—long-acting	(Detrol LA)	4 mg orally qd
Dicyclomine hydrochloride	(Bentyl)	2–30 mg orally tid
Flavoxate hydrochloride	(Urispas)	100–300 mg orally tid
Belladona/opium	(B & O suppository®)	1/3–1 rectally tid

Tolterodine (Detrol) is a competitive muscarinic antagonist that was released for use in the United States in mid-1998. Immediate release tolterodine is administered at 2 mg twice daily, and the extended-release tolterodine at 4 mg once a day. Because of its higher specificity for bladder muscarinic receptors (compared with the salivary gland muscarinic receptors), its systemic and central side effects are significantly reduced and it is far better tolerated than is oxybutynin. Oxybutynin also has an extended-release preparation. For obvious reasons, the compliance with once a day doses is superior to that of multiple dose medications. Brown found that while the efficacy of immediate-release oxybutynin was equivalent to that of extended-release oxybutynin, the incidence of dry mouth was significantly lower for the latter. The incidence of other anticholinergic adverse effects was similar in both groups. A head-to-head study of extended-release preparations of tolterodine and oxybutynin is currently in progress.

TCAs have both anticholinergic and local anesthetic effects, which make them a good choice for treatment of detrusor instability. In addition, the increase in norepinephrine increases α-stimulation at the bladder neck to increase bladder outlet resistance and may theoretically have some effect on the smooth muscle receptors in the bladder body, resulting in smooth muscle relaxation.

Administration of an agent such as 1-desaminocystine-8-D-arginine vasopressin (desmopressin acetate; DDAVP), a synthetic analogue of the antidiuretic hormone, vasopressin, decreases urine production. In this manner, the problem of the bladder instability may be eluded all together, albeit not treated. This drug is primarily used in patients with nocturnal enuresis and diabetes insipidis and is not routinely administered in the therapy of detrusor instability. Adverse effects of DDAVP are rare and usually occur within the first few weeks of therapy. The main risk includes water intoxication and hyponatremia, and therefore, the drug must be used with caution in the elderly, particularly in patients with a history of congestive heart failure.

It is important to obtain a postvoid residual measurement 1 to 2 weeks after these medications are started, especially in patients who had increased residual volumes before the pharmacotherapy was initiated. When residual volumes start to increase, the options are to decrease the dosage or start the patient on clean intermittent catheterization in addition to the medication. A mildly elevated residual volume in the face of improved urinary control, absence of significant frequency of urination, and absence of infections does not need to be treated but should be monitored intermittently to make sure the amount of residual urine does

not continually increase, putting the patient at risk for overflow incontinence and infection.

In summary, failure of one medication is not an indication that all drug therapy will be unsuccessful. Patients may respond to different agents differently. In refractory cases, a combination of agents can be successful. Keep in mind that medical therapy is most successful when combined with behavioral changes, such as dietary adjustments and fluid limitation.

The keys to successful pharmacologic therapy are summarized as follows:

1. Start with a low dosage and increase or decrease the dosage as needed.
2. Tailor the timing and dosage of the medication to the patient's needs.
3. Closely monitor side effects such as constipation and incomplete bladder emptying.
4. Monitor patients for new illnesses or medications that may affect urinary control.
5. Try different drugs or combinations as needed.
6. Refer appropriate patients for specialty evaluation early.
7. Provide written instructions for the patient.

b. Pelvic floor exercises—Exercise programs increase a woman's awareness of her pelvic muscles and how to use voluntary pelvic muscle contractions to her benefit with stressful activities or episodes of urgency. A strong, well-localized pelvic muscle contraction at the time of a strong urge and impending leakage can abort the developing uninhibited bladder contraction reflexively and allow the woman time to walk to the bathroom without leakage. It is impossible to inhibit a bladder contraction and run to the bathroom at the same time.

c. Behavioral modification/bladder training/biofeedback—Unless there is a medical contraindication, fluid limitation in the range of 30–50 ounces per day with avoidance of caffeinated or alcoholic beverages is imperative. Often, patients will increase fluid intake in response to the dry mouth they experience when on anticholinergic medications. Helpful tips for these patients include candy, gum, artificial saliva, or small sips of fluid. In addition, the constipation that is also experienced by many patients taking anticholinergics can be treated with a bulking agent such as psyllium or calcium polycarbophil (eg, Mitrolan, Fibercon).

Bladder training is based on the concept that instability is a result of frequent voiding. Patients are trained to postpone urination and void according to the clock rather than according to the urge to void. Using biofeedback, they are taught to inhibit or resist the sensation of urgency. Initially, the goal is set for urination every 1–2 hours, then gradually increased to 3–4 hours. For patients with instability only at high volumes, timed voiding every 2–3 hours may be helpful in avoiding the uninhibited contractions that result in symptoms of urgency.

Results vary according to the reporting source. Burgio et al studied 197 women with UUI or mixed incontinence with urge as the predominant component; they were randomized to biofeedback, oxybutynin, or placebo. The biofeedback group had the greatest objective and perceived improvement (80.7% and 74.1%, respectively) compared with the medication group (68.5% and 50.9%) and the placebo group (39.4% and 26.9%). Clearly, patients must be compliant and willing to continue the behavioral changes they learn in the program indefinitely.

2. Surgical options—Surgery is the last resort for treatment of urge incontinence. It may be offered to patients who have poor results with medications or are unable to continue medications because of the adverse effects.

a. Augmentation cystoplasty—A patch of ileum or colon may be used to augment the bladder to decrease intravesical pressure and instability and increase bladder capacity. The literature suggests that patients must be counseled on the 30–40% chance of requiring postoperative intermittent catheterization. Success rates for augmentation cystoplasty have been reported to be 69–97%. Risks include a questionable increased risk of developing carcinoma in the bowel patch; gastrointestinal complications including diarrhea, constipation, or bowel obstruction; electrolyte disturbances that vary depending on the bowel segment used; mucus production by the bowel patch; and the possibility of a minimally increased risk of infection. Patients are instructed on periodic irrigation of the mucus from the bladder to minimize the risk of infection or outlet obstruction secondary to a mucous plug. Periodic cystoscopy should be performed to ensure that there are no stones or large mucous plugs within the augmented bladder.

b. Urinary diversion—Urinary diversion or augmentation cystoplasty with creation of an abdominal stoma is a logical consideration for patients who may have difficulty accessing the urethra for catheterization.

c. Sacroneuromodulation—Sacral nerve stimulation has grown in popularity over the past few years as a treatment option for patients with pharmacologically refractory urge incontinence and severe urinary frequency. Sacroneuromodulation involves placement of leads that stimulate the sacral nerves responsible for bladder motor and sensory function. Patients who appear to be candidates undergo a percutaneous test stimulation in the office, during which the leads are placed adjacent to the appropriate nerves under local anesthe-

sia. They are asked to keep a pre-procedural and post-procedural voiding diary, and those who experience significant subjective and objective improvement are candidates for surgical placement of a permanent device (Interstim).

The permanent device is placed subcutaneously through a 4″-5″ incision overlying the sacrum, and the patients are able to control the device via an external mechanism. The surgery requires a 1-night stay in the hospital and minimal recovery. As the research has progressed, the Interstim has interestingly been found to be successful not only in the treatment of patients with urinary frequency and urgency, but also in those with refractory pelvic pain or idiopathic urinary retention.

C. Mixed Urinary Incontinence

Up to 56% of patients with urinary incontinence have components of both SUI and UUI. Nonsurgical therapy aimed at treatment of the urgency component is a very reasonable starting point. However, if this does not provide satisfactory relief of symptoms, and in light of the complex picture with which these patients present, referral of patients with mixed incontinence to a specialist is a proper action.

1. Nonsurgical options—

a. Medications—Medications that increase the bladder outlet resistance and decrease detrusor contractility are ideal. As discussed in previous sections, imipramine has properties that result in both an increase in outlet resistance and in detrusor relaxation. It is therefore an optimal choice for treatment of mixed incontinence with mild to moderate symptoms of stress and/or urgency. Medications may also be tried in conjunction with other nonsurgical treatment options. In fact, nonsurgical therapy alone is typically not successful if the type of SUI involved is intrinsic sphincter deficiency.

b. Behavioral therapy/biofeedback—As discussed above, this involves fluid restriction, avoidance of caffeinated and alcoholic beverages, bladder training, conscious postponement of urination, and pelvic floor exercises. This program can be combined with pharmacologic therapy, often with excellent results.

c. Electrical stimulation—Electrical stimulation is discussed above in the section covering urge incontinence.

2. Surgical options—If a patient's primary complaints consist of stress symptoms and there is urodynamically documented SUI, a sling may be considered. Detrusor instability is alleviated to some degree following anti-incontinence surgery in up to 80% of patients with mixed incontinence.

In extreme cases in which nonsurgical therapy is not adequate to control the patient's symptoms, augmentation cystoplasty with or without urethral bulking injection or sling may be considered. As mentioned above, patients need to be counseled on the necessity for postoperative catheterization.

D. OVERFLOW INCONTINENCE

Treatment of overflow incontinence is important, especially if the patient experiences recurrent urinary tract infections or deterioration of renal function is apparent. The goal of treatment is complete emptying of the bladder. First, the patient's medication profile should be reviewed in consideration of the possibility of urinary retention secondary to anticholinergic or adrenergic effects of medications. Any medications that could be contributing factors should be discontinued, if possible. In the case of persistent retention or when discontinuation of contributing medications is not feasible, the patient should ideally be placed on intermittent catheterization.

1. Nonsurgical options—

a. Medications—In theory, medications that decrease bladder outlet resistance or increase detrusor contractility should promote bladder emptying. However, there is no evidence to support that the available medications accomplish this satisfactorily. Medications that have been tried include bethanechol (Urecholine), although this agent has not been shown to be efficacious.

b. Clean intermittent catheterization—Clean intermittent catheterization is the treatment of choice for overflow incontinence. However, this option requires compliant patients (or caretakers) with the mental capacity and manual dexterity to perform catheterization. In nursing homes, sterile technique may be preferred, albeit not necessarily practical, for the sake of infection control.

c. Indwelling foley catheter or suprapubic tube—Indwelling catheters are a last resort due to the risks of long-term catheters. Complications include urethral damage, infections, stones, and tumor. If a long-term indwelling catheter is necessary despite these risks, a suprapubic cystostomy is preferred to avoid urethral damage. Catheters should be changed monthly.

2. Surgical options—Surgical therapy for treatment of female overflow incontinence is rarely a viable option. However, in the case of bladder outlet obstruction secondary to periurethral scarring or to suture "kinking" the urethra, such as that seen following anti-incontinence surgery, urethrolysis may be performed to free the urethra up and relieve the obstruction. Bladder out-

let obstruction is confirmed by urodynamic studies, ideally with video imaging of the bladder, bladder neck, and urethra, and by pressure-flow studies. The sine qua non of obstruction on a pressure-flow curve is high detrusor pressure, low urinary flow rate, and incomplete bladder emptying. Again, in patients who are unable to catheterize through the urethra, creation of a catheterizable abdominal stoma may be a consideration.

Sacroneuromodulation (discussed above) has recently become a surgical option for patients with idiopathic urinary retention.

E. COMPLEMENTARY THERAPY

Acupuncture is not widely used in the United States, and therefore, the majority of the literature comes from abroad. Kitakoji performed an average of 7 (range 4–12) acupuncture treatments on 11 patients for treatment of an overactive bladder with undetermined follow-up. A needle was inserted bilaterally at a point designated as Zhongliao point BL-33. Nine patients had pre-procedural urge incontinence and 2 had urgency. Urgency resolved in both patients. Five of 9 patients with UUI became dry, and 2 had subjective improvement.

When to Refer to a Specialist

Many cases of urinary incontinence can be diagnosed based on the history, physical examination, and urinalysis alone. Straight-forward incontinence issues, particularly those primarily involving urinary urgency and frequency, can and should initially be managed by a patient's primary care team. Factors that warrant referral to a specialist (female urologist or urogynecologist) are listed below:

1. Hematuria
2. Incomplete bladder emptying
3. History of anti-incontinence or pelvic prolapse surgery that failed to provide relief of symptoms
4. History of radical pelvic surgery
5. History of pelvic irradiation
6. Underlying metabolic or neurologic disease
7. Lack of response to conservative measures for 2–3 months
8. Recurrent symptomatic urinary tract infections
9. Symptomatic pelvic prolapse
10. Surgery planned

Amundsen CL et al: Outcome in 104 pubovaginal slings using freeze dried allograft fascia lata from a single tissue bank. Urology 2000;56:2. [PMID: 11114556]

Appell RA: Surgery for the treatment of overactive bladder. Urology 1998;51(Suppl 2A):27. [PMID: 9495732]

Bo K et al: Pelvic floor muscle exercise for the treatment of female stress urinary incontinence. III. Effects of two different degrees of pelvic floor muscle exercises. Neurourol Urodynam 1990;9:489.

Brown J: Comparison of tolerability and efficacy of once-a-day vs immediate-release oxybutynin chloride in patients with urge urinary incontinence. Oxybutynin XL Study Group, University of California, San Francisco, 1998.

Brown SL, Govier FE: Cadaveric versus autologous fascia lata for the pubovaginal sling: surgical outcomes and patient satisfaction. J Urol 2000;164:1633. [PMID: 11025722]

Buck BE, Malinin TI: Human bone and tissue allografts. Preparation and safety. Clin Orthop 1994;8:303. [PMID: 8194258]

Burgio KL, Robinson JC, Engel BT: The role of biofeedback in Kegel exercise training for stress urinary incontinence. Am J Obstet Gynecol 1986;154:58. [PMID: 3946505]

Buyse G et al: Intravesical oxbutynin for neurogenic bladder dysfunction: less systemic side effects due to reduced first pass metabolism. J Urol 1998;160:892. [PMID: 9720583]

Cammu H, Van Nylen M: Pelvic floor exercises versus vaginal weight cones in genuine stress incontinence. Eur J Obstet Gynecology Reprod Biol 1998;77:89. [PMID: 9550207]

Carbone JM, Kavaler E, Raz S: Disappointing early results with bone anchored cadaveric fascia pubovaginal sling (abstract 736). J Urol 2000;163:166.

Cashman NR: A prion primer. CMAJ 1997;157:1381. [PMID: 9371069]

Cervigni M: Hormonal influences in the lower urinary tract. In: Raz S (editor): Female Urology. WB Saunders and Company, 1996.

Fink RS, Collins WP, Papdaki L: Vaginal oestriol: Effective menopausal therapy not associated with endometrial hyperplasia. J Gynaecol Endocrinol 1985;1–2:1.

Finkbeiner AE: Is bethanechol chloride clinically effective in promoting bladder emptying? A literature review. J Urol 1985;134:443. [PMID: 2863391]

Fitzgerald MP, Mollenhauer J, Brubaker L: Failure of allograft suburethral slings. BJU Int 1999;84:785. [PMID: 10532972]

Gillberg PG, Sundquist S, Nilvebrant L: Comparison of the in vitro and in vivo profiles of tolterodine with those of subtype-selective muscarinic receptor antagonists. Eur J Pharmacol 1998;349:285. [PMID: 9671109]

Haab F et al: Results of the tension-free vaginal tape procedure for the treatment of type II stress urinary incontinence at a minimum followup of 1 year. J Urol 2001;165:159. [PMID: 11125387]

Herschorn S, Radomski SB, Steele DJ: Early experience with intraurethral collagen injections for urinary incontinence. J Urol 1992;148:1797. [PMID: 1433611]

Kato K, Kondo A: Clinical value of vaginal cones for the management of female stress incontinence. Int Urogynecol J Pelvic Floor Dysfunct 1997;8:314. [PMID: 9557998]

Kegel AH: Progressive resistance exercise in the functional restoration of the perineal muscles. Am J Obstet Gynecol 1948;36:238.

Kitakoji H et al: [Effect of acupuncture on the overactive bladder]. Nippon Hinyokika Gakkai Zasshi 1995;86:1514. [PMID: 7474599]

Kobashi KC, Mee SL, Leach GE: A new technique for cystocele repair and transvaginal sling: the cadaveric prolapse repair and sling (CAPS). Urology 2000;56:9. [PMID: 11114557]

Leach GE et al: Female Stress Urinary Incontinence Clinical Guidelines Panel summary report on surgical management of female stress urinary incontinence. The American Urological Association. J Urol 1997;158:875. [PMID: 9258103]

Lightener D et al: A new injectable bulking agent for treatment of stress urinary incontinence: results of a multicenter, randomized, controlled, double-blind study of Durasphere. Urology 2001;58:12. [PMID: 11445471]

Mark SD, Webster GD: Detrusor hyperactivity. In: Raz S (editor): Female Urology. WB Saunders and Company, 1996.

Mattsson LA, Cullberg G: A clinical evaluation of treatment with estriol vaginal cream versus suppository in postmenopausal women. Acta Obstet Gynecol Scand 1983;62:397. [PMID: 6421083]

Morgan TE, Farrow GA, Stewart FE: The Marlex sling operation for the treatment of recurrent stress urinary incontinence: a 16-year review. Am J Obstet Gynecol 1985;151:224. [PMID: 4038585]

Shaker HS, Hassouna M: Sacral nerve root neuromodulation: an effective treatment of refractory urge incontinence. J Urol 1998;159:1516. [PMID: 9554345]

Shortliffe LM et al: Treatment of urinary incontinence by the periurethral implantation of glutaraldehye cross-linked collagen. J Urol 1989;141:538. [PMID: 2918587]

Simonds RJ et al: Transmission of human immunodeficiency virus type 1 from a seronegative organ and tissue donor. N Engl J Med 1992;326:726. [PMID: 1738377]

Staskin DR, Choe JM, Breslin DS: The Gore-tex sling procedure for female sphincteric incontinence: indications, technique, and results. World J Urol 1997;15:295. [PMID: 9372580]

Stein M et al: Biofeedback for the treatment of stress and urge incontinence. J Urol 1995;153:641. [PMID: 7861503]

Tomford WW: Transmission of disease through transplantation of musculoskeletal allografts. J Bone Joint Surg Am 1995;77:1742. [PMID: 7593087]

Ulmsten U, Johnson P, Rezapour M: A three-year follow up of tension free vaginal tape for surgical treatment of female stress urinary incontinence. Br J Obstet Gynaecol 1999;106:345. [PMID: 10426241]

Vandersteen DR, Husmann DA: Treatment of primary nocturnal enuresis persisting into adulthood. J Urol 1999;161:90. [PMID: 10037376]

Weese DL et al: Intravesical oxybutinin chloride: experience with 42 patients. Urology 1993;41:527. [PMID: 8516987]

Wein AJ: Pharmacology of incontinence. Urol Clin North Am 1995;22:557. [PMID: 7645157]

Wilson PD, Borland M: Vaginal cones for the treatment of genuine stress urinary incontinence. Aust N Z J Obstet Gynaecol 1990;30:157. [PMID: 2400361]

Wright EJ et al: Pubovaginal sling using cadaveric allograft fascia for the treatment of intrinsic sphincter deficiency. J Urol 1998;160:759. [PMID: 9720541]

Yamada T et al: The correction of type 2 stress incontinence with polytetrafluoroethylene patch sling: 5-year mean followup. J Urol 1998;160:746. [PMID: 9720537]

Zoedler D, Boeminghaus H: On indication and technique of suspension plastic surgery. Z Urol Nephrol 1965;58:459.

Relevant Web Sites

[American Foundation for Urologic Disease]
http://www.afud. org/conditions/ui.html
[Continence Center at Virginia Mason]
http://www.virginiamason.com/dburology/sec4039.htm
[Food and Drug Administration]
http://www.fda.gov/fdac/features/1997/597_urin.html
[HealthAtoZ]
http://www.healthatoz.com/atoz/incontinence/incontindex.asp
[Mayo Clinic Rochester]
http://www.mayo.edu/geriatrics-rst/incont.html
[National Association for Continence]
www.nafc.org
[National Kidney and Urologic Disorders]
http://www.niddk.nih.gov/health/urolog/pubs/uiwomen/uiwomen.htm
[Tower Urology Institute for Continence]
http://www.towerincontinence.com

Urinary Tract Infections

Catherine S. Thompson, MD

Urinary tract infections are most often the result of bacterial invasion of the urinary tract. Fungal and viral pathogens are much less common. **Bacteriuria** is defined as the presence of bacteria in the urine; however, this finding alone is never diagnostic of a urinary tract infection. Bacteria may be present in uninfected urine if periurethral or vaginal flora contaminate the urine specimen at the time of collection. The term **significant bacteriuria** is used to distinguish contaminated urine from true infection. Depending on the clinical setting and technique of collection, significant bacteriuria can be defined in the following ways:

- At least 10^2 colony-forming units of bacteria per milliliter in a midstream urine sample from a symptomatic woman.
- At least 10^5 colony-forming units of bacteria per milliliter in a midstream urine sample from an asymptomatic woman.
- At least 10^2 colony-forming units of bacteria per milliliter in a symptomatic woman with an indwelling bladder catheter.

Asymptomatic bacteriuria refers to significant bacteriuria in a woman with no symptoms of infection. Asymptomatic infections are particularly common during pregnancy and in older, postmenopausal women.

The term **lower urinary tract infection** includes **cystitis** and **urethritis,** which are infections of the urinary bladder and urethra, respectively. When the kidneys or upper urinary tracts are involved, the term **pyelonephritis** is used. Upper and lower tract infections can be difficult to distinguish on clinical grounds because of significant overlap in presenting symptoms and signs.

Urinary tract infections can be described as either **uncomplicated** or **complicated.** This broad division allows the clinician to design treatment for the infection as well as make plans for follow-up. Complicated infections occur in women with anatomic or functional abnormalities of the urinary tract and can be associated with pathogens that are resistant to conventional antibiotics. The factors that suggest the presence of a complicated urinary tract infection are as follows:

Indwelling bladder catheter
Recent urinary tract instrumentation

Functional or anatomic abnormality of the urinary tract
Diabetes mellitus
Immunosuppression
Recent antimicrobial use
Hospital-acquired infection
Symptoms lasting longer than 7 days.

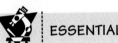 **ESSENTIALS OF DIAGNOSIS**

- *Dysuria, urgency, and frequency.*
- *Colonization of urinary tract by pathogen, usually bacteria.*

General Considerations

In the United States, the annual cost of evaluation and treatment of urinary tract infections in women exceeds $1 billion. This significant health problem is reviewed with an emphasis on pertinent pathophysiology, a diagnostic approach that stresses differential diagnosis, and a discussion of therapeutic options. Infections of the urinary tract occur in women of all ages and affect up to 20% of women during their lifetime. Many will experience multiple or recurrent infections. Infections during the childbearing years are particularly common.

Pathogenesis

Most urinary tract infections develop when fecal uropathogens colonize the vaginal introitus or urethra and ascend into the bladder. The usual result is an inflammatory host response characterized by specific symptoms and pyuria. Women with recurrent urinary tract infections may have an increased susceptibility to vaginal colonization with uropathogens. The risk of developing a urinary tract infection is enhanced by circumstances that propel bacteria from the introital area into the bladder. These include sexual intercourse, use of a contraceptive diaphragm or spermicidal jelly, urinary tract instrumentation, and poor perineal hygiene. The risk of infection also is influenced by intrinsic virulence factors unique to the organism.

Organisms that gain entry into the bladder and establish a lower urinary tract infection may ascend into the upper urinary tract. The risk factors for the development of upper urinary tract infection are incompletely understood. Intrinsic virulence factors of the infecting organism as well as functional or anatomic abnormalities of the urinary tract in the host may increase the risk of upper tract infection.

The vast majority of urinary tract infections are caused by facultative anaerobic gram-negative organisms that colonize the lower gastrointestinal tract. *Escherichia coli* is the most common of these organisms and accounts for 85% of all uncomplicated, community-acquired urinary tract infections. Other enteric gram-negative organisms such as the *Klebsiella* or *Proteus* species are less frequently observed. Gram-positive organisms such as *Staphylococcus saprophyticus* account for 10% of infections. Women with complicated urinary tract infections are infected with *E coli* in 50% of cases. In contrast to simple cystitis, a woman with a complicated urinary tract infection has a higher incidence of infection with gram-negative organisms such as *Pseudomonas, Serratia, Proteus,* or *Klebsiella*. Gram-positive organisms including *Staphylococcus* and enterococci are also recognized pathogens in complicated infections, particularly after instrumentation of the urinary tract.

Clinical Findings

The symptoms of acute lower urinary tract infection (cystitis) are dysuria, urgency, and frequency with or without suprapubic or low back discomfort. Upper tract infection (pyelonephritis) is suggested by the presence of flank pain and a variety of systemic symptoms such as nausea, vomiting, or fever and chills. Differentiation of upper tract infection from simple cystitis may be difficult. Up to one third of women with symptoms suggestive of simple cystitis may have unrecognized involvement of the upper urinary tract. The testing required to distinguish upper from lower tract infection includes such procedures as bladder washout, assay for antibody-coated bacteria (suggestive of upper tract involvement), and selective ureteral catheterization. These procedures are cumbersome, expensive, and have a limited role in the routine management of urinary tract infections. Fortunately, the confirmation of upper tract involvement is rarely necessary.

Differential Diagnosis

Dysuria does not necessarily imply a urinary tract infection. The differential diagnosis includes other conditions such as urethritis caused by *Neisseria gonorrhoeae* or *Chlamydia trachomatis*. Urethritis is the likely diag-

nosis when pyuria without bacteriuria is detected in a woman with dysuria. Other conditions that may confuse the diagnosis include a variety of vaginal infections (*Candida* or *Trichomonas*), herpes simplex infection, genitourinary trauma, or the use of chemical irritants.

The approach to diagnosing a urinary tract infection is simplified by the identification of a specific syndrome that most likely accounts for the clinical presentation. Although there may be overlap in some cases, this approach is useful in evaluation and treatment. Urinary tract infections in women can be categorized broadly as follows: acute uncomplicated cystitis, acute uncomplicated pyelonephritis, complicated urinary tract infection, pregnancy-associated urinary tract infection, urinary tract infection in elderly women, and urinary tract infection with an indwelling bladder catheter.

A. ACUTE UNCOMPLICATED CYSTITIS

The acute, uncomplicated episode of cystitis represents the most common type of urinary tract infection in women. Women of childbearing age are most frequently affected. Sexual intercourse and the use of a contraceptive diaphragm with spermicidal jelly increase the risk of these infections.

1. Diagnosis—Most women are symptomatic with dysuria, frequency, or urgency; often, there is suprapubic or low back discomfort. Pyuria and bacteriuria with or without hematuria are diagnostic findings on urinalysis. The leukocyte esterase dipstick can detect significant pyuria in up to 95% of cases. A urine culture is not necessary in nonpregnant women who present with typical symptoms and findings on urinalysis. A cost-effective approach is to confirm the presence of bacteria and pyuria and institute empiric treatment with oral antibiotics. A follow-up urine culture is not performed unless symptoms persist or recur after treatment. If a urine culture is performed in a symptomatic woman, a colony count of 100 or more (greater than 10^2) colony-forming units of bacteria per milliliter of urine is diagnostic of significant bacteriuria.

2. Treatment—The treatment of uncomplicated cystitis has been simplified by the use of short (3-day) courses of oral antibiotics (Table 26–1). Single-dose therapy is no longer recommended because of lower rates of cure. A 3-day regimen is preferred and is associated with cure rates comparable with a 7-day regimen but without the added cost or drug side effects (rashes, candidal vaginitis, diarrhea) of lengthier treatment. Although resistance to antimicrobials varies from region to region, resistance to trimethoprim and the combination trimethoprim-sulfamethoxazole is generally 5–15% and resistance to fluoroquinolones is generally less than 5%. These agents are the drugs of choice, therefore, for a 3-day regimen. The lower cost of trimetho-

Table 26–1. Three-day oral regimens for the treatment of simple cystitis.[1]

Drug	Dosage
Trimethoprim-sulfamethoxazole DS	160 mg/800 mg q12h
Trimethoprim	100 mg q12h
Ciprofloxacin	250 mg q12h
Levofloxacin	250 mg q24h
Nitrofurantoin monohydrate*	100 mg q12h for 7 days
Amoxicillin clavulanate*	875/125 mg q12h for 7 days

[1]Longer treatment suggested.

prim and trimethoprim-sulfamethoxazole makes this a recommended empiric choice with fluoroquinolones generally reserved for refractory or more complicated cases and for women who are allergic to sulfonamides or trimethoprim. Despite in vitro resistance of some urinary pathogens to trimethoprim-sulfamethoxazole, many episodes of uncomplicated cystitis respond to the drug, presumably due to high concentrations of the antimicrobial achieved in the urine. Nitrofurantoin and amoxicillin-clavulanate can be used to treat uncomplicated urinary tract infection but a longer, 7-day course is suggested when these agents are used.

Recurrent episodes of cystitis can be a problem for some women and are almost always caused by reinfection. Only 10% of women have an anatomic or functional anomaly of the lower urinary tract that predisposes to recurrent, relapsing episodes of cystitis. Recurrent infections should be documented by urine culture and diagnosed as either a **relapse** (infection with the same organism occurring within 2 weeks of initial therapy) or a **reinfection** (infection caused by the same or a different bacterial strain, more than 2 weeks after the last course of antibiotic therapy).

A variety of interventions have been proposed to manage recurrent episodes of cystitis. A true relapse should be treated with a longer course of antibiotics, up to 2–6 weeks, and an anatomic or functional anomaly of the urinary tract should be considered in these cases. An intravenous urogram with or without cystoscopy may be helpful.

For most women, reinfection occurs when a uropathogen colonizes the perineum; anatomic anomalies are rare. The treatment depends on the frequency of the recurrences. Women with fewer than 2 episodes of cystitis in 1 year might be managed with "patient-initiated" therapy. A 3-day regimen of antibiotics, generally trimethoprim-sulfamethoxazole or a fluoroquinolone, is initiated when classic symptoms of infection are

recognized (Table 26–1). For women who have more than 3 infections per year, prophylactic antibiotic regimens can be considered as outlined in Table 26–2. Women who associate their recurrent infections with sexual activity may benefit from postcoital prophylaxis. Women whose recurrences are unrelated to coitus may benefit from daily or thrice weekly prophylaxis with low-dose oral antibiotics.

Postmenopausal women may be affected by recurrent urinary tract infections. Bladder or uterine prolapse may produce incomplete voiding and increase the risk of infection. Prophylactic antimicrobials in selected circumstances may be helpful (Table 26–2).

B. Acute, Uncomplicated Pyelonephritis

Infection of the upper urinary tract (pyelonephritis) presents as a spectrum of illness. Many women have relatively mild symptoms suggestive of simple cystitis. Others have flank discomfort, fever, chills, or nausea and vomiting with or without lower tract symptoms. More than 80% of cases of pyelonephritis are caused by *E coli,* and the remainder of infections is attributed to other gram-negative organisms, enterococci, or *Staphylococcus.* Bacteremia occurs in 15–20% of cases of pyelonephritis.

1. Diagnosis—The unspun urine in women with pyelonephritis contains leukocytes and bacteria. A Gram stain of the urine may be helpful in selecting the antimicrobial therapy; most cases are caused by gram-negative organisms, but enterococcal infection is suggested by the presence of gram-positive cocci on a Gram stain. A urine culture is advised in women with

Table 26–2. Prophylactic antibiotic regimens.[1]

Postcoital prophylaxis: single dose
  Trimethoprim-sulfamethoxazole, 40/200 mg (one half of a single-strength tablet)
  Cephalexin, 250 mg
  Ciprofloxacin, 250 mg
  Norfloxacin, 200 mg
  Nitrofurantoin, 50–100 mg
Daily or 3 times weekly prophylaxis
  Trimethoprim, 100 mg
  Trimethoprim-sulfamethoxazole, 40 mg/200 mg (or 3 times weekly)
  Nitrofurantoin, 50–100 mg
  Norfloxacin, 200 mg
  Ciprofloxacin, 125 mg
  Cephalexin, 250 mg

[1]The specific choice and dosage of antibiotic may vary in patients with impaired renal or hepatic function.

suspected upper tract infection. The distinction between simple cystitis and uncomplicated pyelonephritis may be difficult. A history of pyelonephritis or presence of unusually severe symptoms suggests upper tract infection.

2. Treatment—The management of pyelonephritis differs from that of simple cystitis in the selection and duration of antimicrobial therapy. Nonpregnant women with mild symptoms and no dehydration or gastrointestinal manifestations typically do well with oral antibiotics prescribed on an outpatient basis for 10–14 days. The preferred empiric choice is a fluoroquinolone antibiotic such as ciprofloxacin or levofloxacin. Other choices include trimethoprim-sulfamethoxazole or amoxicillin-clavulanate in the doses outlined in Table 26–1. Women with more severe illness require hospitalization for hydration and intravenous antibiotics. Blood cultures should be obtained. Parenteral therapy as outlined in Table 26–3 is recommended until the patient demonstrates signs of clinical improvement. Oral antibiotics are prescribed subsequently to complete the treatment course of 14 days. The choice of oral agent will depend on the organism and sensitivity pattern. A follow-up urine culture is recommended after completion of therapy.

The symptoms and signs of pyelonephritis should resolve within 72 hours of initiation of antibiotic therapy. Imaging studies of the urinary tract are indicated in women whose symptoms are slow to improve. Occult anatomic anomalies, intrarenal abscess, perinephric abscess, or obstruction may be identified in these settings. Renal ultrasonography, intravenous urography, or computed tomography (CT) of the kidneys may be helpful. Women in whom anomalies are detected on imaging studies are considered to have a complicated infection.

C. COMPLICATED URINARY INFECTIONS

In addition to anatomic anomalies, complicated infections can be associated with an indwelling bladder catheter or with multiresistant or unusual microbial agents. The clinical presentation of a complicated infection is variable, ranging from asymptomatic bacteriuria to life-threatening septicemia.

1. Diagnosis—The diagnosis of a complicated infection is largely one of recognition. Women with one or more of the listed risk factors should be monitored for development of a complicated infection, which requires lengthier treatment and/or additional investigation. A complicated infection can be difficult to recognize if the presenting symptoms and signs are those of a simple, uncomplicated urinary tract infection (either cystitis or pyelonephritis). In other cases, more severe symptoms such as extreme flank discomfort or systemic signs of high fever, lethargy, or confusion provide the clue that a complicated infection may be present. Identification of the woman susceptible to a complicated infection depends on the recognition of risk factors listed previously.

2. Treatment—Treatment with antibiotics, selected on the basis of the results of the urine culture, for a minimum of 14 days is recommended. Parenteral treatment may be indicated for a portion of the treatment course, depending on the clinical setting (Tables 26–3 and 26–4). Anatomic imaging of the urinary tract should be considered in patients who are slow to respond to treatment. A correctable abnormality such as obstruction or the detection of either a renal or perinephric abscess affects the duration and type of treatment. A urine culture obtained after completion of antibiotic therapy is advised in women with a complicated urinary tract infection.

D. URINARY TRACT INFECTIONS DURING PREGNANCY

The detection and treatment of asymptomatic bacteriuria during pregnancy is an important issue in obstetric care. Although asymptomatic bacteriuria complicates only 5–9% of all pregnancies, the infection progresses to a symptomatic urinary tract infection in 20–40% of these women at some point during gestation. The relationship between asymptomatic bacteriuria and a variety of obstetric complications such as prematurity, preterm labor, growth retardation, and maternal hypertension is a controversial issue. There is agreement that screening and treatment of women with asymptomatic bacteriuria during pregnancy is indicated, at least to prevent the development of overt symptomatic urinary tract infection.

Table 26–3. Intravenous treatment of pyelonephritis/complicated urinary tract infection.[1]

Drug[2]	Dosage
Ciprofloxacin	400 mg q12h
Levofloxacin	250–500 mg q24h
Ampicillin/gentamicin	1g q6h/1 mg/kg q8h
Ceftriaxone	1–2 g q24h
Piperacillin	3 g q6h

[1]The specific choice and dosage of antibiotic may vary in patients with impaired renal or hepatic function. Drug levels or other monitoring (eg, creatinine clearance) may be required.
[2]All drugs are given until the patient is afebrile and followed by oral antibiotics to bring the treatment course to 14 days.

Table 26–4. Treatment of urinary tract infection in pregnancy.

Asymptomatic bacteriuria/symptomatic cystitis*:
    Amoxicillin, 250–500 mg q8h × 3 days
    Amoxicillin clavulanate, 250–500 mg q8h × 3 days
    Nitrofurantoin monohydrate, 100 mg q12h × 7 days
    Cephalexin, 250–500 mg q6h × 3 days
    Sulfisoxazole, 1g, followed by 500 mg q6h × 3 days
Prophylactic antibiotic regimens: (for > 2 positive cultures
    Nitrofurantoin 50–100 mg hs
    Cephalexin 250–500 mg hs
Pyelonephritis: 14 day course
Intravenous
    Gentamicin, 1 mg/kg q8h and ampicilin, 1 g q6h
    Ceftriaxone, 1–2 g q24h
    Aztreonam, 1 g q8–12h
    Ticarcillin-clavulanate 3.2 g q8h
Oral†
    Amoxicillin, 500 mg q8h
    Cephalexin, 250–500 mg q6h
    Sulfisoxazole, 500 mg q6h
    Nitrofurantoin monohydrate 100 mg q12h

---

*The specific choice and dosage of antibiotic may vary in patients with impaired renal or hepatic function. Drug levels or other monitoring (eg, creatinine clearance) may be required.
†Oral antibiotics can be substituted for intravenous antibiotics after clinical improvement and sensitivity patterns are known.

The urinary tract undergoes significant change during pregnancy. Hormonal and mechanical factors allow for dilation of the renal collecting system and ureters. These changes predispose women to progression from asymptomatic bacteriuria to symptomatic, and often clinically severe, upper tract infection. Enteric gram-negative bacteria such as *E coli* are the most common organisms cultured from the urine. Less frequently, gram-positive organisms, *Gardnerella vaginalis,* or *Ureaplasma urealyticum* are identified.

1. Screening—Pregnant women should be screened early in gestation for asymptomatic bacteriuria. A quantitative urine culture done during the first trimester and no later than 16 weeks of gestation is recommended. A clean-catch midstream collection is preferred; bladder catheterization is not advised. Significant bacteriuria in an asymptomatic woman is defined by a colony count of greater than 10^5 bacteria per milliliter of urine.

2. Treatment—Treatment is recommended for 3–7 days with an appropriate antibiotic given orally. Amoxicillin has a long safety record and is preferred, but for resistant organisms or patients who are allergic to the drug, nitrofurantoin, sulfisoxazole, and cephalexin are alternatives (Table 26–4). Fluoroquinolone antibiotics should not be used during pregnancy. A follow-up urine culture should be performed one week after antimicrobial treatment is completed. Persistent bacteriuria or relapse of infection during pregnancy can occur in up to 20–30% of women. Serial urine cultures may be needed at monthly intervals during pregnancy; the results guide further courses of oral antibiotic therapy. Suppressive antibiotic regimens for women with more than two positive urine cultures during pregnancy can be considered (Table 26–4). Women who require antibiotic therapy for the duration of pregnancy are likely to have infection of the upper urinary tract and should be evaluated for structural or functional anomalies in the postpartum period.

Symptomatic urinary tract infections develop in 1–2% of all pregnancies. The presentation most closely resembles acute pyelonephritis in nonpregnant women. The typical treatment is hospitalization for intravenous antibiotics, usually ampicillin and an aminoglycoside until culture results are known (Table 26–4). Conversion to oral antibiotics with a total duration of treatment of 14 days is advised. Suppressive antibiotics in lower doses usually are needed until delivery. Failure to respond to standard treatment suggests a complicated urinary infection. Sonography of the urinary tract may be necessary to exclude a renal or perirenal abscess or other anomaly.

E. URINARY TRACT INFECTIONS IN OLDER WOMEN

Bacteriuria in women older than 65 years is common; the prevalence increases with age and approaches 50% by age 80. The incidence of bacteriuria is highest in women living in nursing homes and in women with incomplete bladder emptying, those with fecal incontinence, and those who require bladder catheterization. Bacteriuria in this population can occur sporadically and is often asymptomatic. There is no proven association between asymptomatic bacteriuria in the elderly and increased mortality.

An ascending route of infection via the urethra is the most common cause of bacteriuria in this population. Estrogen deficiency may allow enteric flora to populate the vaginal and periurethral areas. Unfortunately, treatment with exogenous estrogen does not reduce the incidence of urinary tract infection reliably in postmenopausal women.

E coli continues to be the most common infecting organism in this population with other enteric gram-negative rods and enterococci occurring more commonly than staphylococcal infection. Hospitalized elderly women are particularly prone to gram-negative infections other than *E coli.*

1. Diagnosis—The clinical features of urinary tract infections in elderly women are varied. Most women are asymptomatic. Classic lower tract symptoms of dysuria, urgency, and frequency may occur and suggest simple cystitis. Upper tract infection may present with fever and flank discomfort; however, overwhelming sepsis, bacteremia, diminished mental status, and gastrointestinal or respiratory complaints may be the presenting features of pyelonephritis in this population.

2. Treatment—All symptomatic urinary tract infections should be treated. The selection of antimicrobial agents, duration of treatment, and route of administration depends on the clinical setting and whether the presentation most closely resembles simple cystitis, acute uncomplicated pyelonephritis, or a complicated infection. Elderly women with suspected upper tract infection almost always require hospitalization and intravenous antibiotics. Lower tract infections can be managed with 3- to 7-day courses of oral antibiotics.

The management of asymptomatic bacteriuria in elderly women is controversial. The condition is defined as two successive urine cultures with greater than 10^5 (100,000) colony-forming units of bacteria per milliliter. Depending on the clinical setting, either no treatment or no more than a 3-day course of oral antibiotics can be administered. A follow-up urine culture is not necessary, and routine screening for asymptomatic bacteriuria is not recommended in this population.

F. Urinary Tract Infection with Bladder Catheterization

The use of an indwelling bladder catheter is associated with an increasing incidence of urinary tract infection the longer the catheter remains in place. Prophylactic antibiotics are not recommended and are ineffective in preventing infection. If possible, short-term bladder catheterization (fewer than seven days) or in and out bladder catheterization is preferred over the chronic indwelling catheter.

Women who require longer term (more than seven days) indwelling catheters should be monitored for signs and symptoms of cystitis or pyelonephritis but not treated for asymptomatic bacteriuria. Management of the symptomatic patient with intravenous or oral antibiotics depending on the severity of presenting symptoms is recommended (Tables 26–1 and 26–3).

Gupta K, Scholes D, Stamm WE: Increasing prevalence of antimicrobial resistance among uropathogens causing acute uncomplicated cystitis. JAMA 1999;281:736. [PMID: 10052444]

Hooten TM et al: A prospective study of risk factors for symptomatic urinary tract infection in young women. N Engl J Med 1996;335:468. [PMID: 8672152]

Johnson JR, Stamm WE: Urinary tract infections in women: diagnosis and treatment. Ann Intern Med 1989;111:906. [PMID: 2683922]

Patterson TF, Andriole VT: Detection, significance, and therapy of bacteriuria in pregnancy. Update in the managed health care era. Infect Dis Clin North Am 1997;11:593. [PMID: 9378925]

Stamm WE, Hooton TM: Management of urinary tract infections in adults. N Engl J Med 1993;329:1328. [PMID: 8413414]

Warren JW et al: Guidelines for antimicrobial treatment of uncomplicated acute bacterial cystitis and acute pyelonephritis in women. Infectious Diseases Society of America (IDSA). Clin Infect Dis 1999:29:745. [PMID: 10589881]

SECTION VII

Gastrointestinal Disorders

Liver Disease

James E. Bredfeldt, MD

■ GENERAL PRINCIPLES

Most women, who are ultimately identified as having a liver disease, lack any symptoms of a liver disorder or are unaware that they might have an underlying liver condition. Most of the time, a liver disease is suspected when an abnormal elevation of the serum aspartate aminotransferase (AST) and alanine aminotranferase (ALT), or serum alkaline phosphatase (SAP) is found. Usually, these elevations are not great; however, the potential for these abnormalities to reveal a significant liver disorder should not be understated.

Elevated AST & ALT

In the ambulatory care setting, abnormal elevations of the AST and ALT are usually less than 10 times the upper limits of normal and, more commonly, are less than 3 times the upper limits of normal. It is often prudent to exclude a muscle disorder as the cause for this elevation by demonstrating that the creatine phosphokinase level is normal and to confirm the persistence of the AST/ALT elevations by repeating these tests in 4–6 weeks in asymptomatic patients. A careful history is obtained of the patient's current medication use (prescription and otherwise), alcohol ingestion, risk factors for acquiring chronic viral hepatitis B or C, changes in health status (obesity, diabetes mellitus, hyperlipidemias), and family history of liver disorders (Table 27–1). Additional blood testing is then performed to identify or exclude specific liver diseases (Table 27–2).

Elevated Serum Alkaline Phosphatase

Since the elevation of the SAP is often an isolated abnormality with normal AST/ALT levels, it is necessary to demonstrate that the SAP elevation is actually derived from the liver rather from a bone source (Table 27–3). This assessment is best made by testing for either the serum gamma-glutamyltransferase (GGTP) or 5′-nucleotidase level. If these levels are normal, a bone source for the elevated SAP should be explored.

When the SAP is elevated, imaging of the liver by either ultrasonography or computed tomography (CT) is indicated, since hepatic neoplasms and infiltrative diseases are a frequent cause for the SAP elevation. If biliary tract disease is suspected on the basis of typical symptoms but not confirmed by ultrasound or CT scans, a magnetic resonance cholangiopancreatography is a useful, noninvasive examination to evaluate the extrahepatic biliary system. If an obstructive lesion of the biliary system is suspected (such as choledocholithiasis or a biliary stricture) and therapeutic intervention may be needed, an endoscopic retrograde cholangiopancreatography is the indicated procedure.

Liver Biopsy

A percutaneous liver biopsy is an adjunctive means for confirming the diagnosis of liver disease, for providing a histologic staging of the liver disease and for quantitating the hepatic levels of iron and copper in patients with hemochromatosis and Wilson's disease, respectively. A liver biopsy often reveals a clinically significant diagnosis (eg, steatosis, steatohepatitis, cryptogenic cirrhosis, or granulomatosis diseases) in patients with per-

Table 27–1. Differential diagnosis of chronic AST/ALT elevations.

Fatty liver and NASH syndrome
Chronic viral hepatitis
Alcoholic liver disease
Autoimmune hepatitis
Hemochromatosis
Medications
Wilson's disease (in patients younger than 40 years)

NASH, nonalcoholic steatohepatitis.

sistent elevations of the AST/ALT or SAP for more than 6 months and in whom conventional serologic testing has not been diagnostic.

Hepatitis A & B Vaccinations in Chronic Liver Diseases

Prophylactic vaccination against hepatitis A and B in patients with chronic liver disease is safe and effective in preventing infection from these viruses. In patients with chronic hepatitis B, acute coinfection with hepatitis A virus results in higher serum ALT levels, more severe liver disease, and a higher death rate compared with healthy persons infected only with hepatitis A virus. In a similar manner, patients with chronic hepatitis C infection appear to have an increased risk of morbidity and mortality when acutely infected with hepatitis A virus. It also seems that patients with other, nonviral, chronic liver diseases have an increased risk of more severe infection when acutely infected with hepatitis A virus.

Table 27–2. Disease-specific markers.

Disease	Marker
Hepatitis B virus	HBsAg
Hepatitis C virus	Hepatitis C antibody (EIA) Hepatitis C virus RNA by polymerase chain reaction
Autoimmune hepatitis	Antinuclear antibody Anti–smooth-muscle antibody Anti-liver kidney-microsomal antibody
Primary biliary cirrhosis	Antimitochondrial antibody
Hemochromatosis	Serum iron, iron-binding capacity Serum ferritin
Wilson's disease	Serum ceruloplasmin

EIA, enzyme immunoassay.

Table 27–3. Differential diagnosis of elevated serum alkaline phosphatase.

Hepatic
  Neoplasms (benign; malignant [primary, metastatic])
  Fatty liver
  Alcoholic liver disease
  Primary biliary cirrhosis
  Drug-induced hepatotoxicity
  Hepatic granulomas
Biliary tract
  Bile duct obstruction (stones, strictures, neoplasms)
  Primary sclerosing cholangitis
Nonhepatic
  Paget's disease
  Bone metastases
  Physiologic (pregnancy, puberty, aging)

The current vaccination regimens against hepatitis A and B infection include the following: (1) the use of monovalent vaccines against hepatitis A (Havrix or Vaqta) administered at 0 and 6–12 months and hepatitis B (Engerix-B or Recombivax-HB) administered at 0, 1, and 6 months (2) or the newly released combination vaccine for hepatitis A and B (Twinrix) administered at 0, 1, and 6 months.

When to Refer to a Specialist

Most patients who have abnormalities in their liver enzyme levels, whether it is the serum alkaline phosphatase or serum AST/ALT levels, will ultimately have a definitive explanation for these elevations. In the vast majority of the patients, an important and positive impact upon the future health of them may occur. Referral to a gastroenterologist or hepatologist will assist in facilitating the ultimate diagnosis and treatment of the patient. The specialist can determine if a liver biopsy is beneficial in the evaluation of a patient with suspected chronic liver disease, what additional diagnostic modalities are required, and make definitive treatment recommendations. Very often, the support staff within the specialist's office will assist in the further education of the patient about their liver disorder and the treatment modalities. The latter is especially important in the treatment of patients with chronic hepatitis B and C.

Keefe EB: Hepatitis A virus and hepatitis B virus vaccination in patients with chronic liver disease. Clin Perspect Gastroenterol 1999;2:342.

Pratt DS, Kaplan MM: Evaluation of abnormal liver-enzyme results in asymptomatic patients. N Engl J Med 2000;342: 1266. [PMID: 10781624]

■ SPECIFIC LIVER DISEASES

CHRONIC VIRAL HEPATITIS

Chronic viral hepatitis, as a consequence of a hepatitis B virus (HBV) or hepatitis C virus (HCV) infection, may lead to serious health issues. In women, specific health issues are present, including the risk of sexual transmission, the risk of vertical transmission to the neonate, and the risk to the future health of the woman.

Chronic Hepatitis B

While the frequency of chronic hepatitis B is much less in the United States compared with other endemic regions of the world, an estimated 1.25 million people in the United States have chronic hepatitis B. The risk factors for acquiring hepatitis B are listed in Table 27–4.

 ESSENTIALS OF DIAGNOSIS

- *Positive hepatitis B surface antigen (HBsAg) diagnoses HBV.*
- *AST/ALT levels may or not be elevated.*

Diagnosis

Detection of HBsAg indicates that the individual is infected with HBV, regardless of the lack of clinical symptoms or abnormal elevations of AST/ALT. When a chronic hepatitis B infection is identified, demonstration of viral replication is important for treatment recommendations. Replication of HBV is defined as detection of hepatitis B e antigen (HBeAg) and HBV-DNA, the latter being the more sensitive determinant of replication. Most persons with chronic hepatitis B lack liver-specific symptoms, and the infection is often uncovered inadvertently.

Transmission & Prevention

Vertical transmission refers to passage of HBV from an infected mother to the neonate at the time of birth. Vertical transmission of HBV has largely been eliminated through universal, maternal prenatal screening for HBsAg. Once identifying the infected mother, administration of immunoprophylaxis (hepatitis B immune globulin and hepatitis B vaccine) within 24 hours of birth will effectively interrupt transmission of HBV.

Hepatitis B is a sexually transmitted disease. Heterosexual transmission of HBV occurs in at least 25% of regular sexual partners of person known to have an HBV infection. Persons with multiple sexual partners have a 20% prevalence of exposure to HBV, usually defined by the development of antibodies to HBV. Vaccination of regular sexual partners of HBV patients is indicated to prevent acquisition of HBV. Hepatitis B should become a preventable infectious disease through the routine vaccination against HBV. The current initiative of hepatitis B vaccination in children, prior to puberty, should markedly lessen future sexual transmission.

Treatment

Only chronic hepatitis B in the replicative phase is treatable, since all treatment modalities require active replication in order to have any effect. The majority of patients with chronic hepatitis B do not have a replicative infection and are not treatment candidates. The three current treatment regimens used for chronic hepatitis B are interferon alfa-2b, lamivudine, and adefovir dipivoxil. The treatment regimen with interferon alfa-2b is 16 weeks in length and consists of daily, subcutaneous injections of 5 million units each or 10 million units subcutaneously 3 times a week. Thirty-six to 45% of treated patients will convert from HBeAg to anti-HBe with concomitant loss of HBV-DNA, and approximately 25% of those patients eventually will have loss of HBsAg. This is a favorable outcome because there is histologic improvement and lack of future disease progression. Treatment with interferon alfa-2b, however, is associated with a high frequency of side effects, high cost, and positive response in only a minority of treated patients.

Lamivudine, initially used for inhibition of HIV replication, also has antiviral effects against HBV. Lamivudine, 100 mg/d, results in the rapid disappearance of HBV-DNA, but seroconversion to anti-HBe

Table 27–4. Risk factors for acquiring hepatitis virus infection.

Hepatitis B Virus	Hepatitis C Virus
Vertical transmisison	Injection drug use
Sexual transmission	Blood product transfusion
Injection drug use	Sexual transmission
Occupational exposure (health care workers)	Vertical transmission
	Hemodialysis
Nosocomial	Nosocomial
	Miscellaneous (tattooing, body piercing, intra-nasal cocaine use)

only occurs in 15–20% of patients treated for 1 year. In those patients in whom seroconversion to Anti-HBe does not occur, relapse after cessation of therapy is the rule. A significant problem associated with long-term administration is the emergence of lamivudine drug-resistance, mediated through the YMDD mutation, in greater than 50% of treated patients.

Adefovir dipivoxil, 10 mg/d, was recently approved for the treatment of chronic hepatitis B. Preliminary data indicates a marked reduction in HBV-DNA levels, but seroconversion to anti-HBe only occurs in approximately 12% of patients treated for 1 year. The emergence of the YMDD mutation, however, was not observed.

Prognosis

Two factors influence the long-term prognosis of patients with chronic hepatitis B infection. First, progression to cirrhosis leads to the development of portal hypertension and its complications of ascites, variceal hemorrhage, portal-systemic encephalopathy, hepatorenal syndrome, and liver failure. Second, chronic carriage of HBV over many decades predisposes those persons to an inordinately high risk (greater than 200-fold) for hepatocellular carcinoma developing, regardless whether or not cirrhosis is present.

Chronic Hepatitis C

Since the discovery of the HCV genome in 1989 and the subsequent ability to test for HCV infections, knowledge about HCV has grown exponentially. The number of chronic hepatitis C infections in the United States (close to 3 million persons) is even greater than anticipated, and it is unclear if this number is an underestimate. The risk factors for acquiring HCV are listed in Table 27–4.

ESSENTIALS OF DIAGNOSIS

- Positive hepatitis C antibody, confirmed by HCV-RNA by polymerase chain reaction.
- AST/ALT levels may or not be elevated.

Diagnosis

Most persons in whom HCV is diagnosed have no symptoms, are unaware of a prior exposure to viral hepatitis (absence of jaundice) and, almost always, have chronic hepatitis C when it is initially discovered. Many patients with chronic hepatitis C are middle-aged, middle-class persons who had a remote, and often transient, use of injection drugs. Most HCV infections are disclosed by further serologic testing during the evaluation of AST/ALT elevations, life insurance examinations, and volunteer blood donation. The usual test to detect HCV is the hepatitis C antibody (anti-HCV) by EIA (enzyme immunoassay). A positive anti-HCV requires confirmation, usually, by qualitative or quantitative HCV-RNA by polymerase chain reaction. Approximately 25% of anti-HCV–positive patients will have no detectable levels of viremia by HCV-RNA and, therefore, are considered free of an ongoing HCV infection. HCV genotype testing is often performed in patients with chronic hepatitis C infection. At least, 6 major genotypes (or subgroups) are identified worldwide. In the United States, genotypes 1, 2, and 3 are the most common; genotype 1 is identified in 70% of these patients. Genotype is a strong predictor of potential outcomes to antiviral therapy.

A liver biopsy may be a useful diagnostic adjunct, especially in patients with genotype 1. Since many of these patients have had a long duration of infection (20–30 years), the biopsy results will stage the degree of histologic severity and may assist in treatment decisions, especially when advanced histologic changes (bridging fibrosis, for example) are present.

Transmission & Prevention

Vertical transmission of HCV may occur and the rates of this occurrence range from 1% up to 5%. Confirmation of vertical transmission is made by demonstrating the identical maternal genotype in the infant. Maternal factors that might increase the rate of vertical transmission include HIV coinfection, a history of injection drug use, and high levels of maternal viremia. The mode of delivery and breast-feeding have no affect on transmission to the infant. Anecdotal evidence suggests that amniocentesis performed during the third trimester might infect the fetus in utero. In contrast to HBV, no immunoprophylaxis against HCV exists to prevent vertical transmission. At least 6 months should elapse after an infant is born before testing him or her using HCV-RNA. However, there is currently no effective means of treating those neonates who may have unfortunately been infected by vertical transmission.

Heterosexual transmission of HCV may occur. The risk increases directly to the total accumulated lifetime sexual partners. Spouses of patients with chronic hepatitis C infection also have an increased prevalence of chronic hepatitis C infection. The majority of these persons, however, have their own, individual risk factors for acquiring HCV, usually a background of previous injecting drug use; coupled with often different genotypes, the role of direct sexual transmission is diminished. The prevalence of HCV in a spouse lacking an injecting drug use background is 1.5% and increases only as the duration of the marriage exceeds 20 years. Since the risk of future HCV infection in these spouses is low, a firm recommendation for condom use has not been made. A vaccine that is protective against HCV is not forthcoming in the future.

Treatment

The current and standard antiviral therapy for chronic hepatitis C infection is the combination of interferon and ribavirin. "Standard" interferon comes in 2 different chemical forms, interferon alfa-2a and interferon alfa-2b. A "sustained-release" interferon, termed **pegylated interferon,** also has 2 different forms, peginterferon alfa-2a and alfa-2b. The only large, multicenter study of "standard" interferon evaluated interferon alfa-2b, 3 million units 3 times a week as a subcutaneous injection, plus ribavirin 1000 mg/d or 1200 mg/d if the body weight is less or greater than 75 kg, respectively.

The two different pegylated interferons differ in their pharmacologic and chemical properties. Consequently, these differences have lead to different treatment regimens. Peginterferon alfa-2a is administered as a weekly subcutaneous injection of 180 mg each week, and the ribavirin is given as either 1000 mg/d or 1200 mg/d, depending on body weight of less or greater than 75 kg, respectively. The weekly dose of peginterferon alfa-2b is administered according to body weight (refer to the product information for dosing) with 800 mg/d of oral ribavirin.

Treatment outcome is defined as the sustained virologic response in which HCV-RNA remains undetectable 6 months after completion of treatment. A sustained response predicts that 95% or more of these patients will remain free of detectable HCV-RNA in the future and that the liver histology, including fibrosis, will progressively improve. Effectively, these patients are likely "cured" of their chronic viral infection.

The treatment duration and potential treatment outcome are related to the genotypes. Patients having genotype 1 are usually treated for 48 weeks. The sustained virologic response in these patients treated with interferon alfa-2b and ribavirin is in the range of 35%, while treatment with peginterferons and ribavirin is in the range of 45–55%.

Patients who have genotypes 2 and 3 respond considerably better, with a sustained virologic response approaching 80% using either type of interferon and ribavirin. Often, these patients may be treated for 24 weeks. Women who are under the age of 40 years, who have genotypes 2 or 3, and whose HCV-RNA levels are less than 1 million IU/mL may have a predicted sustained virologic response of 90%, or greater.

On the other hand, antiviral treatment requires a considerable dedication by the patient. The treatment duration is quite lengthy, the treatment is cumbersome (injections), the treatment is costly, and the side effects are considerable with a significant impact on quality of life during the treatment. Fertile female patients must practice effective contraception to prevent conception during the treatment course and for an additional 6 months afterward. Ribavirin is highly teratogenic. A monthly pregnancy test during and after treatment for 6 months should be the standard of care. Patients should also abstain from alcohol use during the course of treatment for chronic hepatitis C because alcohol, particularly its abuse, will significantly affect and decrease the response to antiviral therapy.

Prognosis

The natural history of chronic hepatitis C is incomplete. Since most of these patients were infected at a relatively young age (late teens and early 20s), the natural history is important to understand the consequences of having a chronic viral infection for many decades. The degree and rate for liver fibrosis development is a key point in the natural history of chronic hepatitis C. About 25% of patients who have been infected with hepatitis C virus for 30 years will have slow, if any, progression of fibrosis; whether they might progress to cirrhosis in subsequent decades is unknown. Another 15–20% of patients infected with hepatitis C virus for 20–30 years seem to have a rapid progression of fibrosis and are identified as having cirrhosis. Factors that might influence this more rapid progression of fibrosis are alcohol abuse, advancing age, hepatic steatosis, and hepatic iron accumulation.

Patients in whom advanced and decompensated cirrhosis develops are candidates for a liver transplantation. The recipient liver, however, becomes reinfected with HCV and subsequent survival after transplantation is altered. Patients with chronic hepatitis C and cirrhosis have an increased risk for the development of hepatocellular carcinoma.

Alter MJ et al: The prevalence of hepatitis C virus infection in the United States, 1988 through 1994. N Engl J Med 1999: 341:556. [PMID: 10451460]

Conte D et al: Prevalence and clinical course of chronic hepatitis C virus (HCV) infection and rate of HCV vertical transmission in a cohort of 15,250 pregnant women. Hepatology 2000;31:751. [PMID: 10706568]

Komanduri S, Cotler SJ: Hepatitis C. Clin Perspect Gastroenterol 2002;5:91.

Lau DT et al: Long-term therapy of chronic hepatitis B with lamivudine. Hepatology 2000;32:828. [PMID: 11003630]

Lauer GM, Walker BD: Hepatitis C virus infection. N Engl J Med 2001;345:41. [PMID: 11439948]

Lee WM: Hepatitis B virus infection. N Engl J Med 1997;337: 1733. [PMID: 9392700]

Murphy EL et al: Risk factors for hepatitis C virus infection in United States blood donors. NHLBI Retrovirus Epidemiology Donor Study (REDS). Hepatology 2000;31:756. [PMID: 10706569]

Stroffolini T et al: Hepatitis C infection in spouses: sexual transmission or common exposure to the same risk factors? Am J Gastroenterol 2001;96:3138. [PMID: 11721761]

Yeung LT, King SM, Roberts EA: Mother-to-infant transmission of hepatitis C virus. Hepatology 2001;34:223. [PMID: 11481604]

AUTOIMMUNE HEPATITIS

Autoimmune hepatitis is an inflammatory liver disease of unknown etiology and is characterized by hypergammaglobulinemia, the presence of specific autoantibodies, and liver histology of moderately severe chronic hepatitis (Table 27–5). Current evidence points toward a disturbance in the immune function, leading toward an immunologic attack against the liver. Autoimmune hepatitis afflicts predominately women (80% of the cases) and is identified in all ethnic groups. Approximately 100,000 to 200,000 persons in the United States have autoimmune hepatitis.

The clinical manifestations of autoimmune hepatitis may range from mild fatigue to a life-threatening illness with jaundice and liver failure. Autoimmune hepatitis may mimic acute viral hepatitis with the abrupt onset of symptoms and AST/ALT levels exceeding 1000 U/mL; however the presence of hypergammaglobulinemia and autoantibodies are distinctly unusual in acute viral hepatitis. Some common medications, notably nitrofurantoin, may cause a chronic hepatitis that resembles autoimmune hepatitis. Discontinuation of the offending medication leads to resolution of the liver disorder.

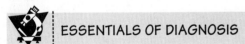

ESSENTIALS OF DIAGNOSIS

- *Significant elevations of AST/ALT, often 10 times the upper limit of normal.*
- *Presence of specific autoantibodies and hypergammaglobulinemia.*
- *Liver biopsy with histologic features of chronic hepatitis, often with increased numbers of plasma cells.*

Diagnosis

The "classic" autoimmune hepatitis, called type 1, is associated with elevated titers of antinuclear antibodies and/or anti-smooth muscle antibodies of 1:80 or greater. This disease is seen in all age groups and is the predominant cause for autoimmune hepatitis in the United States. Frequently, other immunologic diseases (eg, synovitis, thyroiditis, and ulcerative colitis) are identified as concurrent immune diseases. Type 2 autoimmune hepatitis is associated with a detectable anti-liver kidney microsomal antibody type 2. More commonly, this type of autoimmune hepatitis is found in children, ages 2–14 in years, and adults are a distinct minority affected with this disorder. Additional concurrent autoimmune disorders found in type 2 autoimmune hepatitis include: autoimmune thyroiditis, type 1 diabetes mellitus, vitiligo, and autoimmune polyglandular syndrome type 1. Type 3 autoimmune hepatitis is associated with the presence of antibodies against liver soluble antigen/liver pancreas antibodies. This clinical syndrome is very similar to type 1 autoimmune hepatitis but is rarely identified in the United States.

Treatment

Identification of autoimmune hepatitis is vitally important, since some cases are of such severity that prompt institution of corticosteroid therapy may be life-saving. All 3 types of autoimmune hepatitis respond similarly to corticosteroid treatment. Often, azathioprine is added to the treatment regimen as a steroid-sparing drug. Many patients relapse after withdrawal of the immunosuppressive agents, and long-term administration of azathioprine is beneficial for maintaining remission.

Prognosis

Successful treatment results in improvement in 10-year survival of more than 90%, once remission is achieved. Remission, defined as ALT levels < 2 times upper limits of normal or normal, and close to normal liver histology is achieved in 80–85% of treated patients. Immunosuppressive treatment does not "cure" autoimmune hepatitis but mandates a lifelong monitoring and management of the liver disorder. Once remission occurs, the risk for developing cirrhosis is less than 2% per year.

Table 27–5. Diagnosis of autoimmune hepatitis.

Female sex (80% of cases)
Hepatosplenomegaly
Hypergammaglobulinemia
Autoimmune markers (titers of ≥ 1:80)
    Type 1: Antinuclear antibody, Anti-smooth-muscle antibody
    Type 2: Anti-liver kidney microsomal antibody
    Type 3: Anti-soluble liver antigen/liver pancreas
Histologic findings compatible with chronic hepatitis

Al-Khalidi JA, Czaja AJ: Current concepts in the diagnosis, pathogenesis, and treatment of autoimmune hepatitis. Mayo Clin Proc 2001;76:1237. [PMID: 11761505]

PRIMARY BILIARY CIRRHOSIS

Primary biliary cirrhosis (PBC) is a chronic, cholestatic liver disease of unknown cause, although an autoimmune etiology is strongly suggested. PBC is diagnosed almost exclusively (90% or higher) in middle-aged females of all ethnic descents.

 ESSENTIALS OF DIAGNOSIS

- *Elevation of antimitochondrial antibody (AMA) with a titer > 1:80.*
- *Evidence for cholestatic liver disorder (elevated SAP).*
- *Confirmatory liver histology.*

Clinical Findings

More than 80% of patients with PBC have another autoimmune disease: thyroiditis, sicca syndrome, Raynaud's disease, CREST syndrome, celiac disease, or rheumatoid arthritis. The initial clinical presentation of PBC may be subdivided into 3 clinical stages:

(1) Symptomatic stage: The symptomatic stage occurs in the presence of jaundice, pruritus, and fatigue. The SAP level may be quite elevated, and the histologic state of the liver often includes the presence of bridging fibrosis or cirrhosis (histologic stage 3 or 4). This clinical stage is the "classic" presentation for PBC but rarely is encountered today.

(2) Asymptomatic stage: The asymptomatic stage most often is uncovered during the evaluation for elevated SAP when a positive AMA is identified. No symptoms of jaundice or pruritus are present, and the liver biopsy most often shows early histologic abnormalities, similar to those of chronic persistent hepatitis or a mild case of chronic active hepatitis (histologic stage 1 or 2). This presentation is the one most commonly seen today.

(3) Preclinical stage: The preclinical stage is identified in patients who have no symptoms; the SAP level is normal. Because PBC is associated with other autoimmune-related disorders, this stage is often identified by an elevated AMA found during the course of serologic assessment. Symptoms may develop in one third of these patients over the next 5 years. Almost all of these patients will have liver biopsy histology diagnostic of PBC, even though the SAP levels are normal.

Diagnosis

A diagnosis of PBC is made most often in the course of evaluating an elevated SAP level. PBC is associated with an autoantibody, the AMA, which is highly disease-specific when present in titers exceeding 1:80. A liver biopsy is recommended to confirm the diagnosis and to define the histologic stage. Additional assessment of the biliary system may be required if the AMA is negative or the liver biopsy is inconclusive. In this context, an endoscopic retrograde cholangiopancreatography may be indicated.

Treatment

Ursodeoxycholic acid (ursodiol) is the current treatment of PBC. The dosage is 13–15 mg/kg/d. Ursodiol is a safe medication with few side effects that may improve biochemical parameters and slow the histologic progression of the disease. Modeling analysis of ursodiol treatment suggests that it delays progression to cirrhosis for more than 20 years in patients having histologic stages 1 and 2 at the time of the initial diagnosis.

Prognosis

PBC is a progressive liver disease that, in most instances, will eventually evolve into cirrhosis, an event that may take up to several decades. Patients with no symptoms, early histologic stage, and a normal serum bilirubin are expected to have a normal 10-year survival, matched for their age. Once symptoms develop, especially pruritus, and the serum bilirubin level exceeds 2.5 mg/dL, the 5-year prognosis is greatly modified. Patients with PBC who require liver transplantation have a very favorable outcome, compared with other liver diseases.

Heathcote EJ: Management of primary biliary cirrhosis. The American Association for the Study of Liver Diseases practice guidelines. Hepatology 2000;31:1005. [PMID: 10733559]

Heathcote J: Primary biliary cirrhosis. Clin Perspect Gastroenterol 2001;4:39.

HEREDITARY HEMOCHROMATOSIS

Hereditary hemochromatosis is the most common genetic disorder among whites of Western European descent. It is an autosomal recessive disorder with the frequency of homozygosity approaching 1 per 200 in the population. An inappropriate and increased iron absorption in the proximal small intestine leads to massive degrees of parenchymal iron overload in the liver, pancreas, heart, and anterior pituitary gland.

ESSENTIALS OF DIAGNOSIS

- *Abnormal fasting iron studies: transferrin saturation > 45% and/or an elevated serum ferritin level.*
- *Confirmatory gene testing.*

Diagnosis

Any adult having abnormal liver enzyme elevations should be evaluated for hereditary hemochromatosis. It should also be considered in patients with fatigue and arthropathies involving the metacarpal phalangeal joints and hypogonadism. The diagnosis of hereditary hemochromatosis should be suspected on the basis of any abnormally elevated serum iron tests.

A gene test now exists that is readily used when hemochromatosis is suspected. A single point mutation on chromosome 6 results in the abnormal gene, leading to the substitution of tyrosine for cysteine at the 282 amino acid position (the C282Y gene mutation). The gene test evaluates for this C282Y mutation and is present in over 90% of whites with demonstrated iron overload. A second mutation, H63D, does not appear to cause any iron overload disorder.

Although women are protected from iron overload to some degree by pregnancies and menses, homozygote females do develop iron overload with the full phenotypic expression of the disorder. Compared with men of a similar age at the time of diagnosis, the degree of iron overload is less.

A liver biopsy is often performed during the evaluation of hereditary hemochromatosis, since it will confirm the diagnosis by hepatic iron quantitation and determine the presence or absence of significant liver fibrosis. In younger patients (< 40 years in age) with normal AST/ALT levels and a serum ferritin level < 1000 ng/mL, a liver biopsy is not required in patients with documented homozygosity by genetic testing, since it is unlikely that any degree of liver fibrosis or additional end-stage damage in any other organs is present.

The clinical importance of diagnosing hereditary hemochromatosis is to initiate appropriate treatment and for subsequent gene testing of first-degree relatives.

Treatment & Prognosis

The standard treatment of hereditary hemochromatosis is therapeutic phlebotomy, which is the withdrawal of 500 mL of blood, containing 250 mg of iron. Most homozygotes have an excess total body iron in the range of 5–20 g. This treatment is safe and highly effective. Once the patients approach iron depletion, maintenance phletomies, usually 3 to 4 times yearly, are required to prevent the reaccumulation of iron overload. Successful therapeutic phlebotomy prevents progression of the organ damage and leads to a normal 20-year survival in patients who do not have cirrhosis at the time of diagnosis.

Moirand R et al: Clinical features of genetic hemochromatosis in women compared with men. Ann Intern Med 1997;127:105. [PMID: 9229998]

Tavill AS: Diagnosis and management of hemochromatosis. Hepatology 2001;33:1321. [PMID: 11343262]

ALCOHOLIC LIVER DISEASE

Although the manifestations of alcoholic liver disease are similar in women and men, important differences exist. Women appear to be more susceptible to liver injury from alcohol, and the amount of alcohol consumed per day required to produce serious alcoholic liver injury is less than in men. Consumption of 40 g or more of alcohol per day appears to increase the potential for significant alcoholic liver injury that might lead to cirrhosis. Forty grams of alcohol is equivalent to 3 "drinks" of 12 oz beer, 1 5 oz glass of wine, or 1.5 oz of 80 proof spirits; all of which contain approximately 13–14 g of alcohol. Women's greater susceptibility may be related to size and gender differences in alcohol metabolism. Women have a smaller volume of distribution for serum alcohol levels, which leads to higher blood alcohol levels for the equivalent amount of alcohol consumed, compared with men. There also may be differences in the peripheral metabolism of alcohol in women who have lesser concentrations of alcohol dehydrogenase in the stomach, leading to higher concentrations of alcohol delivered to the liver through the portal vein. The duration of alcohol abuse is also important; significant liver injury rarely is found with less than 5 years of abuse, and the risk markedly escalates with 20 years or longer of abuse.

ESSENTIALS OF DIAGNOSIS

- *Risk of alcohol liver disease in women increases when more than 40 g of alcohol are consumed daily.*
- *AST:ALT ratio exceeds 1.5 ("reversed" ratio from other chronic liver diseases).*

• Liver steatosis or steatohepatitis identified on liver biopsy histology.

Diagnosis

Women are less likely than men to be suspected of alcohol abuse; a factor that may delay the diagnosis of alcoholism in women and allow the liver injury to progress to a more advanced stage before it is finally diagnosed. Often, alcohol abuse is covert, and it is only through direct questioning of the patient or the intervention of concerned family members that its existence is revealed. Use of the CAGE questionnaire or the Alcohol Use Disorders Identification Test (AUDIT) often identifies women with alcohol abuse. A liver biopsy is useful to disclose the presence of steatohepatitis (also known as alcoholic hepatitis). This liver disease may be particularly severe when the presence of jaundice, a prolonged prothombin time, and/or portal-systemic encephalopathy is present.

Treatment & Prognosis

The key intervention is abstinence from alcohol and often a very direct approach through inpatient or outpatient therapy is necessary, often with aftercare through Alcoholics Anonymous. Hepatic steatosis will resolve quickly with alcohol abstinence. Patients having severe features of steatohepatitis may require the use of corticosteroids that may be lifesaving. The natural history of alcoholic hepatitis may be different in women, who are more likely to progress to cirrhosis than men, even if they remain abstinent from alcohol.

Patients with chronic hepatitis B or C should be cautioned that abuse of alcohol may worsen the degree of liver injury.

Abittan CS, Lieber CS: Alcoholic liver disease. Clin Perspect Gastroenterol 1999;2:257.

NONALCOHOLIC FATTY LIVER DISEASE

One of the most common causes for asymptomatic elevations in the serum AST/ALT is fatty infiltration of the liver (steatosis). Testing for disease-specific markers can exclude the vast majority of other causes for the abnormally elevated liver enzymes. Once these are ruled out, a clinical diagnosis of steatosis can be made with a high degree of confidence in patients with a combination of obesity, hyperlipidemia (particularly hypertriglyceridemia), and/or glucose intolerance. When liver ultrasonography reveals increased echogenicity, steatosis is the most likely diagnosis and, in the absence of other causes, it may not be necessary to recommend a liver biopsy to confirm the clinical impression.

Nonalcoholic steatohepatitis (NASH) syndrome was initially identified in obese, middle-aged women who often had type 2 diabetes mellitus. The prevalence of NASH syndrome is rising, largely due to the increasing occurrence of obesity in the United States population. Most individuals with NASH syndrome have obesity, type 2 diabetes mellitus, and hyperlipidemia in various combinations. The central metabolic defect for NASH syndrome is insulin resistance, which can be identified in nonobese individuals with NASH syndrome.

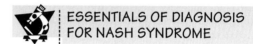

ESSENTIALS OF DIAGNOSIS FOR NASH SYNDROME

• *Histologic picture of steatohepatitis.*
• *Convincing evidence of minimal or no alcohol consumption, < 40 g/wk.*
• *Absence of serologic evidence for chronic viral hepatitis.*

Clinical Findings

Most patients have asymptomatic elevations of the AST/ALT, and radiographic imaging studies are consistent with diffuse fatty infiltration of the liver. The liver histology shows a spectrum, ranging from macrovesicular fatty liver to steatohepatitis with and without fibrosis to cirrhosis.

Treatment

Since NASH syndrome is not a primary liver disease and results from severe underlying metabolic disturbances, treatment is directed toward improvement and correction of these abnormalities. Ursodiol, in a clinical trial, has stabilized the liver biochemical abnormalities.

Prognosis

The long-term prognosis of NASH syndrome is uncertain. It is not known whether medical interventions, such as control of type 2 diabetes mellitus, improvement in lipid abnormalities, or marked weight reduction actually improves the histologic lesion. However, NASH is increasingly recognized as a prominent cause of "cryptogenic" cirrhosis.

Angulo P: Nonalcoholic fatty liver disease. N Engl J Med 2002; 346:1221. [PMID: 11961152]

Sanjal AJ: Nonalcoholic steatohepatitis. Clin Perspect Gastroenterol 2000;3:129.

WILSON'S DISEASE

In patients younger than 40 years, Wilson's disease should be excluded. Wilson's disease is a rare autosomal recessive genetic (frequency of 1 in 40,000) disorder that may present with signs of liver disease or a neurologic disorder. Wilson's disease is characterized by the abnormal accumulation of copper in the liver and central nervous system. The initial laboratory test for Wilson's disease is measurement of the serum ceruloplasmin level. If the serum ceruloplasmin level is low or borderline-low, additional studies are indicated, including a 24-hour urine collection for copper and a slit-lamp examination for Kayser-Fleischer rings. If the diagnosis is suspected, a liver biopsy is indicated to quantitate copper in the liver. This diagnosis is particularly important because treatment with D-penicillamine or zinc acetate prevents many of the serious complications of Wilson's disease.

COMPLEMENTARY THERAPIES & THE LIVER

Complementary and alternative medicine (CAM) use has risen over the last 10 years with close to 50% of interviewed households reporting CAM use and 12% using herbal agents. Physicians cannot readily ignore CAM use in their patients and should inquire about it in a nonconfrontational manner.

Several CAM products are readily used by patients with chronic liver diseases, especially chronic hepatitis C. Silymarin, an extract of silybum marianum (milk thistle), is a frequently used agent by patients with chronic hepatitis C. Randomized clinical trials have not evaluated its clinical efficacy in chronic hepatitis C. Silymarin, however, appears to lack significant side effects.

Glycyrrhizin (licorice root extract) is another CAM agent used in the treatment of chronic liver conditions. No randomized controlled trials on its effectiveness have been reported. Because it has mineralocorticoid activity, its use should be avoided in cirrhotic patients, secondary to worsening of fluid retention and electrolyte disturbances.

Other blended herbal formulations and extracts are used to treat various liver disorders. Rigorous testing of these modalities is lacking.

On the other hand, the easy availability of "natural" herbal agents and vitamins does not imply their safety. Severe and significant hepatic toxicity may result from the uses of some of these compounds.

Two commonly used vitamin compounds may cause hepatotoxicity. First, megadoses of vitamin A may lead to a serious and irreversible liver injury. Daily ingestion of 20,000-25,000 units for 5 or more years or 50,000 units for as short as 2 years may result in significant hepatic fibrosis, leading to portal hypertension. Second, nicotinic acid (niacin) is used as an over-the-counter treatment of hypercholesterolemia. Acute hepatotoxicity may occur after taking 2–4 g/d of sustained-release nicotinic acid for 2–4 weeks.

The list of herbal agents causing hepatotoxicity is ever growing (Table 27–6). An acute liver injury with marked elevations of the AST/ALT is the most common manifestation of herbal hepatotoxicity. A second pattern of liver injury is veno-occlusive disease. This disorder results in the fibrous occlusion of hepatic

Table 27–6. Hepatotoxicity caused by herbal agents.

Herbal Agent	Type of Toxicity
Cascara sagrada	Cholestasis
Celander (chelidonium majus)	AH
Chaparrel leaf (Larrea tridentata)	AH
Germander (Teudrium chamaedrys)	AH
Jin bu huan	AH
Kava (rhizome of pepper plant)	AH
Kombucha mushroom (tea)	AH
Ma-huang (ephedra)	AH
Margosa oil	Microvesicular steatosis
Mistletoe	AH
Pennyroyal (squawmit oil)	AH
Pyrrolizidine alkaloids	
Crotolaria	VOD
Gondolobo herbal tea	VOD
Heliotropium	VOD
Mate (Paraguay) tea	VOD
Symphytum officinale (Comfrey)	VOD
Saw palmetto	Cholestasis
TJ-9	
Dai-saiko-to	AH
Sho-saiko-to	AH
Valerian root and skullcap	AH

AH, acute hepatitis; VOD, veno-occlusive disease.
(Modified from Chitturi, Farrell GC: Herbal hepatotoxicity: an expanding but poorly defined problem. J Gastroenterol Hepatol 2000;15:1093 and from Seefe et al: Hepatology 2001;34:595.

venules, leading to ascites formation and liver failure. Of greater concern is that these compounds can be transported across the placenta with the subsequent development of veno-occlusive disease in the neonate.

The experiences with these easily obtained compounds illustrates the requirement for careful history-taking from patients who present with an unexplained liver disease, since many of these herbal agents may present with a serious liver disorder.

Chitturi S, Farrell GC: Herbal hepatotoxicity: an expanding but poorly defined problem. J Gastroenterol Hepatol 2000;15: 1093. [PMID: 11106086]

Flora K, Benner KG: Treating liver disease with alternative therapy. Clin Perspect Gastroenterol 2001;4:51.

Seefe LB et al: Complementary and alternative medicine in chronic liver disease. Hepatology 2001;34:595. [PMID: 11526548]

Relevant Web Sites

[The American Liver Foundation]
www.liverfoundation.org

Irritable Bowel Syndrome

28

William P. Johnson, MD

ESSENTIALS OF DIAGNOSIS

Based on the recently modified Rome criteria, irritable bowel syndrome (IBS) is defined as the presence of abdominal pain for at least 12 weeks (not necessarily consecutive) in the preceding 12 months that cannot be explained by structural or biochemical abnormalities and has at least two of the following three features:

–Pain relieved with defecation, or

–Onset associated with a change in the form of the stool (loose, watery, or pellet-like), or

–Onset is associated with a change in the frequency of bowel movements (diarrhea or constipation).

General Considerations

Approximately 15% of adults in the United States report symptoms that are consistent with the diagnosis of IBS. IBS is the most common diagnosis made by gastroenterologists in the United States and accounts for 12% of visits to primary care physicians. It is estimated that only 25% of persons with this condition seek medical care for it, and studies suggest that those who seek care are more likely to have behavioral and psychiatric problems than are those who do not seek care. In addition, patients with this diagnosis are at increased risk for other, nongastrointestinal functional disorders such as fibromyalgia and interstitial cystitis. IBS accounts for an estimated $8 billion in direct medical costs and $25 billion in indirect costs annually in the United States alone.

Although IBS was originally described in women of Northern European ancestry, sociocultural studies indicate that this disorder is found in all cultural groups and both genders. There is nothing unique about the way IBS presents in women; however, the disease affects three times as many women as men. Whether this difference reflects a true predominance of the disorder among women or merely the fact that women are more likely to seek medical care has not been determined.

Pathogenesis

Altered bowel motility, visceral hypersensitivity, psychosocial factors, an imbalance in neurotransmitters, and infection have all been proposed as playing a part in the development of IBS. To date, no single conceptual model can explain all cases of the syndrome.

A. ALTERED BOWEL MOTILITY

It is well known that psychological or physical stress as well as ingestion of food may alter the contractility of the colon. A variety of abnormal motility of the small bowel has been described in patients with IBS; however, there is no consistent pattern in those suffering from this disorder. Pain is more frequently associated with irregular motor activity of the small bowel in patients with this syndrome than in normal controls or patients with inflammatory bowel disease.

B. VISCERAL HYPERSENSITIVITY

Patients with IBS experience pain and bloating when balloon-distention studies are performed. These balloons are placed in the rectosigmoid and the ileum, and when inflated, they produce pain and bloating at significantly lower pressures in patients with IBS than in control subjects. This phenomenon has been called **visceral hypersensitivity.** One explanation for this phenomenon is that the sensitivity of receptors in the viscus is altered through recruitment of silent nociceptors in response to ischemia, distention, intraluminal contents, infections, or psychiatric factors. Some data suggest that there is a primary central defect of visceral pain processing. Other data have suggested that hypervigilance rather than true visceral hypersensitivity may be responsible for the low pain threshold in patients with IBS.

C. PSYCHOSOCIAL FACTORS

It is well known that stress can alter motor function in the small bowel and colon in both normal subjects and patients with IBS. At referral centers, the prevalence of psychiatric symptoms such as somatization, depression, and anxiety are much higher in patients with IBS than in control subjects. It has been proposed that experiences in early childhood, especially sexual or physical abuse, may affect the central nervous system and confer a predisposition to a state of hypervigilance.

D. Neurotransmitter Imbalance

Ninety-five percent of serotonin is located in the gastrointestinal tract within enterochromaffin cells, neurons, mast cells, and smooth muscle cells. When serotonin is released, it stimulates extrinsic vagal efferent nerve fibers, resulting in such physiologic responses as intestinal secretion and the peristaltic reflex and this results in such symptoms as nausea, vomiting, abdominal pain, and bloating. There is preliminary evidence that patients with IBS have increased serotonin levels in plasma and in the rectosigmoid colon.

E. Infection and Inflammation

There is convincing evidence that inflammation of the enteric mucosa or neural plexuses initiates or contributes to symptoms associated with IBS. Mucosal inflammatory cytokines may activate peripheral sensitization or hypermotilitiy. There is also some evidence that infectious enteritis may lead to chronic symptoms compatible with IBS.

Prevention

One prevention strategy is to recognize and then modify risk factors for the disease process. The only recognized risk factors for IBS is physical and/or sexual assault in childhood. It is unlikely that internists will see at-risk patients before symptoms develop; however, pediatricians, family practitioners, and emergency department physicians need to be aware of this association. Appropriate referral to a mental health professional may improve clinical outcome.

Clinical Findings

A. Symptoms and Signs

Abdominal discomfort or pain, pain relieved with defecation, change in frequency of bowel movements (constipation and/or diarrhea), change in stool consistency, bloating, and excessive gas are symptoms of IBS. Symptoms may be further classified as pain predominant, diarrhea predominant, and constipation predominant.

- **Pain predominant:** A recent meta-analysis suggests that antispasmodic agents and tricyclic compounds are effective in treating selected patients. Treatment with selective serotonin reuptake inhibitors (SSRIs) has been disappointing. Although not proven, SSRIs that predominately target serotonin may actually increase symptoms, since preliminary data indicate that these patients may have increased levels of serotonin in the plasma and bowel wall. In patients who have pain refractory to treatment with antispasmodics and tricyclic antidepressants, treatment with classic analgesics such as nonsteroidal anti-inflammatory drugs may control pain and improve the quality of life.

- **Diarrhea predominant:** When diarrhea is the predominant symptom, classic antidiarrheal agents such as loperamide and diphenoxylate may help decrease the frequency of bowel movements and improve the consistency of stool. In cases that do not respond to these agents, cholestyramine has been used to bind bile acids that may be responsible for increased secretion and decreased absorption of water in the colon.

- **Constipation predominant:** Increasing fiber consumption is the first step along with adequate water intake (6 glasses per day). Constipation may also be treated with osmotic laxatives such as nonabsorbable carbohydrates (lactulose and sorbitol), milk of magnesia or magnesium citrate, or a polyethylene glycol solution.

Signs of IBS include abdominal distention and pain to abdominal palpation that is out of proportion to the complaint.

B. Laboratory Findings

Routine laboratory tests should include a complete blood cell count, chemistry profile, urinalysis, and thyroid-stimulating hormone measurement. All results should all be normal.

C. Imaging Studies

In patients younger than 50 years with no other risk factors, a flexible sigmoidoscopy alone should be adequate. In patients who are aged 50 or older or who have other risk factors, a colonoscopy should be performed. In patients who have diarrhea predominant IBS, biopsies of the mucosa from the distal colon should be performed to rule out microscopic colitis. In some patients, a barium enema and flexible sigmoidoscopy may be substituted for a colonoscopy.

D. Special Tests

Stool for enteric pathogens, fecal leukocytes, and *Clostridium difficile* toxin should be performed. All results should be negative.

Differential Diagnosis

The diagnosis of IBS is suggested when a patient's symptoms meet the Rome criteria and a complete clinical examination and basic testing is normal. If there are abnormalities on examination and/or testing or if an alarm symptom is present, then IBS becomes a diagnosis of exclusion. Alarm symptoms include evidence of gastrointestinal bleeding such as occult blood in the stool, rectal bleeding, or anemia; anorexia or weight loss; fever; persistent diarrhea causing dehydration or nocturnal symptoms; severe constipation or fecal impaction; a family history of gastrointestinal cancer, inflammatory bowel disease, or celiac sprue; and the onset of symptoms after the age of 50. A number of structural or metabolic abnormalities can cause symptoms similar to IBS, including lactase deficiency; colon cancer; diverticulosis; IBD including microscopic colitis; enteric infection; ischemia; maldigestion or malabsorption; and endometriosis, which is suggested by the presence of pelvic pain at the time of the menstrual period. In the absence of alarm symptoms, the presence of one of these structural or metabolic disorders is very unlikely.

Complications

Most of the complications of IBS will be iatrogenic and related to diagnostic testing and drug therapy. Because many of these patients will have psychosocial concerns, the use of habituating substances like benzodiazepines should be reserved for patients with documented anxiety disorders. It is also possible for patients to restrict their diet so severely that they develop nutritional disorders.

Treatment

A. LIFESTYLE CHANGES

All patients may benefit from a review of their diet; limiting fatty foods, gas-producing vegetables, or products containing sorbitol is recommended. In addition, slowly adding 20–30 g of fiber per day either in the diet

or in the form of supplements such as bran, polycarbophil, or psyllium may relieve constipation.

B. PHARMACOLOGIC

Although many medications have been used to treat IBS, few have been tested in controlled, double-blind studies with adequate statistical power. The commonly used drugs, their doses, and costs are listed in Table 28–1.

C. COMPLEMENTARY THERAPY

The potential benefits of supportive therapy, relaxation exercises, hypnosis, cognitive behavioral therapy, and psychodynamic interpersonal psychotherapy are well recognized. Behavioral feedback has been tried for symptom control but has no lasting effect. There is no convincing evidence that homeopathic therapies such as Asa foetida D3 work or botanic remedies such as aloe vera have any effect on this disorder.

When to Refer to a Specialist

Referral may be appropriate when any of the alarm symptoms listed under differential diagnosis are present. Additional testing that may be obtained before referral include computed tomographic scanning of the abdomen and pelvis, radiographic evaluation of the

Table 28–1. Common medications used to treat irritable bowel syndrome.

Drug	Dose	Cost
Anticholinergic agents		
Dicyclomine	10–40 mg q6h before meals and at bedtime	10 mg (30 caps): $11.48
Hyoscymine	0.125–0.25 mg sublingual q4h	0.125 mg (90 tabs): $52.28
Antidiarrheal agents		
Loperamide	4–8 mg daily in single or divided doses	2 mg (30 caps): $5.65
Diphenoxylate plus atropine	2 tablets 4 times daily	2.5 mg (30 tabs): $19.78
Cholestyramine resin	1 packet (9 g) once or twice daily	4 g (60 packets, 4 g): $60.24
Osmotic laxatives		
Lactulose	15–30 mL daily	480 mL bottle: $27.20
Polyethylene glycol solution	17 g in 240 mL of water daily	1 packet: $13.90
Tricyclic compounds		
Amitriptyline	25–75 mg/d	25 mg (30 tabs): $7.99
Nortriptyline	25–75 mg/d	25 mg (30 tabs): $7.99
Desipramine	25–75 mg/d	25 mg (60 tabs): $7.99

small intestine, and antiendomysial antibody test to screen for celiac sprue.

Prognosis

This disorder is chronic and is highlighted by periods of flares followed by relative quiescence. This disorder does not predispose to any more serious gastrointestinal abnormality.

Drossman DA et al: Sexual and physical abuse and gastrointestinal illness. Ann Intern Med 1995;123:782. [PMID: 7574197]

Horwitz BJ, Fisher RS: The irritable bowel syndrome. N Engl J Med 2001;344:1846. [PMID: 11407347]

Jailwala J, Imperiale TF, Kroenke K: Pharmacologic treatment of the irritable bowel syndrome: a systematic review of randomized, controlled trials. Ann Intern Med 2000;133:136. [PMID: 10896640]

Relevant Web Sites

[National Institute of Diabetes & Digestive & Kidney Diseases] http://www.niddk.nih.gov/health/digest/pubs/irrbowel/irrbowel.htm

SECTION VIII

Cardiovascular Disorders

Risk Factors for Coronary Artery Disease & Their Treatment

29

Edward F. Gibbons, MD

Coronary artery disease (CAD) is the leading cause of death in the United States. Despite a lower overall population prevalence of CAD in women, women and men die of CAD in equal numbers. The death rate from cardiovascular disease (CVD) is nearly twice the death rate from all cancers in women. Risk factors for CAD in women include the postmenopausal state, hyperlipidemia, hypertension, diabetes, smoking, obesity, family history, and use of oral contraceptives in smokers and older women. In addition, a low level of formal education is associated with a higher risk of coronary disease developing in women.

A progressive decline in the death rate from CVD has occurred over the past 25 years, but the slower rate of decline in women compared with men serves to underscore the lethal nature of established coronary disease in women. Modification of risk factors for coronary disease in women is an emerging science; thus far, only cessation of cigarette smoking and cholesterol-lowering drugs (ie, statins) have been shown to confer benefit to women.

ESSENTIALS OF DIAGNOSIS

- *Ischemic coronary disease*
- *Stroke*
- *Congestive heart failure*

General Considerations

CVD is the most common cause of death in women. Yearly, more than 2.5 million women in the United States are hospitalized for cardiovascular disease; 500,000 of these women die annually. Nearly half of these deaths are caused by ischemic coronary disease and the remaining number by stroke, congestive heart failure, or a combination of the three.

CVD as a public health problem in women has been underemphasized when compared with other gender-specific and general diseases. CAD and stroke claim almost twice as many lives as cancers (Figure 29–1). These data show, however, that cancer generally afflicts young women and CAD affects older women. Many more women seek evaluation for cancer prevention than for CVD, despite the higher lifetime risk for heart disease. Fortunately, the overall incidence of CAD and stroke in the general population has fallen progressively over the past 25 years: the coronary death rate has fallen nearly 50% from 1970 to 1990, and the stroke death rate has fallen 57% during the same time period (Figure 29–2). Women as well as men have benefited from this decline in overall age-adjusted mortality, but white women have benefited somewhat less than white men, and black women have benefited less than white men or women or black men (Figure 29–3). The reasons for this general decline in cardiovascular mortality are not clear, but the drop has been attributed to the effects of blood pressure control, reduction of dietary fat, decline in cigarette smoking, and improved care of established coronary disease in myocardial infarction.

The incidence of CAD follows a different pattern in men and women. Although the diagnosis of CAD increases decade by decade in both sexes, women acquire the disease approximately 6–10 years later than men. Because women live longer than men, by the time they reach their eighth or ninth decade of life, their death rate from coronary disease equals that of men of the

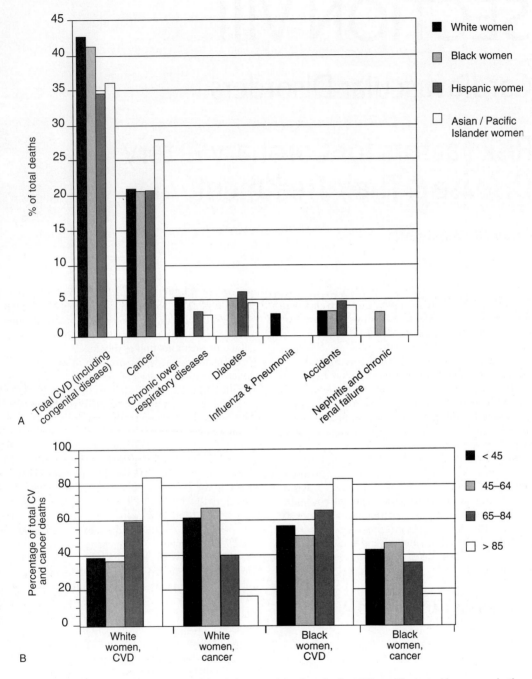

Figure 29–1. The leading causes of death for American females in 1999 are illustrated by age and ethnicity (**A**). The change in cause of mortality with age group for black and white women shifts late after menopause (**B**).

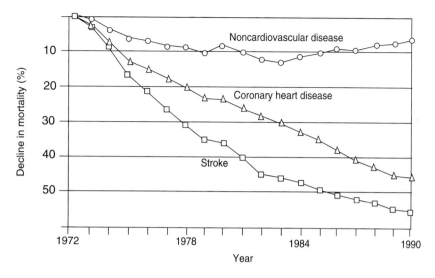

Figure 29–2. Decline in age-adjusted mortality from cardiovascular disease and stroke in the United States since 1972. (Courtesy of National Center for Health Statistics and the National Heart, Lung, and Blood Institute.)

same age. This demographic has resulted in an actual net increase in cardiovascular mortality for women compared with men over the past 20 years (Figure 29–4). The Framingham Heart Study, from its earlier publications over the past 30 years, emphasized the gender differences in presentation with coronary disease. Women were 10 years older than their male counterparts when they sought medical attention for any manifestation of CAD, and they were 20 years older than their male cohorts when they had their first myocardial infarction. In this group, angina was more likely to be present in women than in men (69% versus 30%). Yet within 5 years of the development of angina, myocardial infarction developed in 25% of men and only 14% of women. Even the most recent update from Framingham shows similar gender differences.

Risk Factors

Women and men share most of the risk factors for CAD established by the Framingham study: hypercholesterolemia, hypertension, diabetes, obesity greater than 30% over ideal body weight, family history, and cigarette smoking. Fortunately, the National Cholesterol Education Program (NCEP) has added the postmenopausal state to their list of risk factors for coronary disease in women. The additive effects of these Framingham risk factors apply to both men and women; Figure 29–5 illustrates their multiplicative effect in the Framingham study.

Emerging Risk Factors

Recent studies have suggested a link between elevated levels of some circulating blood elements, and the long-term risk for coronary events. Lipoprotein (a) has a stronger predictive capacity for men than women. Homocysteine levels are generally predictive for coronary and vascular disease and appear to be reduced with B vitamins (folate, pyridoxine, and B_{12}). C-reactive protein, an inflammatory protein, has been found to be present in higher levels in both men and women in whom significant CAD develops. For all of these emerging risk factors, specific treatments and clinical efficacy remain conjecture.

Treatment of Modifiable Risk Factors

CAD develops in the majority of women during the postmenopausal years. As mean survival time of women continues to increase and to exceed that of men, the amount of time a woman spends in the postmenopausal years is clearly increasing. A woman who lives until the age of 85 spends more than one third of her life in the postmenopausal state. Little is known concerning the reasons women under the age of 50 are so well protected against cardiovascular disease, and less is known about how the deterioration of this protection after the age of 50 occurs. There is even less information concerning how to retard or prevent the clinical development of CVD in women. Clinical trials of risk factor intervention prior to myocardial infarction, eg,

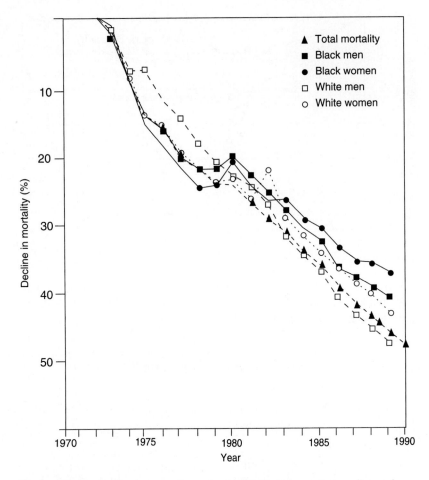

Figure 29–3. Decline in age-adjusted mortality for coronary artery disease by race and gender since 1972. ▲ = total mortality; ■ = black men; ● = black women; ❑ = white men; ○ = white women. (Courtesy of National Center for Health Statistics and the National Heart, Lung, and Blood Institute.)

the MILIS Study, have excluded women by design. Younger women most often are excluded from drug or lifestyle modification studies because of "considerations of childbearing" and because CVD incidence in the short term is so low that statistical design would require enormous numbers of women in treatment arms to provide evidence of a significant risk or benefit. Elderly potential victims of CVD (presently, men and women in near equal numbers) may be excluded because of co-morbidity or "advanced disease." For these and other reasons, including bias, evidence showing that CAD risk factor intervention in women might be effective is far less than for men. However, some guidance data that are available are reviewed here.

A. HORMONE REPLACEMENT THERAPY

Based on current data including the Womens Health Initiative (WHI), HRT cannot be recommended for prevention of CVD.

Selective estrogen replacement modulators (SERMs), such as tamoxifen and raloxifene, are now being studied for their impact on lipids and cardiovascular risk. Raloxifene is being evaluated in ongoing studies to eval-

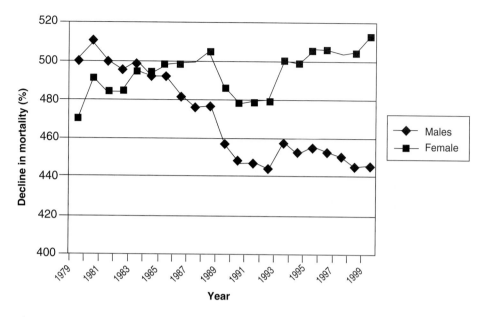

Figure 29–4. The incidence of coronary artery disease in men exceeds that in women until late in life. Although the cardiovascular mortality rate for men has fallen over the past 20 years, women have suffered a rise in total cardiovascular mortality. (Data from the Centers for Disease Control and Prevention and the American Heart Association.)

uate the drug's effect on lipids and markers of cardiovascular risk (MORE study), as well as on myocardial infarction and CVD risk, stroke, breast cancer, and fractures (RUTH study).

The decision to use postmenopausal hormonal therapy must be individualized with the risk of thromboembolism, myocardial infarction, stroke, endometrial carcinoma and higher risk of breast carcinoma, and side effects of the medications. Decision-making must involve the patient and other health care providers to focus on proven methods of CVD risk reduction, osteoporosis prevention and treatment, and reduction of postmenopausal symptoms. Postmenopausal hormones are not recommended to reduce CHD Risk.

B. Hyperlipidemia

The relationship between cholesterol level as a risk factor and treatment risk reduction is generally accepted, although public health issues of cost-effectiveness and population targeting continue to be debated. Both the LRC Study and the Helsinki Study have shown that lipid-lowering drug therapy in high-risk men reduces CAD incidence but not all-cause mortality. Women have been excluded from, or included in insufficient numbers in, primary prevention studies of lipid therapy. It is impossi-

ble to prescribe treatment based on proven benefit because of the lack of substantial prospective, controlled studies of women. The AFCAPS/TexCAPS study suggested, however, that in the 990 women enrolled, a trend toward coronary event reduction was seen with lovastatin and a cholesterol-lowering diet. Of the primary prevention trials available, they have only shown a trend toward coronary event reduction in women (AFCAPS/TexCAPS) or no benefit at all, perhaps because of the overall low short-term event rate in the women enrolled.

No convincing study has demonstrated efficacy of dietary therapy alone in primary CAD prevention in either men or women.

Secondary prevention of CAD morbidity and mortality with lipid-lowering therapy, however, may be valid in both women and men. Angina and recurrent infarction appear to be lessened in degree in men and in the smaller numbers of women with established CAD who have been treated aggressively with lipid-lowering drug therapy.

Several randomized, controlled trials of lipid-lowering statin drugs have included women in secondary prevention. Of the 4444 patients in the Scandinavian Simvastatin Survival Study (4S), 827 were women. In this trial, although total cardiovascular mortality was reduced, the result was only statistically significant in

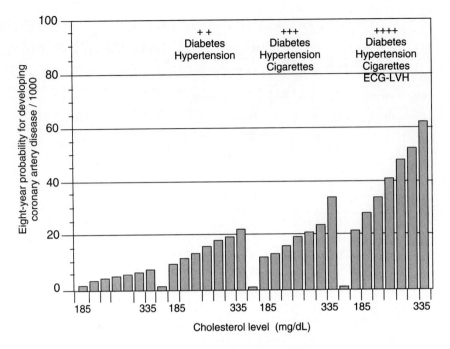

Figure 29–5. Additive effects on the development of coronary artery disease of multiple risk factors: elevated cholesterol, diabetes, hypertension, cigarette smoking, and left ventricular hypertrophy (LVH) on electrocardiogram (ECG). The data are derived for 35-year-old men monitored for 18 years in the Framingham Study, expressed as the 8-year probability of developing coronary heart disease. (Adapted, with permission, from Castelli WP: Epidemiology of coronary heart disease: The Framingham Study. Am J Med 1984;76:4.)

men. Major coronary events, however, were reduced 35% and 34% in men and women, respectively. Similarly, the Cholesterol and Recurrent Events (CARE) study (Figure 29–6) demonstrated a 24% 5-year reduction in fatal myocardial infarction and CHD death for the total population. When gender effect was analyzed, women benefited primarily from a reduction of combined CHD death, nonfatal infarction, and revascularization (46% reduction compared with 20% in males).

The NCEP, Second and Third Reports, places greater emphasis on CAD in women as a problem, postmenopausal state as a risk factor, and female family member with CAD under the age of 65 as a separate risk factor. Although lipoprotein fraction risks have a gender difference, overall CAD risk factors are nearly identical (Table 29–1), and CAD complications and infarction mortality rates are higher in women. Because risk represents a continuum from primary to secondary prevention, a broad public health strategy has been formulated to stratify and treat hyperlipidemia in women.

The Adult Treatment Panel III Guidelines from the NCEP have recently been published. These propose virtually the same strategy for lipid treatment in both men and women, based on short-term and long-term risk of developing CHD. The essential elements of the guideline are summarized in the Box, The Adult Treatment Panel III Guideline Steps in the evaluation and treatment of serum cholesterol.

C. HYPERTENSION

Although women tolerate hypertension for a longer time than men before they show signs of CVD complications, their hypertension accelerates the atherosclerotic process and the risk of myocardial infarction, stroke, and congestive heart failure. The general benefit of antihypertensive therapy has been demonstrated in several large trials. However, the significant reduction in cardiovascular mortality and morbidity has applied most specifically to patients with severe hypertension. Men, who have more atherosclerotic disease, and black

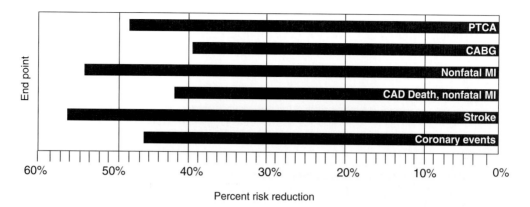

Figure 29–6. The Cholesterol and Recurrent Events Trial (CARE) demonstrated efficacy of cardiac event reduction in its 4159 subjects; 576 of the participants were women. In these women, treatment with pravastatin significantly reduced total coronary events, stroke, death caused by coronary artery disease (CAD), nonfatal myocardial infarction (MI), and the need for revascularization procedures (ie, percutaneous transluminal coronary angioplasty [PTCA] and coronary artery bypass graft [CABG]). (Data from Sacks FM et al: N Engl J Med 1996;335:1001.)

women, whose hypertension takes a more accelerated course, appear to benefit from blood pressure treatment more than white women. White women thus far have appeared to achieve marginal if any reduction in CAD or mortality risk with treatment of mild hypertension. Because the effects of their hypertensive disease take a longer time to become evident, in the treatment trials done so far, the low number of (albeit excess) CAD end points in treated white women may be as much a reflection of treatment toxicity as treatment benefit. However, the major impact in studies to assess CVD risk reduction in hypertensive treatment is in the reduction of incidence of stroke. The fact that stroke risk reduction is significant in all groups is the major justification for therapy of moderate and severe hypertension in women. In addition, the older woman, who frequently has isolated systolic hypertension, has been shown in the Systolic Hypertension in the Elderly Trial to benefit from antihypertensive therapy. In this study, treatment of systolic hypertension (systolic blood pressure above 160 mm Hg) was associated with a 36% reduction in total and nonfatal stroke and a 27% reduction in fatal and nonfatal myocardial infarction, and a similar reduction in the onset of congestive heart failure.

Nonpharmacologic therapy for borderline or mild hypertension in combination with drug therapy for severe hypertension can have beneficial blood pressure lowering effects. These factors include the following:

- Salt restriction to less than 6 g NaCl (2.4 g sodium) daily. This modification is more efficacious in blacks, the elderly, and patients with established hypertension.
- Weight loss to within 10% of ideal weight.
- Restriction of alcohol in women to no more than 0.5 oz daily of ethanol (6 oz of wine, 12 oz of beer, 1 oz of whiskey).
- Moderate exercise (as little as 30 to 45 minutes 5 times weekly of brisk walking).
- Balanced diet for an adequate potassium (90 mmol/d), calcium, and magnesium intake. Supplements are unnecessary if serum levels are normal and not perturbed by diuretic use.
- "Wellness" programs, smoking cessation, stress management, and "heart smart" dieting. The DASH Diet has been shown to reduce blood pressure effectively in both borderline and established hypertension, and

Table 29–1. Coronary artery disease (CAD) risk factor profile in women with hyperlipidemia.

Age > 55 or premature menopause without estrogen therapy
Family history of premature CAD in a male first-degree relative before age 55 or in a female first-degree relative before age 65
Current cigarette smoking
Hypertension, treated or untreated
Low high-density lipoprotein cholesterol (< 50 mg/dL)
Diabetes mellitus

THE ADULT TREATMENT PANEL III (ATP III) GUIDELINE STEPS IN THE EVALUATION AND TREATMENT OF SERUM CHOLESTEROL

Step 1: Determine lipoprotein levels. Obtain complete lipoprotein profile after 9- to 12-hour fast. Note here that the optimal total cholesterol remains below 200 mg/dL, but the definition of low high-density lipoprotein (HDL) has been raised to < 40 mg/dL. Some would argue that the level of low HDL for women should be raised to < 50 mg/dL, but this has not become general policy.

Step 2: Identify presence of clinical atherosclerotic disease that confers high risk for coronary heart disease (CHD) events (CHD risk equivalent). These include clinical CHD, symptomatic carotid artery disease, peripheral arterial disease, and abdominal aortic aneurysm. Since diabetes also confers a high risk for CHD, any diabetic must be included in the high-risk treatment strategy.

Step 3: Determine presence of major risk factors (other than low-density lipoprotein [LDL]). Major risk factors (exclusive of LDL cholesterol) that modify LDL goals include: cigarette smoking, (diabetes is regarded as a CHD risk equivalent), hypertension (blood pressure 140/90 mm Hg or on antihypertensive medication), low HDL cholesterol (< 40 mg/dL), family history of premature CHD (CHD in male first-degree relative younger than 55 years or in female first-degree relative younger than 65 years), age (men 45 years and women 55 years), HDL cholesterol 60 mg/dL counts as a "negative" risk factor (its presence removes one risk factor from the total count).

Step 4: If 2 or more risk factors (other than LDL) are present without CHD or CHD risk equivalent, assess 10-year (short-term) CHD risk. Three levels of risk have been defined: > 20% 10-year risk of developing CHD – CHD risk equivalent; 10–20% 10-year risk of CHD; and < 10% 10-year risk of CHD. The actual calculation of the 10-year risk is cumbersome but can be rapidly done using the ATP III Web site calculator (http://hin.nhlbi.nih.gov/atpiii/calculator.asp?usertype=prof), which is gender-specific. A personal data management tool that can be downloaded is also available.

Step 5: Determine risk category. To do this, first establish LDL goal of therapy, then determine the need for therapeutic lifestyle changes (TLCs), and then determine level for drug consideration (Table 29–6). Note that if the fasting triglyceride exceeds 500 mg/dL, the primary goal of therapy is to reduce triglyceride, then LDL (see Step 9).

Step 6: Initiate TLCs if LDL is above goal. These lifestyle changes include a diet composed of saturated fat < 7% of calories and cholesterol < 200 mg/d. Also, all are advised to consider an increase in viscous (soluble) fiber to (10–25 g/d) and to add plant stanols/sterols (2 g/d) as therapeutic options to enhance LDL lowering. Active attempts at weight control to reduce body mass index toward normal or at least below 27 kg/m^2 are to be encouraged. Increased physical activity to at least 150 minutes per week of moderate exertion should also be added to this regimen.

The comprehensive approach that includes diet and exercise is particularly important to women's lipid profile. Dietary change alone may reduce LDL and raise HDL in men, but dieting alone in women often results in reductions of both LDL and HDL, with a rise of triglyceride. This potentially adverse pattern is exaggerated with rapid acute weight loss and fat restriction. Dietary modification with exercise, however, allows a more favorable lowering of triglyceride and LDL levels and a modest rise of HDL in women according to small studies that have evaluated this process.

As in any hyperlipidemia work-up, secondary causes of hypercholesterolemia should be assessed and, if possible, reversed. Secondary causes include the following: nephrotic syndrome, obstructive liver disease, hypothyroidism, diabetes mellitus, β-blockers, thiazide diuretics, alcohol excess, cyclosporine, corticosteroids, anabolic steroids, androgenic progestins, and retinoid cream for acne.

In addition, 3 months of diet and exercise therapy should be initiated before drug therapy is considered in the asymptomatic patient.

Step 7: Consider adding drug therapy if LDL exceeds levels shown in Table 29–6. Consider using a drug simultaneously with TLCs for CHD and CHD equivalents. Consider adding drug to TLCs after 3 months for other risk categories. For both men and women, the primary target of treatment is the LDL level. A detailed review of drug therapy for hyperlipidemia is beyond the scope of this chapter. Table 29–7 summarizes the drugs, doses, lipoprotein effects, side effects, and contraindications of the agents recommended by the ATP III.

Step 8: Identify metabolic syndrome (Table 29–8) and treat, if present, after 3 months of TLCs. This addition to the ATP III guideline is an important adjunct in the treatment of women with moderate to high risk of long-term CHD, inasmuch as it helps identify a group of women whose aggregate risk must be carefully followed over time, with specific goals of weight reduction, dietary restriction, attention to glucose intolerance, and the need to disengage from a sedentary lifestyle. Treatment of the metabolic syndrome involves (1) addressing the underlying causes (overweight/obesity and physical inactivity) through intensification of weight management and increased physical activity, and (2) treating lipid and nonlipid risk factors if they persist despite initiation of lifestyle therapies. The major therapies to emphasize include treating hypertension, using aspirin for patients with CHD to reduce the prothrombotic state, and treating hypertriglyceridemia and/or low HDL (see Step 9).

Step 9: Treat elevated triglycerides. The ATP III classification of serum triglycerides (mg/dL) is as follows: < 150 is normal, 150–199 is borderline high, 200–499 is high, and 500 is very high.

(continued)

THE ADULT TREATMENT PANEL III (ATP III) GUIDELINE STEPS IN THE EVALUATION AND TREATMENT OF SERUM CHOLESTEROL. (CONTINUED)

Attention to the treatment of elevated triglycerides (150 mg/dL) represents a more concerted effort to reduce the impact of this previously underemphasized risk factor, especially in women. Still, ATP III holds that, in this setting, the primary aim of therapy is to reach the LDL goal, intensify weight management, and increase physical activity. If triglycerides are 200 mg/dL after LDL goal is reached, a new, secondary goal is set for non-HDL cholesterol (total - HDL), 30 mg/dL higher than LDL goal.

Recognizing the risk of high triglyceride with concomitant low HDL, the ATP III has consolidated a new goal of "non-HDL cholesterol" range for each risk category (Table 29–9).

If triglycerides are 200–499 mg/dL after the LDL goal is reached, consider adding a drug if needed to reach non-HDL goal; this may be done either by intensifying therapy with an LDL-lowering drug, or adding nicotinic acid or fibrate to further lower very low density lipoprotein.

If triglycerides are 500 mg/dL or higher, first lower triglycerides to prevent pancreatitis; patients in this category should be advised to adhere to a very low-fat diet (15% of calories from fat), to eliminate alcohol, to engage in weight management and physical activity, and to begin treatment with a fibrate or nicotinic acid.

The treatment of low HDL cholesterol (< 40 mg/dL) is a secondary goal of ATP III. Raising HDL can be accomplished with intensification of weight management and increased physical activity, as well as the use of statins to reach LDL goal. If triglycerides are 200–499 mg/dL, trying to achieve non-HDL goal becomes the next step. Finally, if triglycerides are < 200 mg/dL (isolated low HDL) in CHD or CHD equivalent, consider nicotinic acid or fibrate.

Further recommendations from ATP III specifically regarding women include emphasis on secondary prevention adjuncts in women with CHD, support for extrapolation to women of strategies known to be beneficial to men, based on risk. At each level of CHD risk, estrogen therapy is not recommended to reduce CHD risk.

US Department of Health and Human Services. NIH Publication No. 01-3305, May 2001.

Table 29–6. LDL cholesterol goals and cutpoints for therapeutic lifestyle changes and drug therapy in different risk categories.

Risk Category	LDL Goal	LDL Level at which to Initiate Therapeutic Lifestyle Changes	LDL Level at which to Consider Drug Therapy
CHD or CHD risk equivalents (10-year risk > 20%)	< 100 mg/dL	100 mg/dL	130 mg/dL (100–129 mg/dL: drug optional)[1]
2+ risk factors (10-year risk ≤20%)	< 130 mg/dL	130 mg/dL	10-year risk 10–20%: 130 mg/dL 10-year risk < 10%: 160 mg/dL
0–1 risk factor[2]	< 160 mg/dL	160 mg/dL	190 mg/dL (160–189 mg/dL: LDL-lowering drug optional)

LDL, low-density lipoprotein; CHD, coronary heart disease.

[1]Some authorities recommend use of LDL-lowering drugs in this category if an LDL cholesterol < 100 mg/dL cannot be achieved by therapeutic lifestyle changes. Others prefer use of drugs that primarily modify triglycerides and HDL (eg, nicotinic acid or fibrate). Clinical judgment also may call for deferring drug therapy in this subcategory.

[2]Almost all people with 0–1 risk factor have a 10-year risk< 10%, thus 10-year risk assessment in people with 0–1 risk factor is not necessary.

US Department of Health and Human Services. NIH Publication No. 01-3305, May 2001.

Table 29-7. Drugs used in the treatment of high cholesterol.

Drugs	Daily Doses	Lipid/Lipoprotein Effects	Side Effects	Contraindications
HMG CoA reductase inhibitors (statins)				
Lovastatin Pravastatin Simvastatin Fluvastatin Atorvastatin Cerivastatin	20–80 mg 20–40 mg 20–80 mg 20–80 mg 10–80 mg 0.4–0.8 mg	LDL-C 18–55% HDL-C 5–15% TG 7–30%	Myopathy Increased liver enzymes	**Absolute:** Active or chronic liver disease **Relative:** Concomitant use of certain drugs[1]
Bile acid sequestrants				
Cholestyramine Colestipol Colesevelam	4–16 g 5–20 g 2.6–3.8 g	LDL-C 15–30% HDL-C 3–5% TG No change or increase	Gastrointestinal distress Constipation Decreased absorption of other drugs	**Absolute:** Dysbetalipoproteinemia TG > 400 mg/dL **Relative:** TG > 200 mg/dL
Nicotinic acid				
Immediate release (crystalline) nicotinic acid Extended release nicotinic acid (Niaspan) Sustained-release nicotinic acid	1.5–3 g 1–2 g 1–2 g	LDL-C 5–25% HDL-C 15–35% TG 20–50%	Flushing Hyperglycemia Hyperuricemia (or gout) Upper GI distress Hepatotoxicity	**Absolute:** Chronic liver disease Severe gout **Relative:** Diabetes Hyperuricemia Peptic ulcer disease
Fibric acids				
Gemfibrozil Fenofibrate Clofibrate	600 mg bid 200 mg 1000 mg bid	LDL-C 5–20% (may be increased in patients with high TG) HDL-C 10–20% TG 20–50%	Dyspepsia Gallstones Myopathy	**Absolute:** Severe renal disease Severe hepatic disease

LDL-C, low-density lipoprotein cholesterol; HDL-C, high-density lipoprotein cholesterol; TG, triglyceride.
[1]Cyclosporine, macrolide antibiotics, various antifungal agents, and cytochrome P-450 inhibitors (fibrates and niacin) should be used with appropriate caution.
US Department of Health and Human Services. NIH Publication No. 01-3305, May 2001.

can be recommended to patients to achieve "heart healthy" dietary goals.

- In mild hypertension, 3–6 months of such a program may obviate the need for drug therapy.

The choice of drug therapy for hypertension is a matter of continued debate. The seventh report of the Joint National Committee on Detection, Evaluation, and Treatment of High Blood Pressure (JNC VII) recommends that thiazide diuretics be used as first-line therapy for hypertension, based on population studies demonstrating hypertension mortality reduction with these drugs. ACE inhibitors are recommended for specific applications, such as post–myocardial infarction treatment, reduction of nephropathy and atherosclerotic risk in diabetics (HOPE study), and in congestive heart failure with systolic dysfunction. Therapy should be individualized based on the patient's physiologic status, response to sensible therapy, and minimization of side effects. For example, elderly women with systolic or combined hypertension often have a lower cardiac output with age, higher peripheral resistance, and lower

Table 29–8. Clinical identification of the metabolic syndrome.[1]

Risk Factor	Defining Level
Abdominal obesity[2] Men Women	Waist circumference[2] > 102 cm (> 40 in) > 88 cm (> 35 in)
Triglycerides	150 mg/dL
HDL cholesterol Men Women	 < 40 mg/dL < 50 mg/dL
Blood pressure	130/85 mm Hg
Fasting glucose	110 mg/dL

HDL, high-density lipoprotein.
[1]Any 3 of the below.
[2]Overweight and obesity are associated with insulin resistance and the metabolic syndrome. However, the presence of abdominal obesity is more highly correlated with the metabolic risk factors than is an elevated body mass index. Therefore, the simple measure of waist circumference is recommended to identify the body weight component of the metabolic syndrome.
US Department of Health and Human Services. NIH Publication No. 01-3305, May 2001.

intravascular volume. In addition, they may have depressed autonomic function and reduced renal function with a reduced creatinine clearance. β-Blockers can reduce cardiac output further and contribute to fatigue, lethargy, and depression. In this instance, vasodilators and ACE inhibitors may produce better blood pressure control with fewer side effects. However, if these medications are unsuccessful or not tolerated, calcium channel blockers are also an option. If combination therapy

Table 29–9. Comparison of LDL cholesterol and non-HDL cholesterol goals by risk category.

Risk Category	LDL Goal (mg/dL)	Non-HDL Goal (mg/dL)
CHD and CHD risk equivalent (10-year risk for CHD > 20%)	< 100	< 130
Multiple (2+) risk factors and 10-year risk ≤20%	< 130	< 160
0–1 risk factor	< 160	< 190

LDL, low-density lipoprotein; HDL, high-density lipoprotein; CHD, coronary heart disease.
US Department of Health and Human Services. NIH Publication No. 01-3305, May 2001.

is necessary, the addition of a low-dose diuretic to a vasodilator regimen may be useful.

Young women with mild hypertension tend to have higher cardiac output than older women. They often have normal peripheral resistance and blood volume and increased sympathetic activity. They tend to have a more compliant circulation than men of their age. If a woman's profile fits this clinical description, blood pressure may be treated easily with a low dose of a β-blocker or an ACE inhibitor. Although there is the tendency for β-blockers to lower HDL and raise triglyceride and to promote glucose intolerance, these effects are minimal compared with the long-term benefits of adequate blood pressure control. Black women tend to have an expanded plasma volume and accelerated organ damage, particularly of the kidney, from their hypertension. These women often respond best to diuretics and calcium channel blockers; however, calcium channel blockers may increase cardiovascular risk. Blacks in general tend to respond poorly to β-blockers, with the exception that some may respond better to labetalol, a β-blocker with both α-vasodilating and (weak) β-blocking properties. The JNC VII recommends that black women be treated with β-blockers and ACE inhibitors if other comorbidities urge their use, and that dose of these and appropriate use of diuretics be optimized for blood pressure control.

Obese women tend to have a higher cardiac output because of their increased body surface area, and they tend to have a higher blood volume with normal peripheral resistance. They may be particularly subject to fluid retention with unopposed vasodilation, and as a result, ACE inhibitors may need to be combined with a diuretic. In these patients, β-blockers may slow attempts at weight loss because of their tendency to decrease metabolic rate and may best be used in lower dose combination therapy.

Women with CAD and hypertension may require selective therapy with ACE inhibitors, β-blockers, or both, targeted to the control of heart rate, blood pressure, and symptoms.

Women with congestive heart failure, whether or not hypertension exists, may benefit from ACE inhibitors, especially after a myocardial infarction and particularly if their ejection fraction is below 40%. Further treatment with β-blockers approved for the use of systolic dysfunction (eg, carvedilol, metoprolol, and bisoprolol) is indicated based on the degree of heart failure compensation, etiology, heart rate, and blood pressure. Referral to a cardiologist is often useful in this setting.

Barrett-Connor E et al: Raloxifene and cardiovascular events in osteoporotic postmenopausal women: four-year results from the

MORE (Multiple Outcomes of Raloxifene Evaluation) randomized trial. JAMA 2002;287:847. [PMID: 11851576]

Buller JC et al: Type A behavior pattern, heart disease risk factors, and estrogen replacement therapy in postmenopausal women: the Rancho Bernardo Study. J Womens Health 1998;7:49. [PMID: 9511132]

Grady D et al: Postmenopausal hormone therapy increases risk for venous thromboembolic disease. The Heart and Estrogen/progestin Replacement Study. Ann Intern Med 2000;132:689. [PMID: 10787361]

Hulley S et al: Randomized trial of estrogen plus progestin for secondary prevention of coronary heart disease in postmenopausal women. Heart and Estrogen/progestin Replacement Study (HERS) Research Group. JAMA 1998;280:605. [PMID: 9718051]

Lewis MA: Myocardial infarction and stroke in young women: what is the impact of oral contraceptives? Am J Obstet Gynecol 1998;179(3 Pt 2):S68. [PMID: 9753313]

Simon JA et al: Postmenopausal hormone therapy and risk of stroke: The Heart and Estrogen-progestin Replacement Study (HERS). Circulation 2001;103:638. [PMID: 11156873]

Clinical Findings

A. HYPERLIPIDEMIA

Women demonstrate cholesterol profiles that vary as they age and are significantly different from those of men. Women and men have similar total cholesterol levels up to ages 20–25, after which the levels diverge. Men demonstrate a rise of total cholesterol over the next 20 years, with a subsequent plateau. Women demonstrate a slower increase of total cholesterol, but at ages 45–50, their levels exceed the male average by 20–25 points for the duration of life (Figure 29–7). Total cholesterol level has been correlated with risk for CAD in both women and men. The Framingham study reported that a direct relationship appears to exist between total cholesterol level and annual coronary event rate. The risk of CAD was double in women whose cholesterol levels exceeded 265 mg/dL compared with women whose cholesterol levels were under 205 mg/dL. Data from the Israeli Donolo–Tel Aviv Study show a similar pattern: the incidence of CAD triples among women whose cholesterol levels were greater than 265 mg/dL, compared with those whose cholesterol levels were less than 200 mg/dL. The national Lipid Research Clinics (LRC) study found that women with a total cholesterol of 235 mg/dL had a 70% higher risk of coronary disease than women whose total cholesterol fell below 200 mg/dL.

The total cholesterol level may not be a reliable index of risk for many women, however. Women appear to have a substantially different lipoprotein profile from men. Cholesterol and triglyceride, the major

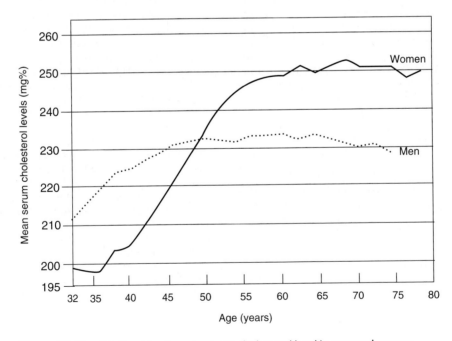

Figure 29–7. Relationship of age to serum cholesterol level in men and women. (Data from the Framingham Heart Study, Examinations 1–10. Department of Health, Education, and Welfare Publication No. [NIH] 74-478, 1973.)

plasma lipids, are solubilized in the bloodstream in envelopes of water-miscible proteins. These lipids are the products of digestion and tissue synthesis, and their concentration in the bloodstream is influenced by both genetic synthetic profiles and dietary intake of cholesterol and fat. In addition, a variety of endocrine and metabolic forces may alter the relative size of these lipid-laden lipoprotein particles. This size differential appears to affect their biochemical activity in that "small" particles appear more active and exert a greater net effect (either atherogenic or atherolytic). The relevant lipoprotein fractions for discussion of coronary risk in women are shown in Table 29–2. It should be emphasized that the measurement of each of these fractions may vary from laboratory to laboratory; unless a clinical laboratory follows national guidelines for the measurement of these lipoproteins, significant errors, particularly in the measurement of high-density lipoprotein (HDL) cholesterol, may occur and lead either to misdiagnosis or to an inability to determine the effects of treatment.

Although total cholesterol levels are higher in men than women after age 20, HDL cholesterol levels are higher in women than men from puberty until menopause, when they may show a decline, along with a rise of total cholesterol. Generally, HDL is higher for women than men throughout life. Thus, with the rise of total cholesterol and a trend for HDL to decrease following menopause, the total cholesterol:HDL ratio in postmenopausal women rises toward that of men. Triglyceride levels in women and men are similar at puberty and rise slowly with age, but they rise more slowly in women than men. By ages 65–70, triglyceride levels are similar in women and men, although they appear to convey a higher risk for women.

The Framingham study has shown that HDL cholesterol is inversely correlated with coronary risk in both men and women and suggests that a low HDL cholesterol level is a more powerful predictor of CAD in women than in men. These studies have suggested that for every 10 mg/dL fall in HDL cholesterol, CAD risk

rises by 40–50%. The Israeli Donolo–Tel Aviv Study found that women with a total cholesterol:HDL ratio of greater than 4.3, regardless of the total cholesterol level, had a 2- to 5-fold increase in CVD risk; this increase occurred even in those with total cholesterol levels less than 200 mg/dL. In addition, women with elevated triglyceride levels have a higher CAD risk independent of total cholesterol; in the Framingham study, women's triglyceride levels tended to be a better predictor for CAD than the level of low-density lipoprotein (LDL) cholesterol. This finding appears to reflect a true gender difference. Of course, an elevated triglyceride level in a patient should prompt an investigation to see if there is an underlying glucose intolerance needing primary attention.

Based on Framingham data and treatment data for hypercholesterolemia from the LRC trial, the NCEP has emphasized diet and drug therapy for hyperlipidemia based largely on male lipid risk profile. The Framingham data have shown that total cholesterol, high LDL, and low HDL (below 35 mg/dL) are CAD risk factors in men; therefore, therapy has been directed toward a reduction of total cholesterol and LDL and an increase of HDL, with minor emphasis on reduction of triglyceride. These recommendations may not be directly applicable to women, however, because the risk profile is different for women. Indeed, LDL has been associated with increased CAD risk in women under age 65, but HDL remains predictive for women both younger and older than 65 years.

Evidence of the magnitude of this difference came from the follow-up study of the LRC. In this study, 1405 women ages 50–69 were followed for an average of 14 years to observe the relationship between lipoprotein levels and CVD death rates (heart disease and stroke). The study presented strong evidence that CVD risk is increased in women with HDL levels less than 50 mg/dL and with triglyceride levels of 200–399 mg/dL; the risk is still higher in women with triglyceride levels greater than 400 mg/dL. CVD risk with total cholesterol level was driven largely by HDL level (ie, only women with HDL less than 50 mg/dL had an increased CVD risk with total cholesterol greater than 240 mg/dL). Also, LDL cholesterol was a poor predictor of CVD risk in women: at all levels of LDL, an HDL level less than 50 mg/dL was a greater risk predictor than was LDL level. HDL and triglyceride levels commonly vary reciprocally in men and in some women (estrogen can increase both). In women with low HDL (less than 50 mg/dL), the triglyceride level is a progressive risk such that women with triglyceride levels greater than 400 mg/dL have a nearly 8-fold increase in risk over women with low HDL and triglyceride levels less than 200 mg/dL. When the risk is adjusted for age, hypertension, diabetes, smoking, history of heart disease, and

Table 29–2. Liproprotein fraction terminology.

Total cholesterol: total of all lipoprotein cholesterol
High-density lipoprotein (HDL) cholesterol: Lipoprotein fraction affecting atherolysis
Very low-density lipoprotein (VLDL) cholesterol: lipoprotein fraction rich in triglycerides
Low-density lipoprotein (LDL) cholesterol: atherogenic lipoprotein fraction
Apolipoprotein A-1: "favorable" lipoprotein subunit of HDL
Apolipoprotein B: "unfavorable" lipoprotein of LDL

estrogen use, women still have independent CVD risks with low HDL and high triglyceride and not necessarily with a high total cholesterol level (Table 29–3).

It should be emphasized that these figures are from 1 large study. Other studies investigating the influence of high levels of triglyceride in a general population have found that the risk is of borderline significance in women. Reciprocally low HDL and high triglyceride levels tend to occur in patients with diabetes and with obesity. Therefore, primary treatment of this lipid abnormality is directed at the treatment of diabetes and obesity.

The influence of LDL on CVD risk in women remains controversial. The Framingham study found a positive association of LDL cholesterol with CVD in women. The Israeli Donolo–Tel Aviv study did not directly evaluate the effect of LDL on CVD rate. Both earlier and later analyses of LRC data show little influence of LDL level on CVD mortality in women. Evidence in men for significant CVD risk with increased levels of both total and LDL cholesterol persists, however; these findings seem to represent a poorly understood gender difference in lipoprotein atherogenicity or susceptibility. Hyperinsulinemia has been targeted as a promoter of atherogenesis in men but not in women and may facilitate LDL deposition to a greater degree in men. There may be subpopulations of women with what has been termed "small dense" LDL, which predisposes, with other constitutional CVD risks, to a higher CVD incidence.

B. Hypertension

Hypertension is defined as a systolic blood pressure of 140 mm Hg or greater or a diastolic blood pressure of 90 mm Hg or greater. The 1994 Census and the Third National Health and Nutrition Examination Survey (NHANES III) report that 1 in 4 American adults is hypertensive. High blood pressure prevalence increases with age, is more common in blacks than whites, and is more common in persons with a lower level of education and a lower socioeconomic status. Hypertension is more common in men than women up to middle age, but in late middle age and the elderly years, women are more likely to be hypertensive than men (Figure 29–8). Hypertension is positively associated in both men and women with both fatal and nonfatal CVD, including CAD, stroke, congestive heart failure, peripheral vascular disease, and renal failure. Morbidity and mortality rise with progressive elevations of both systolic and diastolic blood pressure. Moreover, for any given diastolic blood pressure, the higher the systolic blood pressure, the higher the risk of CVD.

In the Framingham study, diastolic blood pressure was emphasized. In women, diastolic blood pressure of 90–109 mm Hg was associated with a 1.5-fold excess of CVD events, and diastolic blood pressure of greater than 110 was related to a 4-fold excess of CVD events. It is true, however, that women (at least in middle age) tolerate hypertension better than men, with a longer delay in onset of cardiovascular complications. It is probably for this reason that treatment effects for hypertension in women appear to be less than for men.

The Report of the Joint National Committee of Detection, Evaluation, and Treatment of High Blood Pressure (JNC VII) includes recommendations for high blood pressure as a national public health program. These recommendations serve as a useful framework for discussion of hypertension as a risk factor in women. The classification of high blood pressure (Table 29–4) emphasizes both systolic and diastolic blood pressure levels; "prehypertension" blood pressure readings also are targeted and require serial observation to avoid overtreatment and undertreatment of hypertension. The detection and evaluation of hypertension requires much more "hands on" evaluation by the primary physician than does the assessment of hyperlipidemia: the physical examination and physical blood pressure measurement must assess the presence and degree of hypertension, signs of target organ damage, and secondary causes of hypertension or failure of treatment.

Table 29–3. Lipid Research Clinics follow-up study of coronary heart disease (CHD) risk in women.

Lipoprotein Fraction	Relative Risk for CHD
Total cholesterol	
< 200 mg/dL	1.0
200–239 mg/dL	1.11
≥ 240 mg/dL	1.42
High-density lipoprotein cholesterol	
< 50 mg/dL	1.74[1]
≥ 50 mg/dL	1.0
Low-density lipoprotein cholesterol	
< 130 mg/dL	1.0
130–159 mg/dL	0.54
≥ 160 mg/dL	0.80
Triglycerides	
< 200 mg/dL	1.0
200–399 mg/dL	1.65[1]
≥ 400 mg/dL	3.44[1]

Adapted, with permission, from Bass KM: Arch Intern Med 1993;153:2209. Based on Lipid Research Clinics follow-up study analysis of female participants' risk of CHD in 14 years of follow-up.
[1]Result is statistically significant.

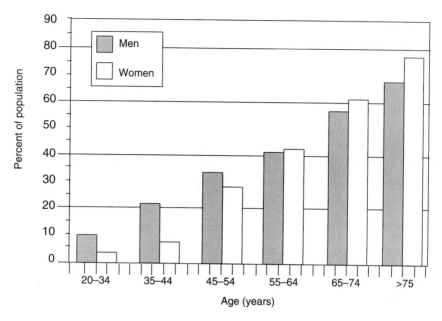

Figure 29–8. Although hypertension is more common in younger men than women, significant hypertension and risk of stroke, myocardial infarction, and congestive heart failure appear for more women late after menopause.

1. Measurement—Despite its elementary nature, blood pressure measurement is subject to some common errors. Blood pressure measurements should be obtained initially in both arms after 5 minutes of rest with appropriate cuff size with a calibrated sphygmomanometer. The systolic reading should correspond to phase I, appearance of Korotkoff sounds, and the diastolic reading should correspond to phase V "disappearance" of Korotkoff sounds. To diagnose hypertension, multiple readings should be obtained, which should coincide within 5 mm Hg. "White coat" hypertension can be documented by having the patient, a relative, or another health care provider measure the blood pressure using similar criteria. At times, ambulatory blood pressure monitoring may be necessary to get an accurate measurement.

Errors in blood pressure measurement may be related to any of the following:

- Defective equipment: bulb cuff mercury level leakage or cuff size too big or too small.
- Patient physiology: pain, anxiety, caffeine or cigarette use within 30 minutes, irregular heart rhythm accentuating systolic blood pressure after an extrasystolic pause, or "rigid vessels" causing overestimation of blood pressure.

- Observer error and bias: improper use of stethoscope over the brachial artery, incorrect speed of inflation or deflation, or improper recording of the figures owing to inability to see the mercury column accurately or to bias in rounding numbers.

The patient's physiologic characteristics may dictate more detailed measurement. Elderly women may have "stiff" arterial vessels that are palpable even with the cuff inflated above systolic blood pressure. "Palpation" of blood pressure here is probably not accurate. Young women, pregnant women, and women with a higher cardiac output (eg, caused by anemia, thyrotoxicosis, or sepsis) have a diastolic blood pressure that corresponds more closely to phase IV "muffling" of Korotkoff sounds.

2. History—A directed medical history should include (1) a family history of high blood pressure, early CAD, stroke, congestive heart failure, diabetes, or hyperlipidemia; (2) a patient history of prior hypertension and onset in relation to puberty, pregnancy, oral contraception, pelvic surgery, and menopause; (3) a history of drug treatment; cardiac, neurologic, or kidney disease; hyperlipidemia, diabetes, or gout; fluid overload; or claudication; (4) a patient profile of weight gain or loss;

Table 29–4. Classification of blood pressure for adults age 18 and older.[1]

Category	Systolic/Diastolic (mm Hg)
Normal[2]	< 120 and < 80
Prehypertension	120–139 or 80–89
Hypertension[3]	
Stage 1	140–159 or 90–99
Stage 2	≥160 or ≥100

[1]For persons not taking antihypertensive drugs and who are not acutely ill. When systolic and diastolic blood pressures fall into different categories, the higher category should be selected to classify the patient's blood pressure status. For example, 160/92 mm Hg should be classified as stage 2 hypertension. Isolated systolic hypertension is defined as systolic blood pressure of 140 mm Hg or greater and diastolic blood pressure below 90 mm Hg and staged appropriately (eg, 170/82 mm Hg is defined as stage 2 isolated systolic hypertension). In addition to classifying stages of hypertension on the basis of average blood pressure levels, clinicians should specify presence or absence of target organ disease and additional risk factors. This specificity is important for risk classification and treatment (see Table 29–5).
[2]Normal blood pressure with respect to cardiovascular risk is below 120/80 mm Hg. However, unusually low readings should be evaluated for clinical significance.
[3]Based on the average of 2 or more readings taken at each of 2 or more visits after an initial screening.
The Seventh Report of the Joint National Committee on prevention, detection, evaluation, and treatment of high blood pressure. NIH Publication No. 03-5233, May 2003.

activity and exercise level; smoking or tobacco chewing; (5) a dietary profile of sodium intake, alcohol use, and fat and cholesterol intake; (6) symptoms that suggest a secondary cause of hypertension; and (7) psychosocial stresses at work and home and from the financial burden of medical care.

3. Physical examination—Physical examination should include (1) blood pressure seated and after standing for 2 minutes; (2) measurement of height and weight and observation and measurement of the body mass index (weight in kilograms/height in meters, squared); (3) fundoscopic examination to assess arterial narrowing, hemorrhage, exudate, and papilledema; (4) neck examination for jugular venous distention, carotid bruits, or thyroid enlargement; (5) cardiac examination for rate, rhythm, S3, S4, murmur of mitral or aortic insufficiency, cardiac enlargement, or apical heave; (6) abdominal examination for vascular bruits, renal enlargement, masses, or aneurysm; (7) peripheral pulse profile and identification of trophic or venous disease; and (8) neurologic examination.

4. Laboratory tests and procedures—For the initial work-up of hypertension, the tests to be considered include complete blood cell count, electrolytes, creatinine, urinalysis, uric acid, calcium, fasting blood sugar, cholesterol, HDL and triglycerides, and if indicated, free T4 and thyroid-stimulating hormone. An electrocardiogram is indicated for assessment of left ventricular hypertrophy and prior infarction. Optional treadmill testing (with echocardiography or nuclear perfusion imaging is indicated [see Chapter 30]) if cardiovascular target organ damage is suspected. If labile or borderline blood pressure is present, measurement of left ventricular mass index by echocardiography is indicated to identify a higher risk "borderline" hypertensive condition with left ventricular mass index greater than 125 g/m^2 of body surface area. At each stage of evaluation, the clinician must be alert to the discovery of target organ damage (Table 29–5).

5. Secondary hypertension—Although 90–95% of hypertension in women is idiopathic or "essential" and often familial in nature, 5–10% of women with hypertension have a secondary, potentially correctable or specifically treatable cause of hypertension. Some of these causes have a predilection for women over men and thus deserve special attention. They should be sought for in women with a negative family history, in children, or in patients with an accelerated or a difficult-to-control pattern of high blood pressure.

6. Renovascular hypertension—Renovascular hypertension resulting from renal artery stenosis is responsible for 2–4% of cases of hypertension. Fibromuscular dysplasia is the underlying cause in 20–50% of cases of renovascular hypertension, more often in younger women; the remainder of cases in older women are attributed to atherosclerotic obstruction in the renal arteries. Medial fibromuscular dysplasia shows an 8:1 female-to-male predominance and is found in middle age (35–52 years), is often bilateral, and causes moderate to severe hypertension. Older women account for 40% of cases of atherosclerotic renal vascular hypertension. The diagnosis may be suspected with identification of a flank or epigastric bruit or deterioration of creatinine level with angiotensin-converting enzyme (ACE) inhibitors, frequently in combination with a negative family history for high blood pressure. The diagnosis is confirmed with spiral computed tomography, magnetic resonance angiography, or duplex ultrasonography (depending on availability and local experience). Treatment with balloon angioplasty with stenting or surgical reconstruction is helpful.

Table 29–5. Cardiovascular risk factor stratification in patients with hypertension.

Risk Stratification Steps
• Determine blood pressure stage
• Determine risk group by major risk factors and TOD/CCD
• Determine treatment recommendations (below)
• Determine goal blood pressure
• Refer to specific treatment recommendations

Major Risk Factors	TOD/CCD (Target Organ Damage/ Clinical Cardiovascular Disease)
• Smoking • Obesity (BMI ≥ 30) • Physical Inactivity • Microalbuminuria or GFR < 60	Heart diseases • LVH • Angina/prior MI • Prior CABG • Heart failure
• Dyslipidemia	Stroke or TIA
• Diabetes mellitus	Nephropathy
• Age >65 years for women, >55 for men	Peripheral arterial disease
• Family history • Women age < 65 • Men age < 55	Hypertensive retinopathy

Blood pressure stages (mm Hg)	Risk group A No major risk factors No TOD/CCD	Risk group B At least 1 major risk factor, not including diabetes No TOD/CCD	Risk group C TOD/CCD and/or diabetes, with or without risk factors
Prehypertension (120–139/80–89)	Lifestyle modification	Lifestyle modification	Drug therapy for those with renal insufficiency or diabetes if > 130/80 Lifestyle modification
Stage 1 (140–159/90–99)	Lifestyle modification (up to 12 months)	Lifestyle modification (up to 6 months) Consider initial drug therapy for those with multiple risk factors	Drug therapy Lifestyle modification
Stage 2 (≥ 160/≥ 100)	Drug therapy Lifestyle modification	Drug therapy Lifestyle modification	Drug therapy Lifestyle modification

Goal Blood Pressure	Clinical Profile
< 140/90 mm Hg	Uncomplicated hypertension, Risk groups A and B; group C except for the following:
< 130/80 mm Hg	Diabetes, renal failure, heart failure

TOD/CCD, target organ damage/clinical cardiovascular disease; LVH, left ventricular hypertrophy; MI, myocardial infarction; CABG, coronary artery bypass grafting; TIA, transient ischemic attack; GFR, glomerular flow rate.

7. Renal parenchymal disease—Renal parenchymal disease caused by hypertension, nephritis, chronic urinary infection, or diabetic nephropathy may not be curable, but control of hypertension with ACE inhibitors or calcium channel blockers may slow progression of chronic renal failure. A history of a single episode of eclampsia during pregnancy does not necessarily predispose to subsequent chronic hypertension, although eclampsia in multiple pregnancies can.

8. Aortic coarctation—Although aortic coarctation has a 2:1 male-to-female predisposition, it is the most common congenital cardiac anomaly of Turner (XO) syndrome in women. Any young woman with upper extremity hypertension should have a leg (popliteal) blood pressure measurement to exclude this diagnosis.

9. Endocrine causes—Mineralocorticoid excess with hypertension, virilization, and hypokalemia caused by 11-β-hydroxylase deficiency is a rare cause of hypertension in young women. The hypertension and hypokalemia are correctable with corticosteroids.

Aldosterone excess, usually due to an adenoma, results in hypokalemic hypochloremic alkalosis, frequently with glucose intolerance; symptoms are referable to the hypertension, hyperglycemia, and alkalosis. Drug or surgical therapy can be effective in eliminating hypertension.

Glucocorticoid excess (Cushing's syndrome) usually results from a pituitary adrenocorticotropic hormone (ACTH) producing adenoma, occurs 6 times more often in women than men, and occurs in the third and fourth decades of life. Less common causes include primary adrenal tumors or malignant tumor–associated ectopic ACTH production. The decision to use drugs, radiotherapy, or surgery depends on consultation with a specialist.

Catecholamine excess caused by pheochromocytoma may be part of a familial multiple endocrine disorder and occurs more frequently in women than men. The manifestations relate to the specific catecholamines produced. Patients may present with flushing, cardiac arrhythmias, chest pain, headache, or syncope. Chronic weight loss, myocardial infarction, cardiomyopathic presentation, "myocarditis," or electrocardiographic abnormalities may be forms of presentation in the absence of discrete "spells." The diagnosis of pheochromocytoma depends on a high index of suspicion and documentation of metanephrine excess in a urine sample, an elevated catecholamine level from an intravenous sample at the time of a "spell," or an elevated plasma chromogranin A level.

Growth hormone excess caused by pituitary adenoma results in hypertension or congestive heart failure in approximately 50% of cases, with other organ manifestations of growth hormone excess or separate endocrine pituitary insufficiency resulting from a tumor compressive effect. The approach to treatment (surgical, chemical, radiation) depends on how advanced the disease is and its morphologic status in the pituitary.

Hyperthyroidism occurs more commonly in women than in men and is associated with hypertension, usually systolic blood pressure elevation from increased cardiac output. Hypothyroidism also results in hypertension, often diastolic blood pressure elevation, caused by elevated peripheral vascular resistance, fluid and sodium retention, and lower cardiac output in the face of elevated peripheral resistance. Hyperparathyroidism is associated with hypertension 60–70% of the time, although removal of the adenoma and normalization of the serum calcium level do not necessarily correct the hypertension completely. When any of these more unusual secondary causes of hypertension are suspected, it is appropriate to refer such a patient to an endocrinologist, nephrologist, or cardiologist, depending on the suspected diagnosis.

C. DIABETES

Established symptomatic or asymptomatic glucose intolerance is a well-known, ominous, and influential risk factor for coronary disease in women. The Framingham study found that women with diabetes have a 5-fold increase in risk for CAD and stroke. The Nurses Health Questionnaire Study noted that diabetes conveyed a 6- to 7-fold, age-adjusted, increased risk of nonfatal myocardial infarction and total cardiovascular mortality and a 3-fold risk of all-cause mortality. The CVD risk is independent of other cardiac risk factors in women and remains a strong risk factor even with diabetes of short recognized duration. But the overall risk of diabetes is magnified 3-fold when hypertension, cigarette smoking, or obesity is present.

Diabetes appears to be a more important risk factor for CVD in women than in men. The Framingham study found that female diabetics had twice the CVD risk of male diabetics. Because of this expressed risk and the higher incidence of obesity, hypertension, and dyslipidemia in female diabetics, therefore, even premenopausal diabetic women lose the protective effect of their premenopausal status. Diabetic women without these comorbidities have a lower CVD rate, but their risk is elevated above that of the general population. The CVD risk in diabetics manifests in an excess incidence of myocardial infarction, congestive heart failure, stroke, and cardiovascular death. The complication rate with myocardial infarction, coronary angioplasty, cardiac surgery, and peripheral vascular surgery also is significantly increased (see Chapter 31).

D. Cigarette Smoking

The Framingham study defined cigarette smoking in men early on as a major risk factor for CAD. Smoking was not defined as a risk in early profiles of Framingham women, probably because smoking incidence in the older woman who manifests CAD was low at the outset of the study in the early 1950s. Since that time, however, cigarette smoking in women has become more common and is associated with excess CVD risk in virtually every population study.

The percentage of men who smoke exceeds that of women. Although the rates of smoking have declined since the 1964 Surgeon General's report, the rate of decline in women has not been nearly as encouraging as in men (6% in women versus 21% in men, and 21% of women continue to smoke; black and white women smoke in equal numbers, but for both races, an educational level below college is associated with more than doubled incidence of smoking. Also, the number of women who begin the habit exceeds that of men, and women's average cigarette consumption has doubled in number. The CAD incidence in women who smoke is particularly enhanced in the premenopausal woman who would otherwise have a low incidence of the disease. The Kaiser-Permanente Walnut Creek Study documented a 3-fold increase in CVD death in premenopausal women who smoke. The Nurses Health Study and other studies have found that the cardiovascular morbidity of smoking is dose-dependent: the risk of premenopausal, nonfatal myocardial infarction is 3 times higher in women who smoke more than 25 cigarettes per day than in those who smoke 15–24 cigarettes per day. Smoking as few as 1 to 4 cigarettes per day increases the risk of CVD death and nonfatal myocardial infarction by a factor of 2.5 over nonsmokers. All health care providers should realize that the risk of nonfatal myocardial infarction in women who both use oral contraceptives and smoke is markedly increased. In women who smoke more than 25 cigarettes per day, the relative risk of nonfatal myocardial infarction has been calculated at 23 versus 4.8 for women who smoke but do not use oral contraceptives.

Similar to the pattern observed in men, cessation of smoking in women reduces the risk of heart disease. The risk of myocardial infarction diminishes to near baseline within 2–5 years of abstinence, and it recently has been shown that the risk reaches baseline by 10 years after cessation of smoking. There is no benefit to switching to low-tar and low-nicotine cigarettes. Based on these observations, it should be a major emphasis of primary care to encourage women to stop smoking, and their risk needs to be placed in context with other risks for coronary disease evolving with age and with the use of oral contraceptives.

E. Obesity

Heart disease and obesity have not always been linked statistically. Early studies eliminated overweight as an independent risk factor. Long-term longitudinal analysis of women in the Framingham study associated obesity with a more than 2-fold increase in CAD, however. In fact, only hypertension and age have been assigned greater risk values in these women. The Nurses Health Study identified obesity of greater than 30% of ideal body weight by Quetelet index to be associated with a relative risk of 3.3 for nonfatal myocardial infarction and CVD death. This risk was only slightly less when adjusted for presence of diabetes, hypertension, or hypercholesterolemia.

In both women and men, the distribution of body fat may be more relevant to CVD risk, especially CAD risk. Women with truncal fat (android habitus) as opposed to hip and thigh fat (gynoid habitus) seem to be at greater risk for CVD complications. The waist:hip ratio has been used to quantify fat distribution. The risk of CVD increases as this ratio increases, with a ratio of 0.8 defined as a threshold for possible aggressive treatment of obesity along with the associated risk factors. The waist:hip ratio also has been used as the criterion for a component of the so-called metabolic syndrome, or "insulin-resistance syndrome," in women. This syndrome is defined as an association of obesity, increased waist:hip ratio, hypertension, and insulin resistance, with hyperinsulinemia, hypertriglyceridemia, low HDL, and hypercholesteremia. It comes as no surprise that patients with this syndrome have an excess of CVD and CAD. That this "phenotype" may be in part genetic and in part acquired has been evaluated by the Women's Twin Study. This study looked at monozygotic twins of which 1 twin showed signs of the metabolic syndrome and found that the clinical expression of the disorder was closely linked to a subclass "phenotype B" of LDL cholesterol. This small, dense LDL cholesterol particle is believed to be more atherogenic and, in association with hypertriglyceridemia and lower HDL, its presence appears to accelerate CAD risk markedly. This manifestation in discordant twins was felt to be acquired with obesity, which magnifies a genetic predisposition to the LDL phenotype B of LDL receptor abnormality. Whether "small, dense LDL" accounts for other manifestations of CVD in women and whether treatment of the insulin resistance and/or the obesity specifically alters this risk remain to be investigated. It is clear, however, that women with central (android) obesity are at a substantial disadvantage in their risk of acquiring premature CAD. The Behavioral Risk Factor Surveillance System (BRFSS) of the Centers for Disease Control and Prevention has documented that for every 1 kg of weight gain, the American population increases type 2 diabetes prevalence by 9%. The risk of nonfatal myocardial infarction and all cause mortality rises progressively with the degree of obesity. Not only does obesity increase the risk of developing hypertension, hyperlipidemia, and type 2 diabetes, but the presence of obesity and its attendant lifestyle accounts for almost 70% of coronary risk.

Approximately 47% of white men and women in the United States are considered overweight, an increase from 40% between 1981 and 1990. But 68% of black women may be overweight, and Hispanics and Pacific Islanders in the United States also are overrepresented in the obese population. Obesity and extreme obesity have likewise become more prevalent (Figure 29–9). This direct impairment of cardiovascular health and associated rise in adult-onset diabetes, has become a major public health issue for the 21st century.

F. FAMILY HISTORY

The influence of a history of premature coronary disease in a first-degree relative is variable for women. In small population studies, the proportion of women with CAD having relatives with CAD ranges from 29% to 48%. In a retrospective study, investigators from The Cleveland Clinic identified a family history of CAD in 54% of women with CAD in whom first-time coronary angiography was to be performed. The Nurses Health Study reported that a parental history of prema-

ture CAD conveys a 2.8-fold age-adjusted relative risk of nonfatal myocardial infarction and a 5-fold risk of fatal CAD in women. This risk was not diminished by adjustment for other risk factors. Family history of premature CAD appears to be an independent risk factor for CAD among women, and premature CAD in a female relative (onset under age 65) has been recognized by the NCEP as a risk factor for both men and women.

G. USE OF ORAL CONTRACEPTIVES

Early reviews of complications of oral contraceptive pills (OCPs) found a disturbingly strong association between the use of these agents and the incidence of myocardial infarction, stroke, and thromboembolic disease. There appeared to be a dose-dependent relationship between the estrogen component and thrombotic potential in women using OCPs. In fact, higher dose estrogens cause significant elevations of plasma fibrinogen and factor 7 and reductions of antithrombin III. In the 1970s, OCPs with a higher estrogen component (50–150 μg) than those currently used posed a relative risk for cardiovascular death which appeared to be related both to the age of the woman and to whether or not she smoked. Older women and women who smoke have a greatly increased risk of CVD when they use oral contraceptives.

In addition to the procoagulant effect (venous effect) of higher dose estrogen, lipid effects and the induction of hypertension may play a role. Estrogen in-

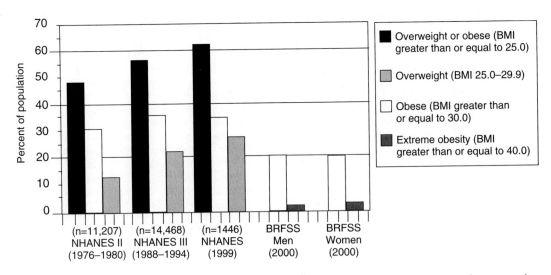

Figure 29–9. The last quarter century has seen a progressive rise in overweight, obesity, and extreme obesity in both men and women, both by direct documentation (NHANES) and self-reporting (BRFSS). (Source: 1999 National Health and Nutrition Examination Survey (NHANES) and, with permission, the Behavioral Risk Factor Surveillance System (BRFSS) in Mokdad et al: JAMA 2001;286:1195.)

creases HDL and triglycerides and decreases LDL, whereas progestins in OCP decrease HDL and increase LDL, with a net effect varying by specific formulation. Most OCPs raise LDL levels. Progestins also may bring out glucose intolerance and hypertension, ie, via arterial disease, in susceptible women. Frank hypertension caused by OCPs is uncommon and is usually mild and reversible within several months of OCP cessation. It is more common in the older or obese OCP user. As a result of earlier adverse CVD effects of OCP, manufacturers have reduced estrogen content from 50–150 μg to 30–35 μg. More recent longitudinal study of women using OCPs with a lower estrogen content and less androgenic progestins suggests that the CVD risk for OCP use has diminished significantly. However, perimenopausal women and women who smoke may still be at increased risk and may need to avail themselves of other methods of contraception. Once OCPs are stopped, prior use does not appear to be a long-term risk factor for the development of CVD.

Although the lower estrogen OCPs appear to have a lower thrombotic potential, individual susceptibility to thromboembolic disease exists, for example, in smokers. Premenopausal women with other CAD risk factors may heighten their risk of CAD with OCPs.

Postmenopausal estrogen replacement appeared in earlier observational studies to reduce a woman's risk of coronary heart disease (CHD) by 35–50%. However, biases inherent to self-reporting of behavior in these studies, as well as recent randomized trials of estrogen use in primary and secondary prevention have called into question the findings of these earlier studies. Results from the Women's Health Initiative (WHI) have shown that estrogen use compared with placebo is associated with an early increased risk of thromboembolism, myocardial infarction, and stroke. The Heart and Estrogen-progestin Replacement Study (HERS), enrolled 2763 postmenopausal women under age 80 with documented CHD, and were given usual dose conjugated estrogen (0.625 mg) and medroxyprogesterone (2.5 mg) or placebo. There was no overall risk reduction in the hormone replacement therapy (HRT) group in either CHD death or nonfatal myocardial infarction. There was, however, a 50% increase in CHD events in the first year of hormone treatment, ameliorated by a moderate risk reduction in year 2 and 3 of the study. Also, more hormone-treated women experienced venous thromboembolism and gallbladder disease than in the placebo arm. The Estrogen Replacement and Atherosclerosis (ERA) trial, like the HERS trial, found an early increase in CHD events, despite a favorable impact on lipoprotein profile. Thus, the American Heart Association recommends that HRT therapy not be used for stroke or heart attack prevention in women.

H. Psychosocial Factors

A review of social patterns since World War II had led some observers to speculate that the increased recognition of CAD in women might be related to their assumption of "male" roles and that women in the workforce may develop more CAD than women who stay home. The Framingham study data lead to an opposite interpretation. In 14 years of follow-up, CAD was found to be unassociated with a woman's fact of employment (at home or commercially). Blue collar working women tended to have more CAD than white collar women, but analysis did not show a statistically significant difference. Marital status or spouse's occupation also did not predict CAD. Educational level has an inverse relationship to the development of CAD, however, such that women with an eighth grade educational level or less appear to have a 4-fold excess incidence of CAD, independent of age, cholesterol level, smoking, blood pressure, weight, or diabetes. This finding deserves further study in a larger cohort, which may be forthcoming from the WHI.

"Type A" personality in men was suggested and then refuted as a CAD risk factor. Women in the Framingham study with type A personality also exhibited an excess incidence of CAD. Some researchers believe that the disruptive type A personality, who is critical, impatient, demeaning, self-important, and somewhat socially isolated, may have a true predisposition to CAD, but the causal link remains obscure.

Aronow WS: Cholesterol 2001. Rationale for lipid-lowering in older patients with or without CAD. Geriatrics 2001;56:22. [PMID: 11582971]

Bandyopadhyay S, Bayer AJ, O'Mahony MS: Age and gender bias in statin trials. QJM 2001;94:127. [PMID: 11259687]

Bass KM et al: Plasma lipoprotein levels as predictors of cardiovascular death in women. Arch Intern Med 1993;153:2209. [PMID: 8215724]

Bolego C, Poli A, Paoletti R: Smoking and gender. Cardiovasc Res 2002;53:568. [PMID: 11861027]

Clearfield M et al: Air Force/Texas Coronary Atherosclerosis Prevention Study (AFCAPS/TexCAPS): efficacy and tolerability of long-term treatment with lovastatin in women. J Womens Health Gend Based Med 2001;10:971. [PMID: 11788107]

Dagenais GR et al: Effects of ramipril on coronary events in high-risk persons: results of the Heart Outcomes Prevention Evaluation Study. Circulation 2001;104:522. [PMID: 11479247]

Downs JR et al: Primary prevention of acute coronary events with lovastatin in men and women with average cholesterol levels: results of AFCAPS/TexCAPS. Air Force/Texas Coronary Atherosclerosis Prevention Study. JAMA 1998;279:1615. [PMID: 9613910]

Fleschler R: Heart-healthy eating. AWHONN Lifelines 1998;2:32. [PMID: 9633305]

Group LIPID Study: Long-term effectiveness and safety of pravastatin in 9014 patients with coronary heart disease and average cholesterol concentrations: the LIPID trial follow-up. Lancet 2002;359:1379. [PMID: 11978335]

Haymart MR, Allen J, Blumenthal RS: Optimal management of dyslipidemia in women and men. J Gend Specif Med 1999; 2:37. [PMID: 11279870]

Kaplan NM: The deadly quartet: Upper body obesity, glucose intolerance, hypertriglyceridemia, and hypertension. Arch Intern Med 1989;149:1514. [PMID: 2662932]

Legato MJ: Dyslipidemia, gender, and the role of high-density lipoprotein cholesterol: implications for therapy. Am J Cardiol 2000;86:15L. [PMID: 11374849]

Lewis SJ et al: Effect of pravastatin on cardiovascular events in women after myocardial infarction: the cholesterol and recurrent events (CARE) trial. J Am Coll Cardiol 1998;32:140. [PMID: 9669262]

Liu S et al: Fruit and vegetable intake and risk of cardiovascular disease: the Women's Health Study. Am J Clin Nutr 2000;72: 922. [PMID: 11010932]

Maki KC et al: Association between elevated plasma fibrinogen and the small, dense low-density lipoprotein phenotype among postmenopausal women. Am J Cardiol 2000;85:451. [PMID: 10728949]

Maron DJ: The epidemiology of low levels of high-density lipoprotein cholesterol in patients with and without coronary artery disease. Am J Cardiol 2000;86:11L. [PMID: 11374848]

Miller M et al: Sex bias and underutilization of lipid-lowering therapy in patients with coronary artery disease at academic medical centers in the United States and Canada. Prospective Randomized Evaluation of the Vascular Effects of Norvasc Trial (PREVENT) Investigators. Arch Intern Med 2000;160: 343. [PMID: 10668836]

Mokdad A et al: The continuing epidemics of obesity and diabetes in the United States. JAMA 2001;286:1195. [PMID: 11559264]

Obarzanek E et al: Effects on blood lipids of a blood pressure-lowering diet: the Dietary Approaches to Stop Hypertension (DASH) Trial. Am J Clin Nutr 2001;74:80. [PMID: 11451721]

Psaty BM et al: Association between blood pressure level and the risk of myocardial infarction, stroke, and total mortality: the cardiovascular health study. Arch Intern Med 2001;161: 1183. [PMID: 11343441]

Sabate J: Nut consumption, vegetarian diets, ischemic heart disease risk, and all-cause mortality: evidence from epidemiologic studies. Am J Clin Nutr 1999;70(3 Suppl):500S. [PMID: 10479222]

Schmitz JM et al: Smoking cessation in women with cardiac risk: a comparative study of two theoretically based therapies. Nicotine Tob Res 1999;1:87. [PMID: 10072392]

Stefanick ML et al: Effects of diet and exercise in men and postmenopausal women with low levels of HDL cholesterol and high levels of LDL cholesterol. N Engl J Med 1998;339:12. [PMID: 9647874]

van der Gaag MS et al: Moderate alcohol consumption and changes in postprandial lipoproteins of premenopausal and postmenopausal women: a diet-controlled, randomized intervention study. J Womens Health Gend Based Med 2000;9:607. [PMID: 10957749]

Wassertheil-Smoller S et al: Hypertension and its treatment in postmenopausal women: baseline data from the Women's Health Initiative. Hypertension 2000;36:780. [PMID: 11082143]

Primary Prevention of Coronary Artery Disease

A. ASPIRIN

The Nurses' Health Study has reported a correlation between taking 1–6 aspirin tablets per week and a lower CAD risk, compared with nonusers of aspirin. In this nonrandomized study, there was a 32% reduction in the incidence of a first myocardial infarction based on this intervention. Although this benefit extended to women who reported taking 1 to 6 aspirin tablets per week, it disappeared in women who took more than 7 aspirin tablets per week. Moreover, those who reported taking more than 15 aspirin per week had a statistically insignificant but nonetheless increased incidence of hemorrhagic stroke. The benefit was limited to women older than 50 years and was greatest among women who smoked and women with hypertension or hypercholesterolemia. The conclusion of the Physician's Health Study that half an aspirin per day may be beneficial cannot be extended to women, because women were not included in that study. Therefore, there is insufficient evidence to recommend prophylactic aspirin therapy for premenopausal women who do not have risk factors for coronary disease as a primary prevention. In women who do have risk factors for coronary disease, including postmenopausal state in combination with diabetes, hypertension, or hypercholesterolemia, the use of 1 aspirin per day may be beneficial, but the risk for hemorrhagic stroke may outweigh this benefit. The WHI is currently studying the effect of 100 mg/d of aspirin in 40,000 female health professionals over the age of 45 to assess the potential benefit of aspirin in primary prevention. However, in women with established cardiovascular disease, including myocardial infarction, stroke, transient ischemic attack, angina and peripheral vascular disease, low dose aspirin (81–325 mg/d) is recommended, based on the results of the Antiplatelet Trialists Collaboration. Recently, Lauer has recommended that the decision to prescribe aspirin for primary prevention follow the similar rules of evidence as are described above for cholesterol treatment. His proposal, for both men and women, is to prescribe aspirin (81–325 mg/d) as secondary prevention for all established coronary disease. Aspirin for primary prevention is indicated when the 10-year risk for cardiac events exceeds 15%, or in well-treated hypertension with end-organ damage or diabetes (10 year risk 7–14%). This strategy aims to optimize the benefit-risk ratio for reduction of cardiac events with the risk of intracerebral hemorrhage.

B. ALCOHOL

The Nurses' Health Study, based on a questionnaire completed by 87,526 female nurses, ages 34–59 years, reported that moderate alcohol consumption appeared to be protective against the risk of nonfatal myocardial infarction, cardiovascular death, and ischemic stroke. Approximately 1 to 2 drinks per day was found to reduce the risk of CAD and ischemic stroke by 40–60%. Other studies have indicated that this finding is likely to be related to the increase in synthesis of subfractions 1 and 2 of HDL cholesterol and intrinsic tissue plasminogen activator. However, there was a statistically nonsignificant but worrisome increased risk of subarachnoid hemorrhage in female nurses who consumed 3 or more drinks per day. It is not recommended that women who do not currently consume alcohol initiate this habit to ameliorate their CAD risk. Those who do drink should be cautioned against excess alcohol consumption and be monitored in relation to its effect on weight, hypertriglyceridemia, and hypertension.

C. VITAMIN E, BETA-CAROTENE, AND OTHER ANTIOXIDANTS

Only vitamin E intake, dietary as well as oral supplementation, has been associated with the reduction of some CVD events in both men and women. In women, this finding comes from a questionnaire derived from the Nurses' Health Study. Nurses who reported increased vitamin E intake had a 30–40% reduction in risk of coronary events. This reduction appeared to be independent of age, smoking status, or other risk factors for coronary disease. This finding needs to be tested specifically, however; cause and effect cannot be construed from the data. It may be that women who reported vitamin E use were exhibiting a healthier lifestyle profile. The WHI is testing the effect of vitamin E as primary prevention with or without aspirin, but the study is still ongoing. The recently published HOPE Trial, 2 × 2 factorial trial of the ACE inhibitor ramipril with or without vitamin E (400 IU/d), did not find a significant benefit for vitamin E (men and women combined), despite the dramatic benefit of ramipril in reducing CVD end points. The safety and efficacy of vitamin E in established coronary disease needs further study. The CHAOS trial found a disparity of benefit for fatal and nonfatal myocardial infarction with vitamin E use. Other antioxidants, such as selenium and beta-carotene, have not been associated with a significant risk reduction of coronary disease in women, either as primary or secondary prevention. Currently the Women's Antioxidant Cardiovascular Study (WACS) is studying the effect of vitamin E, vitamin C, and beta-carotene in 6000 women with established CVD or more than 3 CAD risk factors.

D. SMOKING CESSATION, EXERCISE, AND DIET

Because cigarette smoking is the only reversible CAD risk factor in women that has a proven beneficial effect, cessation of smoking should be emphasized. A program of exercise coupled with diet and weight reduction should be part of a long-term approach to health maintenance. Specific recommendations are found in Chapter 7.

Denke MA: Primary prevention of coronary heart disease in postmenopausal women. Am J Med 1999;107:48S.[PMID: 10484243]

Denke MA: Primary prevention of heart disease in women. Curr Atheroscler Rep 2001;3:136.[PMID: 11177657]

Hennekens CH: Risk factors for coronary heart disease in women. Cardiol Clin 1998;16:1. [PMID: 9507775]

Lauer MS: Clinical practice. Aspirin for primary prevention of coronary events. N Engl J Med 2002;346:1468. [PMID: 12000818]

Lonn E: Epidemiology of ischemic heart disease in women. Can J Cardiol 2001;17:14D. [PMID: 11726992]

Wenger N: Coronary heart disease in women: A "new" problem. Hosp Pract (Nov 15) 1992;59.

Wenger NK, Speroff L, Packard B: Cardiovascular health and disease in women. N Engl J Med 1993;329:247. [PMID: 8316269]

Relevant Web Sites

[Heart Disease in Women Statistics and Guidelines]
http://www. americanheart.org/presenter.jhtml?identifier=2781
[NCEP ATP III Cholesterol Treatment Guidelines]
http://www. nhlbi.nih.gov/guidelines/cholesterol/index.htm
[ATP III 10 year cardiac risk calculator]
http://hin.nhlbi.nih.gov/ atpiii/calculator.asp?usertype=prof
[The JNC VI Guidelines on the treatment of hypertension]
http://www.nhlbi.nih.gov/guidelines/hypertension/jnc6.pdf
[The DASH Diet]
http://rover.nhlbi.nih.gov/health/public/heart/hbp/dash/new_dash.pdf
[Healthy Lifestyle for Women]
http://www.americanheart.org/presenter.jhtml?identifier=1200009

Evaluation of Chest Pain

30

Edward F. Gibbons, MD

The epidemiology of coronary artery disease (CAD) in women attests to its prominence as a public health problem, because of both the large number of women affected and the incomplete understanding of the evolution of serious CAD in women. Because the mortality rate of myocardial infarction (MI) is higher in women than in men, earlier diagnosis and treatment of the manifestations of coronary disease in women are needed. The clinical manifestations of ischemic coronary disease in women must be understood and placed in perspective alongside an understanding of the pitfalls of diagnostic testing for coronary disease, testing that has been designed largely for the diagnosis of coronary disease in men.

■ MANIFESTATIONS OF CAD

ANGINA

ESSENTIALS OF DIAGNOSIS

- *Chronic and reproducible chest tightness, arm, neck, jaw, or upper back pain brought on by exertion or other physiologic stress.*
- *Relieved by rest, nitroglycerin or other antiischemic medication.*
- *With objective findings of coronary ischemia that may not be confirmed by noninvasive testing.*

General Considerations

Angina is much more likely to present in women than men as the initial clinical manifestation of CAD. The 30-year follow-up of men and women in the Framingham Study continues to reflect this earlier trend. Stable and unstable angina account for 54% of initial presentations in women but only 38% of initial presentations in men (Table 30–1). The earlier Framingham data

suggested that men were twice as likely as women to have an MI within 5 years after the onset of angina. The 30-year data give the same impression: men with angina have 2-year and 10-year myocardial rates that are double those in women. CAD death rates and overall mortality rates have been 40–50% higher in men than women at 2 and 10 years after the development of angina. However, survival in women is highly dependent on the age at which angina begins. Women who are in their 50s when angina begins live longer than their male counterparts. Women who are in their 60s when angina begins have a mortality rate comparable with age-matched men (Figure 30–1).

Clinical Findings

There are few specific clinical findings for angina. Physical examination at the time of an anginal episode may demonstrate reversible paradoxic splitting of the second heart sound, a transient ventricular gallop or pulmonary rales, or a transient murmur of mitral regurgitation. The clinical index of suspicion for ischemic coronary disease would be heightened by the presence of uncontrolled hypertension, findings of peripheral vascular disease, carotid disease, abdominal aneurysm, or cutaneous manifestations of hyperlipidemia.

Prognosis

It is not clear whether the stepwise worsening of prognosis is related to aging itself or to the specificity of the diagnosis of CAD, compared with the clinical diagnosis of angina pectoris. Women with angina who were enrolled in the registry of the Coronary Artery Surgery Study (CASS) had a mean age of 54 years, similar to the men, but they were much more likely than men to have atypical or nonexertional chest pain (Table 30–2). Thus, it is not particularly surprising that 50% of these women had no or minimal CAD by angiography, whereas only 17% of the men had trivial coronary disease at angiography (Table 30–3). The pathophysiology of angina in women without angiographic evidence of significant disease has not been adequately explained. Even in women with a high risk-factor profile for CAD

Table 30–1. Initial clinical presentations of coronary heart disease.

Presentation	Men No.	Men %	Women No.	Women %	Total No.	Total %
Angina	291	32	319	47	610	39
Coronary insufficiency*	52	6	50	7	102	6
Recognized myocardial infarction (MI)	267	30	118	18	385	25
Unrecognized MI	140	16	96	14	236	15
Death	145	16	91	14	240	15

*Coronary insufficiency is synonymous with unstable angina.
Reproduced, with permission, from Framingham Heart Study Follow-up Data. Courtesy of J Murabite and the American Heart Association, 1993.

or with typical exertional angina, the incidence of angiographically significant CAD is lower than in men (70% vs 90%). However, if postmenopausal status is added to these features of typical angina pectoris in women, the Cleveland Clinic has shown in a large angiography series that 90% of such women are found to have significant CAD.

These observations call into question the validity of angina as a clinical marker for CAD in women. More-over, if angina is used as a clinical marker without the discrimination of other factors, such as quality of pain, menopausal status, and functional limitation, its presumed benign course may result in underdiagnosis and undertreatment of significant CAD in women. The prognosis of angina becomes diluted when women without significant CAD are included in studies (as in the CASS study), which makes the true prognosis of women with angiographically significant CAD less clear. Also, the migration from atypical to typical symptoms in some women presents a diagnostic dilemma, because population studies have shown that atypical chest pain syndromes appear to be associated with a 5-fold excess of long-term morbidity even in the initial absence of documented CAD. Thus, the distinction between chest pain and clinical exertional angina must be made at the outset; further research is needed to be able to interpret other signs and symptoms of ischemia to allow a more precise diagnosis of CAD in women.

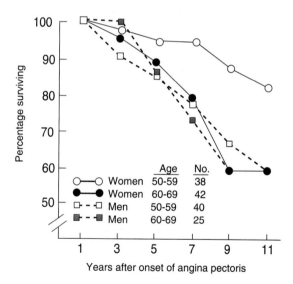

	Age	No.
Women	50-59	38
Women	60-69	42
Men	50-59	40
Men	60-69	25

Years after onset of angina pectoris

Figure 30–1. Survival of men and women after the onset of angina. The postmenopausal state and age greater than 60 years are associated with a worse angina prognosis. (Reproduced, with permission, from Kannel WB, Feinleib M: Natural history of angina pectoris in The Framingham Heart Study. *Am J Cardiol* 1972:29;154.)

Table 30–2. Classification of angina at entry into the Coronary Artery Surgery Study (CASS).

Classification	Male (%)	Female (%)
Definite angina	46	28
unstable	41	52
Probable angina	29	35
unstable	27	31
Probably not angina	9	25
Definitely not angina	2	4
No chest pain	15	7

Reproduced, with permission, from CASS Principal Investigators (authors). The National Heart, Lung, and Blood Institute Coronary Artery Surgery Study (CASS). Circulation 1981; 63(Suppl):1–23.

Table 30–3. Extent of coronary artery disease (CAD) of participants in the Coronary Artery Surgery Study.

Extent of CAD[1]	Male (%)	Female (%)
None	12	40
Mild	5	10
Moderate	4	5
Significant (> 70%)		
1 VD	21	17
2 VD	25	14
3 VD	24	15
Left main (> 50%)	9	4

[1]Extent of disease determined by angiography.
Reproduced, with permission, from CASS Principal Investigators (authors). The National Heart, Lung, and Blood Institute Coronary Artery Surgery Study (CASS). Circulation 1981:63(Suppl I):I–23.

UNSTABLE ANGINA

ESSENTIALS OF DIAGNOSIS

- *New onset of limiting angina, or*
- *Angina at rest or nocturnal angina, or*
- *Prolonged episode of angina or lowered threshold of chronic angina.*

General Considerations

The Framingham Study found no gender differences in unstable angina (prolonged rest pain without MI, in current parlance one of the "acute coronary syndromes," see Chapter 30). This was referred to as "coronary insufficiency," an initial CAD manifestation (see Table 30–1). The CASS enrolled similar numbers of men and women with unstable angina, but of those proceeding to coronary artery surgery, a higher proportion of women than men had a diagnosis of unstable rest angina. Thus, women entered the surgical arm of the study with more advanced disease, which partially explains their higher surgical mortality (see Chapter 31). Unstable angina in the Framingham Study was associated with slightly higher 2-year and much higher 10-year MI and late mortality rates in men than in women. However, these men had a higher incidence of diabetes, smoking, and hypertension than the women at the outset. Other observational surgical and angiographic studies report a higher incidence of women coming to surgery and angiography with unstable angina. Whether this finding reflects a gender-specific predisposition to an unstable pattern or a delay in diagnosis is not certain. A potential delay in angiography for women with unstable angina also may be fueled by the impression that more women than men with unstable angina are found to have normal coronary vessels on angiography. Again, this dilemma requires that more specific diagnostic strategies be developed to define true coronary disease in women with chest pain syndromes.

Clinical Findings

The clinical findings of unstable angina are those of angina in general. Positive findings on physical examination are more likely to be found in women with unstable angina and atherosclerotic risk factors.

Prognosis

The prognosis of unstable angina is dependent on:

- The severity of symptoms
- The acuity of clinical presentation
- Hemodynamic and electrical stability
- Response to treatment of ischemia
- Electrocardiographic signs of ischemia and
- Documentation of serum markers for myocardial necrosis (see Chapter 31).

MYOCARDIAL INFARCTION

ESSENTIALS OF DIAGNOSIS

- *Prolonged chest tightness or angina equivalent symptom (dyspnea, nausea, lightheadedness, syncope).*
- *Associated with serum markers for myocardial necrosis.*
- *With or without new electrocardiographic signs of ischemia or infarction.*

General Considerations

Recognized and unrecognized ("silent") MI in the Framingham Study accounted for 46% of initial CAD events in men but only 32% of initial events in women (see Table 30–1). However, an MI as an initial manifestation of CAD is more likely to be fatal in a woman than in a man (38% vs 25% 1-year mortality rate).

Recognized MI accounts for 66% of MI in men but for only 50–55% in women. Both categories of MI are associated with an excess of early and late recurrences of MI, as well as of cardiovascular and all-cause mortality in women.

Clinical Findings

The recognition and timely treatment of MI in women may be compromised by women's tendency to have (1) less ST-segment deviation with MI, (2) non–Q wave infarction, and (3) more atypical symptoms. A German study showed that *neck and shoulder pain* and *nausea and vomiting* were significantly more likely to be present in women than in men. Other aspects of potential gender bias or gender underdiagnosis are discussed in Chapter 31.

Prognosis

When MI occurs in women, the following adverse variables appear to affect prognosis:

- Higher rate of non–Q wave infarction
- Higher rate of reinfarction at 1 and 2 years
- Higher rate of prior and subsequent congestive heart failure
- Higher rate of myocardial lateral wall and mitral valve rupture (likely age-related)
- Higher rate of post-MI stroke
- Higher 1-year CAD mortality rate (45% vs 10% for men)
- Higher 2-year CAD mortality rate after MI (33% vs 20% for men)
- Higher 10-year overall mortality rate after MI (69% vs 53%, likely age-related)
- Similar 10-year cardiovascular mortality rate (49% vs 41% for men).

Mortality for MI is higher across all age groups in women; the age-adjusted risk of post-MI death across study groups is 40–45% higher for women than men but is 69% higher in black women than white women. Diabetes compounds this risk independent of the size of infarction. Several authors have examined this gender-related difference in mortality and have suggested it can be explained completely on the basis of age and prior comorbidities of diabetes, hypertension, and congestive heart failure. Authors of other studies, in particular the Multicenter Investigation of Limitation of Infarct Size (MILIS) Study, argue for an independent gender-related risk. Whichever interpretation is correct, the average woman with an MI is 40% more likely than a man to die in the hospital.

SUDDEN DEATH

Sudden death accounts for approximately two thirds of coronary deaths and is the single manifestation in 11% of men and 8% of women. Yet, no prior manifestation of the disease was evident in 63% of women who die suddenly with coronary heart disease (CHD). The risk of sudden death occurring as a complication of chronic CAD is twice as likely in men as women, but its risk may be heightened by cigarette smoking and alcohol abuse in women. Sudden death as a manifestation of initial CAD occurs more commonly in women in their 70s than in men in their 50s, possibly because of the greater likelihood of the development of CAD. Complex ventricular ectopy after MI has a worse prognosis for men but not consistently for women. These features have yet to be scrutinized in larger studies set up specifically to look at gender as a risk for sudden death.

LEFT VENTRICULAR DYSFUNCTION

 ESSENTIALS OF DIAGNOSIS

- *Dyspnea, fatigue, or lethargy.*
- *Often but not always associated with physical findings of fluid overload (pulmonary congestion, venous congestion, or ventricular gallop).*
- *Documented by invasive or noninvasive findings of systolic and/or diastolic dysfunction.*

Clinical Findings

Several features of MI complication rates in women may relate to women's underlying risk factors for CAD. Female patients with CAD appear to have more diabetes, hypertension, and hypercholesterolemia than men with CAD. Congestive heart failure complicating MI is more common in women, particularly in black women. Black women have a higher short- and long-term post-MI mortality rate than white women. Curiously, women tend to have a higher left ventricular ejection fraction (LVEF) than men after MI. LVEF is an accurate predictor of survival after MI for both women and men. However, the higher incidence of symptomatic left ventricular dysfunction suggests diastolic dysfunction related to left ventricular hypertrophy and diastolic noncompliance from chronic hypertension and diabetes. Whether this is a sign of myocardial lack of reserve, increased subendocardial ischemia from left ventricular hypertrophy, or silent myocardial ischemia remains to be addressed. If women are more likely than men to have unrecognized MI, the risk of silent ischemia also may be greater. The therapeutic implications of these unanswered questions are likely to have a direct impact on post-MI morbidity and mortality in women.

Prognosis

The prognosis of MI associated with clinical or occult left ventricular dysfunction is significantly worse than that of women without these findings. In-hospital mortality rates for MI complicated by heart failure are increased at least 3-fold, depending on the etiology of the decompensation. An aggressive search for reversible ischemic, valvular, and other mechanical causes of heart failure, as well as early introduction of appropriate pharmacologic therapy are warranted in this setting (see Chapter 31).

■ DIAGNOSIS OF CAD

Because the prevalence of CAD is lower in women than men, any diagnostic test useful for the diagnosis of CAD in men is likely to have less value in women. Even when a test is specifically designed for women, the population of women studied can strongly influence the reliability of the test. For example, tests for CAD in women with typical angina who are postmenopausal or post-MI are bound to have greater sensitivity and specificity than the same tests in an unselected population. A broad, comprehensive strategy is needed to elicit symptoms and reliably find coronary disease in the women at risk for this disease.

Clinical Findings

Of course, a careful history and physical examination should be a part of general health care in women with risk factors for CAD. Women should be asked not only about chest pain, but also about exercise stamina; exertional dyspnea; and exertional neck, throat, and arm tightness or interscapular pain. If such symptoms are present, they may represent true exertional angina. Probable angina refers to a symptom similar to exertional angina but varying in position, precipitant, or duration of pain. Nonischemic chest pain refers to a symptom complex of nonexertional chest pain of atypical duration, association, and precipitation so inconsistent as to raise major doubt concerning its cardiac source. The angiographic prevalence of CAD for each of these categories of chest pain is much lower in women than men even if angina is typical and exertional (Figure 30–2). Even with typical angina, only 62% of women on average have significant CAD on angiography, com-

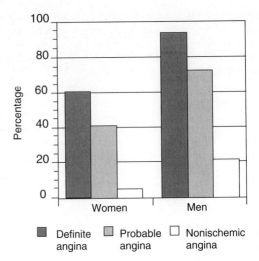

Figure 30–2. The percentage of men and women with angiographically significant CAD, by gender and type of chest pain symptoms. (Reproduced, with permission, from the American Heart Association: CASS registry data. Circulation 1981;63[Suppl I].)

pared with 90–93% of men. The yield is even lower with less typical pain. Multivessel disease or left main coronary disease is seen to occur in only 50% of women with typical angina, 19% of women with probable angina, and 2% of women with nonischemic chest pain. Thus, the clinical history of angina in women has a higher false-positive rate than in men.

ECG Treadmill Testing

All protocols for electrocardiography (ECG) treadmill testing rely on the assessment of the electrocardiographic response to exercise. A response is called positive if the ST segment is depressed 1 mm or more when measured 0.06–0.08 seconds after the J point of the QRS deflection. If baseline ST depression is present, interpretation is more difficult and specificity is lower, but sometimes the result is considered positive if at least 2 mm of ST-segment depression beyond the baseline is seen. Exercise ECG testing was performed as part of the large CASS registry. Although the sensitivity for detecting CAD by this test was similar in men and women (84% vs 80% typical angina), the specificity suffered (71% vs 57% in women) (Table 30–4). Indeed, the less typical the pain, the greater the likelihood that an exercise ECG will be falsely positive (Figure 30–3). A clinical risk score based on gender assigns risk to women (low, < 20%; intermediate, 20–80%; and high, > 80%) based on minor and major determinants (Table 30–5). This scheme can be combined with provocative testing

Table 30–4. Sensitivity and specificity of ECG treadmill testing.

Test	Clinical Pattern	Men		Women	
		Sensitivity (%)	Specificity (%)	Sensitivity (%)	Specificity (%)
Treadmill ECG	Definite angina	84	71	80	57
Normal resting ECG	Probable angina	72	80	67	69
	Nonangina	46	79	22	81
Abnormal resting ECG	Definite angina	90	29	96	22
	Probable angina	85	45	88	33
	Nonangina	90	66	50	41

Reproduced, with permission, from CASS Principal Investigators (authors). The National Heart, Lung, and Blood Institute Coronary Artery Surgery Study (CASS). Circulation 1981;63(Suppl I):I–24.

to increase diagnostic yield of both invasive and noninvasive testing.

In general, ECG exercise testing is marred by false-positive results in women and false-negative results in men. In the CASS registry, when patients were matched for age, sex, and degree of CAD, sensitivity and specificity were similar for men and women. However, other studies looking at the sensitivity of exercise testing (and therefore the percentage of false-negative results) in women have found sensitivity to be 20–30% less for women than men, even when angiographic CAD incidence is comparable. The lower sensitivity of treadmill testing for the diagnosis of CAD in women in several studies may reflect a lower maximal heart rate achieved by women and the lower sensitivity to single-vessel CAD under these circumstances.

For these reasons, there may be a problem in detecting coronary disease in women beyond the difference accounted for by a decreased overall population preva-lence, ie, a non-bayesian pattern. In general, the clinician can have the greatest confidence in a negative ECG treadmill test in a woman with typical exertional angina who achieves high workload on treadmill testing. A considerable number of women in whom a false-positive result is suspected need to be evaluated by additional testing, however. Concern over cost and yield of testing have given rise to several formulas that define exercise treadmill testing as positive when a stratification score is applied to women based on ST-segment depression and exercise performance. The formulation by Robert et al, which integrates ST depression with workload and peak heart rate, increases sensitivity from 59% to 70% and specificity from 72% to 89% and probably deserves wider application. In addition, computer methods for calculating ST heart rate slope have been applied specifically to women and found to achieve a higher specificity with maintenance of sensitivity. The adverse prognostic value of exercise-induced

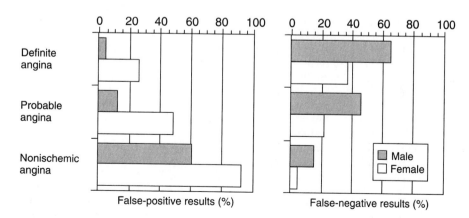

Figure 30–3. Percentage of false-positive and false-negative ECG treadmill tests by type of symptom and gender. (Reproduced, with permission, from the American Heart Association: CASS registry data. Circulation 1981;63[Suppl I].)

Table 30–5. Determinants of CAD in women that have prognostic value for further testing.

Determinants	Risk Level
Minor Age > 65 years Obesity (especially central) Sedentary lifestyle Family history of CAD Other CAD risks	**Low** < 20% likelihood No major; ≤ 1 intermediate or ≤ 2 minor

Intermediate
 Hypertension
 Smoking
 Dyslipidemia (especially
   low HDL cholesterol)
	Intermediate
	 20–80% likelihood
	 1 major or > 1 minor or interme-
	   diate

Major Typical angina Postmenopausal, no HRT Diabetes Peripheral vascular disease	**High** > 80 % likelihood ≥ 2 major or 1 major with ≥ 1 minor or intermediate

CAD, coronary artery disease; HDL, high-density lipoprotein; HRT, hormone replacement therapy.
Diagnostic scheme adapted from Douglas PS and Ginsberg GS, The evaluation of chest pain in women. *N Engl J Med* 1996; 334:1311.

ST-segment depression alone is greater for men than for women, because such a pattern is more likely to represent myocardial ischemia in most men but only in women who are postmenopausal and have CAD risk factors. However, when exercise duration is factored in with ST depression and exercise-induced angina, prognosis can be reliably graded, such that an ischemic pattern with angina at a low workload predicts a poor prognosis and by itself is an indication for coronary angiography. The Duke Treadmill Score, which scores prognosis based on exercise capacity, ST-segment depression, and angina quality, has been found useful in risk stratification and as an indication for more aggressive evaluation and treatment (ie, angiography for high risk) for both men and women.

Score = Exercise time (minutes) − (5 × ST deviation

[mm]) − (4 × exercise angina [0 = none,

1 = nonlimiting, 2 = limiting]).

This score indicates low risk if ≥ 5, and conveys a 1.8% 5-year cardiac mortality rate. Moderate risk (score −10 to +4) conveys a 5.5 % 5-year death rate. High risk (score ≤ -11) is associated with a 13% 5-year mortality rate. This score has been endorsed by the American

College of Cardiology as an initial step in noninvasive testing for women. The higher rate of false-positive results in women with atypical pain has yet to be explained. The ST segment is known to be sensitive to metabolic variables. Left ventricular hypertrophy, thiazide diuretics, digoxin, and hyperventilation can exaggerate the ST segment.

ECG Stress Testing With Cardiac Imaging

A. NUCLEAR PERFUSION TREADMILL TESTING

When thallium perfusion imaging is added to ECG stress testing on treadmill, sensitivity remains in the range of 70–85%, for both men and women, but specificity in women rises in some studies from 60–65% to 80–90%. The test is most useful for "probable" angina or when the baseline electrocardiographic ST segment is abnormal at rest, and it is less useful for nonischemic pain. Studies of more representative general populations than seen in referral centers have shown a disappointing deterioration of specificity in women down to 70%. This result appears to apply to both planar and single-photon emission computed tomography (SPECT) imaging, but it may improve with greater general recognition of breast attenuation artifact. It is important to note that single-vessel disease is diagnosed less often in women (50–60%) than in men (75–85%). The reduced sensitivity appears to be related to a lower heart rate achieved. In some series, single-vessel disease is diagnosed almost equally in women and men, but patients in these series have had a predominance of anterior ischemia, to which thallium has a higher sensitivity in both men and women. The diagnostic yield of thallium imaging in defining multivessel disease is improved if multiple perfusion defects are found and thallium lung uptake (indicative of left ventricular dysfunction) is seen. The diagnostic accuracy of either thallium/sestamibi or sestamibi rest/exercise imaging has been found in selected populations to increase sensitivity of multivessel CAD to 92% with a specificity of at least 75–80%. The enhanced specificity may relate to the coupling of wall motion data to perfusion data. In some centers, this appears to reduce the false-positive rate in women.

B. DIPYRIDAMOLE NUCLEAR PERFUSION IMAGING

By using a pharmacologic "stress" to magnify myocardial perfusion differences, dipyridamole thallium imaging without exercise avoids the heart rate response problem and is applicable to women unable to exercise adequately because of cardiac or noncardiac limitations.

Adenosine may be used instead of dipyridamole; sestamibi may be used instead of thallium. Sensitivity and specificity are somewhat higher for this method than for thallium treadmill testing, depending on the population studied. However, women with single-vessel disease are still underdiagnosed compared with men.

C. STRESS ECHOCARDIOGRAPHY

ECG treadmill testing combined with pre-exercise and postexercise imaging of left ventricular regional and global wall motion by echocardiography assesses left ventricular ischemia and infarction in a way that is complementary to thallium perfusion imaging. In general, the sensitivity and specificity of stress echocardiography are comparable to thallium imaging for CAD detection. In women particularly, this technique has become durably reliable in meta-analysis; single-vessel disease sensitivity and specificity in one series have both been reported to be 80–90%, similar to that of multivessel disease. Although significantly less expensive than thallium imaging, stress echocardiography is technically demanding for the average cardiac ultrasonography laboratory. The study has the potential also to assess coexisting valvular heart disease and define left ventricular hypertrophy in patients with hypertension and a false-positive exercise ECG; also, the method does not involve intravenous infusion or radiation exposure.

D. DOBUTAMINE STRESS ECHOCARDIOGRAPHY

This diagnostic tool is an alternative to dipyridamole thallium imaging with similar indications. Instead of magnifying flow differences with dipyridamole, dobutamine uses its inotropic stimulus in a graded dosing protocol to bring out regional ischemic wall motion abnormalities indicative of coronary artery stenosis. Dobutamine echocardiography provides greater accuracy in predicting CAD in men than treadmill stress ECG and has similar diagnostic and prognostic power for women with suspected CAD.

E. RADIONUCLIDE BLOOD POOL IMAGING

Radionuclide blood pool imaging with stress uses global and some regional left ventricular assessment to diagnose significant CAD. The test is much less sensitive in women than men for the detection of CAD, apparently because the diagnostic usefulness of the test is in identifying multivessel disease by a fall in or failure to increase the LVEF. Men without coronary disease usually raise their LVEF by 20–24%. Normal women do not have this pattern but maintain stroke volume by increasing left ventricular end-diastolic volume with graded exercise. Thus, even normal women by these criteria have a "positive test." This is a pertinent problem, because the large Thrombolysis in Myocardial Infarction-II (TIMI-II) study used exercise blood pool scanning to define ischemia remote from the infarct in evaluating indications for coronary angiography after thrombolytic therapy. Because this approach may be invalid in women, an important aspect of women's post-MI care is uncertain. Dipyridamole nuclear imaging appears to have the greatest usefulness for this purpose, and screening exercise ECG in this high-risk population also has some prognostic usefulness, although its sensitivity is poorly studied.

F. CORONARY CALCIFICATION

Calcification of the coronary vessels may be identified by fluoroscopy of the cardiac shadow and is a useful marker of underlying atherosclerosis. In women, the reported sensitivity of chest fluoroscopy in identifying CAD is 75–80% and the specificity is 83%. Thus, the test might be used for risk stratification of women who have a positive exercise ECG test result. However, the chest fluoroscopy gives no indication of site or degree of ischemia, prior infarct, or left ventricular (LV) dysfunction (as with thallium or stress echocardiography). Its usefulness would be highest with normal results in a woman with "probable" angina and a positive treadmill test. Although it is potentially useful in the work-up, the test is not commonly used. Electron beam computed tomography (EBCT) has become a popular screening method for CAD. With the development of standardized scoring systems, the scans have become reproducible and offer prognostic value with very high score (> 800–1000) when added to traditional Framingham CAD risks. The scans fail to offer an assessment of ischemia, have not been extensively evaluated in women, and are not endorsed by the American Heart Association for routine CAD screening.

Coronary Angiography

Coronary angiography is generally regarded to be the clinical standard for identifying significant CAD. The test is invasive and more expensive than noninvasive testing, but in large centers, it is safe and reliable. The most common measure of coronary stenosis severity is a visual estimate of luminal narrowing. Quantitative computer program measurements of coronary stenosis have become more common and seem to have a closer relationship to the physiologic significance of a lesion as measured by perfusion imaging or positron emission tomography (PET) than do mere "visual estimates." Although the method of quantitative stenosis measurement has not been studied in a large series of women, it may provide more objective assessment of significant coronary disease than visual estimation, because a woman's coronary diameter is significantly smaller than a man's and luminal narrowing may be more difficult to perceive. The recorded threshold of coronary narrowing by angiography is believed to be at least 50% for moderate disease. Severe CAD is defined as one or more stenoses of at least 70–75% or greater than 50% of the left main coronary trunk. Normal or minimal coronary narrowing conveys an excellent prognosis. Moderate coronary narrowing of 50–70% may not be correlated with a worse prognosis unless left main or proximal left anterior descending disease is found, the patient has limiting angina, or thallium perfusion deficit is evident. Also, because coronary stenoses are not uniformly circular and vary in length, an apparent mild stenosis may be hemodynamically important and vice versa. In the coronary angiography descriptions in CASS, women had similar degrees of coronary disease to men, but they had more "tubular, long" stenoses than men. The significance of this difference in terms of women's tendency to present with unstable angina is a provocative aspect that needs further evaluation.

Significant CAD sometimes requires both angiography and stress imaging to define prognosis and suggest treatment. When coronary angiography shows only moderate narrowings of 50–70%, the functional correlates—patient symptoms and treadmill performance—coupled with nuclear perfusion imaging or echocardiography should take priority over anatomic findings in clinical decision making. Thus, the greatest risk to the patient is a positive thallium treadmill test and significant coronary disease by angiography. It has been demonstrated in men that any other combination of results of thallium testing and angiography is associated with excellent long-term survival (Table 30–6). Moderate CAD in an individual with a normal maximal thallium treadmill test or an abnormal thallium test in a patient with convincingly mild CAD on angiography are both associated with a greater than 95% 2- to 3-year survival rate. When both studies are abnormal, long-term survival suffers, and the rates of revascularization and nonfatal MI rise as well. Despite an overall excellent prognosis, each discordant combination is associated

with a 2–3% risk of nonfatal MI, likely related to coronary plaque hemorrhage or in situ thrombosis rather than progression of trivial luminal narrowing. This type of nonfatal MI in a patient with a history of mild coronary disease by angiography is more likely to be seen in women who smoke or take oral contraceptives. Clinicians should recognize that any chest pain syndrome is a morbidity marker, and patients should be instructed to seek attention for a change in symptoms that may herald such an event even when they have been told in the past that they had trivial coronary disease.

EVALUATING CHEST PAIN IN WOMEN WITHOUT ATHEROSCLEROTIC CAD

Each year in the United States, more than 1.5 million people undergo cardiac catheterization, usually with coronary angiography. This procedure is done most often for the evaluation of chest pain. Most cardiac laboratories report normal coronary anatomy in up to 30% of patients, with a higher percentage in women for reasons outlined in the preceding section. These individuals have an excellent prognosis from a coronary standpoint; however, even after the reassuring knowledge of normal coronary anatomy is obtained, chest pain morbidity continues. Up to 70–80% of such individuals continue to have chest pain and to see a physician for this pain. Twenty percent to 70% of these individuals may curtail their activity or employment because of the symptom. Although patients who undergo coronary angiography early in their evaluation are more likely to go back to work on finding out that their coronary anatomy is normal, pain complaints often persist. Subsequent evaluation may be more directed and less expensive, however, once the coronary anatomy has been defined as normal. Long-term, unjustified anti-ischemic medications often can be eliminated.

Such patients require from their clinicians a careful ear in history taking and a proper understanding of the differential diagnosis of chest pain syndromes. Women are more likely than men to have atypical chest pain and thus need such support and insight.

CORONARY ARTERY SPASM

 ESSENTIALS OF DIAGNOSIS

- *Chest tightness, arm, neck, jaw, or upper back pain occurring at rest and/or interrupting sleep.*

Table 30–6. Likelihood of survival based on angiography and thallium perfusion imaging.

Thallium Perfusion Scan Results	Normal Coronary Vessels	Abnormal Coronary Vessels
Normal	96% 7-year survival	98% 2-yr survival (1% nonfatal MI)
Abnormal	97% 3-year survival	86% 5-yr survival (12% nonfatal MI, 35% CABG/PTCA)

MI, myocardial infarction; CABG, coronary artery bypass grafting; PTCA, percutaneous transluminal coronary angioplasty. Compiled from data of Brown, 1963; Cannon, 1992; Kaul, 1988; and Raymond, 1988.

- *Associated with electrocardiographic findings of either ST elevation or depression.*
- *Without angiographic documentation of fixed severe or critical epicardial coronary narrowing.*
- *May be documented on angiography by provocative pharmacologic testing.*

Clinical Findings

Coronary blood flow is regulated by coronary smooth muscle tone, with input from the central nervous system and neuroendocrine stimuli as well as from local factors. Prinzmetal's angina, strictly defined, refers to focal spasm of a coronary vessel at the site of a mild atherosclerotic narrowing. This condition may produce angina at rest, at night, or with exercise; it is more common in men than women. Variant angina is a syndrome of rest, nocturnal, and exertional chest pain with normal epicardial coronary anatomy. This syndrome is more common in persons aged 40–60 years, and it is more common in women than men. Cigarette smokers and women with migraine headaches, esophageal dysmotility, and Raynaud's phenomenon are more likely to have coronary spasm as well. These individuals describe nocturnal awakening with chest pain, a variable onset of effort angina, and angina with cold exposure. Treadmill testing may be positive for ischemia; it is more likely to be so if testing is done in the morning rather than in the afternoon. This difference likely reflects the diurnal variation of coronary artery tone. Holter monitoring or ECG done during pain may show ST-segment elevation or depression and suggest the diagnosis. MI is uncommon, and the prognosis is generally better than that of fixed atherosclerotic coronary disease if the symptoms are controlled. Coronary angiography is frequently necessary to distinguish spasm from fixed CAD, and spasm may be provoked and proved by graded injection of ergonovine maleate during angiography for both variant and Prinzmetal's angina.

Treatment

Nitroglycerin typically relieves the chest pain. Therapy includes chronic nitrates, calcium channel blockers (diltiazem, verapamil) administered at moderate to high dose, cessation of smoking, and avoidance of cold. In addition, women with hyperlipidemia should be treated according to the Adult Treatment Panel (ATP) III guidelines (see Chapter 29), since recent data in men and women suggest that statins improve coronary vasodilation responsiveness over time. β-Blockers may promote coronary spasm in some individuals, just as they exacerbate Raynaud's phenomenon. Their use in such patients for hypertension or arrhythmias should be limited, and the response of chest pain should be judged empirically.

MICROVASCULAR ANGINA

 ESSENTIALS OF DIAGNOSIS

- *Chest tightness, arm, neck, jaw, or upper back pain brought on by exertion or other physiologic stress.*
- *Often associated with noninvasive findings of coronary ischemia, but not associated with epicardial fixed or spastic coronary narrowing.*
- *Responsive to antianginal pharmacologic therapy.*

General Considerations

First described in 1967, microvascular angina became known as syndrome X. This term is still sometimes used, but it should not be confused with the "metabolic syndrome X" of insulin resistance, obesity, hypertension, and hyperinsulinemia. The National Institutes of Health has defined a population of patients with microvascular angina, more commonly women, who have exertional angina, normal epicardial coronary arteries, no focal spasm with ergonovine provocation, and no left ventricular hypertrophy.

Clinical Findings

Microvascular angina responds to nitrate therapy and is often associated with ST-segment depression. Treadmill testing, even with thallium, is inconsistent and often negative in women with this syndrome. Research studies have shown regional or global microvascular coronary flow reserve deficit in some patients. A variety of sophisticated techniques using coronary sinus blood sampling, MRI and PET have indicated that in some patients with the clinical syndrome, there is a documented change in such indicators of ischemia with episodes of pain. Because of the subtlety of this diagnosis, it is often made clinically and based on normal angiographic findings. Support for the diagnosis may be strengthened if ergonovine produces typical chest pain with ECG changes but no focal spasm. Some researchers believe that microvascular angina is a disorder of coronary pain perception rather than coronary ischemia and should be treated symptomatically. Sensitivity to endogenous adenosine, which is believed to be a mediator of perceived myocardial ischemia, has been suggested as a mechanism. However, a subset of patients with microvascular angina who have intermittent or constant left bundle-branch block appear to suffer from a cardiomyopathic process as well, with left ventricular dysfunction appearing after months to years of anginal pain.

Treatment

These individuals should be treated for ischemia and monitored for congestive heart failure and arrhythmias to avert major morbidity and mortality. High-dose calcium channel blockade, nitrates, and occasionally, β-blockers to limit heart rate appear to be the most useful for symptom relief, even in patients without left bundle-branch block.

LEFT VENTRICULAR HYPERTROPHY

 ESSENTIALS OF DIAGNOSIS

- *Hypertrophy of left ventricular myocardium.*
- *Greater than 11 mm on echocardiography.*
- *And underestimated by electrocardiographic signs of hypertrophy.*

Clinical Findings & Treatment

Coronary perfusion to the left ventricular myocardium may be compromised with congenital or acquired left ventricular hypertrophy, elevated left ventricular end-diastolic pressure, or both in combination. Chronic systemic hypertension may lead to both phenomena and compromise subendocardial blood flow. This process may become symptomatic with exertion or tachycardia and cause a form of angina pectoris in the absence of fixed coronary disease. This physiologic picture also may magnify the ischemic potential of mild to moderate coronary disease in women with uncontrolled hypertension. Evaluation should be directed toward documenting the uncontrolled exertional hypertension, quantifying any fixed coronary disease, and controlling hypertension. This angina pattern usually responds to β-blockade, calcium channel blockade, or both in combination.

Asymmetric septal hypertrophy (formerly called IHSS) can exist in women either as a congenital anomaly and familial process or as an acquired process as a result of chronic hypertension. Any obstructive component is exacerbated by dehydration or afterload reduc-

ing agents. With marked hypertrophy, anginal chest pain may occur with exertion or arrhythmias and may even be associated with thallium perfusion abnormalities without associated fixed coronary disease. This phenomenon is diagnosed most easily by cross-sectional and Doppler echocardiography. Hypertension is better managed with β-blockers or verapamil rather than vasodilators or diuretics. Over diuresis can provoke or exacerbate the obstructive component of asymmetric septal hypertrophy.

MYOCARDIAL BRIDGING

 ESSENTIALS OF DIAGNOSIS

- *Dynamic systolic narrowing of an epicardial coronary artery.*
- *Demonstrated on angiography.*

Clinical Findings & Treatment

A myocardial bridge consists of a zone of epicardial myocardium through which a coronary artery dips and by which blood flow may be partially compromised at rapid heart rate during systole. To be considered a cause for angina, the stenosis of the dynamic bridge should be long (10–15 mm) and severe (> 70%). Ideally, the ischemic consequences of a bridge should be documented by perfusion imaging (thallium). Both β-blockers and verapamil, which decrease exercise heart rate and contractility, are effective treatment.

AORTIC VALVE STENOSIS

 ESSENTIALS OF DIAGNOSIS

- *Valvular, subvalvular, or supravalvular aortic narrowing.*
- *Associated with restriction of left ventricular outflow.*
- *And increased potential for myocardial ischemia.*

Clinical Findings

Aortic stenosis of a severe to critical degree has angina as one of its cardinal symptoms. Angina results from increased afterload, as described for left ventricular hypertrophy; in this instance, however, it is related to a fixed obstruction from a narrowed aortic valve orifice. This diagnosis is important to make before treadmill testing, because such testing in patients with critical aortic stenosis can result in circulatory collapse. Echocardiography is the best method for making this assessment. Occasionally, severe or acute aortic insufficiency can cause rest angina, but it is often associated with other signs of heart failure and is an indication for urgent surgery.

AORTIC DISSECTION

 ESSENTIALS OF DIAGNOSIS

- *Intimal disruption of the thoracic and/or abdominal aorta.*
- *Resulting in severe chest, back, or abdominal pain.*
- *With the potential for limb, organ, and cerebrovascular arterial compromise.*
- *Occasionally presenting with syncope or circulatory collapse.*

Clinical Findings & Treatment

Dissection of the thoracic aorta results from a disruption of aortic intima with medial dissection of varying length along a false lumen. Typically, the chest pain produced is acute, severe, and "ripping" in nature as the trajectory of the tear proceeds. Women with Marfan's syndrome can develop aortic dissection in the third trimester of pregnancy and are called the "young dissectors"; it is important to note that dissection can occur in young women with uncontrolled hypertension or Marfan's syndrome even in the absence of pregnancy. Men in their 50s and 60s with hypertension and atherosclerosis are the largest group of dissectors; in the elderly, however, women predominate in aortic dissection, with the same risk factors of hypertension and atherosclerosis. These elderly women may present acutely with chest pain or chronically with a secondary aortic aneurysm and heart failure. Acute aortic dissection is a surgical emergency if the ascending aorta is involved. Prompt cardiologic and cardiac surgical referral is essential. The diagnosis is made most quickly and reliably with transesophageal echocardiography. If this method is unavailable, chest computed tomography (CT) with contrast should be performed.

MITRAL VALVE PROLAPSE

 ESSENTIALS OF DIAGNOSIS

- *Congenital autosomal dominant trait.*
- *Associated with thickening and redundancy of mitral leaflets and chordal apparatus.*
- *With or without mitral regurgitation.*

General Considerations

Mitral valve prolapse (MVP) is a common congenital anomaly. MVP is an overused diagnosis to explain chest pain, particularly in young women. Careful epidemiologic study argues against chest pain as specific to the true congenital MVP independent of documented tachyarrhythmias. Older studies suggesting focal thallium perfusion deficits with MVP have not stood the test of time. Unfortunately, the clinical practice of diagnosing MVP when a young woman has atypical chest pain has led to a false epidemic of MVP, with cases often unsupported by echocardiographic diagnosis. Other causes for chest pain should be sought in women with both undiagnosed murmurs and classic structural MVP.

Clinical Findings & Treatment

True MVP is associated with auscultation findings of an early systolic click that is heard later in systole with physical maneuvers that reduce ventricular volume, such as squatting. A murmur may follow the click and vary in intensity with alterations in systemic arterial afterload and adrenergic state. The murmur becomes holosystolic with severe mitral regurgitation. The complaint of chest pain with MVP should be investigated and treated based on objective findings of any coronary ischemia, arrhythmia, progression of mitral regurgitation, or clues to a noncardiac cause.

PULMONARY HYPERTENSION

 ESSENTIALS OF DIAGNOSIS

- *Elevation of the pulmonary arterial systolic pressure greater than 30 mm Hg and/or mean pulmonary arterial pressure greater than 22 mm Hg at rest.*

Clinical Findings & Treatment

Pulmonary hypertension caused by chronic thromboembolic disease, chronic obstructive pulmonary disease (COPD), collagen vascular disease, or primary pulmonary hypertension may be associated with exertional and rest angina. This anginal syndrome appears to be the result of increased right ventricular afterload and right ventricular hypertrophy. The pain sometimes responds to nitrates, control of systemic hypertension, treatment of hypoxia, and attempts to treat the underlying cause of pulmonary hypertension.

MISCELLANEOUS NONCARDIAC CAUSES

In clinical practice, both the primary clinician and the cardiologist must evaluate noncardiac chest pain in women. Esophageal spasm may produce substernal chest pain radiating to the neck and upper arm, and it may be relieved by nitrates. The pain may be associated with dysphagia for solid foods and cold fluids. Ideally, the diagnosis should be made using strict criteria of esophageal manometry. Diltiazem can be effective treatment. Gastroesophageal reflux can be exertional, particularly in the postprandial time period. Specific questioning and response to treatment with antacids often lead to the diagnosis. Cholelithiasis may result in radiated substernal or epigastric pain that mimics angina in some individuals but is usually nonexertional. This diagnosis may complicate the course in women with CAD or with CAD risk factors; when suspected, it should be documented by ultrasonography and treated. Musculoskeletal, costochondral, or cervical radicular pain or large pendulous breasts may mimic atypical angina, but the pain in these cases is usually positional

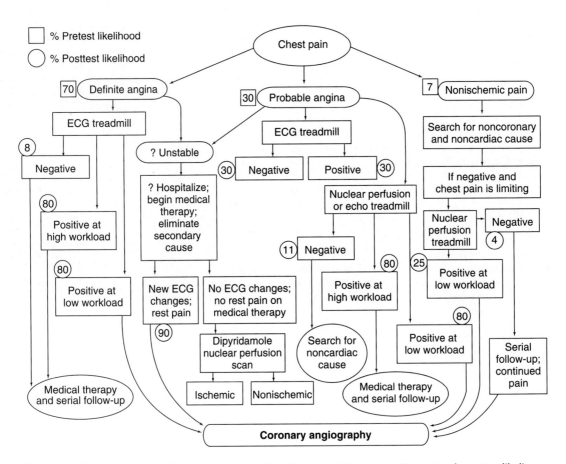

Figure 30–4. Diagnostic algorithm for the evaluation of chest pain in women. Pretest and posttest likelihoods determine the extent of work-up.

or manipulable on examination. Finally, panic disorders can be associated with a multitude of cardiac symptoms including chest pain, palpitations, dyspnea, and dizziness. This disorder should be diagnosed and treated according to strict criteria (see Chapter 10).

DIAGNOSTIC ALGORITHM

The diagnosis of CAD in women is a stepwise process, requiring the input of both clinical pretest diagnostic assessment and posttest likelihood of disease with a positive test result. The clinician's goals are the relief of symptoms, avoidance of MI, and avoidance of unnecessary treatment. The diagnostic algorithm shown in Figure 30–4 synthesizes the concepts explored earlier in the chapter. The rationale for treatment is elaborated on in Chapter 31. Several aspects should be emphasized:

1. Simple ECG treadmill testing is unlikely to improve diagnostic yield with probable angina, but conveys valuable prognostic information for both probable and atypical chest pain; nuclear perfusion treadmill or stress echocardiography is the best first test for atypical chest pain to document true ischemia.

2. Medical therapy should be justified by signs of ischemia.

3. Nonischemic chest pain has a narrow margin of diagnostic yield; even nuclear perfusion imaging was found to increase CAD likelihood only from 7% to 25%; the latter figure is approximately the same as the false-positive rate of thallium imaging in women. If nonischemic chest pain is limiting the patient's lifestyle, coronary angiography may be necessary to refute or confirm the presence of significant coronary disease, particularly in postmenopausal women.

Chae S et al: Identification of extensive coronary artery disease in women by exercise single-photon emission computed tomographic (SPECT) thallium imaging. J Am Coll Cardiol 1993;21:1305. [PMID: 8473634]

Douglas PS, Ginsberg GS: The evaluation of chest pain in women. N Engl J Med 1996;334:1311. [PMID: 8609950]

Fleischmann KE et al: Exercise echocardiography or exercise SPECT imaging? A meta-analysis of diagnostic test performance. J Nucl Cardiol 2000;7:599.

Goldberg R et al: A communitywide perspective of sex differences and temporal trends in the incidence and survival rates after acute myocardial infarction and out-of-hospital deaths caused by coronary heart disease. Circulation 1993;87:1947. [PMID: 8504508]

Greenland P et al: In-hospital and 1-year mortality in 1,524 women after myocardial infarction: Comparison with 4,315 men. Circulation 1991;83:484. [PMID: 1991367]

Kessler KL et al: Examining the prognostic accuracy of exercise treadmill testing in 1617 symptomatic women. Circulation 1996;94:565.

Kong B et al: Comparison of accuracy for detecting coronary artery disease and side-effect profile of dipyridamole thallium-201 myocardial perfusion in women versus men. Am J Cardiol 1992;70:168. [PMID: 1626502]

Mark DB et al: Exercise treadmill score for predicting prognosis in coronary artery disease. Ann Intern Med 1987;106:793. [PMID: 3579066]

Murabito JM et al: Prognosis after the onset of coronary heart disease. An investigation of differences in outcome between the sexes according to initial coronary disease presentation. Circulation 1993;88:2548. [PMID: 8252666]

Opherk D et al: Four-year follow-up study in patients with angina pectoris and normal coronary arteriograms ("syndrome X"). Circulation 1989;80:1610. [PMID: 2598425]

Robert A, Melin J, Detry JM: Logistic discriminant analysis improves diagnostic accuracy of exercise testing for coronary artery disease in women. Circulation 1991;83:1202. [PMID: 2013142]

Rodgers GP et al: American College of Cardiology/American Heart Association clinical competence statement on stress testing: a report of the American College of Cardiology/American Heart Association/American College of Physicians–American Society of Internal Medicine Task Force on Clinical Competence. J Am Coll Cardiol 2000;36:1441. [PMID: 11028516]

Shaw LJ et al: Gender differences in the noninvasive evaluation and management of patients with suspected coronary artery disease. Ann Intern Med 1994;120:559. [PMID: 8116993]

Willich S et al: Unexplained gender differences in clinical symptoms of acute myocardial infarction. J Am Coll Cardiol 1993;21:238A.

Treatment of Coronary Artery Disease

31

Edward F. Gibbons, MD

Women live longer with angina than men do before myocardial infarction (MI) develops, and symptomatic coronary disease develops at an older age. Yet when infarction does develop in women, their complication and mortality rates in most series appear to be higher than in men. Even studies that find no survival disadvantage after age and comorbidity adjustment must be examined in light of the fact that women with coronary artery disease (CAD) are more difficult to treat. Many studies on primary prevention and secondary treatment of CAD have excluded women or excluded sicker women on the basis of age or coexisting diseases. The current approach to treating CAD in women is based on the few studies in which gender is addressed and, by default, on studies in which women appear to do no worse or better than men. An approach to primary prevention of CAD in women is presented in Chapter 29.

ESTABLISHED CORONARY ARTERY DISEASE

Managing Angina Pectoris

A. MEDICAL THERAPY

1. Antianginal drug treatment—There is no information to suggest that one form of antianginal therapy is more useful in the treatment of women than another form. Thus, β-blockers, calcium channel blockers, and nitrates are used in standard practice. The Coronary Artery Surgery Study (CASS) included women treated either surgically or medically, but the study design did not allow for specific evaluation of women. The medical arm of the study had significantly more women than the surgical arm, but this fact probably was related to the lower overall severity of angiographic CAD in the women enrolled. A higher percentage of women than men had normal or mildly diseased coronary arteries. Thus, it is not surprising that men received surgical therapy more often than women. It can only be inferred that women at high risk for poor outcomes with chronic CAD (ischemic at low workload on treadmill testing with left main stenosis, or 3-vessel CAD and left ventricular dysfunction) should be directed toward surgery rather than medical therapy.

If it is true that women are more sensitive than men to fluctuations in coronary vasomotor tone and that this predisposition might be exacerbated with the loss of the protective effect of estrogen, then statin drugs, nitrates, and perhaps calcium channel blockers would be expected to be reasonable medical therapies. However, effective management must account for angina pattern, heart rate, and blood pressure response to exercise so that symptom relief, functional improvement, and objective findings of reduction of ischemia with these agents are achieved. β-Blockers may be useful and should be added to other medical therapy to effect symptom relief, especially in women with hypertension, history of prior MI, resting relative tachycardia, or atrial arrhythmias.

2. Hormone replacement therapy—The introduction of hormone replacement therapy (HRT) for primary or secondary prevention of CAD has not found objective support (see Chapter 29). Observational studies have been confounded with various degrees of observer bias and lack of randomization to HRT or placebo dosing. The Womens Health Initiative (WHI), a large randomized prospective trial, revealed that HRT for primary prevention was associated with an excess of MI, stroke, venous thromboembolism and other adverse outcomes. The American Heart Association does not recommend HRT use for prevention of MI or stroke.

3. Risk factor modification and atherosclerotic regression—Angiographic regression of atherosclerotic plaque in coronary arteries has been used as an index of treatment benefit in several studies of hypercholesterolemia. Although the studies are small, they have shown that significant reductions in low-density lipoprotein (LDL) cholesterol with diet and drug treatment are associated with angiographic regression of disease. A study by Kane that included slightly more women than men, all with familial hypercholesterolemia, showed that both women and men have a significant response to hypolipidemic agents including niacin, bile acid resins, and lovastatin. With these hypocholesterolemic treatments, reduction of LDL, increase of high-density lipoprotein (HDL), and regression of angiographic disease were noted. In fact, regression of disease was more pronounced in women than men in this small series.

Studies of "lifestyle" programs of exercise, vegetarian diet, meditation, and smoking cessation have shown that women have at least as great a potential for atherosclerotic regression as men in this highly motivated population. However, the numbers of women studied have been quite small. Because these effects have been documented in high-risk younger patients, their application to older women needs further study.

B. SURGICAL THERAPY

1. Coronary artery bypass grafting (CABG)—Clinical practice and consensus from surgical studies in the United States and Europe now dictate that CABG is useful for symptomatic relief of limiting angina and for long-term survival when significant left main coronary disease is discovered or significant 3-vessel disease is associated with left ventricular dysfunction. The largest European cooperative study has shown a survival benefit in 3-vessel CAD at all levels of left ventricular function, but this study included men only.

Short- and long-term follow-up data of women undergoing CABG are now available from several large centers. In general, women have a higher operative mortality than men, with equivalent long-term survival. The features that result in these gender patterns are useful to examine, both to understand risk and to forestall treatment bias.

a. Preoperative profile—In the CASS, as well as in studies conducted in Portland, Atlanta, and Cleveland, women coming to CABG were older than men, were more likely to have unstable angina, and if stable, had more limiting angina than men. Women also had more diabetes, hypertension, and congestive heart failure than men before their operation. Men had a higher rate of previous MI, more angiographic CAD, and lower left ventricular ejection fractions than women. Therefore, men had more angiographic risks, and women had more comorbid clinical risks. Men were more likely to be referred for CABG after a positive treadmill test, and women were more likely to be referred based on symptoms refractory to medical therapy and later in the course of their clinical disease and functional deterioration.

b. Operative mortality and graft patency—In separate studies from 1969 to 1991, operative mortality for CABG was found to be consistently higher in women (1.3—8.8%) than in men (0.9—3.0%). The relative risk of CABG mortality in women is 2.2-fold higher than in men. It appears, however, that gender does not play an independent role in CABG mortality; rather, women undergoing CABG are more likely to have clinical and physical predictors of surgical mortality (Table

31–1). These predictors are not contraindications to CABG but factors that increase the risk of postoperative death. When these risk factors are used to explain the higher mortality rate in women, it is found that smaller coronary size, short stature, and severity and instability of clinical disease play a greater role than gender. Despite these considerations, operative mortality is higher for women at all ages studied.

Serial study of CABG mortality at the Cleveland Clinic has shown that, as the general population has aged, so has the CABG population. The CABG mortality rate also has reflected this population trend. At the Cleveland Clinic, the women studied were older, they had more left main and 3-vessel disease than women in earlier surgical series, and they required more urgent surgery. These features generally are related to a more severe clinical profile. It should be noted that left main coronary stenosis occurs equally in men and women; because it is the most ominous angiographic sign, it almost always requires bypass surgery for survival. However, the surgical mortality of left main coronary disease is twice as high in women as in men.

Both acute and long-term graft patency appear to be lower in women than men, which may be related to the size of coronary vessels bypassed (smaller in women) and to a lower percentage of women undergoing left internal mammary artery (LIMA) bypass to the left coronary system. In general, these factors would be expected to reduce symptomatic benefit and short-term survival, but they appear to explain only partially the increased in-hospital mortality rate for CABG among women. Men with small blood vessels and short stature also have an increased incidence of graft closure and a higher mortality rate after bypass surgery. Gender appears not to be a separate risk factor for CABG when age, diabetes, urgency of surgery, and comorbid noncardiac diseases are factored into the analysis; yet these factors are more common in women.

Table 31–1. Predictors of mortality from coronary artery bypass grafting.

Age > 70 years
Functional class 3–4 symptoms
Short stature; body surface area < 1.8 m^2
Unstable angina
Postinfarction angina
Congestive heart failure
Diabetes
Emergency surgery
Angiographic severity of coronary artery disease, especially left main artery > 50%

c. **Long-term survival**—Despite the lower survival rate for women undergoing CABG, women who survive the hospitalization have long-term survival rates nearly identical to those of men. In the CASS, the 6-year mortality rate was 7.9% for men and 8.7% for women. The 10-year mortality rate from the Cleveland Clinic study was 22% for men and 21% for women. A study conducted in Portland, Oregon, of 1979 women and 6927 men after CABG found similar survival rates in men and women at 10, 15, and 18 years. Survival was lower with 3-vessel CAD and left ventricular dysfunction in this series for both men and women. Women tend to die of MI after bypass surgery and from congestive heart failure. Men are more likely than women to die of sudden death or of cancer.

d. **Symptomatic status**—Just as women have angina longer than men before MI and have limiting angina more frequently than men before bypass surgery, they are more likely than men to have angina postoperatively. At 2, 5, and 10 years, women are more likely to have angina than men (40–45% vs 30–35%). However, women report angina to be more manageable than men do and respond in lifestyle questionnaires that they feel their life has been improved after bypass surgery. The fact that, according to most studies, women are less likely to return to work full-time and more likely to retire after CABG may be related to age, financial needs, and other social features rather than anginal status.

2. Percutaneous transluminal coronary angioplasty (PTCA)—

a. **Patient profile**—Indications for PTCA are less well defined for mortality reduction and level of ischemia than they are for CABG. PTCA has grown tremendously over the past 22 years in the United States, and its technical success and refinements appear to have benefited women. PTCA is used for partial or complete coronary revascularization for chronic stable angina, unstable angina, acute MI, postinfarction ischemia, and ischemia after CABG in grafts and native vessels.

A review of early (1978–1981) experience with PTCA in the United States by the National Heart, Lung, and Blood Institute (NHLBI) indicated that women have a lower angiographic success rate and higher in-hospital mortality and complication rates than men. Procedural and technical problems were more likely to occur in women than men and seemed to be related to women's higher risk of acute coronary occlusion, MI, and hypotension with bradycardia. Surviving women had a higher risk of recurrent angina, but they appeared to have lower rates than men of restenosis, mortality, and CABG/PTCA. The higher initial

mortality rate and chronic angina recurrence rate may have led cardiologists to reduce their enthusiasm for PTCA in women.

Although early mortality remained higher in women, based on more recent experience, the overall trend is toward a more encouraging benefit profile. The 1985–1986 NHLBI PTCA registry of 1590 men and 546 women has monitored patients for more than 4 years. In this series, women were older than men once again, and twice as many women as men were older than 65 years. Women had significantly higher rates of hypertension, diabetes, hypercholesterolemia, and prior congestive heart failure, and twice as many women as men had severe coexisting noncardiac disease or were believed to have an inoperable or high-risk surgical profile based on clinical and angiographic features. Women had a higher rate of unstable angina; surprisingly, however, most of this subset of women were under the age of 65. Men had a higher rate of prior MI and bypass surgery and, as a result, a lower ejection fraction than women. The angiographic degree of coronary disease was similar in men and women in this series.

b. **Acute results and complications**—According to a more recent study, a successful result of coronary dilation appears equal in men and women (89% vs 88%), and the clinical success rate (dilation successful with no death, MI, or CABG) is identical at 79%. Complications in the NHLBI series were more common in women (29% vs 20%), however. Major events occurred more commonly in women, with death in 2.6% of women versus 0.3% of men. Women older than 65 had a 5.3% mortality rate. Adverse outcome as defined by death, MI, or emergency CABG was more common in women (9.7% vs 6.3% for men). Nonfatal MI and elective bypass surgery showed no gender difference. Multivariate risk factor analysis showed that age, history of congestive heart failure, diabetes, or multivessel disease conferred a 3- to 5-fold increase in risk; however, women appeared to have a 4- to 5-fold increase in risk based on gender alone. Body size was a risk only regarding short stature and presented a similar risk for men.

The Mayo Clinic review of its PTCA experience between 1988 and 1990 showed no independent risk of PTCA for 860 women, despite a rise in complications and mortality when comparing the results from the 1979–1987 data with the newer data. Several shifts in their PTCA population appeared to account for the rise in PTCA mortality in women from 2.9% to 5.4%. First, both men and women were older, and there was a consistently greater number of risk factors for women, 75% of whom had unstable angina. Second, women had more multivessel disease than in the previous era and matched the men in this regard. Third, and most important, 15% of women and 18% of men had PTCA within 24 hours of an acute MI, representing an expanded, almost routine, application of the procedure. When acute MI patients were excluded, women had a 3% mortality rate overall, still double that of men in the same series; however, disease severity, congestive heart failure, age, and proximal left anterior descending and multivessel disease were more important predictors of mortality than gender.

The most convincing data demonstrating the efficacy of both PTCA and CABG in women comes from the Bypass Angioplasty Revascularization Investigation (BARI). This study enrolled 1829 patients (27% women) with CAD, randomized to PTCA or CABG for symptomatic multivessel CAD. Again, the women enrolled were older and had more congestive heart failure, hypertension, diabetes, and unstable angina than men. Women assigned to CABG had a similar graft number but slightly fewer internal mammary conduits than men. Women assigned to PTCA had more intended target vessels than men. At 5.4 years of follow-up, mortality rates in women (12.8%) and men (12.0%) were similar. The short-term risk of CABG in women was a higher rate of congestive heart failure, with an equal rate to men for death (1.3%) and MI (4.7%). The short-term risk for PTCA for women was congestive heart failure, but rates of death (0.8%), MI (1.2%), emergency CABG, and vessel closure were as low or lower than in men. As in earlier studies, women were more likely to have postprocedure angina initially, but this excess of symptoms in women disappeared by year 5. The authors stress that, for the women in the study, the positive outcome with revascularization is magnified over that for men (relative risk = 0.60) when baseline variables are considered. Moreover, the finding that diabetic subjects do better with CABG than PTCA holds equally for both men and women.

Since the risks for CABG and PTCA in women are similar for in-hospital morbidity and mortality, the potential benefit of revascularization must be evaluated using short- and long-term benefit figures and consideration of symptoms, degree of multivessel coronary disease, and left ventricular dysfunction.

c. Device development—Recent developments in directional coronary atherectomy, intracoronary stent placement, and a variety of laser applications have not shown superior clinical benefit in either men or women. The established efficacy of adjunct antiplatelet (glycoprotein IIb/IIIa inhibitors) and endothelial tissue ingrowth inhibition (radiation brachytherapy) to retard stenosis have contributed to greater long-term vessel patency.

ACC/AHA/ACP-ASIM guidelines for the management of patients with chronic stable angina, with updates: http://www.acc.org/clinical/guidelines/june99/dirlindex.htm

ACC/AHA guideline update for the management of patients with unstable angina and non–ST-segment elevation myocardial infarction. http://www.acc.org/clinical/guidelines/unstable/update_explantext.htm

ACC/AHA guidelines for the management of patients with acute myocardial infarction, with updates. http://www.acc.org/clinical/guidelines/nov96/1999/index.htm

Alexander KP et al: Initiation of hormone replacement therapy after myocardial infarction is associated with more cardiac events during follow-up. J Am Card Cardiol 2001;38:1. [PMID: 11451256]

Bell MR et al: The changing in-hospital mortality of women undergoing percutaneous transluminal coronary angioplasty. JAMA 1993;269:2091. [PMID: 8468762]

Cho L et al: Optimizing percutaneous coronary revascularization in diabetic women: analysis from the EPISTENT trial. J Womens Health Gend Based Med 2000;9:741. [PMID: 11025866]

Eaker ED et al: Comparison of the long-term, postsurgical survival of women and men in the Coronary Artery Surgery Study (CASS). Am Heart J 1989;117:71. [PMID: 2643286]

Frasure-Smith N et al: Gender, depression, and one-year prognosis after myocardial infarction. Psychosom Med 1999;61:26. [PMID: 10024065]

Frishman WH et al: Differences between male and female patients with regard to baseline demographics and clinical outcomes in the Asymptomatic Cardiac Ischemia Pilot (ACIP) Trial. Clin Cardiol 1998;21:184. [PMID: 9541762]

Gallagher EJ, Viscoli CM, Horwitz RI: The relationship of treatment adherence to the risk of death after myocardial infarction in women. JAMA 1993;270:742. [PMID: 8336377]

Goldberg R et al: Age and sex differences in presentation of symptoms among patients with acute coronary disease: the REACT Trial. Rapid Early Action for Coronary Treatment. Coron Artery Dis 2000;11:399. [PMID: 10895406]

Jacobs AK et al: Better outcome for women compared with men undergoing coronary revascularization: a report from the bypass angioplasty revascularization investigation (BARI). Circulation 1998;98:1279. [PMID: 9751675]

Kahn JK et al: Comparison of procedural results and risks of coronary angioplasty in men and women for conditions other than acute myocardial infarction. Am J Cardiol 1992;69:1241. [PMID: 1575199]

Kelsey SF et al: Results of percutaneous transluminal coronary angioplasty in women. 1985ñ1986 National Heart, Lung, and Blood Institute's Coronary Angioplasty Registry. Circulation 1993;87:720. [PMID: 8443892]

Lewis MA: Myocardial infarction and stroke in young women: what is the impact of oral contraceptives? Am J Obstet Gynecol 1998;179(3 Pt 2):S68. [PMID: 9753313]

Limacher MC: Exercise and rehabilitation in women. Indications and outcomes. Cardiol Clin 1998;16:27. [PMID: 9507778]

McSweeney JC: Women's narratives: evolving symptoms of myocardial infarction. J Women Aging 1998;10:67. [PMID: 9870042]

Mosca L et al: Hormone replacement therapy and cardiovascular disease: a statement for healthcare professionals from the

American Heart Association. Circulation 2001;104:499. [PMID: 11468217]

Nohria A, Vaccarino V, Krumholz HM: Gender differences in mortality after myocardial infarction. Why women fare worse than men. Cardiol Clin 1998;16:45. [PMID: 9507780]

O'Connor GT et al: Differences between men and women in hospital mortality associated with coronary artery bypass graft surgery. Circulation 1993;88(part 1):2104. [PMID: 8222104]

Rahimtoola S et al: Survival at 15 to 18 years after coronary bypass surgery for angina in women. Circulation 1993;88(part 2):II71. [PMID: 8222199]

Stone G et al: Primary angioplasty is the preferred therapy for women and the elderly with acute myocardial infarction: Results of the primary angioplasty in myocardial infarction (PAMI) trial. J Am Coll Cardiol 1993;21:330A.

Weintraub W et al: Changing clinical characteristics of coronary surgery patients. Differences between men and women. Circulation 1993;88(part 2):II79. [PMID: 8222200]

Welty F et al: Similar results of percutaneous transluminal coronary angioplasty for women and men with postmyocardial infarction ischemia. J Am Coll Cardiol 1994;23:35. [PMID: 8277093]

ACUTE CORONARY SYNDROMES

Unstable Angina Pectoris

Because unstable angina resulting in necessity for CABG and PTCA presents more commonly in women than in men, it is important to emphasize the role of initial medical therapy prior to or in lieu of revascularization for unstable angina in women.

The syndrome of unstable angina may range from recent onset of limiting chest pain and an acceleration of angina to rest angina refractory to standard medical therapy. Women may seek medical attention later in the clinical course of angina and are overrepresented in PTCA and CABG series with more severe forms of unstable angina. Unstable angina with ST-segment depression or T-wave inversion is associated with a higher risk of infarction and is an indication for aggressive anticoagulation and antianginal therapy. Although no specific gender difference has been reported in the clinical course or in therapeutic response in women with unstable angina, a careful review of the 2 studies in which women were included in the assessment of treatment of unstable angina reveals a nonsignificant higher rate of infarction among women treated either with standard anti-ischemic therapy or with the more effective regimens of aspirin with or without heparin. Nonetheless, women appeared to respond to aggressive antithrombotic therapy in these series in a similar manner to men, with a 50–70% reduction in infarction rate after the development of unstable angina with rest pain.

Unfortunately, the impression that women are more likely to have normal coronary anatomy by angiography in the setting of unstable angina may not benefit women who have angiographic CAD. With a higher mortality rate postinfarction, therefore, women need careful and timely diagnosis and treatment of ischemia if it exists. Their appropriate clinical triage to PTCA or bypass surgery in other series appears related primarily to the knowledge of their coronary anatomy by angiography. This issue is discussed further in the following Gender Bias section.

Any initial evaluation of unstable angina must include a clinical and laboratory survey to exclude the secondary causes of unstable angina, eg, fever, hypoxia, anemia, arrhythmias, uncontrolled hypertension, hyperthyroid state, and volume overload. In the absence of anterior ischemic ECG changes, the therapy of an underlying precipitant to unstable angina frequently allows a delay in or even eliminates entirely the need for more aggressive measures such as angiography, PTCA, or CABG. In the absence of a major secondary cause, primary unstable angina should be treated with heparin (unfractionated if going to intervention, low-molecular-weight heparin otherwise), aspirin, nitrates, and β-blockers. Calcium channel blockers are not considered first-line therapy for unstable angina; in fact, an increase in MI mortality has been associated with the use of simple-release dihydropyridine calcium blockers such as nifedipine. Patients with rest angina with electrocardiographic changes should be treated in a similar manner and most likely will require coronary angiography; this pattern of disease is frequently refractory to continued medical therapy and may require the addition of intravenous glycoprotein IIb/IIIa inhibitors. Aspirin usually is continued with and after heparin therapy to avoid a rebound hypercoagulable state with rebound angina and its risk of infarction. There is no apparent gender difference in response to these agents.

The decision to proceed to angiography is an individual clinical one. Primary unstable angina with rest pain within 48 hours of admission, continued rest pain on medical therapy, or angina with ischemic electrocardiographic changes, particularly in the anterior septal leads, usually warrants angiography. The decision to proceed with PTCA or CABG depends on the identified anatomy, degree of multivessel disease, and left ventricular function. Women with considerable left ventricular dysfunction and multivessel disease are more likely to need CABG, although their morbidity and mortality rates after surgery are higher than in men. In this setting, however, PTCA is believed to carry too high a risk to apply safely with a favorable long-term outcome.

Myocardial Infarction

Most large studies have demonstrated that women who have had an MI have a higher mortality rate than men (see Chapters 29 and 30). Even studies that have not found an independent gender risk for women with MI have shown that in-hospital mortality unadjusted for age is higher in women. Furthermore, mortality in women with MI appears higher than in men at all ages studied. All these data precede the era of intravenous thrombolysis and primary angioplasty for MI, however.

A. THROMBOLYTIC THERAPY

Thrombolytic therapy has been shown in large international trials to promote significant reduction of in-hospital and long-term mortality (Figure 31–1). There is no apparent gender difference in the pharmacologic effects, biochemical response, infarct vessel patency rate, or clinical reperfusion rate. As would be expected, women made up 20–25% of the patients studied in thrombolysis trials. Women in the thrombolysis trials tended to be older and to have more diabetes, hypertension, and antecedent angina as well as a slightly higher rate of prior MI than men. Women also had a higher Killip class of left ventricular dysfunction on admission and received thrombolytic therapy slightly later than men. Women had a higher rate of major and minor hemorrhage than men by a factor of 50–90%. As a consequence, their transfusion requirement was also higher. In most series, women had a higher risk for hemorrhagic and total stroke (by 2- to 3-fold) and a trend toward a higher risk of reinfarction. When corrected for worse baseline clinical characteristics, the use of thrombolytic therapy is still an independent risk factor for hemorrhagic stroke in women, probably somewhat greater for tissue plasminogen activator (t-PA) than for streptokinase.

Mortality rate reduction with thrombolytic therapy is significant for women; it ranges from 19% to 31% for in-hospital mortality and from 10% to 37% at 1-year postinfarction in the published series of thrombolysis trials (Figure 31–1 A and B). Although the absolute reduction in acute mortality is the same in women and men (5–5.5%), the relative reduction in mortality compared with control women is less than in men, ie, more women than men die in the hospital even after thrombolysis. In the International Study of Infarct Survival (ISIS-2)—largest study to date—13,125 men and 3945 women received streptokinase and aspirin. Women had a mortality of 17.5% (placebo control) versus 12.2% (streptokinase), whereas men had a mortality of 12% (placebo control) versus 6.7% (streptokinase). This persistent excess in mortality for women despite treatment with thrombolysis, appears to hold for t-PA as well, with its attendant risk of hemorrhagic and fatal stroke.

This excess in mortality in women even after thrombolysis holds at every age group and is doubled in insulin-dependent diabetic women. Because the control populations in these studies have mortality rates similar to women's statistics in the earlier era, the higher mortality rate after thrombolysis in women has been explained in terms of risk associated with coexisting factors of age, Killip class, reinfarction risk, and stroke risk (Figure 31–1B). There is no gender difference in left ventricular function, infarct vessel site, degree of complex coronary disease, or infarct vessel patency on early angiography. Dosing of t-PA is an issue to be addressed, because the standard dose of 100 mg of frontloaded t-PA for all body weights may be an overdose for small women. Hemorrhagic stroke risk is known to be higher for persons who in earlier trials received 150 mg of t-PA. Weight-adjusted dosing of thrombolytic therapy is now being studied. Current gynecologic opinion is that thrombolytic therapy is not contraindicated in menstruating women, because vaginal bleeding in this setting should be manageable with appropriate gynecologic intervention; however, direct PTCA is preferable if immediate access to PTCA is available.

B. DIRECT PTCA

In large centers with active coronary angiography laboratories, immediate PTCA for acute MI has been feasible. When PTCA was compared with t-PA in the Primary Angioplasty in Myocardial Infarction (PAMI) trial, 107 women and 288 men were randomized to 1 of the 2 groups. PTCA candidates were treated with balloon inflation within 1 hour of presentation of their MI. Overall, there was a nonsignificant trend to lower mortality with PTCA and a marked stroke risk reduction (0% vs 3.5%) with PTCA over t-PA. In women, however, the in-hospital mortality rate was 4% for PTCA and 14% for t-PA (P = .06), and the rate of stroke was 5.3% for t-PA and 0% for PTCA (nonsignificant). Current practice of the optimal management of MI favors the use of primary PTCA with stent placement along with the adjuncts of glycoprotein IIb/IIIa infusion, use of clopidigrel/aspirin, and management of secondary risk.

Although these data are encouraging and help justify the use of PTCA in women and the elderly (who have contraindications to thrombolytic therapy or do not improve with thrombolytic therapy), thrombolytic therapy cannot be abandoned completely. Time is of the essence in achieving reperfusion after MI is diagnosed; most community and tertiary centers do not have immediate PTCA capacity 24 hours a day. Therefore, when it is the only option, thrombolytic therapy should be given to women with acute MI, because it is still associated with a significant reduction in short- and long-term mortality rate.

C. DRUG THERAPY

Because the majority of women with MI currently are not treated with thrombolysis or direct PTCA, adjunctive therapy should be given when appropriate.

A

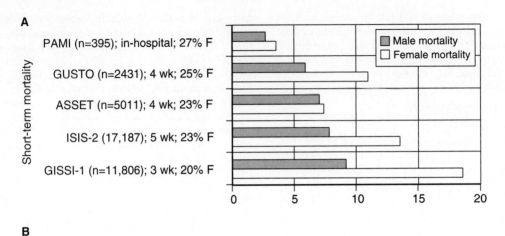

B

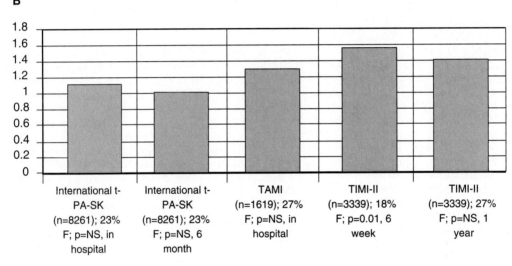

Odds ratio (F:M)

Figure 31–1. **A:** Unadjusted mortality with thrombolysis and primary angioplasty for men and women. GISSI-1, Gruppo Italiano per lo studio della steptochinazi nell'infarto miocardico; ISIS-2, International Study of Infarct Survival-2; ASSET, Anglo-Scandinavian Study of Early Thrombolysis; GUSTO, Global Utilization of Streptokinase and Tissue Plasminogen Activator for Occluded Coronary Arteries; PAMI, Primary Angioplasty in Myocardial Infarction. **B:** Adjusted mortality in thrombolytic trials by gender, showing no significant long-term gender difference adjusted for baseline risks. SK, streptokinase; t-PA, tissue plasminogen activator; TAMI, Thrombolysis and Angioplasty in Myocardial Infarction; TIMI-II, Thrombolysis in Myocardial Infarction.

1. Aspirin—Aspirin given after MI has not been shown to reduce overall mortality in women. Aspirin after MI does reduce the rate of reinfarction and overall cardiovascular mortality by 15%, however, when it is used for cerebrovascular symptoms, unstable angina, or MI. Whether this effect applies equally to women has not been studied. The ISIS-2 study showed that aspirin

alone reduced mortality by 23% compared with thrombolysis (25% reduction) and reduced reinfarction and stroke risk for men and women combined. Thus, until new data argue to the contrary, aspirin should be given in the emergency department to women in whom MI is suspected and continued after discharge in women who suffer an infarction.

2. β-Blockers—Both the Timolol Myocardial Infarction Study and the Beta-Blocker Heart Attack Trial (BHAT) included women and reported reductions as great as or greater than those found in men in mortality and recurrent MI. This finding has applied most convincingly to women with Q-wave infarctions and to individuals whose early course has been complicated by arrhythmia, transient left ventricular dysfunction, or ischemia. The benefit seems to persist for at least 1 year after MI in these higher risk patients, with a 43% mortality rate reduction with continued use of the β-blocker. The mortality rate in women in this trial was doubled by poor compliance with the medication regimen. β-Blockers remain an underused and important, life-saving treatment for those patients having an acute MI. Even in the large trials of thrombolysis, women were less likely than men to receive early and discharge β-blocker and antiplatelet therapy, especially if the MI was a non–Q-wave infarction.

3. Angiotensin-converting enzyme (ACE) inhibitors—The Survival and Ventricular Enlargement (SAVE) trial enrolled men and women with left ventricular dysfunction after MI. Patients were randomized to receive captopril therapy or standard therapy for congestive heart failure and were monitored for complications. Captopril therapy resulted in a 35% reduction of recurrent MI, cardiovascular death, and hospitalization for congestive heart failure. Women, however, appeared to benefit less than men (2% vs 22% mortality reduction). Later studies and a meta-analysis of all post-MI ACE inhibitor treatment have strongly urged the use of ACE inhibitors for women with MI, congestive heart failure with MI, and left ventricular ejection fraction < 40%. ACE inhibitors that last longer than captopril (< 2-h half-life) used in SAVE have been associated with greater clinical benefits than SAVE.

Because women have more congestive heart failure at a higher left ventricular ejection fraction than men after an MI, women who have any degree of global left ventricular dysfunction may benefit from ACE inhibitor therapy early after MI. This finding is most pertinent in the population of women with diabetes and hypertension.

4. Warfarin—Stroke risk after MI is higher in women than men, even without thrombolytic therapy. The stroke risk is related to intracavitary thrombosis in the left ventricle and left atrium rather than hemorrhagic stroke in the group of women who are not given thrombolytic therapy. There has been no gender-specific study of warfarin use after MI despite many studies proposing its general benefit. Warfarin is used currently for women with significant anteroapical hypokinesis or dyskinesis of the left ventricle after MI, and it is used for 2–3 months or indefinitely in the presence of left ventricular aneurysm. In addition, individuals with left ventricular ejection fractions < 30%, particularly with atrial fibrillation or with class IV heart failure, should be treated with warfarin after MI. In this setting, long-term warfarin use with an International Normalized Ratio (INR) goal of 2–3 is felt to reduce the risk of cardioembolic stroke and of venous thromboembolism. It should be noted that estrogen supplements tend to increase the daily warfarin requirement through their stimulation of hepatic synthesis of procoagulant cofactors.

Postinfarction Ischemia

Reduced left ventricular ejection fraction and postinfarction ischemia are the major predictors for mortality and complications in the years after MI in both men and women. Early mortality is greater when ischemia is symptomatic soon after infarction. The detection of post-MI ischemia in women is of great importance, therefore, but has not been rigorously studied. The Thrombolysis in Myocardial Infarction (TIMI-II) study recommended and used exercise radionuclide ventriculography to detect early ischemia after MI in men given t-PA. As discussed in Chapter 30, however, this test may be too insensitive in women to detect ischemia remote from a MI. Therefore, dipyridamole thallium or dobutamine echocardiography after MI needs to be performed in women and the results compared with treadmill testing. This is particularly important after non–Q-wave MI, in which the reinfarction rate in the first year after MI is high, and subsequent mortality in women is excessive. At present, many clinicians perform standard treadmill testing within 3–6 weeks after MI, dipyridamole thallium scanning prior to discharge, or direct coronary angiography for angina recurrence in both men and women after MI.

In a series of 164 women and 341 men studied by Welty et al, PTCA performed for post-MI ischemia produced similar, excellent results for both sexes. Women in this series were older, more likely to have a non–Q-wave MI, and less likely (15% vs 25%) to have received thrombolytic therapy than men. At PTCA, a 90% success rate was achieved, with equivalent low CABG, MI, and death rates (0.6–0.9%). Three-year follow-up showed only a 19% repeat PTCA rate, a 3.6% death rate, and identical reinfarction rates with no differential gender effect. Although this trend is encouraging, patient subsets appropriate for such intervention need to be defined.

CARDIAC REHABILITATION

Formal cardiac rehabilitation is beneficial in men in promoting early return to work after MI and bypass surgery, promoting lifestyle changes to reduce primary risk factors, and identifying and treating these risk factors. Meta-analysis has suggested a trend in men for cardiac rehabilitation to reduce fatal reinfarction rates and cardiac mortality rates. No such data are evident for women. However, fewer women are referred to rehabilitation programs after MI or bypass surgery, and dropout rates are greater and compliance is lower for women. Women are excluded more often from rehabilitation programs for cardiac or medical reasons, yet they have a lower exercise capacity and employment rate than men 1 year after MI or CABG. Psychological studies have shown that lack of emotional support after MI increases the 6- to 12-month mortality risk after MI more for men than for women. Cardiac rehabilitation should be explored for its potential to identify women at higher risk for post-MI ischemia and congestive heart failure and to facilitate a greater functional capacity after MI.

GENDER BIAS

Although angina is the most common presenting form of CAD in women, women are less likely than men to undergo diagnostic study for angina. One large series reported that even when nuclear perfusion studies were done, men were 10 times more likely to have coronary angiography than women (40% vs 4%) after a positive scan. At the time of that series, studies were not necessarily corrected for a woman's potential to exhibit breast thallium attenuation; therefore, current interpretation and appropriate referral may be somewhat better. Regardless, the studies were ordered and interpreted for the purpose of looking for ischemia. The authors of this report conclude that when pretest and posttest likelihood analysis was performed on this population of patients, they would have anticipated only a 2:1 ratio of referral for men versus women based on the positivity of the scan.

In the SAVE trial mentioned previously, coronary angiography was required for participation. Yet women were excluded on this basis more often than men, because angiography was performed, even for postinfarction angina, only half as often in women as in men. Perhaps for similar reasons, women appear to present for CABG and PTCA later and sicker in their course than men, which may contribute to their higher mortality rate with these interventions. However, women do appear to undergo revascularization with PTCA or CABG in equal numbers with men once they have undergone coronary angiography and have "as much disease as a man."

The false impression of the "benign" nature of angina in women may stem from skewed clinical experience or misleading interpretation of the early Framingham and CASS data (see Chapter 29). Similarly, thrombolytic therapy has been given less often to

women than men, both in the 1987–1988 and 1991–1992 series studied. This undertreatment was not accounted for by contraindications to thrombolysis, and bias appeared greatest in women under the age of 50 who had a nonanterior MI. A woman was more likely to receive thrombolytic therapy if her MI was anterior, if she had a history of cardiac disease, or if she had a family history of CAD, in which case there was no gender bias. Patient education programs for women should identify which symptoms are to be interpreted as ischemic or indicative of infarction. Women should be aware of their past history, CAD risk factors, and family history so that they may receive effective treatment if they have the misfortune to have an MI. Simply giving a lucid history may be lifesaving.

It is important to recognize that gender bias may not be malevolent nor universally detrimental. If it is true that men undergo CABG more often on the basis of a positive treadmill test, and women undergo the procedure more often for angina and unstable angina symptoms, it may be that men are overtreated with aggressive revascularization. However, women will be served best when the diagnosis of CAD is made properly and securely and the timing of medical or surgical intervention maximizes survival and functional capacity and minimizes morbidity and mortality.

SUMMARY

Women suffer high morbidity and mortality with the onset of ischemic heart disease. Early diagnosis, appropriate evidence-based intervention, and vigilant follow-up can improve survival and quality of life and relieve symptoms. Appropriate secondary prevention should be introduced, and pharmacologic adjustments made based on risk (Table 31–2).

Eysmann SB, Douglas PS: Reperfusion and revascularization strategies for coronary artery disease in women. JAMA 1992;268: 1903. [PMID: 1404716]

Hachamovitch R et al: Gender-related differences in clinical management after exercise nuclear testing. J Am Card Cardiol 1995;26:1457. [PMID: 7594071]

Kuhn EM, Hartz AJ, Baras M: Correlation of rates of coronary artery bypass surgery, angioplasty and cardiac catheterization in 305 large communities for persons age 65 and older. Health Serv Res 1995;30:425. [PMID: 7649750]

Lincoff AM et al: Thrombolytic therapy for women with myocardial infarction: is there a gender gap? Thrombolysis and Angioplasty in Myocardial Infarction Study Group. J Am Coll Cardiol 1993;22:1780. [PMID: 8245328]

Mark DB et al: Absence of sex bias in the referral of patients for cardiac catheterization. N Engl J Med 1994;330:1101. [PMID: 8133852]

Shaw LJ et al: Prognostic value of noninvasive risk stratification in younger and older patients referred for evaluation of sus-

Table 31–2. Proposed drug strategy for secondary prevention of CAD in women.

Intervention	Goals	Evaluation	Prescriptive
Lipid-lowering	LDL < 100 for CHD/equivalents HDL > 45–50 as secondary goal	Fasting lipid profile (within 24 h admission for MI	TLC Statin Niacin or fibrate if HDL/TG remain risk (see Chapter 29)
Antiplatelet agents	Prevent thrombotic and embolic complications	Monitor for compliance, bleeding risks, and efficacy	Aspirin 81–325 mg/d Clopidogrel for aspirin allergy
β-Blockers	Reduce reinfarction, sudden death, global mortality after MI	Assess for contraindications Evaluate ongoing compliance, response, dosing	Begin within hours of MI hospitalization; continue indefinitely
ACE inhibitors	Reduce morbidity, mortality, reinfarction, and CHF in MI survivors	Assess for contraindications Evaluate ongoing compliance, side effects, and attainment of target dose	Start within days of MI if no hypotension Continue for CHF symptoms, LVEF < 40%, or in diabetic patients In patients at low risk, may stop at 6 wk
HRT	Minimize therapy length for postmenopausal symptoms	Review menstrual status of woman > 40 years Measure follicle-stimulating hormone if unclear	Do not initiate HRT for primary secondary CAD prevention For women with CAD on HRT, collaborate with patient to manage non-CAD benefits If acute CAD event happens, consider discontinuation of HRT or add anticoagulants for thromboembolic risk
OCs	Use lowest therapeutic dose of estrogen/progestin Prevent pregnancy at minimum CAD risk	Establish CAD risk and contraindications for OC candidates	Avoid OC agents in women over 35 who smoke Evaluate lipid and hyperglycemia status before starting OC agents Discontinue OC agents if hypertension develops

CAD, coronary artery disease; LDL, low-density lipoprotein; CHD, coronary heart disease; HDL, high-density lipoprotein; MI, myocardial infarction; TG, triglyceride; ACE, angiotensin-converting enzyme; CHF, congestive heart failure; LVEF, left ventricular ejection fraction; HRT, hormone replacement therapy; OC, oral contraceptives.

pected coronary artery disease. J Am Geriatr Soc 1996;44:1190. [PMID: 8855997]

Travin MI et al: Relation of gender to physician use of test results and to the prognostic value of stress technetium 99m sestamibi myocardial single-photon emission computed tomography scintigraphy. Am Heart J 1997;134:73. [PMID: 9266786]

White HD et al: After correcting for worse baseline characteristics, women treated with thrombolytic therapy for acute myocardial infarction have the same mortality and morbidity as men except for a higher incidence of hemorrhagic stroke. The Investigators of the International Tissue Plasminogen Activator/Streptokinase Mortality Study. Circulation 1993;88:2097. [PMID: 8222103]

Zuanetti G et al: Influence of diabetes on mortality in acute myocardial infarction data from the GISSI-2 study. J Am Coll Cardiol 1993;22:1788. [PMID: 8245329]

Pregnancy & Heart Disease

Michael Longo, MD

Maternal heart disease complicates only 1–2% of all pregnancies but has profound effects on both maternal and fetal outcomes. Rheumatic heart disease remains the most common cardiac condition in pregnant women worldwide, while in the United States and Western world, congenital heart disease (CHD) has recently emerged as the predominant underlying heart condition. Most instances of heart disease in pregnancy are in women with preexisting cardiac conditions. The physiologic stress of pregnancy may unmask previously unrecognized cardiac disease. A normal pregnancy may produce signs and symptoms that mimic cardiac disease making it difficult for both primary care physicians and specialists to differentiate between normal and pathologic conditions. This chapter will review the normal hemodynamic changes of pregnancy and highlight the most frequently encountered cardiac conditions, with a particular focus on diagnosis and management. The use of cardiovascular drugs in pregnancy will also be discussed.

Normal Hemodynamic Changes in Pregnancy

The major hemodynamic changes in pregnancy include a marked increase in cardiac output and blood volume with a reduction in systemic vascular resistance (SVR). These changes begin within the first few weeks of pregnancy, peak in the second trimester, and plateau until delivery (Table 32–1). Plasma volume increases steadily throughout pregnancy on average 40–50% above baseline levels. Red blood cell mass also increases but less than plasma volume resulting in the physiologic or dilutional anemia of pregnancy with the average hematocrit in the 30–32% range. Cardiac output increases 30–50% above prepregnancy levels. This is achieved in early pregnancy primarily via an increase in stroke volume and in later pregnancy by an increase in heart rate. Near the end of gestation, maternal cardiac output is significantly affected by changes in body position. With a supine position the gravid uterus compresses the inferior vena cava, thus decreasing venous return and cardiac output. Assuming a left lateral decubitus position helps to relieve or minimize this obstruction. During labor and delivery, cardiac output increases an additional 20–25%. SVR significantly decreases due to direct vasodilation and the creation of a low resistance

circuit by the gravid uterus. This results in a decrease in systolic blood pressure on average 10 mm Hg reaching its nadir during the second trimester. Diastolic blood pressure decreases even further resulting in a widening of the pulse pressure. Heart rate increases on average 10–20 beats per minute.

Hunter S, Robson SC: Adaptation of the maternal heart in pregnancy. Br Heart J 1992;68:540. [PMID: 1467047]

Clinical Findings

A. Symptoms and Signs

The expanded blood volume and hyperdynamic circulation of pregnancy may produce signs and symptoms that appear to represent cardiac disease but are more often normal findings. Breathlessness, decreased exercise tolerance, easy fatigability, palpitations and lightheadedness are frequently experienced during a normal pregnancy. On the other hand, paroxysmal nocturnal dyspnea, chest pain, hemoptysis, syncope, and anasarca with or without proteinuria should be considered abnormal and warrant further evaluation. Common physical examination findings normally found in pregnancy include prominent jugular venous pulsations, a prominent laterally displaced ventricular impulse, loud heart sounds, and a third heart sound that is present in more than 80% of pregnant women near term. Systolic ejection murmurs at the left sternal border can be heard in nearly all pregnant women resulting from increased blood flow into the pulmonary trunk. Soft systolic murmurs due to mild mitral or tricuspid regurgitation are also common. Mammary soufflés, systolic or continuous murmurs heard over the breasts in the third trimester or postpartum in lactating women, are frequently heard. Bibasilar rales due to atelectasis from compression by the gravid uterus and peripheral edema are also common findings in a normal pregnancy. Diastolic murmurs, grade III and above systolic murmurs, a fourth heart sound, or fixed splitting of the second heart sound are abnormal findings and should be further investigated with echocardiography.

B. Special Tests

Maternal cardiac testing must balance the potential benefits of the information obtained against possible risks. Protecting the fetus from ionizing radiation is a

Table 32–1. Hemodynamic changes during normal pregnancy.

Parameter	Trimester		
	First	*Second*	*Third*
Blood volume	↑	↑↑	↑↑↑
Cardiac output	↑	↑↑ to ↑↑↑	↑↑↑ to ↑↑
Stroke volume	↑	↑↑↑	↑, ↔, or ↓
Heart rate	↑	↑↑	↑↑ to ↑↑↑
Systolic blood pressure	↔	↓	↔
Diastolic blood pressure	↓	↓↓	↓
Pulse pressure	↑	↑↑	↔
Systemic vascular resistance	↓	↓↓↓	↓↓

↔, no change compared with nonpregnant level; ↑, small increase; ↑↑, moderate increase; ↑↑↑, large increase; ↓, small decrease; ↓↓, moderate decrease; ↓↓↓, large decrease.
(Reproduced with permission from Braunwald E: *Heart Disease*, 5th ed. WB Saunders Company, 1997:1843.)

primary concern. The potential harmful effects of ionizing radiation are dependent on the stage of fetal development and the dose of radiation. Proper shielding of the abdomen is always required.

Echocardiography is generally considered the test of choice for evaluating cardiac disease in pregnancy. There is no evidence to suggest that soundwaves are harmful to the fetus and echocardiography provides useful information about ventricular function, valvular structure and function, intracardiac shunting, and pulmonary artery pressures. Common findings in a normal pregnancy include mild four-chamber enlargement, mild pulmonic and tricuspid regurgitation (90%), mild mitral regurgitation (30%), and a small pericardial effusion.

Chest radiography may occasionally be required during pregnancy. While the dose of radiation to which the fetus is exposed is small, the procedure is best avoided unless the information cannot be obtained by other means. Maternal adaptation to pregnancy leads to changes in the chest radiograph that may mimic cardiac disease and must be interpreted with caution. Cardiomegaly, increased pulmonary markings, and straightening of the left heart border are all common findings during a normal pregnancy.

The safety of maternal stress testing in pregnancy has not been fully established. Stress testing may be necessary to evaluate ischemic heart disease or to assess functional capacity in pregnant women with cardiac disease. The use of a low level protocol limiting heart rate response to less than 140 beats per minute or 75% of the predicted maximum heart rate is recommended for the safety of the fetus. Diagnostic results may be limited because of the presence of resting ST-segment and T-wave abnormalities in pregnant women and the increased rate of false-positive results of exercise electrocardiography in all women. Radionuclide imaging with agents such as sestamibi or thallium is best avoided since the safety of these agents in pregnancy is unclear at this time.

Coronary angiography is generally reserved for emergent situations such as acute myocardial infarction. The dose of radiation to the fetus is relatively high. Steps taken to limit fetal exposure include using a brachial rather than femoral artery approach, shielding the abdomen, and minimizing fluoroscopy time.

Connelly MS et al: Canadian Consensus Conference on adult congenital heart disease 1996. Can J Cardiol 1998;14:395. [PMID: 9551034]

Hunter S, Robson SC: Adaptation of the maternal heart in pregnancy. Br Heart J 1992;68:540. [PMID: 1467047]

Mishra M, Chambers JB, Jackson G: Murmurs in pregnancy: an audit by echocardiography. BMJ 1992;304:1413. [PMID: 1628016]

Risk Assessment

Maternal and fetal mortality is strongly correlated with New York Heart Association (NYHA) functional class of the mother prior to pregnancy. Women who are asymptomatic or minimally symptomatic (eg, class I or II) generally tolerate pregnancy well. However, for women in NYHA class IV, maternal and fetal mortality approaches 50%. Previously asymptomatic women may experience a dramatic deterioration in functional class during pregnancy depending on the type of underlying cardiac abnormality. Conditions associated with severe left heart obstruction (eg, aortic stenosis, mitral stenosis, and hypertrophic obstructive cardiomyopathy) and severe pulmonary hypertension are poorly tolerated due to the inability to increase cardiac output. Left ventricular ejection fraction (LVEF) < 40% and a maternal history of congestive heart failure (CHF), stroke, or arrhythmias are also predictive of adverse cardiac events during pregnancy. The overall risk of pregnancy in women with cardiovascular disease is outlined in Table 32–2.

Presbitero P et al: Pregnancy in cyanotic congenital heart disease. Outcome of mother and fetus. Circulation 1994;89:2673. [PMID: 8205680]

Siu SC et al: Risk and predictors for pregnancy-related complications in women with heart disease. Circulation 1997;96: 2789. [PMID: 9386139]

Table 32–2. Risk classification with pregnancy.

High risk
Pulmonary hypertension
Functional class III–IV
Marfan syndrome
Cyanotic congenital heart disease
Severe aortic or mitral stenosis
Left ventricular ejection fraction < 35%
Prosthetic heart valves
Previous peripartum cardiomyopathy

Intermediate risk
Large left to right shunts
Moderate aortic or mitral stenosis
Uncorrected aortic coarctation

Low risk
Small left to right shunts
Aortic or mitral regurgitation with normal left ventricular
  ejection fraction
Mitral valve prolapse
Corrected congenital heart disease

Whittemore R, Hobbins JC, Engle MA: Pregnancy and outcome in women with and without surgical treatment of congenital heart disease. Am J Cardiol 1982;50:641. [PMID: 7113941]

Zuber M et al: Outcome of pregnancy in women with congenital shunt lesions. Heart 1999;81:271. [PMID: 10026351]

Valvular Diseases

A. Mitral Stenosis

Rheumatic mitral stenosis is the most common hemodynamically significant valvular abnormality encountered in pregnant women. A previously asymptomatic woman can rapidly decompensate during pregnancy. Elevated cardiac output, blood volume and heart rate lead to an increased gradient across the stenotic mitral valve causing higher left atrial pressures and pulmonary edema. Symptoms include dyspnea, orthopnea, paroxysmal nocturnal dyspnea, and hemoptysis. Heart failure can develop at any time but the most critical periods are during the third trimester, labor and delivery, and postpartum when heart rate and cardiac output are at maximal levels. Atrial fibrillation may develop and lead to sudden deterioration due to a rapid ventricular response. The risk of thromboembolism is increased. The aim of treatment is to reduce heart rate and blood volume by the restriction of physical activities and by the administration of β-blockers and diuretics as needed. Most pregnant women with mild to moderate mitral stenosis respond to appropriate treatment. Mitral balloon valvuloplasty has been successfully performed in

pregnant women and is preferred over mitral commissurotomy in patients refractory to medical therapy.

B. Aortic Stenosis

Hemodynamically significant aortic stenosis is rare in women of childbearing age. The most common causes are congenital from a bicuspid aortic valve or rheumatic heart disease. As with mitral stenosis, mild to moderate aortic stenosis is fairly well tolerated in pregnancy. Severe aortic stenosis (aortic valve area < 1.0 cm^2 or mean gradient > 50 mm Hg) is poorly tolerated due to the fixed cardiac output, and aortic valve replacement is indicated prior to pregnancy even in asymptomatic women. The most common symptoms are angina and dyspnea. Hypotension is particularly dangerous and can cause syncope or even sudden cardiac death.

C. Mitral and Aortic Regurgitation

Regurgitant valvular disease is usually well tolerated in pregnancy because the reduction in SVR favors forward flow and reduces the degree of regurgitation. The increase in heart rate with pregnancy shortens diastole and thus reduces the degree of aortic insufficiency. Mitral valve prolapse (MVP) is the most common cause of mitral regurgitation in pregnancy. Although MVP may slightly increase the risk of arrhythmias and predispose to endocarditis, it has not been shown to adversely affect maternal or fetal outcomes. While not uniformly agreed upon, many experts recommend antibiotic prophylaxis for labor and delivery in women with MVP with thickened leaflets and associated mitral regurgitation.

Avila WS et al: Course of pregnancy and puerperium in women with mitral valve stenosis. Rev Assoc Med Bras 1992;38:195. [PMID: 1340375]

Connelly MS et al: Canadian Consensus Conference on adult congenital heart disease 1996. Can J Cardiol 1998;14:395. [PMID: 9551034]

Farhat MB et al: Percutaneous balloon mitral valvuloplasty in eight women with severe mitral stenosis during pregnancy. Am J Cardiol 1994;73:398.

Lao TT et al: Congenital aortic stenosis and pregnancy—a reappraisal. Am J Obstet Gynecol 1993;169:540. [PMID: 8372858]

Patti G et al: Myocardial infarction during pregnancy and postpartum: a review. G Ital Cardiol 1999;29:333. [PMID: 10231682]

Cardiomyopathies

A. Peripartum Cardiomyopathy (PPC)

PPC is a rare form of cardiomyopathy that results in CHF in the last month of pregnancy, or within 5 months of delivery, in the absence of a recognizable cause. Peak occurrence is 1 month postpartum. While the cause of PPC is unknown, several factors have been implicated including myocarditis, hormonal effects, nutritional deficiencies, small vessel disease, genetic susceptibility, and abnormal immunologic responses to fetal or viral antigens. The incidence of PPC is estimated at 1 in 3000–4000 live births in the United States. Risk factors include advanced maternal age (older than 30 years), multiparity, multiple gestations, African-American heritage, and prolonged tocolytic therapy. Symptoms result from CHF with dyspnea, cough, and orthopnea predominating. Palpitations and vague chest or abdominal pain are common and often misleading symptoms. The timing of the onset of symptoms provides important diagnostic clues. PPC is rare before 36 weeks gestation while women with underlying cardiovascular disease most often develop symptoms in the second or early third trimester. Furthermore, the hyperdynamic circulation of pregnancy and effects of the gravid uterus resolve rapidly postpartum. Thus, persistent or worsening heart failure in the last month of pregnancy or early postpartum strongly suggest PPC. Echocardiography most commonly demonstrates four-chamber cardiac enlargement with a marked reduction in LVEF. The clinical course is highly variable ranging from asymptomatic left ventricular dysfunction to florid CHF and early death. While LVEF returns to normal usually within 6 months of diagnosis in 50% of cases, reported mortality with PPC remains high at 25–50%. The majority of deaths occur within the first 3 months postpartum as a result of progressive CHF, ventricular arrhythmias, or thromboembolic complications. Treatment of PPC is standard heart failure therapy with sodium restriction, diuretics, afterload reduction (eg, hydralazine prepartum, and angiotensin-converting enzyme inhibitors postpartum), β-blockers, and anticoagulants because of the high risk of peripheral embolization. The role of immunosuppressive therapy remains unclear. Heart transplantation has been successfully performed in patients refractory to medical therapy. Relapse with subsequent pregnancies frequently occurs. Most experts agree that pregnancy is contraindicated in women with a history of PPC and persistent left ventricular dysfunction.

B. HYPERTROPHIC CARDIOMYOPATHY

Hypertrophic cardiomyopathy is generally well tolerated in pregnancy due to balanced effects on outflow obstruction from the reduction in SVR and increase in plasma volume. Symptoms during pregnancy include chest pain, dyspnea, and syncope. Delivery is a particularly vulnerable time due to decreased preload from venal caval obstruction and the Valsalva maneuver and the compensatory tachycardia from a variety of causes.

Hypovolemia worsens the situation. β-Blockers are used to treat symptomatic patients.

Connelly MS et al: Canadian Consensus Conference on adult congenital heart disease 1996. Can J Cardiol 1998;14:395. [PMID: 9551034]

Hunter S, Robson SC: Adaptation of the maternal heart in pregnancy. Br Heart J 1992;68:540. [PMID: 1467047]

Midei MC et al: Peripartum myocarditis and cardiomyopathy. Circulation 1990;81:922. [PMID: 2306840]

Patti G et al: Myocardial infarction during pregnancy and postpartum: a review. G Ital Cardiol 1999;29:333. [PMID: 10231682]

Acute Coronary Syndromes

Myocardial infarction may complicate pregnancy even though coronary artery disease is rare in women of childbearing age. Coronary dissection is the most common cause involving the left anterior descending artery in 80% of cases. The typical presentation involves the abrupt onset of typical anginal chest pain late in the third trimester or early postpartum. Thrombosis due to the hypercoagulable state of pregnancy; coronary spasm, which may be induced by oxytocin or ergot derivatives; embolism; and atherosclerotic plaque rupture must also be considered. Therapy of acute infarction in pregnancy is similar to the nonpregnant state taking both maternal and fetal risks into consideration. Primary angioplasty is generally preferred over thrombolytic therapy due to hemorrhagic risks. The use of low-dose aspirin, heparin, nitrates, and β-blockers appear safe if indicated.

Patti G et al: Myocardial infarction during pregnancy and postpartum: a review. G Ital Cardiol 1999;29:333. [PMID: 10231682]

Hypertension in Pregnancy

Hypertensive disorders in pregnancy include chronic hypertension (HTN), gestational HTN, preeclampsia or pregnancy-induced HTN, and preeclampsia superimposed on chronic HTN. Chronic HTN is defined as blood pressure > 140/90 mm Hg before the 20th week of pregnancy or after 12 weeks postpartum. Transient HTN is elevated blood pressure during pregnancy in the absence of preexisting HTN or other signs of preeclampsia. While HTN increases the risk of maternal and fetal morbidity and mortality including abruptio placentae, cerebral hemorrhage, intrauterine growth retardation (IUGR) and premature labor, the treatment of mild to moderate HTN remains controversial largely because outcomes are not improved with therapy. Generally accepted indications for treatment include diastolic blood pressure consistently greater than 100 mm

Hg, systolic blood pressure > 160–180 mm Hg or signs of end-organ damage. Methyldopa and hydralazine have been the most extensively studied and are considered first-line agents. β-Blockers are good alternatives especially when used late in pregnancy. Experience with using calcium channel blockers is growing.

Preeclampsia is the development of HTN after 20 weeks of gestation in association with proteinuria and/or edema. Seizures in the setting of preeclampsia indicate eclampsia. HTN is usually the earliest sign of preeclampsia with gradual increases during the latter stages of pregnancy. True HTN, blood pressure > 140/90 is rare until the third trimester. Preeclampsia complicates 5–8% of pregnancies in the United States and is the leading cause of maternal mortality after thromboembolic disease. Young primagravidas (younger than 20 years) are at the greatest risk. Other women at risk are older multiparas (older than 35 years), and those with chronic HTN, multiple gestations, and a family history of preeclampsia. The only definitive treatment is delivery of the fetus. Pharmacologic therapy is targeted at blood pressure control and the prevention of seizures. Severe HTN usually requires hospitalization and parenteral therapy with hydralazine or labetalol, which are the preferred agents. Long-term prognosis is usually favorable because of the self-limited nature and rapid resolution of HTN after delivery and a low risk of chronic HTN developing or of recurrence in future pregnancies.

Barrilleaux PS, Martin JN Jr: Hypertension therapy during pregnancy. Clin Obstet Gynecol 2002;45:22. [PMID: 11862056]

National High Blood Pressure Education Program Working Group Report on High Blood Pressure in Pregnancy. Am J Obstet Gynecol 1990;163:1689.

Congenital Heart Disease

Recent advances in the medical and surgical treatment of CHD have enabled the majority of affected women to reach reproductive years. While the incidence of CHD in the general population is only 0.5%, there is approximately a 5% chance of CHD in the offspring of a woman with CHD. Pregnancy is usually well tolerated in asymptomatic women with acyanotic CHD. Poor maternal and fetal outcomes are expected with pulmonary HTN, cyanosis, and maternal functional class III or IV. The greatest risk is with pulmonary HTN, particularly with Eisenmenger's syndrome as the hemodynamic changes of pregnancy are poorly tolerated due to the high fixed pulmonary resistance and the inability to increase cardiac output. In this condition, maternal and fetal mortality approach 50%, and pregnancy is thus considered contraindicated. Maternal cyanosis places the fetus at high risk for IUGR, prematurity, and spontaneous abortion. Even a mild degree of cyanosis is of concern as right-to-left shunting increases during pregnancy due to the decrease in SVR, leading to further reductions in maternal oxygen saturation.

A. ATRIAL SEPTAL DEFECTS

Atrial septal defects (ASD) is the most common form of CHD encountered in pregnancy. Left-to-right shunts (eg, ASD, ventriculoseptal defect, and patent ductus arteriosus) are generally well tolerated due to the reduction in SVR. The overall risk is related to the size of the shunt and degree of pulmonary HTN. With ASD, there is an increased risk of paradoxical embolism and supraventricular arrhythmias.

B. AORTIC COARCTATION

Aortic coarctation is most often corrected before a woman reaches reproductive age. It is commonly associated with a bicuspid aortic valve. The maternal mortality rate with uncorrected coarctation is 3–4%. In pregnancy, there is an increased risk of aortic dissection, infective endocarditis, cerebral hemorrhage, CHF, and hypertensive complications. The management of HTN with coarctation is complicated by the risk of precipitating hypotension distal to the site of the narrowing thus compromising fetal blood flow. IUGR and prematurity are common. β-Blockers may be used to treat both the HTN and reduce the risk of aortic dissection.

C. MARFAN'S SYNDROME

Marfan's syndrome is genetically transmitted as an autosomal dominant trait with a 50% chance of being transmitted to the offspring. Pregnancy increases the risk of aortic dilatation, dissection, and rupture. Women with preexisting aortic dilatation are at greatest risk and an aortic root diameter greater than 4 cm is considered a contraindication to pregnancy. Periodic echocardiographic assessment of the aortic root is recommended. Treatment includes restriction of physical activities and the use of β-blockers to decrease the risk of aortic dilatation and dissection.

D. TETROLOGY OF FALLOT (TOF)

TOF is the most common cause of cyanotic CHD encountered in pregnancy. Most women with surgically corrected TOF and normal oxygen saturations tolerate pregnancy without difficulty. In women with uncorrected TOF, or only palliative repair, pregnancy increases right-to-left shunting, worsening cyanosis. Pregnancy is contraindicated when the woman has hematocrit > 65%, oxygen saturation < 70%, pulmonary HTN, or a maternal history of syncope.

Coleman JM et al: Congenital heart disease in pregnancy. Cardiol Rev 2000;8:166. [PMID: 11174890]

Connelly MS et al: Canadian Consensus Conference on adult congenital heart disease 1996. Can J Cardiol 1998;14:395. [PMID: 9551034]

Gleicher N et al: Eisenmenger's syndrome and pregnancy. Obstet Gynecol Surv 1979;34:721. [PMID: 503376]

Presbitero P et al: Pregnancy in cyanotic congenital heart disease. Outcome of mother and fetus. Circulation 1994;89:2673. [PMID: 8205680]

Siu SC et al: Risk and predictors for pregnancy-related complications in women with heart disease. Circulation 1997;96:2789. [PMID: 9386139]

Zuber M et al: Outcome of pregnancy in women with congenital shunt lesions. Heart 1999;81:271. [PMID: 10026351]

Cardiovascular Drugs in Pregnancy

Since most cardiovascular drugs cross the placenta and may pose harmful effects on the fetus, the risk-benefit ratio must be carefully evaluated before use in pregnant women. Table 32–3 outlines the safety and adverse effect profile of cardiac drugs in pregnancy.

A. ANGIOTENSIN-CONVERTING ENZYME INHIBITORS

Angiotensin-converting enzyme (ACE) inhibitors are contraindicated in pregnancy due to an increased risk of congenital malformations (skull and limb bones),

Table 32–3. Effects of cardiovascular drugs taken during pregnancy.

Drug	Potential Fetal Adverse Effects	Safety
Warfarin	Fetal hemorrhage in utero, embryopathy, central nervous system abnormalities	Unsafe
Heparin	None reported	Safe
Digoxin	Low birth weight	Safe
Quinidine	Toxic dose may induce preterm labor and damage to the eighth cranial nerve	Safe
Procainamide	None reported	[1]
Disopyramide	May initiate uterine contractions	[1]
Lidocaine	In high blood levels and fetal acidosis may cause central nervous system depression	Safe
Mexiletine	Fetal bradycardia, IUGR, low Apgar score, neonatal hypoglycemia, bradycardia, and hypothyroidism	[1]
Flecainide	One reported fetal death	[1]
Propafanone	None reported	[1]
Adenosine	None reported. Limited use during the first trimester	Safe
Amiodarone	IUGR, prematurity, hypothyroidism	Unsafe
Calcium antagonists	Fetal distress due to maternal hypotension	[1]
β-Blockers	IUGR, apnea at birth, bradycardia, hypoglycemia, hyperbilirubinemia, initiation of uterine contractions	Safe
Hydralazine	None reported	Safe
Sodium nitroprusside	Potential thiocyanate toxicity with high dose, fetal mortality in animal studies	Potentially unsafe
Organic nitrates	Fetal heart rate deceleration and bradycardia	[1]
ACE inhibitors	Skull ossification defect, IUGR, prematurity, low birth weight, oligohydramnios, neonatal renal failure, anemia and death, limb contractures, patent ductus arteriosus	Unsafe
Diuretic agents	Impairment of uterine blood flow, thrombocytopenia, jaundice, hyponatremia, bradycardia	Potentially unsafe

IUGR, intrauterine growth retardation; ACE, angiotensin-converting enzyme.
[1]To date only limited information is available, and safety during pregnancy cannot be established.
(Reproduced with permission Bonow RO et al: ACC/AHA Guidelines for the management of patients with valvular heart disease. JACC 1998:32;1547.)

IUGR, neonatal anuric renal failure, and death. There are no data on the use of angiotensin-II receptor antagonists and given a similar mechanism of action to ACE inhibitors, they are best avoided in pregnancy.

B. ANTIARRHYTHMICS

Adenosine has been successfully used to treat supraventricular tachycardia (SVT) without adverse maternal or fetal events. Chronic treatment of SVT in pregnancy is more difficult. Quinidine has been the most widely studied and appears safe, although elevated levels can cause premature labor and fetal thrombocytopenia. Amiodarone may result in fetal hypothyroidism and is generally reserved to treat arrhythmias refractory to other agents. Lidocaine is the agent of choice for the treatment of ventricular arrhythmias.

C. β-BLOCKERS

The use of β-blockers in pregnancy is growing although there are limited data regarding their use. Short-term use appears safe but chronic use in pregnancy is associated with IUGR and respiratory distress. Neonates exposed to β-blockers must be observed for the development of bradycardia and hypoglycemia. β-Blockers are most commonly used in the treatment of HTN, arrhythmias, and hypertrophic cardiomyopathy.

D. CALCIUM CHANNEL BLOCKERS

There is limited information on the use of calcium channel blockers in pregnancy, although they appear to be safe. Using nifedipine to treat HTN and preeclampsia has become more common in recent years.

E. DIURETICS

Diuretics may cause a reduction in placental blood flow, which limits their usefulness. Furosemide is used to treat CHF refractory to sodium restriction.

F. HYDRALAZINE AND METHYLDOPA

These agents have been extensively studied and are not associated with congenital abnormalities. Methyldopa is generally considered the first-line agent for chronic HTN in pregnancy. Hydralazine is the vasodilator of choice for managing CHF during pregnancy and frequently used in the management of HTN and preeclampsia.

G. ANTICOAGULATION

Anticoagulation during pregnancy has been referred to as "double jeopardy," because it places the mother and fetus at risk for both thrombotic and hemorrhagic complications. The risk of valve thrombosis or other life-threatening complications during pregnancy is approximately 10% in women with mechanical heart valves. The greatest risk is with mechanical heart valves in the mitral position. Coumadin appears superior to heparin

in reducing maternal thromboembolic and bleeding complications, but is a known teratogen. Fetal exposure to coumadin during the first trimester results in a 15–30% incidence of fetal embryopathy, a syndrome of multiple fetal malformations including nasal hypoplasia, saddle nose deformity, and stippled epiphysis. Central nervous system abnormalities including blindness may occur due to fetal hemorrhage and scarring. High rates of spontaneous abortions and stillbirths are also observed. Heparin, on the other hand, does not cross the placenta and has rarely been associated with still-

Table 32–4. Recommendations for anticoagulation during pregnancy in patients with mechanical prosthetic valves: weeks 1 through 35.

Indication	Class
The decision whether to use heparin during the first trimester or to continue oral anticoagulation throughout pregnancy should be made after full discussion with the patient and her partner: if she chooses to change to heparin for the fist trimester, she should be made aware that heparin is less safe for her, with a higher rate of both thrombosis and bleeding, and that any risk to the mother also jeopardizes the baby.[1]	I
High-risk women (a history of thromboembolism or an older generation mechanical prosthesis in the mitral position) who choose not to take warfarin during the first trimester should receive continuous unfractionated heparin intravenously in a dose to prolong the midinterval (6 hours after dosing) activated partial thromboplastin time to 2 to 3 times control. Transition to warfarin can occur thereafter.	I
In patients receiving warfarin, international normalized ratio should be maintained between 2.0 and 3.0 with the lowest possible dose of warfarin, and low-dose aspirin should be added.	IIa
Women at low risk (no history of thromboembolism, newer low-profile prosthesis) may be managed with adjusted-dose subcutaneous heparin (17,500 to 20,000 U bid) to prolong the midinterval (6 hours after dosing) activated partial thromboplastin time to 2 to 3 times control.	IIb

[1]From the European Society of Cardiology Guidelines for Prevention of Thromboembolic Events in Valvular Heart Disease. (Reproduced with permission from Bonow RO et al: ACC/AHA Guidelines for the management of patients with valvular heart disease. JACC 1988;32:1549.)

birth or prematurity. The optimal management of anti-coagulation during pregnancy remains controversial. Strategies include the following:

1. Subcutaneous heparin in the first trimester followed by coumadin
2. Coumadin alone
3. Subcutaneous heparin alone

The American Heart Association and American College of Cardiology recommendations for anticoagulation during pregnancy are outlined in Table 32–4.

Coumadin should be discontinued before term and replaced with heparin in anticipation of labor. Whatever approach is adopted, the use of anticoagulation in pregnancy is associated with a 30–35% risk of maternal or fetal complications.

ACC/AHA Guidelines for the management of patients with valvular heart disease. A report of the American College of Cardiology/American Heart Association. Task Force on Practice Guidelines (Committee on Management of Patients with Valvular Heart Disease). J Am Coll Cardiol 1998;32:1486. [PMID: 9809971]

Elkayam UR: Anticoagulation in pregnant women with prosthetic heart valves: a double jeopardy. J Am Coll Cardiol 1996;27:1704. [PMID: 8636557]

Gohlke-Barwolf C et al: Guidelines for prevention of thromboembolic events in valvular heart disease. Study Group of the Working Group on Valvular Heart Disease of the European Society of Cardiology. Eur Heart J 1995;16:1320. [PMID: 8746900]

Joglar JA, Page RL: Antiarrhythmic drugs in pregnancy. Curr Opin Cardiol 2001;16:40. [PMID: 11124717]

Nightingale SL: From the Food and Drug Administration. JAMA 1992;267:2445. [PMID: 1349355]

Relevant Web Sites

[American Heart Association]
www.americanheart.org
[Heart Disease Online]
www.heartdiseaseonline.com/article/pregnancy.shtml
[Adult Congenital Heart Association]
www.achaheart.org/newsletter/pregnancy.php
[Merck]
www.merck.com/pubs/mmanual/section18/chapter251/251b.htm
[Heart Center Online]
www.heartcenteronline.com

SECTION IX

Infectious Diseases

HIV Infection

Roger W. Bush, MD

The HIV epidemic has brought sharp focus to the social, economic, and medical conditions of women. Heterosexual contact and drug use, alone and in combination, expose women to HIV infection often without their awareness of risk at the time of exposure or clinical presentation. Providers must be vigilant for HIV risk and manifestations because HIV infection is often diagnosed later in women than in other groups. High transmission rates in adolescents and young adults, vertical transmission, and social conditions that promote high-risk behaviors confound control of the HIV epidemic. As the HIV epidemic continues beyond the risk behaviors, geographic areas, and demographic groups initially described, health care providers are confronted with HIV infection, including its prevention, treatment, and continuing care.

General Considerations

A. EPIDEMIOLOGY

In the years before 1988, 7% of AIDS cases reported in the United States occurred in women. Between July 1998 and June 1999, women and teenage girls (older than 13 years) constituted 23% of all adults and adolescents with HIV and AIDS in North America. However, AIDS cases and deaths probably exceeded these figures. Worldwide, 43% of approximately 33 million HIV-infected adults are women. Infected women are more likely to live in developing countries, have poorer access to treatment, and often have dependent children and family members.

The addition of highly active antiretroviral therapy (HAART) to the treatment armamentarium has significantly decreased morbidity and mortality in women with AIDS. Therefore, many more women are living with HIV and AIDS. Early in the epidemic, women with AIDS were few in number and usually were infected through injection drug use rather than heterosexual

contact. Since 1992, however, more women with AIDS have acquired infection through heterosexual activity than through injection drug use. Women younger than 30 years are infected as adolescents.

B. PRESENTATION IN WOMEN

Progression of HIV disease in women is quite similar to that of men. For any given CD4 count, women tend to have an HIV RNA level 30–50% lower than infected men, and women suffer faster progression to AIDS and death than men with similar HIV RNA levels. Whether gender is the cause of these differences or whether the lower socioeconomic circumstances of women is the cause has not been determined.

In addition to facing gynecologic and pregnancy-related problems, women with AIDS get the same opportunistic infections as men. Risk behaviors that result in HIV infection dictate opportunistic diseases; the gender does not. For example, Kaposi's sarcoma is rare in women and limited to those who have had sex with bisexual men. Herpes simplex virus and cytomegalovirus (CMV) infection, wasting, and esophageal candidiasis may be more common in women than men. *Pneumocystis carinii* pneumonia (PCP) is still the most common opportunistic illness in both genders. When the data are controlled for race, ethnicity, and mode of transmission, most AIDS-defining conditions are of equal prevalence in women and men. Although the clinical course of PCP is similar in women and men, women may have greater hospital mortality from the disease than men, possibly because of inadequate access to providers experienced in its treatment.

Risk Factors for Transmission

Race and ethnicity are not risk factors, but they serve as markers of socioeconomic status and access to medical care; therefore, they identify groups at high risk for

HIV infection such as blacks and Hispanics. Black and Hispanic women constitute 80% of AIDS cases in women.

The social blights of crack cocaine and injection drug use often are associated, directly or indirectly, with HIV, especially in the Northeast region of the United States and in women older than 30. In 1992, injection drug use was the predominant mode of HIV transmission for women in the Northeast. Of HIV infections attributed to heterosexual contact, most (56.8%) involved sex with an injection drug user. Risk factors such as anal intercourse, genital ulcers, syphilis, sex without condoms, multiple sexual contacts, oral (nonbarrier) contraceptive use, and high viral load of male contacts increase the male-to-female transmission rate. Sex with high-risk men and survival sex (trading sex for money, shelter, food, or drugs) are also important risk behaviors. Unfortunately, many women with HIV and their health care providers are unaware of their condition, because women often are diagnosed with HIV at or near their death. To make an early diagnosis of HIV infection, it is imperative for providers to ask patients about drug use and sexual behaviors since 1978. Because many women are unaware of their risk even when questioned, risk-based screening may miss 50–60% of infected women.

The risk of vertical HIV infection (mother to child) is 13–15% in Europe, 15–30% in the United States, and 25–52% in developing countries. The risk of increased vertical transmission is correlated with high viral load, high CD8 lymphocyte levels, low CD4 lymphocyte levels, placental inflammation/disruption, invasive fetal monitoring, vaginal delivery, episiotomy, fever, and premature birth. Some experts suspect that 50% of vertical transmission occurs perinatally; therefore, all infants should be regarded as uninfected while in labor and be protected from maternal secretions. Women in the United States should avoid breast-feeding if they can afford bottle-feeding, because breast-feeding increases vertical transmission risk by 14%. Issues of economics and water purity make bottle-feeding less desirable in the developing world. Prenatal care may reduce the rate of vertical transmission.

HIV Testing

Women who have been determined to be at risk should be counseled concerning how tests are performed and the meaning of positive and negative test results. Issues of confidentiality, anonymity, and voluntary disclosure should be addressed frankly. After careful risk assessment and pretest counseling, a screening enzyme-linked immunosorbent assay (ELISA) or a rapid diagnostic test approved by the US Food and Drug Administration should be offered, and a time should be arranged for test results to be delivered in person. Pretest and posttest counseling sessions are strategic opportunities for advice on modifying behaviors to avoid additional exposures and transmission.

If the initial ELISA is positive, the test should be repeated and then confirmed with a Western blot. If the test result is indeterminate, is unexpectedly positive or negative, or there is any doubt about test validity, it should be repeated with a new sample.

Prevention

The low socioeconomic status of many women at risk for HIV makes prevention difficult. Elimination of risk behaviors is the only available definitive prevention strategy. Knowledge of what motivates and influences behavior and effective counseling practices are the fundamental tools of prevention. Many communities can provide substance abuse treatment, detection and treatment of all sexually transmitted diseases, needle exchange programs for injection drug users, frank sexual safety education, prenatal care for expectant HIV-infected mothers, and promotion of condom use.

Women are often tested because of illness, sexual contact, or blood donation; many do not perceive that they are at risk. Most women are infected during heterosexual contact (40–55%), often without condoms, or from either injecting drugs (42%) or a sexual partner who injected drugs. HIV prevention programs have failed to reach women as well as they have male heterosexuals at risk for HIV infection. Fewer prevention messages are specifically targeted at women, many messages are too euphemistic to be effective, and women often are not in control of condom use or their sexual exposures. Ideally, methods for prevention of HIV and other sexually transmitted diseases would be controlled by women and have high efficacy. Condoms have the highest theoretic preventive efficacy, but diaphragms and spermicides are controlled by women and therefore likely to be more effective. However, microbicidal activity of spermicides is suspect and unreliable. Only 18% of women report that their male partners use condoms for any reason. Intravaginal pouches (female condoms) may offer a level of protection similar to condoms, are woman-controlled, and appear to be acceptable in use; however, they cost approximately $2.50 each. All these methods should be promoted, along with limiting and carefully selecting partners. Women must do their best to persuade male sexual partners to use condoms. If for any reason sex without condoms occurs, a spermicide and latex barrier should be used.

Postexposure prophylaxis with antiretroviral medications may reduce the likelihood of HIV infection after an exposure. Evidence for efficacy is primarily from occupational exposures. Postexposure prophylaxis should be restricted to patients with high-risk exposures within 72 hours of contact with the contagion.

Clinical Findings

The initial physical examination should be comprehensive, with particular attention to the weight, mouth, pelvic examination, and mental status examination. Weight trends provide a useful index of progression of disease and response to therapy, and weight loss greater than 10% of body weight constitutes "wasting syndrome," an AIDS-defining illness particularly common in women. Thrush, oral ulcers, and oral hairy leukoplakia are common findings, whereas Kaposi's sarcoma is unusual in women. These examinations should be performed at each visit. A fundoscopic examination should be done every 3–6 months, with the clinician looking for the hemorrhage and yellow-white spots commonly seen in CMV retinitis. Papanicolaou (Pap) smears should be done at least every 6 months, with early gynecologic referral if atypia, dysplasia, or squamous intraepithelial lesion (SIL) is found, or if there is a history of untreated SIL. The clinician should remain vigilant for mental disorders; depression, dementia, encephalopathy, central nervous system toxoplasmosis, lymphoma, and drug or alcohol abuse are encountered frequently.

A. Symptoms and Signs

The most common and serious infections among HIV-infected women are pneumococcal pneumonia, sepsis, and tuberculosis. Gynecologic conditions are common HIV-associated clinical problems and often occur before the patient is aware of her HIV infection or exposure. Cervical dysplasia and cancer became AIDS-defining illnesses in January 1993. Nearly half (49%) of sexually active adults have been infected with human papillomavirus, and HIV-infected women have even higher prevalence. Women with both HIV and human papillomavirus infection have an increased risk of cervical disease, and cervical cancer is more aggressive when accompanied by HIV infection, particularly when HIV disease is advanced. HIV infection is often otherwise asymptomatic in women who present with cervical cancer.

Candida vulvovaginitis is the most common gynecologic problem of HIV-infected women and was the initial clinical manifestation of 38% of women in one series. It can cause painful ulcerations that are refractory to topical treatment, particularly in severely immunocompromised hosts. Similarly, herpes genitalis can be severe, widespread, and refractory to treatment. Syphilis is increasing in incidence, and coinfection with HIV is common. The clinical course of syphilis in HIV-infected patients is telescoped in that neurosyphilis can

occur early after infection. Such genital ulcers are common in those at risk for HIV, can be signs of HIV infection, and can increase sexual transmission of HIV.

The presence of HIV-related symptoms may have important prognostic implications; therefore, the review of systems should include early symptoms of HIV infection, such as fevers, night sweats, diarrhea, weight loss, lymphadenopathy, thrush, vaginitis, and skin changes, as well as all the following items:

Past or present sexually transmitted diseases

Past or present pelvic inflammatory disease

Recurrent or severe vulvovaginal candidiasis

Sepsis or recurrent bacterial pneumonia

Herpes zoster

Tuberculosis

Unexplained persistent constitutional symptoms

Hepatitis B markers

Autoimmune thrombocytopenic purpura

Cervical dysplasia or genital warts

Genital ulcers

Unexplained diarrhea

Fever and thrush are independent predictors of early progression to PCP and should lead to prophylactic antibiotic therapy for the disease. The patient's medical history should determine whether tuberculosis or sexually transmitted diseases (eg, genital warts, cervical dysplasia, herpes, and syphilis) has ever been diagnosed; reproductive history should include the determination of contraception method. Immunization history, travel, diet, drug and alcohol history, and a review of urgent social needs and supports are also important issues to be addressed.

B. Laboratory Findings

After diagnosis of HIV infection, baseline clinical and laboratory data should be obtained. The clinician's goal is to collect a comprehensive database, provide staging and prognostic information, and formulate a treatment plan. The patient, however, often needs counseling, empathy, and reassurance. With a simple structure to follow and with practice, both agendas can be met.

The laboratory evaluation must be tailored to the patient, practice circumstances, and laboratory capabilities. The following list of initial tests and vaccines for HIV-infected women provides a guideline for the clinician:

CD4 lymphocyte count

Quantitative viral load assay

Complete blood cell count and platelets

Chemistry panel to survey for hepatic, renal, or metabolic abnormalities

Purified protein derivative (PPD-5TU) and anergy panel (yearly if patient is positive for PPD and not anergic)

Lipid profile

Serologic test for syphilis (yearly)

Toxoplasma IgG

Hepatitis B & C serologic study (hepatitis B core antibody and hepatitis C screening antibody test)

Pap smear (every 6 months)

Screening for chlamydia and gonorrhea infections

Vaccinations: pneumococcus once, influenza yearly, diphtheria-tetanus every 10 years, hepatitis B if not immune

If symptomatic, obtain a chest radiograph

T-cell subsets are useful prognostically, but they are notoriously variable from day to day and laboratory to laboratory. Every reasonable effort should be made to have serial subsets drawn at the same time of day, at the same menstrual stage, and not during or immediately after an acute illness. Many HIV-related infections are reactivation illnesses; therefore, tuberculin testing, syphilis serologic tests, and *Toxoplasma* antibody status can guide the practitioner diagnostically when an acute illness occurs. CD4 lymphocyte counts are the most prognostically useful laboratory index, yet similar levels do not necessarily reflect identical risk of progression.

Opportunistic diseases usually do not occur in patients with CD4 lymphocyte counts greater than 0.25×10^9/L. Although these counts are incomplete in their predictive value, they help the clinician anticipate progression of disease and survival.

In general, asymptomatic patients with CD4 counts greater than 0.50×10^9/L should be monitored every 6 months; symptomatic patients with CD4 counts between 0.20 and 0.50×10^9/L should be seen every 3–6 months, and patients with fewer than 0.20×10^9/L CD4 cells should be monitored according to their disease activity.

Evaluation & Monitoring

The occurrence of AIDS-indicator diseases is strongly associated with degree of immunosuppression but not with gender or risk group. Tables 33–1 and 33–2 outline the AIDS case definition and indicator conditions. Major infectious illnesses that are not in the 1993 AIDS case definition are related to immune compromise as well, but they also are related to injection drug use, probably caused by ongoing needle use, alcohol use, and poor living conditions.

One way to start an initial interview is with an open-ended question about why the patient took the test for HIV infection, followed by some exploration of her social milieu. An explicit history of risks and current practices, an estimate of the likely duration of infection, identification of contacts and children who may be infected, and a review of symptoms may follow. Disclosure to children, other family members, and child care providers as well as reproductive counseling are features of HIV care for women that are foreign to many HIV care providers. These are difficult tasks that may elicit fears of rejection and loss. Once women understand the risks that their loved ones may bear and the benefit of early medical intervention, however, they are usually eager to cooperate.

Table 33–1. AIDS surveillance case definition for adolescents and adults: 1993.

	Clinical Categories		
CD4 Cell Categories	**A** Asymptomatic, or PGL or Acute HIV Infection	**B** Symptomatic[2] (not A or C)	**C**[1] AIDS Indicator Condition (1987)
1) > 500/µL (≥ 29%)	A1	B1	C1
2) 200–499/µL (14% to 28%)	A2	B2	C2
3) < 200/µL (< 14%)	A3	B3	C3

PGL, persistent generalized lymphadenopathy.

[1]All patients in categories A3, B3, and C1-3 are defined as having AIDS based on the presence of an AIDS-indicator condition (Table 33–2) and/or a CD4 cell count < 200/µL.

[2]Symptomatic conditions not included in Category C that are a) attributed to HIV infection or indicative of a defect in cell-mediated immunity, or b) considered to have a clinical course or management that is complicated by HIV infection. Examples of B conditions include but are not limited to bacillary angiomatosis; thrush; vulvovaginal candidiasis that is persistent, frequent, or poorly responsive to therapy; cervical dysplasia (moderate or severe); cervical carcinoma in situ; constitutional symptoms such as fever (38.5° C) or diarrhea > 1 month; oral hairy leukoplakia; herpes zoster involving 2 episodes or > 1 dermatome; idiopathic thrombocytopenic purpura (ITP); listeriosis; pelvic inflammatory disease (PID) (especially if complicated by a tubo-ovarian abscess); and peripheral neuropathy.

Table 33–2. Indicator conditions in case definition of AIDS (adults)—1997.[1]

Candidiasis of esophagus, trachea, bronchi, or lungs—3846 (16%)

Cervical cancer, invasive [2,3]—144 (0.6%)

Coccidioidomycosis, extrapulmonary[2]—74 (0.3%)

Cryptococcosis, extrapulmonary—1168 (5%)

Cryptosporidiosis with diarrhea > 1 month—314 (1.3%)

CMV of any organ other than liver, spleen, or lymph nodes; eye—1638 (7%)

Herpes simplex with mucocutaneous ulcer > 1 month or bronchitis, pneumonitis, esophagitis—1250 (5%)

Histoplasmosis, extrapulmonary[2]—208 (0.9%)

HIV-associated dementia[2]: Disabling cognitive and/or other dysfunction interfering with occupation or activities of daily living—1196 (5%)

HIV-associated wasting[2]: Involuntary weight loss > 10% of baseline plus chronic diarrhea (≥ 2 loose stools/day ≥ 30 days) or chronic weakness and documented enigmatic fever ≥ 30 days—4212 (18%)

Isoporosis with diarrhea > 1 month[2]—22 (0.1%)

Kaposi's sarcoma in patient under 60 yrs (or over 60 yrs[2])—1500 (7%)

Lymphoma, Burkitt's—162 (0.7%), immunoblastic—518 (2.3%), primary CNS—170 (0.7%)

Mycobacterium avium, disseminated—1124 (5%)

Mycobacterium tuberculosis, pulmonary—1621 (7%), extra-pulmonary—491 (2%)

Pneumocystis carinii pneumonia—9145 (38%)

Pneumonia, recurrent-bacterial (≥ 2 episodes in 12 months)[2,3]—1347 (5%)

Progressive multifocal leukoencephalopathy—213 (1%)

Salmonella septicemia (nontyphoid), recurrent[2]—68 (0.3%)

Toxoplasmosis of internal organ—1073 (4%)

Wasting syndrome due to HIV (as defined above—HIV-associated wasting) (18%)

CMV, cytomegalovirus; CNS, central nervous system.

[1]Indicates frequency as the AIDS-indicator condition among 23,527 reported cases in adults for 1997. The AIDS diagnosis was based on CD4 count in an additional 36,643 or 61% of the 60,161 total cases. Numbers indicate sum of definitive and presumptive diagnosis for stated condition. The number in parentheses is the percentage of all patients reported with an AIDS-defining diagnosis: these do not total 100%, since some had a dual diagnosis.

[2]Requires positive HIV serology.

[3]Added in the revised case definition, 1993.

Advance directives regarding life-sustaining treatments, durable power-of-attorney for health care, and guardianship of dependent children should be addressed as soon as rapport allows. Most patients appreciate the affirmation of control over their own care and are glad to have the opportunity to discuss treatment goals, although negative emotional responses such as fear and hopelessness can occur initially.

Treatment

Management of women with HIV infection should be in the context of comprehensive, longitudinal, patient-centered care given by primary care providers, in regular consultation with clinicians experienced and expert in care of HIV-infected patients. Patients who require fiberoptic bronchoscopy; cancer treatment planning; or treatment for complex, rare infectious complications often require subspecialty consultation. The value of a close doctor-patient relationship cannot be overstated, and evidence clearly shows that being patients of experienced and expert HIV care providers confers survival advantage to patients. Multidisciplinary teams may include social workers, mental health professionals, nutritionists, rehabilitation specialists, and pharmacists.

A. ANTIRETROVIRALS

Antiretroviral therapy is a complex and fast-changing area; expert consultation should be freely accessed. Potent antiretroviral therapy has dramatically impacted the clinical course of HIV infection, reduced hospitalization rates and costs, and prolonged and improved life and function for many patients in the developed world. All of the 15 or so currently available antiretroviral agents have roles in the treatment of HIV infection, but they must be used in combination, have many drug and disease interactions, and are frequently toxic. These are treatments that should be used carefully in the context of comprehensive primary care and HIV expertise, with patients sharing in decision-making. These choices must be made with awareness of benefits, toxicities, drug resistance, adherence, uncertainty, and expense. Patients must be educated about treatment options and their impact on quality of life. Clear, validated algorithms are not feasible, although broad, evidence-based guidelines are available.

Initiation of antiretroviral therapy should be considered for symptomatic patients and for patients with CD4 cell counts less than 0.35×10^9/L. Antiretroviral therapy may delay progression to AIDS, reduce incidence of opportunistic infections, and prolong life in many patients. Antiretroviral therapy is not recommended for patients with stable CD4 counts of more than 0.50×10^9/L and is of uncertain, temporary (12–24 months or less) benefit for asymptomatic patients with CD4 counts of 0.20–0.50×10^9/L.

Recommendations and guidelines for antiretroviral treatment are frequently updated by the Department of Health and Human Services Panel on Clinical Practices for Treatment of HIV Infection (Table 33–3).

B. GYNECOLOGIC CARE

Vaginal symptoms and sexually transmitted diseases often herald HIV infection and must be taken seriously in all women. HIV testing should be offered to all sexu-

Table 33–3. Indications for the initiation of antiretroviral therapy in the patient infected with HIV-1.

Clinical Category	CD4+ T Cell Count	Plasma HIV RNA	Recommendation
Symptomatic (AIDS, severe symptoms)	Any value	Any value	Treat
Asymptomatic, AIDS	CD4+ T cells < 200/μL	Any value	Treat
Asymptomatic	CD4+ T cells > 200 μL but < 350/μL	Any value	Treatment should generally be offered although controversy exists.
Asymptomatic	CD4+ T cells > 350/μL	> 55,000 (by bDNA or RT-PCR)	Some experts would recommend initiating therapy, recognizing that the 3-year-risk of developing AIDS in untreated patients is > 30% and some would defer therapy and monitor CD4+ T cell counts more frequently.
Asymptomatic	CD4+ T cells > 350/μL	< 55,000 (by bDNA or RT-PCR)	Many experts would defer therapy and observe, recognizing that the 3-year risk of developing AIDS in untreated patients is < 15%.

RT-PCR, reverse transcription polymerase chain reaction.
Source: Adapted from DHHS 2002.

ally active women and promoted for women with any risk factors or suggestive clinical problems, such as severe yeast vaginitis, cervical dysplasia, or invasive cervical carcinoma. As mentioned, HIV-infected women should receive Pap smears every 6 months, with prompt referral to gynecologic specialists if SIL is identified, because cervical dysplasia progresses rapidly in these patients.

Standard therapies for yeast vaginitis are often effective, and they can be used as periodic maintenance treatment when frequent recurrences are a problem. Unusually severe or recalcitrant cases usually can be controlled with systemic ketoconazole or fluconazole.

Fertility and reproductive issues are complex and difficult for women with HIV infection. Because most children are infected perinatally and prenatal care may reduce vertical transmission, prenatal testing has been advocated. Contraception and abortion decisions are complicated by increased risk of pregnancy for the mother, the likelihood she would not live to raise the child, and the frequent absence of other suitable childcare. HIV-infected women may want to continue a pregnancy but fear potential outcomes so much that they seek termination, which may be difficult to arrange.

C. PREGNANCY CARE

Because pregnancy does not appear to accelerate progression of HIV disease in the mother, treatment of pregnant women should not be significantly different from that of nonpregnant women. CD4 lymphocyte counts and viral load assays should be determined at the time of presentation for prenatal care or at delivery for women who receive no prenatal care. Pregnant women usually should be offered antiretroviral treatment to preserve the mother's health and to prevent vertical transmission. In 1994, results from ACTG 076, a randomized, double-blind, placebo-controlled clinical trial of zidovudine (ZDV) treatment for pregnant women with CD4 counts of 0.20×10^9/L or greater and no clinical indications for antepartum ZDV therapy showed an 8.3% vertical (mother to child) transmission rate when the mother took ZDV, 500 mg/d orally, initiated in the second or third trimester, and 1 mg/kg/h intravenously during labor. The vertical transmission rate in the placebo group was 25.5%. No significant short-term side effects were seen in mothers or infants. On the basis of this study, pregnant women with HIV infection should be offered second- and third-trimester antepartum and intrapartum ZDV therapy, in a context of expert consultation. A substantial (8.3 ± 4.5%) risk of transmission persists even with treatment, so women must be counseled that this intervention does not make pregnancy free of risk for the infant. Although the effect of ZDV on the fetus is unknown, delaying treatment may put the fetus at increased risk for HIV infection and put the mother at increased risk for progression, which could endanger both mother and fetus. Other antiretroviral agents have also been shown to be effective in preventing vertical transmission. Women considered at risk for opportunistic infections also should receive prophylactic therapy for PCP and toxoplasmosis with trimethoprim-sulfamethoxazole. Some providers prefer aerosolized pentamidine because of the risk of kernicterus in premature infants exposed to sulfamethoxazole.

D. Prevention of Opportunistic Illness

Primary (for those with CD4 count less than $0.20 \times 10^9/L$) and secondary PCP prophylaxis is justified by strong evidence of reduced incidence and prolonged survival at a reasonable cost. Trimethoprim-sulfamethoxazole is the first-line, most effective agent and should be promoted actively, even if only as small a dose as 3 double-strength tablets a week can be tolerated. It also may prevent *Toxoplasma* and gram-positive bacterial infection. Dapsone rarely cross-reacts in patients allergic to sulfa and is more effective as well as much less expensive than inhaled pentamidine.

Secondary prophylaxis (maintenance therapy) of infection with *Cryptococcus, Toxoplasma,* recurrent herpes simplex, CMV, and tuberculosis (for 12 months in all PPD-positive patients) is imperative. Early pneumococcal and annual influenza vaccination may be useful, and hepatitis B vaccination for unexposed women is advised. In addition to preventing the psychological and physiologic stress of opportunistic disease, prevention and early detection of treatable complications may slow HIV disease progression.

Prognosis

Women with HIV infection can expect excellent longevity and functional status, if they have access to experienced HIV care providers, adhere to HAART, and respond completely with viral suppression and immune reconstitution. About 80% of HAART-naïve, adherent patients benefit with a durable, complete response. Initial treatment in the setting of profound immunocompromise produces a less durable response. Nonresponders frequently have psychosocial and socioeconomic barriers to access and adherence.

Metabolic complications of HIV disease and HAART will develop in a significant minority of responders. These adverse effects include insulin resistance, hyperlipidemia, fat redistribution (dorsocervical fat pad, central and visceral obesity, wasting of extremities, temporal, and buccal areas), and diabetes mellitus.

Anderson JR: A Guide to the Clinical Care of Women with HIV. 2001 edition. US Department of Health and Human Services, Health Resources and Services Administration, HIV/AIDS Bureau. This and subsequent editions also available at http://www.hab.hrsa.gov

Bartlett JG, Gallant JE: Medical Management of HIV Infection. 2001-2002 edition. Johns Hopkins University. Available for review or online ordering at http://hopkins-aids.edu

HIV/AIDS Treatment Information Service: 1-800-HIV-0440 (1-800-448-0440) http://www.hivatis.org

To obtain materials for women with HIV, or more information about women and HIV, contact the CDC National Prevention Information network at 1-800-458-5231.

Relevant Web Sites

[AIDSinfo includes guidelines and links to excellent federal resources.]
http://www.aidsinfo.nih.gov
[AIDSmap]
http://www.aidsmap.com/
[Gay Men's Health Crisis]
http://www.gmhc.org/
[AIDS Education Global Information Service]
http://www.aegis.com/
[International Association of Physicians in AIDS Care]
http://www.iapac.org/
AIDS Treatment News
[http://www.immunet.org/immunet/home.nsf/page/homepage]
[JAMA HIV/AIDS Resource Center]
http://www.ama-assn.org/special/hiv/hivhome.htm
[Johns Hopkins AIDS Service]
http://www.hopkins-aids.edu/

Sexually Transmitted Infections & Pelvic Inflammatory Disease

34

David E. Soper, MD

Sexually transmitted infections (STIs) affect more than 15 million people in the United States each year. Current figures suggest that 1 of 4 and perhaps as many as 1 of 2 people will contract an STI at some time in their lives. The groups most affected by STIs include women; teenagers; the poor; and members of minority groups, especially blacks. The annual cost associated with STIs and their complications has been estimated to be more than $16 billion.

Women are more susceptible to STIs and have a harder time being diagnosed than men because the infections are often asymptomatic in women. The clinical manifestations of STIs are due to the ability of most pathogens to elicit an inflammatory response from the host. For this reason, the primary clinical sign of infection with an STI is the presence of pus, an accumulation of polymorphonuclear white blood cells. The detection of this inflammation is the clinical challenge. Because so many women with STIs are asymptomatic, screening for selective STIs is important. The prevalence of STIs in a patient population should influence the decision to screen. Women with one STI are often infected with others.

It should be noted that HIV infection modifies the presentation and response to therapy of patients with STIs. All patients with STIs should be offered serologic testing for HIV infection.

DISEASES CHARACTERIZED BY ABNORMAL VAGINAL DISCHARGE

 ESSENTIALS OF DIAGNOSIS

- *Evaluate appearance of vaginal secretions.*
- *Measure the pH of vaginal secretions.*
- *Examine vaginal secretions with microscopy for clue cells, motile trichomonads, fungal elements, and white blood cells.*
- *Obtain whiff test (add 10% potassium hydroxide to the vaginal secretions to detect a fishy odor).*
- *Perform vaginal yeast culture (for women with vaginitis symptoms but negative microscopy results).*
- *Evaluate the cervix for erythema, friability, and mucopus.*
- *Test for* Chlamydia trachomatis *and* Neisseria gonorrhoeae *if mucopus present.*

General Considerations

Trichomoniasis and chlamydia are 2 of the most common STIs in the United States (Table 34–1). Bacterial vaginosis is a genital infection that is not sexually transmitted but is associated with sexual intercourse.

Traditional STI risk factors appear to be correlate to the probability of encountering an infected partner; other factors influence the probability of infection if exposed or the probability of manifesting disease if infected. Major sexual behavioral risk factors for STIs appear to include (1) multiple sex partners, (2) high rates of acquisition of new sexual partners within specific time periods, (3) high rates of partner change, (4) contact with casual sexual partners, and (5) risky sexual practices (eg, rectal intercourse). Alcohol and drug use produce situational modification of sexual behavior or health care behavior. Health care behaviors that can reduce the risk of acquiring STIs or prevent complications include the use of condoms for prophylaxis, early consultation for diagnosis and treatment, compliance with therapy, and partner referral. Absence of such behaviors can be regarded as risk factors for STIs. Douching represents a behavior that, although undertaken for "feminine hygiene," increases the risk of bacterial vaginosis as well as pelvic inflammatory disease (PID) and its sequelae.

Other indicators of risk include young age, single marital status, membership in particular ethnic groups, and urban residence. These risk indicators are correlates of sexual behavior, disease prevalence in sex partners, and health-seeking behaviors. Age also may affect host susceptibility in that the prevalence of cervical ectopy is

Table 34–1. Sexually transmitted infections in the United States.

Infection	Incidence (Estimated number of new cases every year)	Prevalence (Estimated number of people currently infected)
Chlamydia	3 million	2 million
Gonorrhea[1]	650,000	Not available
Syphilis[1]	70,000	Not available
Herpes	1 million	45 million
Human papillomavirus	5.5 million	20 million
Hepatitis B	120,000	417,000
Trichomoniasis[1]	5 million	Not available
Bacterial vaginosis[1,2]	Not available	Not available

[1]No recent surveys on national prevalence of gonorrhea, syphilis, trichomoniasis or bacterial vaginosis have been conducted.
[2]Bacterial vaginosis is a genital infection that is not sexually transmitted but is associated with sexual intercourse.
(Source: Cates W: et al. Sex Trans Dis 1999;26:S2.)

higher in young women and may increase a woman's susceptibility to gonorrhea, chlamydia, and HIV.

Prevention

The screening of women for chlamydial infections is a critical component in a *Chlamydia* prevention program. Seventy-five percent of women with chlamydial infection are asymptomatic and the infection may persist for extended periods of time. Many women of reproductive age undergo pelvic examination during visits for routine health care or because of illness. During these examinations, specimens can be obtained for screening tests for *Chlamydia*.

Women who should be screened for chlamydial infection include adolescents, those undergoing induced abortion, those attending sexually transmitted infection clinics, and women in detention facilities. Screening at family planning and prenatal care clinics is particularly cost-effective because of the large numbers of sexually active young women who undergo pelvic examinations. Other groups of women who should be tested for *Chlamydia* include those who have mucopurulent cervicitis (MPC) and those who are sexually active and younger than 20 years of age. In addition, women between 20 and 24 years of age who meet either of the following criteria and women older than 24 years who meet both of the criteria should be screened: (1) inconsistent use of barrier contraception and (2) having a new sex partner or more than one sex partner during the last 3 months. Screening should be repeated at least annually.

Gonococcal infections also are often asymptomatic in women. For this reason, a primary measure for controlling gonorrhea has been the screening of high-risk women. Because gonorrhea tends to be spread by a core group, screening the general population is not as effective as screening women with specific risk factors for the infection. Women with a history of gonorrhea, commercial sex workers, young women, and the homeless are considered at greater risk for gonorrhea.

Clinical Findings

Symptoms associated with vaginitis include an abnormal vaginal discharge, vulvar itching or irritation, and a fishy vaginal odor. The 3 common diseases characterized by vaginitis are bacterial vaginosis, vulvovaginal candidiasis, and trichomonas vaginitis.

The diagnosis of vaginitis is made with 4 clinical tests. These tests include an assessment of the appearance of the vaginal discharge, the pH of the vaginal secretions, microscopy of the vaginal secretions, and the whiff test. The whiff test is positive when the addition of potassium hydroxide to the vaginal secretions results in the volatilization of organic amines (trimethylamine), causing a fishy odor.

Women with bacterial vaginosis have a thin, homogeneous discharge, a pH greater than 4.5, microscopy showing clue cells, and a positive whiff test.

Vulvovaginal candidiasis is characterized by vulvar erythema and a cottage cheese–like vaginal discharge. The vaginal pH is normal (< 4.5). Microscopy of the vaginal secretions should show the presence of fungal elements. The whiff test is negative. A vaginal yeast culture should be performed in women complaining of vulvovaginal symptoms consistent with yeast vaginitis but have a normal microscopy of the vaginal secretions. If these patients also have a normal vulvovaginal examination, it is unlikely that they have vaginitis caused by *Candida* infection.

Diagnosis of trichomoniasis is based on the appearance of motile trichomonads during microscopy of the vaginal secretions. Women with vaginal trichomoniasis commonly show evidence of concurrent bacterial vaginosis.

MPC is characterized by a yellow or green endocervical exudate. The condition is asymptomatic among many women, but some experience an abnormal vaginal discharge, abnormal vaginal bleeding especially after coitus, and pelvic cramping. The cervix may be friable (bleeds easily when touched with a cotton swab), erythematous, and edematous. MPC can be caused by *C trachomatis* or *N gonorrhoeae,* although in most cases neither organism can be detected. Bacterial vaginosis is commonly associated with MPC. A Gram stain of the cervical mucus confirms a predominance of leukocytes, usually greater than 10–30 per oil immersion field.

Differential Diagnosis

It is particularly important to consider the cervix as a possible source of the complaint. In addition, mixed infections are not uncommon. Trichomonas vaginitis and/or MPC are commonly present when microscopy of the vaginal secretions reveals leukorrhea (leukocytes outnumber the vaginal epithelial cells) in association with the findings consistent with bacterial vaginosis.

As many as 10% of women presenting with a chief complaint of an abnormal vaginal discharge will have no disease. The clinician's ability to confidently confirm the presence of normal vaginal flora with microscopy of the vaginal secretions (lactobacilli predominance) can prevent unnecessary and arbitrary treatment.

Complications

Serious problems can result from STIs, including PID, infertility, ectopic pregnancy, cervical cancer, and transmission of STI to offspring during pregnancy or childbirth. Perinatal and neonatal STIs can cause spontaneous abortion, stillbirth, infant death, premature delivery, mental retardation, blindness, and low birth weight.

Treatment

The principal goal of treating vaginitis is to relieve vulvovaginal symptoms and signs. In patients with trichomoniasis, prevention of transmission is also a goal of therapy. Treatment regimens for bacterial vaginosis and trichomoniasis are noted in Tables 34–2 and 34–3. Treatment regimens for vulvovaginal candidiasis are described in Table 48-2 (Diseases of Vulva & Vagina).

Regimens for treating MPC caused by *C trachomatis* or *N gonorrhoeae* infections are noted in Tables 34–4 and 34–5, respectively. Because of the high prevalence of coinfection with *C trachomatis* among patients with gonococcal infection, presumptive treatment for *Chlamydia* in patients being treated for gonorrhea is appropriate, particularly if no diagnostic test for *C trachomatis* infection has been performed.

Many antibiotics are safe and effective for treating gonorrhea—eradicating *N gonorrhoeae*, ending the possibility of further transmission, relieving symptoms, and reducing the chances of sequelae. Selection of a treatment regimen for *N gonorrhoeae* infection requires consideration of the anatomic site of infection, resistance of *N gonorrhoeae* strains to antimicrobials, possibility of coinfection with *C trachomatis*, and side effects and costs of the various treatment regimens. In clinical trials, the recommended regimens cured more than

Table 34–2. Regimens for the treatment of bacterial vaginosis.

Recommended regimens
Metronidazole 500 mg orally twice a day for 7 days
    or
Metronidazole gel, 0.75%, one full applicator (5 g) intravaginally, once a day for 5 days
    or
Clindamycin cream, 2%, one full applicator (5 g) intravaginally at bedtime for 7 days

Alternative regimens
Metronidazole 2 g orally in a single dose
    or
Clindamycin 300 mg orally twice a day for 7 days
    or
Clindamycin ovules 100 g intravaginally once at bedtime for 3 days

Pregnancy
Metronidazole 250 mg orally 3 times a day for 7 days
    or
Clindamycin 300 mg orally twice a day for 7 days

95% of anal and genital infections; any of the regimens may be used for uncomplicated anal or genital infection. Published studies have indicated that both ceftriaxone, 125 mg, and ciprofloxacin, 500 mg, can cure more than 90% of pharyngeal infections.

Cefixime is an oral cephalosporin alternative to parenteral ceftriaxone. Ciprofloxacin or ofloxacin (or levofloxacin) are quinolones and can be used as oral agents for the treatment of gonorrhea. Both quinolones are contraindicated for pregnant or nursing women and for persons younger than 18 years.

A test of cure is not necessary for women treated with the recommended regimens. Women with persistent symptoms should be evaluated by culture for *N gonorrhoeae,* and any gonococci isolated should be tested for antimicrobial susceptibility. Infections following therapy with the regimens mentioned usually are due to reinfection. Persistent symptoms also may be caused by *C trachomatis.*

Table 34–3. Regimens for the treatment of vaginal trichomoniasis.

Recommended regimen
Metronidazole 2 g orally in a single dose

Alternative regimen
Metronidazole 500 mg twice a day for 7 days

Table 34–4. Regimens for the treatment of chlamydial infections.

Recommend regimens
    Azithromycin 1 g orally in a single dose
        or
    Doxycycline 100 mg orally twice a day for 7 days[1]

Alternative regimens
    Erythromycin base 500 mg orally 4 times a day for 7 days
        or
    Erythromycin ethylsuccinate 800 mg orally 4 times a day
        for 7 days[1]
        or
    Ofloxacin 300 mg orally twice a day for 7 days[1]
    Levofloxacin 500 mg orally for 7 days[1]

---

[1]Avoid during pregnancy.

Sex partners should be evaluated and treated for uncomplicated lower genital tract infection with *N gonorrhoeae* and *C trachomatis*. Patients should be instructed to avoid coitus until both the patient and partner or partners are cured. In the absence of a test of cure, abstinence should continue until treatment is completed and the patient is asymptomatic.

When to Refer to a Specialist

Patients with persistent symptoms and/or signs of disease despite treatment for a confirmed diagnosis should be referred for further evaluation. Recurrent vulvovaginal candidiasis can be due to non-albicans *Candida,* which tend to be resistant to commonly used azole antifungals. Recurrent bacterial vaginosis is due to the failure of protective hydrogen peroxide–producing lactobacilli to recolonize the vagina. Persistent trichomonas vaginitis despite metronidazole therapy suggests resistance.

Table 34–5. Recommended regimens for the treatment of gonorrhea.

Cefixime 400 mg orally in a single dose
    or
Ceftriaxone 125 mg IM in a single dose
    or
Ciprofloxacin 500 mg orally in a single dose
    or
Ofloxacin 400 mg orally in a single dose
    or
Levofloxacin 250 mg orally in a single dose
PLUS, if chlamydial infection not ruled out, Azithromycin 1 g
    orally in a single dose
    or
    Doxycycline 100 mg orally twice daily for 7 days

Prognosis

Diseases characterized by an abnormal vaginal discharge can be easily diagnosed in the office, and appropriate therapy can be prescribed for the patient. The prognosis is excellent. Problems can arise when diagnoses are not confirmed by clinical examination or tests and therapy become empiric.

DISEASES CHARACTERIZED BY GENITAL ULCERS

 ESSENTIALS OF DIAGNOSIS

- *Inspection of ulcer morphology.*
- *Serology for syphilis.*
- *Culture for herpes simplex virus (HSV).*
- *Type specific HSV serology in women with a negative herpes culture.*

General Considerations

A. EPIDEMIOLOGY

Up to 30% of first episode cases of genital herpes are caused by HSV-1, and recurrences are much less frequent for genital HSV-1 infection than genital HSV-2 infection. Therefore, the distinction between virus types influences the prognosis and counseling. For these reasons, the diagnosis of genital herpes usually should be confirmed by laboratory testing. Both virologic tests and type-specific serologic tests for HSV-specific glycoprotein G are available.

Since 1990, syphilis rates have declined 88% to 2.5 cases per 100,000 people in 1999. Screening with the low-cost nontreponemal tests such as the rapid plasma reagin (RPR) is appropriate for women who are likely to have had multiple sex partners for short periods of time and patients seen for STIs other than syphilis.

B. PRESENTATION IN WOMEN

Genital herpes, the most common cause of genital ulcer disease in the United States, is characterized by a prodrome of paresthesias 12–48 hours before the appearance of blisters. The mean incubation period is 7 days. The severity of first episodes of genital herpes depends on whether the patient has been exposed previously to HSV. Women with no preexisting antibody to HSV have severe disease with large numbers of vesicles and systemic signs of infection including fever and lymphadenopathy. No systemic signs are noted in patients with preexisting antibody to HSV. A common symptom accompanying an outbreak of genital herpes is dysuria. This dysuria is external in nature (splash dysuria). Patients who do not respond to urinary tract antiseptics for a presumptive diagnosis (many times prescribed over the phone) of lower urinary tract infection should be examined to rule out genital herpes. Despite the association of genital herpes with the symptoms described, most infected women have no symptoms and are unaware of their infection. Some women have symptoms shortly after infection and then never again. Most infected women never have recurrent genital lesions.

Syphilis is the second most common cause of genital ulcer disease. The mean incubation period is 3 weeks, and primary disease is characterized by a solitary ulcer called a **chancre.** Secondary syphilis usually occurs about 4–10 weeks after the chancre appears and may manifest as a flu-like syndrome and generalized lymphadenopathy. Most diagnoses of syphilis are made by serologic screening.

Chancroid is rare in the United States. This genital ulcer disease tends to be limited to commercial sex workers and other women who are at very high risk for STIs. Ulcers are usually few (1 to 3) and are associated with unilateral, tender lymphadenopathy.

Lymphogranuloma venereum (LGV) is also rare in the United States. Most patients do not notice this subtle ulcer, which may be described better as a fissure.

Prevention

Women with gonorrhea should be screened for syphilis by serologic study when gonorrhea is first detected. Gonorrhea treatments that include ceftriaxone or a 7-day regimen of doxycycline or erythromycin may cure incubating syphilis, but few data relevant to this topic are available. Pregnant women should undergo routine serologic screening as a means of preventing congenital syphilis.

Transmission of genital herpes usually occurs from an asymptomatic sexual contact who may be unaware that they are infected. The use of condoms should be suggested for future sexual exposures. Women should alert their obstetricians concerning a history of genital herpes so that strategies for the prevention of neonatal transmission can be considered.

Clinical Findings

Grouped vesicles on an erythematous base are the hallmark of genital herpes. These vesicles rupture, leaving multiple shallow and painful ulcerations. Primary first-episode disease (no preexisting antibody to HSV) is severe, with multiple painful vesicles and associated lymphadenopathy, myalgia, headache, and fever (see Figure 48–11). The lesions last 2–3 weeks. Nonprimary first-

episode and recurrent genital herpes (preexisting antibody to HSV present) present a much milder clinical picture (see Figure 48–12). These patients have many fewer vesicles usually clustered unilaterally on the vulva and disappearing within 3–4 days.

The chancre associated with syphilis is surprisingly painless; it has smooth margins and a firm, palpable (indurated) border (see Figure 48–13). The ulcer base is clean with a serous, not purulent, exudate. Atypical ulcers are common, especially when associated with secondary infection. In women, the external genitalia are the most common site for ulcers. Ulcers may occur in the vagina and on the cervix. Bilateral lymphadenopathy is common.

The most prominent feature of secondary syphilis is a generalized maculopapular rash affecting the trunk and limbs, including the palms of the hands and soles of the feet. Condylomata lata, fleshy lesions with a pearly gray appearance, may occur on the genitalia.

Chancroid ulcers are painful and tend to be deep, "beefy," and purulent; they usually have an irregular, undermined border. These ulcers have a ragged appearance and can reach the size of a quarter. Lymphadenitis may result in local suppuration and rupture of a lymph node with drainage of pus unilaterally.

The ulcer associated with LGV is transient, shallow, and painless and precedes the appearance of bilateral inguinal lymphadenopathy by 7–30 days. The inguinal lymphadenopathy occurs as a result of multiple enlarged, matted, and tender nodes, which coalesce and result in what has been referred to as the groove sign.

Differential Diagnosis

Despite the imprecision of the clinical diagnosis of genital ulcer disease, several presentations are highly suggestive of specific diagnoses:

1. A nonpainful and minimally tender ulcer that is not accompanied by inguinal adenopathy is likely to be syphilis, especially if the ulcer is indurated.

2. Grouped vesicles mixed with small ulcers, particularly in a patient with a history of such lesions, are almost pathognomonic of genital herpes.

3. One to 3 extremely painful ulcers, accompanied by tender inguinal lymphadenopathy, are unlikely to be anything except chancroid; if the adenopathy is fluctuant, the diagnosis is secured.

4. An inguinal bubo accompanied by 1 or several ulcers is most likely to be chancroid; if there is no ulcer, the most likely diagnosis is LGV.

In addition to a serologic test for syphilis, a test for HSV should be performed in all patients with genital ulcer disease. In areas where chancroid is common, a Gram stain of ulcer exudate may suggest the diagnosis by showing gram-negative rods in a "school of fish" arrangement. These lesions also should be cultured for *Haemophilus ducreyi.* If buboes are present, a diagnostic and therapeutic aspiration through intact skin (not through inflamed skin, for fear of fistula formation) should be performed. The aspirate should be cultured for *H ducreyi* and *C trachomatis.*

Complications

Genital herpes has special relevance in pregnancy. Active lesions found when a patient presents in labor are an indication for cesarean delivery. This prevents exposure of the neonate to viral shedding and therefore prevents vertical transmission of herpes. Antepartum cultures to detect asymptomatic viral shedding are not recommended.

Treatment

Genital herpes is a viral disease that can be recurrent and has no cure. Systemic antiviral therapy (acyclovir, famciclovir, or valacyclovir) provides partial control of symptoms and signs of a first clinical episode and may suppress recurrences. Antiviral therapy does not prevent the establishment of latent infection and therefore does not prevent recurrent episodes of genital herpes. Topical therapy is substantially less effective than oral therapy, and its use is discouraged. Most women with recurrent genital lesions receive no benefit from intermittent therapy for recurrent episodes unless therapy can be initiated during the prodrome or within 2 days of the onset of lesions. Because recurrent disease tends to be associated with a milder and shorter course of lesions, antiviral therapy generally is not recommended for women with recurrent disease except for use in suppression.

The recommended regimens for treatment of genital herpes are noted in Table 34–6. Patients desiring therapy for recurrent episodes receive shorter courses of therapy than those having a first episode. Daily suppressive therapy reduces the number of recurrences by 75% in patients who have frequent recurrences. Intravenous therapy should be offered to patients with severe disease or with complications of infection necessitating hospitalization, eg, disseminated infection, hepatitis, pneumonitis.

Patients should be advised to refrain from sexual contact while lesions are present and be informed of the natural history of the disease and risk for subsequent transmission.

Parenteral penicillin G is the preferred drug for treatment of all stages of syphilis. The preparations used (eg, benzathine penicillin), the dosage, and the length of treatment depend on the stage and clinical manifestations of the disease. Parenteral penicillin is the

Table 34–6. Recommended regimens for the treatment of genital herpes.

First clinical episode
Acyclovir 400 mg orally 3 times a day for 7–10 days
or
Acyclovir 200 mg orally 5 times a day for 7–10 days
or
Famciclovir 250 mg orally 3 times a day for 7–10 days
or
Valacyclovir 1 g orally twice a day for 7–10 days
Suppressive therapy of recurrent genital herpes
Acyclovir 400 mg orally twice a day
or
Famciclovir 250 mg orally twice a day
or
Valacyclovir 500 mg orally once a day
or
Valacyclovir 1 g orally once a day

only therapy with documented efficacy for neurosyphilis and for syphilis during pregnancy. Patients with neurosyphilis and pregnant women with syphilis in any stage who report penicillin allergy almost always should be treated with penicillin, preceded by desensitization if necessary. Skin testing for penicillin allergy is helpful since most patients with a history of penicillin allergy have a negative skin test result.

The Jarisch-Herxheimer reaction is an acute febrile reaction, accompanied by headache, myalgia, and other symptoms, that may occur within the first 24 hours after any therapy for syphilis. This reaction is common among patients with early syphilis. Antipyretics are recommended, but there is no proven method for prevention. Recommended regimens for the treatment of the various stages of syphilis are listed in Table 34–7.

Table 34–7. Treatment regimens for syphilis.

Stage	Treatment Regimen
Primary, secondary, or early latent[1]	Benzathine penicillin, 2.4 million units IM
Late latent[2] or late	Benzathine penicillin 2.4 million units IM for 3 doses at 1-week intervals (total = 7.2 million units)
Neurosyphilis	Aqueous penicillin G 18–24 million units daily administered as 3–4 million units IV every 4 hours or continuous infusion, for 10–14 days

[1]Asymptomatic syphilis of less than 1 year in duration.
[2]Asymptomatic syphilis of greater than 1 year in duration.

Quinolones are not active against *Treponema pallidum*. Persons exposed to a patient with syphilis should be evaluated clinically and serologically and treated, even if they are seronegative.

Successful treatment of chancroid cures infection, resolves clinical symptoms, and prevents transmission to others. Recommended regimens for the therapy of chancroid are listed in Table 34–8.

Treatment of LGV cures infection and prevents ongoing tissue damage, although the tissue reaction can result in scarring. Buboes may require aspiration or incision and drainage through intact skin. Doxycycline is the preferred treatment (Table 34–9).

When to Refer to a Specialist

The patient with a genital ulcer that does not respond to antimicrobial therapy should undergo additional evaluation. A biopsy of this ulcer should be performed to rule out squamous cell carcinoma.

It should be noted that HIV infection modifies the presentation and response to therapy of patients with STIs. Patients with genital ulcer disease and HIV infection resulting in immunosuppression are at risk for disseminated disease. Moreover, the lesions tend to be larger and more atypical in their presentation. Clinicians should consider management of these patients in conjunction with an infectious disease specialist. All patients with STIs, particularly genital ulcer disease, should be offered serologic testing for HIV infection.

Prognosis

Management of genital ulcer disease is straightforward and effective. However, the latency of HSV is well known. Patients with genital herpes may have recurrent outbreaks of vesicles as well as experience asymptomatic shedding. This may occur despite early therapy of primary infections with antiviral agents. Most patients diagnosed with a primary episode of genital herpes will be asymptomatic for increasing intervals as the time from

Table 34–8. Recommended regimens for chancroid.

Azithromycin 1 g orally in a single dose
  or
Ceftriaxone 250 mg IM in a single dose
  or
Ciprofloxacin 500 mg orally twice a day for 3 days
  or
Erythromycin base 500 mg orally 3 times a day for 7 days

Table 34–9. Regimens for lymphogranuloma venereum.

Recommended regimen
  Doxycycline 100 mg orally twice a day for 21 days

Alternative regimen
  Erythromycin base 500 mg orally 4 times a day for 21 days

---

infection lengthens. However, most women with genital herpes infection have never had symptoms at all.

DISEASES CHARACTERIZED BY ACUTE DYSURIA

 ESSENTIALS OF DIAGNOSIS

- *History of acute dysuria.*
- *Urinalysis showing pyuria.*
- *Urine culture.*
- *Evaluation of the cervix for erythema, friability, and mucopus.*
- *Tests for* C trachomatis *and* N gonorrhoeae.

General Considerations

Cystitis is characterized by the acute onset of internal dysuria. There may be associated irritative bladder symptoms including urgency and frequency. Occasionally, hematuria is noted or the patient will complain of cloudy, foul-smelling urine.

Urethritis, or inflammation of the urethra, is caused by infection characterized by the discharge of mucoid or purulent material and by burning during urination. In women, dysuria is the most common symptom; urethral discharge may be noticed as a vaginal discharge or may be asymptomatic. There may be a history of a new sex partner.

Clinical Findings

The patient may have suprapubic tenderness and/or bladder tenderness on bimanual examination. A urinalysis shows evidence of pyuria. Urine culture identifies an acute urethral syndrome caused by coliform bacteria or *Staphylococcus saprophyticus*. Urine culture often shows colony counts between 100 and 10,000 colony forming units per milliliter in these cases. In the symptomatic patient, these bacterial concentrations are significant. In high-risk patients and those with a negative urine culture, urethral infection with either *C trachomatis* or *N gonorrhoeae* should be considered and tests for these organisms performed. Pelvic examination may show evidence of MPC.

Differential Diagnosis

Although the most common cause of acute dysuria or urgency in women is bacterial cystitis secondary to coliform bacteria, 65% of women with a negative urine culture will have a chlamydial infection. Urethral infection with *N gonorrhoeae* is another cause of acute dysuria in women.

Treatment

It is not uncommon for clinicians to treat women with acute dysuria and pyuria with antimicrobial therapy appropriate for an uncomplicated lower urinary tract infection. Many of these antimicrobials such as nitrofurantoin have insufficient activity against *Chlamydia* and the gonococcus. It is appropriate to consider the STIs as a cause of these symptoms, especially in high-risk women.

Ideally, patients with MPC should have cervical specimens tested for chlamydia and gonorrhea before they are treated. Treating such women empirically without testing is a reasonable approach, but one must remember that sex partners need to be treated as well. It may be more difficult to involve the sex partner in the treatment program without proof of an STI.

When to Refer to a Specialist

Women with acute urethritis or cystitis respond promptly to therapy. However, if the symptoms become chronic, further evaluation is in order. Patients with urethral syndrome symptoms, usually chronic and not associated with pyuria, require cystoscopy and the consideration of alternative diagnoses including interstitial cystitis.

Prognosis

Women treated with the appropriate antibiotic regimen can expect total resolution of symptoms and signs of infection. Patients note an improvement in symptoms within 2 days if treated with an antimicrobial alone. Concurrent treatment with a urinary analgesic such as

pyridium can produce a more prompt cessation of symptoms.

HUMAN PAPILLOMAVIRUS INFECTION

 ESSENTIALS OF DIAGNOSIS

- *Inspection of the vulva for both exophytic and flat warts.*
- *Cervical cytology if none exists within the past 12 months.*
- *Biopsy pigmented lesions or those unresponsive to therapy.*

General Considerations

Exophytic genital and anal warts are benign growths most commonly caused by human papillomavirus (HPV) types 6 and 11. Research indicates that approximately 1% of sexually active adults have external genital warts (EGW). These estimates are based on select studies showing an incidence of 1.5% in female college students treated in student health clinics to 13% in some STI clinics. The total incidence in the United States of HPV infection is much higher: most women with HPV have no visible lesions and are asymptomatic. HPV types 16, 18, 31, 33, and 35 have been associated with squamous intraepithelial lesions of the cervix and cervical cancer.

The Papanicolaou (Pap) smear is not an effective screening test for STIs. However, a significant proportion of abnormal Pap smears are representative of subclinical genital HPV infection. Whenever a woman has a pelvic examination for STI screening, the health care provider should inquire about the result of her last Pap smear and should emphasize the importance of yearly Pap smears. A Pap smear should be performed for any woman has not had one during the previous 12 months.

Clinical Findings

Most genital warts are seen in young adults. The mean age of onset for women is between 16 and 25 years. Women with EGW may note small lesions about the vaginal introitus. EGW generally occur first at the posterior fourchette and adjacent labia; they also may appear on the perineum or perianal area. Occasionally, warts can be seen on the cervix.

Differential Diagnosis

Condylomata acuminata (or EGW) are soft, fleshy, vascular lesions first noticed on the vulva. They must be differentiated from condylomata lata, a manifestation of secondary syphilis. In addition, there are epithelial papillae and small sebaceous glands common on the vulva as well as fibroepithelial polyps that can be confused with EGW. Consideration of vulvar intraepithelial neoplasia, especially in women with persistent lesions, is important. Vulvar biopsy and serologic testing for syphilis should be performed when there is a question concerning the diagnosis.

Treatment

The goal of therapy is removal of exophytic warts and eradication of the signs and symptoms of infection. No therapy has been shown to eradicate HPV infection. It is speculated that HPV infection may persist throughout a patient's lifetime in a dormant state and become infectious intermittently. It has been suggested that genital warts are more infectious than subclinical infection and that the risk of subsequent transmission of HPV can be decreased by removal of the warts. Recurrences of genital warts result more commonly from reactivation of subclinical HPV infection than from reinfection by a sex partner. The effect of treatment on the natural history of genital warts is unknown.

Treatment of genital warts should be guided by patient preference. Expensive therapies, toxic therapies, and procedures that result in scarring should be avoided. Limited numbers of external genital and perianal warts can be treated with cryotherapy with liquid nitrogen or cryoprobe or with electrodesiccation or electrocautery. Topical therapy with imiquimod 5% cream (an immune modulator) or podofilox 0.5% solution or gel are patient-applied therapies. Topical therapy with podophyllin 10–25%, and trichloroacetic acid 80–90% are provider-administered therapies. These chemical treatments should be repeated weekly for as long as lesions persist or for 6 applications. Lesions persisting for longer than 6 weeks should be treated with other therapies; biopsy should be considered in such patients to rule out intraepithelial neoplasia.

Examination of sex partners is not necessary because the role of reinfection is believed to be minimal. However, sex partners with obvious warts should be counseled to seek treatment because the disease is contagious. The use of condoms may reduce the chance of transmission to new partners who may be uninfected.

When to Refer to a Specialist

Patients with persistent disease or those with unusually large genital warts should be referred to a specialist.

Many women in this category will also be immunocompromised patients due to other underlying diseases (eg, lymphoma) or medications (eg, chemotherapy).

Prognosis

Most women with mild cytologic abnormalities on Pap smear will show gradual resolution during the year of follow-up. Most patients with EGW respond well to a provider-administered or patient-administered compound. Recurrence of EGW, however, is not uncommon.

PUBIC LICE & SCABIES

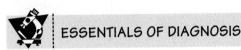 ESSENTIALS OF DIAGNOSIS

- *Predominant symptom is pruritus for both diagnoses.*
- *Microscopy aids diagnosis.*

Clinical Findings

Patients with pediculosis pubis (pubic lice) usually seek medical attention because of pruritus or because they notice lice on pubic hair. In addition, many women present for treatment because their sex partners are suspicious of infection. The predominant symptom of scabies is also pruritus.

Both adult lice and their eggs (nits) are seen easily by the naked eye. On examination of the vulva, lice may be perceived as scabs over what first appear to be excoriations. Nits may be seen on the hairs. Microscopic analysis of the pubic hair can confirm the presence of both adult lice and nits.

Scabies most commonly affect the hands, with characteristic lesions occurring mainly on the finger webs. Women may have eczematous lesions on the breast or papular lesions on the abdomen (particularly around the umbilicus) and on the lower buttocks in the crease where they join the thigh. Skin scrapings of the unexcoriated papules or burrows can confirm the diagnosis. Microscopy confirms the presence of the mite. A shave biopsy of a suspicious papule also may be performed to obtain material for microscopy.

Treatment

The recommended regimens for the treatment of lice and scabies are noted in Tables 34–10 and 34–11, respectively. Sex partners within the past month should be treated.

Table 34–10. Recommended regimens for pediculosis pubis (pubic lice).

Permethrin 1% cream rinse applied to affected areas and washed off after 10 minutes
or
Lindane 1% shampoo applied for 4 minutes to the affected area and then washed off[1]
or
Pyrethrins with piperonyl butoxide applied to the affected area and washed off after 10 minutes

[1]Avoid in pregnant or lactating women.

PELVIC INFLAMMATORY DISEASE

 ESSENTIALS OF DIAGNOSIS

- *Any genitourinary tract symptom including pain, abnormal vaginal bleeding or discharge, or lower urinary tract symptoms.*
- *Microscopy of the vaginal secretions shows leukorrhea.*
- *MPC is present.*
- *Bimanual pelvic examination confirms pelvic organ tenderness: uterus, adnexa, or both.*

General Considerations

Traditionally, the diagnosis of PID has been applied to patients presenting with lower abdominal pain. It is now well recognized that pain is not necessarily present in patients with PID. Any of the genitourinary symptoms previously described that lead the clinician to consider the presence of chlamydia or gonorrhea should be considered symptoms compatible with a diagnosis of

Table 34–11. Regimens for treatment of scabies.

Recommended regimen
Permethrin cream (5%) applied to all areas of the body from the neck down and washed off after 8–14 hours

Alternative regimen
Lindane (1%) 1 oz of lotion or 30 g of cream applied thinly to all areas of the body from the neck down and thoroughly washed off after 8 hours
Or
Ivermectin in 2 doses of (200 µg/kg) separated by 2 weeks

PID. Lower genital tract symptoms of dysuria, urgency, and abnormal vaginal discharge may herald the onset of PID. In addition, symptoms suggesting peritoneal irritation such as pelvic pain should be considered suggestive of PID. Abnormal uterine bleeding, especially breakthrough bleeding in patients taking oral contraceptives, may indicate the presence of endometritis and therefore also is suggestive of PID. Classic symptoms associated with clinically severe PID include fever and lower abdominal pain. Chlamydia screening programs have been effective in decreasing the incidence of PID.

Clinical Findings

It is important to appreciate the clinical signs associated with the diagnosis of PID. These signs result from the ascending inflammation present in patients with PID. The most important sign is leukorrhea, which is present when microscopy of the vaginal secretions reveals a predominance of leukocytes. Uterine tenderness and cervical motion tenderness and/or adnexal tenderness (usually bilateral but possibly unilateral) reflect the presence of inflammation in the upper genital tract.

If an adnexal mass is found during bimanual pelvic examination and other criteria for the diagnosis of PID are present, the patient should be presumed to have a tuboovarian abscess (TOA). Ultrasonography can be used to characterize the adnexal mass.

Endometrial biopsy can be used to confirm the presence of upper genital tract inflammation (endometritis). Additional findings of elevated temperature; abdominal tenderness with or without rebound; leukocytosis; and positive tests for chlamydia, gonorrhea, or both, help increase the specificity of the diagnosis.

Differential Diagnosis

The differential diagnosis of women with PID includes other causes of acute pelvic pain. These include appendicitis, a ruptured ovarian cyst or ovarian torsion, and ectopic pregnancy. Evaluation of the lower genital tract is helpful in discriminating among these diagnoses. Women with PID will have leukorrhea with or without bacterial vaginosis, while the clinician can expect the young woman with appendicitis to have normal vaginal flora without leukocytes.

Treatment

PID treatment regimens must provide empiric, broad-spectrum coverage of likely pathogens. Antimicrobial coverage should include *N gonorrhoeae*, *C trachomatis*, gram-negative facultative bacteria, anaerobes, and streptococci (Tables 34–12 and 34–13). Because PID may be due to a polymicrobial flora, a longer duration of therapy is needed than for monoetiologic infections.

Table 34–12. Oral treatment of pelvic inflammatory disease.

Regimen A
Ofloxacin 400 mg orally twice a day for 14 days (or levo-floxacin 500 mg orally once daily)
WITH or WITHOUT
Metronidazole 500 mg orally twice a day for 14 days[1]

Regimen B
Ceftriaxone 250 mg IM once
PLUS
Doxycycline 100 mg orally twice a day for 14 days
WITH or WITHOUT
Metronidazole 500 mg orally twice a day for 14 days[1]

---

[1]Add metronidazole if patient has evidence of bacterial vaginosis.

Table 34–13. Parenteral treatment of pelvic inflammatory disease.

Regimen A
Cefotetan 2 g IV every 12 hours or cefoxitin 2 g IV every 6 hours
PLUS
Doxycycline 100 mg orally every 12 hours once patient is tolerating oral intake

Regimen B
Clindamycin 900 mg IV every 8 hours
PLUS
Gentamicin loading dose IV (2 mg/kg of body weight) followed by a maintenance dose (1.5 mg/kg) every 8 hours. Single daily dosing may be substituted.

Generally speaking, women with mild clinical disease who are able to tolerate oral therapy can be treated as outpatients. Patients with severe clinical disease should be admitted for observation. Outpatients should be reevaluated in 72 hours to ensure that there is clinical improvement. Hospitalized patients should be treated as inpatients until their fever has resolved, the white blood cell count has normalized, and abdominal and bimanual pelvic examinations reveal marked amelioration of pelvic organ tenderness with the absence of rebound tenderness. For patients who do not respond to antibiotic therapy, further diagnostic work-up, surgical intervention, or both is required.

Patients with TOA should be admitted to the hospital for observation and parenteral antibiotic therapy. Either of the parenteral regimens given in Table 34–13 is acceptable. Failure to respond to therapy suggests the need for surgical drainage.

Sex partners of women with PID should be evaluated and treated for lower genital tract infection by *N gonorrhoeae* and *C trachomatis*.

When to Refer to a Specialist

As in the STIs discussed in this chapter, referral for PID is warranted when the diagnosis is uncertain or treatment is unsuccessful. The majority of women treated with an outpatient regimen for PID will improve and become asymptomatic. Women with a diagnosis of recurrent PID commonly have another diagnosis. This is particularly true if the patient has no history of chlamydia or gonorrhea and has no evidence of leukorrhea when evaluating the lower genital tract secretions. Diagnostic laparoscopy will confirm the presence of endometriosis in many of these women.

Cates W et al: Estimates of the incidence and prevalence of sexually transmitted diseases in the United States. Sex Trans Dis 1999;26:S2.

Holmes KK et al: *Sexually Transmitted Diseases,* 3rd ed. McGraw-Hill, 1999.

Sexually transmitted disease treatment guidelines 2002. Centers for Disease Control and Prevention. MMWR 2002;51(RR-6):1. [PMID: 12184549]

Relevant Web Sites

[Centers for Disease Control and Prevention. Easy access to treatment guidelines, epidemiologic data and other valuable information concerning STIs.]
www.cdc.gov

SECTION X
Hematologic & Oncologic Disorders

Breast Cancer

35

Judy M. Cheng, MD, PhD & Hope S. Rugo, MD

ESSENTIALS OF DIAGNOSIS

- *Microcalcifications may represent preinvasive ductal carcinoma in situ (DCIS).*
- *Five to 10% of cases can be attributed to identifiable inherited genetic mutations.*
- *Typical presentations include a palpable breast lump or an abnormal mammogram with microcalcifications or a spiculated mass.*
- *Less typical presentations include diffuse areas of breast thickening, nipple inversion, dimpling, bloody nipple discharge, axillary lymphadenopathy, or diffuse swelling and erythema of the breast.*

General Considerations

Carcinoma of the breast is the most common cancer in women in the United States, accounting for 31% of all female cancers. Breast cancer represents 16% of cancer deaths in women, a number exceeded only by lung cancer. An estimated 205,000 new cases of invasive breast cancer and 40,000 deaths from breast cancer will occur in women in the United States in 2002. Approximately 1 of 8 women in this country, or about 12–13% of the population, will be diagnosed with breast cancer during her lifetime, with a 3–4% risk of dying of this disease. Although breast cancer is predominantly a disease of women, there will be approximately 1500 new cases of breast cancer in men and approximately 400 deaths in the United States during the same time period. There is striking variation in the incidence of breast cancer throughout the world. The highest incidence is seen in Europe, Australia, and North America, and the lowest incidence is in Asia and Latin America. Environmental and lifestyle factors may play at least a part in these differences in incidence; women who migrate from low-risk countries such as Japan to high-risk countries such as the United States experience an increasing risk over the next two generations.

Racial susceptibility may also play a small role. There is also significant variation in breast cancer incidence through the United States, with one of the highest rates occurring in Northern California. The reasons for this geographic variation in incidence are unknown but again are likely related to environmental and lifestyle factors. Ongoing research is attempting to identify specific environmental risk factors that might impact the incidence of breast cancer starting from an early age (see risk factors below).

In the United States, data from the Surveillance, Epidemiology, and End Results (SEER) program of the National Cancer Institute, show a stable incidence of breast cancer over the last decade, preceded by a rise in incidence from the 1940s through the early 1990s of approximately 1% per year. The incidence at this time is approximately double what it was in 1940. When the incidence of cancer per 100,000 women is calculated, the slow, gradual rise in incidence was confined predominantly to postmenopausal women. Why did the incidence increase and then level off? It has been estimated that half of the increased incidence over the last 50 years is caused by increased longevity, due to the fact that breast cancer is largely a disease of older women. Other contributory factors include changes in lifestyle that have occurred in society since World War II. The average age of menarche has gradually dropped, likely due to improved nutrition, women are delaying childbirth, breast-feeding is generally less common, and the use of postmenopausal hormone replacement therapy has become more common (although this may change

319

with recent data, see following section on Hormonal Factors). All these factors are known to increase the risk of breast cancer (see the following section, Risk Factors). The relatively steeper rise in incidence seen in the 1980s most likely reflects increased detection of prevalent cancers through improved access to and widespread acceptance of screening mammography. Improved screening is also responsible for the increase in incidence of early-stage invasive breast cancer and DCIS and decrease in incidence of larger tumors and more locally advanced disease. Probably due to a combination of mammographic detection of earlier, more curable cancers as well as routine use of tamoxifen as a treatment for early-stage disease, the mortality rate from invasive breast cancer has declined by 1% to 2% per year over the last decade.

Harris JR et al (editors): *Diseases of the Breast.* 2nd ed. Philadelphia: Lippincott Williams & Wilkins, 2000. (In depth textbook covering a wide range of topics in breast cancer.)

Hulley S et al: Noncardiovascular disease outcomes during 6.8 years of hormone therapy: Heart and Estrogen/progestin Replacement Study follow-up (HERS II). JAMA 2002;288:58. [PMID: 12090863]

Risk Factors

Multiple risk factors predispose a patient to breast cancer and there does not appear to be a single predominant cause such as smoking resulting in lung cancer. Female gender and increasing age are the most definitive risk factors; breast cancer is overall quite rare in women under the age of 30 with a significant increase in risk with each additional decade of life. Sixty-five percent of all breast cancers occur in women aged 55 and older; in contrast, only 13% occur in women under the age of 45 (Table 35–1). Multiple genetic, dietary, environmental, and hormonal factors also contribute to the incidence. Breast cancer, like other malignant diseases, is caused by alterations in *somatic* genes, or genes that are present in differentiated tissues. Mutations in DNA including acti-

Table 35–1. New breast cancer cases, 1995–1999.

Age	Percent of Cases
20–34	2.1%
35–44	11%
45–54	21.6%
55–64	20.4%
65–85+	44.9%

Data taken from http://seer.cancer.gov/csr/1973_1999/breast.pdf

vation of oncogenes, inactivation of tumor-suppressor genes, or alterations in programmed cell death (apoptosis) pathways result in unregulated cell growth and the ability of cells to invade normal tissues, stimulate new blood vessel growth, and escape the bodies normal immune defense system. Current research is focusing on identifying the genetic alterations and resulting change in cell signals that result in the process of malignant cell development. Understanding the genetics of breast cancer will also help elucidate mechanisms for biologic differences in individual cancers, both in patterns of growth and response to therapy. *Germ-line* or inherited genetic alterations that increase susceptibility to breast cancer are discussed below.

A. RACE AND CULTURAL FACTORS

The geographic variation in incidence is at least partly due to lifestyle differences between populations. The complexity of the analysis of such differences is underscored by the fact that there are many covariables. For example, the average Japanese woman, compared with the average North American woman, not only eats a diet lower in fat but also eats a different spectrum of food entirely. Japanese women also tend to mature later, have a leaner body habitus, and appear to have a lower endogenous estradiol level than American women. When Asian women immigrate to the United States, their risk increases but remains less than Asian women born in the United States. Even within the United States, there are differences in incidence both between racial groups and geographic areas. The lifetime risk of breast cancer developing in black women is 1 in 10 compared with 1 in 8 for white women, although with a higher mortality rate overall and stage for stage (Table 35–2). While mortality rates for both black and white women are decreasing, the rate of decline is much lower in the black population. The reason for the relatively higher mortality in black women is unknown but is at least partially related to more aggressive biologic disease and less access to screening and medical care. Asian and Hispanic American women also seem to have lower rates of cancer than white women. The incidence of breast cancer in various racial groups is shown in Figure 35–1. There appear to be geographic differences in the incidence of breast cancer in the United States. Pockets of higher risk areas have been associated with higher socioeconomic status, differences in reproductive choices, genetic variation, diet, environmental exposures or other factors although the relative contribution of specific risk factors is not well understood.

B. HEREDITY

1. Family history—Family history is a well-established risk factor for breast cancer. When assessing a

Table 35–2. Breast cancer incidence and mortality.

	Incidence per year per 100,000 1992–1998	Mortality per year per 100,000 1992–1998	Lifetime Risk of Invasive Cancer	Lifetime Risk of Dying of Breast Cancer
All women	132	29.7	13.3%	3.12%
White women	137	29.3	13.95%	3.12%
Black women	121	37.3	10.21%	3.39%

(Lifetime risk estimates based on 1997–1999 data; data taken from http://seer.cancer.gov/csr/1973_1999/breast.pdf)

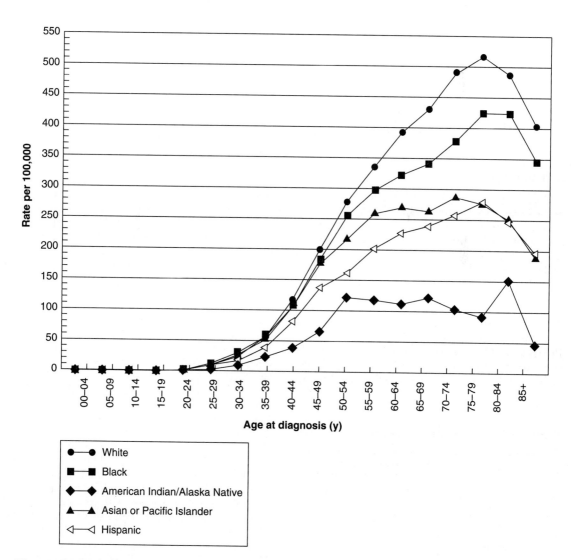

Figure 35–1. Breast cancer incidence from 1992–1999 by age and race. (Data from http://seer.cancer.gov/faststats/html/inc_breast.html)

person's risk of breast cancer based on a family history, it is important to recognize that there is enormous variation in risk depending on the specifics of the cancer history in the extended family. It is important to take a full multi-generational history since cancers in extended family members may identify familial syndromes associated with a very high risk (see below) for development of a variety of cancers. This has important impact on screening recommendations as well as consideration for preventive measures. For evaluating routine risk of breast cancer, only first-degree relatives are considered. If a first-degree relative had breast cancer, the relative lifetime risk of developing breast cancer is 1.8-fold that of the general population. This risk increases with each additional affected relative, including siblings. The Gail model is 1 way to calculate the probable risk of breast cancer for an individual over the next 5 years and over that person's lifetime that takes into account a patient's family history and well as other well-defined risk factors. Six factors are considered in this model:

1. Current age of the patient
2. Race
3. Age at menarche
4. Age of first birth
5. Number of first-degree relatives with breast cancer
6. Number of previous breast biopsies with increased weight given to biopsies showing atypical hyperplasia.

The Gail model was first proposed in 1989 and data from large prospective and observational studies have been used to validate its predictive accuracy. One problem with using this model to predict risk and test the subsequent impact of preventive measures is that it tends to overestimate risk in younger and higher-risk patients and, correspondingly, underestimate risk in older and lower-risk patients. However, overall, the Gail model has been found to perform reasonably well, with an expected to observed case ratio of 1.03 (95% confidence interval of 0.88 to 1.21) in a large validation study in 1999 performed by the National Surgical Adjuvant Breast and Bowel Project (NSABP), a national cooperative oncology research group. Other smaller validation studies also show a high predictive value in patients with a positive family history who underwent annual mammographic screening. The Gail model is now routinely used as a risk assessment tool to identify women at moderate risk for breast cancer as well as patients who may be candidates to participate in clinical trials. Women at higher risk should be referred to high-risk programs for counseling or screening and possible preventive treatments.

2. Inherited genetic mutations—Genetic susceptibility is the strongest known risk factor in women or men

with very strong family histories of cancer. Specific details about family history, including cancers occurring in multiple generations and at a young age, less common cancers, and more than one cancer in a single relative, should trigger further evaluation with consideration for referral to genetic counseling and possible genetic testing. Appropriate evaluation may have a significant impact on screening and preventive measures that may, in turn, reduce the risk of cancer incidence and death in an individual. In the early 1990s, genetic linkage studies of families that had high rates of breast and ovarian cancer identified 3 mutations in 2 genes referred to as BRCA1 and BRCA2 that are associated with hereditary breast and ovarian cancers, as well as an increased risk of other cancers. These mutations are inherited in an autosomal dominant mode, (eg, each offspring of an affected individual has a 50:50 chance of inheriting the faulty gene). For a woman who inherits the mutated gene, the lifetime risk of breast cancer is about 55–85% for BRCA1 and 40–85% for BRCA2. For a woman in the same family who does not inherit the gene, the risk of breast cancer is that of the rest of population, 12–13%. Overall, these 2 genes account for less than 1% of all cases of breast cancer. Most women with sporadic, nonhereditary cases of breast cancer do not have mutations in BRCA1 or BRCA2. However, in patients of Ashkenazi Jewish descent, even in those with weak family histories, BRCA1 or BRCA2 mutations account for a much higher percentage of cancers, up to 20–40% for patients with a diagnosis under the age of 50. In non-Jewish populations, the incidence of BRCA1 or BRCA2 mutations is also higher in patients with a diagnosis under the age of 30 or with family histories containing multiple cases of early breast cancer, a single case of ovarian cancer, or male breast cancer. Individuals with this background should be referred for genetic counseling. Genetic testing should only be done in the setting of appropriate counseling by trained individuals.

There are increasing options for prophylaxis and screening for women with known BRCA1 or BRCA2 mutations. Prophylactic mastectomy and/or oophorectomy significantly decreases the risk of subsequent cancer but obviously has a major impact on lifestyle and quality of life. Oophorectomy in premenopausal women who have completed childbearing decreases the subsequent risk of breast cancer, and new screening measures may improve detection of early stage and noninvasive cancers. Patients with inherited mutations should also have increased surveillance for cancer of the colon and skin.

There are a number of other rare familial syndromes associated with an increased risk of breast cancer. The Li-Fraumeni syndrome, characterized by a familial clustering of breast cancer in women, soft-tissue and bone sarcomas in children, acute leukemia, brain tumors, and adrenocortical carcinomas, is caused by a germ-line mutation in the p53 tumor-suppressor gene. Women in such families who inherit the faulty gene have a lifetime risk of breast cancer of greater than 50-fold. Other rare familial syndromes have been identified. In some families, there is an increased susceptibility to breast, colon, and other epithelial tumors (Lynch syndrome type II, which may be a variant of hereditary nonpolyposis colorectal cancer (HNPCC). These families have abnormal genes responsible for DNA mismatch repair. Cowden disease and Peutz-Jeghers syndrome, rare syndromes characterized by multiple hamartomas, are also associated with increased risk of breast cancer. Overall, these rare familial syndromes as a group account for less than 1% of all breast cancers.

C. HORMONAL FACTORS

The breast epithelium is sensitive to stimulation by estrogen. Early menarche, late menopause, nulliparity, and delayed childbearing are associated with an increased risk of breast cancer. It is likely that early menarche and late menopause increase the risk by increasing the lifetime exposure of the breast epithelium to the proliferative effect of estrogen due to the increased number of menstrual cycles. Women with increased breast density appear to have a slightly higher risk of developing breast cancer; this has been attributed to relatively higher levels of circulating estrogen. Reduction in breast density is being used as a possible short-term surrogate marker of effectiveness (reduction of subsequent risk of breast cancer) in several large prevention trials testing new hormonal agents.

Women who have children at a younger age appear to be at a reduced risk of developing breast cancer. Whereas a woman who has her first child after age 35 may have a relative risk of breast cancer of 1.2, a woman who has a child while in her early teens or women with multiple full-term pregnancies have a relative risk as low as 0.4. This appears to be related to relatively less exposure to ovarian cycles of estrogen; oophorectomy at an early age (as well as early natural menopause) is also associated with reduced subsequent risk of breast cancer. A recent, large, population-based study has demonstrated significant impact from longer durations of breast-feeding on reduction of breast cancer risk. Women who breast-fed for longer than 9 months with each infant were found to have the lowest overall risk of breast cancer, with a 4–5% relative risk reduction for every 12 months of lifetime breast-feeding. Interestingly, this risk reduction is independent of the 7% relative risk reduction with each birth, and it appears to be much stronger. Breast-feeding clearly has many benefits to the child as well, and increased practice of breast-feeding for at least 9 months duration

may have an impact on overall breast cancer rates in the population.

1. Hormone replacement therapy (HRT)—For the past decade, tens of millions of women have been treated with exogenous estrogen for perimenopausal hot flashes and for primary prevention of osteoporosis and cardiovascular disease. From observational studies including the Nurses Health Study, an increased risk of breast cancer was suggested in long-term users (5 years or more) of combined hormonal therapy. However, this risk was deemed acceptable given strong observational data that HRT significantly reduced the risk of cardiovascular disease and mortality. Recently, two randomized, controlled trials have brought this practice into question. In 2000, the Heart and Estrogen Replacement Study (HERS), a randomized trial of estrogen plus progestin versus placebo in women with known coronary artery disease, found a short-term increase in cardiovascular events, and a 27% increase in breast cancer in women taking HRT during 6.8 years of follow-up. The Women's Health Initiative (WHI) is a randomized, controlled, primary prevention study of HRT (combined estrogen and progesterone [Prempro] versus placebo in women with an intact uterus and estrogen alone [Premarin] versus placebo in women who do not have a uterus) in healthy postmenopausal women. In August 2002, at a median follow-up of 5.2 years, the WHI study reported both an increase in cardiovascular disease as well as a 26% increase in the incidence of breast cancer in women taking Prempro, a combination of estrogen and progesterone. The absolute increase was approximately 0.4% at 5 years, or 8 additional cases of breast cancer per year for every 10,000 women receiving HRT. The estrogen/progestin arm of the WHI trial was prematurely terminated due to these findings, although the study remains open for women enrolled on the estrogen alone arm until the trial's end points are reached. These randomized trials appear to confirm a small increase in the risk of invasive breast cancer with long-term use of combination HRT. It is important to note that there is not yet survival data from these studies. Breast cancer that develops on HRT has been found to be generally associated with a more favorable prognosis than breast cancer in general; until survival data is available the true impact of HRT remains unclear.

2. Oral contraceptives—Oral contraceptives, in contrast, have generally not been shown to increase the risk of breast cancer. The Cancer and Steroid Hormone Study in 1986 appeared to exonerate oral contraceptive pills, most commonly an estrogen and progesterone combination, from contributing to breast cancer risk. In recent years, multiple studies have been done to determine whether any subsets of women who have taken oral contraceptives are at increased risk. A large case-control study of over 9000 women published in 2002 confirms that there is no increased risk for current or former users. There was no evidence that use of oral contraceptives interacted with other breast cancer risks such as family or gynecologic history. In contrast, women with a family history of breast cancer who took high-dose estrogen pills before 1975 appear to have a slightly increased risk of breast cancer later in life. At this time, it is reasonable to conclude that use of current oral contraceptive pills for several years does not increase the risk of breast cancer.

D. ENVIRONMENTAL EXPOSURE

Exposure to ionizing radiation is clearly associated with an increased risk of breast cancer. There was an increased incidence of breast cancer among women who survived the atomic bombing of Hiroshima, and young women who were treated with mantle radiation for Hodgkin's disease have been found to have a significantly increased risk of breast cancer later in life, often while they are still younger than 40. Reanalysis of old data on long-term consequences of exposure to fluoroscopy for tuberculosis showed that women who were under age 25 when they were exposed had a small increased risk of breast cancer, whereas older women did not. The radiation sensitivity of the breast epithelium clearly decreases with age, and it should be emphasized that the radiation risk of screening mammography in women is extremely small.

Much less clear is the role of chemicals or agents as carcinogens. Much research has focused on organochlorines, which include DDT, dioxin and polychlorinated biphenyls (PCBs). These agents are mutagenic in laboratory studies and, in some instances, have been shown to have weak estrogenic activity. However, studies comparing levels of various organochlorines in body tissues in women with and without breast cancer have not been able to show a clear increase in subsequent risk, with previous studies reporting conflict data on the role of polycyclic hydrocarbons and cancer risk. A large study sponsored by the National Cancer Institute, the Long Island Breast Cancer Study Project, attempted to explore the role of environmental exposure to chemicals and risk of breast cancer. Results published in August 2002 showed no correlation between serum levels of DDT, PCBs, or other organochlorines and risk of breast cancer. A 1.5-fold increase in risk was seen in women with the highest levels of polycyclic aromatic hydrocarbons, chemicals which are found in combustion by-products, cigarette smoke, and smoked foods, although no correlation was found with smoking or other specific environmental exposures. This risk still was much lower than that of established risk factors such as family history. The results of the Long Island

study are not definitive due to the difficulty in tracing exposure from a variety of environmental sources over a woman's lifetime. To date however, there is no conclusive link between environmental exposures and breast cancer risk.

E. ALCOHOL AND DIET

Several studies have looked at the relationship between alcohol intake and the incidence of breast cancer. Initially controversial, there appears to be growing evidence for a small increased risk with moderate alcohol intake. A recent study indicated that the relative risk was greatest in women who averaged 2 or 3 alcoholic drinks per day compared with those with no alcohol consumption. Although the relative risk has been reported to be only be 1.2- to 1.4-fold that of non-drinkers, alcohol intake is a potentially modifiable risk factor. The increase in incidence may be related to higher endogenous circulating estrogen levels in women following alcohol ingestion.

The hypothesis that a high-fat diet is associated with an increased risk of breast cancer first came from epidemiologic studies showing that the incidence of breast cancer across the world correlated with the per capita fat intake in the countries studied. Large cohort studies examining fat intake, fiber, and antioxidant vitamins over time have not been able to correlate risk with diet. In the Nurses Health Study conducted by the Harvard School of Public Health in which 89,000 nurses were surveyed about diet and other lifestyle factors, there was no increased risk of breast cancer associated with a high-fat diet. A small inverse correlation was seen with high intake of fruits and vegetables; there was no effect on risk from varied dietary fiber intake. The increased risk with low fruit and vegetable consumption has not been confirmed in other studies. However, other health benefits exist in increasing fruit and vegetable intake and, as with alcohol intake, this is another modifiable risk factor. One of the goals of the WHI is to conduct a prospective study of the effects of diet modification on a variety of diseases including breast cancer.

F. PROLIFERATIVE BREAST DISEASE AND A PREVIOUS HISTORY OF INVASIVE BREAST CANCER

A personal history of proliferative breast disease on breast biopsy, such as atypical ductal hyperplasia, increases the risk of developing cancer as does a previous history of in situ or invasive cancer. In a landmark study in 1985, Dupont and Page identified histologic subtypes of benign breast lesions that are associated with a subsequent increase in the risk of breast cancer. Women with 10,542 consecutive benign breast biopsies were followed for a median of 17 years, and the relative risk of breast cancer in these women was compared with that of a population of case-matched women without a history of breast biopsy. The majority of lesions were classified pathologically as "nonproliferative," including fibrocystic and papillary apocrine changes; women with these diagnoses did not have an increased risk of breast cancer compared with women in the control group. However, women whose biopsies revealed proliferative abnormalities, including atypical hyperplasia and carcinoma in situ were found to be at increased risk for the development of invasive cancer (see following Pathology section). A previous history of invasive breast cancer results in a risk of subsequent breast cancer of about 0.8% per year, for a lifetime risk of approximately 15%. The risk is higher with younger age at diagnosis of first cancer and is complicated by the difficulty separating local recurrences from new cancers.

Dupont WD, Page DL: Risk factors for breast cancer in women with proliferative breast disease. N Engl J Med 1985; 312:146.

Gail MH et al: Projecting individualized probabilities of developing breast cancer for white females who are being examined annually. J Natl Cancer Inst 1989;81:1879. [PMID: 2593165]

Gammon MD et al: Environmental toxins and breast cancer on Long Island. II. Organochlorine compound levels in blood. Cancer Epidemiol Biomarkers Prev 2002;11:686. [PMID: 12163320]

Gammon MD et al: Environmental toxins and breast cancer on Long Island. I. Polycyclic aromatic hydrocarbon DNA adducts. Cancer Epidemiol Biomarkers Prev 2002;11:677. [PMID: 12163319]

Hulley S et al: Noncardiovascular disease outcomes during 6.8 years of hormone therapy: Heart and Estrogen/progestin Replacement Study follow-up (HERS II). JAMA 2002;288:58. [PMID: 12090863]

Marchbanks PA et al: Oral contraceptives and the risk of breast cancer. N Engl J Med 2002;346:2025. [PMID: 12087137]

Risks and benefits of estrogen plus progestin in healthy postmenopausal women: principal results From the Women's Health Initiative randomized controlled trial. JAMA 2002; 288:321. [PMID: 12117397]

Sakorafas GH, Krespis E, Pavlakis G: Risk estimation for breast cancer development: a clinical perspective. Surg Oncol 2002; 10:183. [PMID: 12020673]

Smith-Warner SA et al: Alcohol and breast cancer in women: a pooled analysis of cohort studies. JAMA 1998;279:535. [PMID: 9480365]

Pathology

A. The Normal Breast

The mammalian breast, or mammary gland, consists of a specialized branching epithelial ductal system nestled in stroma; its purpose is to conduct milk from the alveoli to the nipple during lactation. Prepubescent girls already have a rudimentary ductal network that undergoes further growth and differentiation during puberty to become the adult breast. Additional differentiation occurs during pregnancy and lactation accompanied by milk formation, followed by regression of the alveoli and ducts after lactation ceases. The specialized stroma in which the ducts and lobules lie is largely composed of fat (Figure 35–2). The density of breast is related to the percentage of fat versus stroma and appears to correlate with levels of circulating estrogen. Women with higher circulating estrogen in menopause have been found to have a lower ratio of fat versus stroma, or dense breasts on mammography. Increased density contributes to breast cancer risk by being a surrogate marker for increased estrogen, as well as making mammographic detection of early malignancy more difficult. With rare exceptions, including primary lymphomas and sarcomas (phylloides tumors) of the breast, malignant tumors of the breast arise from the epithelial ducts or lobules.

B. Premalignant Lesions

Although a majority of breast biopsies, particularly in younger women, are benign, some of these benign conditions of the breast appear to be associated with an increase in subsequent risk of invasive or in situ breast cancer. In general, these conditions involve excessive proliferation of the epithelial cells lining the ducts or lobules. Epithelial hyperplasia, sometimes classified as usual ductal hyperplasia or hyperplasia without atypia, is a proliferation of normal cells in the epithelial lining, associated with a very small if any increase in the relative risk of future breast cancer (1.5- to 2-fold). Sclerosing adenosis and fibroadenomas also are categorized as proliferative lesions without atypia and with little if any increase in risk of cancer. If the cells in the multi-layered epithelium have acquired histologic atypia, the condition is termed **atypical ductal hyperplasia (ADH)**. Atypical lobular hyperplasia (ALH) is a related condition with involvement of the lobular units. Both share some pathologic characteristics with carcinoma in situ, but they do meet the diagnostic criteria for **lobular carcinoma in situ (LCIS)** or DCIS and are not considered malignant. However, studies have shown a 4- to 5-fold increased risk with ADH and a 5- to 6-fold increased risk with ALH of subsequent development of invasive cancer. These proliferative lesions are often bilateral and carry a higher future cancer risk at any site in either breast, regardless of where the initial lesion was identified on biopsy. Young women with a diagnosis of atypical hyperplasia should be referred to high-risk programs for discussion of preventive strategies and close monitoring.

C. Carcinoma In Situ

1. Lobular carcinoma in situ—LCIS is generally an incidental finding on biopsy that only occasionally presents as a mass or mammographic finding. LCIS is often found extensively throughout both breasts. Like

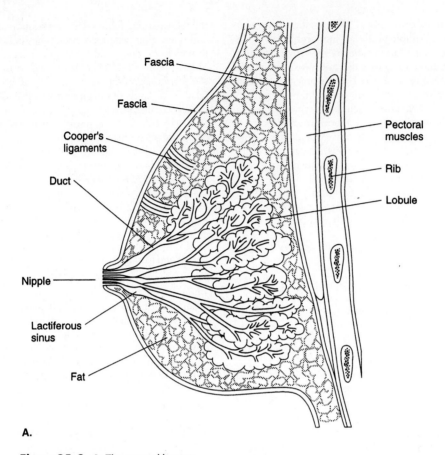

Figure 35–2. A: The normal breast.

atypical hyperplasia, its presence confers an increased risk of future invasive cancer in either breast, and subsequent cancers can be of ductal or lobular histology. Patients with LCIS on breast biopsy have a 7- to 10-fold lifetime relative risk of developing invasive cancer, although this is lower than patients with more aggressive forms of DCIS (see below). In the past, some breast surgeons recommended bilateral mastectomy as primary treatment for LCIS; however, this is not considered standard or required therapy for this noninvasive and non–life-threatening lesion. There is no indication that cancers arising in a background of LCIS are more aggressive than other breast cancers. Careful breast examination with annual mammography is a reasonable monitoring schedule for a patient with LCIS; chemoprevention should also be considered.

2. Ductal carcinoma in situ—Unlike ADH or LCIS, DCIS usually presents as a focal process. It may arise in a breast with preexisting proliferative epithelial changes,

or it may be found de novo. Pathologically, DCIS has the appearance of more advanced ductal cell proliferation, with the cells frequently filling the whole lumen of the affected ducts. Cellular necrosis and calcium deposits are often present. These calcium deposits appear as microcalcifications on mammography. Extensive DCIS refers to larger lesions that may encompass the majority of the breast, and may be associated with small areas of invasive cancer termed "microinvasion." Because of the heterogeneity of the lesions pathologically, DCIS is classified by nuclear grade and presence of necrosis and histologic pattern such as comedo or papillary; these features can affect propensity for recurrence after excision.

Epidemiologic and genetic data support DCIS as a precursor lesion to invasive cancer, with atypical hyperplasia as perhaps the first step in a multi-step process toward more biologically aggressive disease (Figure 35–3). Before the advent of screening mammography, pure DCIS comprised less than 2% of breast cancers

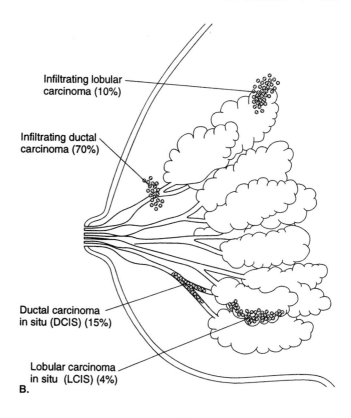

Infiltrating lobular
carcinoma (10%)

Infiltrating ductal
carcinoma (70%)

Ductal carcinoma
in situ (DCIS) (15%)

Figure 35–2. **B:** Subtypes of breast cancer.
(Courtesy of I. Kuter, MD, DPhil.)

Lobular carcinoma
in situ (LCIS) (4%)

B.

and presented typically as a palpable lump. Currently, with the prevalence of mammography, approximately 15–20% of all breast cancers are pure DCIS. It is unlikely that this increase in DCIS is due to the discovery of lesions that would never become clinically significant as the incidence of invasive cancers has declined during the same time period. Based on limited data in women with untreated DCIS, if pure DCIS is not detected and removed, it has a high probability of developing into an

invasive cancer with a 20–50% incidence over 10–15 years. Invasive cancer is commonly associated with varying amounts of DCIS, and 50% of local recurrences following primary treatment for pure DCIS will be invasive cancers. Genetic studies have revealed similar changes in DCIS and subsequent invasive cancer in the same breast, suggesting that they originate from the same cells. Untreated DCIS may continue to grow and spread through the branching ductal system of the

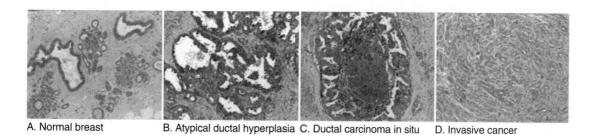

A. Normal breast   B. Atypical ductal hyperplasia   C. Ductal carcinoma in situ   D. Invasive cancer

Figure 35–3. Theory of pathologic progression of breast cancer from normal epithelium (**A**) to atypical ductal hyperplasia (**B**) to ductal carcinoma in situ (**C**) and finally to invasive cancer (**D**). (Reprinted with permission from Britt-marie Ljung, MD, Professor of Pathology, University of California, San Francisco.)

breast in an insidious, indolent fashion rather than evolve into an invasive cancer. In contrast to invasive cancer, however, even extensive DCIS is not lethal; a simple mastectomy is 99% curative with the majority of localized lesions managed by lumpectomy. However, it is important to rule out microinvasive cancer in patients with extensive DCIS; these patients should be considered for node evaluation as well as systemic therapy depending on the size and aggressiveness of the invasive component (see Treatment section).

D. Invasive Cancer

Breast cancer cells arise predominantly in the terminal ducts. When cancer cells migrate upward and fill the ducts, they are termed **ductal carcinomas** whereas if they migrate into the lobules, they are termed **lobular carcinomas.** The main subtypes of breast cancer and their cells of origin are shown in Figure 35–2. The majority of breast cancer is infiltrating or invasive ductal carcinoma, constituting approximately 70–80% of all cases. Lobular carcinomas account for an additional 10–20%, and the remainder are composed of a mix of histopathologic subtypes with differing clinical and prognostic features.

Invasive ductal carcinomas, the most common type, often arise from preexisting DCIS. The cancer cells invade and infiltrate the basement membrane under the epithelial lining, with subsequent movement of cells out of the duct or lobule and into the surrounding stroma. Invasive cancer is defined by cells that have acquired the ability to invade stroma as well as to migrate into adjacent lymphatics and blood vessels. This process allows the spread of tumor cells outside of the breast, into surrounding and distant sites, resulting in metastases. Invasive lobular carcinoma spreads via lymphatic channels and blood vessels just as invasive ductal carcinoma does, but it has specific features that differentiate it from ductal carcinoma. Lobular carcinoma cells characteristically invade the stroma in a single-file pattern without disrupting the architecture of the gland. As a result of this pattern of spread, the disease may present as a vague area of diffuse thickening in the breast rather than as a discrete mass. Unlike infiltrating ductal carcinomas, lobular carcinomas are not usually associated with calcifications. Lobular carcinoma is the most common reason for a false-negative mammogram, and fine-needle aspirations (FNA) may also be negative due to interspersion of cancer cells in normal breast tissue. Overall, infiltrating lobular carcinomas are more difficult to diagnose than infiltrating ductal carcinomas, and for that reason may more frequently present at a later stage than ductal cancers. Interestingly, the biology of lobular cancers also appears to be distinct from ductal cancers. Essentially, all lobular carcinomas are hormone receptor positive, whereas only two thirds of

ductal carcinomas are hormone receptor positive. The pleomorphic variant represents about 5% of lobular cancers and is usually hormone receptor negative and particularly aggressive. Lobular carcinomas often have a different pattern of metastasis than infiltrating ductal carcinomas, with metastases occurring in relatively unusual sites such as bone marrow and lymph nodes. In addition, lobular carcinomas may metastasize as nodules or masses on the serosal surface of the bowel or around the ureters with resulting bowel or ureteral obstruction. This can complicate diagnosis of metastatic disease.

Rarer histologic variants of ductal carcinoma include mucinous and tubular carcinomas. Mucinous carcinoma is characterized by extracellular mucin production, metastasizes less frequently, and has a more favorable prognosis than classic invasive ductal carcinoma. Tubular carcinoma tends to recapitulate ductal structure after spreading into the stroma and is associated with a particular good prognosis.

Inflammatory breast cancer is a poorly differentiated infiltrating ductal carcinoma that invades dermal lymphatics. Diagnosis is made by the clinical appearance of the breast, including generalized edema and 'peau d'orange,' characterized by marginated erythema, skin thickening, and prominent pores. Mammography is often nondiagnostic, showing only a diffuse increase in the parenchymal pattern without a visible mass. Although pathologic demonstration of skin involvement as well as lymphatic invasion by cancer cells is commonly found in inflammatory breast cancer, the diagnosis is made by finding classic clinical features on examination and pathologic confirmation is not required.

Paget's disease is a ductal carcinoma involving the nipple. Clinically, it resembles eczema of the nipple. It may be completely in situ, with an excellent prognosis following local treatment. Less commonly, Paget's disease may be associated with a mass in the breast representing invasive cancer. In this case, the prognosis is that of the associated infiltrating carcinoma.

Harris JR et al (editors): *Diseases of the Breast.* 2nd ed. Philadelphia: Lippincott Williams & Wilkins, 2000. (In depth textbook covering a wide range of topics in breast cancer.)

Hulley S et al: Noncardiovascular disease outcomes during 6.8 years of hormone therapy: Heart and Estrogen/progestin Replacement Study follow-up (HERS II). JAMA 2002;288:58. [PMID: 12090863]

Wickerham DL: Ductal carcinoma-in-situ. J Clin Oncol 2001;19: 98S. [PMID: 11560982]

Clinical Findings

A. Symptoms and Signs

The typical finding of cancer on physical examination is a palpable mass. Other suspicious symptoms and signs of cancer include nipple inversion, dimpling of the breast, bloody or clear nipple discharge, new axillary lymphadenopathy, or occasionally breast pain. Invasive lobular cancer may present as diffuse thickening of the breast without a definite mass. Occasionally, breast cancer presents as diffuse erythema and edema of the breast (peau d'orange). This clinical finding is diagnostic of inflammatory breast cancer and is associated with extensive infiltration of lymphatic channels by cancer cells. Patients will often have breast pain and palpable axillary adenopathy. This high risk and poor prognosis malignancy is often confused with mastitis, delaying diagnosis and treatment during long courses of antibiotics. Mild erythema of the breast may be seen with invasive breast cancer, particularly following biopsies, and should not be confused with inflammatory disease. Occasionally, isolated axillary lymphadenopathy will be the only clinical finding, without a clinical or radiographically evident breast lesion. If biopsy proves nodal involvement with adenocarcinoma, occult breast cancer should be ruled out. The primary lesion may be high in the axillary tail or in extramammary breast tissue in the axilla. Sensitive imaging, such as specialized magnetic resonance imaging scanning of the breast, may help identify the occult primary. However, breast cancer can occur in an isolated axillary lymph node without occult breast cancer even on extensive testing. This presentation is likely due to breast cells that have migrated to the axillary nodes. It is important that the primary tumor site be confirmed; lung cancer is the second most common adenocarcinoma to present as an axillary lymph node. Usually the tissue of origin can be determined by pathologic staining for characteristic antigens, although chest computed tomography can be done to look for an occult primary tumor of the lung before definitive breast surgery is undertaken. The finding of positive estrogen receptors strongly points to a primary tumor of the breast; tumors of the ovary should also be ruled out. Rarely, breast cancer presents with symptoms secondary to systemic metastases, such as bone or abdominal pain, due to a primary occult tumor of the breast.

B. IMAGING STUDIES

Mammography, breast self-examination (BSE), and a clinical breast examination (CBE) by a health care provider are screening modalities for the detection of breast cancer. Multiple randomized trials, including the HIP (Health Insurance Plan) of New York trial, multiple Swedish trials, and the Canada National Breast Screening Study, have been conducted over the past 30 years to study the benefits of screening mammography. These trials all clearly indicated a reduction in breast cancer mortality of 20–25% when mammograms were conducted every 1–2 years for women over the age of

50. The benefit is lower among women aged 40–49 because of the reduced incidence of breast cancer in that age group. However, a meta-analysis done in 2001 has created controversy over the value of screening mammography by questioning both the mortality benefit and the validity of many studies. Most experts still favor regular mammographic screening as a means of detecting earlier stage and more curable cancers. Current recommendations from the US Preventive Services Task Force are to screen all women over the age of 40 every 1–2 years. Other groups, including the American Cancer Society, agree that annual mammography screening should be recommended to all women age 40 and older.

There is little evidence-based data to support BSE or routine or regular CBE as a means to decreasing breast cancer mortality. However, both are believed to be important screening tools as 10–15% of new cancers are undetectable on mammography. Monthly BSE involves educating patients to do self-examinations during the same time of the menstrual cycle each month to avoid confusing normal hormonal changes in the breast with pathology. Regular self-examination allows patients to learn their normal baseline and bring new changes to their physician's attention. Likewise, with CBE, regular examinations may help in detecting mammographically silent lesions increasing the possibility of earlier detection than waiting for incidental discovery. A recent study examined the benefit of BSE in Shanghai, China and found no difference in mortality in women who performed regular BSE compared with women who had regular CBE by a trained practitioner. The results of this study are not widely applicable to US women. In the United States, a combination of mammography, BSE, and CBE have been advocated as the best combined methods of early detection. The Shanghai study further supports this multi-modal approach as opposed to using a single procedure alone for breast cancer screening.

A normal mammogram clearly does not rule out the presence of an invasive cancer. Approximately 10–15% of cancers are mammographically invisible; this is more common in women with dense breasts or with lobular histology. Ultrasonography can be used to further evaluate a palpable lesion and will also distinguish solid lesions from more benign fluid-filled cysts but is not useful for routine screening. Current research is evaluating more sensitive techniques for radiographic detection of breast cancer, particularly in women at high-risk. Digital mammography provides clear images that can be digitally stored, allowing easy data transfer and comparison with prior films. Unfortunately, it is not more sensitive overall than standard mammography at detecting neoplasms. It will likely be the primary detection system in the future due to the ease of data storage and retrieval. Magnetic resonance imaging of the breast is a very sensitive technique that is being widely tested in high-risk women and appears quite promising; however, the risk of false-positive results is likely to increase significantly as more sensitive testing is performed. Newer techniques require testing in populations at high-risk to determine the effect of screening on subsequent mortality from cancer.

One interesting newer screening technique being tested in higher risk women is ductal lavage. In this procedure, a small tube is placed in the opening of a duct in the nipple, and fluid is washed into the duct and then examined for the presence of atypical cells. The benefits of this technically difficult procedure have yet to be demonstrated, and currently this technique can only detect lesions that are present in the lumen of the duct (in situ). Difficulty cannulating the duct, the specific duct evaluated and the quality of the fluid all impact the sensitivity and specificity of ductal lavage.

Harris JR et al (editors): *Diseases of the Breast.* 2nd ed. Philadelphia: Lippincott Williams & Wilkins, 2000. (In depth textbook covering a wide range of topics in breast cancer.)

Hulley S et al: Noncardiovascular disease outcomes during 6.8 years of hormone therapy: Heart and Estrogen/progestin Replacement Study follow-up (HERS II). JAMA 2002;288:58. [PMID: 12090863]

Humphrey LL et al: Breast cancer screening: a summary of the evidence for the US Preventive Services Task Force. Ann Intern Med 2002;137(5 Part 1):347. [PMID: 12204020]

Nystrom L et al: Long-term effects of mammography screening: updated overview of the Swedish randomised trials. Lancet 2002;359:909. [PMID: 11918907]

Diagnosis

Evaluation of a palpable mass in the breast usually does not require an open biopsy. In addition, an initial open biopsy may create poorer cosmetic results and complicate the approach and landmarks at the time of definitive surgery. The easiest initial approach is to obtain an FNA. Cytology from FNA can confirm the presence of malignant cells, and if necessary, markers such as hormone receptors can be obtained by additional staining. Although FNA is a very sensitive test, a negative result does not rule out cancer in the setting of a clinical suspicious lesion and additional testing should be performed. Lobular cancer presenting as a diffuse lesion may be more difficult to diagnose by FNA, and cytology may not be able to distinguish an invasive from a noninvasive cancer. If a diagnosis cannot be made by FNA, or the results are suspicious but not confirmatory, a core needle biopsy with or without mammographic guidance can be done. Core needle biopsies are performed in the clinic with local anesthesia with a specialized biopsy tool. This procedure is less invasive than an excisional biopsy, results in a tiny scar, and usually

gives a specimen with all necessary histologic data. Evaluation of a nonpalpable, mammographic abnormality can often be accomplished by a needle localization or stereotactic core biopsy. Using 3-dimensional mammographic guidance, a wire is positioned so that its tip is at the site of the suspicious lesion. The surgeon then uses the wire to guide the core biopsy needle. Rarely, an excisional biopsy is done when a highly suspicious lesion does not yield adequate pathologic data by other techniques; or the lesion is too deep for the core biopsy needle. In this case, the surgeon follows the wire and excises around its tip or simply performs an open biopsy if the lesion is palpable. Most patients can be spared multiple surgical procedures prior to definitive surgery using this approach. Testing for estrogen- and progesterone-receptor studies and expression of the HER-2/neu oncogene is usually reserved for the final surgical specimen unless systemic therapy prior to surgery is planned (neoadjuvant therapy). Treatment and prognosis are affected by the status of these markers.

Staging

Breast cancer is staged by the internationally accepted tumor/nodes/metastasis (TNM) system that has recently been significantly revised to more accurately reflect prognosis. The new staging system will be adopted in the United States in January of 2003. The **clinical stage** applies to the extent of disease as assessed by physical examination and radiologic studies. The **pathologic stage** applies to the extent of disease found by examination of the breast tissue and lymph nodes removed at the time of surgery. A simplified version of the new staging system published by the American Joint Committee on Cancer (AJCC) demonstrating pathologic stage is presented in Table 35–3.

Stage I cancers must be less than 2 cm with negative lymph nodes. Stage II cancers either measure between 2 and 5 cm or have 1 to 3 involved axillary lymph nodes. Stage III cancers include a primary tumor larger than 5 cm, smaller tumors with 4 or more nodes involved, tumors with axillary lymph nodes that are stuck to each other (matted) or to the chest wall, tumors associated with involved internal mammary or supraclavicular lymph nodes, or tumors that extend to the chest wall or skin. Inflammatory breast cancers are included in the more advanced stage III category. Stage IV cancers have any size tumor or nodal status but also have distant metastases.

There are several major changes from the previous staging criteria published in 1997, intended to improve uniformity of reporting and estimates of prognosis by stage. In the past, the presence of any positive axillary lymph node was called stage II disease. This could in-

Table 35–3. The TNM staging system for breast cancer.

Primary tumor (T)

T0	No evidence of primary tumor
Tis	Carcinoma in situ
T1	Tumor 2 cm or less in greatest dimension
T2	Tumor between 2 and 5 cm in greatest dimension
T3	Tumor more than 5 cm in greatest dimension
T4	Tumor of any size with any of the following: extension to chest wall, edema or ulceration of the skin of the breast, satellite skin nodules confined to the same breast, inflammatory carcinoma.

Regional lymph nodes (N) (by pathologic staging)

NX	Regional lymph nodes cannot be assessed
N0	No regional lymph node metastases
N0 (i+)	Isolated tumor cells positive by immunohistochemistry only in sentinel node < 0.2 mm
N1 (mic)	Micrometastases > 0.2 mm but < = 2 mm
N1	Metastases to 1–3 axillary lymph nodes
N2	Metastases to 4–9 axillary lymph nodes or to internal mammary nodes in the absence of axillary lymph nodes
N3	Metastases to 10 or more axillary lymph nodes, or fewer axillary lymph nodes with internal mammary nodal involvement, or metastases to ipsilateral infraclavicular or supraclavicular nodes.

Distant metastases

Mx	Presence of distant metastasis not assessed
M0	No distant metastasis
M1	Distant metastasis

Stage grouping

Stage 0	Tis	N0	M0
Stage I	T1	N0	M0
Stage IIa	T0, T1	N1	M0
	T2	N0	M0
Stage IIb	T2	N1	M0
	T3	N0	M0
Stage IIIa	T0, T1, T2	N2	M0
	T3	N1, N2	M0
Stage IIIb	T4	Any N	M0
	Any T	N3	M0
Stage IV	Any T	Any N	M1

(AJCC Cancer Staging Manual, Springer-Verlag New York, Inc., 6th edition, 2002)

clude diseases with such diverse prognoses as a tumor with 1 positive node and a tumor with 40 positive nodes! The new staging criteria now separates 1–3 positive nodes as N1 (stage II) and 4 or more nodes as N2 (stage III). In addition, long-term follow-up indicates that some patients with an involved supraclavicular node at the time of initial presentation may enjoy long-term, disease-free survival. Therefore, a positive supraclavicular node is now classified as N3 disease (stage IIIb), rather than a metastasis. Immunohistochemical staining for cytokeratin in the axillary lymph node has improved the sensitivity of detection of malignant cells to such an extent that the prognostic value of these tests is unclear. The new staging system reflects this concern, classifying a single node with isolated tumor cells measuring less than 0.2 mm as N0(i+), microscopic involvement of node measuring between 0.2 mm and 2.0 mm as N1(mi), and all others as clearly positive nodes. Hopefully this will help clarify extent of node involvement as well as allow prospective assessment of the impact of minimal axillary node involvement on prognosis. In general, staging is used to grossly estimate prognosis and as a basis for inclusion in clinical trials. Clearly, biologic factors play a critical role as well in determining prognosis and treatment and are outlined below.

Greene FL et al (editors): AJCC (American Joint Committee on Cancer) Cancer Staging Manual. 6th ed. New York: Springer-Verlag New York, Inc., 2002.

Singletary SE et al: Revision of the American Joint Committee on Cancer staging system for breast cancer. J Clin Oncol 2002; 20:3628. [PMID: 12202663]

Prognosis

Table 35–4 shows the survival rates (up to 5 years) of women with breast cancer as a function of race and extent of disease at diagnosis. Survival at 10 years is approximately 70–80% in patients with stage I breast cancer, approximately 50–60% in patients with stage II cancer, approximately 30% in stage III, and less than 10% in stage IV.

Carcinoma in situ is confined to the ducts or lobules and, by definition, does not invade stroma including adjacent blood and lymphatic vessels. Therefore, metastases are rare and are thought to be due to occult invasive cancer. The risk of local recurrence in women who have had breast-conserving surgery is a function of extent of disease, age at diagnosis, and aggressiveness of the lesion, measured by nuclear grade (see below). Survival at 10 years is 98–99%.

In contrast, even stage I invasive breast cancer is associated with a low but continuing risk of recurrence and death, confirming the systemic nature of this seem-

Table 35–4. Five-year survival rates of women with breast cancer by stage at presentation.

	All women	White women	Black women
All stages	86%	88%	73%
Localized	97%	97%	89%
Regional	78%	80%	65%
Distant	23%	24%	15%

SEER Staging definitions: Localized: primary tumor only and node-negative; Regional: node-positive or T4 tumor by AJCC criteria; Distant: metastatic disease by 5th edition AJCC definition. (SEER data 1992–1999 taken from http://seer.cancer.gov/csr/1973_1999/breast.pdf)

ingly localized disease. Recent research has looked at the bone marrow as a harbinger of occult microscopic disease. Although these results need to be confirmed, occult malignant cells were found even in patients with stage I disease, and the presence of cells appeared to predict a higher subsequent risk of recurrence and death from cancer. Further research is required to understand the value and impact of specialized testing such as this.

Prognostic factors at the time of diagnosis that impact both risk of recurrence and death as well as treatment choices include the presence and number of involved axillary lymph nodes, the size and grade of the primary tumor, results of biologic factors including estrogen and progesterone receptors (ER and PR), and the HER2/neu oncoprotein, and the age and general health of the patient. The single most important prognostic factor is involvement of the axillary nodes, with a worse prognosis associated with a single positive node. Extent of node involvement is important as well; it appears that microscopic involvement of only 1 lymph node carries only a slightly worse prognosis than negative axillary nodes. In contrast, 4 or more positive lymph nodes carry a much worse prognosis than that of only 1 to 3 positive nodes. Women who have 10 or more positive lymph nodes have a particularly poor prognosis with a 20% or lower 5-year survival.

Other prognostic factors are important, and particularly for women with negative axillary lymph nodes. Tumor size is one of the most important, although tumor grade may modify this risk assessment. In general, women who have a tumor that measures less than 1 cm with negative axillary lymph nodes have a greater than 95% chance of a 10-year disease-free survival. As the tumor size approaches 2 cm, the chance of being disease free at 10 years drops to about 70%. Histologic tumor grade is determined by a scoring system of 3 pathologic findings by the modified Scarff-Bloom-

Richardson scoring system: a score of 1–3 is given for tubule and papillae formation (how close the cancer looks to normal breast tissue), for nuclear grade (how homogeneous, small and round the nucleus appears) and for mitoses (how many are counted per high-powered field); a higher number indicates greater abnormality. A score of 3–5 is low grade, or well differentiated; a score of 6–7 is intermediate grade, or moderately well differentiated; and a score of 8–9 is high grade, or poorly differentiated.

Grade I cancers typically occur in older women, are often hormone receptor positive, and have a better than average prognosis for tumor size. In contrast, grade II and III cancers tend to be more aggressive, rapidly growing tumors that are more frequently found in younger women and are associated with a poorer prognosis than might be expected for tumor size or extent of nodal involvement.

Other important prognostic factors that affect decisions regarding treatment and prognosis include expression of ER and/or PR, HER2/neu gene amplification or protein overexpression, and the presence of lymphatic or blood vessel invasion. ER and PR expression in the tumor are detected by immunohistochemical staining and reported as both a percent of positive cells out of the total evaluated, and as an intensity of staining. Although in the past a level below 10% was considered negative, it is now recognized that even patients with very low-level positivity for hormone receptors may respond to hormonal therapy. Therefore, it is critical to know the actual percent of positive cells, rather than just a negative or positive result. Cancers that are hormone receptor positive tend to be slower growing, with a better prognosis. Recurrences also generally occur later than receptor negative tumors, with a low but steady rate of metastases diagnosed more than 10 years following primary diagnosis. In addition, hormone receptor positive tumors are responsive to adjuvant hormonal therapy (see Treatment section below), which has an enormous impact on risks of recurrence and death.

One of the most exciting developments in understanding breast cancer over the past 2 decades has been a greater understanding of biologic factors that impact prognosis and treatment decisions and have resulted in the development of novel targeted therapeutics. The only biologic factor other than hormone receptors currently understood well enough for clinical use is overexpression of the growth-factor receptor HER2/neu, which is associated with amplification of the HER2/neu gene. This poor prognosis factor is found in approximately 20% of breast cancers and is more often associated with higher histologic grade and hormone receptor negativity (although 30–40% are positive for ER and/or PR). HER2/neu positive cancers are particularly sensitive to systemic chemotherapy that includes anthracyclines (eg, doxorubicin), and data indicates that use of anthracycline containing adjuvant chemotherapy may to some degree counter the poorer prognosis associated with this subtype of breast cancer. Additional treatment considerations associated with HER2 positive cancers are discussed in the Treatment section below. HER2/neu positivity is generally determined by immunohistochemical staining for the receptor; 0–1+ is considered negative, 2+ is indeterminate, and 3+ appears to be clearly positive. Patients with a 2+ result should have testing for gene amplification to confirm positivity using fluorescent in situ hybridization (FISH) as only 20% will be truly positive. HER2/neu is an important prognostic factor that has significant prognostic and treatment implications; it is important that all cancers at diagnosis be evaluated for overexpression.

Other cellular and molecular factors have been evaluated for their role in determining prognosis or progression of cancer, but no one single factor has emerged other than HER2/neu at this time that has the same degree of impact. There is intense interest in identifying new factors that can be used to develop additional targeted therapeutic strategies and current research is aggressively pursuing this goal.

Invasion of lymph or blood vessels in the tumor specimen has been associated with a higher risk of local recurrence, as has extension of cancer outside of the capsule of an axillary lymph node. These findings might impact decisions regarding radiation therapy to improve local control (see Treatment section). Currently, most clinical decisions regarding prognosis and the need for adjuvant treatment are made on the basis of lymph-node status, tumor grade and size, hormone-receptor status, HER2/neu status, and clinical factors such as the patient's age and comorbidities.

Haffty BG et al: Outcome of conservatively managed early-onset breast cancer by BRCA1/2 status. Lancet 2002;359:1471. [PMID: 11988246]

Treatment

A. Ductal Carcinoma In Situ (DCIS)

Before the era of screening mammography, DCIS was uncommon and generally presented as a palpable mass. It is now the most frequent reason for an abnormal mammogram, and appropriate management remains controversial. Similar to invasive breast cancer, traditional treatment in the past for DCIS was simple mastectomy without additional therapy. Mastectomy results in cure rates of about 99% for this noninvasive malignancy, with mortality at 10 years at 1–2% (primarily due to occult invasive disease). Currently, mastectomy for DCIS is reserved for extensive disease or for women who either do not want or are not candidates for breast

irradiation. The appropriate management of localized DCIS now consists of resection with breast irradiation. Local excision without radiation results in a significant risk of local recurrence due to spread of cancer cells along the ductal tree, with 50% of recurrences being invasive disease. Depending on the extent and nuclear grade of the DCIS, local recurrence rates may exceed 40% over a 10 years. Radiation significantly reduces that risk. The NSABP B-17 study evaluated the role of radiation therapy in local control of DCIS. Patients underwent local excision, then were randomized either to radiation or no additional therapy. With a median follow-up of over 7 years, the rate of local recurrence in the group having lumpectomy alone was approximately 28%, with half of these recurrences presenting as invasive cancers. Radiation reduced this rate to about 12%, with only one fourth (approximately 4%) of these recurrences representing invasive cancers.

The role of surgical margin width has developed increasing significance based on recent research indicating an extremely low local recurrence rate following local excision of DCIS without radiation when the margin width of normal surrounding breast tissue exceeds 1 cm. In carefully selected patients, this approach can be used to avoid local radiation therapy as well as mastectomy in the management of DCIS, although ongoing research is attempting to identify the most appropriate candidates. It is likely to be most effective in localized and lower grade lesions.

Hormonal receptors are not traditionally measured in DCIS, although this may change in the future. However, interest arose in the use of tamoxifen to reduce local recurrence of DCIS after it appeared that local recurrence of DCIS associated with invasive cancer were decreased by adjuvant use of this hormonal agent. NSABP B-24 was a large randomized trial that randomized patients with DCIS alone following lumpectomy and radiation to 5 years of tamoxifen or placebo. In this hallmark study, tamoxifen reduced the local recurrence rates for DCIS by 20%, for invasive cancer by 50%. This included rates of contralateral disease as well. Current work is focusing on identifying patients who are most likely to benefit from adjuvant tamoxifen following local excision of DCIS. Tamoxifen does not appear to replace radiation therapy, however, in terms of local disease control.

At this time, there is no single standard therapy for patients with DCIS. Surgically, the goal is to achieve negative surgical margins; given the heterogeneity of DCIS, treatment options should be individualized to best reduce the risk of future invasive cancer.

B. Invasive Breast Cancer

1. Treatment of the primary tumor—The Halsted radical mastectomy was an important advance in the treatment of breast cancer at the turn of the last century because it spared women from dying with fungating masses on the chest; however, even this aggressive surgery failed to prevent women with breast cancer from dying of systemic metastases. The goal of surgery now is to provide local disease control; it is now understood that metastases are due to early systemic spread of cells through the bloodstream and lymphatics. Modified radical mastectomy, which preserves the muscles of the chest wall, has been shown to be equivalent to the more radical Halsted approach and was the standard surgical treatment for operable breast cancer until recently. Lumpectomy or partial mastectomy "tylectomy," (or "quadrantectomy"), where only the tumor and small amount of surrounding tissue is removed, has recently been shown to be equivalent to mastectomy in terms of long-term survival. Lumpectomy alone is associated with high local recurrence rates of 30–40%; the addition of radiation therapy reduces local recurrence rates to only 5–10%. A local recurrence following lumpectomy and radiation is usually successfully treated with modified radical mastectomy. Unfortunately, breast conservation therapy (BCT) is still underused, despite confirmation of the above results in two large randomized trials with long-term follow-up. BCT offers women preservation of breast tissue and nipple sensation, and should be discussed with every woman eligible for this procedure. The recommended technique for breast conservation includes local excision of the primary tumor with clear surgical margins, followed by breast irradiation to 4500–5000 cGy with or without a boost. Adjuvant chemotherapy is usually given prior to radiation (see below). Recent studies have suggested that women over the age of 70 with small, low-grade tumors may not benefit significantly from the addition of radiation therapy. Due to a relatively shorter expected survival, and low likelihood of local recurrence as well as mortality from local recurrence, radiation may provide relatively less benefit than for younger women.

There are specific situations in which breast conservation is not recommended, including women with a higher likelihood of local recurrence, with larger or inflammatory cancers, or women at increased risk for radiation toxicity. Women with multifocal disease in different quadrants of the breast; associated extensive DCIS; inflammatory cancer; or contraindications to full-dose radiation such as early-stage pregnancy, previous irradiation, or a history of collagen vascular disease (CVD) should not be treated with BCT. Isolated cases of severe local toxicity in women with CVD who received breast or chest wall radiation have been reported, with sloughing of the chest wall. It is unclear which patients are at risk for this complication, or how pervasive the effect is. For this reason, patients with CVD are generally not treated with radiation.

If a mastectomy is the primary definitive surgery, chest wall radiation is given only for patients with a high risk of local recurrence. Many studies have shown that radiation to the chest wall after mastectomy can reduce local recurrence risk but does not affect survival. However, there are higher risk situations when radiation may be particularly useful. This includes women with a positive or very close resection margin, skeletal muscle (chest wall) involvement, a very large primary tumor ($\geq$ 5 cm), or extensive invasion of lymph vessels with cancer cells.

Women with large primary tumors may not be candidates for BCT, or lumpectomy may result in poor cosmetic results. Preoperative or 'neoadjuvant' chemotherapy has been shown to improve rates of BCT, and the result of treatment provides important prognostic information based on surgical results. A large randomized trial (NSABP B-18) demonstrated the safety of neoadjuvant chemotherapy with no difference in overall survival based on the timing of chemotherapy. These results further emphasize the importance of systemic therapy in the treatment of localized breast cancer. Neoadjuvant chemotherapy results in tumor shrinkage in about 80% of cases, and should be considered for larger tumors (see Adjuvant Therapy below). Neoadjuvant hormonal therapy may be used in older patients with hormone receptor positive disease who are not candidates for chemotherapy.

2. Treatment of Axillary Lymph Nodes—The ipsilateral axillary lymph nodes drain the majority of lymphatics from the breast and may be the first site of metastases from a primary tumor. Although it is now clear that microscopic cells may hide in a variety of areas including the bone marrow and internal mammary nodes, the presence of cells in the axillary nodes is still the most important determining prognosis and appropriate adjuvant therapy.

The standard technique for evaluating the axillary nodes until quite recently has been full axillary dissection. This involves sampling axillary nodes at 3 levels, from the lowest to highest areas in the axilla. Generally, an adequate sampling required removing 8 to 10 nodes. However, this procedure can result in significant morbidity, including immediate postoperative pain and fluid accumulation, with subsequent local anesthesia or hyperesthesia, and a long-term risk of lymphedema (chronic swelling of the arm). The risk of neurologic impairment and lymphedema is related to the extent of axillary surgery as well as to radiation of the axilla.

Removing axillary nodes that are not involved with cancer has no clear therapeutic benefit, therefore there has been interest in finding ways to predict axillary involvement without sampling multiple nodes. A novel technique of sampling the first draining axillary lymph node, or sentinel node, has been developed that appears to be highly sensitive in predicting additional node involvement. The procedure involves injection of radioactive colloid or blue dye at the tumor site, with identification and resection of the node or nodes that drain the tumor bed. The sentinel lymph node is identified in the majority of cancer surgeries, although the surgeon must be trained and experienced in this technique. A pathologically negative sentinel node is highly predictive of a subsequently negative axillary dissection and this potentially morbid procedure can be avoided. In qualified hands, the sentinel lymph node biopsy accurately represents the remaining nodes 95% of the time. Sentinel lymph node biopsy is contraindicated in patients with clinically palpable nodes; its use in patients who have received neoadjuvant chemotherapy appears promising and is under investigation. The morbidity from sentinel node dissection is significantly less than that from a full dissection, and in particular the rate of lymphedema is very low (although the risk is not completely eliminated).

Radiation therapy to the axilla is also an important treatment modality, and in specific situations not only significantly reduces the risk of local recurrence, but possibly the risk of distant recurrence as well. Two large trials demonstrated a lower incidence of distant metastases and improved survival in patients with 4 or more involved axillary lymph nodes who were treated with axillary field radiation. The benefit in women with 1 to 3 involved nodes was less clear; radiation in this setting is still under investigation. Other reasons for axillary radiation include disease associate with a high risk of local recurrence including extension of tumor outside of the capsule of the axillary node, or a single very large node replaced with tumor. Women with negative axillary nodes or with minimal involvement of the axilla do not require axillary radiation, which increases the risks associated with axillary dissection. Generally, chest wall or breast radiation ports include the lower part of the axilla in the most lateral portion of the field. The use of radiation as a substitute for axillary sampling is being studied; at the present time, radiation is not considered as an alternative for pathologic assessment.

C. Adjuvant Chemotherapy

It is clear that systemic spread of breast cancer cells occurs early, while the primary tumor is still small. The concept behind adjuvant treatment is to target these 'microscopic' metastases and prevent the development of established macroscopic metastatic disease. The first trials studied single agents for short, perioperative courses with the rationale that the cells were shed systemically at the time of surgery, but these treatments have evolved to include combinations of non–cross-resistant chemotherapy given for longer durations following primary surgery.

Initial studies were designed to assess effects of combinations of chemotherapy in women at the highest risk for relapse, defined as premenopausal women with node-positive breast cancer. These initial studies, as well as subsequent trials with more active combinations, demonstrated significant improvement in both disease-free and overall survival. Analysis of multiple randomized trials has definitively shown that the benefits of adjuvant chemotherapy are, to some degree, independent of menopausal status. More recent studies have also demonstrated benefit from adjuvant chemotherapy in higher risk node-negative cancers (see below).

The 'Early Breast Cancer Trialists' Collaborative Group (EBCTCG, also known as the 'Oxford Overview' due to the location of the meeting) has published periodic meta-analyses of randomized adjuvant chemotherapy trials since 1985, with the most recent published results in 1998 and a publication pending from the 2000 meeting. The results published in 1998 from the 1995 Overview represented a meta-analysis of over 40 randomized trials including 18,000 women worldwide. These data confirm the benefits of both chemotherapy and hormonal therapy in premenopausal and postmenopausal women with early-stage breast cancer. Overall, chemotherapy results in about a 33% reduction in risk of recurrence, and a 25% reduction in risk of death. It is clear, however, that the degree of benefit is based on the individual tumor risks and biologic factors as well as the patient's age and general health.

The benefits of adjuvant chemotherapy overall are slightly lower in postmenopausal women although still significant because of a predominance of hormone receptor positive less aggressive disease in this group of women. When the postmenopausal group was broken down by age, it was noted that women between 50 and 59 benefited from the chemotherapy more than those who were 60–69 years old, although not as much as those who were younger than 50 years. Relatively few women over the age of 70 were included in these trials, and no significant difference in recurrence or mortality was seen. It is likely that these differences are due to the contributing impact of comorbid illnesses with increasing age, as well as an increase in the proportion of less aggressive cancers with increasing age. Due to the widespread dissemination of this data, chemotherapy is being offered to more women in the 50- to 70-year-old age group than in the past and to selected women with very high risk disease over the age of 70.

Prospective randomized trials have shown that both premenopausal and postmenopausal women with 'node negative' early-stage breast cancer may derive a significant benefit from adjuvant chemotherapy. Women with negative lymph nodes were found to experience the same relative reduction in recurrence and mortality as women with positive lymph nodes, but because the absolute recurrence and mortality rates are smaller, the absolute benefits are also smaller with approximately a 6% absolute mortality benefit in premenopausal women and a 2% benefit in postmenopausal women. One of the most difficult questions now is to decide which patients with negative axillary lymph nodes should receive adjuvant chemotherapy. Currently, selection is based on biologic factors associated with a higher risk of recurrence. Calculation of benefit is based on relative reductions in risk of recurrence and mortality; consequently, the higher the risk of recurrence, the greater the degree of possible benefit. Possibility of benefit in any situation must be weighed against the risks and toxicities of treatment. In addition, the benefits of adjuvant hormonal therapy must also be taken into consideration when assessing the benefits of chemotherapy. A postmenopausal woman with a small, low grade, estrogen receptor-positive cancer with negative lymph nodes is likely to have less than a 5% risk of recurrence following surgery and radiation, with the possible addition of adjuvant hormonal therapy. In this situation, addition of chemotherapy would not be considered beneficial. In contrast, a younger woman with negative lymph nodes with a higher grade tumor, or a tumor larger than 2 cm may have a 10-year disease-free survival of only 70–80%, regardless of hormone receptor status. In this situation, the use of chemotherapy provides a significant impact on recurrence risk and is generally recommended. This is particularly true in the setting of hormone receptor negative disease, when the only option for risk reduction is chemotherapy.

Currently, decisions on whom to offer adjuvant chemotherapy are based on tumor size, grade, nodal status, estrogen-receptor status, and the patient's age, performance status, and other medical conditions. Patients' preferences and understanding of the risks and benefits of therapy are critical in arriving at an acceptable treatment plan. Computer-based models using data obtained from the National Cancer Institute's SEER database as well as the Oxford Overview are now available to aid in decision analyses and provide information regarding 10-year risk of recurrence and mortality as well as benefits from chemotherapy, hormonal therapy, and the combination. These decision tools are designed to provide general rather than specific information; the data is based on population rather than individual data and is limited by information provided in large randomized clinical trials. Inasmuch as this information is continually changing, limitations must be taken into consideration.

D. CHEMOTHERAPY REGIMENS FOR EARLY-STAGE DISEASE

The combination chemotherapy regimen CMF (cyclophosphamide, methotrexate, 5-fluorouracil) given for 6 cycles over 6 months, was the standard adjuvant chemotherapy regimen for breast cancer until recently, when treatment began to shift toward anthracycline-containing regimens. Data from the 1998 and 2000 Oxford Overview confirmed a small, but statistically significant advantage of anthracycline-containing regimens—including doxorubicin (Adriamycin) and epirubicin (Ellence)—over CMF in risk of recurrence and mortality for node-positive breast cancers. The absolute gain in survival on average favoring anthracyclines was 4% for node positive at 10 years, with a trend of 1.7% for node negative at 5 years. This large meta-analysis was also able to show that prolonged administration of these regimens for up to 1 year was not better than a 4–6 month adjuvant course.

Typical regimens include CAF (cyclophosphamide, doxorubicin, fluorouracil), AC (cyclophosphamide, doxorubicin) and CEF (cyclophosphamide, epirubicin, and fluorouracil). Epirubicin is a newer anthracycline with lower cardiac toxicity than doxorubicin that is particularly popular in Europe and Canada. One large Canadian study showed a benefit from CEF compared with CMF, increasing interest in use of this anthracycline. Most chemotherapy regimens are given intravenously in cycles repeated every 3 to 4 weeks for 4–6 cycles over 3–6 months. Classic CMF and CAF include oral cyclophosphamide for 2 weeks out of each 4-week cycle. AC became the most popular adjuvant chemotherapy regimen following a large randomized trial showing equivalent results to CMF. This particular regimen is given every 3 weeks for a total of 4 cycles, so that treatment is completed in only 3 months.

Although AC clearly results in reduction in risks of recurrence and death from early-stage cancers, there has been great interest in exploring different agents and combinations to further reduce the risk of death from early-stage cancers. Following success of a newer class of agents, the taxanes, in the treatment of metastatic breast cancer, these agents were tested in the adjuvant setting either following AC or in combination. In patients with node-positive disease, the addition of the taxane, paclitaxel (Taxol), following AC, improves both disease-free and overall survival. There may be a differential response with the primary benefit in hormone receptor negative disease, although this data remains unclear. A recent study demonstrated a small bit of significant improvement in disease-free and overall survival with no excess toxicity when these chemotherapy agents are given every 2 weeks ("dose-dense") compared with standard every 3-week dosing. The 2-week regimen requires myeloid growth factor support, with a significant increase in cost, and data are early at 3 to 4 years median follow-up. Preliminary data using a combination of AC with a newer taxane, docetaxel, given every 3 weeks showed a significant reduction in the risk of relapse and mortality although with significantly greater toxicity than sequential treatment. In this trial, it appeared that the greatest benefit was in women with 1 to 3 positive axillary nodes, or those with HER2 overexpressing disease. In contrast, there does not appear to be a benefit from escalating doses of doxorubicin or cyclophosphamide. Ongoing trials are attempting to delineate the most appropriate combination and setting for taxane containing adjuvant therapy, and results in high-risk node negative disease should be available in the next year or two.

1. Side effects of adjuvant chemotherapy—Toxicity from adjuvant chemotherapy is regimen- and agent-specific but in general includes reversible alopecia, nausea and vomiting, mouth sores, diarrhea or constipation, fatigue, and bone marrow suppression with neutropenia and anemia. The majority of the most unpleasant side effects can now be reduced in severity or eliminated with the use of appropriate premedications and support following treatment. The newer antiemetics are highly effective, particularly when given in conjunction with dexamethasone. Both myeloid and erythroid growth factors (eg, GCSF, erythropoietin) given by subcutaneous injection are available to prevent or treat chemotherapy-induced bone marrow suppression, significantly reducing the risk of febrile neutropenia and hospitalization following treatment. Treatment of anemia in the adjuvant setting has been shown to improve quality-of-life measures. Long-acting growth factors have been recently approved that reduce the number of required injections in appropriately selected patients. Treatment-related mortality is exceedingly rare in the adjuvant setting and is generally due to serious infections from untreated febrile neutropenia. It is critical that patients receiving adjuvant chemotherapy be instructed on possible risks of treatment and appropriate management.

The taxanes are associated with unique toxicities including short-term myalgias for the first few days following treatment, peripheral neuropathy that usually completely or almost completely resolves in the months following cessation of treatment, and edema. The use of pretreatment corticosteroids has reduced the problem of edema, and premedications are commonly given to reduce the risk of allergic reactions, which are particularly common with the first dose of taxane therapy.

There is no known treatment that reliably prevents chemotherapy-induced alopecia. Caps that cool the scalp have been tested but are not approved for use in the United States due to concerns about an increase in the risk of scalp metastases. These side effects completely reverse following completion of chemotherapy.

Long-term toxicities of adjuvant chemotherapy include amenorrhea and infertility. All chemotherapy regimens have been associated with short-term, chemotherapy-induced amenorrhea. In younger women, and depending on the particular chemotherapy regimen, menses usually return although the risk of infertility is unknown. Women over the age of 35 at the time of treatment have an increased risk of chemotherapy-induced permanent menopause, with rates ranging from 30% to 60%. The use of ovarian suppression as a way to maintain ovarian function in young women for whom fertility is a significant concern appears promising and is under investigation. However, there is also evidence that suppression of ovarian function may have a therapeutic role in the treatment of early-stage disease by suppressing estrogen levels.

Other toxicities include a risk of secondary acute leukemia of approximately less than 1% at 10 years, although recent data indicates that the risk of acute leukemia from current chemotherapy treatment regimens may not be any higher than the risk in the general population. Anthracycline-containing regimens used in standard doses and in women with normal myocardia are associated with a less than 1.5% risk of congestive heart failure. These short-term and long-term toxicities need to be considered in treating patients with low risks of recurrence and whose absolute benefit is small.

2. Special topics in adjuvant therapy—Retrospective analyses of several trials indicate that the poorer prognosis of HER2+ breast cancers may be abrogated by the use of anthracycline-containing adjuvant chemotherapy. Anthracycline regimens are considered a standard treatment for these higher risk tumors. In addition, there is great international interest in testing the monoclonal antibody, trastuzumab (Herceptin) in the adjuvant setting to reduce relapse and death from HER2+ disease. Trastuzumab is currently approved for the treatment of metastatic breast cancer overexpressing HER2/neu. In the United States alone, 3 large randomized trials are ongoing for node-positive breast cancer and will include high-risk node-negative disease as well in the near future. The major side effect of trastuzumab is a reduction in ejection fraction; this agent should not be given concurrently with anthracyclines or outside of the setting of a randomized clinical trial in early-stage disease.

In the late 1980s, investigators began to explore the use of very high doses of chemotherapy to overcome chemotherapy resistance in metastatic breast cancer. With encouraging early results, trials expanded to include the highest risk node-positive disease in the adjuvant setting, women with 10 or more involved axillary lymph nodes. The doses of chemotherapy were high enough that autologous bone marrow and subsequently stem cell transplant or rescue were required to offset toxicity. For almost a decade, high-dose chemotherapy with stem cell rescue or stem cell transplantation was routinely prescribed for women with 10 or more positive nodes. Mortality from this treatment was variable, ranging from about 2% to up to 10% and appeared to be dependent on the experience of the institution, the chemotherapy regimen, and the patient population. The enthusiasm for this toxic and expensive therapy was based on results of phase II trials in highly selected patients. By the late 1990s, results of large randomized trials in both the adjuvant and metastatic setting showed a lack of benefit of this treatment approach; several trials are still ongoing. Although it is still possible that a subset of patients may benefit from this approach, therapy should only be given in the setting of a randomized clinical trial directed toward answering this question.

E. ADJUVANT HORMONAL THERAPY

The rate of hormone receptor positivity in breast cancer increases with increasing age at diagnosis, and about two thirds of breast cancer cases will overexpress either estrogen or progesterone receptors or both. Probably the greatest advance in the treatment of early-stage breast cancer over the last 2 decades has been the use of the selective estrogen receptor modulator (SERM), tamoxifen. Tamoxifen binds to the estrogen receptor and blocks the ability of estrogen to bind to the receptor, therefore blocking estrogen-related cell signaling. Estrogen receptor binding leads to cell growth and proliferation in hormone receptor positive cancers. Multiple randomized clinical trials involving over 30,000 women have been performed over the past 30 years evaluating the use of adjuvant tamoxifen. These studies have shown that tamoxifen significantly decreases mortality and recurrence of hormone receptor positive breast cancer. Five years of therapy at 20 mg/d decreases recurrences by about half and overall mortality by about one third, with an 8% absolute reduction in mortality at 10 years. This benefit is seen in node-positive (an 11% absolute mortality benefit) and node-negative disease (a 6% absolute mortality benefit) and in both premenopausal and postmenopausal women. In patients treated with adjuvant chemotherapy, the benefit of tamoxifen is independent and additive to any reduction in recurrence or mortality risk gained from chemotherapy. Studies also have demonstrated that 5 years of therapy is optimal compared with 1 or 2 years and that longer duration therapy up to 10 years does not further improve disease-free or overall survival and may be detrimental due to increased risk of toxicity (see Side Effects below).

Patients with tumors that are estrogen and/or progesterone positive at any level are eligible for and may benefit from adjuvant hormonal therapy. Response rates based on extent of hormone positivity have been estimated from treatment of metastatic disease; the highest and most durable response rates have been seen in tumors that are strongly positive for both receptors. However, responses may be seen even in tumors that are only minimally positive for either ER or PR.

1. Side effects of adjuvant tamoxifen—Despite the benefits of tamoxifen, side effects remain a significant problem. Common initial side effects include hot flashes, insomnia, vaginal discharge and dryness, and irregular menstrual bleeding. Hot flashes and insomnia can be particularly difficult to tolerate; if these side effects are not treated, they can lead to discontinuation of therapy. A randomized trial found the antidepressant venlafaxine (Effexor) was more effective at reducing the frequency and intensity of hot flashes, the doses were lower than those used for depression at 25 mg twice a day. Other medications that are used include clonidine, herbal preparations, and vitamin E although none have been shown to have a significant effect over placebo. Vaginal dryness can often be effectively managed with the Estring, a flexible ring impregnated with estradiol that is placed against the cervix and results in slow release of local hormone over 3 months. Very little, if any, estradiol is released into the circulation. Topical estrogen and testosterone have also been used with improvement in symptoms. Other less common problems include weight gain and joint pains.

The side effects from tamoxifen are thought to be due to differential effects of this SERM in different tissues. While tamoxifen has antiestrogenic properties in breast tissue, it has proestrogenic, and growth-promoting properties in other tissues. This includes maintenance of bone mineral density with the beneficial effect of preventing osteoporosis as well as the dangerous property of stimulating proliferation of the lining of the uterus, and inducing blood clots in susceptible individuals. Tamoxifen therapy has been associated with an increase in the risk of endometrial polyps as well as both adenocarcinoma and sarcoma of the endometrium. These endometrial malignancies are exceedingly rare and are almost never seen in premenopausal women. Although tamoxifen increases the risk of endometrial cancer 4-fold with 5 years of therapy, in women under the age of 70 this risk is still generally under 1–1.5%. In the EBCTCG analysis of tamoxifen in all adjuvant trials through 1998, this increase in endometrial cancer was still significantly less than the decrease in recurrent breast cancer. Deaths from endometrial cancer due to tamoxifen were 1–2 per 1000 over 10 years, also not enough to offset the overall mortality benefit. For patients in whom the benefit from tamoxifen is substantial, the small risk of endometrial cancer should not deter use of the drug. Vaginal bleeding associated with early-stage disease is the presenting complaint in the majority of women;

this symptom should be evaluated carefully in any woman on tamoxifen with vaginal ultrasound to assess endometrial thickness and an endometrial biopsy. An acceptable endometrial thickness on ultrasound has not clearly been established for women on tamoxifen therapy as the therapy itself causes edema of the endometrium resulting in an abnormal endometrial stripe. Using postmenopausal criteria of < 5 mm as an acceptable cut-off generally means that most women receiving tamoxifen will need a biopsy for definitive diagnosis. A side effect more commonly seen in premenopausal women is ovarian cysts. Rarely, women on tamoxifen will develop pain associated with hemorrhage into an enlarging cyst. Other possible complications of ovarian cysts include cyst rupture or torsion of the cyst requiring surgery.

The second serious toxicity from tamoxifen is the risk of venous thromboembolic disease. Although the absolute incidence in studies has been small, tamoxifen does increase the incidence of deep venous thromboses and pulmonary emboli 1.5- to 2-fold. This risk increases in the postmenopausal population and with patient age, with significant risks only seen in women over the age of 70. In the adjuvant trial analysis by the EBCTCG though, no clear increase in deaths due to thromboembolic events was identified. Other than patient age, it appears that an additional risk factor for tamoxifen-related thromboses is a genetic predisposition to blood clots. Women with mutations in prothrombin, or with less common mutations in protein factors C and S, have an increased risk of blood clots that appears to be significantly higher in the presence of estrogen. Due to tamoxifen's ability to act like an estrogen, hypercoagulability may be worsened in patients with this predisposition. Therefore, tamoxifen has been generally contraindicated without concurrent anticoagulation in patients with a significant personal or family history of thromboembolic events. Screening for common mutations can be performed in women who are at risk before starting therapy, although now an alternative to adjuvant tamoxifen exists for patients in this setting.

2. Aromatase inhibitors—There has long been interest in finding alternative treatment options to tamoxifen, due to a variety of factors including the issue of acquired resistance to estrogen receptor blockade, the side effect profile, and the ability of tamoxifen to act like an estrogen in certain tissues and perhaps in breast cancer cells with prolonged use. In postmenopausal women, lower levels of estrogen are produced by peripheral aromatization, the conversion of adrenal androgens to estrogen via the aromatase enzyme in other tissues. Three highly specific and potent inhibitors of the aromatase enzyme are now approved for the treatment of postmenopausal metastatic breast cancer. Anastrozole

has been recently approved for use in the adjuvant setting in postmenopausal women. The approval of anastrozole was based on preliminary data from the ATAC trial, a large randomized trial of over 9000 women in which the aromatase inhibitor was compared with tamoxifen or the combination of the two drugs. At 3 years of follow-up, treatment with anastrozole resulted in fewer relapses, specifically in women who had not received adjuvant chemotherapy. The majority of impact was in reduction of new breast cancers, and there is no survival data at this early date.

Aromatase inhibitors have a slightly different toxicity profile than tamoxifen. Treatment appears to result in fewer hot flashes (although they still occur), more joint pain, and perhaps an increase in osteoporosis. There does not appear to be an increased risk of endometrial cancer or blood clots. Due to the early nature of this data and concern regarding unknown long-term side effect, caution has been recommended in the use of aromatase inhibitors in the adjuvant setting. National recommendations are to still consider tamoxifen as the gold standard, but to consider anastrozole use in women who are either intolerant to tamoxifen or who have absolute contraindications to its use. Multiple randomized trials are ongoing comparing all 3 aromatase inhibitors (anastrozole, letrozole, and exemestane) with tamoxifen. Additional studies are evaluating the impact of these agents following 5 years of tamoxifen to reduce late relapses. Over the next several years, further data should emerge on the long-term impact of aromatase inhibitors on breast cancer mortality.

3. Special topics in hormonal therapy—Very young women with hormone receptor positive early-stage breast cancer are thought to have a particularly poor prognosis, despite aggressive adjuvant therapy. A variety of clinical trials have shown a reduction in relapse among women in whom chemotherapy-induced menopause developed, presumably due to a significant decrease in circulating estrogen levels. For that reason, there has been intense interest in the study of short-term ovarian suppression in premenopausal women with high-risk breast cancer using gonadotropin releasing hormone agonists (GnRHa). Two large studies will test the benefits of ovarian suppression with either tamoxifen or the aromatase inhibitor exemestane following adjuvant chemotherapy in premenopausal women with early-stage disease.

F. Neoadjuvant Therapy

Neoadjuvant therapy, or chemotherapy or hormonal therapy given before surgery for operable breast cancer, has an increasing role in the management of locally advanced breast cancer. A large randomized trial compared treatment before or after surgery with the chemotherapy combination AC and found an increased rate of breast conservation surgery in women receiving treatment before surgery. There was no difference in overall or disease-free survival; however, the approximately 13% of women who had no evidence of invasive breast cancer remaining at the time of surgery enjoyed a substantially improved prognosis compared with women who did not have a complete remission. Therefore, response to neoadjuvant chemotherapy appears to have prognostic value as well as increasing the rate of breast conservation.

Preliminary results of a recently completed randomized trial, NSABP B-27, indicate that extending neoadjuvant therapy with an additional 3 months of taxane therapy to a total of 6 months of preoperative chemotherapy doubles the number of women who have a complete remission of invasive breast cancer and also increases the number of women with negative axillary nodes. Survival data is not yet available, but additional studies are investigating the use of various combinations, sequences, and schedules of chemotherapy to further improve these results. Current trials have also included serial biopsies of the breast tumor to assess genetic changes that might predict either responsiveness or resistance to specific types of treatment. Hopefully these studies will allow further development of treatments targeted to specific tumor types in the future.

Disadvantages of neoadjuvant therapy include a potential for inaccurate staging; generally this does not affect treatment choices following surgery. Neoadjuvant chemotherapy has also been used to convert inoperable tumors to operable tumors (see section below).

Neoadjuvant hormonal therapy can be used to treat larger tumors in older women who either refuse or who are unable to receive chemotherapy. The majority of these tumors are hormone receptor positive; however, it is very important to check receptor status before a treatment decision has been made. Several clinical trials have shown improvement in breast conservation rates following neoadjuvant hormonal therapy, and one randomized trial demonstrated superiority of the aromatase inhibitor letrozole over tamoxifen in terms of reduction of tumor size and ability to undergo breast-conserving surgery. Neoadjuvant hormonal therapy is an important treatment option, and should be considered in older women with larger tumors. Additional studies are evaluating the effects of hormonal therapy in this setting.

G. Inflammatory and Locally Advanced Breast Cancer

Inflammatory breast cancer generally has an extremely poor prognosis. Cancer associated with extensive invasion of dermal lymphatics, with invasion of the skeletal muscle of or fixed to the chest wall, or with fixed or matted axillary nodes is considered inoperable due to

difficulty achieving clean surgical margins and very high rates of local recurrence. Neoadjuvant chemotherapy is the preferred initial treatment for inflammatory or locally advanced unresectable disease, with the hope that resection will eventually be feasible. Response rates up to 80% are seen, and in many cases mastectomy is possible. It is important that radiation be used following surgery to reduce the high risk of local recurrence. One small series has reported reasonable long-term disease control with chemotherapy followed by radiation, suggesting that surgery may not be required in every case. Patients with hormone receptor positive disease should also receive 5 years of adjuvant hormonal therapy. Despite this aggressive treatment approach, 10-year disease-free survival for inflammatory disease is at best in the 30% range, and clearly this is an area where greater understanding of the biologic factors resulting in early spread via lymphatics is required. Patients with fixed or matted axillary nodes or a tumor that invades the chest wall may still enjoy reasonable 10-year disease-free survival rates if their tumor demonstrates significant response to neoadjuvant therapy.

H. Treatment of Local Recurrence and Metastatic Disease

Recurrence of cancer in a breast treated conservatively with lumpectomy and irradiation is usually treated successfully with salvage mastectomy. Repeat excision has been shown to have a high local failure rate, and irradiation is usually not possible due to the possibility of significant tissue damage. When recurrence is localized to the breast, cancer-related mortality is not significantly altered from that of the original diagnosis. It may be difficult to determine whether the cancer represents an in breast recurrence or a new primary breast cancer; tumor markers and comparison of the pathology can often help and should be routinely performed since this significantly impacts decisions regarding systemic therapy.

Local or chest wall recurrence following mastectomy has a much worse prognosis and is associated with a high incidence of systemic recurrences, up to 90% at 10 years. Chest wall recurrence usually involves skin and/or muscle as there is no remaining breast tissue and is considered metastatic disease. Patients who present with chest wall recurrence should be completely staged to rule out distant metastases. A small subset of women with local recurrence and no evidence of distant spread may benefit from aggressive treatment, which may include chest-wall resection and irradiation with potential for long-term disease-free survival. Chemotherapy has not been shown to improve outcome in resectable disease but is given for palliation for more extensive involvement. Hormonal therapy is also useful for patients with hormone receptor positive disease. Patients with isolated axillary recurrences can also be successfully treated with resection and radiation (if the area was not previously irradiated) with some long-term benefit.

Unfortunately, most relapses are systemic. The most common sites of involvement are the bones and bone marrow, lungs, pleura, liver, lymph nodes, and brain. Metastatic breast cancer is considered incurable; however, significant palliation and prolongation of life can be obtained with systemic therapy. The goal of treatment is improvement of quality as well as quantity of life, and toxicity must be carefully evaluated with each therapeutic option. The median survival in patients with metastatic breast cancer is about 3 years; however, it ranges from several months to several years, with 5–10% of patients alive at 10 years. Duration of survival is largely determined by the biology and responsiveness of the individual cancer. In general, younger patients with hormone receptor negative, HER2/neu negative disease and extensive visceral involvement have the poorest survival, particularly if the relapse occurred within 1 year of completing adjuvant therapy. In contrast, postmenopausal women with hormone receptor positive disease involving only bones may have a much more indolent course, with survival in some cases for longer than 10 years.

Treatment options for metastatic disease include systemic chemotherapy, either given in combination or as sequential single agents, the antibody trastuzumab, and sequential hormonal therapies. The choice of treatment depends on the hormonal and HER2 status of the tumor, presence of visceral metastases, and the patient's medical condition and willingness to tolerate toxicities of therapy.

Hormone receptor positive disease is generally initially treated with hormonal therapy. The mean time to an objective response is 2 months, and the mean duration of response is 1–2 years, although many patients may experience longer response durations. If the disease responds to first-line hormonal therapy, there is a strong chance of a response to second-line and even third-line hormonal therapy. Until quite recently, tamoxifen was the first-line hormonal therapy of choice in the metastatic setting for premenopausal and postmenopausal women. For postmenopausal women, new options for hormonal therapy include the potent aromatase inhibitors (letrozole, anastrozole, exemestane). As first-line therapy, studies have shown equal or better responses to these agents than tamoxifen in the metastatic setting; however, survival was not affected by initial treatment choice. Fulvestrant is a new antiestrogen that directly blocks the estrogen receptor without the estrogen-like effects of tamoxifen. This newly approved drug has been shown to be equivalent to anastrozole in women whose disease has progressed despite treatment with tamoxifen. The aromatase inhibitors are given by mouth on a daily basis; fulvestrant is given by intramuscular injection once a month. The progestin megestrol acetate may also be effective in the later treatment of hormone responsive metastatic disease; although its side effect profile is not as good as other newer agents, it can improve appetite in patients who are anorectic.

Premenopausal women do not benefit from aromatase inhibitors unless their ovaries are suppressed or removed, and fulvestrant has not yet been evaluated in this setting. The use of ovarian suppression with GnRH agonists or oophorectomy is an effective hormonal therapy. Some studies have shown improved response rates and survival when tamoxifen was given concurrently with ovarian suppression as first-line therapy for metastatic disease.

Chemotherapy is another option for systemic treatment. It is the treatment of choice for women with ER-negative cancers or women with rapidly progressive disease. Although more aggressive regimens utilizing combinations of chemotherapy drugs can result in higher response rates than single agents, there is substantially more toxicity without improvement in overall survival. In general, either less toxic combinations or sequential single agents are preferred unless a rapid response is required for particularly aggressive disease. A wide range of active agents, from older drug combinations such as CMF or AC, to active single-agents such as the taxanes (paclitaxel and docetaxel) and epirubicin are available. Newer active drugs include liposomal doxorubicin (doxorubicin encased in a liposome to decrease toxicity and improve drug delivery and half-life), capecitabine (an oral prodrug of 5-fluorouracil), vinorelbine, gemcitabine, and platinum salts (cisplatin and carboplatin). These agents are effective as single agents with tolerable toxicity and are usually administered on a weekly basis. In the first-line setting, the most highly active agents are usually given with responses in the 40–60% range although duration of response may only last 6 months.

For HER2/neu positive disease, the combination of chemotherapy with the antibody trastuzumab has been shown to significantly prolong survival compared with chemotherapy alone. Patients with relatively asymptomatic HER2/neu positive metastatic disease may benefit from treatment with trastuzumab alone. The most serious adverse effect of trastuzumab is cardiac toxicity with 10–15% having some degree of cardiac dysfunction and 2% having clinically significant heart failure; this risk is increased 2- to 3-fold if the drug is given in combination with an anthracycline.

The choice of second-line therapy depends on response to prior treatment. Response rates to each subsequent chemotherapy regimen are generally lower and of shorter duration than the prior episode, although not easily predictable for any given patient. When to continue treatment or whether to wait for cancer-related symptoms or significant progression of disease by imaging or examination is a very individual decision for the patient and her oncologist. Current research is focusing on the addition of novel targeted agents to standard chemotherapy regimens, although it is not yet clear how these agents will be used effectively.

I. SUPPORTIVE CARE

Inasmuch as the goal of treatment for metastatic disease is palliation, careful attention must be paid to symptom control throughout the course of disease. Painful bone lesions can be treated with radiation to not only control pain but also prevent pathologic fractures. The bisphosphonates pamidronate and zoledronate have been shown to reduce bone pain from metastases as well as delay time to bone problems such as fracture or need for radiation. They are given by monthly intravenous infusion in patients with known bone involvement. The erythroid growth factor, erythropoietin, may be used to combat the effects of anemia and improve anemia related fatigue. Other agents are also being tested to treat cancer-related fatigue, which can be disabling. Anorexia can often be successfully treated with high doses of megestrol acetate or the oral form of THC from marijuana, marinol. Management of pain can be difficult, but newer long-acting narcotics with short-acting drugs for break-through pain are the most effective approach.

In addition to supporting physical symptoms, psychosocial support is also important. Support groups as well as counseling regarding end-of-life decisions can make this very difficult period of life more tolerable. Organizations such as the American Cancer Society can offer help with transportation costs. The decision to stop active treatment of advanced breast cancer is a difficult one, and must be made together with the patient's family and oncologist. In this situation, the primary care physician can play an invaluable role, providing both advice and support to the patient and patient's family. Hospice services can also be of tremendous help, and eliminate the need for clinic visits that can be exhausting and painful.

Anastrozole alone or in combination with tamoxifen versus tamoxifen alone for adjuvant treatment of postmenopausal women with early breast cancer: first results of the ATAC randomised trial. Lancet 2002;359:2131. [PMID: 12090977]

Breast cancer and breast-feeding: collaborative reanalysis of individual data from 47 epidemiological studies in 30 countries, including 50302 women with breast cancer and 96973 women without the disease. Lancet 2002;360:187. [PMID: 12133652]

Costantino JP et al: Validation studies for models projecting the risk of invasive and total breast cancer incidence. J Natl Cancer Inst 1999;91:1541. [PMID: 10491430]

Fisher B et al: Lumpectomy and radiation therapy for the treatment of intraductal breast cancer: findings from National Surgical Adjuvant Breast and Bowel Project B-17. J Clin Oncol 1998; 16:441. [PMID: 9469327]

Fisher B et al: Tamoxifen in treatment of intraductal breast cancer: National Surgical Adjuvant Breast and Bowel Project B-24 randomised controlled trial. Lancet 1999;353:1993. [PMID: 10376613]

Fraile M et al: Sentinel node biopsy as a practical alternative to axillary lymph node dissection in breast cancer patients: an approach to its validity. Ann Oncol 2000;11:701. [PMID: 10942059]

Polychemotherapy for early breast cancer: an overview of the randomised trials. Early Breast Cancer Trialists' Collaborative Group. Lancet 1998;352:930. [PMID: 9752815]

Schwartz GF, Giuliano AE, Veronesi U: Proceedings of the consensus conference on the role of sentinel lymph node biopsy in carcinoma of the breast, April 19–22, 2001, Philadelphia, Pennsylvania. Cancer 2002;94:2542. [PMID: 12173319]

Slamon DJ et al: Use of chemotherapy plus a monoclonal antibody against HER2 for metastatic breast cancer that overexpresses HER2. N Engl J Med 2001;344:783. [PMID: 11248153]

Tamoxifen for early breast cancer: an overview of the randomised trials. Early Breast Cancer Trialists' Collaborative Group. Lancet 1998;351:1451. [PMID: 960580]

Follow-Up

A patient who has undergone primary therapy for local breast cancer needs to be monitored for new cancers in the contralateral breast and, if treated with breast-conserving therapy, recurrences in the ipsilateral breast. In addition, patients on hormonal therapy are monitored so that possible side effects or toxicities can be managed. Usually the patient is seen and examined every 3–4 months for 2 years, every 6 months for a total of 5 years, then yearly. Regular mammography should be performed, with a baseline approximately 6 months after completion of radiation therapy.

Regular examinations for local or regional recurrence and breast imaging with mammography are important parts of the follow-up for a woman diagnosed with early-stage breast cancer because these procedures aid in early detection of curable lesions. In contrast, screening for metastatic disease with routine chest films, bone scans, liver scans, and blood tests is not recommended as the early detection of asymptomatic metastases does not affect overall survival or outcome from metastatic disease. Noninvasive assessments for metastases include a detailed review of systems; a thorough general physical examination looking especially for adenopathy, chest-wall lesions, pleural effusions, hepatomegaly, bony tenderness, or neurologic dysfunction. Imaging studies should be performed to evaluate new symptoms, such as persistent cough, new bone pain, or neurologic symptoms. Laboratory testing, including alkaline phosphatase or liver function tests to screen for bone and liver abnormalities, should be done to further aid in the evaluation symptoms. The use of blood tumor markers such as carcinoembryonic antigen (CEA) or the breast cancer markers CA 15-3 and CA 27.29, are not recommended as screening tests for recurrent disease. Markers may be elevated for a variety of benign reasons; they do not rise with localized, curable disease, and they may be normal in the setting of widespread metastatic disease. In addition, testing can be associated with significant patient anxiety, as well as inappropriate treatment. Until the time that early detection of metastatic disease impacts survival, regular testing of tumor markers should be discouraged. Patients should undergo screening for other malignancies following standard guidelines for their age.

Patients with a previous diagnosis of early-stage breast cancer are generally recommended to avoid supplemental estrogen and progesterone due to concern regarding increasing the risk of relapse or new cancers. However, little information is known about hormone replacement in this setting. Given the data showing an increase in the risk of primary breast cancer in women taking estrogen and progesterone replacement following menopause, it seems prudent to avoid hormones except in situations where quality of life is severely affected and other methods of treating menopausal symptoms have been ineffective.

Issues of Pregnancy & Breast Cancer

Breast cancer occurring during pregnancy has been thought to have a worse prognosis than average; in fact, stage for stage the prognosis is probably not worse than the same disease in a woman who is not pregnant. However, cancers diagnosed during pregnancy tend to present at an advanced stage, and with poorer prognostic biologic features. The breast swelling that accompanies pregnancy makes it more difficult to detect masses, and the pregnancy or lactating breast is hypervascular, which may aid in distribution of metastatic cells. Pregnant patients with newly diagnosed breast cancer face unique challenges to therapy. No treatment is known to be safe in the first trimester of pregnancy, and depending on the stage of breast cancer and the individual woman, consideration should be given to termination of very early pregnancies in this situation. However, it appears to be relatively safe to administer certain chemotherapeutic agents, such as doxorubicin and cyclophosphamide, in the second and third trimesters although rates of fetal demise may be elevated. Radiation therapy is contraindicated throughout pregnancy, making lumpectomy a bad option if the patient is diagnosed early in pregnancy. Careful discussion of treatment options is very important.

In the past, there has been concern that pregnancy following a diagnosis of early-stage breast cancer with its accompanying elevated hormonal levels might trigger recurrence. Recent studies of women who had successful pregnancies following early-stage breast cancer, albeit representing limited numbers, have not shown a significant impact of pregnancy on relapse or survival. In addition to small numbers, this data is limited by the fact that the women who became pregnant tended to have the earliest stage and best prognosis disease. Advice to a woman who desires to become pregnant should be based on common sense; the advisability of pregnancy depends at least to some degree on the statistical likelihood of recurrence and the potential dilemmas posed by the need to treat a recurrence during pregnancy.

Chemoprevention

Prevention of breast cancer is clearly a desirable goal. Recent efforts have been aimed at inhibiting proliferation of breast tissue by modifying hormonal effects on growth. To this end, a large randomized trial, NSABP P-1, was conducted in the mid 1990s to assess the role of tamoxifen in the primary prevention of breast cancer. This was based on the observed benefit of tamoxifen as secondary prevention in patients treated for localized breast cancer. In this pivotal trial, 13,388 women at moderate risk for breast cancer were randomized to 20 mg/d of tamoxifen versus placebo for 5 years. Eligible women included those over the age of 60 or between the ages of 35 and 59 with a 5-year predicted risk of cancer using the Gail model of at least 1.66% or women with a previous diagnosis of LCIS. Three quarters of the study participants had a 5-year predicted risk of 2% or greater. At 6 years of follow-up, tamoxifen was shown to reduce the incidence of invasive breast cancer by 50%. When cancers were stratified by estrogen-receptor status, a decrease was only seen in estrogen-receptor positive tumors; equal numbers of estrogen-receptor negative tumors were seen in both groups. Tamoxifen was shown to have a beneficial effect on bone density, decreasing the incidence of osteoporosis-related fractures. Similar to the data from adjuvant trials, the incidence of endometrial cancer was increased 2.5-fold, and thromboembolic events were increased 2- to 3-fold. There were no deaths in this study attributable to endometrial cancer, which were all stage I. Deaths from pulmonary emboli were seen in the tamoxifen arm, all in postmenopausal women. Two smaller randomized trials in Europe did not show a primary prevention benefit from tamoxifen although differences in the study population and compliance could potentially explain their negative outcomes. Based on these data, tamoxifen for 5 years is a reasonable option for patients at high risk for breast cancer, but the decision must take into account the known risks associated with its use. An ongoing second primary prevention trial (the STAR trial) is randomizing postmenopausal women to receive either tamoxifen or raloxifene (another SERM). Raloxifene has been approved for use in the treatment of osteoporosis and has some antiestrogenic properties in breast tissue. Unlike tamoxifen though, it does not promote endometrial proliferation and is unlikely to result in an increased risk for endometrial cancer. There are a number of ongoing trials testing the use of aromatase inhibitors in postmenopausal women at high risk for breast cancer, and in women with a history of DCIS. With advances in hormonal therapy, it is likely that continued progress will be made in finding safe interventions for the prevention of breast cancer.

Fisher B et al: Tamoxifen for prevention of breast cancer: report of the National Surgical Adjuvant Breast and Bowel Project P-1 Study. J Natl Cancer Inst 1998;90:1371. [PMID: 9747868]

Kinsinger LS et al: Chemoprevention of breast cancer: a summary of the evidence for the US Preventive Services Task Force. Ann Intern Med 2002;137:59. [PMID: 12093250]

Rhodes DJ: Identifying and counseling women at increased risk for breast cancer. Mayo Clin Proc 2002;77:355. [PMID: 11936931]

Relevant Web Sites

[National Comprehensive Cancer Network site providing up to date treatment guidelines and information for patients and physicians for many cancers.]

www.nccn.org

[Surveillance and Epidemiology and End Results site: Large database on incidence and mortality for the United States.]

seer.cancer.gov

[National Cancer Institute web site with general information and links to many other sites.]

www.nci.nih.gov/cancer_information

Venous Thromboembolic Disease 36

Alison Stopeck, MD, & Deborah Fuchs, MD

ESSENTIALS OF DIAGNOSIS

- *Swollen, erythematous tender extremity.*
- *Shortness of breath, tachycardia, pleuritic chest pain, hemoptysis.*
- *Confirmatory radiologic study (eg, ventilation-perfusion scan, spiral computed tomography, ultrasonography, or angiography).*

General Considerations

Thrombotic disease is the leading cause of death in the United States, outnumbering cancer deaths approximately 3-fold. Venous thromboembolism (VTE) occurs an estimated 600,000 episodes per year; however, a projected two thirds of these events are undiagnosed. Pulmonary embolism (PE) remains the most common cause of preventable death in hospitalized patients. For these reasons, understanding VTE pathophysiology, prophylactic measures, and therapy options is imperative. Treating and preventing VTE in women presents unique issues. Estrogen therapies, pregnancy, and hereditary thrombophilias interact synergistically to potentiate a woman's risk of VTE, VTE recurrence, and can effect treatment options. Recent advances in understanding thrombophilia have improved the clinician's ability to predict which patients are at risk for thrombosis and initiate appropriate prophylactic therapy. The myriad of new anticoagulants now available have revolutionized the ability of physicians to treat patients safely and effectively.

Pathogenesis & Risk Factors

In 1856, the German pathologist Virchow postulated 3 main predictors for thrombosis: venous stasis, hypercoagulability (changes in clotting factors or inhibitors), and vascular injury (endothelial damage). Endothelial damage is the most important factor in arterial thrombosis. Such damage exposes subendothelial collagen to circulating factors, most notably von Willebrand factor, that precipitate platelet adhesion and tissue factor release, thus initiating coagulation. In the venous system,

stasis and hypercoagulability are the main causes of thrombosis. Venous stasis prevents clearance of activated clotting factors and influx of endogenous inhibitors.

Table 36–1 lists the genetic and acquired hypercoagulable states. In most patients with VTE, more than 1 risk factor is identified (eg, thrombosis develops in a young woman with factor V Leiden after beginning to take oral contraceptives). In general, the more risk factors a patient has, the higher the likelihood of a thrombotic event. Recognizing existing hypercoagulable states is important for determining appropriate treatment, prophylaxis, and counseling of patients.

The major natural anticoagulants, antithrombin, protein C, and protein S are directed against the formation or action of thrombin. Antithrombin, formerly known as antithrombin III, inactivates thrombin and other serine proteases, including FVIIa, FXIIa, FXIa, FXa, and FIXa, via irreversible binding to the active site. Heparins, natural (heparan sulfate from the endothelium) or exogenous, enhance the inhibitory activity of antithrombin 1000-fold. The protein C inhibitory pathway is initiated when thrombin binds thrombomodulin, allowing this complex to activate protein C. Activated protein C, in the presence of its cofactor, protein S, proteolytically inactivates factors Va and VIIIa, thereby dampening the coagulation cascade.

A. HEREDITARY HYPERCOAGULABLE STATES

Factor V (FV) Leiden mutation represents the most common inherited thrombotic disorder accounting for approximately 20–50% of recurrent thrombosis (Table 36–2). During normal hemostasis, FVa is inactivated via proteolysis by activated protein C (APC). A single point mutation in the FV gene results in the substitution of glutamine for arginine at amino acid residue 506. This alteration in the FV molecule prevents APC cleavage of the peptide bond that under normal circumstances results in FVa inactivation. This leads to decreased responsiveness when APC is added to standard clotting tests (ie, the activated partial thromboplastin time [APTT]) termed "APC resistance." The FV Leiden mutation (R506Q substitution) accounts for greater than 90% of cases of APC resistance as diagnosed by clotting tests. It is inherited in an autosomal manner with heterozygotes having a 5- to 10-fold in-

Table 36–1. Hypercoagulable states.

Genetic
  Factor V Leiden (activated protein C resistance)
  Prothrombin gene mutation
  Elevated factor VIII level
  Antithrombin deficiency
  Protein C deficiency
  Protein S deficiency
  Homocysteinemia
Acquired
  Malignancy
  Surgery
  Pregnancy/Puerperium
  Estrogen therapy/oral contraceptives
  Antiphospholipid antibody syndrome/lupus anticoagulant
  Diabetes
  Polycythemia vera/essential thrombocythemia
  Nephrotic syndrome
  Disseminated intravascular coagulation (chronic)
  Inflammatory bowel disease
  Paroxysmal nocturnal hematuria
Venous stasis/endothelial injury
  Immobility
  Obesity
  Indwelling venous catheter
  Trauma
  Hip fracture
  Congestive heart failure

Table 36–3. Frequency of factor V Leiden mutation in United States by ethnicity.

Ethnic Origin	Percentage of Cases of Factor V Leiden Mutation
White	5.3
Hispanic	2.2
Black	1.4
Native American	1.3
Asian	0.46

creased risk of thrombosis and homozygotes a 50- to 100-fold increased risk. This mutation demonstrates variable frequencies in ethnic groups (Table 36–3). Testing for the FV Leiden mutation by polymerase chain reaction (PCR) is specific for the R506Q substitution and will not detect other causes of APC resistance, including acquired conditions or as yet unidentified mutations.

The prothrombin gene mutation accounts for approximately 10% of inherited thrombosis and is the second most common cause of hereditary thrombophilia in persons of European descent. A guanine to adenosine substitution at nucleotide position 20210 in

Table 36–2. Hereditary thrombophilias.

Defect	Number of Known Mutations	Incidence		Relative Risk of DVT
		Normal Population	Hypercoagulable State[1]	
Prothrombin gene mutation	1	2–4%	20%	2–4
Factor V Leiden	1	2–15%		
Heterozygote			20–50%	5–10
Homozygote				50–100
Protein C, Heterozygote	> 160	0.3%	5–10%	7
Protein S, Heterozygote	> 130	< 1%	5–10%	6–10
Antithrombin	> 120	0.02%	5–10%	10–20
Heterozygote		0.05–1.0%		
Hyperhomocysteinemia	[2]	10%	20%	2–3
MTHFR	1	4–5%		

DVT, deep venous thrombosis; MTHFR, methylene tetrahydrofolate reductase.
[1]patients with family history or personal history of DVT or pulmonary embolism.
[2]Involves multiple genes and mutations.

the untranslated region of the prothrombin gene leads to elevated prothrombin levels that promote enhanced thrombin generation and increase the risk of a thrombotic event 2- to 3-fold.

Antithrombin is an inhibitor of the activated serine proteases (thrombin [FIIa], FIXa, FXa, FXIa, FXIIa). Homozygous antithrombin deficiency is not observed and is thought to be lethal in utero, attesting to the importance of this inhibitor in hemostasis. Known mutations result in either qualitative or quantitative defects and confer relative heparin resistance. Patients with heparin resistance (ie, requiring larger than usual quantities of heparin for therapeutic anticoagulation) should prompt evaluation for antithrombin abnormalities. Antithrombin deficiency has a prevalence of approximately 1% in patients with VTE. The odds ratio for thrombosis is 10- to 20-fold, which is greater than that seen in the more common hereditary thrombophilias.

Protein C and S are vitamin K–dependent plasma glycoproteins that are synthesized predominantly in the liver. Other sites of protein S synthesis include endothelial cells and megakaryocytes. Protein C is cleaved by the thrombin-thrombomodulin complex to form APC, which in the presence of protein S, calcium, and phospholipid, proteolytically inactivates FVa and FVIIIa. Acquired protein C deficiency is commonly seen in vitamin K deficiency (oral anticoagulants or nutritional), liver disease, and disseminated intravascular coagulopathy (DIC).

Protein S functions as a nonenzymatic cofactor for APC in the inactivation of FVa and FVIIIa and may directly inhibit the tenase and prothrombinase complexes. Active protein S circulates free in the blood and accounts for 40% of total protein S. The inactive form (60%) is bound to C4-binding protein (C4BP). C4BP is an acute phase reactant and can be increased in many conditions including pregnancy, inflammatory bowel disease, and infection. In these situations, the elevated protein binds a higher percentage of protein S thereby causing a secondary decrease in protein S activity. Acquired deficiencies of protein S occur in vitamin K deficiency, liver disease, DIC, nephrotic syndrome, and pregnancy. Deficiencies in protein C and protein S are autosomally inherited.

B. ANTIPHOSPHOLIPID ANTIBODIES

Antiphospholipid antibodies include a variety of autoantibodies that occur in the setting of autoimmune disease or as reactions to drugs or infections. Clinically significant antibodies are usually classified as primary (primary antiphospholipid syndrome) when occurring without a known inciting agent or disease or secondary when occurring in association with a known disorder, most commonly systemic lupus erythematosus. Anti-

phospholipid antibodies are recognized as a major cause of both venous and arterial thromboembolic events. The designation of antiphospholipid antibody is a misnomer as most of the antibodies are directed against phospholipid binding proteins (ie, β_2-glycoprotein I or prothrombin). These are nonspecific inhibitors, as they are not directed against a specific factor and are rarely associated with hemorrhagic disorders. Antiphospholipid antibodies can be divided into 2 broad categories based on the testing methodology used to detect them, lupus anticoagulants (LAC) inhibit phospholipid-dependent clotting based studies; and anticardiolipin antibodies (ACA) are detected by solid-phase enzyme-linked immunosorbent assays (ELISAs). The presence of these autoantibodies associated with clinical features including arterial, venous, or small-vessel thrombosis, recurrent fetal loss, autoimmune thrombocytopenia, livedo reticularis, skin ulceration, or hemolytic anemia characterize the antiphospholipid syndrome. Pregnancy complications known to be associated with antiphospholipid antibodies include spontaneous abortions (typically after week 10), fetal growth retardation or demise, placental abruption, and preeclampsia. The consensus criteria for the diagnosis of antiphospholipid antibody syndrome include at least 1 clinical manifestation of venous or arterial thrombosis or pregnancy complication in association with positive laboratory testing. Infection-associated antibodies are usually transient, low-titer (usually IgM) and clinically insignificant. In vivo, the mechanism of antiphospholipid antibody-induced thrombosis is unknown, but various hypotheses include endothelial cell activation, inhibition of APC, and/or increased prothrombin binding to phospholipid surfaces.

Antiphospholipid antibodies are a heterogeneous group of autoantibodies (IgG > IgM > IgA) that often interfere with in vitro, phospholipid-dependent coagulation tests, most commonly the APTT or dilute Russel's viper venom time, resulting in prolongation. Due to the heterogeneous nature of the antibodies and the different sensitivities of the testing reagents, multiple tests may need to be performed to confirm the presence of an LAC. The APTT alone is not a reliable screening test for LAC. If an LAC is suspected and the APTT is normal, additional clotting based tests designed to accentuate the effects of an LAC, such as dilute Russel's viper venom time or dilute prothrombin time, should be performed. In addition, all positive tests should be confirmed at least 6 weeks apart as transient antiphospholipid antibodies are seldom clinically relevant. Identification and confirmation of an LAC requires 3 steps: (1) prolongation of a phospholipid-dependent clotting test, (2) mixing studies with normal plasma to demonstrate an inhibitor pattern rather than a factor deficiency, and (3) neutralization of this inhibitory effect by phospholipids added to the test system (ie, platelet neutralization procedure). In this procedure, added excess phospholipid binds the LAC, thus neutralizing it and allowing the clotting time to correct toward normal.

Elevated levels of ACAs by ELISA testing can also be used for diagnosing antiphospholipid antibody syndromes. In general, IgG, IgA, and IgM levels are assayed with higher titers of the IgG or IgM subtype being more commonly associated with clinical sequelae. LACs are thought to be more predictive of thrombotic complications than positive ACA titers. Concordance between ACA and clotting-based LAC testing is only 60–80% and thus both ELISA and clotting-based studies are recommended for excluding antiphospholipid antibody syndromes. Antibodies directed against other phospholipids including β_2-glycoprotein I, phosphatidylethanolamine, and phosphatidylserine have also been reported to be associated with antiphospholipid antibody syndromes and can be obtained commercially if the aforementioned testing is negative and clinical suspicion remains high.

Asymptomatic patients found incidentally to have LAC (ie, after evaluation for a prolonged APTT) should not be treated expectantly, but rather aggressively treated with prophylaxis in moderate- or high-risk situations. The incidence of developing a subsequent thrombosis in this group of patients is unknown. Reducing or eliminating arterial and venous thrombotic risk factors, ie, smoking, oral contraceptives, hormone replacement therapy (HRT), obesity, hyperhomocysteinemia is reasonable as there is data to suggest that antiphospholipid antibody-associated thrombosis occurs most commonly in the setting of other precipitating risks.

C. HYPERHOMOCYSTEINEMIA

Hyperhomocysteinemia is a risk factor for premature peripheral vascular disease, Alzheimer's disease, and arterial and venous thrombosis. Methionine is a by-product of protein metabolism that is metabolized to homocysteine. Two enzymes, cystathionine B-synthase (CBS) and methylene tetrahydrofolate reductase (MTHFR), and 3 vitamins (B_{12}, B_6, and folic acid) are involved in the regulation of homocysteine levels. Both genetic (mutations in CBS or MTHFR) and nongenetic factors (vitamin B_{12}, B_6, or folic acid deficiencies, smoking, increasing age, renal failure, and hypothyroidism) impair homocysteine metabolism leading to elevated levels of homocysteine. It has been shown that elevated homocysteine levels lead to vascular smooth muscle proliferation, lipid peroxidation, and vascular matrix damage resulting in atherogenesis. In addition, vascular endothelial injury mediated by homocysteine renders the endothelial surface prothrombotic. Thus, hyperhomocysteinemia is an independent risk factor for acute myocardial infarction, coronary heart disease, and peripheral vascular disease. In the Leiden Thrombophilia Study, the odds ratio for VTE was increased to 2.5 in patients with plasma homocysteine levels > 18 μmol/L (normal < 10 μmol/L). Plasma levels of homocysteine are determined in morning fasting blood samples using high-performance liquid chromatography (HPLC) or immunoassay.

D. ELEVATED FACTOR LEVELS

A recent association has been described between elevated factor levels and thrombosis, particularly with FVIII, FIX, FXI, and fibrinogen. Patients with elevated FVIII levels may also be at increased risk for recurrent venous thrombosis. Elevated FXI levels may be a risk factor for venous thrombosis by increasing thrombin production and subsequent protection of fibrin from proteolysis.

E. ESTROGENS

Throughout a woman's life, there are fluctuations in VTE risk secondary to changes in the estrogen and progesterone environment. Whether it be through pregnancy, oral contraceptive pills (OCPs), HRT, or the use of a specific estrogen response modifier (SERMs) for treatment or prevention of breast cancer, it will be important to advise her appropriately about her risk of VTE (Table 36–4). All estrogens increase factor VIII and von Willebrand factor levels, resulting in increased risk of VTE. This risk extends not only to the occurrence of spontaneous VTE, but also increases the recurrence rate of VTE, and in particular, markedly increases the risk of VTE in patients with hereditary thrombophilias.

All oral contraceptive formulations have been associated with increased risk of thrombosis, with the risk varying by the specific estrogen and progestin dosing

Table 36–4. Risk of venous thromboembolism with hormone therapies.

Therapy	Relative Risk	Estimated Events per 10,000 Patients[1]
None	1	10
Hormone replacement therapy	2–4	20–40
Tamoxifen/raloxifene	3–7	30–70
Chemotherapy plus tamoxifen	5–15	50–150

[1]In 60-year-old women.

(Table 36–5). In first generation OCPs, ethinyl estradiol was typically 50 mg or higher, and the progestin was typically norethindrone. The risk of VTE was approximately 10-fold higher in women taking these first generation OCPs compared with women of similar age not using OCPs. In an effort to decrease the risk of thrombosis, second generation OCPs with lower estradiol concentrations between 35 mg and 50 mg were introduced. The decrease in estrogen dosing resulted in a decrease in the risk of VTE to 3- to 4-fold. More recently, third generation OCPs have been introduced containing less than 35 mg of estradiol, but with new progestins including desogestrel, gestodene, and norgestimate. These third-generation OCPs have been found to have an increased risk of VTE compared with second-generation OCPs and are generally thought to have a 6- to 8-fold increased risk of VTE. This risk also seems to be additive with other risk factors and perhaps even synergistic with hereditary thrombophilias. In several small studies, women who are heterozygous for the FV Leiden mutation and/or prothrombin gene mutation have markedly increased risks of VTE after initiating therapy with OCPs or HRT. In particular, patients who are heterozygous for FV Leiden had a 35-fold increased risk of VTE after initiating OCPs. Recently, elevated factor VIII levels have also been associated with a 2-fold increased risk of thrombosis, with concomitant OCP use increasing this risk to approximately 10-fold. Despite this pronounced increase in VTE risk, routine screening of all women for common hereditary thrombophilias before starting OCPs or HRT is not cost-effective secondary to the relative rarity of these thrombophilias. However, women with a prior history of VTE or a family history suggesting a hereditary thrombophilia should be considered for thrombophilia screening before initiating hormonal therapies. In patients found to have a hereditary thrombophilia, referral to a hematologist or physician well-versed in thrombophilia is recommended for a careful discussion of the risks and benefits of HRT. Other options including bisphosphonates for osteopenia and venlafaxine (Effexor) for hot flashes can be offered as alternative therapies for postmenopausal symptoms and complications.

Advising women with thrombophilias on birth control methods can be challenging. As pregnancy itself increases a normal woman's risk of thrombosis 5- to 6-fold, avoiding an unwanted pregnancy is particularly advantageous for women with hereditary thrombophilias. Unfortunately, few methods of contraception have the efficacy of OCPs. In general, progestin-only contraceptives have a far lower risk of VTE compared with estrogen and progestin combinations. Increased risks or odd ratios of 1.3–2.19 have been found with progestin-only contraceptives. When used at higher doses, similar to estrogens, a dose-dependent increase in the risk of VTE has been observed. It is unclear whether the increase in VTE is secondary to the indications for the higher dose progestins or a dose-dependent effect of the progestins themselves.

Postcoital contraception with either a combination ethinyl estradiol plus levonorgestrel taken 12 hours apart for 2 doses within 72 hours of unprotected intercourse or levonorgestrel at a slightly higher dose taken in a similar manner has not been associated with an increased risk of VTE. This suggests that short-term hormone therapy has little effect on VTE risk and is a reasonable method of contraception for women having infrequent intercourse.

Effective methods of contraception are particularly important in patients with thrombophilias who are currently on long-term warfarin therapy. Warfarin is a known teratogen, particularly during the first 12 weeks of pregnancy. As progestin-only containing contraceptives often produce irregular menstrual bleeding, more frequent pregnancy testing may be warranted in these patients who are currently receiving warfarin therapy.

The use of HRT in perimenopausal and postmenopausal women has recently become more controversial. Recent studies, including the Heart and Estrogen/Replacement Study (HERS), suggest an increased risk of VTE in women receiving HRT without confirming a decreased risk of cardiovascular events. In particular, in the HERS study of women with a history of coronary artery disease, the risk of cardiovascular events was increased during the first year of observation with a decrease in cardiovascular events during years 4

Table 36–5. Risk of VTE with oral contraceptives.

OCP	Ethinyl Estradiol	Progesterone	Increase in VTE Risk
First generation	> 50 mg	Various	> 10-fold
Second generation	35–50 mg	Levonorgestrel	3- to 6-fold
Third generation	≤ 35 mg	Desogestrel, gestodene, norgestimate	6- to 8-fold

VTE, venous thromboembolism; OCP, oral contraceptive pills.

and 5 of follow-up. The increased risk of VTE persisted throughout the study period, although it was highest during the first year of HRT use. The Women's Health Initiative, which is currently evaluating cardiovascular events as well as VTE episodes in healthy women receiving estrogen replacement therapy also found an increased incidence of cardiovascular events in women receiving HRT in the first 2 years of follow-up. As HRT may increase the risk of cardiac events in the short-term, but decrease the risk over a longer time frame, further follow-up of this very large cohort of healthy women is necessary for defining the role of HRT in decreasing cardiovascular risk.

F. PREGNANCY

The problem of VTE in pregnancy warrants special discussion, as thromboembolic disease is the leading cause of maternal death in the United States. The incidence of VTE is 1 in every 1000 to 2000 pregnancies. Several physiologic changes during pregnancy act to increase coagulability including increased levels of clotting factors (fibrinogen, FVII, FVIII, FIX, FX), decreased active (free) protein S levels, and decreased fibrinolysis secondary to increased levels of plasminogen activator inhibitors. In addition, increased plasma volume and uterine compression on the pelvic veins leads to venous stasis (maximum at 34 weeks) and trauma to the pelvic vasculature during delivery produces endothelial damage. As a result of these collective effects, pregnancy increases VTE risk 5- to 6-fold. Other known factors that increase a woman's risk of pregnancy-related or puerperium VTE include (1) uterine sepsis (acquired protein C deficiency), (2) cesarean section (especially emergent), (3) complicated delivery, (4) gravida > 4, (5) increased maternal age, (6) prolonged bedrest during pregnancy, (7) previous thrombosis while taking OCPs or during a prior pregnancy, (8) preeclampsia, (9) hereditary thrombophilia, or (10) antiphosholipid antibody syndrome.

G. MALIGNANCY

Thromboembolism is a well-recognized complication of cancer. Thromboembolic complications include arterial embolism, DIC, and VTE. The pathogenesis of thromboembolism in cancer is poorly understood. Hemostatic disturbances include coagulation cascade activation, platelet activation, and inhibition of the fibrinolytic system. Tissue factor, which activates FVII in the first step of the extrinsic pathway, is frequently expressed on malignant cells and thought to play a major role in cancer-induced hypercoagulability. Other cascade activating factors directly produced by tumor cells include cancer procoagulant (directly activates FX) and cytokines. Compounding these tumor-related prothrombotic factors are additional risk factors such as chemotherapy, surgery, immobilization, direct venous obstruction by the tumor, and indwelling catheters. Patients with more extensive cancer (ie, advanced stage) or receiving concomitant chemotherapy with hormonal therapy (ie, tamoxifen) are at particularly high risk. Oncologic surgery is extensive and complicated, which often leads to prolonged immobilization, endothelial damage, and possible release of tumor expressed procoagulants during tumor manipulation. Consequently, VTE prophylaxis is crucial.

Gerhardt A et al: Prothrombin and factor V mutations in women with a history of thrombosis during pregnancy and the puerperium. N Engl J Med 2000;342:374. [PMID: 10666427]

Lane DA, Grant PJ: Role of hemostatic gene polymorphisms in venous and arterial thrombotic disease. Blood 2000;95:1517. [PMID: 10688804]

Levine JS, Branch DW, Rauch J: The antiphospholipid syndrome. N Engl J Med 2002;346:752. [PMID: 11882732]

Maartinelli I et al: Mutations in coagulation factors in women with unexplained late fetal loss. N Engl J Med 2000;343:1015. [PMID: 11018168]

Rosendaal FR: Venous thrombosis: a multicausal disease. Lancet 1999;353:1167. [PMID: 10209995]

Seligsohn U, Lubetsky A: Genetic susceptibility to venous thrombosis. N Engl J Med 2001;344:1222. [PMID: 11309638]

Vandenbroucke JP et al: Oral contraceptives and the risk of venous thrombosis. N Engl J Med 2001;344:1527. [PMID: 11357157]

Prevention

Prophylaxis is the most cost-effective way to reduce the negative impact of thrombosis. Despite the plethora of trials documenting the efficacy of both mechanical and pharmacologic therapies in decreasing the incidence of postoperative deep venous thrombosis (DVT) and PE, there are still wide practice variations in initiating prophylaxis. Most studies suggest that only one third of hospitalized patients receive appropriate prophylaxis as judged by standard prophylaxis guidelines, ie, The ACCP Consensus Conference on Antithrombotic Therapy. The reasons physicians avoid prophylaxis are multifactorial including fear of increased postoperative bleeding and wound hematomas, underestimation of risk (thrombotic complications develop in many patients after they have been discharged), and the costs of thromboprophylaxis. These concerns do not justify inadequate prophylaxis but rather confirm the importance of estimating every patient's risk individually and providing appropriate prophylaxis.

Methods of prophylaxis are generally divided into mechanical or pharmacologic. Mechanical therapies are designed to improve venous return and decrease endothelial damage and include graduated elastic compression stockings and intermittent pneumatic compression. Mechanical methods do not increase the risk of postoperative bleeding and thus are ideal for patients in whom anticoagulation therapy is contraindicated.

Pharmacologic methods of prophylaxis include low-dose unfractionated heparin at 5000 units SQ every 8 or 12 hours, low-molecular-weight heparin (LMWH) on either a once a day or twice a day dosing, warfarin targeted to an international normalized ratio (INR) of 2.0–3.0, and aspirin. In general, in patients at increased risk for bleeding, intermittent pneumatic compression should be initiated intraoperatively and continued until the patient is fully ambulatory. In patients in whom pharmacologic thromboprophylaxis is to be initiated, this should be started as soon as it is considered hemodynamically safe, and preferably within 8–12 hours postoperatively. Newer data suggest that initiating prophylaxis within 6 hours postoperatively may be more effective but will minimally increase the risk of postoperative bleeding. In general, levels of LMWH > 3400 U/d and starting prophylaxis preoperatively or within 6 hours after surgery are associated with improved prophylaxis at a cost of slightly higher bleeding rates. Absolute contraindications to early initiation of heparin prophylaxis include intracranial bleeding, spinal cord injury associated with perispinal hematoma, ongoing or uncontrolled bleeding, and an uncorrected coagulopathy. Recommended thromboprophylactic regimens for medical and surgical patients are presented in Tables 36–6 and 36–7, respectively.

When evaluating surgical risk, one must consider both the patient's individual characteristics as well as the operation (Tables 36–7, 36–8, and 36–9). Patient characteristics that portend greater risk include increasing age, obesity, active malignancy, prior history of VTE, known hereditary thrombophilia, family history of thrombosis, estrogen use, and varicose veins. The duration of the surgery, particularly longer than 2 hours; general anesthesia for more than 30 minutes; preoperative and postoperative immobility; level of hydration; sepsis; and abdominal, pelvic, or lower extremity surgery are additional risk factors for postoperative VTE. Gynecologic surgery for both benign and particularly malignant diseases carry significant VTE risks of 14–38% without postoperative prophylaxis. In general, patients considered at low risk for VTE are recommended to have early ambulation plus or minus graduated elastic compression stockings as their only form of prophylaxis. Conversely, patients at the highest risk for VTE should receive intermittent pneumatic compression combined with LMWH or adjusted-dose warfarin targeting an INR of 2.5.

Patients receiving spinal or epidural anesthesia are a special population as perispinal hematoma is a rare but catastrophic complication. The US Food and Drug Administration (FDA) issued a warning regarding the risk

Table 36–6. ACCP recommended regimens for VTE prophylaxis.

Method	Description
LDUH	Unfractionated heparin 5000 U SC q8–12h
ADH	Start unfractionated heparin at 3500 U SC q8h and adjust to maintain midinterval APTT at high normal value
LMWH	**General surgery, moderate risk** Dalteparin 2500 U SC preoperatively then daily Enoxaparin 20 mg SC preoperatively then daily Tinzaparin 3500 U SC preoperatively then daily
	General surgery, high risk (including orthopedic surgery) Dalteparin 2500 U SC 6–8h postoperatively then 5000 U SC daily Danaparoid 7500 U SC preoperatively and then q12h postoperatively Enoxaparin 40 mg SC preoperatively then daily or 30 mg SC q12h startin 8–12h postoperatively Tinzaparin 4500 U SC preoperatively then daily or 75 U/kg SC daily starting 12–24h postoperatively Fondaparinux 2.5 mg SC starting 6 h postoperatively[1]
	High Risk Medical Patients Dalteparin 2500 U SC daily Danaparoid 750 U SC q12h Enoxaparin 40 mg SC daily
Warfarin	Start 5 mg daily dose day of or day after surgery and adjust to INR 2.0–3.0
IPC/GEC	Start intraoperatively and continue until ambulatory

ACCP, American College of Chest Physicians; LDUH, low-dose unfractionated heparin; ADH, adjusted dose unfractionated heparin; LMWH, low-molecular-weight heparin; INR, international normalized ratio; IPC, intermittent pneumatic compression; GEC, graduated elastic compression stockings.
[1]Recently approved by the US Food and Drug Administration for prophylaxis after orthopedic surgery.

of perispinal hematoma in 43 US patients receiving predominantly enoxaparin as prophylaxis after orthopedic procedures. Risk factors associated with this complication included traumatic catheter insertion, blood return from the catheter, use of continuous epidural catheters, concurrent medications that increase bleeding tendencies, and female gender. Thus, in general LMWH and unfractionated heparin should be used in caution in patients with spinal anesthesia with insertion

Table 36–7. Surgical risk categories and recommended prophylaxis.

Risk Category	Definition	Recommended Prophylaxis
Low	Minor surgery in patients younger than 40 years without additional risk factors	Aggressive mobilization
Moderate	Minor surgery in patients older than 40 years without additional risk factors Minor surgery in patients of any age with additional risk factors Major surgery in patients younger than 40 years without additional risk factors	LDUH q12h LMWH GEC or IPC
High	Major surgery in patients older than 40 years Major surgery in patients of any age with additional risk factors Minor surgery in patients older than 60 years or with additional risk factors	LDUH q8h LMWH IPC
Very high	Major surgery in patients older than 40 years with additional risk factors of prior VTE, cancer, hereditary thrombophilia Hip or knee arthroplasty Hip fracture Major trauma Spinal cord injury	LMWH Coumadin IPC/GEC ADH

LDUH, low-dose unfractionated heparin; LMWH, low-molecular-weight heparin; GEC, graduated elastic compression; IPC, intermittent pneumatic compression; ADH, adjusted-dose unfractionated heparin.

or removal of the catheter delayed to 12 and preferably 24 hours after a prophylactic heparin injection. Heparin prophylaxis should probably be avoided in patients with renal insufficiency who may have delayed LMWH clearance, patients with traumatic or bloody lumbar puncture, patients receiving aspirin or other platelet inhibitors, and patients with known bleeding tendencies. Diagnostic imaging and surgeons capable of decompressing a spinal hematoma should also be available emergently.

Medical patients should be considered for prophylaxis in all situations, and ideally, they should be given prophylactic therapy if they have any of the following diagnoses: stroke, myocardial infarction, congestive heart failure, chronic obstructive pulmonary disease, or infection in association with another risk factor. Studies suggest that medical patients are at moderate to high risk for VTE with incidences ranging from 10% to 60%. Cancer patients have a 2- to 3-fold increased inci-

dence of VTE compared with patients with similar risk without cancer. In addition, VTE diagnosis is often difficult in cancer patients secondary to chronic leg edema and abnormal chest films, while anticoagulation with warfarin is complicated by frequent antibiotic use, chemotherapy, poor diet, and can be less efficacious than in noncancer patients. Thus, all hospitalized cancer patients should be considered at moderate to very high risk and given prophylaxis accordingly. The use of daily warfarin (1 mg) or subcutaneous LMWH has been shown to decrease the risk of catheter-related thrombosis and sepsis in randomized prospective trials and should be used routinely unless contraindicated.

The length of VTE prophylaxis is controversial, particularly as the duration of hospital stays decrease. In general, trials of postoperative prophylaxis after orthopedic procedures have included 7–10 days of prophylaxis. Seven days should be considered the minimum duration of prophylaxis for patients in the high risk or very high risk categories. In patients with the highest risk, including patients taking estrogen replacement therapy undergoing orthopedic procedures, prolonged prophylaxis for up to 35 days is probably cost-efficient and worth consideration. Multiple studies in patients following orthopedic surgery and recently following abdominal/gynecologic surgery for cancer have documented the efficacy of long-term prophylaxis with LMWH or coumadin (INR target 2.5) in decreasing the incidence of radiographically documented DVT by 50–60%. As these therapies are associated with a mildly increased risk of bleeding and require monitoring of the INR for coumadin therapy or the platelet count with heparin therapy, they are

Table 36–8. Surgical risk of VTE without prophylaxis.

Risk Level	Calf Vein VTE	Proximal Vein VTE	Clincal PE	Fatal PE
Low	2%	0.4%	0.2%	0.002%
Moderate	10–20%	2–4%	1–2%	0.1–0.4%
High	20–40%	4–8%	2–4%	0.4–1.0%
Very high	40–80%	10–20%	4–10%	1–5%

VTE, venous thromboembolism; PE, pulmonary embolism.

Table 36–9. Risk categories for prophylaxis in hospitalized patients.

Risk Factor	Score
Age > 70 years	+3
History of VTE	+3
Inherited thrombophilia	+3
Age 60–70 years	+2
Malignancy	+2
Major surgery (> 2 h)	+2
CHF/MI	+2
Severe infection/sepsis	+2
Patient confined to bed > 72 h	+2
Multiple trauma	+2
Hip fracture or total joint replacement	+2
Age > 40 but < 60 years	+1
Pregnancy or puerperium	+1
Obesity (> 2% IBW)	+1
OCPs, estrogen use	+1
Varicose veins	+1
Inflammatory bowel disease	+1
Family history of DVT	+1
Leg swelling, ulcers, stasis	+1
Central venous access	+1

VTE, venous thromboembolism; CHF, congestive heart failure; MI, myocardial infarction; IBW, ideal body weight; OCP, oral contraceptive pills; DVT, deep venous thrombosis.
1, low risk; 2, moderate risk; 3–4, high risk; > 5, very high risk.

considered most appropriate for patients with multiple risk factors for postoperative DVT.

While aspirin is a questionable and insufficient form of prophylaxis when used alone after orthopedic surgery, the results of the Pulmonary Embolism Prevention (PEP) trial confirm that aspirin can decrease the risk of VTE approximately 20–30%. In addition, long-term aspirin use is easy to administer, inexpensive, and thus a reasonable option for long-term (post-discharge) prophylaxis in patients without additional risk factors suggesting higher intensity prophylaxis would be required.

In studies assessing the pharmacoeconomics of prophylaxis, including extended duration, the broad application of prophylaxis is highly cost-effective and currently the only proven means to avoid the acute and chronic morbidity of VTE. Implementation of prophylaxis guidelines and protocols should be a goal of every hospital and health care provider.

New anticoagulants often are first tested in the prophylaxis setting. Fondaparinux, a synthetic analogue of the pentasaccharide of heparin required for binding to antithrombin, has recently been tested in over 7000 patients receiving orthopedic prophylaxis. In these trials, a single daily subcutaneous dose of 2.5 mg of fondaparinux starting 6 hours postoperatively was compared with once a day preoperative or twice a day postoperative enoxaparin. A single end point of VTE incidence as determined by bilateral venograms between days 5 and 11 prior to hospital discharge was used in all studies. Fondaparinux prophylaxis decreased the incidence of proximal and total VTE with a relative risk reduction of 50% compared with enoxaparin. Bleeding complications were not significantly increased, although there was a slight trend toward increased bleeding with fondaparinux. Based on these studies, fondaparinux (Arixtra) has gained US FDA approval for prophylaxis after surgery for hip fracture or hip/knee arthroplasty.

Geerts WH et al: Prevention of venous thromboembolism. Chest 2001;119(Suppl 1):132S. [PMID: 11157647]

Clinical Findings

A. SCREENING

The initial evaluation of a patient with VTE includes a thorough history and physical examination; stool should be tested for occult blood. Special attention to potential predisposing factors including malignancy, obesity, immobility, myeloproliferative disorders, vascular disease, trauma, and antiphospholipid antibody syndrome is warranted to exclude acquired causes.

Pregnancy or the puerperium state may be the triggering factor precipitating an initial VTE in a patient with a hereditary thrombophilia. FV Leiden; prothrombin gene mutation; hyperhomocysteinemia; and protein C, protein S, and antithrombin deficiencies have also been implicated in obstetric complications including preeclampsia, fetal demise, and placental abruption. Thus, indications for screening for hereditary thrombophilias and for the presence of antiphospholipid antibodies include patients with recurrent fetal demise (≥ 3), and perhaps even severe preeclampsia if these early reports are confirmed in additional clinical trials. Hopefully, the increased awareness of hypercoagulability with pregnancy complications will lead to clinical trials designed to optimize safe and efficacious prophylaxis for these women.

Familiarity with the physiologic changes of pregnancy is also important when considering testing. Levels of free protein S can decline by 40% and protein C and factor VIII levels are elevated during pregnancy. Therefore, it is recommended that testing be performed 3 months after delivery. Molecular testing can be performed at any time.

The question of whether to screen patients who have idiopathic VTE for an occult malignancy is controversial. Extensive screening is costly and can be associated with potential morbidity. In addition, it is unclear if diagnosing the malignancy at the time of the presenting VTE would have a significant impact on cancer-related mortality or morbidity. In several studies, extensive screening has resulted in earlier detection of malignancies. Clinical clues that suggest an underlying occult malignancy include recurrent VTE in patients without a family history of VTE, recurrence or propagation of a DVT while on therapeutic warfarin, age younger than 45 years, and superficial as well as deep thrombophlebitis (Trousseau's syndrome). The most common tumors associated with hypercoagulable states are mucin-secreting adenocarcinomas (lung, gastrointestinal, and pancreas). Thus, abdominal computed tomography (CT) scans detect the majority of occult malignancies and should be considered in patients who present with idiopathic VTE. In most cases, the history, physical examination, laboratory evaluation, chest radiographs, stool guaiac, and routine cancer screening appropriate for age (ie, mammogram in women over 40, colonoscopy in patients over 50, and prostate specific antigen testing in men over 50) is sufficient to suggest the suspected malignancy.

The clinical signs and symptoms of DVT and PE have both a low sensitivity and specificity for the diagnoses. Thus, objective testing is always necessary to confirm the diagnosis. Autopsy experience and prophylaxis trials prove that a large percentage of patients remain asymptomatic. For these reasons, a high level of suspicion is also required.

B. Imaging Studies

1. Ultrasonography—For diagnosing DVT, the venogram remains the gold standard, although it is seldom used in the United States for this purpose. Instead, the cornerstone of diagnosis has become the venous ultrasound for diagnosing proximal DVT in the extremities. Because the clinical findings of DVT—pain, swelling, and erythema of the involved extremity—can be caused by many other etiologies, including superficial thrombophlebitis, cellulitis, ruptured muscle or tendon, muscle strain, ruptured popliteal cyst, vasculitis, lymphedema, and acute or chronic venous stasis, DVT is not confirmed in approximately 70% of patients in whom these classic signs and symptoms are present. Real-time B-mode ultrasound is the most common noninvasive test available in the United States.

This test is highly accurate for diagnosing proximal vein thrombosis, especially in the common femoral and popliteal veins in symptomatic patients. The test is fast, relatively inexpensive, widely available and has a sensitivity and specificity greater than 95% in several series involving symptomatic patients. Isolated calf vein thrombosis (approximately 10–15% of cases) may be missed by ultrasound and can propagate to the proximal veins approximately 25% of the time. Therefore, when using ultrasonography as the sole diagnostic method, serial testing over 7–10 days should be performed in patients with an initially normal test result and a moderate or high pretest probability (PTP) of DVT. Randomized studies have confirmed the safety of withholding anticoagulation therapy based on serial normal ultrasonograms with an acceptable 1.3% risk of developing VTE complications over 3 months of follow-up. Femoral vein DVT in the upper thigh may also be hard to visualize in some patients, and the sensitivity of ultrasound drops significantly (40–50%) in asymptomatic patients. Duplex ultrasonography adds Doppler imaging to standard compression criteria for diagnosing a thrombus. Doppler analysis allows for better imaging of the femoral vein and thus slightly improved sensitivity and specificity, but is more expensive, time-consuming, and operator dependent.

2. Ventilation-perfusion scans—The value of the ventilation perfusion (V̇/Q̇) scan in diagnosing acute PE was established by the PIOPED (Prospective Investigation of the Pulmonary Embolism Diagnosis) study. In this landmark study, 933 patients with suspected PE were studied prospectively by V̇/Q̇ scanning with 81% undergoing confirmatory pulmonary angiography. In this multicenter trial, central radiographic review was used to classify V̇/Q̇ scans as high probability, intermediate probability, low probability, and near normal/normal. Results of this trial confirmed the high positive predictive value associated with high-probability scans (88%), high negative predictive value of a near normal or normal scans (96%), and the importance of combining the V̇/Q̇ scan interpretation with a PTP or clinical assessment of the patient's likelihood of having a diagnosis of PE. The study also demonstrated that the positive predictive value of high probability scans was significantly lower in patients with a prior history of PE (74% compared with 91% in patients without a prior history of PE) and the need for additional diagnostic evaluation in patients with intermediate and low probability scans (Table 36–10). Subsequently, additional publications have strengthened the predictive power and reproducibility of the PIOPED results by further defining criteria for interpreting V̇/Q̇ scans as well as the PTP for PE (Table 36–11). Unfortunately, these studies have also confirmed that only a few subsets of

Table 36–10. Probability of PE determined by V̇/Q̇ scan plus clinical assessment.

V̇/Q̇ Scan Category	Clinical Assessment (PTP)		
	High	Moderate	Low
High probability	96–97%	84–88%	56–82%
Intermediate probability	45–66%	28–37%	16–25%
Low probability	21–40%	12–16%	4%
Near normal/normal	0%	0–6%	0–2%

PE, pulmonary embolism; V̇/Q̇, ventilation-perfusion; PTP, pretest probability.
(Adapted from PIOPED study.)

patients ie, those with normal perfusion scans, high probability V̇/Q̇ scans combined with high clinical suspicion, and low probability V̇/Q̇ scans combined with a low clinical suspicion (low PTP), have sufficient sensitivity and specificity to avoid further diagnostic testing. Thus, a significant proportion of patients who have a high or moderate PTP of PE will need additional testing for diagnosis.

Approximately 50–70% of patients with PE are found to have proximal DVTs. Thus, one approach for diagnosing PE in patients with indeterminate V̇/Q̇ scans is to perform bilateral noninvasive testing for proximal DVT. In this setting, a positive abnormal ultrasonogram suggests the need for anticoagulation therapy, which provides adequate therapy for both the DVT and presumed PE. An initial normal ultrasono-

Table 36–11. Model for predicting PTP for PE.

Clinical Feature	PTP Score
Signs or symptoms of DVT	+3
Pulse > 100 beats per minute	+1.5
Hemoptysis	+1
Active cancer	+1
Bedridden > 3 days or major surgery within 4 weeks	+1.5
History of prior PE or DVT	+1.5
PE is the most likely diagnosis	+3

PTP, pretest probability; PE, pulmonary embolism; DVT, deep venous thrombosis.
Score: < 2, low; 2–6, moderate; > 6, high.
(Adapted from Wells PS et al: Thromb Haemost 2000;83:416.)

gram indicates the need for additional testing. In patients with compromised cardiopulmonary status who are believed to be unsafe to send home without anticoagulation therapy, pulmonary angiography based on the perfusion scan results is reasonable to confirm or refute the diagnosis. In patients with reasonable cardiopulmonary function, repeated negative compression ultrasounds over the next 7–10 days is also considered a reasonable strategy with an acceptably low risk to the patient.

3. Spiral CT scans—Largely because of the inconvenience of obtaining V̇/Q̇ scans outside the normal working hours of the nuclear medicine department, spiral or helical CT scans have gained acceptance as an alternative method for diagnosing PE. Two systematic reviews of spiral CTs note methodologic problems in studies evaluating spiral CT for diagnosing PE, including failing to meet criteria for adequately evaluating sensitivity and specificity. Currently, there is no prospective study in which anticoagulation therapy is withheld based solely on a normal spiral CT, without further testing for VTE. Thus, the safety of withholding anticoagulation therapy in patients based on a normal spiral CT alone is uncertain.

Recently, 2 prospective studies testing the validity of spiral CT in the diagnosis of PE have been performed. In both of these studies, the sensitivity of spiral CT was found to be approximately 70%. In addition, the specificity was found to be between 84% and 91%. These studies also delineated the importance of the anatomic level of the PE when using spiral CT for diagnosis. The sensitivity of diagnosis with spiral CT was far greater when diagnosing thrombosis in segmental or larger vessels, and fell to only 21% when the thrombosis was lodged in a subsegmental pulmonary vessel. In addition, a significant false-positive rate of 38% was observed when evaluating segmental vessels as opposed to 0% in the main pulmonary arteries. Thus, from these recent prospective trials, it is possible to conclude that a normal spiral CT does not exclude PE, particularly in the subsegmental vessels. There are limited data on the safety of withholding treatment based on a normal result, and spiral CT should not be used as the sole diagnostic test when the only positive result is in a segmental artery or smaller. A positive spiral CT result in a lobar or main artery can probably be used alone as an indication for therapy.

C. LABORATORY FINDINGS

1. Initial laboratory tests—The initial laboratory evaluation should include a complete blood cell count, chemistries including renal and liver function panels, and baseline prothrombin time (PT) and APTT. Additional laboratory evaluation should be considered in subsets of patients including those in whom other risk factors do not exist, ie, idiopathic VTE. Candidates for testing for an inherited thrombophilia include those in whom the first thrombosis developed at a young age (younger than 50 years), who have recurrent thrombosis, who have thrombosis at an unusual site (ie, mesenteric, portal, or cerebral veins), who have a life-threatening event, and/or have a family history of VTE. Laboratory evaluation to determine the cause for the hypercoagulable state often aids in determining the choice and length of therapy and prophylaxis, risk of recurrence, and risk to family members.

Acute thromboembolic events can alter levels of the natural procoagulants and anticoagulants. Therefore, it is recommended that the initial laboratory evaluation (Table 36–12) be performed 3–6 months after the initial event when possible. In addition, heparin and coumadin can effect testing for inhibitors or deficiencies of the clotting system. In general, a normal test at the time of the acute VTE rules out a hereditary deficiency, but a low value necessitates confirmatory testing 3–6 months after the acute event. In addition, all functional studies of clotting factors or inhibitors should be confirmed over time prior to labeling a patient with a hereditary deficiency. Gene testing by PCR methods can be performed at any time and are not affected by acute events or therapies and thus seldom need to be repeated. Laboratory evaluation for hereditary thrombophilias can be an expensive endeavor with long-term consequences to the patient and their family, therefore consideration of risk factors, ethnicity, and timing is necessary for cost-effective testing (Table 36–13).

Table 36–12. Laboratory testing for hypercoagulable state.

Initial evaluation
  Activated protein C resistance/factor V Leiden mutation
  Prothrombin gene mutation
  Plasma homocysteine
  Factor VIII level
  Lupus anticoagulant (by 2 clotting based tests; ie, DRVVT and APTT)
  Anticardiolipin antibodies
If above negative, then test for deficiencies of the following:
  Protein C
  Protein S
  Antithrombin

DRVVT, dilute Russel's viper venom time; APTT, activated partial thromboplastin time.

2. D-dimer assay—Another recent test that has gained popularity in patients with suspected VTE is the D-dimer assay. Elevated D-dimer levels suggest ongoing clot formation and dissolution. The assay is most often used to stratify patients into high and low risk groups. Patients with elevated D-dimer levels are considered high risk and undergo further diagnostic radiographic studies to confirm a DVT or PE while patients with low PTP and normal D-dimer levels are assumed not to have a VTE, and other etiologies for their symptoms are pursued. Imperative in using the D-dimer assay is an understanding of the various types of assays currently available for D-dimer quantitation. D-dimer is a specific degradation product formed by cross-linked fibrin. There are currently 3 types of assays used in quantitating D-dimers. These include the ELISA, whole blood agglutination assay (simpliRED), and latex agglutination assay. Of these 3 assays, only the ELISA and whole blood agglutination assay have sufficient sensitivity for excluding DVT. First-generation latex agglutination tests should not be used for this purpose. Second-generation latex agglutination testing using automated microparticle assays have sufficient negative predictive value to exclude DVT. The popularity of D-dimer assays to exclude VTE primarily stems from the ease of obtaining results since the assay can be performed quickly at the bedside or in the coagulation laboratory. In addition, there are significant cost-savings compared with spiral CT, or even ultrasound, if the diagnosis can be excluded without additional testing.

In using the D-dimer assay in predicting VTE, it is important to realize that a positive test is not diagnostic of VTE, since it is a relatively nonspecific test. In addition, the D-dimer should only be used in the setting of a PTP assessment. The PTP divides patients into different categories, depending on their probability of having a VTE. As both the positive and negative predictive values of a diagnostic test are dependent on disease prevalence, the negative predictive value of the D-dimer assay is determined by the patient's PTP. The PTP assessment is based on the presenting signs and symptoms of the patient. In addition, it evaluates other risk factors such as cancer, immobilization, and major surgery, in determining a PTP of the patient having a VTE. Tables 36–11 and 36–14 show clinical models for both PE and DVT. Using these models, a low, moderate, or high PTP can be assigned to most patients on presentation to the emergency department. Once a PTP has been assigned, the negative predictive value of the various D-dimer assays can be determined. In general, a low PTP implies an approximately 5% probability of the patient having a VTE, compared with an approximately 25% probability in those with a moderate PTP, and an approximately

Table 36–13. Hypercoagulable testing.

Test	Cost ($US)	Coumadin	Heparin	Pregnancy	Liver Disease	Acute VTE
FV Leiden						
PCR based	87–290	NE	NE	NE	NE	NE
Clotting based[1]	21–71	NE	NE	NE	NE	NE
PT Gene PCR	84–280	NE	NE	NE	NE	NE
LAC						
DRVVT	14–49	Evaluable	Unevaluable	NE	Evaluable	NE
ACA	39–130	NE	NE	NE	NE	NE
Homocysteine	21–70	NE	NE	↓	NE	NE
Protein S						
Total	14–47	↓	NE	↓	↓	↓
Functional	40–134	↓	NE	↓	↓	↓
Protein C						
Total	14–47	↓	NE	NE or ↑	↓	↓
Antithrombin						
Enzymatic	24–80	↑/NE	↓	NE/↓	↓	↓
Antigenic	22–76	↑/NE	↓	NE/↓	↓	↓
Factor VIII		NE	NE	↑	↑	↑

VTE, venous thromboembolism; FV, factor V; PCR, polymerase chain reaction; PT, prothrombin; LAC, lupus anticoagulant; DRVVT, dilute Russel's viper venom time; ACA, anticardiolipin antibodies; NE, no effect.
↓, decreased; ↑, increased.
[1]Assumes use of factor V deficient plasma.

75% probability in patients with a high PTP. In the low PTP group, a negative D-dimer assay has approximately a 99% negative predictive value, which is comparable to serial Doppler ultrasounds or normal V̇/Q̇ scans. In patients with a moderate PTP, a negative D-dimer assay has a negative predictive value ranging from 93% to 98%, while in the high PTP group the negative predictive values falls to an unacceptable 60–87% range, without additional diagnostic testing (Table 36–15). For example, in cancer patients who have a relatively high PTP, negative D-dimer assays have a negative predictive value of < 80% compared with the 97–99% value in patients without cancer. Thus, understanding and calculating the PTP is crucial for interpreting the results of D-dimer assays.

Perrier A et al: Performance of helical computed tomography in unselected outpatients with suspected pulmonary embolism. Ann Intern Med 2001;135:88. [PMID: 11453707]

Value of the ventilation/perfusion scan in acute pulmonary embolism. Results of the prospective investigation of pulmonary embolism diagnosis (PIOPED). The PIOPED Investigators. JAMA 1990;263:2753. [PMID: 2332918]

Diagnosis

A. VTE DURING PREGNANCY

Diagnosing VTE is often difficult in the pregnant patient because leg swelling and pain are common complaints. One clinical clue is that pregnancy-related DVT most commonly involves the left iliofemoral veins (72%) and the left leg 90% of the time. Thus, the evaluation should start with an ultrasound of the left leg. If the ultrasound is normal and clinical suspicion is high, a limited venogram with abdominal shielding is indicated; this results in < 0.05 rads exposure to the fetus. If clinical suspicion is moderate, serial testing or a limited venogram are both reasonable options.

Table 36–14. Model for predicting pretest probability for DVT.

Clinical Feature	Score
Active cancer	+1
Paralysis, immobilization of LE	+1
Bedridden > 3 days	+1
Surgery within 4 weeks	+1
Localized tenderness along a venous distribution	+1
Entire leg swollen or > 4 cm swelling compared with asymptomatic leg	+1
Pitting edema	+1
Collateral superficial veins	+1
Alternative diagnosis as likely as DVT	–2

DVT, deep venous thrombosis; LE, lower extremity. Score: < 1, low; 1–2, moderate; > 2, high.
Adapted from Wells PS et al: Lancet 1997;350:1795.

D-dimers are almost always positive in pregnancy and are thus of little value in diagnosing pregnancy-related or puerperium VTE.

B. RECURRENT VTE

Diagnosing recurrent VTE is particularly challenging because post-phlebitic symptoms, including chronic swelling, pain, and leg discoloration, develop in 25–50% of patients. Because these signs and symptoms develop over months to years, distinguishing an evolving post-phlebitic syndrome from a recurrent VTE can be problematic. Risk factors for post-phlebitic syndrome include larger thrombus, more proximal thrombus, especially DVT involving the iliofemoral veins, obesity, and recurrent thromboses. In patients prone to

Table 36–15. Negative predictive value of D-dimer assay in diagnosing VTE based on PTP.

D-dimer Assay	Low PTP	Moderate PTP	High PTP
ELISA	99%	98%	87%
Whole blood agglutination assay	99%	93%	61%
2nd generation Latex agglutination assay	99%	98%	81%

VTE, venous thromboembolism; PTP, pretest probability; ELISA, enzyme-linked immunosorbent assay.

post-phlebitic symptoms as well as those with ongoing risk factors that increase the risk of recurrence (ie, hereditary thrombophilias and antiphospholipid antibody syndromes), it is reasonable, if not preferable, to obtain follow-up imaging studies at 3 and 6 months post DVT to document regression or persistence of the thrombus. A recurrent VTE often has important therapeutic consequences to the patient as it will necessitate a longer course, if not lifelong anticoagulation therapy, an increase in the targeted INR with a concomitant increase in bleeding complications, or a switch from coumadin to parenteral heparin therapy. Thus, it is often clinically important to differentiate between recurrent VTE and post-phlebitic syndrome. A new positive finding on either ultrasound or V/Q scan documents a new recurrence, but a positive result in an area that was previously positive and had never reverted to normal is inconclusive. A venogram can be helpful in documenting the appearance of an acute thrombus, but often the venogram will also be inconclusive, especially if there is no prior study for comparison. The D-dimer assay has recently been studied in this difficult patient population. Again, a baseline negative D-dimer assay 3 months after the initial VTE is important as well as calculating each patient's PTP. In 1 prospective study, a 100% negative predictive value was found in the group of patients with a low PTP and negative D-dimer assay (0/29 patients had a recurrent DVT over 3 months of follow-up), with a negative predictive value of 91% in the group as a whole.

van der Meer FJ et al: The Leiden Thrombophilia Study (LETS). Thromb Hemost 1997;78:631. [PMID: 9198229]

Wells PS et al: Value of assessment of pretest probability of deep-vein thrombosis in clinical management. Lancet 1997;350:1795. [PMID: 9428249]

Complications of VTE

Complications of VTE include death, recurrence, and post-phlebitic syndrome. A study of 355 patients with venography-proven DVT had an 8-year death rate of 30% with the highest mortality rate in the first year. A similar study of patients who presented with PE demonstrated a 1-year mortality rate of 23.1%. Surprisingly, recurrence of VTE accounts for a minority of deaths with only a small proportion of patients (~2%) dying of PE when appropriate doses of heparin and warfarin therapy are promptly initiated. The predominant cause of death in most studies is malignancy.

Post-Phlebitic Syndrome

Symptoms of post-phlebitic syndrome include skin discoloration, edema, leg swelling, difficulty walking, discomfort, and ulceration. The reported incidence varies but is typically between 25% and 50%, with larger, recurrent, and more proximal thromboses having a higher incidence. Ulceration occurs in approximately 2–10% of patients within 10 years after DVT. Compression stocking use after DVT can reduce development of post-phlebitic complications by 50%. Recently, small studies have reported that LMWHs are slightly superior to coumadin in reducing post-phlebitic complications.

Treatment

Treatment of proximal DVT and symptomatic or asymptomatic PE is generally similar. At presentation, all patients with moderate or high PTP should initially receive heparin until the diagnosis has been ruled out. If the diagnosis is confirmed, patients should be treated with either unfractionated heparin or LMWH.

A. HEPARIN

1. Unfractionated heparin—Unfractionated heparin can be administered as a continuous infusion or as a bolus subcutaneously administered injection on an every 12 hour schedule. In general, continuous intravenous infusion is the more common administration schedule because monitoring is easier, risk of bleeding lower, and therapeutic anticoagulation more dependably obtained. Maintaining therapeutic anticoagulation is the most important factor for preventing recurrent VTE. Therapeutic heparin levels have been determined in animal models as a plasma heparin concentration between 0.2 and 0.4 IU/mL by protamine titration. As this test is not readily available in most coagulation laboratories, the APTT is the most commonly used test for monitoring heparin. In general, an APTT greater than 1.5 times the control value corresponds to a plasma heparin level of 0.2 IU/mL. Several studies have verified

the effectiveness of weight-based normograms or protocols for monitoring and maintaining heparin in the therapeutic range. These protocols are generally based on frequent APTT monitoring (every 6 hours until stable), rapid APTT turn-around time, and immediate changes in heparin dosing based on the obtained APTT during the first few days of heparin therapy. An example of one such protocol is Table 36–16.

2. Low-molecular-weight heparins—LMWHs are the newest class of drugs to be approved for inpatient and outpatient therapy of DVT and PE. Over the last several years, they have come to supplant the use of unfractionated heparin in these disease states. Currently there are 3 LMWHs that are FDA-approved and commercially available in the United States: enoxaparin (Lovenox), dalteparin (Fragmin), and tinzaparin (Innohep). Heparins are a heterogeneous group of glycosaminoglycans, consisting of alternating saccharide residues of uronic acid and glucosamine. Heparins function by binding to antithrombin and increasing antithrombin's inhibition of thrombin and factor Xa. A pentasaccharide fragment of heparin is essential for interacting with antithrombin and inhibiting activated factor X. Longer polysaccharide molecules of over 16 saccharide units are necessary to enhance antithrombin's inhibition of thrombin. Thus, unfractionated heparins inhibit thrombin and activated factor X equally, while LMWHs are composed of shorter polysaccharide fragments that preferentially inhibit activated factor X. Because of the more homogenous, shorter structure of LMWHs, they have more uniform bioavailability, excretion, and decreased binding to platelets, endothelial cells, and monocytes compared with unfractionated heparin. These properties lead to a preferable pharmacokinetic profile whereby LMWHs can be safely administered subcutaneously on either a once or twice a day basis without routine monitoring of the APTT, or anti-

Table 36–16. Example of a heparin protocol.

Initial unfractionated heparin dosing: Loading dose 80 IU/kg, maintenance infusion to start at 18 IU/kg/h			
APTT (sec)	**Dose Change U/kg/h**	**Additional Action**	**Next APTT h[1]**
< 35 (< 1.2 × mean normal)	+4	Rebolus with 80 IU/kg	6
35–45 (1.2–1.5 × mean normal)	+2	Rebolus with 40 IU/kg	6
46–70 (1.5–2.3 × mean normal)	0	0	6
71–90 (2.3–3.0 × mean normal)	–2	0	6
> 90 (> 3.0 × mean normal)	–3	Stop infusion x 1 h	6

APTT, activated partial thromboplastin time.
[1]Repeat APTT every 6 hours for the first 24 hours and then every morning if therapeutic.

Xa levels. In fact, the plasma level of anti-Xa activity does not appear to correlate with antithrombotic effectiveness in either animal models or human clinical trials. Thus, anti-Xa monitoring is not recommended except when treating special populations. Because of their preferential anti-Xa effects, neither the PT or APTT are reliable measures of the anticoagulant effects of LMWHs. In addition, unlike unfractionated heparin, which can be neutralized by protamine sulfate, LMWHs are only partially to minimally effected by protamine and currently no antidote is available for excessive anticoagulation or bleeding. Thus, in patients with higher risks of bleeding, unfractionated heparin is the safer anticoagulant choice.

There are in vitro and in vivo differences that can be demonstrated among the LMWH products with regard to neutralization by protamine sulfate, half-life elimination, and tissue factor pathway inhibitor (TFPI) release. For these reasons, different LMWHs should not be used interchangeably, and dosing must be administered at the recommended dose for each particular drug product. Differences between the LMWHs are also found with regard to antithrombin activity. To date, no clinical trial of DVT treatment or orthopedic prophylaxis that has directly compared 2 different LMWH preparations has found a significant difference in the incidence of death or recurrent VTE. However, most of these studies have been small and underpowered to show minor differences between the LMWH preparations, and it is doubtful that sufficiently large clinical trials will be performed to differentiate between these agents. Consequently, evidence-based literature supports the use of each LMWH only at the FDA-approved indication and dose.

Multiple prospective, randomized trials have now been published verifying the safety and efficacy of LMWHs as outpatient or inpatient therapy for DVT or asymptomatic PE or inpatient therapy for symptomatic PE. While these studies generally show parity between LMWH and inpatient continuous infusion therapy with unfractionated heparin, meta-analyses have consistently shown slightly improved outcomes with respect to VTE recurrence, major bleeding, and thrombocytopenia in favor of LMWHs. Pharmacoeconomic analyses have also shown that outpatient therapy with LMWHs offers substantial cost-savings over inpatient therapy with unfractionated heparin. This is true even after accounting for the 5- to 10-fold increased cost of LMWHs and the added expense of home health visits for close follow-up of patients discharged immediately from the emergency department. An estimated 70% of patients qualify for outpatient VTE therapy using standardized selection criteria and protocols, significant health cost savings are possible (Tables 36–17 and 36–18).

Table 36–17. Outpatient management of VTE.

Suspicion of VTE
CBC with platelet count, PT/PTT at baseline
IV heparin bolus 5000 U
Initiate testing for VTE (ie, Doppler scans of LE, ventilation–perfusion scan)
Start LMWH
Start coumadin 5 mg/d (if not at increased risk of bleeding)
Arrange for outpatient PT/INR and platelet count monitoring on days 3 and 5
Evaluate patient in follow-up at day 5 or 7
Stop LMWH when INR > 2 on 2 consecutive readings

VTE, venous thromboembolism; CBC, complete blood cell; PT, prothrombin time; PTT, partial thromboplastin time; LE, lower extremity; LMWH, low-molecular-weight heparin; INR, International normalized ratio.

B. INITIATING ORAL WARFARIN THERAPY

Warfarin should be initiated on day 1 after achieving therapeutic doses of LMWH or unfractionated heparin. The rationale for initiating warfarin therapy as soon as possible is to limit the time on heparin, and consequently reduce the chance of developing heparin-induced thrombocytopenia (HIT). Thus, unless there is a contraindication to warfarin therapy, it should be initiated within 24 hours of starting heparin therapy. The initial dose of warfarin should generally be 5 mg/d. This dose should be adjusted according to the INR response. Daily and baseline INRs should be obtained during the initiation of warfarin therapy until a stable INR and dose is determined. The use of a higher warfarin loading

Table 36–18. Exclusion/inclusion criteria for outpatient management of VTE.

Does patient have a proven DVT?
If so, are there contraindications to anticoagulation or history of HIT?
If not, does patient require inpatient therapy?
Extensive iliofemoral DVT
Concomitant symptomatic PE
Concomitant disease (ie, CHF, CRF)
History of GI bleed, bleeding diathesis, heme positive stool
Noncompliant, homeless, injecting drug abuser, alcoholic
Home resources, drug unavailable
If yes to any question except number 1, then inpatient therapy is recommended.

VTE, venous thromboembolism; DVT, deep venous thrombosis; HIT, heparin-induced thrombocytopenia; PE, pulmonary embolism; CHF, congestive heart failure; CRF, chronic renal failure; GI, gastrointestinal.

dose appears unnecessary—and may even be contraindicated—because large warfarin loading doses have been associated with excessive early anticoagulation and precipitous declines in protein C, which may be associated with coumadin necrosis and a transient acquired hypercoagulable state. In addition, there are no data suggesting that a higher warfarin loading dose shortens the time required to achieve a stable and/or therapeutic INR. In some patient populations, a lower initial warfarin dose of 2–3 mg/d should be used, including those patients with a history of protein C or S deficiency, liver dysfunction, or after heart valve replacement.

The effectiveness and safety of warfarin is largely based on maintaining the INR in a therapeutic range. Anticoagulation clinics have been shown to be superior to individual practitioner monitoring or physician-directed care. Self-management by patients using portable monitors has also been shown to be effective with an increase in the time in the therapeutic range compared with physician-directed monitoring. In addition, patients expressed increased satisfaction with the use of self-testing and self-management of warfarin in several clinical trials comparing patient self-management to anticoagulation clinics or physician-directed care.

C. Anticoagulation in Special Populations

1. Antiphospholipid antibodies—Patients with antiphospholipid antibodies and thrombotic complications require long-term anticoagulant therapy because they have high rates of recurrence (up to 80%) in several series. Monitoring of therapy can be difficult as the clotting-based tests used may be prolonged due to the antiphospholipid antibodies. In this situation, the risk of thrombosis may be increased if anticoagulation is not adequate. In patients who present with a VTE and a prolonged APTT, LMWHs are an excellent choice for initial anticoagulation therapy since monitoring is not required. Unfractionated heparin therapy can be monitored with an anti-Xa heparin assay. In patients with baseline prolonged prothrombin times, warfarin therapy can be monitored by determining factor X levels (targeting a FX level of 15–20%). Patients with antiphospholipid antibodies and a prolonged PT should also be screened for acquired factor II deficiency, which has been described in this patient population and associated with increased bleeding risks.

2. Renal insufficiency—Heparin is cleared from the circulation by 2 mechanisms. The first results in rapid clearance of heparin from the blood in a dose-dependent and saturable manner as a result of heparin binding to plasma proteins and blood cells. The second mechanism is slower through elimination by the kidney. Thus, lower doses of heparin are cleared more rapidly and clearance is variable between individuals. LMWHs undergo predominantly renal elimination as

they bind far less to plasma proteins and blood cells. Consequently, renal insufficiency is a relative contraindication to LMWH use without additional anti-factor Xa monitoring. In all large trials to date using LMWH as therapy for DVT in an inpatient or outpatient setting, patients with creatinine clearance less than 30 mL/min have been excluded. In smaller trials of LMWHs in patients with varying levels of renal insufficiency, plasma half-life is prolonged and clearance decreased even in patients with mild renal insufficiency as defined by creatinine clearance of 50–80 mL/min or serum creatinine greater than 2 mg/dL. Thus, anti-factor Xa levels should be available in real-time when administering LMWHs at therapeutic doses to patients with renal insufficiency to avoid increased anticoagulant effects and prevent excessive bleeding. General recommendations include obtaining anti-factor Xa levels 4 hours after the third morning dose of the LMWH and adjusting the dose targeting the anti-factor Xa level to 0.5–1.0 IU/mL with every 12-hour dosing and 1–2 IU/mL with once daily dosing. The LMWH dose should be adjusted up or down by 20% with retesting after 3 doses as required. If anti-factor Xa levels are not available expeditiously, unfractionated heparin with standard APTT monitoring should be used in treating patients with renal insufficiency.

3. Obesity—Obese patients are another special population when considering inpatient or outpatient weight-based therapy with LMWHs. To date, trials have treated patients at their actual body weight up to 150 kg. Mean trough anti-factor Xa levels have been poorly correlated with body weight and thus decisions on dosing patients over 150 kg is controversial. In morbidly obese patients, real-time monitoring of anti-factor Xa levels is recommended when administering weight-based LMWHs until further safety and efficacy data are available for this group of patients. Treatment with unfractionated heparin with standard APTT monitoring is currently the preferred option in patients with morbid obesity.

4. Pregnancy—Heparin in always the drug of choice as an anticoagulant during pregnancy. Warfarin is a known teratogen, especially during the 6th to 12th week of gestation. Because warfarin crosses the placenta, it can also cause significant bleeding in the fetus and neonate. Warfarin is not secreted in breast milk and thus is safe to administer after delivery. Heparin is safe throughout the pregnancy and postpartum period; it does not cross the placenta and is not secreted in breast milk. The main risks associated with heparin use during pregnancy include an increased risk of osteoporosis and a 2% incidence of clinical bleeding. As plasma volume and plasma proteins change throughout pregnancy, monitoring is required during each trimester to ensure adequate anticoagulation. In general, requirements for heparin increase as the pregnancy progresses. Heparin should be stopped 24 hours prior to inducing labor and can be reinitiated 6 hours postpartum if the patient is clinically and hemodynamically stable. In cases of emergent delivery, APTT monitoring for unfractionated heparin should be used and protamine administered to reverse anticoagulant effects of unfractionated heparin.

In the most recent American College of Chest Physicians (ACCP) consensus conference on antithrombotic therapy, LMWHs were recommended for the first time as an anticoagulation option for pregnant patients requiring prophylaxis (prior history of VTE, thrombophilia, increased risk of pregnancy loss) or treatment of acute VTE. While there have been no randomized trials comparing unfractionated heparin and LMWH in pregnant women, there have been small trials suggesting LMWHs may have equal efficacy and a lower risk of osteoporosis associated with their use. LMWH dosing also must be monitored during pregnancy as clearance increases as the pregnancy progresses. Therefore, when administering weight-based LMWH for treating acute VTE, anti-factor Xa levels should be monitored 4 hours after the morning dose to achieve an anti-Xa level of 0.5–1.2 U/mL. LMWH should also be stopped 24 hours prior to inducing labor or initiating epidural or spinal anesthesia. Unlike the situation with unfractionated heparin, LMWHs are only partially reversed with protamine sulfate and no antidote exists for emergent anticoagulant reversal. Thus, many obstetricians favor switching patients from LMWH to unfractionated heparin late in the third trimester.

Importantly, LMWHs are contraindicated in pregnant patients with mechanical heart valves as several deaths secondary to valve thrombosis have recently been reported. Prophylaxis of pregnant women with mechanical heart valves is a particularly vexing problem. Warfarin targeting an INR of 3.0 appears to be the most effective agent in the European literature, but increases the risk of an embryopathy. Subcutaneous unfractionated heparin with twice a day dosing is a reasonable alternative but needs to be administered at adequate doses (ie, targeting the 6-h postinjection APTT to at least twice control), monitored throughout the pregnancy, and significantly increases bone loss during the pregnancy.

How best to treat patients with antiphospholipid antibodies and recurrent fetal loss is another controversial area. Prednisone seems to offer no benefit. Current strategies from small trials suggest the addition of aspirin plus unfractionated heparin or LMWH at prophylactic doses improves fetal survival, decreases maternal complications, and does not significantly increase the risk of hemorrhage.

D. THROMBOLYTIC THERAPY

Thrombolytic agents directly activate plasminogen to plasmin which then lyses fibrin in the thrombus. This leads to a more rapid dissolution of clots, hemodynamic improvement after massive PE, and decreased pain and swelling in the thrombosed extremity. Multiple trials have documented improved lysis of the thrombus after treatment with a thrombolytic agent compared with heparin therapy alone, but none has shown an improvement in mortality. Because of the consistent 1–2% rate of intracranial hemorrhage associated with thrombolytics and the lack of a survival advantage associated with their use, thrombolytic therapy is generally reserved for patients with hemodynamically significant PE or younger patients with massive ileofemoral DVT in an effort to prevent severe post-phlebitic syndromes. Absolute contraindications to thrombolytic therapy include recent surgery and known bleeding disorders with relative contraindications including older age, hypertension, and recent aspirin use. Three thrombolytic regimens are currently approved for use in PE (Table 36–19). Monitoring is generally not required for tissue plasminogen activator (tPA) therapy. For streptokinase or urokinase infusions, a prolongation of the thrombin time or APTT by 10 seconds 2–4 hours after starting the infusion is recommended. It is considered safe to initiate intravenous heparin therapy once the thrombin time or APTT is less than 2 times normal.

D. INFERIOR VENA CAVA FILTERS

For patients with an absolute contraindication to anticoagulation or with recurrent PE despite adequate anticoagulation, placement of an inferior vena cava (IVC) filter should be considered. Other possible indications for IVC filters include massive hemodynamically compromising PE and surgical pulmonary embolectomy. The most common IVC interruption is the Greenfield filter, which is inserted via the internal jugular or

Table 36–19. Thrombolytic regimens for pulmonary embolism.

Agent	Regimen
Streptokinase	250,000 IU loading dose over 30 min followed by 100,000 IU/h for 24 h
Urokinase	4400 IU/kg loading dose over 10 min followed by 2200 IU/kg/h for 12 h
Tissue plasminogen activator	100 mg continuous IV infusion over 2h

femoral vein and then advanced into the IVC under ultrasonic or fluoroscopic guidance. In a prospective randomized study, IVC filters were effective in reducing the rate of PE following a DVT in the first 3 months following diagnosis. Unfortunately, the initial protection afforded by IVC filters was counterbalanced by a subsequent increased rate of recurrent thrombotic complications at and distal to the IVC filter. Thus, in patients who undergo IVC filter placement, indefinite anticoagulation should be strongly considered, particularly in patients with only a transient contraindication to anticoagulation therapy.

F. SUPERFICIAL AND CALF VEIN THROMBOSIS

Patients with symptomatic calf vein thrombosis should generally receive therapeutic anticoagulation with heparin followed by warfarin therapy for 3–6 months. For patients with increased bleeding risks, anticoagulation therapy can be withheld and serial ultrasounds performed over the following 10–14 days to exclude proximal clot propagation requiring full dose anticoagulation.

In patients with physical examinations suggestive of a superficial thrombophlebitis, ultrasound examination should be performed to rule out involvement of the deep venous system. In particular, thrombosis of the greater saphenous vein can be associated with extension into the common femoral vein in 10% of patients with complications including documented PE. Symptomatic therapy with nonsteroidal anti-inflammatory drugs and warm soaks is usually sufficient in patients without additional risk factors or involvement of the deep veins. Recurrent episodes suggest the presence of an underlying malignancy or hereditary thrombophilia (ie, FV Leiden) and additional testing should be initiated.

G. COMPLEMENTARY THERAPY

Many medications, including prescription and over-the-counter (including alternative therapies), interact with coumadin to either counteract or potentiate its anticoagulant effect, resulting in potential thrombosis or bleeding, respectively. Coumadin has a narrow therapeutic index and is metabolized extensively through the P-450 system. Thus, the addition of almost any agent can effect its metabolism and the INR. Mechanisms of interaction include reduced clotting factor synthesis, competitive antagonism (vitamin K), enzyme induction, and enzyme inhibition. Some drugs may act by more than 1 mechanism. The majority of patients using alternative therapies do not report this to their health care providers. Therefore, it is critical to obtain a thorough medication history including herbal remedies prior to institution of oral anticoagulant therapy and during anticoagulation monitoring. Patients should also be instructed not to initiate any therapies, including over-the-counter without discussion. In addition, monitoring of the INR should be obtained upon any change in medication usage (addition, discontinuation, or change in dosage). The true risks of adverse interactions of warfarin with many herbal remedies are unknown because most of these are anecdotal. Potential and documented interactions of herbal remedies with coumadin are listed in Table 36–20.

As previously described, hyperhomocysteinemia is a risk factor for arterial and venous thrombosis. Two thirds of all cases are associated with vitamin deficiencies in folate, vitamin B_{12}, or vitamin B_6. Cigarette smoking, hypothyroidism, and OCPs are known to alter the bioavailability of these vitamins and thus may lead to hyperhomocysteinemia. In 1996, the FDA required that enriched grain foods be fortified with folic acid (140 µg/100 g) in an effort to decrease the incidence of congenital neural tube defects. Following this mandate, there has been a 48% reduction in the number of people with high homocysteine levels (> 13 µmol/L). Elevated levels of homocysteine can be reduced in most patients by supplementation of vitamins involved in methionine metabolism. Daily recommended vitamin supplementation for decreasing plasma homocysteine levels are 1–5 mg of folic acid, 0.4 mg of hydroxycobalamin (vitamin B_{12}), and 15–50 mg of pyridoxine (vitamin B_6).

Table 36–20. Herbal remedies with potential warfarin interaction.

Possible increase in warfarin's effects	
Arnica	Devil's claw
Astragalus	Dong quai
Black cohosh	Feverfew
Cholestin	Papain
Danshen	Vitamin E

Possible decrease in warfarin's effects	
Coenzyme Q	Guar Gum
Ginseng	Physillium
Goldenseal	St. John's Wort
Green Tea	

Potential increase in risk of bleeding		
Angelica root	Chamomile	Parsley
Arnica flower	Clove	Passionflower herb
Anise	Fenugreek	Poplar
Asafoetida	Garlic	Quassia
Bogbean	Ginkgo	Red Clover
Borage seed oil	Goldenseal	Rue
Bromelain	Horse chestnut	Sweet clover
Capsicum	Licorice root	Turmeric
Celery	Lovage root	Willow bark

Gould MK et al: Low-molecular-weight heparins compared with unfractionated heparin for treatment of acute deep venous thrombosis. A meta-analysis of randomized controlled trials. Ann Intern Med 1999;130:800. [PMID: 10366369]

Heck AM, Dewitt BA, Lukes AL: Potential interactions between alternative therapies and warfarin. Am J Health Syst Pharm 2000;57:1221. [PMID: 10902065]

Complications of Therapy

A. HEPARIN-INDUCED THROMBOCYTOPENIA

The most catastrophic complication of heparin therapy and perhaps the most important drug-induced thrombocytopenia that clinicians must treat is HIT. HIT is classified as 2 distinct entities: HIT I and HIT II. The benign, usually asymptomatic form (HIT I) is seen within 1–5 days of initiating heparin therapy and is characterized by a mild thrombocytopenia (≤ 20% drop in baseline platelet count). This form of HIT occurs in about 10–20% of patients exposed to heparin and is self-limiting, benign, and requires no therapy.

HIT II is potentially life-threatening and frequently associated with venous and arterial thrombosis when unrecognized and untreated. As there is no easily available test for conclusively diagnosing this type of HIT, recognizing the clinical scenario is most important for treating patients and preventing morbidity and mortality. HIT should be suspected in patients in whom thrombocytopenia develops while receiving heparin or with a history of recent heparin use. HIT II can develop with any heparin administration, including subcutaneous and catheter flushes. In general, intravenous therapy has a greater incidence than subcutaneous administration, bovine heparin appears to be more immunogenic than porcine, and this complication develops more commonly in patients receiving heparin after orthopedic surgeries rather than patients hospitalized for nonsurgical admissions. LMWH also has a decreased incidence of HIT compared with unfractionated heparin. When using porcine unfractionated heparin there is an approximately 4- to 7-fold increased risk of HIT compared with LMWH (3–5% vs 0.75%).

HIT II typically develops 5–11 days after initiating heparin therapy unless the patient has had recent previous exposure to heparin, in which case thrombocytopenia may be evident within hours. The thrombocytopenia is more severe with platelet counts less than 100,000/μL or decreased 50% from baseline although the median platelet count tends to be 50,000–60,000/μL. HIT II is immunologically mediated and is due to antibodies (usually IgG) reactive against a complex of heparin and platelet factor 4 (PF4). Binding of the HIT antibody to PF4-heparin complexes results in platelet activation via platelet Fc gamma receptors. The activated platelets bind fibrinogen, recruit other platelets, and initiate primary clot formation. Endothe-lial cells can also be activated by the HIT antibody to express tissue factor, generate thrombin, and further trigger the clotting cascade. HIT II is different from other immunologically mediated thrombocytopenias in that hemorrhage rarely develops. In a study of postoperative orthopedic patients treated with unfractionated heparin, HIT developed in 5% of patients, with approximately half of these patients suffering HIT-associated thrombosis. The mortality rate associated with untreated HIT is approximately 30% with a 50% morbidity rate.

Treatment of HIT II includes stopping all heparin exposure (line flushes, heparin-coated catheters, and prophylactic and therapeutic heparin) as well as initiating antithrombin therapy. Exposure to less than 10 U of heparin per day is usually sufficient to sustain the thrombocytopenia and risk for thrombosis. Platelet counts generally normalize within 7–10 days after the cessation of heparin and tend to rise more quickly in patients treated with antithrombin therapies. The risk of new thromboembolic events falls rapidly as the platelet count rises. Warfarin therapy alone is contraindicated as it leads to a precipitous fall in protein C levels and a transient imbalance between procoagulant and anticoagulant proteins. Progressive thrombosis and even skin necrosis and venous limb gangrene have been described in this setting. LMWH is likewise contraindicated as there is a high degree of cross-reactivity (90%) with unfractionated heparin that may lead to persistent or recurrent thrombocytopenia and thrombosis. VTE is the most common thrombotic complication, but arterial thrombosis can also be seen, particularly in areas of recent vascular trauma. Some experts propose screening patients with clinically suspected HIT for DVT of the lower extremities using objective imaging modalities to rule out subclinical disease. Despite discontinuing heparin, a thromboembolic event will ultimately develop in 50% of patients with serologically confirmed HIT if left untreated. Thus, all patients with suspected or diagnosed HIT should receive antithrombin therapy as outlined in Table 36–21. Currently, argatroban and hirudin are the only FDA-approved therapies for HIT. Danaparoid has been used extensively in Europe and Canada and has the advantage of being available in subcutaneous as well as intravenous, and prophylactic as well as therapeutic dosing. In general, patients who present with VTE and HIT should receive therapeutic dosing while patients who present without a VTE and HIT can be treated with prophylactic doses of danaparoid to prevent VTE occurrence. In patients with newly diagnosed VTE who will need at least 3 months of anticoagulation therapy, warfarin therapy can be initiated after full dose anticoagulation has been achieved with either hirudin or argatroban. Both of these agents effect PT monitoring of warfarin and thus the warfarin

Table 36–21. Anticoagulants safely used in heparin-induced thrombocytopenia.

Agent	Route	Loading Dose	Maintenance Dose	Clearance	Monitoring
Danaparoid (therapeutic)	IV	2250 U bolus followed by 400 U/h × 4 h, then 300 U/h × 4 h (for people 50–90 kg)	150–200 U/h (anti-Xa levels 0.5–0.8 U/mL if monitoring)	Renal	None
Danaparoid (prophylaxis)	SC	750 U/kg q12h or q8h		Renal	None
Argatroban[1]	IV	2 µg/kg/min	To maintain APTT 1.5–3.0 × baseline (not to exceed 100s)	Liver	Yes INR
Hirudin[1]	IV	0.4 mg/kg bolus	0.15 mg/kg/h to maintain APTT 1.5–2.5 × normal	Renal	Yes INR

APTT, activated partial thromboplastin time.
[1]FDA-approved.

dose needs to be adjusted per the algorithm included in each package insert. Hirudin and danaparoid dosing should be adjusted in patients with renal insufficiency and argatroban dosing adjusted in patients with significant liver dysfunction.

Thrombocytopenia can occur rapidly in patients with a history of prior HIT or heparin exposure due either to residual circulating HIT antibodies or an anamnestic antibody response. It is believed that the antibodies formed during previous exposure, within the last 100 days, are the cause of rapid-onset HIT. However, if over 100 days has lapsed since the last exposure to heparin, the HIT antibody appears to disappear and thus clinically significant antibodies will not be formed for 5 days. Some experts in HIT have tested this hypothesis in patients requiring cardiopulmonary bypass surgery and brief heparin exposure. In these patients, it appears to be safe to proceed with a brief heparin exposure, ie, during cardiac or vascular surgery, if a preoperative ELISA test for HIT antibodies is negative and alternative anticoagulation is started after the surgery.

B. HEMORRHAGIC RISKS AND REVERSAL OF ANTICOAGULATION

Bleeding is the major complication of anticoagulation therapy and is directly related to the level of the INR or APTT. The risk of bleeding associated with heparin therapy increases with dose and with concurrent thrombolytic therapy or antiplatelet therapy. In addition, bleeding has been shown to be higher in patients with the following risk factors: trauma, recent surgery (within last 10 days), history of bleeding disorders, advanced age, recent stroke, and hypertension. Rapid neutralization of unfractionated heparin can be achieved by intravenous administration of protamine sulfate. Protamine, a cationic protein derived from fish sperm, binds avidly to the strongly anionic heparin. Each milligram of pro-

tamine can reverse 100 U of heparin. Calculation of the appropriate dose of protamine is based on the amount of unfractionated heparin given in the preceding few hours assuming a half-life of heparin of 60 minutes. Neutralization of subcutaneously administered heparin may require repeated protamine injections. Protamine may cause transient hypotension, particularly when given rapidly. Normalization of the APTT and thrombin time are used to verify neutralization.

The risk of hemorrhage associated with oral anticoagulants is related to intensity of anticoagulation, patient characteristics, drug interactions, and length of therapy.

Levels of the INR > 4.0–4.5 are particularly associated with higher risks of bleeding. The most common reasons for excessive anticoagulation include interference by concomitant medications, particularly antibiotics and over-the-counter herbal remedies, the presence of comorbid illnesses, particularly congestive heart failure and renal failure, dietary changes, and viral illnesses associated with diarrhea. Patients who are currently receiving warfarin therapy and who have an elevated INR should be evaluated for active bleeding. Patients with active or major bleeding should receive fresh frozen plasma (FFP) in combination with intravenous vitamin K. In patients who have a prolonged INR but are without signs of active bleeding, the warfarin should be withheld and oral vitamin K should be administered at a dose dependent on the INR level. In patients who need prolonged anticoagulation on warfarin, small doses of vitamin K (ie, 1 mg) are often sufficient to rapidly correct the INR yet allow for warfarin therapy to be reinitiated quickly and effectively. Responses to oral or intravenous vitamin K can be observed as quickly as 8–12 hours but are typically seen within 24 hours of administration. Further decreases in the INR may occur over the next 48 hours after administration of a single vitamin K dose. Vitamin K may be administered intravenously, subcutaneously, or orally. Intravenous vitamin K rapidly and reliably reduces INR values. Complications of intravenous vitamin K therapy include anaphylaxis, warfarin resistance, and skin reactions. Adverse reactions are more common with higher doses of intravenously administered vitamin K. Rarely is it necessary to intravenously administer more than 1–2 mg of vitamin K slowly, over 30 minutes. Subcutaneous vitamin K appears to be less effective than either oral or intravenously administered drug.

Orally administered vitamin K is not associated with anaphylactoid or skin reactions. In a trial of 92 patients with INR values between 4.5 and 10, patients had their warfarin held and were randomized to receive 1 mg of oral vitamin K versus placebo. Of the patients receiving the vitamin K, 56% had an INR between 1.8 and 3.2, 24 hours following study drug. Only 20% of placebo patients who held their coumadin therapy obtained an INR value within this range. In addition, none of the patients who received oral vitamin K had an increase in their INR, compared with 9% of the placebo group. Higher doses of oral vitamin K need to be administered to patients with cholestatic liver disease and elevated INRs, and oral doses up to 20 mg have been used effectively in these patients.

In patients with catastrophic hemorrhage secondary to excess warfarin anticoagulation, prothrombin complex concentrates can be used. Prothrombin complex concentrates have a more rapid and complete reversal of warfarin-induced anticoagulation compared with FFP. In addition, they do not carry the fluid consequences of several units of FFP and can be administered rapidly, as they do not require thawing. The use of prothrombin complex concentrates has been limited secondary to fears of thrombotic complications. Thrombotic complications are thought to be secondary to activated clotting factors contained in the concentrates that are not cleared efficiently, particularly in patients with liver dysfunction.

If oral anticoagulation therapy is discontinued temporarily, 5–7 days is required for the INR to normalize. Despite normalization of the INR, depression of other coagulation factors (especially factors II and X which have longer half-lives) often still exist, and thus normal hemostasis may still be impaired. There is also substantial variation between individuals depending on their liver function and age, which may also affect the fall of their INR and normalization of hemostasis.

Hemorrhagic skin necrosis is due to the short half-life of protein C relative to that of the other vitamin K clotting factors II, VII, IX, and X. This may result in a period of hypercoagulability that lasts until the activities of these factors fall. Skin necrosis can be seen in pa-

tients with an underlying protein C or S deficiency, antithrombin deficiency, lupus anticoagulants, and those who receive high loading doses of warfarin. If skin necrosis develops on coumadin, the drug should be discontinued immediately and heparin started.

Despite the many limitations of warfarin therapy—including the need for close monitoring, numerous drug and dietary interactions, and variability between patients—the increasing indications for long-term anticoagulation, ease of oral administration, and inexpensiveness of the drug suggests warfarin therapy will remain the mainstay of long-term anticoagulation for at least the next several years. Alternative antithrombotic agents, including oral antithrombins and oral heparins, are currently being tested in the clinic. These agents have several advantages over coumadin including the lack of necessity for monitoring, inconsequential dietary or medication interactions, and they are not metabolized by the P-450 system. Several large clinical trials are currently evaluating oral antithrombins in both the prophylaxis and treatment settings. These agents hold high promise if their clinical efficacy is proven and their costs are not prohibitive.

Duration of Anticoagulation after Initial VTE

The risk of recurrent VTE is highest within the first year after diagnosis. Treatment reduces the risk but does not eliminate it. A study published in 1995 observed 902 patients with DVT for 2 years and found a 13.7% VTE recurrence rate. There was a significant difference in VTE recurrence based on length of oral anticoagulation therapy with 6 months (9.5% recurrence rate) being superior to 6 weeks (18.1% recurrence rate) of warfarin therapy. Shortening the duration of anticoagulation from the standard 3–6 months to 4–6 weeks is associated with at least a 2-fold increase in the risk of recurrent VTE. This increased risk of VTE recurrence occurs even in patients whose risk factor for thrombosis was transient and reversible, ie, surgery. Patients who have a continuing risk factor for thrombosis are at an even higher risk for recurrence than patients who have a transient or reversible risk factor.

The optimal duration of anticoagulation for patients after an initial idiopathic VTE is also controversial. In a study published by Kearon et al, patients with a first episode of idiopathic VTE were treated with 3 months of warfarin and then randomized to an additional 2 years of placebo or warfarin therapy targeting an INR of 2.5. The study was terminated prematurely at the interim analysis when a statistically significant decrease in recurrent VTE was observed in the group receiving prolonged coumadin therapy. Seventeen patients, or 27.4% per patient-year in the placebo group had recurrent VTE compared with only 1 patient (1.3% per patient-year) in the coumadin-treated group. Extended coumadin therapy had resulted in a 95% reduction in the risk of recurrent VTE. The risk of major bleeding was slightly increased in the extended coumadin therapy group (3.8% vs 0% per year in the patients receiving placebo). Other studies have also documented a rebound increase in the recurrence rate of VTE after discontinuing anticoagulation therapy after 3, 6, or even 12 months of therapy.

In patients with a known thrombophilia, the risk of recurrence seems to be significantly higher in patients with an acquired antiphospholipid antibody or LAC-type inhibitor. The recurrence rate associated with the more common hereditary thrombophilias, heterozygous FV Leiden or prothrombin gene mutation, appears to be much lower and thus the need for lifelong or lengthy anticoagulation in this group of patients is controversial. Additive risk factors such as homozygous FV Leiden, or a combination of 2 hereditary thrombophilias, are associated with an increased risk of recurrence, and long-term anticoagulation is recommended in these patients unless otherwise contraindicated. Factors to be considered when determining an individual's risks and benefits of long-term anticoagulation include the location of the thrombosis, severity of the initial thrombotic event, and the patient's inherent risk factors for bleeding. For example, patients with large iliofemoral DVTs, cerebral vein thrombosis, or symptomatic PE should be considered for long-term anticoagulation as they are at higher risk for recurrence and chronic morbidity from a recurrence than patients with isolated distal DVTs. Patient characteristics including renal insufficiency, congestive heart failure, age older than 75, hypertension, and history of previous gastrointestinal bleeding are associated with an increased annual risk of bleeding.

Kearon C et al: A comparison of three months of anticoagulation with extended anticoagulation for a first episode of idiopathic venous thromboembolism. N Engl J Med 1999;340:901. [PMID: 10089183]

When to Refer to a Specialist

Physicians trained in primary care or internal medicine should be able to easily manage the majority of patients with VTE, including their diagnosis, treatment, and long-term follow-up. Special circumstances that should prompt referral to a specialist include patients with recurrent VTE, younger patients with idiopathic VTE after evaluation, patients who require alternative anticoagulation approaches after failing warfarin therapy, patients who present with unusual thromboses or widespread thrombosis, and patients who require genetic counseling for hereditary thrombophilias. Patients in whom unexpected or rare complications develop from anticoagulation therapy (including massive hemorrhage requiring rapid reversal, HIT, or coumadin skin necrosis) may benefit from consultation with a hematologist trained in coagulation. Patients with severe postphlebitic syndromes or pulmonary hypertension should be considered for referral to vascular surgeons and pulmonologists, respectively. Pregnant women with a history of VTE, a hereditary thrombophilia, or recurrent spontaneous abortions secondary to an antiphospholipid antibody should be monitored by high risk obstetricians well-versed in anticoagulation therapy and its complications or in association with a coagulation specialist. Difficulty maintaining the INR in the therapeutic range is a risk factor for recurrent VTE and is often corrected by referral to an anticoagulation clinic or point of care home warfarin monitoring. Lastly, a specialist should be consulted for any patient whose clinical course or response to therapy is confusing or unexpected.

Relevant Web Sites

[A quick reference guide for clinicians summarizing the results of the sixth ACCP consensus conference on antithrombotic therapy.]

www.chestnet.org

[Created by the Council on Anticoagulation Advancement through Scientific Evidence to provide access to the latest research, case studies, slide presentations on anticoagulation therapy.]

www.casse.org

[Details drug interactions.]

www.drugdigest.org

SECTION XI

Other Common Disorders

Hematologic Complications of Pregnancy

37

David M. Aboulafia, MD

Under normal conditions, the quantities of circulating blood cells, platelets, and plasma proteins in a woman's body are regulated within a relatively narrow physiologic range. Pregnancy represents a challenge to the body's homeostatic reserves. The hematologic consequences of this challenge may be negligible, as in mild to moderate iron deficiency, incidental thrombocytopenia of pregnancy, or the induction of an asymptomatic hypercoagulable state. The consequences are more serious when the woman is faced with anemia-induced high-output cardiac failure, pulmonary embolism, life-threatening thrombocytopenia, or uncontrolled bleeding post-delivery.

One difficulty in evaluating hematologic abnormalities during pregnancy is distinguishing normal physiologic changes that occur routinely from uncommon pathologic events that occur only occasionally. This challenge is heightened because laboratory values change in pregnancy, and their interpretation requires an understanding of the hematologic changes of pregnancy (Table 37–1). Furthermore, any therapeutic decisions must be examined for their dual effects on both the mother and the fetus.

The clinical features, diagnosis, and management of the most commonly encountered hematologic disorders of pregnancy are reviewed in this chapter. The hypercoagulable state induced by pregnancy and the treatment of pregnancy-associated thrombosis are discussed in Chapter 36.

ANEMIA

Anemia is the most common hematologic problem in pregnancy, as either a component of a primary underlying hematologic condition or as a secondary consequence of pregnancy. Its frequency is heavily influenced by the socioeconomic circumstances of the mother, because nutrition and prenatal care contribute greatly to the overall incidence of this complication.

The physiologic expansion of the expectant mother's blood volume consists of an increase in plasma volume (25–60%) beginning at approximately 6 weeks of gestation and continuing until the 24th week, at which time there is a more gradual rise. The red blood cell (RBC) mass also increases during this time but at a slower rate (20–30%); this "hydremia" of pregnancy results in a decline in hematocrit (HCT) to the 30–32% range, necessitating a revision downward in the limits of a normal hemoglobin level to 10 g/dL (Table 37–1). The precise stimuli leading to the increase in plasma volume and RBC mass are unknown, although alterations in various hormones, such as progesterone and erythropoietin, and the development of placental vascular shunts may be important in this process. A reduction in blood viscosity results in decreased peripheral resistance and may offset the effects of increased levels of fibrinogen and enhanced RBC aggregation during the later stages of pregnancy.

As opposed to this "physiologic" anemia of pregnancy, the true anemias of pregnancy represent a genuine reduction in RBC mass and not merely a dilution of the RBC mass. These anemias most often are a consequence of iron or folate deficiency; more rarely, anemias of pregnancy are caused by other factors, such as hemolysis, infections, or very rarely, malignancy or aplastic anemia.

Duffy TP: Hematologic aspects of pregnancy. In: Hoffman R et al (editors). *Hematology: Basic Principles and Practice,* 3rd ed. Churchill Livingstone; 2000;2374.

Table 37–1. Hematologic laboratory values.

Test	Nonpregnant Women	Pregnant Women
White blood cell count	4000–10, 500/µL	9000–15,500/µL
Hemoglobin	12.5–14 g/dL	10–13 g/dL
Platelets	150,000–400,000/µL	125,000–400,000/µL
Reticulocyte count	0.5–1%	1–2.5%
Total iron-binding capacity	250–300 µg/dL	280–400 µg/dL
Transferrin saturation	25–35%	15–30%
Serum ferritin	75–100 µg/L	55–70 µg/L
Serum folate	6.5–19.6 µg/mL	4–10 µg/mL

IRON DEFICIENCY ANEMIA

Iron deficiency anemia (IDA), the most common type of anemia in pregnancy, occurs when there is insufficient iron to support normal RBC production. In some developing countries, as many as 83% of anemic pregnant women have iron deficiency; in inner-city pregnant women in the United States, 50% may have IDA even though prenatal iron is prescribed. The average menstruating woman requires 15–20 mg of absorbable iron in her daily diet to compensate for the loss of approximately 2 mg/d (from urine, stool, and skin); more is lost if she is pregnant. These figures translate into an average daily requirement of 4 mg of iron during the early stages of pregnancy; the requirement reaches 6.6–8.4 mg/d at term. Because this amount is more than can be supplied by even the most iron-rich diets, supplements are necessary to avoid iron deficiency.

For many women, dietary sources are especially iron-poor. A variety of social, economic, and cultural factors are important in determining the quantity and quality of the food supply. Even among fairly homogeneous groups, factors such as menstrual blood loss and amount of animal protein consumed are variable.

Duffy TP: Hematologic aspects of pregnancy. In: Burrow GN, Duffy TP (editors). *Medical Complications of Pregnancy*, 5th ed. WB Saunders; 1999;79.

Frenkel EP, Yardley DA: Clinical and laboratory features and sequelae of deficiency of folic acid (folate) and vitamin B_{12} (cobalamin) in pregnancy and gynecology. Hematol Oncol Clin North Am 2000;14:1079. [PMID: 11005035]

Graves BW, Barger MK: A "conservative" approach to iron supplementation during pregnancy. J Midwifery Womens Health 2001;46:159. [PMID: 11480748]

Rosenberg IH: Folic acid and neural-tube defects—time for action? N Engl J Med 1992;327:1875. [PMID: 1448126]

Routine iron supplementation during pregnancy: Policy statement. US Preventive Services Task Force. JAMA 1993;270:2846. [PMID: 8133625]

Sifakis S, Pharmakides G: Anemia in pregnancy. Ann N Y Acad Sci 2000;900:125. [PMID: 10818399]

Stein ML, Gunston KD, May RM: Iron dextran in the treatment of iron-deficiency anaemia of pregnancy. Haematological response and incidence of side-effects. S Afr Med J 1991;79:195. [PMID: 1996436]

Clinical Findings & Diagnosis

Because the symptoms of mild IDA are insidious and nonspecific, they are not of great value. When the hemoglobin level falls below 9 g/dL, however, IDA should be suspected. Careful physical examination may detect the acute or chronic effects of IDA including pallor, glossitis, stomatitis, patchy alopecia, or koilonychia. High-output congestive heart failure may be seen rarely with extreme anemia.

In pregnant patients, a diagnostic evaluation begins with a careful history which, if available, includes previous hematologic values in the prepregnant state and a detailed family history. Some patients may have an exaggerated, yet tolerable, decrease in hemoglobin during pregnancy, a phenomenon that is most common in the hemoglobinopathy states. The evaluation continues with morphologic classification using the RBC mean corpuscular volume (MCV) and the blood smear. In clear-cut instances of IDA, a peripheral blood smear will contain small hypochromic RBCs of various sizes and shapes. In pregnancy-associated IDA, microcytosis is not always seen because the MCV usually rises slightly in pregnancy. The normal reticulocyte count is 1%. If the feedback erythropoietin loop between the kidney and bone marrow is intact, evolving anemia should lead to a compensatory and macrocytic reticulocytosis. Failure to mount an appropriate reticulocytosis in the setting of anemia indicates a hyporegenerative state, most commonly seen with iron and folate deficiency. An inadequate reticulocyte response also accompanies erythropoietin-deficient erythropoiesis, the cause of anemia that accompanies progressive renal failure (Table 37–2). The reticulocyte count and MCV refine the possible causes of anemia and help determine whether additional blood tests are required.

Laboratory diagnosis of IDA in pregnancy may be complicated further by the observation that total iron-binding capacity (TIBC) increases in pregnancy even when iron stores are normal. To enable a better interpretation of laboratory indices of anemia, serum iron, TIBC, and ferritin levels should be obtained and reviewed in aggregate. Serum iron levels less than 30

Table 37–2. Anemia during pregnancy.

1. True anemia versus physiologic anemia or hydremia of pregnancy (Hgb < 10g/dL).
2. Elevated blood loss = blood loss or hemolysis.
3. Diminished reticulocyte count = red blood cell hypoproliferation, usually iron or folate deficiency.
4. Low MCV < 80 fl = iron deficiency anemia; confirm with serum ferritin.
5. High MCV > 95 fl = folate deficiency; conform with RBC folate.
6. Normal MCV 80–95 fl = possible combined deficiency; evaluate with RBC red cell distribution width.

Hgb, hemoglobin; MCV, mean corpuscular volume; fl, femtoliter; RBC, red blood cell.

μg/dL, TIBC greater than 450 μg/dL, and plasma ferritin levels less than 10 μg/L are the most reliable laboratory indicators of IDA. If immune-mediated hemolysis is present, a direct and indirect Coombs' test may return positive. The presence of urine hemosiderin and undetectable serum haptoglobin are indicative of intravascular hemolysis. A urine analysis and rectal examination with stool occult blood test are sometimes overlooked but essential to perform in all anemic patients to evaluate for potential genitorectal sources of blood loss. For complex cases or those not responding to iron therapy, the gold standard among hematologists is to obtain a bone marrow aspirate and biopsy to assess for iron stores and to rule out more unusual causes of anemia, such as myelodysplasia, aplastic anemia, leukemia, or lymphoma.

Differential Diagnosis

Folate deficiency also may complicate pregnancy because of a similar increase in demand for this essential cofactor in nucleic acid synthesis. Total body folate stores are small and short-lived, and nausea and vomiting may significantly impair the intake of folate. Folate deficiency is more frequent with twin pregnancies and with multiparity, the latter being associated with repeated states of negative folate balance. Alcohol consumption interferes with folate metabolism and cigarette smoking also places stress on the availability of folate. Drugs interfering with the absorption and metabolism of folic acid, such as phenytoin, trimethoprim, and nitrofurantoin, can aggravate folate deficiency further. Strict vegans also may develop overt folate deficiency during pregnancy.

The assessment of folate status in pregnancy, like that of iron, must take into account the expected decline in serum folate levels occurring in normal pregnancy; at term, the levels are only half of the early pregnancy values. The observed decline in serum folate levels is believed to be, in part, a dilutional effect caused by plasma volume expansion. A normal serum folate level is helpful in ruling out folate deficiency as a cause of anemia, and a fasting serum folate level of less than 3 ng/mL is considered diagnostic of folic acid deficiency. Uncomplicated folate deficiency typically leads to a macrocytic anemia, hypersegmented neutrophils, and varying degrees of leukopenia and thrombocytopenia, but the expected elevation in RBC MCV may be masked if IDA is also present. A deficiency of both these nutrients may produce a normocytic anemia, although the presence of hypersegmented polymorphonuclear cells may be a clue to diagnosing folate deficiency. Finding a dimorphic population of small and large RBCs on peripheral blood smear should alert the clinician to a possible combined nutritional deficiency. In such instances the RBC distribution width will be widened considerably.

Folate deficiency in pregnancy is accompanied by a 3- to 4-fold increase in occurrence of spina bifida in the fetus. Most prenatal vitamins contain folate in addition to iron. Pregnant women should receive 0.5–1 mg/d of folate. The salutary effects of vitamins and the importance of obtaining an accurate dietary history are underscored by the recommendation of the US Food and Drug Administration that all pregnant women should take multivitamin supplements.

During pregnancy, there is a progressive decline in the serum cobalamin (B$_{12}$) level, but the availability of maternal stores and the low fetal requirement for this vitamin mean that pregnancy has little effect on overall cobalamin status. Pernicious anemia is usually a disease of older women, and women who have significant cobalamin deficiency are often infertile. Cobalamin deficiency, in the absence of strict adherence to a vegetarian diet or a history of prior gastrectomy or ileal disease, should not be considered an important cause of anemia during pregnancy.

Among the most common non-nutritional causes of hypoproliferative anemia encountered in pregnant women is the anemia associated with chronic disease, or inflammatory block. Rheumatoid arthritis, chronic renal failure, and insulin-dependent diabetes mellitus are examples of diseases associated with mild to moderate anemia. In these conditions, serum iron may be low or normal, but unlike in IDA, the TIBC will be low and ferritin levels will be elevated. Erythropoietin is effective in ameliorating the anemia of inflammatory block, and its use is preferred over blood transfusions in nonemergent situations.

A more exaggerated decrease in hemoglobin during pregnancy commonly develops in patients with thalassemia trait compared with that of normal controls.

This decrease is attributable to an expansion in plasma volume and has no ill effects on the mother or fetus. The work-up of heterozygous thalassemia, which is common in some Mediterranean, Asian, and African populations, may provide a diagnostic challenge and usually requires the assistance of a hematologist.

Treatment

Because IDA is the most common type of anemia in pregnancy, some experts recommend empiric iron therapy without further testing if no other cause is suggested by history, physical examination, and by review of the peripheral blood smear. Three to 4 325-mg ferrous sulfate tablets per day (60–180 mg of elemental iron) taken without food is sufficient to ensure maximal hemoglobin regeneration. Within 4–6 weeks of treatment, the HCT should normalize to a level expected as a result of blood volume expansion, with the increase beginning at 2 weeks. An increase in the reticulocyte count 5–10 days after the initiation of iron therapy provides even earlier evidence for improved RBC production. If there is minimal or no rise in the HCT in 4–6 weeks or the reticulocyte count remains depressed after 10 days, further investigation is necessary. For patients who are intolerant of oral therapy, parenteral iron is an alternative. Intravenous iron can be associated with significant toxicity, particularly for those women with autoimmune disorders. The product insert should be read and a hematologist consulted before parenteral iron is recommended. Because patients may experience significant infusion-related side effects, nurses experienced in the delivery of parenteral iron should administer the medication and monitor the patient during each infusion.

The recommendation to provide all pregnant women with iron supplements is based largely on the following assumptions:

1. IDA in the mother is potentially harmful to the mother, fetus, and newborn.
2. The use of iron supplements can reduce perinatal morbidity.
3. The potential benefits of iron supplements outweigh their adverse effects.

A critical review of the available literature, however, challenges the assumptions that routine iron supplementation during pregnancy improves clinical outcomes for the mother, fetus, and newborn. A recent meta-analysis of twenty controlled trials of iron supplementation for pregnant women showed that there was a substantial reduction of women with hemoglobin levels below 10 or 10.5 g/dL in late pregnancy. Iron supplementation, however, had no detectable effect on any substantive measures of either maternal or fetal outcome. For women in economically developed countries who are generally clinically healthy and have access to adequate nutrition, the benefits of iron supplement remain unclear, and there may be risks. Further research of this issue must include large and more carefully designed randomized and prospective clinical trials before definitive conclusions can be reached about the effectiveness of routine iron supplementation.

Unlike B_{12}, folate stores within the body are marginal. Consequently, folate supplementation has become a standard component of prenatal care. Most prenatal vitamins contain 1 mg folate, an ample amount to fulfill the escalated folate needs of pregnancy. A 5-mg supplement is recommended for patients with hemolytic disorders such as sickle cell anemia (SCA) or thalassemia.

SICKLE CELL ANEMIA

Sickle cell disease is endemic to black people of both northern and sub-Saharan African descent and is the most common inherited form of anemia complicating pregnancy. In the United States, approximately 8% of the black population carries the sickle hemoglobin (Hgb S) gene; 0.15% of black newborns are homozygous (Hgb S-S) and suffer from sickle cell anemia (SCA). The most common heterozygote sickle genotypes are Hgb S-A (sickle cell trait), Hgb S-B thal (sickle-beta thalassemia), and Hgb S-C.

The biochemical basis for the abnormal, premature sickling of RBCs in Hgb S-S is a genetic point mutation resulting in the substitution of valine for glutamic acid on the beta-hemoglobin chain. This single beta-hemoglobin chain alteration leads to RBC membrane distortion with resultant obstruction of capillary blood flow. It also contributes to a characteristic hemoglobin electrophoretic mobility that facilitates laboratory distinction between the various hemoglobinopathies.

Obstruction of blood vessels causes worsening hypoxemia that serves to perpetuate and aggravate RBC sickling. Patients with SCA experience painful vaso-occlusive crises resulting in severe skeletal, abdominal, and chest pain syndromes often associated with fever. The spleen is the most susceptible organ to sickle-induced injury because of its highly vascularized tissue. Because of repetitive microinfarcts, the spleen eventually is rendered small, fibrotic and without function. The presence of an enlarged spleen raises the possibility of a superimposed thalassemia. Other organs at risk for ischemic damage include the heart, lungs, kidneys, eyes, long bones, and brain. Infection, hypoxemia, acidosis, and dehydration are just a few factors that can precipitate a painful crisis and trigger end-organ damage.

Clinical Findings & Diagnosis

Although morbidity and mortality among women with SCA has improved substantially over the past 2 decades, there is still a higher incidence of pneumonia, choLecystitis, pulmonary emboli, retinal hemorrhage, preeclampsia, and pyelonephritis compared with the general population. Hyposplenism, decreased serum IgM, reduced opsonization activity, impaired phagocytosis, and poor general nutrition contribute greatly to the increased risk of infection. The greatest threat to the pregnant woman with SCA is acute chest syndrome, in which a pulmonary infiltrate with fever leads to hypoxemia. These infiltrates, previously believed to be infectious in origin, are now thought to have an in situ sickling or embolized necrotic marrow from sickled bones as their etiology. The fetus of a woman with SCA is also at increased risk for perinatal complications including spontaneous abortion, preterm delivery, intrauterine growth retardation, and stillbirth. The cause of neonatal death is obscure, but it may sometimes result from vaso-occlusion of the placenta; the postpartum findings are those of intrapartum anoxia.

Because of routine screening hemoglobin electrophoresis in families known to be at risk as well as the development of clinical complications at an early age, most women with sickle cell disease are diagnosed before pregnancy. Rarely, patients become symptomatic for the first time during pregnancy with painful crisis, infection, or overt infarction. Anemia is typically normocytic, with HCT below 25% and a reticulocyte count greater than 10%. On peripheral blood smear, characteristic sickle cells, target cells and, because of splenic hypofunction, Howell-Jolly bodies are present. A total bilirubin value between 3 and 5 mg/dL is primarily unconjugated, reflecting the presence of brisk RBC hemolysis. An elevation in alkaline phosphatase and conjugated bilirubin should trigger an evaluation to rule out cholelithiasis, a common complication in patients with hyperproliferative anemia.

It is important to screen all black and other at-risk patients by hemoglobin electrophoresis to detect the asymptomatic carrier state and arrange for genetic counseling. Input from a team of various experts, including a genetic counselor, obstetrician, hematologist, nutritionist, pediatrician, and primary care provider, helps ensure the best possible outcome. Testing the father for carrier status allows for better risk assessment of the fetus. Amniocentesis, chorionic villus sampling, and cordocentesis (umbilical vein cannulation and aspiration) allow for in utero diagnosis with the aid of new advances in molecular biology.

Treatment

The decrease in maternal and perinatal morbidity and mortality among pregnant SCA patients is due in part to the coordinated efforts of obstetricians and hematologists working as a team. Because toxemia and preterm labor and prematurity are increased in frequency, patients should be taught to recognize the subtle prodromal symptoms and signs including headache, right upper quadrant pain, scotoma, cramping, lower abdominal pressure, edema of hands and feet, and mucovaginal discharge, which might predict early onset of complications. If acute or chronic events related to SCA or obstetric-related complications are identified, they should be treated promptly.

The enthusiasm for prophylactic exchange transfusions for all pregnant women with sickle cell disease has waned and given way to watchful anticipation of the patient's course by hematologist and obstetrician in consultation. (An exchange transfusion is when the same amount of blood that has been withdrawn is equal to the amount of packed red blood cells given by transfusion.) The advantage of exchange transfusion is that it increases the level of hemoglobin A in the blood. This results in improved oxygen-carrying capacity and a decreased percentage of sickled hemoglobin. Disadvantages include the risks of viral infection (ie, HIV, hepatitis B and C, cytomegalovirus, and human T-cell leukemia/lymphoma virus [HTLV-I-II]), transfusion reaction, allosensitization, and further contribution to preexisting iron overload.

There is a high risk of stillbirth, abortion, and fetal growth retardation in pregnancies of hemoglobin S-S mothers who have not received transfusion. However, some investigators have speculated that poor prenatal care in this often socioeconomically disadvantaged group may be a more important factor leading to fetal morbidity and mortality. Because of the increased risks to the fetus, fetal assessment, biophysical profiles, or contraction stress tests should begin at 32 weeks of gestation. Serial ultrasonography is performed to assess for intrauterine growth retardation.

Pain crisis in pregnancy is managed as in nonpregnant patients with oxygen, hydration, and adequate analgesia. Transfusions are reserved for any acceleration of the sickling disorder itself, worsening anemia (HCT below 18%), or obstetric complications. Because of ongoing hemolysis, 5 mg of folic acid is prescribed routinely to avoid a reticulocytopenic megaloblastic crisis. Some pregnant sickle cell patients may also need iron supplementation; they can be identified by evaluating serum iron, TIBC, and ferritin levels. Newer strategies aimed at preventing vaso-occlusive complications, such as pain crisis, in the nonpregnant state include the use of butyrate preparations, hydroxyurea, erythropoietin, high-dose intravenous methylprednisolone, gene therapy, and bone marrow transplantation. The most extensively studied of these treatments, hydroxyurea, decreases intracellular hemoglobin polymerization and erythrocyte sickling by increasing the levels of fetal hemoglobin. Its use is not recommended during pregnancy and both female and male patients should be counseled regarding the importance of contraception while taking this drug.

Management of women with SCA during delivery is controversial. Many physicians continue to advocate exchange transfusions if general anesthesia is contemplated; the potential for an anesthetic accident with hypoxemia is the rationale for this recommendation. Epidural anesthesia reduces this risk, but hypotension secondary to venous pooling may develop. Attention to adequate fluid repletion, use of pneumatic stockings or pressure leg wraps, and left-sided positioning of the mother to reduce inferior vena cava compression are routine strategies to minimize blood pressure fluctuations. Standard care also includes frequent monitoring for fetal distress. Oxytocin and induction anesthesia are safe during labor, and early ambulation is introduced postpartum to reduce the risk of thromboembolism. For patients who choose to terminate pregnancy, most abortion methods are well tolerated. Hypertonic saline injections are contraindicated because they may precipitate RBC sickling, but hypotonic urea can be used. If abortion is to be performed, it is best done early in pregnancy.

Potential complications and concerns that are relevant for pregnant women with sickle cell disease are applicable to individuals with other interacting hemoglobins that can participate in the sickling process, ie, Hgb S-C, Hgb S-B-thal, and Hgb S-E. In contrast, sickle cell trait poses no increase in maternal morbidity with the exception of a higher incidence of kidney and bladder infections and, rarely, splenic infarction. Because of their higher risk of urinary tract infections, women with sickle cell trait should be screened and treated if asymptomatic bacteruria is detected.

Buetler E: The sickle diseases and related disorders. In: Buetler E, et al (editors). *Williams Hematology,* 6th edition. New York: McGraw-Hill; 2001:581.

Koshy M et al: Prophylactic red-cell transfusions in pregnant patients with sickle cell disease. A randomized, cooperative study. N Engl J Med 1988;319:1447. [PMID: 3054555]

Platt OS et al: Mortality in sickle cell disease. Life expectancy and risk factors for early death. N Engl J Med 1994;330:1639. [PMID: 7993409]

Pollack CV Jr: Emergencies in sickle cell disease. Emerg Med Clin North Am 1993;11:365. [PMID: 8491111]

Smith JA et al: Pregnancy in sickle cell disease: experience of the Cooperative Study of Sickle Cell Disease. Obstet Gynecol 1996;87:199. [PMID: 8559523]

Wayne AS, Kevy SV, Nathan DG: Transfusion management of sickle cell disease. Blood 1993;81:1109. [PMID: 8443373]

LEUKOCYTOSIS

Total white blood cell (WBC) counts rise in pregnancy mainly because of an absolute increase in the number of neutrophils. Neutrophilia usually is discovered during the second month and progresses gradually before plateauing in the second or third trimester. The average peak is at the upper limits of nonpregnant normal, with WBC counts of approximately 9000/μL; however, WBC counts of up to 18,000/μL occasionally are noted in normal pregnant women during the third trimester. Total WBC counts within the normal range of nonpregnant women are to be expected by the sixth postpartum day, provided no complications supervene.

Clinical Findings & Diagnosis

Plasma cortisol, which is known to stimulate demargination of neutrophils in other circumstances, rises substantially during pregnancy and is the substance presumed to be most responsible for neutrophilia in pregnancy. When a modest elevation in neutrophils is discovered during pregnancy, a diagnostic evaluation is rarely necessary. A normal physical examination in an afebrile and asymptomatic woman is usually sufficient to rule out infection. Leukocyte Döhle bodies (blue cytoplasmic inclusions consisting of rough endoplasmic reticulum) and metamyelocytes frequently are seen in sepsis as well as pregnancy, and their presence alone is not an indication for additional blood tests or cultures.

Differential Diagnosis

Distinguishing the neutrophilia of pregnancy from leukemia usually is not a difficult problem. Bone marrow biopsy and aspirate, histochemical stains, chromosome analysis, polymerase chain reaction–based technology to detect oncogene expression, and WBC flow cytometric analysis help identify the rare pregnancy complicated by the chronic or acute forms of leukemia.

Many of the studies required to evaluate the extent and nature of leukemia or lymphoma can be safely carried out in a pregnant patient. Specifically, history and physical examination, laboratory tests, bone marrow biopsy, lymph node biopsy, and ultrasound studies pose little risk. However, interpreting the tests must take into consideration the changes associated with pregnancy, and physical assessment of the abdomen is complicated as the pregnancy progresses. Most experts believe that a chest radiograph is safe in pregnancy but that computed tomographic scans and radionuclide imaging studies in pregnancy should be avoided if possible.

When leukemia does occur during pregnancy, difficult decisions are presented by the anticipated toxic effects of chemotherapy on mother and fetus (the most active stage of fetal organogenesis is during the first trimester) as well as the long-term prospects for survival. Although a number of case reports detail successful, uncomplicated births following chemotherapy for acute leukemia, the most common outcomes are abortion and fetal loss. Leukapheresis may serve as an effective stopgap measure to control WBC counts in chronic leukemia until after delivery and thus delay the use of drugs that are potentially immunosuppressive and teratogenic. Invariably, input from consultants from the various disciplines of hematology and oncology, reproductive medicine, obstetrics, neonatology, medical ethics, psychiatry, and medical social work are brought to bear on a course of action that may have immediate repercussions for both the mother and fetus. The variables associated with the patient's mores, clinical status, and type of malignancy all need to be taken into account in planning management.

Armitage JO: Lymphoma and leukemia in pregnancy. In: Schecter GP, et al (editors). Hematology 1999: American Society of Hematology Education program book. American Society of Hematology 1999:497.

Duffy TP: Hematologic aspects of pregnancy. In: Hoffman R et al (editors). *Hematology: Basic Principles and Practice,* 3rd ed. Churchill Livingstone; 2000:2374.

THROMBOCYTOPENIA

During late pregnancy, many healthy women become thrombocytopenic, defined by a platelet count below 150,000/μL. The reasons why mild thrombocytopenia occurs during normal pregnancy are complex. Alterations in plasma volume probably result in a "dilutional thrombocytopenia." Increased platelet consumption related to low-grade disseminated intravascular coagulation (DIC) within the uteroplacental circulation also contributes to mild thrombocytopenia. A lowering of the platelet count during pregnancy may be a physiologic adaptation allowing preservation of the uteroplacental interface. Following delivery, mild thrombocytopenia resolves spontaneously.

In a large, prospective study of more than 6000 pregnant women, approximately 8% had mild thrombocytopenia at term, yet no adverse results were experienced by the women or their infants. Because a platelet count in the range of 75,000–150,000/μL in an otherwise uncomplicated pregnancy rarely causes clinical complications, restraint should be exercised in evaluating and treating patients with isolated and mild thrombocytopenia. The cause of thrombocytopenia should not be overlooked, however, when platelet counts are less than 75,000/μL, when other cell lines are affected, or when medical problems supervene. Finding and eliminating the cause has special significance, because bleeding complications can threaten both mother and fetus and may influence the method of delivery and define the infant's needs for postnatal care.

Aster RH: "Gestational" thrombocytopenia: a plea for conservative management. N Engl J Med 1990;323:264. [PMID: 2366835]

Burrows RF: Platelet disorders in pregnancy. Curr Opin Obstet Gynecol 2001;13:115. [PMID: 11315863]

Burrows RF, Kelton JG: Fetal thrombocytopenia and its relation to maternal thrombocytopenia. N Engl J Med 1993;329:1463. [PMID: 8413457]

Burrows RF, Kelton JG: Thrombocytopenia at delivery: a prospective study of 6715 deliveries. Am J Obstet Gynecol 1990; 162:731. [PMID: 2316579]

Fischer J, Dietl J, Goelz R: Fetal and maternal thrombocytopenia. N Engl J Med 1994;330:940. [PMID: 8114878]

McCrae KR, Samuels P, Schreiber AD: Pregnancy-associated thrombocytopenia: pathogenesis and management. Blood 1992;80:2697. [PMID: 1450402]

Samuels P et al: Estimation of the risk of thrombocytopenia in the offspring of pregnant women with presumed immune thrombocytopenia purpura. N Engl J Med 1990;323:229. [PMID: 2366833]

IMMUNE THROMBOCYTOPENIC PURPURA

Immune thrombocytopenic purpura (ITP) is characterized by a decreased platelet count caused by splenic sequestration mediated by antiplatelet antibodies. It is relatively common during pregnancy, occurring once or twice in 1000 deliveries. Although pregnancy is not discouraged in women with preexisting ITP, maternal and fetal complications can occur, and additional monitoring and therapy may be needed.

ITP can be classified based on its chronicity. The acute form typically affects children more often than adults and occurs following a viral illness. Thrombocytopenia and purpura usually develop within 1–2 weeks of a viral prodrome, affect males and females with equal frequency, and are self-limiting. Chronic ITP is more likely to affect young women and, as suggested by its designation, is longer lasting. Platelet counts usually remain low; remission refers to absence of purpura rather than normality of the platelet count. In pregnancy-associated ITP, maternal death is rare, and morbidity correlates with the severity of thrombocytopenia. Postpartum hemorrhage caused by cervical or vaginal laceration is the most common thrombocytopenic complication. The aspect of ITP that is unique to pregnant patients is that the fetus may be affected by the disorder. Although maternal platelet-associated IgG antibodies can cross the uteroplacental barrier and affect fetal platelets, significant fetal thrombocytopenia at or following delivery (50,000/μL) occurs in only 10–15% of instances and is rarely associated with significant morbidity.

Clinical Findings & Diagnosis

If thrombocytopenia develops in the first half of pregnancy, it is unlikely to be pregnancy-associated and more likely to be ITP. A healthy woman who is found, on the basis of routine laboratory studies, to have isolated thrombocytopenia, normal-appearing or mildly enlarged platelets on peripheral blood smear, and a bone marrow containing normal or increased numbers of megakaryocytes presumably has ITP. Most patients with platelet counts less than 30,000–50,000/μL offer a history of easy bruising and findings of petechiae, epistaxis, or gingival oozing. Overt hemorrhage is uncommon, however, unless the platelet count is below 20,000/μL. Physical examination is otherwise unremarkable, and the presence of significant lymphadenopathy or splenomegaly should call into question the diagnosis of ITP. Patients with ITP of pregnancy need the usual investigations at the start of pregnancy, including thyroid function tests, HIV serology, as well as a careful review of the peripheral blood smear to exclude clumping which could lead to a falsely low platelet count. Tests for anticardiolipin antibody and lupus anticoagulant are sometimes useful, particularly if there is a history of thrombosis or fetal demise. Assays for platelet-associated antibody, however, are rarely helpful in establishing the diagnosis of ITP; the antibody is not always detected and may not correlate with clinical findings.

Differential Diagnosis

Other causes of thrombocytopenia during pregnancy include infection with HIV or other viruses, neoplasms, aplastic anemia, and vitamin deficiency. Eclampsia and related syndromes, such as the syndrome of hemolysis with elevated liver enzymes and low platelet count (HELLP), DIC, and autoimmune disorders, must be excluded by laboratory and clinical evaluation. A careful drug history should also be elicited; a number of drugs used commonly during pregnancy may cause thrombocytopenia (Table 37–3). Two drug-induced syndromes relatively unique to pregnancy deserve mention: (1) acute cocaine ingestion has been associated with the transient development of a syndrome resembling severe preeclampsia and may be accompanied by profound thrombocytopenia; and (2) neonatal thrombocytopenia may occur in the infants of women who have taken thiazide diuretics or hydralazine, which are used occasionally to manage pregnancy-induced hypertension.

Treatment

Treatment for ITP during pregnancy typically is initiated once platelet counts fall below 30,000/μL throughout pregnancy and below 50,000/μL near term. Prednisone at a dose of 1–1.5 mg/kg/d is the treatment of choice. Eighty percent of women with acute ITP respond to this regimen with a rise in platelet counts within 10–14 days. If the patient does not respond

Table 37–3. Drugs occasionally associated with thrombocytopenia in pregnancy.

Class	Drug
Cytotoxic agents	Nitrogen mustard
	Cyclophosphamide
	5-Fluorouracil
	Methotrexate
Antacids	Cimetidine
	Ranitidine
	Nizatidine
	Omeprazole
Diuretics	Chlorothiazide
Antihypertensives	Hydralazine
Antibiotics	Penicillin
	Sulfa-containing drugs
Oral hypoglycemics	Sulfonamides
	Tolbutamide
	Glyburide
Anticonvulsants/hypnotics/ antiemetics	Chlorpropamide
	Diazepam
	Diphenylhydantoin
	Chlorpromazine
Pain modulators	Acetaminophen
Miscellaneous	Gold salts
	Heparin
	Heroin
	Cocaine
	Alcohol
	Cancer chemotherapy

within 2–4 weeks or if there are relative contraindications to use of steroids (eg, poorly controlled diabetes, active psychiatric problems, or labile hypertension), high-dose intravenous immunoglobulin (IVIG) is infused to raise maternal platelet counts. IVIG presumably imparts a beneficial effect on platelet counts by blocking the maternal reticuloendothelial receptor uptake of IgG-coated platelets. The usual total dose is 1–2 g/kg divided into daily doses given over 1–5 days. Although a response is seen within days, platelet increases are usually short-lived, and therapy may need to be repeated as often as every 2–3 weeks.

Although splenectomy can be performed safely in the second trimester of pregnancy, it usually can be avoided because of the ready availability and success of steroids and IVIG. Other drugs that are used occasionally for nonpregnancy-associated ITP, such as cyclophosphamide, vincristine, and azathioprine, usually are held in reserve during pregnancy because of concerns regarding their immunosuppressive or teratogenic potential. For patients with symptomatic and refractory thrombocytopenia, cytotoxic chemotherapy and rituximab monoclonal antibody infusions have been used with some success, although experience in the pregnant female is lacking. Danazol, 200 mg orally 3 times daily, is prescribed occasionally; however, platelet count increases are not consistent, and concern for possible hepatotoxicity mandates that liver enzymes be monitored periodically. Experience with anti-D immunoglobin in pregnant women is limited although this may be a viable alternative for those who are Rh positive. Platelet transfusions are of limited benefit because of their rapid elimination from the circulation. As a result, they are used only in the setting of life-threatening or difficult-to-control hemorrhage. Drugs that inhibit platelet aggregation such as aspirin and other nonsteroidal anti-inflammatory drugs (NSAIDs) should be avoided; women should not receive intramuscular injections because they can lead to painful hematomas. Patients with platelet counts less than 30,000/μL are reminded to use soft-bristled toothbrushes, dental floss, or metal razors with care. Opinions vary regarding how far a platelet count can fall before it is unsafe to recommend epidural anesthesia. Most anesthesiologists will favor a platelet count greater than 50,000–100,000/μL before agreeing to place an epidural catheter.

A major area of controversy in the field of maternal thrombocytopenia is how best to manage the fetus. In theory, head trauma associated with the passage of the fetus through the birth canal during labor and delivery could precipitate a devastating intracranial hemorrhage. Efforts to predict or influence fetal platelet counts by looking at the maternal platelet count, assaying for platelet-associated IgG, and providing the mother with corticosteroids have, however, proved to be unreliable. More recently, scalp blood sampling has been used to assess fetal platelet counts directly. The value of this test is compromised by the need for adequate cervical dilatation before the procedure is performed and the possibility of inaccuracy owing to dilution with amniotic fluid or clotting of the sample. Umbilical vein sampling may be a more accurate means of assessing fetal platelet counts but most experts contend that the risks associated with the procedure outweigh the risk of intracranial hemorrhage due to ITP.

There is disagreement as to what risk maternal ITP poses to the fetus. Severe fetal thrombocytopenia (platelet level below 20,000/μL) rarely occurs; the incidence may be in the range of 4%. Consequently, the risk of intracranial hemorrhage or other major bleeding complications is less than 1%, but this risk is higher than among infants born from mothers without ITP. Although there is still support for giving corticosteroids and IVIG to ITP-affected mothers during the 3 weeks before delivery for their effect on the fetus, no studies have shown convincingly a reliable benefit to the fetus.

In the absence of a simple, accurate method to determine or influence fetal platelet counts, cesarean section often has been recommended, in the hope of protecting the fetus from bleeding during labor and delivery. Unfortunately, there are no studies indicating that the risk of intracranial bleeding is reduced by the use of cesarean section, and current practice has shifted so as not to alter the mode of delivery.

Once the fetus is delivered, the neonate's platelet count should be monitored for several days. Cranial ultrasonography is performed to evaluate intracranial bleeding in infants with low platelet counts. IVIG, corticosteroids or both are often given in the setting of fetal platelet counts less than 30,000/μL. In the setting of severe bleeding, platelet transfusions are administered. Exchange transfusion is rarely needed and reserved for the most difficult cases. Thrombocytopenia in the infant generally resolves within a few weeks of delivery. Mothers with ITP may breast-feed their infants.

Because the state-of-the-art is evolving rapidly for women and their neonates with ITP, expert consultation from a hematologist, neonatologist, obstetrician, and anesthesiologist, all experienced in these matters, is essential.

Cines DB, Blanchette VS: Immune thrombocytopenic purpura. N Engl J Med 2002;346:995. [PMID: 11919310]

Cook RL et al: Immune thrombocytopenic purpura in pregnancy: a reappraisal of management. Obstet Gynecol 1991;78:578. [PMID: 1923158]

PREECLAMPSIA- & ECLAMPSIA-RELATED HEMATOLOGIC ABNORMALITIES

Preeclampsia is a frequent complication occurring in as many as 5–13% of pregnancies. Thrombocytopenia develops in 15–50% of patients with preeclampsia, making preeclampsia a common cause of significant thrombocytopenia. Most commonly, these patients are primigravidas in their third trimester. The pathogenesis of preeclampsia-associated thrombocytopenia is uncertain. Patients with preeclampsia and thrombocytopenia have large mean platelet volumes and increased megakaryocytes. Suggested reasons for low platelet counts include increased consumption of platelets owing to damaged or activated endothelium, alterations in thrombin generation, and enhanced sequestration of platelets caused by the deposition of IgG or circulating immune complexes on their cell surface.

Clinical Findings & Diagnosis

The diagnosis of preeclampsia is established by an increase in blood pressure to at least 140/90 mm Hg, accompanied by edema, proteinuria greater than 0.3 g/24 h or 10 mg/dL in at least 2 random specimens collected 6 hours apart, or both. Preeclampsia is observed most often in women who are younger than 20 or older than 30 years.

In mild preeclampsia, alterations in HCT usually are not seen. In severe preeclampsia, a reduction in plasma volume may be reflected by a rapid increase in the HCT (hemoconcentration) over 5–10 days. Severe eclampsia can also cause anemia due to intravascular/mechanical hemolysis induced by increased sheer stress as RBCs traverse the microvasculature. This traumatic hemolysis leads to the presence of helmet cells, shistocytes, and microspherocytes on the peripheral blood smear, elevated lactate dehydrogenase (LDH), and diminished serum haptoglobin due to binding with free hemoglobin.

In more than 20% of patients with severe preeclampsia, consumption of procoagulants takes place, with some evidence of DIC (antithrombin III deficiency, reduced protein C and S, and presence of fibrin degradation products [FDPs]). Although the cause of eclampsia is not always known, platelet-endothelial activation is universally present and is manifest by altered angiotensin II sensitivity in conjunction with platelet activation and consumption. Antiplatelet antibodies are not present, therefore fetal ITP is not a concern. Rather, thrombocytopenia in eclampsia has its major risks in placental disruption and fetal loss.

Differential Diagnosis

When thrombocytopenia occurs in a patient in whom classic signs of preeclampsia (edema, followed by hypertension and proteinuria) or eclampsia (seizures/ coma) are developing, the cause of the thrombocytopenia is usually evident. Thrombocytopenia also may accompany hepatic forms of toxemia in which the usual signs of preeclampsia are absent. Acute fatty liver of pregnancy is one of these variants; clinical attention is drawn to liver abnormalities including profound elevations in transaminases along with less impressive rises in bilirubin and alkaline phosphatase. The hematologic alterations in pregnancy may extend to encompass the HELLP syndrome. Criteria for diagnosis include (1) microangiopathic hemolytic anemia with schistocytes on the peripheral blood film; (2) bilirubin above 1.2 g/dL, LDH above 600 U/L, and serum aspartate aminotransferase (AST) at least 70 U/L; and (3) platelet count less than 100,000/μL. Because many patients with HELLP also manifest hypertension and proteinuria, there is clinical overlap with eclampsia.

Thrombotic thrombocytopenic purpura (TTP) and the hemolytic uremic syndrome are additional disorders characterized by microangiopathic hemolytic anemia and severe thrombocytopenia, sometimes in the setting of fever, renal insufficiency, and fluctuating mental status changes. Although both diseases are rare in pregnancy, they should be considered when evaluating a pregnant patient with thrombocytopenia, for with prompt initiation of plasmapheresis, medical outcomes in TTP may be vastly improved. Commercial test kits to assay for von Willebrand's factor (vWF) cleavage protein have recently become available and offer the hope of improved diagnostic accuracy in distinguishing TTP from the other microangiopathic processes that lead to low platelet counts. When treating pregnant women who have platelet counts less than 75,000/μL, input from a hematologist should be requested.

Treatment

Management of eclampsia usually consists of delivery of the infant when this is possible based on its maturity. The high frequency of thrombocytopenia and the early onset of thrombocytopenia suggested that antiplatelet agents such as aspirin could be effective. However, recent large multicenter trials that have included over 25,000 women have not demonstrated benefit of aspirin compared with placebo in high-risk, moderate-risk, or low-risk pregnant women. Because heparin may enhance the bleeding tendency, its use should be avoided. Rather, platelet transfusions are ordered just before delivery in an effort to maintain platelet numbers greater than 20,000–50,000/μL, especially if cesarean section is contemplated, or at higher platelet counts if there are signs of increased bleeding or bruising.

Although significant bleeding usually does not occur in patients with preeclampsia, minor bleeding and postoperative oozing are common. Occasionally, bleeding is the result of a coagulopathy such as DIC.

Davis GL: Hemostatic changes associated with normal and abnormal pregnancies. Clin Lab Sci 2000;13:223. [PMID: 11586509]

Nizzi FA Jr, Mues G: Hemorrhagic problems in obstetrics exclusive of disseminated intravascular coagulation. Hematol Oncol Clin North Am 2000;14:1171. [PMID: 11005040]

Saphier CJ, Repke JT: Hemolysis, elevated liver enzymes, and low platelets (HELLP) syndrome: a review of diagnosis and management. Semin Perinatol 1998;22:118. [PMID: 9638906]

DISSEMINATED INTRAVASCULAR COAGULATION

DIC is an acquired syndrome of laboratory and clinical findings in which proteins important in coagulation are consumed and the fibrinolytic system is activated. It is a frequent cause of abnormal bleeding and, less commonly, thrombosis in obstetric patients. Activation of the coagulation system has been associated with abruptio placentae, sepsis, retained intrauterine fetal death, and amniotic fluid embolus. Other causes of DIC include liver disease, trauma, and hypovolemic shock. Common to many of these conditions is the release of a thromboplastin or endotoxin-like substance into the circulation, resulting in intravascular clotting and fibrin formation in the microvasculature (Figure 37–1).

The coagulation factors most readily consumed in DIC include platelets, prothrombin, factor V, and factor VIII. The body has a finite capacity to replace these factors, which are critical to clot formation. When procoagulants are consumed, a bleeding diathesis may ensue. Activation of the fibrinolytic system produces FDPs, which interfere with normal clotting mechanisms. Systemic manifestations include endothelial damage with increased vascular permeability, hemorrhage, and end-organ ischemia.

The obstetric diseases associated with DIC can be divided into 3 major groups based on the mechanisms by which the primary disease initiates vascular clotting. DIC is triggered in the first group by the intravascular infusion of tissue thromboplastins. Abruptio placentae and the dead fetus syndrome fall into this grouping. In the dead fetus syndrome, consumption occurs slowly over a period of days to weeks. With abruptio placentae, consumption is rapid and fulminant, and the chief complication is hemorrhage.

A second group of pathologic conditions causing DIC includes those associated with endothelial damage. An example already reviewed is eclampsia or preeclampsia.

A third group of conditions associated with DIC encompasses nonspecific or indirect effects of certain diseases. This group includes amniotic fluid embolus, gram-negative sepsis, and saline abortion. Amniotic fluid embolism is usually fatal (85% mortality rate), more as a result of cardiovascular collapse than of its hemorrhagic complications. This life-threatening entity occurs most frequently during difficult deliveries in multiparous women. Hypoxemia, shock, and hemorrhage in this setting should suggest the diagnosis. The prototype for sepsis causing DIC is clostridial infection. This aftermath of septic abortions also is characterized by severe intravascular hemolysis attributed to the direct bacterial by-product attack of lecithinase on the RBC membrane.

Clinical Findings & Diagnosis

The signs and symptoms of DIC are those of the underlying disease with the addition of hemorrhage, thrombosis, or both. Hypotension from hemorrhage and/or bradykinin release, red cell lysis from complement activation, and uterine atony are variably present. Acute DIC most often is associated with bleeding, and chronic DIC is associated with thrombotic complications. Acute DIC poses a great risk to the mother, with intracranial hemorrhage the most worrisome complication. Thrombotic presentations may be neurologic, with seizures, delirium, or coma, or they may be dermatologic, with focal ischemia and superficial gangrene. Thrombosis of the renal vasculature can cause cortical necrosis and renal failure. Infarcts and emboli represent

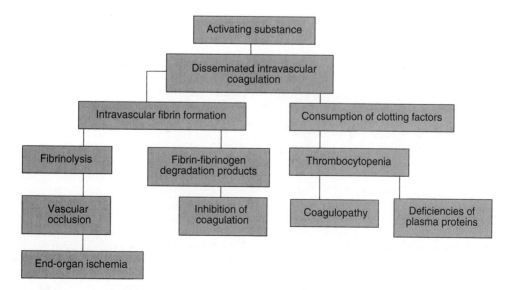

Figure 37–1. Pathophysiology of disseminated intravascular coagulation.

pulmonary vascular obstruction, whereas phlebitis and extremity gangrene are the result of thrombosis of peripheral blood vessels. DIC must be considered a possibility in any obstetric patient presenting with risk factors as noted or who has unexplained bleeding or thrombosis.

The laboratory diagnosis of acute DIC is usually clear (Table 37–4). As RBCs are forced through the obstructed microvasculature, they are sheared. Consequently, schistocytes and helmet cells are seen on peripheral blood smear. Thrombocytopenia is invariably present. Fibrinogen, which usually is elevated to supranormal levels in uncomplicated pregnancy, is low or low-normal (less than 250 mg/dL), and circulating FDPs are elevated. The prothrombin time (PT) and partial thromboplastin time (PTT) are prolonged in most cases. If intravascular hemolysis is sufficiently brisk, hemoglobinuria occurs, and serum haptoglobin levels decline to absent or barely detectable levels. Like fibrinogen, serum haptoglobin is an acute-phase reactant and is elevated in uncomplicated pregnancies. The diagnosis of amniotic fluid embolism usually is made in the setting of DIC and cardiopulmonary collapse. The condition is most likely to occur in the setting of prolonged labor in a multiparous woman. The diagnosis can be confirmed by demonstrating amniotic fluid components in blood obtained from the pulmonary vascular current. Monoclonal antibodies reactive against these components are available to make a more secure diagnosis of this condition.

The laboratory diagnosis of chronic DIC may prove more subtle and require the expertise of a hematologist to interpret.

Differential Diagnosis

Various clinical disorders not associated with DIC can result in an acquired bleeding diathesis and significant

Table 37–4. Typical laboratory findings in acute disseminated intravascular coagulation.

Laboratory Test	Result
Platelet count	Decreased
Fibrinogen	Decreased
Antithrombin III	Decreased
Prothrombin time	Usually prolonged
Activated partial thromboplastin time	Usually prolonged
Fibrinogen-fibrin degradation products	Increased
Schistocytes on peripheral blood smear	Present

hemostatic laboratory abnormalities. Thrombocytopenia may be due to a bone marrow failure state, an infiltrative bone marrow process such as leukemia or lymphoma, endothelial-mediated platelet activation such as vasculitis or TTP, or immunologic destruction. Platelet counts may fall in the septic patient, but in the patient with platelet counts less than 50,000/μL, DIC is most likely.

The rare syndrome of primary fibrinolysis may require the expertise of a hematologist to diagnose. It can occur with the independent generation of plasmin without concomitant thrombin generation. Such patients can have a low fibrinogen, prolonged screening assays, and elevated FDPs. In addition, patients with liver disease and primary fibrinolysis with portal hypertension may have thrombocytopenia secondary to splenic sequestration. A euglobulin clot lysis test will, however, be significantly shortened, and the protamine paracoagulation assay is negative for fibrinogen monomer.

Treatment

Of major importance in the management of a patient with DIC is recognizing and treating the underlying cause. In the obstetric arena, in particular, treating the underlying cause produces profound improvement in hematologic and clinical parameters. Chronic DIC is now infrequently a problem because its principal cause, fetal death in utero, is recognized easily; coagulation abnormalities tend to rapidly normalize after oxytocin induction of delivery and blood component therapy.

Treatment of acute DIC triggered by abruptio placentae consists of delivery of the infant under the coverage of the appropriate blood components—platelets, cryoprecipitate, and fresh frozen plasma. Guidelines for the replacement of blood products include maintenance of a HCT of 20–25%, normovolemia reflected by a urinary output of greater than 30 mL/h, a platelet count in excess of 20,000/μL, and a fibrinogen level of greater than 100 mg/mL. Abruptio placentae has reemerged as an important cause of DIC because of its causal relationship to cocaine abuse.

Treatment of amniotic fluid embolism is focused on vigorous supportive therapy directed toward gas exchange with mechanical respiratory assistance and intravascular fluid and pressor infusions to maintain adequate cardiac output. In patients in whom continued entry of amniotic debris may be contributing to intravascular clotting, heparin may be a reasonable adjunct to therapy. Because heparin may exacerbate bleeding and possibly thrombocytopenia, it should be used in the coagulopathic patient under direction of the consulting hematologist.

During the second trimester, saline-induced abortions often result in mild DIC. Most of these patients do not have clinical signs of bleeding, although brisk oozing is sometimes seen at delivery. This complication is short-lived and disappears after the fetus is delivered. In the rare instance in which bleeding persists and fibrinogen or platelet counts are low, the patient should be treated appropriately with cryoprecipitate and platelet transfusions to correct the deficiency. If vaginal bleeding occurs in the face of normal hemostatic factors, however, the bleeding may be due to retention of fetal products rather than a systemic hemostatic defect.

Bick RL: Syndromes of disseminated intravascular coagulation in obstetrics, pregnancy, and gynecology. Objective criteria for diagnosis and management. Hematol Oncol Clin North Am 2000;14:999. [PMID: 11005032]

Lurie S, Feinstein M, Mamet Y: Disseminated intravascular coagulopathy in pregnancy: thorough comprehension of etiology and management reduces obstetricians' stress. Arch Gynecol Obstet 2000;263:126. [PMID: 10763841]

VON WILLEBRAND'S DISEASE

von Willebrand's disease (vWD) is an inherited qualitative or quantitative abnormality of vWF. vWF functions in 2 ways: (1) as an adhesive protein that permits efficient binding of platelets to the endothelium and (2) as a carrier molecule for factor VIII. vWD is the most common coagulopathy that causes problems during pregnancy and delivery. Abnormalities in vWF most commonly are inherited in an autosomal dominant or autosomal recessive fashion with variable penetrance, although they may be acquired also.

Structurally, vWF consists of a series of multimers. Cross-immunoelectrophoretic experiments reveal variable mobility of the multimers, with the smallest multimers having the most rapid mobility. The clinical relevance of these multimer fractions is the apparent relationship between size and hemostatic efficacy. Larger multimeric fractions are the most functionally active, and deficiencies of these factors frequently result in a prolonged bleeding time.

Clinical Findings & Diagnosis

The clinical symptoms among patients with vWD vary greatly. In the usual heterozygous form, defects of primary hemostasis are seen including bruising, epistaxis, gingival oozing, and gastrointestinal blood loss. For some vWD patients, bleeding may not occur except during episodes of added hemostatic stress such as seen with the inadvertent use of NSAIDs. In female patients, the only clue to this condition may be a history of menorrhagia, and frequently, postextraction and posttraumatic bleeding is moderately prolonged. Among females who present with menorrhagia, the prevalence of vWD ranges between 7% and 20%. Homozygous or doubly heterozygous patients may experience severe

bleeding such as postsurgical bleeding, hemarthrosis or, more rarely, uncontrollable gastrointestinal hemorrhage. Many persons with vWD are not diagnosed until adulthood. Bleeding symptoms show considerable variability within a family as well as in an individual on different occasions.

vWD is phenotypically heterogenous and classified into 3 different types (Table 37–5). Type I has a mild reduction in quantity of apparently normal vWF, with a normal multimeric profile; type II and its subgroups have qualitative abnormalities in vWF, either in function or in electrophoretic multimer distribution; and type III is characterized by absent levels of vWF. Clinical severity varies by group, with type III the most severe.

The laboratory diagnosis of vWD is complex and should be undertaken with the assistance of a hematologist or coagulation technician. The criteria for the laboratory diagnosis of vWD include quantitative and qualitative abnormalities of vWF. Because several of the clinical and laboratory findings mimic those of hemophilia (eg, easy bruisability, postprocedure hemorrhage, prolonged PTT, and reduced factor VIII levels), it may be necessary to perform tests for vWD in persons with decreased factor VIII levels and no clear evidence of sex-linked bleeding history. A prolonged bleeding time is characteristic of vWD; in hemophilia, bleeding is a function of reduced factor VIII or factor IX levels, but platelet function (in the absence of recent NSAID use) is normal.

Prolongation of the bleeding time is not specific for vWD; it can be observed in a myriad of platelet and vessel wall abnormalities. In vWD, the bleeding time is abnormal because platelet adherence to subendothe-

Table 37–5. Current classification of von Willebrand's disease.

Type	Description
I	Partial quantitative deficiency of vWF
II	Qualitative deficiency of vWF
IIA	Decreased platelet-dependent vWF function, with lack of high molecular weight multimers (HMWM)
IIB	Increased vWF platelet-dependent vWF function, with normal multimeric structure
IIM	Decreased platelet-dependent vWF function, with normal multimeric structure
IIN	Decreased vWF affinity for factor VIII
III	Complete deficiency of vWF

vWF, von Willebrand's factor.

lium is compromised, thus preventing a normal hemostatic plug. Rarely, bleeding times in vWD remain normal; further testing is recommended if there is a personal or family history of hemorrhage. In the type I variant, in particular, there is an increase in factor VIII coagulant and antigen levels during pregnancy. The PTT and thrombin time are usually normal, although modest elevations in PTT are seen when factor VIII is decreased secondary to the decline in vWF.

Patients with type I vWD may be partially protected during pregnancy because factor VIII and vWF levels increase, often to near-normal levels; therefore, immediate postpartum hemorrhage is an infrequent occurrence. There remains a risk of bleeding after delivery in these women because of the rapid return of the coagulant levels to a nonpregnant, deficient state. The caregiver must be aware that hemorrhage can occur up to 5 weeks postpartum. In type II vWD, in which a qualitative defect in vWF exists, increased levels of vWF during pregnancy may not translate into normalization of the bleeding time. Thrombocytopenia may occur in type IIB disease, presumably because of the increased concentration of more reactive, high-molecular-weight multimers of vWF. Thrombocytopenia and clotting during pregnancy are grounds for thinking about this entity along with the lupus anticoagulant and pregnancy antiphospholipid syndrome.

Treatment

Desmopressin is a synthetic analog of vasopressin and provides temporary benefit to patients with type I vWD by inducing release of vWF from endothelial stores. It has little oxytocic activity and can be used in the early period of pregnancy in women with low factor VIII levels to prevent bleeding at the time of invasive procedures, such as chorionic villus sampling and amniocentesis. Its use is limited by the development of tachyphylaxis after repeated administration. In persons with type II vWD, response to desmopressin is limited and unpredictable. In persons with type IIB vWD, administration of desmopressin can accentuate thrombocytopenia, further aggravating the bleeding problem. Persons with type III vWD do not respond to desmopressin.

Two other types of nontransfusional therapy are sometimes used postpartum in the management of vWD: synthetic antifibrinolytic amino acids and preparations containing both estrogen and progestin. Antifibrinolytic amino acids interfere with the lysis of newly formed clots by saturating the binding sites of plasminogen, thereby preventing its attachment to fibrin and making plasminogen unavailable to activation within the forming clot. Estrogens, synthetic or natural, increase vWF levels, but the response is variable.

Traditionally, cryoprecipitate infusions have been the treatment of choice for patients with all subtypes of vWD who are actively hemorrhaging. Single-donor cryoprecipitate has all the fractions of vWF found in normal plasma. Bleeding usually is arrested once factor VIII procoagulant activity and vWF levels of 50% of normal are achieved. Because the therapeutic effects last approximately 4 hours, cryoprecipitate must be reinfused to maintain normal hemostatic control.

Humate-P® is a stable, purified, sterile, lypholized concentrate of factor VIII prepared from pooled human plasma, which contains vWF. It has been used instead of cryoprecipitate to stop bleeding. Because it is heated to 60 °C for 10 hours, several DNA viruses (cytomegalovirus, herpes, hepatitis B) and RNA viruses (rubella, mumps, measles, and poliomyelitis) are inactivated. While the use of this compound is not approved by the US Food and Drug Administration for the treatment of vWD, there are reports of the use of Humate-P in the treatment of pregnant patients with type IIB disease, and other patients unresponsive to desmopressin.

While there have been no randomized prospective trials of epidural/spinal anesthesia in women with vWF, there are several reports of uncomplicated needle placement in laboring patients. A reasonable option would be to maintain vWF within the normal range with either desmopressin, Humate-P, or cryoprecipitate prior to needle placement and removal. Early consultation with the hematologist and the anesthesiologist should be sought to establish placement criteria.

Figure 37–2 represents an algorithm for the postpartum management of the vWD patient. Elective procedures such as circumcision should be delayed until the disease status of the neonate is known. Maternal vWF generally returns to baseline values within 1 to 3 days. There is no universally agreed upon standard for how long postpartum replacement therapy should be given. In general, replacement therapy is continued for 7–10 days for all patients not responsive to desmopressin. Oral contraceptives containing a synthetic estrogen and a progestin are useful in reducing the severity of menorrhagia in women with vWD, even in those with severe type III. Factor VIII and vWF levels are not significantly modified by this treatment; hence, efficacy is thought to be mediated by the changes induced by oral contraceptives on the endometrium that make it less likely to bleed severely at time of menstruation.

Duffy TP: Hematologic aspects of pregnancy. In: Hoffman R et al (editors). *Hematology: Basic Principles and Practice*, 3rd ed. Churchill Livingstone; 2000:2374.

Duffy TP: Hematologic aspects of pregnancy. In: Burrow GN, Duffy TP (editors). *Medical Complications of Pregnancy*, 5th ed. WB Saunders; 1999:79.

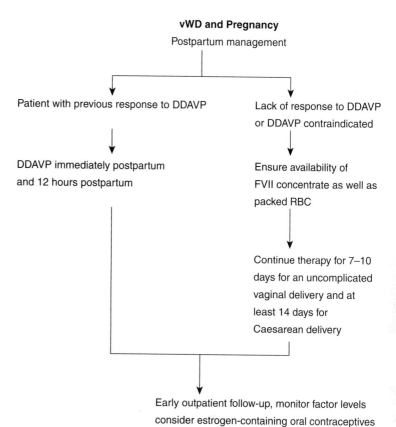

Figure 37–2. Postpartum management of vWD.

Kouides PA: Obstetric and gynaecological aspects of von Willebrand's disease. Best Pract Res Clin Haematol 2001;14:381. [PMID: 11686106]

Mannucci PM: How I treat patients with von Willebrand's disease. Blood 2001;97:1915. [PMID: 11264151]

Roque H, Funai E, Lockwood CJ: von Willebrand disease and pregnancy. J Matern Fetal Med 2000;9:257. [PMID: 11132579]

Roque H, Funai E, Lockwood CJ: Hemostatic problems before, during and after delivery. J Perinat Med 2001;29:241.

When to Refer to a Specialist

When sorting out hematologic issues in the pregnant woman, it is essential to be aware of the physiologic changes in pregnancy that affect hematologic laboratory parameters. Although the treatment and obstetric management of most hematologic disorders is well established, controversy exists concerning conditions such as ITP, DIC, and sickle cell disease. In addition, therapies chosen to manage a maternal problem must be modulated according to their potential for damage to the fetus. To ensure optimal health of the pregnant woman and fetus, a hematologist should be consulted in the evaluation of patients with moderate to severe thrombocytopenia, anemia that is not responsive to iron supplementation, or a prior history of moderate to severe bleeding after surgical procedures.

SECTION XII

Neurologic Disorders

Headache

38

David Likosky, MD & Laird G. Patterson, MD

MIGRAINE

The cause of migraine (MG), a ubiquitous disorder, is obscure. There is no universally accepted definition of the condition. In 1988, the International Headache Society published criteria that are useful for gathering data and assessing treatment; however, the criteria are too complex for everyday use. MG can be defined generally as paroxysmal or periodic recurrent attacks of headache, frequently unilateral, and often preceded by or associated with widespread premonitory systemic or neurologic symptoms. MG is no longer classified as common or classic but rather as MG without aura and MG with aura (see the following section, Migrainous Aura).

ESSENTIALS OF DIAGNOSIS

- *Strong family history.*
- *Pattern altered by hormonal factors including menses, pregnancy, menopause, ingestion of oral contraceptives, and hormone replacement therapy.*
- *Existence of endogenous and exogenous triggering factors.*
- *Consisting of a prodrome, aura (15–20% of patients), headache, associated symptoms, and postdrome.*
- *Headache responds to medications that have agonist and antagonist actions at the serotonin (5-HT) receptor site.*

General Considerations

Although the heterogeneity makes prevalence difficult to estimate, studies suggest that MG occurs in 18% of women and 6% of men. Peak onset is in the third and fourth decades. Prevalence of MG seems to increase steadily from childhood until approximately age 40 and then decrease beginning in the fifth decade. Although MG tends to resolve with age, it continues into old age in 25% of patients. Migraineurs have a strong family history of MG; 50–60% identify first-degree relatives as affected. The risk of developing MG is especially high if the condition is present in both parents.

Migraine prevalence is inversely related to household income and is not related to intelligence test scores or socioeconomic class. Migraineurs with higher intelligence test scores and in higher socioeconomic groups, however, are more likely to consult a physician.

Pathogenesis

Any attempt to explain the cause of MG must encompass all of its features including trigger factors, prodrome, aura, headache, associated systemic and neurologic symptoms, and the aftermath, or postdrome. Earlier, vasomotor theories did not adequately explain this conflation of events. Although an exact cause remains elusive, reproducible changes in brain biochemistry and physiology have been documented repeatedly.

Serotonin has been recognized for a long time to be a neurotransmitter of interest in MG. Platelet serotonin levels fall dramatically prior to an attack and rise later. A variety of 5-HT receptors populate the intracranial and extracranial vasculature, and their activation produces both vasoconstriction and vasodilation. Serotonin acts as a regulatory neurotransmitter in the endogenous pain control pathway and stimulates peripheral nociceptive nerve terminals. It is important in the regulation of mood, appetite, and sleep. Several drugs affecting serotonin release and uptake may cause headache, and anti-MG drugs have an agonist or antagonist function at the 5-HT receptors.

Brainstem areas such as the locus ceruleus and dorsal raphe nuclei innervate intracranial vasculature and may influence its reactivity. Stimulation of these centers may initiate some of the hemodynamic and vascular changes that occur during MG; however, the factors that initially activate neurons in these nuclei are unknown.

A corollary to the brainstem neural hypothesis of MG is the observation that the aura is associated with spread of a transient depolarizing wave beginning posteriorly and propagating anteriorly across the cortical surface. During this event, neurons are depolarized; repolarization is delayed; and transient, reversible fluxes in potassium, sodium, and calcium can be measured. During the aura, oligemia has been measured, and soon thereafter, hyperemia occurs. The inciting event is not known, although projections from the brainstem nuclei may stimulate the cortex and cortical vessels and disrupt normal neurophysiologic and vasomotor function.

Headache is another feature of MG that is not explained easily, contrary to earlier theory, cephalgia begins before vasodilatation. Unknown triggers stimulate trigeminal afferents in vessel walls and generate nociceptive impulses. Neuropeptides (eg, substance P and bradykinin) are released within the vascular endothelium causing plasma extravasation, inflammation, and persistent pain. The frontal and occipitocervical distribution of the trigeminal nerve is coincidentally the distribution of MG pain.

Although no single theory accounts for all of the phases of MG, it appears certain that neural and vascular components both are necessary and that serotonin is an important mediator of the neurovascular events that culminate as the MG phenomenon. Advances in functional imaging with magnetic resonance imaging (MRI) and positron emission tomography scanning as well as noninvasive transcranial magnetic stimulation hold promise in unraveling the nature of MG.

Clinical Findings

The diagnosis of MG relies almost exclusively on the patient's history because there are no tests that support the diagnosis. A careful search for the typical features aids in characterizing a syndrome that may have seemed vague to the patient or other examiners and allows for appropriate therapy. Essential aspects of the headache evaluation are listed in Table 38–1.

Table 38–1. Headache/migraine history.

Chronology
    Age and circumstances of onset
    Frequency and duration
    Timing (day, week, month, season)
Pain descriptors
    Location and radiation
    Course and severity
    Character of pain
Precipitating factors
    Exogenous
    Endogenous
Aggravating factors
    Exertion
    Position, movement
    Valsalva maneuver
Associated systemic and neurologic features
    Prodrome
    Aura
    Headache
    Postdrome
Past and present therapy
    Nonpharmacologic
    Pharmacologic
        Drug, dose, duration
        Combinations
    Response to therapy
    Abuse or overuse
Other illnesses
Personal history
    Occupation
    Family situation
    Habits
    Emotional state
    Biorhythms
        Sleep
        Eating habits
    Family history of migraine or other headaches

A. History

Many patients mistakenly believe that they have several different varieties of headache when they experience occipitocervical pain on one occasion; sharp stabbing pains on another; and intense, throbbing hemicranial pain on a third. In fact, these headaches are all part of the MG syndrome. The misattribution of allergy as a cause of headache is due to the mistaken impression that foods cause headache through allergic rather than biochemical mechanisms. Sinus disease, ophthalmologic and dental conditions, and temporomandibular joint syndrome are often mistakenly considered causes of headaches that are of migrainous origin.

The circumstances of the first recognized attack, premonitory symptoms, aura (if any), and temporal profile of the headache itself with its associated features are all important in identifying a headache as migrainous or not. Pain location, quality, and severity should be determined. The episodic nature and associated features of the MG syndrome best define it, and these symptoms should be sought in detail. The patient's memory of the attacks may be inaccurate, and only specific questioning may elicit the necessary information.

It is important to know the particulars of past headache treatments. Medications and combinations of medications, doses, duration of therapeutic trials, and treatment response all should be detailed, because patients commonly take subtherapeutic doses for inappropriately short periods. Presumed side effects that prevented the use of effective drugs may turn out to have been insignificant or misattributed, and another trial may be initiated. Prior nonpharmacologic interventions and their benefits are also important to know about before a new treatment strategy is designed.

The patient's occupation, with its stresses or exposure to triggering factors, may contribute to the MG syndrome. Family difficulties; poor health habits, particularly smoking and excessive drinking; overuse of caffeine; sleep disruptions; and situations that produce wide emotional swings all provoke MG. Other illnesses often have an impact on MG either because of medications required for their treatment or because of the illness itself. Head injuries can precipitate or aggravate migrainous headache. Withdrawal from prescription or illicit drugs as well as caffeine can cause headache as well.

A search for familial MG should consist of more than an inquiry as to whether or not other family members have headaches. Patients often mistakenly attribute familial headaches to sinus disease, allergy, or head injury, or may state that a relative with headaches was told that the problem was not MG. Further questioning often discloses that family members who were thought to have nonmigrainous headache may have had MG syndrome.

B. Physical Examination

The interictal physical examination usually is normal. If patients are examined during the attack, they are pale and diaphoretic, appear acutely ill, are sitting or lying in a darkened room when the examiner enters, and may vomit during the course of the evaluation. Blood pressure elevation and tachycardia are often present. Facial flushing, tearing, conjunctival injection, nasal stuffiness, and even unilateral ptosis and miosis may be encountered. Patients who have mentioned focal swelling of the scalp, periorbital tissues, or face may demonstrate

that finding. Some patients appear reluctant to answer questions, may seem dazed or confused, or may even have a hemiparesis, hemisensory abnormalities, aphasia, or brainstem signs such as disconjugate gaze, nystagmus, dysarthria, ataxia, paresis, or sensory loss.

C. Symptoms and Signs

The heterogeneity of MG symptoms implies a widespread disruption of normal physiologic function that is not confined to the brain and cerebral vessels. Migraine with aura constitutes only 15–20% of all MG. Many migraineurs who experience aura have attacks that are aura-free. In addition, the aura can occur without headache. Whether or not the various forms of MG are the same disorder, they share many of the same clinical, biochemical, and electrophysiologic characteristics.

1. The prodrome—Migraineurs may have vague premonitory or prodromal experiences preceding their headache by 24–48 hours. These include insidious changes in mood, behavior, and appetite; fatigue; gastrointestinal disturbances; and fluid retention. Mild confusion, irritability, elation, depression, or anxiety can also can be part of the prodrome.

2. Triggers or precipitants—A multiplicity of exogenous triggering factors are recognized by MG patients (Table 38–2). Endogenous genetic and biologic factors also may initiate an attack. Foods containing biogenic amines or additives such as monosodium glutamate, nitrites, or aspartame are major precipitants. Biogenic amines are concentrated principally in cheese, dairy products, chocolate, seafood, and citrus fruits. Alcohol (in particular, red wine) may contain impurities or biogenic amines. Physical factors such as exertion, glare, or bright or flashing lights may evoke headache. Many patients are sensitive to loud noises, odors, or changes in barometric pressure. Disruption of eating and sleeping routines, stress, and letdown from stress are all disturbances of biologic rhythm that can initiate attack. Head trauma, especially in young patients with familial MG, may trigger a series of attacks. Medications are often responsible for the onset or perpetuation of an episode (Table 38–3).

Migraineurs often cannot identify a consistent relationship between a triggering factor and the development of headache. In addition, with the passage of time and changes in the MG pattern, patients become sensitive to factors to which they previously were resistant. Precipitants may induce changes in vascular reactivity, neurotransmitter function, or receptor sensitivity that eventuate in the MG attack. Therefore, while identification of precipitants may be helpful, it is rare to be able to markedly alter MG by avoiding triggers.

3. Migrainous aura—An aura is a well-defined neurologic symptom that is often, but not always, followed

Table 38–2. Triggering factors for migraine.

Diet
   Processed, fermented, preserved foods
   Bioactive amines
     Phenylmethylamine—chocolate
     Tyramine—red wine, cheese
     Octopamine—citrus fruits
   Additives
     Monosodium glutemate (MSG)
     Nitrites, nitrates
     Aspartame
     Excess salt
   Beverages
     Alcohol
     Caffeine (withdrawal)
Physical/environmental factors
   Exertion
   Heat, cold
   Visual stimulus—glare, flashing lights
   Noise
   Odors, fumes
     Solvents
     Hydrocarbons
     Perfumes
     Smoke
   Barometric pressure
     Weather change
     High altitude
   Head trauma
Psychological factors
   Stress, stress letdown
   Depression
   Anxiety
Biorhythm disturbances
   Sleep disruption, deprivation
   Weekends, holidays
   Fasting, overeating
   Time-zone changes
Hormonal changes
   Menses, ovulation
   Pregnancy
   Menopause
Medications (see Table 38–3)
Other systemic symptoms
   Fever
   Dehydration
   Dialysis
   Anemia

Table 38–3. Medication triggers.

Illicit drugs
   Cocaine
   Amphetamines
Antibiotics
   Griseofulvin
   Trimethoprim
Antihypertensives
   Captopril
   Minoxidil
   Nifedipine
   Reserpine
Nitrates
   Isosorbide dinitrate
   Trinitroglycerine
Hormones
   Estrogen
   Oral contraceptives
   Danazol
   Medroxy progesterone acetate (Depo-Provera)
Nonsteroidal anti-inflammatory drugs (NSAIDs)
   Indomethacin
   Ibuprofen
H_2-receptor antagonists
   Cimetidine
   Ranitidine
Miscellaneous
   Vitamin A derivatives
   Abuse or overuse of over-the-counter drugs

by headache. The most common aura is either a negative (absence of vision) or a scintillating scotoma marching slowly across the visual field. Unilateral face and arm paresthesias, lateralized mild weakness or clumsiness, language and cognitive impairment, alterations in consciousness such as dreamlike states, depersonalization, and distortions of the visual environment all have been reported. Vertigo; olfactory or gustatory sensations; and nonspecific intracranial, visceral, or abdominal sensations occur independently or accompany other, better-defined symptoms. Auras persist for minutes to as long as an hour and may vary in intensity and duration from one attack to another.

Complicated MG is a term reserved for episodes of headache with an aura of severe unilateral paralysis, aphasia, and sensory or visual loss. Deficits may be prolonged or persistent. **Basilar MG,** an unusual entity that occurs in young persons, includes a variety of brainstem and cerebellar symptoms, viz, dramatic changes in the visual fields, diplopia, dysarthria or anarthria, vertigo, ataxia, and weakness or numbness. Transient unresponsiveness, syncope, or a confusional state may accompany basilar MG.

4. Headache characteristics—Headache that follows an aura may occur as the aura is resolving or any time 1–2 hours later. Migrainous head pain is often unilateral (strictly so in 50% of adults) and may switch sides during different episodes. Headache typically begins unilaterally in the occipitocervical region and radiates anteriorly, but it is frequently holocranial from the onset. Pain frequently radiates to the orbit or retroorbital area and face, particularly the cheek or jaw, or even to shoulders and arms. Headaches are usually contralateral to the aura. Head pain is sometimes sharply localized and accompanied by focal scalp tenderness. Cervical paraspinous and trapezius soreness or tenderness may precede a full headache.

MG pain may be throbbing and pulsatile or simply dull and aching in character. At times, an intense, pounding headache is relieved by vomiting. Pain may be incapacitating and only partially attenuated by lying quietly in a dark room. Physical activity, jolting, or Valsalva maneuver intensifies the pain. Headache may last from a few minutes to as long as several days; a nagging, dull, cephalgia or scalp tenderness may persist even after the primary headache has resolved. Discrete jabbing, sharp, ice pick–like pains may be superimposed on the headache or continue after it has resolved.

5. Associated symptoms—Although headache is the salient feature of an MG attack, other associated symptoms may be even more disabling. Patients experience phonophobia and photophobia of varying severity, and they may have an aversion to smells that are normally pleasurable. Nausea or vomiting complicates the headache in more than 50% of cases. Vomiting may intensify the headache or may provide relief. If vomiting is severe and prolonged, it causes dehydration and electrolyte depletion, further aggravating the condition. Diarrhea and bowel hyperactivity can be prodromal symptoms but often occur during the headache. Gastric emptying is usually slowed. Light-headedness, severe orthostatic dizziness, or even syncope may accompany attacks. Patients can experience a vague sense of disequilibrium or even have true vertigo.

During an attack, it is common for patients to feel mildly disoriented or confused, and concentration is poor. Mood changes overwhelm many patients; they may become agitated, tearful, irritable, hostile, and easily angered, or they may withdraw and desire seclusion or isolation. Lassitude, enervation, drowsiness, and an overwhelming sleepiness appear during and after the peak of the headache. In severe cases, there may be extreme disorganization of thought processes, depersonalization, and impaired memory or even amnesia.

Other ictal changes include signs of vasomotor instability such as flushing, pallor, diaphoresis, and unilateral swelling of the face, periorbital tissues, or scalp.

Although more commonly seen in cluster headaches, unilateral ptosis, miosis, conjunctival injection, and nasal congestion may be evident with strongly unilateral migraine. Temperature dysregulation and elevation of blood pressure may be recorded during the episode. Many female patients experience fluid retention prior to the attack and later undergo a diuresis.

6. Postdromal symptoms—Premonitory and ictal symptoms often obscure the postdromal or postictal phase. Some patients note that sleep restores a feeling of well-being; however, many continue to feel mentally dull and slightly dazed, with mild head discomfort, for 24–48 hours afterward. For 1–2 days or even a week, patients may note listlessness, fatigue, somnolence, and a subdued or depressed mood. Cognitive function, including concentration and memory, may remain impaired, although some patients emerge from an attack feeling refreshed, elated, and energetic. Enhanced appetite can occur, but nausea, often in association with the smell of certain foods, can persist for several days.

7. Headache patterns—MG peaks between the ages of 20 and 40. In many patients, MG develops in early childhood, becomes latent, and reemerges in early or mid adulthood. The frequency of attacks varies considerably. There may be lengthy periods without headaches, followed by a clustering or grouping of headaches. Some patients have predictable episodic cephalgia (eg, during the menstrual cycle). MG typically worsens during the first trimester of pregnancy and improves thereafter. Others have headache only when they fail to avoid a known trigger factor. Migraineurs may go for months or years without experiencing an attack, but when they do have one, it can be severe and prolonged. Headache duration averages 12–72 hours, but it can be briefer, and headaches can persist for a week or more. Headache-free intervals are the norm between attacks, but ice pick pains or dull, chronic daily headache (CDH) may complicate the interictal period. Discrete MG attacks with interposed CDH often result from overuse of ergotamines, triptans or over-the-counter (OTC) medications—so called "rebound" headache. The migraine pattern may change during the childbearing years and perimenopausally.

Episodes often occur at or near the same time of day, week, or month. Some patients are awakened with headache in the middle of the night or in early morning, possibly during rapid eye movement sleep. Others note attacks at the end or beginning of a workweek. Vacations or holidays are other likely periods of risk, and a clustering of attacks may disrupt major holiday periods. Migraineurs who travel frequently and cross multiple time zones may experience headache because of a change in their usual diurnal pattern.

D. LABORATORY FINDINGS

Blood tests are unnecessary in the investigation of typical MG, but they can be important in evaluating alternative causes of headache such as temporal arteritis or a systemic illness. Occasionally, patients have a dramatic aura accompanying their headache that is suggestive of a seizure disorder; such patients need an electroencephalogram to help differentiate MG aura from the aura of a seizure disorder. Lumbar puncture (LP) usually is reserved for patients in whom subarachnoid hemorrhage, infection, or intracranial hypertension is suspected. It is necessary if a previously asymptomatic patient experiences a fulminating headache even though it may have some of the features of MG.

E. IMAGING STUDIES

Imaging studies are appropriate only if there is confusion about the diagnosis. Computed tomography (CT) with and without contrast or MRI and magnetic resonance angiography may be useful depending on the situation. When MG is clearly the cause of a patient's symptoms, imaging studies are not needed. Percutaneous angiography is performed rarely now that magnetic resonance angiography is available. Some patients cannot be dissuaded from pursuing testing, because they want to know the cause of their headaches. Neuropsychiatric testing may be helpful in validating complaints of persistent cognitive dysfunction but is a lengthy procedure.

Variations & Complications of Migraine

A. CHRONIC DAILY HEADACHE

This condition occurs often in patients with prior attacks of MG in whom there has been transformation from episodic headache with headache-free intervals to daily headache with superimposed attacks of MG. In this group, there usually is a strong family history of MG, and hormonal changes are a triggering factor; many patients report associated gastrointestinal and neurologic symptoms. Transformation of MG to CDH is common in mid life or during the perimenopausal years. Tobacco use may contribute to CDH of this and other types.

A second group of patients with CDH have had episodic tension-type headache, which may have been associated with cervical and pericranial tenderness. The headaches may be intermittent initially and transform gradually into CDH, although some patients have headaches that are daily in occurrence from the onset. Associated features are rare, but photophobia and nausea can occur. Patients with chronic tension-type headache do not have a history of episodic MG-type headache with clear-cut attacks and associated migrainous features.

A third group of patients with CDH have symptoms related to viral infections, particularly Epstein-Barr. Following the onset of headaches, prolonged CDH, often self-limited, occurs. Symptoms may continue for months.

There are several distinctive clinical features of CDH. There is an increased incidence of depression. Medication overuse is common and includes excessive ingestion of OTC medications such as aspirin, acetaminophen, and headache preparations containing caffeine. Medications may be overprescribed, contributing to dependency and analgesic rebound. It must be remembered that some medications used for prophylactic therapy can produce headache that resembles CDH as a side effect.

The headache caused by analgesic rebound or medication overuse varies in location and severity. It often is precipitated by minimal activity or stress, and many patients become irritable, cannot concentrate, complain of sleep-related difficulties, awaken in the morning with severe headache, and become physically inactive and socially withdrawn.

Among the consequences of continued medication overuse are reduction or nullification of the effectiveness of other symptomatic and prophylactic therapies. The headache is perpetuated by the continued use of medication, and short periods of withdrawal or partial reduction in the frequency or dosage of medication does not result in significant improvement and often results in marked discomfort discouraging further attempts.

Management of CDH can be difficult and requires a multidisciplinary or multimodal approach. Complete discontinuation of the offending medications is mandatory if the headache cycle is to be interrupted. Judicious and temporary use of benzodiazepines to help patients taper and discontinue the offending drugs may be necessary. Stress management, biofeedback, other forms of counseling, and a vigorous exercise program should be instituted if appropriate. Patients should be instructed clearly on the deleterious effects of medication overuse.

Prophylactic treatment can begin with a reasonable chance for effectiveness once patients have been withdrawn successfully from their medications. These patients need close follow-up care and continued monitoring of their medication use.

The prognosis of CDH is somewhat discouraging. Despite attempts to withdraw medication, initiate changes in lifestyle, and institute effective prophylaxis, at least one third of patients continue to experience headache. There is a discouraging relapse rate if patients are not carefully monitored. Some authors believe these patients get little or no relief despite all the changes that are made and resume their previous habits of medication overuse. In refractory cases, there may be some advantage in enrolling patients in a pain clinic or a specialized headache clinic for intense outpatient or inpatient therapy.

B. Status Migrainosus

Status migrainosus (SM) is defined as a continuous severe headache lasting longer than 72 hours with less than 4 hours during that period (not counting sleep) of headache-free time with or without treatment. In addition to the usual triggering factors, viral or other febrile illness or a minor head injury may precede the development of SM. Even when the inciting event remits, the headache may continue. Changes in hormonal status such as menopause or changes in the menstrual cycle may be associated with SM in susceptible persons.

Features of SM in addition to intractability and long duration include sleep deprivation (which undoubtedly aggravates the headache); nausea; vomiting; dehydration; and behavioral changes such as irritability, agitation, and withdrawal. Often, multiple attempts to control the headache have failed, and patients may have complicated the situation by self-medication with other drugs or alcohol in an attempt to control the headache. When a patient has SM, a careful search should be made for other causes of severe unremitting headache, such as infection, subarachnoid hemorrhage, or a space-occupying lesion, although these conditions often are clinically apparent and uncommon. A thorough history and neurologic examination is the key to these diagnoses.

Treatment of SM often requires hospitalization for rehydration and intravenous medication. Dihydroergotamine mesylate (DHE) (0.5 mg) and metoclopramide (10 mg) can be administered intravenously over a 2–3 minute period, and repeated every 8 hours if the initial dose provides temporary relief of the headache. Higher doses of DHE (0.75–1 mg) may be given if the lower dose is not effective and nausea is not a limiting side effect. This schedule of DHE and metoclopramide may be continued until the headache is relieved completely but should not exceed 3 days. Treatment of other complications, such as electrolyte disturbances and dehydration, and the addition of intravenous methylprednisolone or dexamethasone may help terminate SM. On an outpatient basis, a short burst of oral corticosteroids may abort the episode.

C. Cerebrovascular Complications

Persistence of neurologic deficits and abnormal imaging studies that suggest cerebral ischemia occur in some patients with MG. It has been estimated that approximately 10% of cases of stroke seen in patients under age 40 are related to an attack of MG. The incidence is significantly higher in women by a factor of 3 or 4. Strokes occur more often in patients who have a discrete, intense aura associated with their headache. Smoking and hypertension increase the risk of MG-related stroke. It is not clear whether oral contraceptives are associated with an increased incidence of migrainous stroke because study results are conflicting.

The pathophysiology of MG stroke is not completely understood. Cerebral imaging and blood flow studies demonstrate persistent hypoperfusion and ischemia, but whether these are caused by vasospasm or whether neural activity influences the perfusion abnormalities is yet to be determined. There may be an increase in platelet aggregation, and a hypercoagulable state may contribute to the ischemic process. The clinical features of the stroke often resemble the symptoms of a previous aura. Stroke often occurs during the course of an MG attack or may begin with the aura. Other causes of stroke must be excluded even in young patients who have MG. Medications that intensify vasoconstriction are among the factors thought to precipitate MG stroke. The ergotamines and triptans have been of concern, although no direct evidence exists that they cause stroke. Trauma and arteriography sometimes are identified as precipitating causes of stroke in migraineurs.

Stroke is most common in the posterior cerebral circulation, although middle cerebral artery branch ischemia is also seen. Patients may have monocular symptoms caused by retinal infarction. A variety of visual, somatosensory, motor, and cognitive changes have been reported with MG stroke. Fortunately, recovery is often good, although it may be incomplete.

Patients who have severe aura and in whom stroke is a concern should avoid vasoconstrictor therapy and undergo long-term treatment with verapamil and aspirin. They should be encouraged strongly to discontinue any adverse lifestyle habits such as smoking and any medications that may be harmful such as oral contraceptives. If stroke occurs, evaluation for other causes should be undertaken. Neurologic consultation should be strongly considered for determination of appropriate work-up and choice of anticoagulation.

D. Migraine and the Hormonal Cycle

1. Menstrual MG—Menstrual MG affects approximately 60% of female MG sufferers, in whom some or all of their headaches are related to the menstrual cycle. Most attacks occur during the first 2–3 days preceding the onset of menstruation or during the first or second day of the menses. The timing is consistent for individual patients. Headaches are frequently severe; are somewhat longer lasting than other forms of MG, persisting for 2–3 days; and are accompanied by nausea and vomiting. Most of the attacks occur without aura, although patients who have MG with aura at other times often experience aura with menstrual MG.

Menstrual MG may be absent for several cycles only to occur repetitively for several subsequent cycles before remitting again. In women whose menstrual cycle is irregular, headaches are unpredictable. Other women may have headache only during ovulation at mid cycle, although both mid- and end-of-cycle headaches can coexist in the same patient. The onset of menstrual MG often coincides with menarche. The age of onset seems to be slightly younger than that of MG that is not related to the menstrual cycle.

The role of hormones in the genesis of menstrual MG is not fully understood; however, it is clear that headache is associated with a rapid fall in plasma estradiol levels. Progesterone fluctuations do not play a significant role. Absolute estrogen levels are not as important as the rate and degree of their fall.

Artificially maintaining a high estrogen level during the menstrual period may delay headaches until the estrogen level falls. Other hormones that have been studied include prostaglandins, prolactin, and the endorphins, but their roles in the genesis of menstrual MG are unclear.

Treatment of menstrual MG depends on the patient's history. If an attack of MG is similar to other attacks occurring during the month, the timing represents menstrual worsening of the underlying MG, and treatment is no different than for other forms of MG. MG that is purely menstrual can be resistant to therapy.

If headache is predictable, prophylactic therapy begun 1 week before onset of menses and continued for the week afterward allows for intermittent rather than daily therapy. At times, however, daily therapy may be necessary. Low dose ergots can be used around the time of menstruation. Prostaglandin inhibitors are another consideration. Conventional abortive and prophylactic medications are largely effective. Calcium channel blockers, which often require considerable time to exert their effect, are less likely to be successful. Although diuretics might seem useful because the premenstrual period often is associated with fluid retention, they generally are not helpful.

Because of the relationship between headache and the drop in estrogen levels, hormonal manipulation has been attempted to prevent menstrual MG; however, there has not been a consistent response. Although oral estrogen replacement is usually ineffective, the use of transdermal estradiol may suppress symptoms possibly due to more stable levels as the headache correlates with estrogen withdrawal. Estrogen therapy usually delays the onset of headache rather than eliminating it. Androgens, tamoxifen, and bromocriptine mesylate all have been tried, but reports of success have been anecdotal only.

Overall, the best approach to therapy is restricted prophylaxis in patients who have predictable menses

and headaches. A combination of naproxen and ergotamine tartrate begun 3–4 days prior to the predicted onset of an attack is often best, and more complicated regimens may be unnecessary. Indeed, naproxen itself may be sufficient.

2. Oral contraceptive use—An increased incidence of headache in previously headache-free women and aggravation of existing MG are reported by 20–50% of patients taking oral contraceptives. As might be expected, the attacks tend to occur during the period when medication is not taken, when estrogen levels are falling.

One third of patients taking oral contraceptives report improvement in their headache syndromes, but most patients experience no change. If onset of MG occurs with oral contraceptive use, it is generally during the earlier cycles, but it can emerge after months or even years of use. On occasion, headaches may be related to a change in the type of oral contraceptive. A family history of MG is absent in up to 60% of women in whom symptoms develop with oral contraceptive use, making it difficult to predict who might be at risk.

Guidelines for the use of oral contraceptives are not formally established, and many contraindications are relative. Family history, as noted, is not a good predictor of risk, but a strong family history of MG may be a relative contraindication. If new-onset MG that develops early in the course of oral contraceptive use is severe, disruptive, or associated with significant neurologic dysfunction, the patient should discontinue the drug.

Patients with preexisting MG who have marked aggravation of their symptoms may respond best to a lower dose oral contraceptive or to withdrawal rather than an attempt to treat the headache and continue the oral contraceptive. Stroke risk is difficult to assess; however, there is some suggestion that patients with severe and prolonged aura or neurologic symptoms should discontinue oral contraceptives because stroke sometimes occurs in this group. Change in the pattern of MG from headache without aura to headache with aura may define another subgroup of patients who should discontinue oral contraceptives. The rate of migrainous infarction is greater in patients with risk factors such as smoking, hypertension, or lipid disorders, and these factors are strong contraindications to use of oral contraceptives.

Treatment of patients with oral contraceptive–related MG clearly involves withdrawal of the offending agent. If the headache persists, taking 6 months to a year to resolve, routine symptomatic or prophylactic MG therapy is used.

3. Pregnancy and the postpartum period—Pregnancy usually has a beneficial effect on MG, and suppression or resolution of the attacks is seen in 50–90% of cases. Improvement often begins during the last 2 trimesters; migraine can worsen during the first trimester. It is much less likely that a patient will have worsening of attacks during pregnancy. In 10–15% of cases, MG makes its initial appearance in the first trimester of pregnancy. Uncommonly, MG may mark the onset of preeclampsia or eclampsia. Some patients with MG have a less well-defined headache at the onset of their pregnancy, which later resolves. Nonspecific, limited peripartum headache is also frequent in migraineurs. Elevated hormone levels may play a role in the genesis of pregnancy-related MG, and the rapid fall associated with delivery may be the cause of postpartum headaches.

Treatment of MG during pregnancy rarely requires prophylaxis or significant amounts of abortive or symptomatic medication, because patients often are able to cope with the pain. If medication must be used, small doses of acetaminophen or codeine are relatively safe. Nondrug therapies should be emphasized. If prophylaxis is required, β-blockers and amitriptyline are acceptable. For acute, severe headache, injections of meperidine and antinauseants such as metoclopramide, if used infrequently, are deemed safe. Intravenous or oral corticosteroids given on rare occasions for persistent headache also are not associated with complications.

Other causes of headache during pregnancy besides MG should be considered. Hypertension, pseudotumor, subarachnoid hemorrhage caused by aneurysm or arteriovenous malformation, expanding tumors (particularly of the pituitary gland or meningiomas), and *Listeria monocytogenes* infection all are possible causes of headache during pregnancy and may need to be excluded by appropriate studies before MG therapy is instituted.

If headaches requiring treatment recur during the postpartum period in a nursing mother, consideration must be given to concentrations of anti-MG drugs in breast milk. Aspirin and the ergotamines are likely to be present at high levels. Medications that are considered safe include acetaminophen, most of the nonsteroidal anti-inflammatory drugs (NSAIDs), β-blockers, calcium channel blockers, and codeine.

Headache in some patients may be refractory to treatment because of lifestyle changes, such as sleep disruption or deprivation, that occur with mothering an infant. It may be necessary to discontinue nursing if the mother is incapacitated by headache.

4. Menopause—Although MG may disappear during menopause, it may make its initial appearance, change character, or worsen in some patients. A change in MG may precede menopause by 5 or more years, possibly because of hormonal changes that ultimately lead to cessation of the menses.

The course of MG often is altered by the need for hormone replacement therapy (HRT). Although it may be associated with improvement in the MG syndrome, HRT often produces no change or even a marked worsening of MG, and it may be responsible for a dramatic alteration in the character of the headache. Excessive use of OTC medications may be largely responsible for the changing character of the headache.

Treatment of menopausal and postmenopausal MG relies on the medications previously outlined. Attempts to manipulate the hormonal status of the patient by HRT or by more drastic measures such as hysterectomy generally have failed. Occasionally, shifting the dosage and type of HRT or changing from a cyclic regimen to a continuous regimen may be beneficial. Discontinuing oral HRT and using the transdermal delivery route may improve symptoms in some patients. The lowest possible dosage of estrogen necessary to maintain the desired effect or a change in the type of estrogen may diminish or eliminate the headaches. If hormonal manipulation is not effective, routine anti-MG prophylaxis or symptomatic therapy can be used.

Treatment

A. GENERAL PRINCIPLES

The goal of MG therapy, whether aimed at alleviating the acute attack or preventing recurrent attacks, is the reduction in headache frequency, severity, and duration, and in associated symptoms. Complete success is not always achieved, however, and symptom reduction rather than absolute relief may be the best that can be accomplished. Many migraineurs have tried numerous OTC and prescription medications and had numerous physician interactions and remain discouraged. They need to be made aware that headache therapy is a long-term process. A good doctor-patient relationship is critical to the success of any treatment program.

The foundation of any treatment plan is nonpharmacologic management. This aspect includes alterations in adverse lifestyle practices; identification and elimination of triggering factors; and a review of the social, familial, and occupational situation of the patient to determine what changes will enhance the success of a headache management program.

Pharmacologic treatment strategy depends on a variety of considerations such as the frequency and severity of the MG syndrome. Infrequent headache, even though severe, may not warrant preventive therapy if it can be managed with abortive and symptomatic medications. Patients with fewer than 2–4 headaches a month usually do not require prophylactic medication. However, frequent headaches or headaches that are infrequent but severe and disruptive require the addition of prophylactic therapy. Patients who have transient physical manifestations such as hemiparesis, and those who have stroke should uniformly receive prophylactic therapy. Migraineurs are more likely, in general to have a stroke—particularly seen in women under age 45 and in patients with aura. Therefore, patients with severe aura (weakness, aphasia, etc) are generally given prophylaxis.

Patients who have an identifiable prodrome or aura often respond well to abortive medication, because they can take it early in the course of the episode before symptoms are fully developed. Delayed use of abortive medications is generally ineffective and may even contribute to the headache. The route of administration for acute therapy must be chosen on the basis of convenience, suitability, and patient acceptability.

Because gastric emptying time often is delayed or vomiting intervenes, oral administration frequently is impossible. Use of an antiemetic such as metoclopramide (acts at a subtype of the serotonin receptor) prior to other medication may improve tolerance of the oral route, however. Rectal administration gives the best absorption of medication and avoids the problem of vomiting. Nasal and inhalant forms of medication are now available as are rapidly dissolving oral formulations. Self-administered subcutaneous injection of various medications is an option for patients willing to learn self-injection techniques.

The physician must be aware of such contraindications to medications as pregnancy, concomitant diseases, or interactions with other medications. Most drugs should not be used by pregnant patients. Cardiovascular, gastrointestinal, hepatic, renal, or pulmonary disease precludes the use of many anti-MG drugs. Potential adverse interactions with drugs used to treat systemic illnesses may limit treatment choices.

Prophylactic therapy is reserved for patients with frequent or severe disruptive headache or for those in whom acute therapy has failed or is contraindicated. It is important for patients taking prophylactic medications to record treatment effects to guide changes in medication in complicated or resistant cases. It should be emphasized to patients that prophylactic therapy is not a cure; it is considered effective if it reduces the frequency, severity, and duration of the MG episode or enhances the benefits of symptomatic therapy. Preventive therapy is selected with careful attention to drug safety and is used at the lowest effective dose. Encouragement is necessary, as prophylactic treatment may take some time to titrate to an effective dose.

Minor side effects may emerge with administration of prophylactic drugs; in many cases, however, patients adapt with continued use. If side effects remit, patients should be encouraged to continue.

Cost is a consideration when devising a treatment plan. Although many medications are generic and inexpensive, visits to the emergency department, newer medications, and some prophylactic medications are expensive.

B. Nonpharmacologic Treatment

Lifestyle changes may be difficult to enact, but they should be pursued. Stress reduction may be accomplished through counseling. Job changes and family therapy may eliminate some obstacles to headache improvement without resorting to medication.

Personal habits are important to explore. Smoking or other forms of tobacco use not only are potential triggering factors for MG, but also negate the effects of symptomatic and prophylactic therapy. These habits must be discontinued before therapy can succeed.

Dietary factors often are known and avoided, but it may take further questioning to identify obscure items in the diet that also trigger headache. So-called elimination diets, which attempt to eliminate all foods that might potentially cause headache, are generally not effective.

Management of biorhythm disturbances, such as unconventional eating habits, sleep disruption, and frequent time zone changes, improves many MG patients. An aerobic exercise program may aid in eliminating symptoms of MG (if they are not precipitated or aggravated by exercise).

Other techniques such as biofeedback, manipulative therapy, physical therapy, massage, and acupressure have been tried, but adequate studies validating their use are not available; anecdotal and testimonial evidence of success can be found. There have been a number of trials looking at the role of acupuncture in treating headache (both MG as well as other types). A recent Cochrane review summarized by saying that there was supportive but "not fully convincing" evidence.

C. Treatment of the Acute Attack

Treatment of the acute attack has 2 phases. If there is any warning prior to the headache, abortive therapy is used. If headache occurs without warning and is the only harbinger of the attack, abortive therapy may be less useful, and purely symptomatic therapy in an attempt to suppress the headache is the treatment employed.

Medications used for the abortive treatment of acute MG (Table 38–4) share the characteristic of agonist activity at 5-HT$_1$-receptor sites. To be effective, abortive therapy must be used as soon as possible after a warning, and the dosage must be adequate to suppress the headache. Frequently, patients either are misinstructed or are reluctant to take an adequate dose of medication and lose the opportunity to abort the attack. The ergot-

Table 38–4. Abortive therapy for migraine.

Drug	Route	Dosage
Ergotamine and caffeine, 1 mg	PO	2 mg at onset; repeat 1–2 mg q$\frac{1}{2}$–1 h; limit: 4 mg/d, 6 mg/wk
Ergotamine and caffeine, 2 mg	PR	1–2 mg at onset; repeat in $\frac{1}{2}$–1 h; limit: 4 mg/d, 6 mg/wk
Ergotamine, 2 mg	SL	2 mg at onset; repeat in 1 h; limit: 4 mg/d, 6 mg/wk
Isometheptene and acetaminophen	PO	2 caps at onset; repeat q$\frac{1}{2}$–1 h × 2
Dichloralphenazone, acetyl salicylic acid, and caffeine	PO	2–3 tabs at onset; repeat q3–4 h
Naproxen sodium, 550 mg	PO	550–775 mg at onset; repeat 550 mg q4 h × 2
Ibuprofen, 400 mg	PO	400–1200 mg at onset; repeat 400–800 mg q3–4 h
Metoclopramide, 10 mg	PO	10 mg at onset; repeat 10 mg q4–6 h
Butorphanol, 1 mg	NS	1 mg (one spray) at onset; repeat q1–2 h × 4
Dihydroergotamine, 1 mg	SQ	0.5–1 mg 1 h × 3
Naratriptan, 1 mg, 2.5 mg	PO	1–2.5 mg at onset; may repeat once after 4 h; limit: 5 mg/24 h
Almotriptan, 6.25 mg, 12.5 mg	PO	6–12.5 mg at onset; may repeat after 2 h; limit: 2 doses/24 h
Sumatriptan, 6 mg 5 mg, 20 mg 25 mg, 50 mg, 100 mg	SQ NS PO	6 mg; may repeat after 1 h; limit: 12 mg/24 h May repeat after 2 h; limit: 40 mg/24 h 25–100 mg; may repeat after 2 h; limit 200 mg/24 h
Rizatriptan, 5 mg, 10 mg	Tab and disintegrating form	5–10 mg; may repeat after 2 h; limit: 30 mg/24 h
Zolmitriptan, 2.5 mg, 5 mg	Tab and disintegrating form	2.5 mg tab; may repeat after 2 h; limit: 10 mg/24 h

amines (with or without caffeine) are effective abortive medications in patients who tolerate them. The oral route is used frequently but absorption may be poor, and ergotamine may contribute to nausea and vomiting. Rapid and higher drug levels are achieved with the rectal route.

A combination of a vasoconstrictor (isometheptene), a mild sedative (dichloralphenazone), and acetaminophen is also a reliable abortive medication and produces less nausea than the ergotamine-caffeine combination (Table 38–5). Subcutaneous or intranasal DHE prevents headache and is not associated with significant rebound or nausea. It can be given later in the cycle and still suppress symptoms.

The triptans are a revolutionary new class of 5-HT receptor agonist that function as an abortive. Although generally well regarded, their drawbacks are expense, and unacceptable side effects in some patients. There is a tendency to rebound with all migraine medications—triptan percentages range as high as 40%. Thorough familiarity with the class is recommended before use because of their potential for marked vasoconstriction. The triptans have been excellent medications for many

patients who previously did not respond to other therapy. Indeed, some consider headache response to a triptan to be necessary for the diagnosis of migraine. Currently, triptans are available as injectable, inhalant, oral, and dissolving wafer forms. There are a number of different triptans available with some difference in time of action, efficacy, and rate of rebound. Some patients find one or another to be more useful; therefore, if results are poor with one, consider a trial with another. Any of the medications discussed in this section may need to be administered with an antinauseant.

Symptomatic therapy is used if patients experience no warning prior to the headache or as an adjunct to abortive therapy. Simple measures should be given an adequate trial before more complicated and expensive medications, with a greater potential for side effects, are prescribed. Aspirin and NSAIDs such as ibuprofen and naproxen sodium are simple but effective symptomatic drugs and can also be used prophylactically.

Combination prescription and nonprescription medications such as aspirin or acetaminophen with caffeine and/or butalbital seem to be more effective than single analgesics in many patients. The addition of bu-

Table 38-5. Symptomatic therapy for migraine.

Drug	Route	Dosage
Naproxen sodium	PO	550–775 mg q4–6 h
Ibuprofen	PO	600–800 mg q4–6 h
Ketorolac	PO	10 mg qid
	IM	60 mg q4 h × 2
Acetylsalicylic acid, acetaminophen, caffeine, butalbital	PO	1–2 tabs q4–6 h
Analgesic-narcotic combination	PO	Use as directed for acute headache; monitor use
Promethazine	PO, PR, IM	50–100 mg q4–6 h
Hydroxyzine	PO, IM	50 mg q4–6 h
Prochlorperazine	PO, PR, IM	10–25 mg q4–6 h
Dihydrotryotamine	IV, SQ, IM	0.5–1 mg q6–8 h
Meperidine	IM	75–125 mg q3–4 h × 2; use with antiemetic; limit 2–4 injections/m; monitor use
Dexamethasone	IV	10–16 mg; may repeat q6–8 h × 1

talbital introduces the potential for abuse. Patients who experience frequent headaches may overuse these medications, and rebound headaches may develop as a complication. Restricted use of opioids is appropriate for patients who have no more than 2 or 3 headaches per month.

Some patients respond well to low-dose propranolol taken at the time of the headache. Twenty milligrams every 4 hours in combination with a simple analgesic may eliminate the headache completely. Patients who fail to respond to self-administered abortive and symptomatic measures may have intractable headache with vomiting and dehydration and must be treated in the office or emergency department. Patients can receive DHE intramuscularly or intravenously in combination with a parenteral antiemetic.

Ketorolac, 60 mg intramuscularly, relieves headache in some patients. Triptan administration should be monitored to avoid overuse and severe rebound headache. Parenteral antiemetics and opioids relieve headache in many patients, although there may be rebound. Opioids should be given in adequate doses but used selectively and monitored rigorously because of their potential for abuse. Meperidine, 75–125 mg, and an antiemetic such as promethazine or prochlorperazine can be given concomitantly. If patients experience repeated headache and initial emergency department therapy does not control symptoms, intravenous dexamethasone, 10–20 mg, eventually may terminate the attack. Intranasal lidocaine is one appealing alternative given the mild side effect profile. A small amount of 4% lidocaine is applied inside the nares and is thought to anesthetize the trigeminal nerve. There have been multiple studies performed and most have found benefit.

D. Prophylactic Therapy

Prophylactic treatment aims to decrease the frequency and severity of attacks that occur more than 2–4 times per month or are severe enough to be disruptive. It also may improve the effectiveness of symptomatic therapy if headaches break through the protective barrier of a prophylactic regimen. The prophylactic medications have a variety of biologic effects, making it impossible to attribute their success to any one mechanism. Most of the effective prophylactic drugs appear to have antagonist activity at the 5-HT$_2$–receptor site. There are no definitive guidelines for the selection of one medication over another, but side effects, patient tolerance, effective dosage, and cost are considerations that make it important to individualize treatment. Preventive therapy is considered successful if it reduces the frequency, duration, and intensity of the attacks by 50% or more. If stabilization and control are established after a period of treatment of 6 months to 1 year, medications can be discontinued slowly, and there may be a prolonged remission.

The most successful of the drugs available for prophylactic therapy include β-blockers, calcium channel blockers, and tricyclic antidepressants (TCA) (Table 38–6). Either monotherapy or combination therapy with these prophylactic agents is effective in 50–70% of patients.

1. β-Blockers—β-Blockers are perhaps the most widely used agents. Propranolol, nadolol, and atenolol are all effective. The nonselective β-blockers are more highly regarded than the selective group, but they may have more side effects. Low-dose regular-acting or long-acting treatment is preferred, and the dosage should be increased gradually until an effect is apparent or side effects intervene. If there is no significant response after 6–8 weeks of treatment at the maximal dosage, a different β-blocker

Table 38–6. Prophylactic therapy for migraine.

Drug	Daily Doses
β-Blockers	
Propranolol	60–160 mg
Nadolol	40–180 mg
Atenolol	50–100 mg
Calcium channel blockers	
Verapamil	120–480 mg
Nifedipine	20–80 mg
Tricyclic antidepressants	
Amitriptyline	10–100 mg
Imipramine	25–100 mg
Nortriptyline	25–100 mg
Protriptyline	10–40 mg
Doxepin	25–100 mg
Other antidepressants	
Trazodone	50–100 mg
Fluoxetine	20–40 mg
Phenelzine	15–45 mg
5-HT-receptor-influencing drugs	
Methysergide	4–8 mg
Cyproheptadine	4–12 mg
Ergotamine, belladonna, phenobarbital	1–2 tab
Nonsteroidal anti-inflammatory drugs	
Naproxen	250–750 mg
Ketoprofen	50–150 mg
Endomethacin	50–150 mg
Miscellaneous drugs	
Divalproex sodium	500–1500 mg
Lithium	300–900 mg
Anticonvulsants[1]	
Valproic acid	500–1500 mg[1]
Phenytoin	200–500 mg[1]
Carbamezepine	800–1200 mg[1]
Gabapentin	300–3600 mg
Topiramate	400–800 mg[1]

[1]Requires close laboratory monitoring.

may be tried. Caution must be used so that hypotension and bradycardia do not occur. Some patients note lassitude, depression, poor endurance, and weight gain, although the medications are well tolerated by most patients, especially at lower doses. The β-blockers should be used with caution in patients with asthma, insulin-dependent diabetes, and heart failure, and in those who are already taking other antihypertensive agents.

2. Calcium channel blockers—Verapamil is the most effective of the calcium channel blockers. Dosages ranging from 40–240 mg twice daily can be effective. The long-acting preparation is quite effective, although the dosage may need to be split because 24-hour prophylaxis may not be achieved with single-dose therapy. For the response to verapamil to be evaluated thoroughly, patients need to take the maximal dosage for at least 4–6 weeks.

Although initial aggravation of headache may occur, the verapamil should be continued if the headaches are not disabling because improvement often follows. Prolonged aura or complicated MG may be treated more effectively by calcium channel blockers than by other agents. In addition to hypotension, side effects of verapamil include constipation and fluid retention. Although other calcium channel blockers may be useful at times, they may cause or aggravate headaches.

3. Tricyclic antidepressants—The prophylactic effect of the TCAs is independent of any antidepressant activity. The best medications for headache are amitriptyline, doxepin, and imipramine, which inhibit serotonin reuptake and block the 5-HT$_2$ receptor. The more adrenergic TCAs such as nortriptyline and desipramine are used if the other TCAs fail. The selective serotonin reuptake inhibitors such as fluoxetine have not fulfilled their initial promise as prophylactic agents and in some cases seem to cause or intensify headache. As with the β-blockers, lack of effectiveness of one TCA does not preclude switching to another.

Side effects that limit the use of TCAs include drowsiness, dry mouth, constipation, urinary dysfunction, and weight gain. They are contraindicated in patients with hypertension or significant cardiovascular disease. Some of the less bothersome side effects often disappear with continued use; if the drug is started at a low dosage and gradually increased, some of the side effects can be avoided altogether. TCAs are effective at lower dosages than those used for depression, and dosages above 75–100 mg of amitriptyline or its equivalent provide little added benefit. When given once a day before bedtime, TCAs are particularly effective against headache that awakens patients from sleep.

4. Other 5-HT$_2$-receptor antagonists—Methysergide, cyproheptadine, and the ergotamines may be tried if drugs in the major 3 categories for prophylaxis have failed. Methysergide is one of the oldest anti-MG preparations, but its use has been limited because of fear of tissue fibrosis and potential for idiosyncratic coronary artery spasm.

Cyproheptadine is a relatively safe drug with drowsiness and weight gain as its only major side effects. It is more useful as an adjunctive drug than a primary therapeutic agent. The ergotamines are not only effective for abortive therapy but they also act as prophylactic agents when taken once daily in low doses.

5. Nonsteroidal anti-inflammatory drugs—NSAIDs can be given alone or in combination with other classes of drugs for MG prophylaxis. Their usefulness may be limited by gastrointestinal or renal side effects. Naproxen, ketoprofen, fenoprofen, and indomethacin are all effective. It has been noted that 325 mg of aspirin at bedtime sometimes has a prophylactic effect.

6. Anticonvulsants—Anticonvulsants such as sodium valproate, phenytoin, and carbamezepine are being used more commonly as prophylaxis. Newer anticonvulsants such as gabapentin and topiramate may also be useful. One needs to be familiar with side effects, titration schedules, and need for laboratory monitoring with these medications. However, they can often be used at lower doses than those prescribed for seizures. While there are risks for cognitive and other side effects, these medications are often very well tolerated and can be quite useful.

7. Other drugs—Several other medications are reserved for prophylaxis in refractory cases. Lithium, 300 mg 2–3 times daily, sometimes prevents cyclic MG. Lithium levels require careful monitoring, and the drug should not be used in patients with renal or cardiac disease.

Phenelzine, a monoamine oxidase inhibitor (MAOI), also may be tried when other medications fail. With MAOIs, the diet must be restricted to prevent exogenous vasoactive amine ingestion. Sympathomimetics should be avoided. Narcotics, particularly meperidine, should never be administered to patients taking MAOIs because death has been reported. Other drugs to be avoided when MAOIs are taken include fluoxetine, β-blockers, and calcium channel blockers because of the potential for severe hypotension. Patients with hypertension or hepatic, cardiovascular, or renal disease should not be treated with MAOIs.

Drugs that are likely to cause dependency, including the opiates and the benzodiazepines, should not be used on a chronic basis. Many of these medications as well as OTC analgesics are overused by patients who experience frequent MG attacks and cause rebound headache or the failure of prophylactic therapy.

8. Combination therapy—In cases that are refractory to single drug therapy, combination therapy provides added treatment flexibility. The best combinations are a β-blocker or calcium channel blocker and a TCA or valproate. Cyproheptadine, an NSAID, or lithium also can be used as a second-line drug in combination with any of the aforementioned medications. When combination therapy is used, lower dosages of both medications are generally preferable. Adding a third drug rarely provides additional benefit.

9. Riboflavin—Riboflavin may have a role as MG prophylaxis. One randomized trial has been performed with

a 59% response rate. The dose used was fairly high (400 mg) but few patients had side effects. Given the benign nature of this treatment, it may warrant consideration although further studies are pending. In one study, magnesium at 600 mg/d reduced frequency of MG by 41%. Diarrhea, however, occurred in 18% of patients. For patients who prefer a more "natural" approach to prophylaxis, this may well be another viable alternative.

Prognosis

Forty percent of children in whom MG develops between ages 7 and 15 may be in remission by age 30; after prolonged MG-free intervals, however, some experience recurrence. At least one third of such children have no remission at any time. The prognosis for remission tends to be better in boys than in girls.

There is controversy about the mortality rate of MG patients compared with the general population. Some studies have suggested a higher and others a lower rate.

IDIOPATHIC INTRACRANIAL HYPERTENSION

Idiopathic intracranial hypertension (IIH), also known as pseudotumor cerebri, is a condition of elevated intracranial pressure documented by LP. Neurologic examination is unremarkable with the exception of papilledema and possible sixth-nerve oculomotor dysfunction. Imaging studies show no evidence of ventricular enlargement, meningeal thickening, inflammation, or space-occupying lesion.

ESSENTIALS OF DIAGNOSIS

- *Increased cerebrospinal fluid (CSF) pressure documented by LP.*
- *Papilledema.*
- *Normal imaging studies.*
- *More common among women (female:male ratio, 8:1).*
- *Associated obesity and endocrine disturbances.*
- *Headache and visual disturbances are often the only symptoms.*

General Considerations

IIH has an overall prevalence of 1 in 100,000. In obese women between the ages of 20 and 44 who weigh more than 20% above their ideal weight, the incidence rises dramatically to nearly 20 in 100,000.

Patients with IIH often have endocrine disturbances, and menstrual irregularities are common. Corticosteroid abnormalities, thyroid disease, disorders of the hypothalamic-pituitary axis, and hypoparathyroidism or pseudohypoparathyroidism all have been reported. The incidence is high in obese young women, and recent weight gain and obesity are common in the year prior to the onset of symptoms. Use of numerous medications, drugs, and supplements has been reported in association with IIH, including tetracycline, nitrofurantoin, indomethacin, oral contraceptives, vitamin A, isotretinoin, and corticosteroids.

The cause of IIH is not known, although several mechanisms have been proposed. These include increased outflow resistance leading to a decrease in CSF absorption via the arachnoid villi, excess brain water content, and elevated intracranial blood volume. None of these mechanisms have been confirmed in all cases of IIH.

Clinical Findings

A. Physical Examination

Papilledema is almost always present in IIH, although it can be subtle with blurring only of the upper and lower disk margins or absence of spontaneous venous pulsations. Long-standing papilledema may be associated with optic atrophy. Sixth-nerve dysfunction, although uncommon, is the only oculomotor abnormality. Visual field defects such as enlarged blind spots or diminished peripheral vision presumably are due to disk edema.

B. Symptoms and Signs

Headache is the symptom that usually provokes patients to seek medical evaluation. The headache is nondescript and can be either throbbing or nonthrobbing in character; it may be holocranial and worse in the reclining position. Visual disturbances are frequent and may include fixed visual field defects, transient visual obscurations, or even visual loss. Patients may comment on a "halo" around lights at night. Diplopia, if present, usually is due to a sixth-nerve paresis. Patients often complain of tinnitus or other intracranial noises. Focal neurologic symptoms generally are not reported; if they are, they raise the possibility of a different cause of headache.

C. Laboratory Findings

Laboratory studies are usually normal, although endocrine or calcium metabolism abnormalities may be detected. LP should document a pressure of at least 250 mm of H_2O; however, lower levels, particularly in thinner patients, may indicate disease. Pressures above 180 but below 250 are in the equivocal range. All CSF studies should be negative.

D. Imaging Studies

Imaging studies disclose no abnormalities except for possible decrease in ventricular size. Transependymal absorption can be evident on both CT and MRI (decreased density seen around the ventricles on CT). Increased pressure on the suprasellar leptomeninges may be associated with the empty-sella syndrome.

Treatment

Because many patients with IIH are obese or have experienced recent weight gain, weight loss and maintenance of ideal body weight often reverse the process. A diagnostic LP can be permanently therapeutic, but repeat LPs may be needed to manage recurrent pressure elevation. Carbonic anhydrase inhibitors or loop diuretics may relieve cerebral edema, although carefully controlled studies documenting their effectiveness are not available. Steroid pulse therapy sometimes controls severe symptoms temporarily. Digoxin decreases CSF production, but there is a paucity of evidence in treating IIH.

Surgery is a last resort; lumboperitoneal or ventriculoperitoneal shunt restores normal CSF pressure. Fenestration of the optic nerve sheath also is advocated as a method of surgically lowering the CSF pressure. The primary goal is to avoid loss of vision.

Prognosis

IIH is a self-limiting condition in many patients; once it remits, however, there is a recurrence rate of approximately 10%. Some patients enter a phase of chronic IIH with gradual worsening of vision and may be unaware of gradual visual field deterioration unless formal evaluation is performed. It is estimated that permanent visual disturbances occur in 25% of patients with IIH. Blindness, formerly seen in 10% of patients, is now a rare complication.

Pregnancy & IIH

Onset of IIH during pregnancy is usually in the first trimester. Nonpharmacologic treatment of IIH during pregnancy is similar to management of IIH in nongravid patients. If medication is absolutely necessary because weight control and serial LPs have not controlled the pressure, acetazolamide or corticosteroids can be used after 20 weeks of gestation. Therapeutic abortion almost never is indicated. Visual fields should be monitored carefully during pregnancy if there are visual complaints. The recurrence rate in subsequent pregnancies is low.

COITAL HEADACHE

ESSENTIALS OF DIAGNOSIS

- Precipitated by sexual activity or exertion.
- May recur with repeated sexual activity or other exertion if not treated but is usually self-limited.

Clinical Findings

This headache is precipitated by sexual activity, including arousal, intercourse, and masturbation. It seems to occur more frequently in patients with an MG diathesis. Onset can be sudden or may be gradual, with the headache building in severity. It often resolves after release of tension; however, it may persist in the occipitonuchal area and be accompanied by tenderness of the cervical muscles. Although the headache can recur subsequently, it frequently remits spontaneously. Diagnosis is usually not difficult in typical cases; however, other causes of explosive headaches, such as subarachnoid hemorrhage or sudden increase in intracranial pressure resulting from ventricular occlusion, may need to be ruled out.

Treatment

Medication is sometimes effective in preventing recurrent coital headache. Anti-inflammatory medications such as indomethacin or naproxen taken during a 24- to 48-hour period before anticipated sexual activity or exertion may prevent the headache. β-Blockers and verapamil are useful prophylactic medications in patients who suffer frequent, recurrent attacks.

Prognosis

Headache accompanying sexual activity or exertion usually spontaneously remits. Such headaches are almost never due to underlying disease and are self-limited.

CHRONIC PAROXYSMAL HEMICRANIA

ESSENTIALS OF DIAGNOSIS

- Hemicranial, frequent, and brief but often severe headaches.
- Absolute response to indomethacin.

General Considerations

Chronic paroxysmal hemicrania (CPH) is a rare disorder with a predominance in women; the female:male ratio is 7:1. Mean onset is in the third and fourth decades.

Clinical Findings

Findings during a period of headache are similar to those in cluster headache. Patients have lacrimation, miosis, ptosis, conjunctival injection, unilateral nasal congestion, and rhinorrhea. Unilateral periorbital edema on the symptomatic side may occur.

The headache of CPH is unilateral and almost always is confined to the same side. Pain is throbbing or pulsatile, but it can be sharp and localized to the periorbital region. Multiple attacks occur in the course of a 24-hour period, lasting from a few minutes to as long as an hour. Nocturnal attacks are uncommon in this type of headache. The menstrual cycle has a variable effect on the occurrence of the CPH; the fact that the headache almost invariably diminishes during pregnancy, however, indicates some hormonal relationship. Whereas its counterpart, cluster headache, occurs more frequently in smokers, patients with CPH have no increased incidence of smoking. Also, cluster headache has a male predominance. Other differences from cluster headaches include the higher attack frequency and shorter duration of CPH. Patients with cluster headaches tend to have little pain between attacks, whereas CPH often is associated with a lingering discomfort in the affected area between attacks.

Treatment

CPH may be defined by its absolute response to indomethacin. Dosages of 150 mg/d for several days suppress the headache, but continued treatment is often necessary at a lower dose (25–100 mg/d). After 2–4 weeks of therapy, long-lasting remission may occur. Other medications are not likely to provide relief.

When to Refer to a Specialist

Neurologic consultation can be quite useful in headache that is difficult to diagnose and/or treat. Atypical features of the headache (eg, marked severity, late age of onset, and motor or sensory complaint) may prompt appropriate referral. Often a headache specialist will be able to diagnose an unusual headache syndrome some of which have very specific and effective therapy. Cephalgia, which is very difficult to treat should also be referred. Neurologic consultation may be sought in patients using large or frequent doses of narcotics or vasoconstrictors. If a clinician is uncomfortable using unfamiliar anticonvulsants, or other prophylactics, additional sources of expertise may be helpful. Often, a one-time consultation will provide enough information to help confirm a diagnosis and suggest a course of treatment.

Boyle CA: Management of menstrual migraine. Neurology 1999;53(4 Suppl 1):S14. [PMID: 10487508]

Evans RW, Lipton RB: Topics in migraine management: a survey of headache specialists highlights some controversies. Neurol Clin 2001;19:1. [PMID: 1141758]

Goadsby PJ, Lipton RB, Ferrari MD: Migraine—current understanding and treatment. N Engl J Med 2002;346:257. [PMID: 11807151]

Hu XH et al: Burden of migraine in the United States: disability and economic costs. Arch Intern Med 1999;159:813. [PMID: 10219926]

Lay CL, Mascellino AM: Menstrual migraine: diagnosis and treatment. Curr Pain Headache Rep 2001;5:195. [PMID: 11252155]

Lipton RB et al: Efficacy and safety of acetaminophen, aspirin, and caffeine in alleviating migraine headache pain: three double-blind, randomized, placebo-controlled trials. Arch Neurol 1998;55:210. [PMID: 9482363]

Maizels M et al: Intranasal lidocaine for treatment of migraine: a randomized, double-blind, controlled trial. JAMA 1996;276:319. [PMID: 8656545]

Mathew NT, Kurman R, Perez F: Drug induced refractory headache–clinical features and management. Headache 1990; 30:634. [PMID: 2272811]

Melchart D et al: Acupuncture for idiopathic headache. Cochrane Database Syst Rev 2001;(1):CD001218. [PMID: 11279710]

Peikert A, Wilimzig C, Kohne-Volland R: Prophylaxis of migraine with oral magnesium: results from a prospective, multi-center, placebo-controlled and double-blind randomized study. Cephalalgia 1996;16:257. [PMID: 8792038]

Radhakrishnan K et al: Idiopathic intracranial hypertension. Mayo Clin Proc 1994;69:169. [PMID: 8309269]

Raskin NH: Serotonin receptors and headache. N Engl J Med 1991;325:353. [PMID: 1647497]

Schoenen J, Jacquy J, Lenaerts M: Effectiveness of high-dose riboflavin in migraine prophylaxis. A randomized controlled trial. Neurology 1998;50:466. [PMID: 9484373]

Sheftell FD: Chronic daily headache. Neurology 1992; 42(3 Suppl 2):32. [PMID: 1557189]

Silberstein SD: Preventive treatment of migraine: an overview. Cephalalgia 1997;17:67. [PMID: 9137840]

Silberstein S: Shared mechanisms and comorbidities in neurologic and psychiatric disorders. Headache 2001;41:S11. [PMID: 11903535]

Silberstein SD, Lipton RB: Overview of diagnosis and treatment of migraine. Neurology 1994;44(10 Suppl 7):S6. [PMID: 7969947]

Silberstein SD, Merriam GR: Estrogens, progestins, and headache. Neurology 1991;41:786. [PMID: 2046918]

Treatment of migraine attacks with sumatriptan. The Subcutaneous Sumatriptan International Study Group. N Engl J Med 1991;325:316. [PMID: 1647495]

Tzourio C et al: Migraine and risk of ischaemic stroke: a case-control study. BMJ 1993;307:289. [PMID: 8374374]

Vijayan N: Symptomatic chronic paroxysmal hemicrania. Cephalalgia 1992;12:111. [PMID: 1290485]

Relevant Web Sites

http://www.ama-assn.org/special/migraine/migraine.htm
http://www.migraines.org

Multiple Sclerosis

39

Barbara S. Giesser, MD

Multiple sclerosis (MS) is the most common demyelinating disorder of the central nervous system (CNS) and is among the leading causes of disability among young adults. As is the case with most other "autoimmune" diseases, the majority of persons with MS are women. This gender bias affects disease management and may hold important implications for pathogenesis and future treatment strategies as well.

ESSENTIALS OF DIAGNOSIS

- *Objective evidence of CNS white matter lesions.*
- *Separation in time and space.*
- *No alternative explanation.*

General Considerations

Currently, an estimated 350,000 individuals in the United States have MS; of these 75% are women. The disease usually manifests itself between the ages of 15 and 50, with a peak incidence in the third decade, although onset before age 15 and after age 60 is well documented. The most common initial presentation is the relapsing-remitting form, with clear episodes of disease exacerbation and remission. (An exacerbation is defined as the appearance of new neurologic signs and/or symptoms, or clear worsening of preexisting signs and symptoms, that lasts at least 24 hours). Patients with the relapsing-remitting form of the disease tend to average 1–2 attacks annually. At least half of these patients will transition into the secondary progressive form within 10 years after onset with insidious disease progression over time, and less distinct periods of relapse and recovery. The primary progressive form of the disease is marked by frank progression from onset, although there may be periods of superimposed relapses, with some return to baseline. The primary progressive form tends to occur more often in men and at a somewhat older age of onset than patients with the relapsing-remitting form of disease. The progressive relapsing designation refers to those patients who begin with progressive disease and have superimposed relapses, with or without recovery.

The incidence of MS is highest among whites, particularly those of Northern European or Scandinavian ancestry. Incidence is also higher in colder climates. Furthermore, there are data that suggest that risk of developing MS may be influenced by migration, and that moving from a high-risk area to a low-risk one before age 15 decreases the person's overall lifetime risk. The specific environmental factors influencing disease development have not yet been determined, but one possibility is that exposure to infectious agents at a critical time in life may play a role in triggering the disease in genetically predisposed persons.

Genetic factors are clearly involved in the pathogenesis of MS, including the genes that determine major histocompatibility type II loci, although the exact genotype(s) that confer(s) susceptibility is as yet unknown. Approximately 15–20% of persons with MS have an affected family member.

Lublin FD, Reingold SC: Defining the clinical course of multiple sclerosis: results of an international survey. National Multiple Sclerosis Society (USA) Advisory Committee on Clinical Trials of New Agents in Multiple Sclerosis. Neurology 1996;46:907. [PMID: 8780061] (The paper that defined the current classifications of the different clinical courses of MS.)

Noseworthy JH et al: Multiple sclerosis. N Engl J Med 2000; 343:938. [PMID: 11006371] (An excellent overview of the epidemiology, genetics, pathology, and treatment of MS.)

Whetten-Goldstein K et al: A comprehensive assessment of the cost of multiple sclerosis in the United States. Mult Scler 1998;4:419. [PMID: 9839302]

Pathogenesis

The essential pathophysiology of MS involves an immune response directed against the brain, spinal cord, and optic nerve, which are normally immunologically privileged sites. Immune cells in the periphery become sensitized to a CNS antigen, which then allows these activated T cells to breach the blood-brain barrier and initiate an immune cascade within the CNS. Injury to myelin, oligodendrocytes, and axons occurs via direct cell-mediated responses, antibody- and complement-mediated destruction, and myelinotoxin cytokines. Relapses are more likely to be characterized by inflammation, compared with progressive forms of the disease where other mechanisms of damage may be involved.

Although demyelination is the hallmark of the disease, axonal injury is common, may occur early, and is associated with permanent disability. Recent reports have indicated that there are several distinct immunopathophysiologic subtypes that occur in the MS population, but that only 1 pathophysiologic process occurs in a given patient. This implies that it may eventually be possible to tailor therapies to a particular pathophysiology.

Neuroimaging studies have documented that disease activity, as characterized by the appearance of new or enhancing lesions on magnetic resonance imaging (MRI) is ongoing, even in the absence of frank clinical relapses. Furthermore, spectroscopy studies indicate that axonal damage can be present in areas of "normal appearing" cerebral white matter. This information underscores the need for early diagnosis and prompt treatment with disease modifying agents (DMAs).

Lucchinetti C et al: Heterogeneity of multiple sclerosis lesions: implications for the pathogenesis of demyelination. Ann Neurol 2000;47:707. [PMID: 10852536] (An important paper that describes the different pathologic subtypes found in MS.)

Trapp BD et al: Axonal transection in the lesions of multiple sclerosis. N Engl J Med 1998;338:278. [PMID: 9445407] (This paper underscores that axonal damage in MS is prevalent and can occur early.)

Clinical Findings

The most common presenting complaints in MS are sensory, (ie, numbness and paresthesias); motor manifestations are seen almost as often initially, usually presenting as a paraparesis or monoparesis. However, an acute hemiparesis simulating a stroke may also occur. Optic neuritis as an initial symptom occurs in about 15% of patients. Studies indicate that if an MRI of the brain is normal at the time of first-episode optic neuritis or other monosymptomatic presentation, clinically definite MS will develop in less than 20% of patients within 5 years. Other presenting symptoms may include diplopia, ataxia, tremor, and fatigue. Fatigue is in fact the most prevalent symptom in persons with MS, occurring in up to 85% of individuals with the disease. Genitourinary symptoms as a presenting symptom occur only about 5% of the time but are eventually present in 80–90% of the MS population. The most frequent complaints are urinary urgency, frequency, hesitancy, nocturia, and incontinence. Bowel disturbances include constipation, tenesmus, and incontinence. Sexual dysfunction is a problem for both sexes, and includes erectile dysfunction, anorgasmia, loss of sensation, dyspareunia, and decreased libido.

Pain is very common in MS and is represented by a number of different syndromes. The most common is neuropathic pain (ie, felt as prickling, burning, stabbing, itching, or deep aching dysesthesias). Trigeminal neuralgia is not uncommon in persons with MS, and other stabbing or lancinating dysesthesias in the face or head may also occur. Pain may also result from spasticity or musculoskeletal conditions.

Unusual symptoms of MS include seizures, dystonia, non-scotomatous visual field defects, and aphasia.

Findings on examination generally include signs of upper motor neuron dysfunction, sensory deficit, cerebellar or brainstem findings, and optic/oculomotor abnormalities (Table 39–1).

Cognitive impairment occurs in at least 50% of persons with MS and may range from minimal disturbance, such as occasional word finding difficulty, to disability to such a degree that the individual needs 24-hour supervision. Common complaints by the patient may include word-finding difficulty, impaired short-term memory, or difficulty learning new tasks or executing previously learned tasks. In addition, the caregiver or family may report decreased awareness of deficit, poor compliance with medication regimens, irritability and personality changes, or emotional lability. Depression is higher among persons with MS than the general population and may be chronic or episodic.

Andrews KL, Husmann DA: Bladder dysfunction and management in multiple sclerosis. Mayo Clinic Proc 1997;72:1176. [PMID: 9413302] (A review of the types of bladder dysfunction seen in MS patients and treatment approaches.)

Table 39–1. Common signs in multiple sclerosis.

Upper motor neuron
 Weakness
 Spasticity
 Hyperreflexia
 Extensor Babinski response
Sensory deficit
 Numbness
 Decreased vibration/position
 Sensory level
 Hyperesthesia/allodynia
Brainstem
 Nystagmus
  Internuclear ophthalmoplegia
 Dysarthria
 Dysphagia
Cerebellar
 Intention tremor
 Ataxia
Optic
 Decreased visual acuity
 Optic disc pallor
 Afferent pupillary defect

Barkhof F et al: Comparison of MRI criteria at first presentation to predict conversion to clinically definite multiple sclerosis. Brain 1997;120:2059. [PMID: 9397021]

Moulin DE, Foley KM, Ebers GC: Pain syndromes in multiple sclerosis. Neurology 1988;38:1830. [PMID: 2973568] (A classic paper describing the different pain syndromes seen in patients with MS.)

Diagnosis

The sine qua non for making the diagnosis of MS is to establish the presence of CNS white matter lesions separated in time and space. MRI, presence of cerebrospinal fluid abnormalities, and lesions detected by evoked-potential testing are helpful in establishing the presence of such lesions. All patients in whom the diagnosis of MS is being considered should have at least 1 cerebral MRI, and it may be necessary to image the spinal cord as well. Approximately 90–95% of persons with MS will have cerebral evidence of demyelination on MRI. The diagnosis of MS may not be made on MRI findings alone. It is important to keep in mind other conditions—such as migraine, vasculitis, or ischemia—that may produce "white spots" on MRI. Some findings on MRI will help establish a diagnosis of MS (Table 39–2 and Figures 39–1 and 39–2).

Approximately 85–90% of patients with definite MS will have abnormal cerebrospinal fluid, as indicated by the presence of oligoclonal bands (that are not present in the serum) and/or an increased IgG index, indicating increased intrathecal production of immunoglobulin. Similarly, visual evoked potentials and somatosensory evoked potentials are abnormal in up to 90% of patients with definite MS and are sensitive, noninvasive indicators of subclinical lesions that may be used to demonstrate separation in space.

Because there is no pathognomonic sign or laboratory test for MS, it is important to rule out the common conditions that may mimic the clinical presentation (Table 39–3). Clues that may alert the clinician that MS is *not* the likely diagnosis include strong family history

Table 39–2. Findings on MRI consistent with multiple sclerosis.

At least 4 white matter lesions
   3 lesions if 1 is periventricular
Lesions in posterior fossa or peri-callosal
Lesions perpendicular to ventricles ("Dawson's fingers")
At least 3 mm in diameter

MRI, magnetic resonance imaging.
(Adapted, with permission, from Paty DW et al 1988 and Barkhoff 1997.)

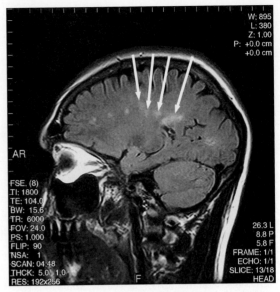

A

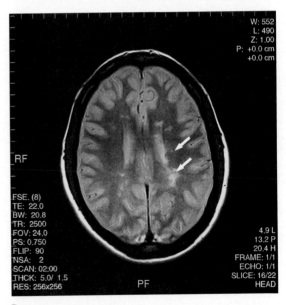

B

Figure 39–1. Typical white matter lesions of multiple sclerosis in the peri-callosal area. **A:** Lateral view. **B:** Caudal view.

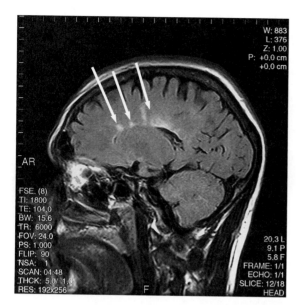

Figure 39–2. "Dawson's fingers."

Table 39–3. Common differential diagnoses in multiple sclerosis.

Collagen vascular/vasculitis
  Systemic lupus erythematosus
  Behçet's syndrome
  Sjögren's disease
  CNS vasculitis
  Sarcoidosis
Vitamin B$_{12}$ deficiency
Neoplastic/structural
Arteriovenous malformation
Infectious
  HIV
  Lyme disease
  Syphilis
  HTLV I
Antiphospholipid syndromes
Neurodegenerative diseases
  Spinocerebellar degenerations
  Adrenoleukodystrophy
Acute disseminated encephalomyelitis
Toxic/metabolic
  Hypothyroidism
  Heavy metal intoxication
  Cigeratoa intoxication
MS variants
  Devic's (neuromyelitis optica)
  Marburg's
  Schilder's disease
  Balo's concentric sclerosis

CNS, central nervous system; HTLV I, human T-cell lymphotropic virus type 1.

of neurologic disease, unifocal disease, absence of genitourinary, sensory or oculomotor/optic involvement, or systemic symptoms such as joint swelling or rash.

Brex P et al: A longitudinal study of abnormalities on MRI and disability from multiple sclerosis. N Engl J Med 2002;346:158. [PMID: 11796849] (These studies indicate long-term risk of developing MS and disability based on MRI findings at presentation.)

McDonald WI et al: Recommended diagnostic criteria for multiple sclerosis: guidelines from the International Panel on the diagnosis of multiple sclerosis. Ann Neurol 2001:50:121. [PMID: 11456302] (The most recent diagnostic guidelines, which incorporate MRI findings into criteria.)

Paty DW et al: MRI in the diagnosis of MS: a prospective study with comparison of clinical evaluation, evoked potentials, oligoclonal banding, and CT. Neurology 1988;38:180. [PMID: 3340277]

Multiple Sclerosis & Hormonal Influences

MS is primarily a disease of young, premenopausal women. As such, it would be expected that there would be profound interactions between the disease and reproductive function.

The precise interaction of gender and immunopathology in MS is not yet clear, but it is well documented that sex hormones are potent immunomodulators. Estrogen may promote a Th1 (pro-inflammatory) or Th2 (anti-inflammatory) cytokine profile depending on concentration, with higher concentrations favoring a Th2 profile. Administration of progesterone and testosterone in both in vitro and animal models of MS appear to shift cytokine responses to a Th2 response. In addition, administration of estriol ameliorates disease in the animal model of MS, experimental autoimmune encephalomyelitis and has been shown to improve MRI and clinical parameters in a pilot study of women with MS. This may explain, in part, the fluctuation in neurologic status that is seen in women with MS during periods of changing hormonal environments (vide infra).

A. PREGNANCY

In general, MS does not affect fertility or lead to an increase in congenital malformations or miscarriages. Extensive prospective and retrospective studies of women with MS have documented that relapse rates are decreased during pregnancy, with the most pronounced decrease during the third trimester. This is at least in part due to the production of many immunosuppressive substances including estriol, progesterone, cortisone, and alpha feto-protein. There is an increase in relapses during the first 3–6 months postpartum, but this transiently increased relapse rate does not produce an increase in long-term disability compared with a nulliparous cohort. There are limited data that suggest that pregnancy may even have a relative protective effect and delay disease onset.

While pregnancy appears to have salutory effects on MS itself, some neurologic symptoms may be aggravated during pregnancy. These include fatigue, ataxia, bladder and bowel dysfunction, and impaired mobility.

Women with MS who wish to become pregnant should be advised that compared with the general population there is a 20–50% increase in risk of MS developing in their offspring but that the absolute risk is itself low (1–5%).

Most of the pharmacologic agents that are used to manage MS are not indicated for use during pregnancy (Table 39–4). Similarly, the DMAs are also not approved for use in pregnant women, and a patient may have to choose between starting disease modifying therapy or starting a family. A conservative recommendation would be for the patient to discontinue use of DMA for at least 1–2 menstrual cycles before attempting to conceive. It is not known whether DMAs are excreted in breast milk, and currently their use is not advised in women who wish to breast-feed. Breast-feeding itself has not been associated with increased relapses.

B. MENSES AND MENOPAUSE

Although pregnancy has been well studied in MS, there are very few studies about the neurologic status of women with MS at different phases of the menstrual cycle. Limited data indicate that a majority of women with MS who were studied do notice an association between their periods and neurologic symptoms. In self-report studies, this association was most often reported to be a worsening of neurologic symptoms occurring a few days before the onset of menses. Larger scale studies with objective markers are needed to confirm these observations.

There are no large scale or prospective studies that have examined the interaction between MS and menopause. To date, there are no data to indicate that women with MS should not use hormone replacement therapy if medically indicated.

C. CONTRACEPTION

Although older studies reported a slightly lower risk of MS developing among women who used oral contraceptives, more recent data do not support any association between oral contraceptive use and risk of MS.

Table 39–4. Pregnancy risk categories of drugs used to manage multiple sclerosis.

Drug	Indication	Risk Category
Corticosteroids	Acute attack[1]	C
Baclofen	Spasticity	C
Tizanidine	Spasticity	C
Amantadine	Fatigue[1]	C
Modafinil	Fatigue[1]	C
Amitriptyline	Mood, pain[1], bladder[1]	C
Gabapentin	Seizures, pain[1], spasticity[1]	C
Fluoxetine	Mood, fatigue[1]	C
Oxybutynin	Bladder	C
Tolterodine	Bladder	C
Benzodiazepines	Anxiety, spasticity[1]	D
Carbamazepine	Seizures, pain[1], dystonia[1]	C
Beta-interferon 1-a	DMA	C
Beta-interferon 1-b	DMA	C
Glatiramer acetate	DMA	B
Immunosuppressants		
Azathioprine[1]		D
Cyclophosphamide[1]		D
Methotrexate[1]		X
Mitoxantrone		D

DMA, disease modifying agent.
[1]No FDA indication for this use or no indication for this use in multiple sclerosis.

Some drugs that are used for symptom management of MS (eg, anticonvulsants) may interfere with oral contraceptive action. In addition, barrier methods of contraception may be difficult to use for a woman who has incoordination or impaired sensation.

Dalal M, Kim S, Voskuhl RR: Testosterone therapy ameliorates experimental autoimmune encephalomyelitis and induces a T helper 2 bias in the autoantigen-specific T lymphocyte response. J Immunol 1997;159:3. [PMID: 9200430]

Damek DM, Shuster EA: Pregnancy and multiple sclerosis. Mayo Clinic Proc 1997;72:977. [PMID: 9379704] (An excellent and comprehensive review of studies of pregnancy in women with MS.)

Gilmore W, Weiner LP, Correale J: Effect of estradiol on cytokine secretion by proteolipid protein-specific T cell clones isolated from multiple sclerosis patients and normal control subjects. J Immunol 1997;158:446. [PMID: 8977221]

Kim S et al: Estriol ameliorates autoimmune demyelinating disease: implications for multiple sclerosis. Neurology 1999;52:1230. [PMID: 10214749] (This paper was one of the first to demonstrate the therapeutic effects of sex hormones in the animal model of MS.)

Sicotte NL et al: Treatment of multiple sclerosis with the pregnancy hormone estriol. Ann Neurol 2002;52:421. [PMID: 12325070]

Whitacre CC, Reingold SC, O'Looney PA: A gender gap in autoimmunity. Science 1999;283:1277. [PMID: 10084932] (A brief summary of current knowledge about the interaction between the neural, endocrine, and immune systems.)

Zorgdrager A, De Keyser J: Menstrually related worsening of symptoms in multiple sclerosis. J Neurol Sci 1997;149:95. [PMID: 9168172]

Psychosocial Issues

Any chronic illness affects not only the patient but also their significant others and other family members. For women with MS, the issues are complex and range from change in self-image to alteration in roles as spouse, parent, sexual partner, or income provider.

A. CHANGE IN IMAGE

MS can affect a woman's self-perception, even if there are no outwardly visible changes. Symptoms, especially the "invisible" symptoms of pain, fatigue, cognitive dysfunction or spasticity, can affect her functioning in many spheres and may lead to feelings of inadequacy. Increasing physical disability and visible consequences of this (such as change in appearance or grooming or need for assistive devices) may foster a perception that she is no longer sufficiently desirable to her sexual partner.

B. CHANGE IN ROLES

In many households, women assume the bulk of parenting duties. The mother with MS may have to delegate large parts of her parenting role to others and may require care herself. This can obviously put a strain on marital relationships and indeed divorce rates are several times higher among persons with MS compared with the general population.

C. UNEMPLOYMENT

Studies have reported that over 70% of persons with MS are out of the workforce by 10 years after diagnosis. Women with MS are more likely to quit the workforce than men with MS. Loss of employment-related income has been estimated to account for over 50% of the financial costs of MS. Loss of employment may also contribute to difficulty in obtaining health insurance and hinder access to health care.

D. ACCESS TO HEALTH CARE

A recent study has demonstrated that women with MS have lower rates of routine gynecologic screening such as mammograms and Papanicolaou smears, with mobility directly correlated with access to services. There are multifactorial reasons for this, including inadequate social support systems (eg, childcare), access to health care providers, access to facilities and equipment, and difficulties in obtaining insurance.

E. VIOLENCE AND ABUSE

Domestic violence is the leading cause of injury in women between the ages of 18 and 44, and persons with disabilities are at increased risk. Abuse may take the form of actual battery, exploitation or theft, inadequate care, or caregiver "burn-out." There is little literature about this in the MS population, but 1 study did find that abuse is common among persons with MS and that abuse is more common against patients who are more disabled and cognitively impaired.

F. DEPRESSION

Depression has been reported to occur in over half of the MS population, and women are more at risk than men. Depression may compound other disabling symptoms of MS such as fatigue or cognitive impairment. It has been reported that suicide as a cause of death occurs in the MS population at a rate several times that of age-matched controls in the general population. In addition, treatment with beta-interferon 1-b has been associated with depression in a small percentage of MS patients.

Cheng E et al: Mobility impairments and use of preventive services in women with multiple sclerosis: observational study. BMJ 2001;323:968. [PMID: 11679386]

Conomy J, Miller D, Van Hook S: A study of domestic violence in persons affected by MS. Ann of Neurology 1991;30(2):318A.

Sadnovick AD et al: Depression and multiple sclerosis. Neurology 1996;46:628. [PMID: 8618657]

Treatment

A. SYMPTOM MANAGEMENT

The goals of treating a person with MS are to ameliorate symptoms, improve function, avoid complications, and improve quality of life. There are many pharmacologic, rehabilitative, and psychosocial interventions that may be used to achieve these goals.

Pharmacologic treatment of acute exacerbations is usually done with a short course of high-dose corticosteroids. Intravenous methylprednisolone may be given in divided doses of 1000 mg/d for 3–5 days with an optional brief oral taper to follow. This may be done on an outpatient or in-hospital basis. For milder attacks, a 1- to 2-week course of oral prednisone or dexamethasone is often effective and well tolerated. In treating any acute change in neurologic status, it is important to rule out any infection (eg, urinary) that may have triggered the episode. Appropriate treatment for any infection should be initiated before beginning therapy with corticosteroids.

Table 39–5 summarizes the more common symptoms of MS and their pharmacologic management. A key point to remember in the management of MS is to involve the patient as much as possible in treatment decisions and encourage them to be responsible for monitoring medication efficacy and side effects.

Persons with MS are at increased risk for osteoporosis. Factors predisposing to this include decreased mobility, corticosteroid use, and poor nutrition. Women with MS may incur additional risk due to natural loss of estrogen with aging.

B. DISEASE MODIFYING AGENTS

Beta-interferon 1-b (Betaseron), the first DMA approved by the US Food and Drug Administration for treatment of MS, was introduced in 1993. Beta-interferon 1-a (Avonex) and glatiramer acetate (Copaxone) were approved in 1996. Beta-interferon 1-a (Rebif) was approved in the United States in early 2002, although it has been available in Europe and Canada for several years. Beta-interferon 1-a and beta-interferon 1-b are recombinant forms of a naturally occurring cytokine; glatiramer acetate is a synthetic polypeptide. These agents differ in their routes of administration and side effects (Table 39–6). Beta-interferon appears to have a number of immunomodulatory actions, including decreasing antigen presentation, inhibiting trafficking of activated immune cells across the blood-brain barrier, and inducing anti-inflammatory cytokines. Glatiramer acetate is believed to act by competitively binding to the myelin basic protein receptor on T cells, and inducing a shift from Th1 (pro-inflammatory) cytokine profile to Th2 (anti-inflammatory), with migration of Th2 cells into the CNS.

In double-blind, placebo-controlled trials in patients with relapsing-remitting MS, the DMA have been shown to reduce the number and severity of exacerbations and increase the time between first and second relapses and increase the amount of time that is relapse free. In addition, they reduce the number of new lesions occurring on cerebral MRI. The efficacy of the beta-interferons appears to be dose and frequency related, and to date, they have been demonstrated to have a more robust effect in reducing numbers of new gadolinium-enhancing lesions on MRI than glatiramer acetate. Limited studies to demonstrate efficacy in pa-

Table 39–5. Management of multiple sclerosis symptoms.

Symptom	Drug	Usual Dose	Side Effects
Spasticity	Baclofen	10–80 mg/d and/or prn	Sedation, weakness
	Tizanidine	4–32 mg/d	Sedation, hypotension
	Benzodiazepine	2–10 mg/d and/or prn	Sedation, tolerance
Fatigue	Amantadine[1]	100–200 mg/d	Insomnia, anticholinergic
	Modafinil[1]	100–200 mg/d	Insomnia, headache
	Pemoline[1]	18.75–37.5 mg/d	Palpitations, insomnia
Pain	Amitriptyline[1]	25–100 mg/d or prn	Sedation, anticholinergic
	Gabapentin[1]	100–1500 mg/d or prn	Sedation
	Carbamezepine	200–1000 mg/d or prn	Sedation, nausea, ataxia
Urinary urgency	Oxybutynin	5–20 mg/d	Urinary retention, anticholinergic
	Tolterodine	2–6 mg/d	Urinary retention, anticholinergic
	Pro-pantheline	15–45 mg/d	Urinary retention, anticholinergic
	Imipramine[1]	25–100 mg/hs	Urinary retention, anticholinergic
Urinary retention	Tamsulosin[1]	0.4 mg/d	Hypotension
Constipation	Fiber, sodium docusate	As directed	Bloating, diarrhea
	Laxatives		
Sexual dysfunction	Sildenafil[1]	50 mg prn	Headache, flushing, angina

[1]No FDA indication for this use or not indicated for this use in multiple sclerosis.

Table 39–6. Characteristics of disease modifying agents (DMAs).

Characteristics	DMA			
	Avonex (Beta-interferon 1-a)	**Betaseron (Beta-interferon 1-b)**	**Copaxone (Glatiramer acetate)**	**Rebif (Beta-interferon 1-a)**
Formulation	Recombinant form of natural protein	Recombinant form of natural protein	Synthetic polymer	Recombinant form of natural protein
Administration	30 μg IM weekly (1 mL)	250 μg SQ every other day (1 mL)	20 mg SQ daily (1 mL)	44 μg SQ (0.5 mL) 3 times per week
Side effects (clinical)	Fever, chills, malaise	Fever, chills, myalgias, menstrual irregularities, site reactions	Site reactions, idiosyncratic vasovagal reaction	Fever, chills, myalgias, site reactions
Side effects (laboratory)	Leukopenia, thrombocytopenia, liver enzyme elevation	Leukopenia, thrombocytopenia, liver enzyme elevation	No hematologic or hepatic toxicity	Leukopenia, thrombocytopenia, liver enzyme elevation

tients with secondary progressive disease have been less conclusive. One study has reported efficacy of early treatment with beta-interferon 1-a in delaying the conversion to clinically definite MS in patients with clinically isolated syndromes and an abnormal MRI. A consensus statement released by the National MS Society in 1998 suggested that DMA be offered to all patients with a confirmed diagnosis of relapsing-remitting MS as early as possible and that treatment should not necessarily be limited by age or degree of disability.

The main side effects of beta-interferon include a "flu-like" syndrome consisting of fever, chills, myalgias, and malaise. This can be greatly ameliorated or avoided in most patients by gradual dose escalation when initiating therapy and concomitant use of acetaminophen or ibuprofen. In addition, complete blood cell and platelet counts and liver function tests should be monitored periodically because of potential for leukopenia, thrombocytopenia, or hepatic enzyme elevation. Use of glatiramer acetate is associated with a 15% incidence of an idiosyncratic vasovagal reaction, which includes flushing, palpitations, dyspnea, and anxiety. This is a benign, self-limiting occurrence that generally subsides in 15–20 minutes but is unpredictable and may be recurrent. There are no drug interactions between DMAs and other drugs used to manage MS or other commonly used agents such as oral contraceptives or hormone replacement therapy.

Side effects of the DMA that may be of particular concern to women include a statistically significant incidence of menstrual irregularities seen in the clinical trials with beta-interferon 1-b (compared with placebo), the abortifactant properties of beta-interferon, and cosmetic considerations due to site injection reactions with beta-interferon 1-b (Betaseron), beta-inter-

feron 1-a (Rebif), and glatiramer acetate (Copaxone). Monitoring for efficacy of DMA would include periodic evaluations of neurologic status and function and repeat MRI.

Late in 2000, an immunosuppressant agent, mitoxantrone (Novantrone) was approved for treatment of secondary progressive, progressive relapsing, and "worsening relapsing-remitting" MS. Mitoxantrone is an anthracene compound originally approved to treat certain cancers. It has been demonstrated to reduce MRI lesion burden and delay disability in patients with progressive MS. In addition to bone marrow suppression, and concomitant risk of infection, mitoxantrone treatment carries with it a risk of irreversible cardiotoxicity, which is dose related. Current guidelines indicate that a cumulative lifetime dose of 140 mg/m^2 should not be exceeded. Mitoxantrone also produces menstrual irregularity, may impair fertility, and has been associated with permanent amenorrhea in some women.

C. REHABILITATION

Rehabilitative services are an important part of treatment. Acute rehabilitative intervention may be indicated at the time of a decline in function due to an exacerbation. In addition, a regular exercise program is important for persons with MS to maintain adequate muscle tone, improve flexibility, increase or maintain endurance, and promote maximum safety and efficiency in ambulation and mobility. Occupational therapy is indicated to maximize function in activities of daily living and is also invaluable for energy conservation techniques. Speech therapy can also assess swallowing and cognitive function. Psychological counseling and support may be indicated not only for the patient but also for family and caregivers as well. A referral to vocational rehabilitative services may extend the income-producing time available to a patient.

Cosman F et al: Fracture history and bone loss in patients with MS. Neurology 1998;51:1161. [PMID: 9781548]

Goodin DS et al: Disease modifying therapies in multiple sclerosis: report of the Therapeutics and Technology Assessment Subcommittee of the American Academy of Neurology and the MS Council for Clinical Practice Guidelines. Neurology 2002;58:169. [PMID: 11805241] (A review of the different clinical trials of DMA in MS.)

Millefiorini E et al: Randomized, placebo-controlled trial of mitoxantrone in relapsing-remitting multiple sclerosis: 24-month clinical and MRI outcome. J Neurol 1997;244:153. [PMID: 9050955]

Stolp-Smith KA et al: Management of impairment, disability and handicap due to multiple sclerosis. Mayo Clinic Proc 1997;72:1184. [PMID: 9413303] (A comprehensive review of treatment strategies.)

When to Refer to a Specialist

Any patient in whom the clinical presentation or radiologic findings suggest MS should be referred to a neurologist for diagnosis confirmation and treatment plan. Regular neurologic evaluation is important in assessing neurologic status, monitoring disease progression, and evaluating efficacy of treatment.

Prognosis

While one of the more constant features of MS is its unpredictability, there are certain prognostic indicators. Few attacks in the first several years after onset, monosymptomatic attacks, complete recovery from attacks, a paucity of motor, cerebellar or brainstem findings early on, and small MRI lesion burden tend to augur a somewhat better prognosis. Studies to date indicate that overall about 50% of all patients in whom MS is diagnosed will need to walk with a cane 15 years after onset. However, most of the data concerning the natural history and course of MS have been collected before widespread use of DMAs, and it remains to be seen how these treatments will affect long-term course and disability.

Relevant Web Sites

[National MS Society. A comprehensive resource for both patients and health professionals.]

www.nmss.org

SECTION XIII

Pulmonary Disorders

Asthma

40

Joyce Lammert, MD, PhD & Erica Pascarelli, MD

ESSENTIALS OF DIAGNOSIS

- *Documented reversible airflow obstruction.*
- *History of persistent symptoms.*
- *Exclusion of alternative diagnoses.*

General Considerations

A. EPIDEMIOLOGY

There are approximately 14 million people in the United States who have asthma. Asthma is most common in childhood, declines in the late teens, and then increases steadily into the 70s. Asthma prevalence, rates of hospitalization, and mortality rates appear to be on the rise in many countries. Results from the National Health Interview Survey (NHIS) showed an increase in asthma prevalence in the United States of 29% from 1980 to 1987. In persons younger than 20, rates increased by 42% for the whole group and 69% for females.

Low income has been found to be a strong independent predictor of asthma prevalence and outcome. A variety of complex social factors may explain this finding, including increased exposure to allergens and irritants such as tobacco smoke, a less nutritional diet, and lack of medical care.

B. PRESENTATION IN WOMEN

Sex differences in asthma prevalence and morbidity have been reported in many countries and persist when adjusted for socioeconomic status and environmental exposures. During childhood, boys have a significantly higher risk of developing asthma than do girls, and asthmatic males have a higher rate of hospitalization. After puberty, the risk is higher in women than men. The smaller airway diameters in women as well as hormonal factors are believed to play a role.

Premenstrual exacerbations of asthma have been reported in up to 40% of females. The underlying mechanisms are not well understood but may include increased airway inflammation and cyclic changes in β-adrenergic receptor regulation. Asthma during pregnancy improves in roughly one third, stays the same in one third, and worsens in one third. After the 36th week, asthma symptoms occur less frequently and are less severe in most women.

Pathogenesis

In 1892, William Osler described asthma as a special form of inflammation of the airways. In the last 10 years, bronchoscopy studies have confirmed Osler's impression. Biopsy studies have demonstrated significant inflammation even in patients with mild asthma. Bronchoalveolar lavage fluid contains eosinophils, macrophages, activated T cells, and interleukins important in IgE production and the recruitment of inflammatory cells. There is an association between the degree of inflammation and the degree of bronchial hyperreactivity. Most important, the inflammation appears to lead to airway remodeling with thickening of the airway walls and increases in the adventitia and smooth muscle. The result is that asthmatic patients have a greater decline in lung function with age than nonasthmatic persons. Early recognition and treatment of the underlying inflammation has, as a result, become the focus of asthma treatment.

Clinical Findings

A. SYMPTOMS AND SIGNS

Symptoms of asthma can include dyspnea, wheezing, chest tightness, and cough. Although wheezing is common, an isolated cough has been shown to be associated with bronchial hyperreactivity in up to one third of cases. Factors that influence the symptoms of asthma can include allergen exposure, respiratory tract infections, physical activity, weather, the menstrual cycle, aeroirritants, medications, and gastroesophageal reflux. Time of day is also important with symptoms typically worse at night.

Physical signs of asthma depend on the degree of obstruction present. The examination may be unremarkable, or findings may include tachypnea, tachycardia, pulsus paradoxus, diaphoresis, the use of accessory muscles, prolongation of the expiratory phase, and wheezing or rhonchi on auscultation. Associated conditions include rhinitis due to allergen exposure, polyposis, chronic sinusitis, or atopic dermatitis. Classic allergic findings on nasal examination include enlarged moist pale turbinates with clear watery discharge.

B. LABORATORY FINDINGS

Eosinophil counts and total IgE levels are not diagnostic of asthma. They can be helpful if allergic bronchopulmonary aspergillosis, eosinophilic pneumonia, or Churg-Strauss syndrome is being considered. Sputum analysis is helpful only when ruling out a secondary infection.

C. IMAGING

Chest radiographs are usually normal in uncomplicated asthma. Chest radiographs are indicated when there are acute or chronic changes in symptoms. Findings can include infiltrates, atelectasis, pneumothorax, or pneumomediastinum. A limited cut computed tomography scan of the sinuses is indicated if persistent upper respiratory symptoms seem to be complicating asthma control.

D. PULMONARY FUNCTION TESTING

Pulmonary function testing can help establish the diagnosis, indicate disease severity, and can be used in monitoring the clinical course. An improvement in the forced expiratory volume in 1 second of 12% following β-agonist treatment is generally accepted as diagnostic. The National Institutes of Health (NIH) Expert Panel suggests spirometry tests be done at least every 1 to 2 years to assess the maintenance of airway function. Normal pulmonary function tests do not rule out asthma and inhalation challenge with methacholine or histamine can be used if the diagnosis is uncertain. The diffusion capacity is generally normal or elevated in asthma and is helpful in differentiating between asthma and emphysema.

E. SPECIAL TESTS

Asthmatic patients with persistent symptoms who require daily medications should be evaluated for allergen sensitivity. This can be done with skin testing or in vitro testing.

Differential Diagnosis

- Chronic obstructive pulmonary disease
- Pulmonary embolus
- Congestive heart failure
- Laryngeal dysfunction/vocal cord dysfunction
- Drug reaction (eg, cough with angiotensin-converting enzyme [ACE] inhibitor)
- Pulmonary infiltrates with eosinophilia
- Gastroesophageal reflux
- Mechanical obstruction
- Allergic bronchopulmonary aspergillosis
- Hyperventilation/anxiety

Treatment

The goals of the treatment of asthma are to prevent chronic symptoms, maintain near normal pulmonary function, maintain normal activity levels, and prevent acute exacerbations.

A. GENERAL APPROACH

Education is the first step. The patient needs to understand the nature of the disease, the role of triggers, and the purpose of medications. Metered dose inhalers should be used with spacers to improve deposition of the drug into the lungs. Inhaler and spacer technique should be taught and periodically reevaluated. Avoidance of clinically significant triggers is important in improving control. Peak flow meters and symptom diaries can help with early recognition of an asthma exacerbation. All patients should have a written action plan with step-up and step-down therapy based on NIH guidelines of asthma severity (Tables 40–1 and 40–2). The chronic treatment plan needs to be simple to ensure long-term compliance. Patients should be seen by their physician at 1- to 6-month intervals to review asthma control and consider step-down therapy. All patients with asthma should be considered for annual influenza vaccination.

B. MEDICATIONS

1. Long-term control medications—The concept that asthma is a chronic disorder with recurrent episodes is reflected in the categorization of asthma

Table 40–1. Classification of asthma severity.

Category	Symptoms	Nighttime Symptoms	Lung Function
Severe persistent	Continual Limited physical activity Frequent exacerbations	Frequent	FEV_1 or PEF < 60% predicted, PEF variability > 30%
Moderate persistent	Daily symptoms Daily use of β-agonist Exacerbation > 2 times per week	> 1 time per week	FEV_1 or PEF > 60 to < 80% predicted, PEF variability > 30%
Mild persistent	Symptoms > 2 times per week but < 1 time per day	> 2 times per month	FEV_1 or PEF > 80% predicted, PEF variability 20–30%
Mild intermittent	Symptoms < 2 times per week Asymptomatic and normal PFTs between exacerbations Brief exacerbations	< 2 times per month	FEV_1 or PEF > 80% predicted, PEF variability < 20%

FEV_1, forced expiratory volume in 1 second; PEF, peak expiratory flow; PFTs, pulmonary function tests.
(From The National Heart, Lung, and Blood Institute, National Institutes of Health: Expert Report Panel 2: guidelines for the diagnosis and management of asthma. July 1997.)

medications into long-term control medications that treat the underlying inflammation and quick-relief medications. Long-term control medications are taken daily in order to prevent an exacerbation (Table 40–3). Inhaled corticosteroids are the mainstay of long-term therapy for asthma. Bronchial biopsies of patients with asthma who use inhaled corticosteroids show a marked reduction in the number of mast cells and eosinophils and a clearing of epithelial desquamation. Local adverse side effects can include oropharyngeal candidiasis, dysphonia, and cough, all of which can be reduced by

using a spacer and rinsing the mouth after use. High-dose inhaled corticosteroids can contribute to osteoporosis and patients on high-dose inhaled corticosteroids and/or intermittent systemic corticosteroids should be monitored with periodic bone density scanning. Cromolyn and nedocromil are alternative anti-inflammatory medications with minimum side effects that can be used as alternative therapies for mild asthma. Agents that modify the leukotriene pathway have also been shown to reduce airway inflammation in short-term studies. Inhaled corticosteroids appear to be more effective than the leukotriene modifers in the few short-term studies that have compared efficacy.

Long-acting β-agonists and the methylxanthines are useful for better control of nighttime symptoms. A combination of a long acting β-agonist (salmeterol) and an inhaled corticosteroid (fluticasone) recently became available. The combination of the 2 appears to be more effective than using a higher dose of inhaled corticosteroid.

2. Quick-relief medications—β-Adrenergic agonists relax smooth muscle in the airway and may modulate mediator release from mast cells and basophils. They are the primary medications for treatment of acute bronchospasm. Inhaled therapy is preferred over oral therapy because it has a more rapid onset of action, achieves a similar therapeutic effect, and has fewer systemic side effects. Most of the currently available agents

Table 40–2. Asthma treatment guidelines.

Mild intermittent
  No daily medication
Mild persistent
  Low-dose inhaled corticosteroid, or
  Cromolyn/nedocromil, or
  Leukotriene modifier
Moderate persistent
  Medium-dose inhaled corticosteroid, or
  Low to medium dose inhaled corticosteroid plus long-acting $β_2$-agonist
Severe persistent
  High-dose inhaled corticosteroid plus long-acting $β_2$-agonist plus oral corticosteroid

Table 40–3. Long-term control medications.

Drug	Available Preparation	Medium Adult Dose Per day
Inhaled corticosteroids		
Beclomethasone dipropionate		504–840 µg
Beclovent	MDI: 42 µg/puff	12–20 puffs
Vanceril	MDI: 42 µg/puff	12–20 puffs
Vanceril DS	MDI: 84 µg/puff	6–10 puffs
Budesonide		400–600 µg
Pulmicort Turbuhaler	DPI: 200 µg/puff	2–3 inhalations
Flunisolide		1000–2000 µg
Aerobid	MDI: 250 µg/puff	4–8 puffs
Fluticasone		264–600 µg
Flovent	MDI: 44, 110, 220 µg/puff	2–6 puffs (110)
	DPI: 50, 100, 250 µg/puff	3–6 inhalations (100)
Triamcinolone acetonide		
Azmacort	MDI: 100 µg/puff	8–12 puffs
Other agents		
Cromolyn sodium		4800–12,800 µg
Intal	MDI: 800 µg/puff	6–16 puffs
Nedocromil sodium		7–28 mg
Tilade	MDI: 1.75 mg/puff	4–16 puffs
Zileuton		
Zyflo	600 mg qid	
Montelukast		
Singulair	10 mg qhs	
Zafirlukast		
Accolate	20 mg bid	
Theophylline	10 mg/kg of body weight	
Salmeterol		
Serevent	MDI: 42 µg bid	
Fluticasone/ Salmeterol		
Advair	DPI: 100/50; 250/50; 500/50	1 puff bid

MDI, metered dose inhaler; DPI, dry powder inhaler.

(albuterol, terbutaline, pirbuterol) have a 4- to 6-hour duration of action. The anticholinergic ipratropium bromide may provide additive benefit to β-agonists in severe exacerbations. If a β-adrenergic agent is being used on a regular basis twice a week, it is suggested that an anti-inflammatory medication be started. For moderate to severe exacerbations, systemic corticosteroids are used. The dose and length of treatment need to be individualized based on clinical response.

C. TREATMENT IN PREGNANCY

Up to 10% of women of childbearing age have bronchial asthma, and studies suggest that up to 4% of pregnancies are complicated by asthma.

Most studies of the outcome of pregnancy in women with asthma have found that the major variable predicting outcome is how well the asthma is controlled. Both maternal and fetal complications can occur in patients with uncontrolled asthma. Undertreatment of asthma because of fears about the effects of medication is a major problem in the management of asthma in pregnancy. Goals for the treatment of asthma during pregnancy are exactly the same as for nonpregnant women.

Pregnant women with asthma should avoid exposure to both allergens and nonspecific irritants. Exposure to tobacco smoke should be eliminated. Smoking has been shown to cause low-birth-weight infants, and this effect may be additive if maternal asthma flares secondary to smoke exposure. Immunotherapy can be continued at the dose achieved before pregnancy unless the patient has experienced frequent reactions. It is recommended that immunotherapy not be started during pregnancy. Influenza vaccine is recommended for pregnant patients with moderate or severe asthma.

Women with asthma should be followed regularly during pregnancy. They should have regular objective measurements of pulmonary function and facilitated access to the health care provider for increased symptoms. Many women experience some dyspnea during pregnancy, which is believed to be associated with the progressive increase in progesterone. Pulmonary function tests help sort out dyspnea of pregnancy from true asthma flares. These tests also allow the health care provider to identify patients with minimal symptoms but significant obstruction that might have an impact on the pregnancy.

Most retrospective studies of the adverse outcomes associated with the use of asthma medications during pregnancy have had negative or inconclusive results. In contrast, there are well-performed studies that have shown adverse outcomes of hypoxemia on the fetus. Patients need to be reassured that asthma medications are not only safe and necessary but also help ensure a healthy outcome of the pregnancy. All patients with persistent asthma should receive an anti-inflammatory and short-acting β-agonist rescue therapy as needed.

D. Complementary Therapy

There are very few studies that have looked at the efficacy of alternative therapies such as acupuncture, homeopathy, and herbal medications in the treatment of asthma. Patients should be encouraged to continue the use of conventional medical therapy until better studies allow the determination of possible benefits.

When to Refer to a Specialist

Referral to a specialist is indicated under the following circumstances:

1. A patient has symptoms of asthma but examination and pulmonary function tests are unremarkable or the signs and symptoms are atypical

2. Multiple visits to the emergency department or hospitalizations have taken place or the patient has had a life-threatening exacerbation

3. The patient is not meeting the goals of asthma therapy

4. Additional diagnostic testing is needed, such as allergy testing or provocation challenge

5. The family or patient needs ongoing education or close follow-up

6. The patient requires frequent use of systemic corticosteroids.

Prognosis

Most studies that have looked at the natural history of asthma were performed before inhaled corticosteroids were available. Because these medications reduce bronchial hyperreactivity and the inflammatory infiltrate normally seen in asthma, they might have the potential to alter the course of the disease. Remission rates are highest during adolescence and are lowest in those with severe disease in whom fixed obstruction develops.

Asthma mortality appears to be increasing in the United States. From 1980 to 1987, total asthma deaths rose from 2891 to 4360 or from 1.3 to 1.7 per 100,000. Rates increased 2-fold in women compared with men. Mortality is high in children, the elderly, urban dwellers, blacks, and those in lower socioeconomic groups. These increases remain after taking into account changes in disease coding.

Becklake MR, Kauffmann F: Gender differences in airway behavior over the human life span. Thorax 1999;54:1119. [PMID: 10567633]

Busse W, Lemanske R: Asthma. N Engl J Med 2001;344:1257. [PMID: 11172168]

Frew AJ, Plummeridge MJ: Alternative agents in asthma. J Allergy Clin Immunol 2001;108:3. [PMID: 11447376]

Naureckas ET, Solway J: Mild asthma. N Engl J Med 2001; 345:1257. [PMID: 11680447]

National Heart, Lung, and Blood Institute; National Institutes of Health: Expert Report Panel 2: guidelines for the diagnosis and management of asthma. July 1997.

Schatz M: Interrelationships between asthma and pregnancy: a literature review. J Allergy Clin Immunol 1999;103:S330.

Relevant Web Sites

http://www.nhlbi.nih.gov/guidelines/asthma/asthmagdln.pdf
http://www.lungusa.org/asthma
http://www.aaai.org

SECTION XIV

Dermatologic Disorders

Dermatologic Disorders

41

Suseela Narra, MD

ACNE

General Considerations

Acne is a pervasive, and for some persons, a persistent condition. Adolescents are the most frequently affected but acne can persist well into the third or fourth decade. It is a multifactorial disease involving the sebaceous follicles. Sebaceous glands are found attached to hair follicles all over the skin except on the palms and soles which have no hair follicles. Sebaceous glands are the largest and most numerous on the scalp and the face. The hair associated with these glands on the face is often very small. In general, patients with acne have larger sebaceous glands and produce more sebum.

Clinical Findings

The primary site of acne is the face, but it can also occur on the trunk. Acne lesions include comedones (blackheads and whiteheads), inflamed papules, and pustules. Rarely, there can also be large nodules. The primary event is follicular plugging leading to a comedone formation. Inflammation in the comedones, often caused by extracellular products secreted by follicular bacteria *Propionibacterium acnes,* then leads to inflammatory papules and pustules. Androgenic hormones are thought to play a role in acne by increasing sebaceous gland size and sebum production. Testosterone and adrenal androgens can stimulate the sebaceous gland, although testosterone is more potent in this regard.

Treatment

Treatment of acne can be challenging. Cleansing only has a limited role as surface oils and surface bacteria are thought not to play an important role. In order for cleansers and topical agents to be effective, they have to reduce oils and bacteria within the follicle. Benzoyl peroxide and topical antibiotics such as erythromycin and clindamycin are all effective in reducing bacteria counts. Unless combined with benzoyl peroxide, monotherapy with topical antibiotics leads to emergence of bacterial resistance in a short duration. Other topical agents such as tretinoin, adapalene, and salicylic acid are effective in preventing comedone formation by altering the follicular epithelium. When acne is unresponsive to topical agents, systemic antibiotics are the next line of therapy. Common antibiotics used in acne therapy include tetracycline (500 mg twice a day), doxycycline (100 mg twice a day), and minocycline (100 mg twice a day). The above-mentioned antibiotics cannot be used by nursing or pregnant women. They also cannot be used in children younger than 13 years. Oral erythromycin (500 mg twice a day) is an option in these patients. As acne improves after several months of treatment, the dosing can be tapered to once a day and then finally discontinued.

Oral contraceptive pills (OCPs) are also helpful in acne treatment as they can decrease serum levels of the male hormone testosterone. Estrogens increase serum levels of sex hormone binding globulin which "soaks" up serum free testosterone. Reduced levels of serum testosterone result in reduced hormonal stimulation of the sebaceous glands and fewer acne lesions. Estrogens also inhibit sebum production but at much higher doses than normally found in OCPs. Second-generation progestins (norgestimate, desogestrel, and gestodene) have low intrinsic androgenic activity and OCPs containing these agents are preferred in female patients suffering from acne. OCPs are especially useful in women who note exacerbations of acne in relation to their menstrual cycle.

In severe cases of acne unresponsive to routine therapy, the oral retinoid isotretinoin can make a dramatic difference. Isotretinoin is usually administered as a

20-week course and requires monthly blood work and doctor's visits. Although the mechanism of action of isotretinoin is not entirely clear, it is known that isotretinoin decreases the activity of sebaceous glands, decreases *P acnes* count, has anti-inflammatory action and alters follicular keratinization. Treatment with isotretinoin can result in prolonged and often permanent remissions of acne. The most concerning aspect of isotretinoin therapy is its effect on the fetus. It interferes with organogenesis and can cause severe birth defects. Strict adherence to double contraception is a must during therapy.

Shalita AR: Acne revisited. Arch Dermatol 1994;130:363. [PMID: 8129417]

Strauss JS, Thiboutot DM: Diseases of the Sebaceous Glands. In: Freedberg IM et al (editors): *Fitzpatrick's Dermatology in General Medicine,* vol II, 5th ed. McGraw Hill, 1999.

ROSACEA

Clinical Findings

Rosacea is a chronic condition of the mid face that is most common in fair-skinned individuals. It is more common in women than men, but men tend to have the more severe manifestations. The 3 cardinal features are redness, groups of small blood vessels, and papulopustules. Initially, rosacea presents as prolonged episodes of blushing and flushing in reaction to stimuli such as alcohol, topical irritants, spicy foods, hot drinks, heat, cold, and the sun. Episodic flushing and blushing eventually leads to permanent redness. Although the face is the most affected, the neck, V of the chest, and the upper back can also be involved. Eventually, small blood vessels start to appear as do groups of red papules and pustules. A few unlucky patients progress on to the advanced stage of rosacea, which consists of tissue hypertrophy resulting in rhinophyma. The etiology of rosacea remains unclear.

Treatment

Rosacea is a treatable but not curable condition. Avoidance of the trigger factors mentioned above is of paramount importance. Topical metronidazole is an effective treatment for the papular and pustular component. It is less effective for the redness. Other effective topical agents include sulfur-based medicines and topical retinoids such as tretinoin and adapalene. Topical retinoids should be used with caution as they can sometimes worsen rosacea because of their propensity to irritate the skin. Oral therapy with systemic antibiotics such as tetracycline, doxycycline, and minocycline are also effective in controlling the flares of rosacea. The dosing is the same as for acne therapy. Antibiotics can be tapered as the rosacea improves, normally after 4 to 6 weeks of therapy. Topical agents should be continued to maintain the remissions.

Medications are not effective for fine telangiectasias. They can be destroyed using laser or electrodessication. More than 1 treatment session may be necessary and recurrence is common. However, the cosmetic appearance can be significantly improved with these modalities. Rhinophyma responds to surgical intervention only.

Plewig G, Jansen T: Rosacea. In: Freedberg IM et al (editors): *Fitzpatrick's Dermatology in General Medicine,* vol I 5th ed. McGraw Hill, 1999.

Wilkin JK: Rosacea. Pathophysiology and treatment. Arch Dermatol 1994;130:359. [PMID: 8129416]

MELASMA

General Considerations

Melasma is a fairly common condition in women of childbearing age. However, men can also be affected. It is more common among persons of Latin and Asian ancestry but is present in all races. The majority of cases correspond to pregnancy and OCP use. The progestational component of the OCPs appears to be the more likely culprit rather than the estrogenic component.

Clinical Findings

Melasma presents as strikingly symmetric brownish patches with reticulated appearance. It appears exclusively in sun-exposed areas. The most common pattern is involvement of the central face including the nose, cheeks, forehead, upper lip, and chin. Less common patterns involve just the malar cheeks and the nose or the mandibular pattern, which involves just the jaw line. Melasma can also affect the neck and forearms. It is exacerbated by sun exposure, pregnancy, OCPs, and certain anti-epilepsy drugs.

Treatment

Sunblocks and sun avoidance are of the utmost importance in melasma treatment. Sunblock with SPF 30 is preferable. Treatment with bleaching creams containing 4% hydroquinone is very effective in reducing the pigmentation. Addition of topical tretinoin or alphahydroxy acid creams can enhance results by allowing better penetration of hydroquinone. However, it can take 2 months to see improvement and up to 6 months to get satisfactory results. More aggressive treatments include chemical peels and laser treatment.

Torres JE, Sanchez JL: Melasma and Other Disorders of Hyperpigmentation. In: Arndt KA et al (editors): *Cutaneous Medicine and Surgery,* vol II. WB Saunders and Company, 1996.

INTERTRIGO

Clinical Findings

Intertrigo is an inflammatory dermatitis occurring in areas with apposition of 2 skin surfaces. Common areas in which intertrigo occurs include the axilla area, inframammary area, inguinal area, perianal area, interdigital webs, and in abdominal pannus folds. It is more common in hot and humid climates and in the obese. The affected body folds develop redness and maceration secondary to constant friction, heat, and moisture. The maceration allows secondary infection with bacteria and yeast.

Treatment

The acute dermatitis can be treated with a low to mid potency topical corticosteroid such as hydrocortisone cream 1% or triamcinolone cream 0.025%, combined with an antifungal cream such as miconazole or clotrimazole. Recurrences are likely unless the affected area is kept dry. The areas should be thoroughly dried after bathing and application of powder (eg, Zeasorb) helps absorb moisture during the day. Cotton undergarments also help in absorbing moisture. Application of antiperspirant sprays in the affected areas is also helpful.

Dannaker CJ: Responses to friction and hydration. In: Arndt KA et al (editors): *Cutaneous Medicine and Surgery,* vol II. WB Saunders and Company, 1996.

HIRSUTISM

General Considerations

Defining hirsutism is extremely difficult. There exists a large individual and racial variation in the amount and pattern of body hair. The perception of what is considered "normal" amount of hair in postpubertal women is often heavily influenced by cultural and cosmetic factors. From a medical perspective, only a small percentage of those complaining of excess hair will have any worrisome underlying pathology.

Clinical Findings

The diagnosis of excess body hair is made by a patient's history and clinical examination. In addition to hirsutism, other signs of hyperandrogenism include extensive, treatment-resistant acne, alopecia, menstrual disturbances and, in severe cases, virilization. The goal of evaluating patients with hirsutism is not to confirm the diagnosis but to identify underlying hyperandrogenism and its significance. In pursuing this goal and in deciding which laboratory examinations are appropriate, patients can be divided into several categories.

Category I consists of women with long-standing hirsutism, alopecia, or treatment-resistant acne. Most of these women have either "idiopathic" or "familial" hyperandrogenism. There are no signs of infertility or menstrual disturbances. Although the chance of finding abnormal plasma androgens is low, laboratory examination of total testosterone and dehydroepiandrosterone sulfate (DHEAS) is reasonable.

Category II consists of "complicated" hirsutism, acne, or alopecia. This group differs from the first in that the cutaneous findings are more severe and have either a rapid onset or progressive worsening. The initial evaluation would consist of the same tests as in category I, but the threshold of suspicion should be much lower. If any of the values are abnormal, consultation with an endocrinologist should be obtained for further testing to determine the source of androgens. Some authors suggest that in this group of patients, further evaluation for cortisol excess might be routinely indicated as well. Possible sources of androgens could be Cushing's syndrome or late-onset congenital adrenal hyperplasia (CAH).

Patients in category III have menstrual dysfunction as the characteristic feature in addition to other signs of hyperandrogenism discussed above. Menstrual dysfunction includes highly irregular or infrequent periods, amenorrhea and infertility. It is felt that most of these women will have polycystic ovary syndrome (PCOS) (see Chapter 20).

Frank virilization constitutes category IV. Virilization refers to development of hirsutism on the shoulders or back, clitoromegaly, deepening of voice, or onset of a muscular body habitus. These findings always indicate severe androgen abnormality and necessitate the search for an androgen secreting tumor. A referral to an endocrinologist or gynecologist is always indicated in this situation.

Treatment

The treatment of neoplastic causes of hyperandrogenism could involve surgery, radiation therapy, or chemotherapy. It will not be discussed further as it does not usually involve primary care practitioners. The treatment of nonneoplastic causes of hirsutism (ie, acne and alopecia) falls into 3 broad categories: adrenal suppression, ovarian suppression, and androgen antagonism.

The treatment for all varieties of CAH is adrenal suppression with corticosteroid replacement, usually with dexamethasone. There is evidence that dexamethasone therapy can be discontinued after 1 year with 85% of patients showing no recurrence. A sufficiently high dose of dexamethasone will also suppress adrenal androgen production in patients without CAH. Such nonspecific suppression can improve hirsutism and acne. A test dose can be performed using 0.5 mg dexamethasone 4 times a day for 2 days. A DHAS concentration less than 400 ng/mL indicates adequate adrenal suppression. However, long-term adrenal suppression has many side effects and is not recommended.

OCPs are a relatively safe and simple method of ovarian suppression in patients with no contraindications. They are the first-line of therapy for PCOS but have also been shown to be useful in "idiopathic" hirsutism. OCPs can also be used in combination with antiandrogens or other forms of therapy. There are several mechanisms by which OCPs can be helpful in hirsutism. The combination of estrogen and progestin suppresses pituitary gonadotropin secretion. This reduces both androgen and estrogen synthesis by the ovary. Estrogen also opposes the effect of androgen on the hair follicle itself. Some studies have shown 75% of patients with idiopathic "hirsutism" to show improvement with OCPs. Women with recent onset of hirsutism respond best whereas those with long-standing hirsutism seldom show much improvement.

Androgen antagonists are used to treat "idiopathic" hirsutism when neither the ovary nor the adrenal glands have been shown to be the source of increased androgenic activity. These medications block the effects of testosterone by competitively binding to target cell androgen receptors. Spironolactone is often the drug of choice for hirsutism accompanied by normal menses. It has also been used for treatment-resistant acne and alopecia. Spironolactone works by interfering with testosterone synthesis, suppressing 5α-reductase activity, increasing peripheral conversion of testosterone to estradiol, and competing with dihydrotestosterone (DHT) for the androgen receptor. The dosage ranges from 50 to 200 mg/d. Side effects include menorrhagia, teratogenicity, and hyperkalemia. Flutamide and finasteride both have been shown to be helpful in hirsutism as well, especially in combination with other agents such as OCPs. Flutamide is a nonsteroidal, selective antiandrogen without progestational, estrogenic, corticoid, or antigonadotrophic activity. Because it has been associated with severe hepatitis, use of flutamide is limited. Finasteride is a 5α-reductase inhibitor indicated for male pattern baldness, which has been shown to have limited success in treating hirsutism. All the antiandrogenic agents have the potential for feminization of the fetus and should be used only with strict contraceptive measures in women of childbearing age.

Weight loss has also been shown to be beneficial to some degree in all women with hyperandrogenism regardless of the presence of PCOS; the degree of hyperandrogenism; and the magnitude, degree, and distribution of obesity. A restricted caloric intake (1000 calorie/d) resulted in decreased levels of circulating testosterone and circulating androstenedione whereas the levels of estradiol, luteinizing hormone, follicle-stimulating hormone, DHAS, and sex hormone-binding globulin remained unchanged.

Cosmetic removal of terminal hair includes depilatory creams, shaving, plucking, waxing, and electrolysis. Repeated shaving can result in the appearance of coarse hair similar to that in men and plucking leads to the eventual development of ingrown hairs and folliculitis. Depilatory creams and waxing give a more cosmetically acceptable result on the face. Electrolysis is often advertised as permanent, but it is not. Laser hair removal is a more recent method that has become very popular. After a series of 3 to 5 treatments, there is a marked decrease in the amount of hair present. Few studies are available to assess long-term effectiveness. Eflornithine HCl 13.9% (Vaniqa) is a new topical agent approved for decreasing terminal hair on the upper lip. It is an inhibitor of the follicular enzyme ornithine decarboxylase. Long-term use results in gradual decrease in the quantity of facial hair. Upon discontinuation of therapy, hair often reverts to pretreatment levels.

Women should be advised that they may not see improvement with medical therapies for 3 to 6 months. In addition, excess hair needs to be removed by mechanical means after about 6 months of therapy. It should also be noted that upon discontinuation of medical therapy, the degree of hirsutism starts to increase and can return to pretreatment levels.

Dawber RP, Sinclair RD: Hirsuties. Clin Dermatol 2001;19:189. [PMID: 11397598]

Sperling LC, Heimer WL 2nd: Androgen biology as a basis for the diagnosis and treatment of androgenic disorders in women. II. J Am Acad Dermatol 1993;28:901. [PMID: 8496453]

■ SUPERFICIAL FUNGAL INFECTIONS

TINEA VERSICOLOR

General Considerations

Tinea versicolor is a superficial fungal infection caused by the yeast *Malassezia furfur*. It is more common in adolescents and young adults who perspire profusely. Warm climate exacerbates this condition; it is most frequently found in tropical and subtropical climates. Men and women are equally affected and there is no racial predilection.

Clinical Findings

Tinea versicolor generally presents as an asymptomatic, scaly eruption. It mainly involves the sebaceous areas such as the sternal region, abdomen, upper back, neck, and pubis. The face is usually spared. Lesions can be hyperpigmented and/or hypopigmented. They are erythematous, fawn- or salmon-colored, scaly macules. In more advanced cases, these discrete macules can coalesce into large patches. When it is symptomatic, pruritus, exacerbated by sweating, is the most common complaint. The diagnosis is confirmed by potassium hydroxide (KOH) preparation.

Treatment

Topical regimens are usually satisfactory in most cases. Selenium sulfide 2.5% can be applied to the entire trunk for 10–15 minutes for 14 days. This can be repeated once a week after the initial treatment for prevention of recurrences. Other topical agents that are effective include the azole class of medications and the allylamines. In more severe cases, treatment with 400 mg of ketoconazole administered as a single dose and repeated in 7 days is effective. Persistence of pigmentation changes does not necessarily indicate treatment failure; it may take several months for normal pigmentation to return. It is important for the patient to realize that tinea versicolor can be a recurring problem in susceptible individuals. Use of selenium sulfide as mentioned above or daily use of zinc pyrithione (eg, ZNP) bar soap might be indicated in individuals with frequent recurrences.

DERMATOPHYTOSIS

General Considerations

The general term "tinea" refers to dermatophyte infection. Dermatophytes produce infection in all cutaneous appendageal structures including skin, nails, and hair. Although generally benign, they can produce more severe infections in immunocompromised individuals.

Clinical Findings

Tinea corporis is a superficial dermatophytic infection of the trunk and extremities. *Trichophyton rubrum* is the most common dermatophyte causing tinea corporis. It can spread from human to human, animal to human, or soil to human. It is more prevalent in tropical climates. Tinea corporis typically presents as an annular, erythematous, scaly patch. The border is often elevated and can show follicular pustules and follicular accentuation. The lesions can be single or multiple. Predisposing factors include immunodeficiency states,

immunosuppressive medications, diabetes mellitus, and atopy. Individuals at risk include athletes, veterinarians, and animal handlers. Definitive diagnosis is made by a KOH preparation that shows septate hyphae. A fungal culture would also establish the diagnosis but can take 2–4 weeks to yield the final result.

Tinea pedis is dermatophyte infection of the feet. Infection is rare before puberty. It has 3 presentations: moccasin, interdigital, and inflammatory. Moccasin tinea pedis presents as scaling and erythema on the plantar surface extending on to the lateral and medial aspects of the foot. Inflammatory tinea pedis has vesicles and bullae and can involve a limited or extensive area. This variant is often mistaken for dyshidrotic eczema. Scale, crusting, and maceration in the interdigital areas are the presenting signs of the interdigital variant. Bacteria and yeast secondarily infect the macerated area and produce cheesy, malodorous lesions.

Tinea capitis is infection of the hair follicles of the scalp. It is much more frequent in children but can be seen in adults. It can present as diffuse scaling with or without erythema. Hair breakage occurs 1–2 mm above the scalp due to weakening of the hair shaft from fungal invasion. Extensive cases of tinea capitis can cause large areas of scarring and result in permanent alopecia.

Tinea unguium is infection of the nail unit by fungi. When the infecting agent is a dermatophyte, tinea unguium is the correct terminology. Onychomycosis refers to dermatophyte and nondermatophyte infection of the nail unit. Dermatophytes cause over 90% of nail unit infections, with *Candida albicans* and other molds accounting for the rest of the infections. Predisposing factors include tinea pedis, communal bathing, hyperhidrosis, trauma, diabetes, and immunodeficiency. Clinical appearance of the nail plate includes thickening, discoloration, onycholysis, and subungual debris. Psoriasis and lichen planus can resemble tinea unguium and can be differentiated by performing a fungal culture.

Treatment

Uncomplicated cases of tinea corporis and tinea pedis can be treated with topical antifungal agents including the imidazoles, triazoles, and allylamines. Oral agents can be used in more extensive cases. Griseofulvin, the azole family, and terbinafine have all been shown to be effective against dermatophytes in multiple studies. It should be noted that only griseofulvin and ketoconazole are actually approved by the US Food and Drug Administration for treatment of tinea corporis and tinea pedis.

Tinea unguium and tinea capitis require oral therapy. Griseofulvin is still the mainstay of therapy for tinea capitis. Itraconazole and terbinafine are increasingly being studied for tinea capitis with encouraging results, but the exact dosing and duration of treatment have not been fully established. Itraconazole and terbinafine are the only oral agents approved for onychomycosis. Itraconazole can be administered as continuous dosing or pulse dosing. Pulse dosing has so far been approved only for fingernail onychomycosis. Hence for fingernail onychomycosis, itraconazole can be administered 200 mg orally daily for 6 weeks or 200 mg twice daily for 1 week followed by a second pulse 4 weeks later. Toenail onychomycosis is treated with 12 weeks of itraconazole 200 mg daily. Terbinafine is administered in a continuous dosing schedule at 250 mg daily for a period of 6 weeks for fingernail onychomycosis or 12 weeks for toenail infection. Ciclopiroxolamine nail lacquer is the only topical agent approved for treatment of onychomycosis. Although its effectiveness is significantly less than that of the oral agents, it also does not have the systemic complications associated with oral agents.

SCABIES

General Considerations

Scabies is infestation with the mite *Sarcoptes scabiei var humanus.* It is spread by close skin-to-skin contact. Increased severity of infestation leads to easier transmission. It affects both sexes and all age groups equally.

Clinical Findings

Pruritus is often the presenting symptom and it tends to be the worst at night. Lesions often begin on the hands and involve the interdigital webs and lateral aspects of the fingers. Commonly affected areas include the flexor surfaces of the wrist and elbows and the anterior axillary folds. Penile involvement is very common and can present as papules, nodules, or ulcers. The typical lesion consists of an excoriated, erythematous papule adjacent to a wavy dirty line that represents the burrow.

Variants of scabies include nodular scabies and crusted (Norwegian) scabies. Nodular scabies presents as large reddish brown, pruritic nodules frequently found on male genitalia and in groin and axillary regions. It is thought to represent a hypersensitivity reaction to retained mite parts or antigens. Crusted scabies appears as a widespread scaling eruption concentrated on hands and feet with nail dystrophy. It is extremely contagious and more common in immunodeficient individuals. Diagnosis of scabies can be confirmed by identification of the mite, eggs, or fecal pellet under the microscope. An unexcoriated papule or burrow is scraped with a 15 blade and transferred to a slide. Min-

eral oil is then placed on the slide before examining the specimen.

Treatment

There are several scabicidal agents that offer excellent results. Permethrin cream 5% is a safe and effective treatment. The cream should be applied to the entire body and removed after 10 hours. A second application in 1 week should follow. There are no reported cases of resistance. Infants younger than 2 months of age and pregnant women should not use this medicine. Lindane 1% is also effective and is applied the same way as permethrin, except that it should be washed off after 8 hours. Lindane can cause central nervous system toxicity if misused. It should not be used in infants, children, pregnant or nursing women or in those with seizure disorders or other neurologic diseases. Precipitated sulfur (6%) in petrolatum is safe for infants under the age of 2 months and for pregnant or lactating women. It is applied nightly for 3 sequential nights and washed off thoroughly 24 hours after the last application. Close contacts should also be treated. At the end of therapy, bed linens, towels, and undergarments should be thoroughly washed and dried using the hot cycles.

Elewski BE: Common Superficial Mycoses. In: Arndt KA et al (editors): *Cutaneous Medicine and Surgery,* vol II. WB Saunders and Company, 1996.

Elewski BE: The Dermatophytoses. In: Arndt KA et al (editors): *Cutaneous Medicine and Surgery,* vol II. WB Saunders and Company, 1996.

Elewski BE: Tinea capitis: a current perspective. J Am Acad Dermatol 2000;42:1. [PMID: 10607315]

Meinking TL, Taplin D: Safety of permethrin vs lindane for the treatment of scabies. Arch Dermatol 1996;132:959. [PMID: 8712847]

Orkin M, Maibach HI: Scabies and Pediculosis. In: Freedberg IM et al (editors): *Fitzpatrick's Dermatology in General Medicine,* vol I, 5th ed. McGraw Hill, 1999.

Rand S: Overview: The treatment of dermatophytosis. J Am Acad Dermatol 2000;43:S104. [PMID: 11044285]

■ EPITHELIAL CYSTS

SEBACEOUS CYSTS

Clinical Findings

Clinically, "cysts" are any dome-shaped lesions that contain expressible material. Cysts can be classified according to cyst lining and cyst contents histologically. Sebaceous cysts arise from the infundibular portion of the pilosebaceous unit. They occur primarily on the neck, chest, face, and especially on the periauricular areas. Interestingly, this distribution correlates to that of acne vulgaris, and patients with acne have a higher rate of developing sebaceous cysts. The genitalia are another common site for development of sebaceous cysts. Calcification is frequently seen in genital cysts. The typical presentation is that of a flesh-colored nodule that can be several millimeters to several centimeters in size. Frequently a small punctum can be seen. This indicates the site of the cyst's connection to the overlying epidermis.

Complications

Cyst rupture is the most common complication. This results in spilling of cyst contents into the dermis and leads to suppuration, granuloma formulation, and granulation tissue formation with chronic inflammation. Presenting signs are erythema and tenderness localized to the cyst. Infected cysts present with erythema that extends well beyond the cyst and tenderness as well. Fluctuance and spontaneous drainage of purulent material may be present.

Treatment

Definitive treatment of cysts is excision of the sac and its contents. Simple expression of the cyst contents frequently leads to recurrence. Inflamed cysts can be injected with intralesional triamcinolone and excised after the inflammation has subsided. Treatment of infected cysts includes incision and drainage and systemic antibiotics that cover *Staphylococcus aureus*.

MILIA

Clinical Findings

Milia are small, white to yellow papules mainly located on the face with predilection for the periorbital region. Adults and children are equally affected. Many patients have a history of using powder cosmetics or cleansing granules. It is thought that the abrasive nature of these materials invaginates portions of the vellus follicular ostia leading to milia formation.

Treatment

Milia are easily expressed by nicking the surface of the small papules and compressing them between 2 cotton-tipped swabs. Use of topical retinoids can help in preventing formation of new lesions.

Bhawan J, McGillis TS: Cysts of Epithelial Adnexal Origin. In: Arndt KA et al (editors): *Cutaneous Medicine and Surgery*, vol II. WB Saunders and Company, 1996.

■ BENIGN GROWTHS

SEBORRHEIC KERATOSES

Clinical Findings

Seborrheic keratoses are the most common cutaneous neoplasms. They are macular or papular lesions that vary in size from 1 mm to several centimeters. They range in color from waxy yellow to dark brown. The surface can be flat or can have a velvety, verrucous appearance often with a greasy, hyperkeratotic scale. Seborrheic keratoses are unusual in children but increase in size and number with increasing age. They can occur in any anatomic location and are equally common among men and women. Seborrheic keratoses are mostly asymptomatic but are sometimes pruritic. They can also become inflamed and painful if they are constantly rubbed by clothing or jewelry.

Differential Diagnosis

The heavily pigmented papular lesions are often mistaken for malignant melanoma. Although melanoma is also dark in pigmentation, it usually does not have a velvety or verrucous appearance as do seborrheic keratoses. Differentiation between flat pigmented seborrheic keratoses and melanocytic nevi can be difficult clinically as well. In the genital area, condyloma accuminata and seborrheic keratoses are often indistinguishable clinically and histologically. DNA analysis has shown that 53% of seborrheic keratoses in the genital area were positive for human papillomavirus (HPV) DNA whereas only 3% of nongenital seborrheic keratoses contained HPV DNA.

Treatment

Multiple flat to slightly raised lesions can be treated with liquid nitrogen if they are symptomatic to the patient. Light electrodessication followed by wiping the area with gauze is also effective for slightly elevated lesions. Thicker lesions need more aggressive therapy. Prolonged liquid nitrogen application is an option but might not be tolerated by the patient without local anesthesia. Another option is aggressive curettage with or without preceding electrodessication. This procedure also requires local anesthesia.

CHERRY ANGIOMAS

Clinical Findings

Cherry angiomas are easily identified dome-shaped, red papules that are a few millimeters in diameter. Histologic examination shows cherry angiomas to consist mainly of ectatic blood vessels. They arise in young to middle-aged adults and become more numerous with age. The skin of the abdomen is most frequently involved, but any skin surface can be involved. Cherry angiomas are usually asymptomatic but can sometimes bleed or become inflamed.

Treatment

Symptomatic lesions can be treated by shave excision or electrocautery. Laser treatment by pulsed-dye laser or KTP laser is also effective.

DERMATOFIBROMAS

Clinical Findings

Dermatofibroma is a common fibrohistiocytic growth. It appears as a round to oval firm nodule with a dermal component that is attached to the overlying skin, responsible for the "pucker sign" when pinched. It is a slow growing lesion that can range in size from several millimeters to several centimeters. Color of the lesions range from reddish brown to dusky brown and rarely to black if there is a large vascular component. Young to middle-aged adults have the highest predilection for developing dermatofibromas. There is no racial predilection. The extremities are the most commonly affected site, with legs of women being especially prone to developing dermatofibromas. Trauma from shaving or other minor trauma is thought to contribute to the preponderance of the lesions on female legs. Lesions can be solitary, but in 20% of cases they are multiple.

Differential Diagnosis

Dermatofibromas are mistaken for many different entities. Lightly pigmented lesions are confused with scars, keloids, xanthomas, and neurofibromas. Darkly pigmented lesions can resemble atypical nevi, melanoma, or Kaposi's sarcoma.

Treatment

Treatment is indicated only if the lesions become symptomatic. Presence of the dermal component renders the lesions more difficult to eradicate with superficial destruction. A shave excision will remove the protuberant portion. There will be a remnant firm area, but it will give relief to patients who find that the protuberant lesions interfere with shaving. An adequate histologic sample can also be obtained with this method. Cryosurgery with liquid nitrogen can also be effective for smaller lesions. Larger symptomatic lesions require excision to the level of subcutaneous fat.

Fish FS, Kamino H: Fibrous Neoplasms. In: Arndt KA et al (editors): *Cutaneous Medicine and Surgery,* vol II. WB Saunders and Company, 1996.

Smoller BR, Graham G: Benign Neoplasms of the Epidermis. In: Arndt KA et al (editors): *Cutaneous Medicine and Surgery,* vol II. WB Saunders and Company, 1996.

■ PRECANCEROUS GROWTHS

ACTINIC KERATOSES

General Considerations

Actinic keratoses are scaly patches that occur in sun-exposed areas and are common precursors to squamous cell cancer (SCC) of the skin. They have a low rate of malignant transformation but are a good indicator of patients who might develop nonmelanoma skin cancer. Increased risk of actinic keratoses is indicated by older age, blue eyes, and childhood freckling. Decreasing sunlight exposure during childhood can decrease the incidence of actinic keratoses and SCCs.

Clinical Findings

Actinic keratoses are present on sun-exposed body regions in middle-aged or older people. They are often multiple in number. They appear as skin-colored to reddish brown to yellowish black macules with scaliness and feel rough to touch. They can cause itching, tenderness, and crusting.

Treatment

Treatment of actinic keratoses is indicated to decrease discomfort and more importantly to prevent malignant conversion. Frequently used modalities include destruction with liquid nitrogen or topical 5-fluorouracil cream.

Leshin B, White WL: Malignant Neoplasms of Keratinocytes. In: Arndt KA et al (editors): *Cutaneous Medicine and Surgery,* vol II. WB Saunders and Company, 1996.

■ MALIGNANT GROWTHS

BASAL CELL CARCINOMA

Pathogenesis

Basal cell carcinoma (BCC) is a malignancy of the epithelial cells, and it is the most frequent cancer in man.

BCC is closely related to chronic ultraviolet radiation exposure. Those with extensive occupational or recreational sun exposure are the most frequently affected. Fair skinned individuals who burn easily are the most susceptible. Over 99% of persons in whom BCC develops are white and those who are of Scot, Celtic, or Scandinavian ancestry are especially susceptible.

Clinical Findings

BCC most frequently presents on the face as a dome-shaped pearly, waxy, translucent growth with tiny blood vessels. This nodular variant can become ulcerated and crusted. BCC can also present insidiously with a scar-like appearance, and it is termed "morpheaform basal cell." Any unexplained atrophic scars in sun-exposed areas should raise suspicion. Morpheaform BCC can be hard to detect initially, and at the time of diagnosis, it can extend over a large area. Superficial BCC commonly arises on the trunk and extremities and presents as a red and scaly patch.

Complications

BCC rarely metastasizes to other sites but can cause extensive local tissue destruction and deformity. The rate of metastasis is estimated to range from 0.0028% to 0.1% and is often from untreated or inadequately treated lesions. The metatypical (basosquamous) variant of BCC has a higher rate of metastasis. The lung, bone, lymph nodes, and liver are common sites of metastasis. Metastasis, although extremely rare, can result in death.

Differential Diagnosis

Nodular BCC can resemble nonpigmented melanocytic nevus, SCC, pyogenic granuloma, merkel cell carcinoma, or seborrheic keratosis. Pigmented BCC can resemble malignant melanoma. Superficial BCC can be mistaken for actinic keratosis, Bowen's disease, psoriasis, or chronic cutaneous lupus erythematosus. Morpheaform BCC, as already mentioned, can present insidiously as a scar.

Treatment

The initial step should always be a biopsy that establishes the diagnosis of BCC as well the histologic subtype. Nodular and superficial BCCs can be treated with excision or electrodessication and curettage. Aggressive subtypes require Mohs micrographic surgery, which ensures histologic margin clearance at the time of excision.

SQUAMOUS CELL CARCINOMA

General Considerations

SCC is the second most common form of skin cancer. It is a malignancy of the keratinocytes and most commonly arises in areas of chronic sun exposure. SCC has a higher rate of metastasis than BCC, although it is still not that common.

Pathogenesis

SCC has a multifactorial etiology. The single most important factor is chronic exposure to ultraviolet light. It is more common in whites than in blacks or Asians, and individuals who burn easily are at a higher risk. Other etiologies of SCC include chronic arsenic exposure, exposure to x-radiation, and occupational exposure to some hydrocarbons. HPV plays a role in the development of SCC as does depressed immunity secondary to underlying disease or medications. Transplant patients have a high rate of SCC because of their long-term dependence on immunosuppressive agents.

Clinical Findings

SCC often presents as crusty or scaly growth on sun-damaged skin. The lesions sometimes are red.

Treatment

Treatment options include excision, electrodessication and curettage, or excision with margin control (Mohs). Important factors that determine the treatment choice include size of the tumor, depth of invasion, and location. Excision is the treatment of choice, but superficial SCC can be treated with electrodessication and curettage. High risk SCCs include tumors that invade deeply and tumors located on the lip, ear, temple, or genitalia. In these cases, Mohs surgery is indicated to achieve complete margin clearance.

MELANOMA

General Considerations

Melanoma is a malignancy of melanocytes. The incidence of melanoma is increasing more rapidly than for any other cancer. From 1935 to 1987, the incidence of melanoma in the United States increased from 1.2 to 10.4 cases per 100,000 persons. Individual risk in the United States has increased from 1/1500 in the year 1935 to 1/75 in the year 2000.

Pathogenesis

Significant amount of **data** exist to support the theory that exposure to solar radiation is the major cause of cutaneous melanomas in light-skinned individuals. In whites, melanoma incidence is inversely proportional to the latitude of residence, and by extension, the dose of ultraviolet radiation. Blacks living in a similar geographic region have one tenth to one twentieth the incidence of melanoma as whites. Among whites, lighter-pigmented individuals have higher incidence. Ultraviolet radiation from phototherapy using psoralen plus ultraviolet A also increases the incidence of melanoma. Tendency to sunburn and little tendency to tan constitute a higher risk for developing melanoma.

Family history also plays a significant role. Patients with a family history of melanoma have an elevated risk of developing melanoma. Melanomas develop in these patients at an earlier age, and there is a higher chance of multiple primary melanomas developing. Regular screening skin examinations are extremely important in this subgroup.

Clinical Findings

Visual skin examination is the most important step in melanoma detection. Melanoma can occur anywhere on the skin surface. When it occurs on hard to monitor areas such as the back, it can escape patient detection until it is too late. Hence, routine visual inspection by spouses, nurses, or physicians is important. Pigmented lesions should be inspected with ABCD guidelines: A, asymmetry; B, border irregularity; C, color (variegation or dark black color); and D, diameter greater than 0.6 cm. A history of new pigmented lesions or change in an existing one are both suspicious symptoms and should be evaluated thoroughly. Changes can include change in the color, size, shape, or surface. Pain or other discomfort is rare except in advanced lesions.

The clinical presentation of melanoma depends on the subtype that is present. Lentigo maligna is a superficial growth that commonly occurs on the head and neck in the background of sun-damaged skin. It is more common in patients in the fifth decade or older. It begins as a tan or brown patch with irregular borders and slowly enlarges over time. Over time it can develop raised areas, which indicate deeper invasion. Superficial spreading melanoma can occur anywhere on the skin. It grows more rapidly than lentigo maligna and is more common in the fourth decade. It often arises in a long-

Table 41–1. Melanoma TNM classification.

T Classification	Thickness	Ulceration Status
T1	≤ 1.0 mm	a: Without ulceration and level II/III b: With ulceration or level IV/V
T2	1.01–2.0 mm	a: Without ulceration b: With ulceration
T3	2.01–4.0 mm	a: Without ulceration b: With ulceration
T4	> 4.0 mm	a: Without ulceration b: With ulceration

N Classification	No. of Metastatic Nodes	Nodal Metastatic Mass
N1	1 node	a: micrometastasis[1] b: macrometastasis[2]
N2	2–3 nodes	a: micrometastasis[1] b: macrometastasis[2] c: in transit met(s)/satellite(s) without metastatic nodes
N3	4 or more metastatic nodes, or matted nodes, or in transit met(s)/satellite(s) with metastatic node(s)	

M Classification	Site	Serum Lactate Dehydrogenase
M1a	Distant skin, subcutaneous, or nodal metastases	Normal
M1b	Lung metastases	Normal
M1c	All other visceral metastases	Normal
	Any distant metastasis	Elevated

[1]Micrometastases are diagnosed after sentinel or elective lymphadenectomy.
[2]Macrometastases are defined as clinically detectable nodal metastases confirmed by therapeutic lymphadenectomy or when nodal metastasis exhibits gross extracapsular extension.

Table 41–2. Proposed stage groupings for cutaneous melanoma.

	Clinical Staging[1]			Pathologic Staging[2]		
	T	N	M	T	N	M
O	Tis	N0	M0	Tis	N0	M0
IA	T1a	N0	M0	T1a	N0	M0
IB	T1b	N0	M0	T1b	N0	M0
	T2a	N0	M0	T2a	N0	M0
IIA	T2b	N0	M0	T2b	N0	M0
	T3a	N0	M0	T3a	N0	M0
IIB	T3b	N0	M0	T3b	N0	M0
	T4a	N0	M0	T4a	N0	M0
IIC	T4b	N0	M0	T4b	N0	M0
III[3]	Any T	N1	M0			
		N2				
		N3				
IIIA				T1-4a	N1a	M0
				T1-4a	N2a	M0
IIIB				T1-4b	N1a	M0
				T14b	N2a	M0
				T1-4a	N1b	M0
				T1-4a	N2b	M0
				T1-4a/b	N2c	M0
IIIC				T1-4b	N1b	M0
				T1-4b	N2b	M0
				Any T	N3	M0
IV	Any T	Any N	Any M1	Any T	Any N	Any M1

[1]Clinical staging includes microstaging of the primary melanoma and clinical/radiologic evaluation for metastases. By convention, it should be used after complete excision of the primary melanoma with clinical assessment for regional and distant metastases.

[2]Pathologic staging includes microstaging of the primary melanoma and pathologic information about the regional lymph nodes after partial or complete lymphadenectomy. Pathologic stage 0 or stage 1A patients are the exception; they do not require pathologic evaluation of their lymph nodes.

[3]There are no stage III subgroups for clinical staging.

standing nevus. There is a great variation in its appearance with patches having colors of pink, red, brown, tan, and black. Raised areas indicate deeper invasion. Nodular melanoma appears as a raised bump and is most common on the trunk in men and on the legs in women. Acral lentiginous melanoma is found on the palms or soles or in nail beds and is the most frequent type of melanoma in nonwhites. It presents as a dark brown or black patch with irregular borders and can develop raised areas as well.

Treatment

Treatment of melanoma includes excision of the primary lesion and ancillary work-up to stage the disease. The thickness of the melanoma is the most important factor in determining the prognosis and it determines what the appropriate work-up should include. The most recent melanoma staging takes into account the tumor thickness, presence or absence of ulceration, presence or absence of nodal metastases, and the presence or absence of distant metastases. Tables 41–1 and 41–2 show the melanoma TNM classification and the staging guidelines. A thorough skin examination, physical examination to assess any nodal involvement, chest radiography, and laboratory examination including complete blood cell count, liver function tests, and metabolic panel are indicated for all patients diagnosed with melanoma. For those with stage 0 or stage IA, no further work-up is necessary. Although still controversial, all other stages require sentinel node biopsy to evaluate for micrometastasis to lymph nodes. Those with positive lymph node metastasis or distant metastasis are candidates for interferon alpha-2b therapy.

Balch CM et al: Final version of the American Joint Committee on Cancer staging system for cutaneous melanoma. J Clin Oncol 2001;19:3635. [PMID: 11504745]

Gershenwald JE et al: Multi-institutional melanoma lymphatic mapping experience: the prognostic value of sentinel lymph node status in 612 stage I or II melanoma patients. J Clin Oncol 1999;17:976. [PMID: 10071292]

Langley RGB et al: Neoplasms: Cutaneous Melanoma. In: Freedberg IM et al (editors): *Fitzpatrick's Dermatology in General Medicine,* vol I, 5th ed. McGraw Hill, 1999.

Leshin B, White WL: Malignant Neoplasms of Keratinocytes. In: Arndt KA et al (editors): *Cutaneous Medicine and Surgery,* vol II. WB Saunders and Company, 1996.

Miller DL, Weinstock MA: Nonmelanoma skin cancer in the United States: incidence. J Am Acad Dermatol 1994;30:774. [PMID: 8176018]

Schwartz RA, Stoll HL: Squamous Cell Carcinoma. In: Freedberg IM et al (editors): *Fitzpatrick's Dermatology in General Medicine,* vol I, 5th ed. McGraw Hill, 1999.

SECTION XV

Musculoskeletal Disorders

Fibromyalgia & Myofascial Pain | 42

Donald H. Lieberman, MD

Fibromyalgia (FM) is a syndrome of heightened pain perception. The cause is unknown, although recent research is beginning to uncover neurohormonal and other abnormalities in patients with FM. There remains no identifiable cause, and no specific treatment is universally beneficial. The diagnosis is a clinical one; laboratory findings are only useful in ruling out other diseases. Exercise combined with medications that affect pain perception, sleep, and depression can improve the outcome in FM. Understanding and treating chronic pain has become a major challenge in contemporary medicine. This is reflected in the growing number of "pain clinics" across the United States, most of which have long waiting lists.

Musculoskeletal pain has an enormous impact on our society and costs the United States billions of dollars each year in direct health care costs and productivity. Chronic pain and arthritis is found in 14–26% of the adult population. Approximately 15% of lost workdays result from musculoskeletal pain disorders.

Chronic pain has traditionally been misunderstood. Many physicians believe it to be an extension of acute pain and treat it (unsuccessfully) as such. Few physicians complete their medical residencies with competency in chronic pain management. There is a continuum from transient local pain to chronic intractable widespread pain. FM is a syndrome along this continuum.

Although diffuse pain is the defining symptom in FM, it is associated with a long list of other complaints. There are critics of the concept that FM is a distinct entity and believe it is no different than chronic widespread pain with a high tender point count. FM is perceived by some clinicians as a somatic syndrome of psychogenic origin. There remain others who do not think FM exists at all! Since pain and physical signs (tender points) are entirely subjective with no hard evidence of underlying abnormalities, skepticism has con-

tinued. Many physicians view the diagnosis as more of an enabler than a disabler. Recently, numerous papers have defined neurochemical, neuroendocrine, and imaging findings that have strengthened the view that FM is not a psychogenic disease but an amalgam of interrelated abnormalities.

 ESSENTIALS OF DIAGNOSIS

- *Widespread pain involving all 4 quadrants of the body and the axial skeleton.*
- *Pain is present for at least 3 months.*
- *Eleven of 18 positive trigger points on examination.*
- *Fatigue.*
- *Sleep disorders.*

General Considerations

A. EPIDEMIOLOGY

Almost 4 million Americans suffer from this common condition. The estimated prevalence of FM in the general population is 2% overall, 3.4% for women, and 0.5% for men. This makes FM twice as common as rheumatoid arthritis and places it second on the list of most common diagnoses in rheumatology clinics. Prevalence increases with age. The peak prevalence in a study conducted in Wichita, Kansas, United States was 60–79 years, affecting more than 7% of women. In a study conducted in Ontario, Canada the peak prevalence was in the 55- to 64-year-old group.

It has been suggested that FM is becoming an epidemic. This assumption has limitations. There is an increasing awareness of FM. It has been reported widely in the media, has been an Internet favorite, and more patients with widespread pain are referred to specialists. This also makes the referral clinic population appear significantly larger than the general population. The greater proportion of females in the clinic population may result from more women seeking medical care in general.

A report by Wolfe et al showed that the female FM prevalence appears to increase steadily through the eighth decade. The same study showed an association with divorce, failure to complete high school, and low household income.

B. PRESENTATION IN WOMEN

Studies done in humans have shown that females have a lower pain threshold and tolerance. In addition, they have a higher sensitivity to various noxious stimuli. Interestingly, chronic *regional* pain has been reported to have a similar prevalence in men and women.

Changes in pain throughout the menstrual cycle have been evaluated. Increased tenderness (greater number of tender points) was demonstrated in the postmenstrual (follicular) phase of the cycle compared with the intermenstrual (luteal) phase in normally cycling women. This variation was not found in users of oral contraceptives. This supports the role of hormonal influence in modulating pain perception.

The incidence of FM is dramatically higher in women and often begins with menopause. This has led to the study of the role gonadal steroids may play in the development of FM. Hormonal status may play a part in disturbing the hypothalamic-pituitary-adrenal (HPA) axis, which is now known to play a role in FM. Almost all postmenopausal women develop HPA axis dysregulation during depression. Premenopausal women appear to be relatively resistant to changes in HPA axis function in depressive states. Estrogen impairs glucocorticoid negative feedback leading to increases in HPA axis reactivity. When estrogenic stimulation diminishes around menopause, the function of the HPA axis decreases; whether this contributes to or helps sustain FM is speculative.

Benjamin S et al: The association between chronic widespread pain and mental disorder: a population-based study. Arthritis Rheum 2000;43:561. [PMID: 10728749]

Buskila D: Fibromyalgia, chronic fatigue syndrome, and myofascial pain syndrome. Curr Opin Rheumatol 2000;12:113. [PMID: 10751014]

Buskila D, Neumann L: Fibromyalgia syndrome (FM) and nonarticular tenderness in relatives of patients with FM. J Rheumatol 1997;24:941. [PMID: 9150086]

Crofford LJ, Clauw DJ: Fibromyalgia: where are we a decade after the American College of Rheumatology classification criteria

were developed. Arthritis Rheum 2002;46:1136. [PMID: 12115214]

Goldenberg DL: Fibromyalgia syndrome a decade later: what have we learned? Arch Intern Med 1999;159:777. [PMID: 10219923]

White KP, Harth M: Classification, epidemiology, and natural history of fibromyalgia. Curr Pain Headache Rep 2001;5:320. [PMID: 11403735]

Wolfe F et al: Work and disability status of persons with fibromyalgia. J Rheumatol 1997;24:1171. [PMID: 9195528]

Wolfe F et al: The American College of Rheumatology 1990 Criteria for the Classification of Fibromyalgia. Report of the Multicenter Criteria Committee. Arthritis Rheum 1990;33:160. [PMID: 2306288]

Pathogenesis

A. MUSCLE

Since FM is characterized by widespread muscle pain, many investigators over the past 10 years have focused on muscle abnormalities. Muscle abnormalities can be structural, metabolic, or functional. These abnormalities correlate with disturbances in the neurologic and endocrine systems. Serum levels of muscle enzymes and electromyographic findings are normal. Reviews of muscle biopsies have revealed a spectrum of descriptions from mild changes to abnormal mitochondria, reduced capillaries, thickened endothelium, ragged red fibers and, most recently, type II fiber atrophy. The theory that both intrinsic muscle abnormalities and extrinsic factors involving the nervous and endocrine systems account for the pain in FM is gaining support.

Intrinsic factors include disturbances in microcirculation, ischemia, and decreased adenosine triphosphate (ATP) concentration. Abnormally thickened capillaries with decreased blood flow through muscle could lead to decreased oxygenation, resulting in decreased ATP synthesis.

Park et al have used P-31 magnetic resonance spectroscopy to evaluate the biochemical status of muscle. Concentrations of inorganic phosphate, phosphocreatine (PCr), ATP, and phosphodiesters were measured during rest and exercise in FM patients. Measurements showed that patients with FM had significantly lower (15%) PCr and ATP levels than normal controls at rest. During exercise, at 25% of maximum voluntary contraction, the PCr and ATP levels were also significantly lower in patients with FM. Pain was inversely correlated with ATP levels during exercise. This study provides objective evidence for metabolic abnormalities that correlate with clinical symptoms in patients with FM.

B. NEUROTRANSMITTERS

Changes in the activities of neurotransmitters along central pain pathways may be involved in the pathogenesis of FM. Increased levels of substance P (a peptide neurotransmitter) and activated serotonin metabolites in the cerebrospinal fluid have been demonstrated. Liew et al found increased concentrations of nerve growth factor (NGF) in patients with FM. NGF appears to be involved in inflammation and hyperalgesia. When NGF is injected intravenously, muscle pain results in a dose-dependent manner. Interestingly, this affects women more than men. It is unclear whether increased NGF concentration is a factor in the pathogenesis of FM or part of the mechanism underlying the symptoms of chronic musculoskeletal pain. This finding does suggest a central mechanism involving abnormalities in neuropeptides.

C. Hypothalamic-Pituitary-Adrenal Axis

Impaired functioning of the HPA axis has been seen in FM. Compared with normal controls, 24-hour levels of free cortisol in urine are low in patients with FM. Morning cortisol levels are normal and evening cortisol levels are elevated in patients with FM. Most patients with FM have nonrestorative sleep. Growth hormone (GH) is maximally secreted during stages 3 and 4 of non–rapid eye movement sleep. Therefore, patients with FM may have impaired GH secretion. Low levels of insulin-like growth factor-1 (IGF-1) have been observed in FM. This may be a consequence of impaired GH secretion and therefore a secondary phenomenon. Park has suggested that "disturbances in the HPA axis may amplify and promote the extent and intensity of neurotransmitter imbalance." The deficits in GH, IGF-1, and thyroid-stimulating hormone curtail ATP production and muscle tissue repair following exercise and exertion.

Paiva et al have demonstrated that serum levels of IGF-1 are diminished in a substantial percentage of patients with FM. They showed that treatment with GH leads to improvement in symptoms. In their most recent study, they demonstrated that failure of the GH axis to respond to an exercise stress is attributed to increased levels of somatostatin. Administering pyridostigmine reversed the impaired response. Because pyridostigmine is known to reduce somatastatin tone, it is surmised that the defective GH response to exercise in patients with FM probably results from increased levels of somatastatin. The reason for increased levels of somatastatin is unknown. The authors suggest that the regulatory mechanisms are localized in the central nervous system. The altered response to stress strengthens the evidence that central mechanisms are involved in the pathophysiology of FM.

Other authors stress that the HPA axis activity may be independently altered by comorbid conditions such as mood disorders or chronic fatigue syndrome. This alteration could make certain populations more vulnerable to FM.

Figure 42–1 is a diagram of *proposed* interactions of peripheral and central factors leading to pain and muscle dysfunction in FM.

D. Central Sensitization

Central sensitization has been defined by Yunus and Inanici as "an exaggerated response of the central nervous system to a peripheral stimulus that is normally painful (hyperalgesia) or non-nociceptive such as touch (allodynia), denoting hyperexcitablity and hypersensitivity of the CNS neurons. Another characteristic of central sensitization is the prolongation or persistence of pain." The details of this important phenomenon is beyond the scope of this chapter but can be found in *Myofascial Pain and Fibromyalgia* by Raichlin and Raichlin.

There is a family of central sensitivity syndromes that includes FM, chronic fatigue syndrome, irritable bowel syndrome, tension-type headaches, migraine, multiple chemical sensitivity, primary dysmenorrhea, periodic limb movement disorder, restless legs syndrome, temporomandibular pain and dysfunction syndrome, and regional fibromyalgia/myofascial pain syndrome.

Central sensitivity syndromes share many common clinical characteristics such as gender, age distribution, symptoms, and the lack of demonstrable structural abnormalities. It must be emphasized that these syndromes are not synonymous with psychiatric illness.

Bennett RM: Emerging concepts in the neurobiology of chronic pain: evidence of abnormal sensory processing in fibromyalgia. Mayo Clin Proc 1999;74:385. [PMID: 10221469]

Bennett RM, Clark SC, Walczyk J: A randomized, double-blind, placebo-controlled study of growth hormone in the treatment of fibromyalgia. Am J Med 1998;104:227. [PMID: 9552084]

Giovengo SL, Russell IJ, Larson AA: Increased concentrations of nerve growth factor in cerebrospinal fluid of patients with fibromyalgia. J Rheumatol 1999;26:1564. [PMID: 10405946]

Paiva ES et al: Impaired growth hormone secretion in fibromyalgia patients: evidence for augmented hypothalamic somatastatin tone. Arthritis Rheum 2002;46:1344. [PMID: 12115242]

Park JH, Niermann KJ, Olsen N: Evidence for metabolic abnormalities in the muscles of patients with fibromyalgia. Curr Rheumatol Rep 2000;2:131. [PMID: 11123050]

Yunus MB, Inanici F: Fibromyalgia syndrome: Clinical features, diagnosis, and biopathophysiologic mechanisms. In: *Myofascial Pain and Fibromyalgia, Trigger Point Management*, 2e. Mosby, 2002.

Clinical Findings

Clinical factors associated with FM in the general population are decreased pain threshold, "pain all over," subjective joint swelling, paresthesias, morning stiffness lasting longer than 15 minutes, sleep disturbance, fa-

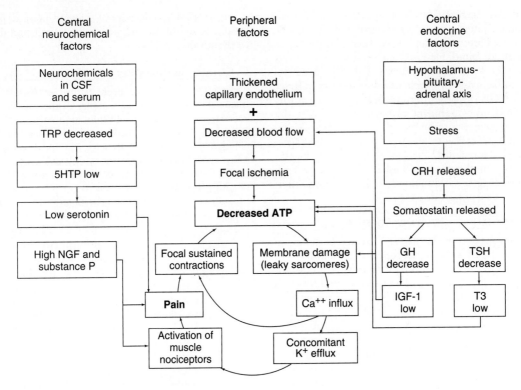

Central
neurochemical
factors

Peripheral
factors

Central
endocrine
factors

Figure 42–1. Proposed interactions of peripheral and central factors that lead to pain and muscle dysfunction in fibromyalgia. (Reproduced with permission from Park JH, Niermann KJ, Olse N: Evidence for metabolic abnormalities in the muscles of patients with fibromyalgia. Curr Rheumatol Rep 2000;2:13140.)

tigue, irritable bowel syndrome, moderate or severe impairment on a health assessment questionnaire, increased pain, fair and poor self-reported health status, and moderate and marked dissatisfaction with health.

Psychological factors included somatization, anxiety, depression, increased global severity of psychiatric illness, history of past or current depression, prior hospitalization for depression, and family history of depression.

Familial aggregation of FM has been reported with first-degree relatives of people with FM displaying the disease with a greater than expected frequency.

Trauma (mostly physical) has been reported to precede the onset of FM in 25% of patients.

The classification criteria for FM developed by the American College of Rheumatology were not intended for diagnosing disease in individual patients but were developed to provide investigators with a homogenous group of patients to study. FM has become a popular syndrome. There are more than 20 full-length "self-help" books available and the Internet is flooded with

web sites on this disorder. Some sites are reputable and provide up-to-date useful information, while others tout useless treatments and misinformation. Many patients arrive at the office "self diagnosed" asking for confirmation or prescriptions. Countless others have undergone extensive work-ups for arthritis, neurologic disease, thyroid disease, cardiac abnormalities, and psychiatric disease. Diagnosis requires a careful history, physical examination, and judicious use of laboratory testing.

A. HISTORY

To fulfill the criteria for FM a patient must have a history of widespread pain involving all 4 quadrants of the body and the axial skeleton (cervical spine, anterior chest, thoracic spine, or low back. In addition, the patient must report pain in 11 of 18 "tender points" (Figure 42–2). Pain caused by the application of 4 kg/cm (pressure that is adequate enough to cause the examiners nail bed to blanche) is considered "positive." Pain should be present for at least 3 months.

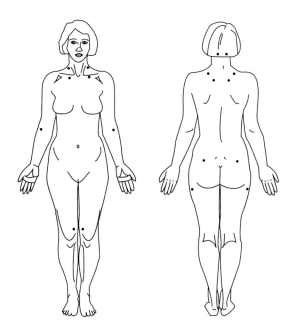

Figure 42–2. Tender points in patients with fibromyalgia.

In addition to widespread pain and muscle tenderness, the most characteristic symptoms of FM are sleep disturbances, fatigue, and morning stiffness. These symptoms are seen in 75% of patient's with FM, although the simultaneous presence of all 3 is not necessary for diagnosis. Fatigue is experienced in 90% of patient's with FM.

Pain is the most common symptom of FM. It is usually present in all 4 limbs. Pain can be almost anywhere but is more common in the axial skeleton, either in the upper or lower back. Pain in the anterior chest is sometimes confused with cardiac pain. Some patients have a more peripheral presentation and feel they have arthritis. Pain may be aggravated by cold or humid weather, poor sleep, noise, anxiety, stress, and overuse.

Sleep disturbances are prominent in FM. Sleep encephalograms show an intrusion of alpha waves during stage 4, non–rapid eye movement sleep. Because alpha activity is part of arousal, the patient experiences a wakeful arousal pattern during periods of what should be deep, restful sleep. This pattern causes nonrestorative sleep, which may influence the ability to modulate pain, contributing to a lower pain threshold. A recent study has identified 3 distinct patterns of alpha activity in FM: phasic alpha (50%), tonic alpha (20%), and low alpha (30%). Phasic alpha sleep activity was the pattern that correlated best with clinical manifestations of FM. Some studies have found sleep apnea to be common in

men with FM. Restless leg syndrome has also been reported. It is unknown whether disturbance of non–rapid eye movement sleep leads to FM or is a consequence of this disorder.

Fatigue and sleep disturbances are almost universal in FM and their absence should initiate a search for another diagnosis.

Primary FM by definition has no underlying known precipitating event. **Secondary** FM occurs after physical or emotional trauma, which may be minor in nature. Infection (particularly viral) may trigger FM. (FM has been reported to occur after infection with coxsackievirus, parvovirus, and HIV.)

FM often coexists with other syndromes such as headaches, irritable bowel syndrome, restless legs syndrome, depression, and chronic fatigue syndrome. Each of these syndromes includes an array of symptoms such as facial pain, Raynaud's phenomenon, dysmenorrhea, sicca symptoms, urinary frequency, dizziness, and disturbances in concentration.

Patients should be asked about current drug use. Certain antivirals and lipid-lowering drugs can cause myalgias. In addition, many patients use herbs and supplements and often do not offer this information unless specifically asked.

B. PHYSICAL EXAMINATION

Physical examination is unremarkable except for tender points. Tender points, however, do not define the typical pain of FM. It is likely that many physicians apply too much or too little pressure and often apply this pressure in the wrong areas. The previous concept of using "control points" (areas that should not be tender) has been abandoned. Patients with FM appear to be more sensitive to pain throughout their entire body, which underscores the limitations of defining trigger points.

The skin of a patient with FM may be mottled or "net-like" in appearance. Raynaud's phenomenon is often reported. It was present in only 15% of patients, but it was highly specific (95%) in the multicenter criteria study of FM.

C. LABORATORY FINDINGS

An erythrocyte sedimentation rate (or C-reactive protein), thyroid-stimulating hormone, and complete blood cell count are helpful in most patients. Since most patients have had symptoms for 5 to 7 years before a diagnosis has been made, some physician's include kidney and liver function studies, muscle enzymes, and electromyography for completeness.

Unless there is evidence to suggest an autoimmune disorder, serologic studies such as antinuclear antibodies or rheumatoid factor are of little use and have a low predictive value. In addition, when the studies are positive in low titer, they may confuse the issue and deflect attention from the diagnosis.

D. IMAGING STUDIES

Radiographs are not indicated because FM has no structural abnormalities.

E. NEUROENDOCRINE STUDIES

Although an increasing number of neuroendocrine tests are abnormal in FM, none of these studies is either sensitive enough or specific to the diagnosis.

Wolfe F: What use are fibromyalgia control points? J Rheumatol 1998;25:546. [PMID: 9517779]

Differential Diagnosis

FM has the characteristic symptoms of widespread pain, fatigue, and sleep disturbance. It should be kept in mind that other diseases need not be excluded in making the diagnosis and may occur concurrently. Treating the concurrent disease will not ameliorate the symptoms of FM. It is extremely important to identify comorbid diseases so that they are adequately treated. Table 42–1 lists the appropriate testing for conditions that may simulate or confound the diagnosis of FM.

Treatment

In order to treat FM, the physician must believe it is a real syndrome. Many physicians still believe that FM is imaginary and represents a depressed or manipulative patient. Since many patients have become frustrated over time, they are often angry; this compromises the doctor-patient relationship from the outset.

Many well-respected rheumatology clinics will see the patient for an initial consultation to confirm the diagnosis and exclude other conditions. Patients are then referred back to the primary care physician. This attitude may be a response to the large volume of patients with FM and the paucity of effective treatment modalities.

Once the diagnosis of FM is established, the patient must understand that there is no clear treatment algorithm that results in relief. An empathetic but realistic approach should promise no cure and emphasize that treatment is by trial and error, is lifelong, and is rarely completely satisfactory. Education of the patient should stress the point that FM is not crippling, is not fatal, and can be managed. The patient will require the support of family, friends, employers, and the physician. Constant complaining and self-victimization will eventually alienate those who are most needed for support.

There has been a reluctance and even a warning not to label patients as having FM, since this can create "illness behavior" and a need for disability. A recent com-

Table 42–1. Conditions that simulate or confound the diagnosis of fibromyalgia.

Condition	Investigation
Arthritis (autoimmune and osteoarthritis)	Objective swelling, laboratory markers, roentgenograms
Polymyalgia rheumatica	ESR, anemia
Myopathy	Weakness, increased muscle enzymes
Hepatitis C	LFTs, antibody
Sleep apnea	Sleep study, careful history
Cervical stenosis	Roentgenograms, MRI, electromyography, neurologic examination
Chest pain	Electrocardiography, stress test, chest roentgenograms
Back pain	Roentgenograms, MRI
Hypothyroidism	TSH, T4
Malignancy	History, ESR, imaging studies, laboratory tests
Medications (lipid-lowering, antivirals)	Medication history
Viral infection	Titers for parvovirus, cocksackie-virus, and HIV
Malingering	Common sense

ESR, erythrocyte sedimentation rate; LFTs, liver function tests; MRI, magnetic resonance imaging; TSH, thyroid-stimulating hormone.

munity study appears to refute this concept since there was no worsening of pain, fatigue, or other symptoms in a group of patients who were labeled with FM from the outset and monitored over time. A diagnosis is very helpful to many patients and terminates their extensive search for the cause of their symptoms. Figure 42–3 is a suggested treatment algorithm.

A. PHARMACOLOGIC

1. Tricyclic antidepressants—The beneficial effects of tricyclic antidepressants in FM may be related to their ability to inhibit reuptake of serotonin and possibly norepinephrine.

Amitriptyline has been the most widely studied drug in this class. Only 25–30% of patients experience clinically significant improvement. The relief is only modest and decreases with time. In addition, side effects are seen in up to 20% of patients because of sedative and anticholinergic properties. Most physicians start with 10 mg

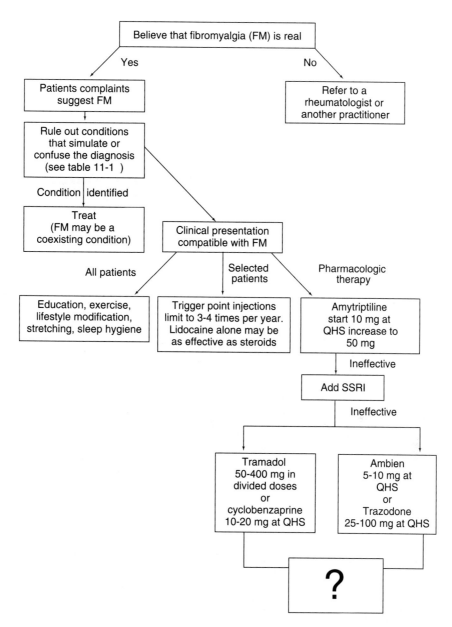

Figure 42–3. Algorithm for managing fibromyalgia.

at bedtime and increase up to 50 mg if needed. Mean scores of pain, sleep, global assessment, and tender point scores all improved with amitriptyline therapy. Amitriptyline should be used with caution in patients with urinary retention and narrow-angle glaucoma.

Cyclobenzaprine is a tricyclic agent that is chemically similar to amitriptyline and has been traditionally marketed as a muscle relaxant. Although it has only modest efficacy in FM and its use is limited by its anticholinergic effects, certain subgroups seem to do well, and it is worth a trial. It produces more consistent improvement in sleep time than in pain relief. The starting dose is 10 mg at bedtime. It can be increased to 20 mg. Daytime use is limited due to drowsiness.

2. Selective serotonin reuptake inhibitors (SSRIs)—
These agents have been studied with conflicting results. One study on fluoxetine concluded it was not effective in FM. A second study showed that both fluoxetine and amitriptyline were effective and were more effective in combination than either drug alone. Single trials of other SSRIs have shown some benefit.

A recent meta-analysis of antidepressants showed they were efficacious in treating many of the symptoms of FM. Patients were 4 times as likely to report overall improvement in well being, with moderate reductions in sleep disturbance, fatigue, and pain but not trigger points.

3. Analgesics—Tramadol (Ultram) is a centrally acting analgesic, with both μ-opioid receptor binding and noradrenaline (norepinephrine) and serotonin reuptake inhibition. Trials have confirmed its efficacy and safety in relief of pain. Dosage ranges from 50–400 mg/d.

Trazodone (Desyrel) and zolpidem (Ambien) may benefit some patients with insomnia who are intolerant to the tricyclics.

Nonsteroidal anti-inflammatory drugs (NSAIDs) are not effective. Since FM is not accompanied by inflammation, this is not surprising, and continuous use of these drugs can cause gastrointestinal and renal toxicity in addition to edema and hypertension. Despite this observation, over 90% of patients with FM are taking anti-inflammatory agents. Relief from minor arthritis or dysmenorrhea may explain their continued usage.

Simple analgesics such as acetaminophen are not very effective. When patients were asked to compare relief from acetaminophen with NSAIDs, the majority reported acetaminophen to be less effective.

Prednisone is not effective and has multiple adverse effects.

Gabapentin a central analgesic and antiseizure medication helpful for neuralgia may show some efficacy but has not been evaluated for FM.

Soma compound is a combination of carisoprodol (200 mg), acetaminophen, and caffeine. In an 8-week study of its use in FM, it was significantly better than placebo in relieving pain and improving sleep as well as increasing the pressure pain threshold.

4. Opioids—Opioids are not required for the majority of patients with FM. Some physicians never prescribe narcotics for these patients. Some physicians will prescribe opioids for a small number of refractory cases, while others reserve using opioids for flares. The decision to use opioids should not be made because of patient pressure or physician frustration. On the other hand, opiates are the most effective medications for managing most chronic pain states. Many physicians have avoided opioids because of medicolegal reasons.

Ignorance regarding the propensity to cause addiction, physical dependence, and tolerance is fading with physician education and recent encouragement to use these drugs without the fear of penalty.

B. NONPHARMACOLOGIC

1. Exercise—Patients with FM often have kinesophobia. This fear of movement causes increased muscle pain and joint stiffness resulting in a vicious circle. Aerobic exercise has been shown to be more effective than stretching. Aerobic exercise 3 times per week can reduce tender point tenderness. Although overall pain may decrease, sleep disturbance and fatigue are unaffected. Many patients have postexertion exacerbation of symptoms. Low level aerobic fitness should be encouraged (walking). Some patients can achieve long-term aerobic capacity and decrease the need for medication.

One recent study compared trainability of the neuromuscular system of women with FM and healthy women. Both groups had similar trainability, lending support to the theory that FM has a central rather than a peripheral (muscular) basis.

Another study confirmed that cardiorespiratory fitness in female patients with FM is similar to healthy controls, but the **perceived** exertion scores were higher.

2. Diet—Investigators have found that between 26% and 40% of patients with FM attempt dietary changes. Foods may be eliminated or added to the diet.

Brain tryptophan is low in FM. Protein rich foods have been reported to lower brain tryptophan. A vegetarian diet was tried to decrease symptoms without success. One study of a very strict Vegan diet for 3 months did decrease pain.

3. Sleep hygiene—In addition to the pharmacologic interventions to improve sleep, the patient can make lifestyle adjustments that are beneficial. Patients should go to sleep and wake up at same time every day. Caffeine and alcohol should not be used before bedtime. The bed should be used for sleeping, not for watching television. Ear plugs may be helpful if outside noise is disruptive. Drugs that disrupt sleep, such as appetite suppressants, antiemetics, and sedative hypnotics, should be avoided.

4. Biofeedback—Abnormal electromyographic activity and reduced muscle sensitivity have been reported in FM. Electromyography feedback has been studied and its role in uncertain. Exercise training combined with biofeedback resulted in a greater benefit and longer lasting results than either modality alone.

5. Hypnotherapy—Patients with FM experienced greater benefit from hypnotherapy than physical therapy. The benefit was in pain, fatigue, and global assessment.

6. Acupuncture—Very few studies have been conducted on the effect of acupuncture therapy in FM. Electroacupuncture may be beneficial but may not correlate with traditional acupuncture. The National Institutes of Health consensus statement on acupuncture concluded that in some situations, including FM, "acupuncture may be useful as an adjunct treatment or an acceptable alternative or may be included in a comprehensive management program."

7. Interdisciplinary programs—Structured programs reduce some symptoms with the most severely affected benefiting the most.

Tender-point injections with or without corticosteroids may provide **temporary** relief. Many physicians use 1% lidocaine without the addition of corticosteroids since there is no evidence that the addition of corticosteroids is more effective (Figure 42–3).

C. COMPLEMENTARY THERAPY

Complementary and alternative medical therapies have been defined as "those interventions neither taught widely at US medical schools nor generally available in US hospitals." Complementary therapies refer to unconventional treatments used in conjunction with a traditional treatment plan. Eisenberg et al have reported that there are now more office visits made seeking complementary and alternative therapies in the United States than for the services of conventional primary care physicians.

Many patients with FM are frustrated by the lack of relief from traditional medicine and are willing to try a wide variety of remedies. A recent study revealed that sales of vitamins, minerals, and herbs as well as other supplements is over $10 billion per year. These therapies are not regulated by the US Food and Drug Administration and therefore remain experimental and unproved. The contents, potency, and side effects of alternative remedies cannot be guaranteed and may be dangerous. The physician must emphasize to the patient that herbals cannot be removed from the market unless they are proved harmful! Patients should always be asked about their use of supplements, vitamins, and herbs because they often do not offer this information. Patients often feel it is not important for the doctor to know or feel the physician will disapprove or discourage use of such use.

S-adenosylmethionine is a naturally occurring active derivative of methionine. Antidepressant, analgesic, and anti-inflammatory properties have been identified. Only short-duration studies have been done, with mixed results concerning effectiveness. Since FM is not considered an inflammatory disease, it is likely that any efficacy seen is secondary to the antidepressant or analgesic property of the compound. One study showed no effectiveness.

Magnesium and malic acid are available in a combination tablet, Super Malic. This preparation contains 200 mg malic acid and 50 mg magnesium. One theory of pain in FM postulates a deficiency of ATP. Both magnesium and malic acid are involved in the generation of mitochondrial ATP. In a 4-week study administering 3 tablets twice daily, pain and tenderness were not significantly improved. There were improvements, however, in the 6-month open-label extension administering 6 tablets twice daily. Further studies are needed to determine long-term efficacy.

Guafenesin, a popular treatment for FM, was touted as a cure for some time. Studies have shown it has no effect.

GH injected on a daily basis to 22 women with low IGF-1 levels for 9 months resulted in an improvement in their symptoms and number of tender points. No patients had complete remission of their symptoms. Patients did not see improvement until after 6 months of therapy. Almost one third of the patients developed carpal tunnel syndrome (usually seen in the early stages of therapy.) The cost-benefit ratio prohibits widespread use since GH costs more than $1500 per month.

There was no difference in response using magnetic fields compared with sham or usual care groups. Cognitive-behavioral treatment has been reported to be of some benefit.

Abeles M, Watermann J, Maestrello S: Tender point injections in fibromyalgia (abstract). Arthritis Rheum 1997;40(Suppl): S187.

Bennett RM, TPS-FM Study Group: A blinded, placebo-controlled evaluation of Tramadol in the management of fibromyalgia pain. J Musculoskeletal Pain 1998;6(Suppl 2):146.

Buckelew SP et al: Biofeedback/relaxation training and exercise interventions for fibromyalgia: a prospective trial. Arthritis Care Res 1998;11:196. [PMID: 9782811]

Eisenberg DM et al: Trends in alternative medicine use in the United States, 1990–1997: results of a follow-up national survey. JAMA 1998;280:1569. [PMID: 9820257]

Wolfe F, Zhao S, Lane N: Preference for nonsteroidal antiinflammatory drugs over acetaminophen by rheumatic disease patients: a survey of 1,799 patients with osteoarthritis, rheumatoid arthritis, and fibromyalgia. Arthritis Rheum 2000; 43:378. [PMID: 10693878]

When to Refer to a Specialist

Many patients have concurrent illnesses, both psychiatric and medical, that make the diagnosis more challenging. FM is present in 10–40% of patients with systemic lupus erythematosis and in 10–30% of patients with rheumatoid arthritis. Differentiating a flare of a connective tissue disease from FM is often difficult, and referral to a rheumatologist is both cost-effective and helpful to the patient.

A. PHYSIATRIST

Patients who do not respond to conventional therapy within a month may benefit from a consultation with a physiatrist. Physiatrists are often leaders of multidisciplinary teams that include physical and occupational therapists as well as psychologists and vocational counselors. In addition, they can prescribe the most appropriate exercise programs. In cases where symptoms begin after a motor vehicle or work-related injury, a physiatrist will be invaluable because he or she is familiar with litigation and worker's compensation.

B. PSYCHOTHERAPIST

Approximately 20–40% of people with FM seen in tertiary centers have identifiable **current** mood disorders. The lifetime incidence of psychiatric comorbidities in patients with FM from tertiary care centers ranges from 40% to 70%.

The number of patients with major depression is probably not much higher than that seen in rheumatoid arthritis and in healthy controls. It should therefore be remembered that most patients with FM (even in tertiary referral clinics) do not have a current psychiatric illness.

Psychological assessment and treatment may be helpful in patients who have severe symptoms, those with poor coping skills, and those with anger and hostility. Pain management techniques that can be learned include various coping and relaxation techniques, pacing, and identification of activities that exacerbate symptoms. Because interpersonal relationships may be affected, the involvement of relatives or partners in counseling is recommended. Many of the psychological aspects of FM are the sequelae of chronic pain rather than of significant psychopathologic conditions.

Treatment of uncomplicated depression involves counseling and use of antidepressants. The low doses of antidepressants frequently used for their analgesic or sleep modulating effects are not adequate treatment for depression, although they may alleviate some of the symptoms of FM. Higher doses of tricyclics or SSRIs may be helpful. Successful treatment of depression frequently is accompanied by decreased pain levels in patients with chronic pain, but pain relief may not occur in FM even with treatment of depression.

Prognosis

The prognosis is generally favorable, although 10–30% of patients describe being work impaired. Factors associated with a better prognosis are higher level of education, younger age, early diagnosis, and greater time spent exercising. Poor prognosis is associated with initial severity, depression, and multiple tender points. Table 42–2 shows long-term prognosis of patients with FM.

There is a sharp contrast between community-based studies and medical center outcomes. Patients in the community with chronic pain have better outcomes than patients in tertiary referral centers. In general, complete remissions are rare, although 1 report from Australia reported 25% of patients to be in remission 2 years after diagnosis. The study did not use the current criteria for FM. In the longest study, 29 patients were surveyed 1, 3, and 14 years after diagnosis; 19 (66%) of 29 felt better 14 years after diagnosis and 16 (73%) of 22 thought that their symptoms interfered little with work. In a recent study from Canada, one third of patients monitored for 3 years experienced a reduction in pain by at least 30% from baseline, as well as better outcomes in overall status of FM. In addition, medica-

Table 42–2. Long-term prognosis in fibromyalgia.

Study	N	Setting	Female, %	Mean age (range), y	Follow-up, y	Remissions[1] %
Kennedy and Felson [91]	29	Specialty clinic	86.2	43.5 (—)	10	0
Bengtsson and Backnman [92]	49	Specialty clinic	—		8	"rare"
Ledingham et al. [93]	72	Specialty clinic	90.3	52 (18–81)	4	2.8
Granges et al. [94]	44	Specialty clinic	84.1	35.7 (15–61)	2	24.2
Felson and Goldenberg [95]	39	Specialty clinic	84.6	44.1 (—)	2	0
Papageorgiou et al. [97]	79	General population	94	48.6 (24–86)	1.5	6.3

[1]Remissions defined as resolution of chronic widespread pain.
(Reproduced with permission from White KP, Harth M: Classification, epidemiology, and Natural history of fibromyalgia Current Pain and Headache Reports 2001; August 5, p 320–329.

tion use decreased, whereas the use of alternative products increased.

Relevant Web Sites

[The Arthritis Foundation]
http://www.arthritis.org/
[American Fibromyalgia Syndrome Association]
http://afsafund.org/

[The Oregon Fibromyalgia Foundation]
http://www.myalgia.com/
[Fibromyalgia Network]
http://fmnetnews.com/
[A database of natural remedy brands that have been independently tested]
http://www.ConsumerLab.com/

Sports Medicine

Margot Putukian, MD

More and more girls and women are becoming physically active, taking part in organized athletics, and enjoying a healthy, active lifestyle. Involvement in sport is beneficial not only for improving health and decreasing risk factors for disease, but also for personal development and mental well being. Although the medical care of athletes does not differ significantly from that of the general population, there are some considerations that make athletes a special population. Female athletes have specific issues to deal with such as exercise in pregnancy, menstrual dysfunction, and eating disorders as well as nutritional and musculoskeletal factors.

Exercise can play a role in decreasing the risk factors for coronary heart disease, with its effect on the lipid profile, body mass index, and diabetes mellitus. Because coronary heart disease is the leading cause of death among women, accounting for 28% of all fatalities, an exercise program is an essential component of preventive and rehabilitative medicine for women. For many individuals, exercise also provides an opportunity for social interaction and personal growth.

The physiologic responses to strengthening and conditioning are the same in women and men, as are the types of muscle fibers utilized and the ability to metabolize fat. Although there is an absolute difference in some of these variables, such as maximal oxygen uptake, these differences disappear when related to lean body weight. Similarly, although the absolute increase in muscle size in response to strength training is larger in men than women, it is the same when lean body mass is taken into account. Relative changes in other physiologic variables in response to exercise, such as heart size, volume, and metabolism, are similar in men and women.

Although it is clear that the benefits of exercise and competitive athletics transcend gender, it is unclear what the effects are of competitive exercise on the female reproductive, endocrinologic, and musculoskeletal systems. Most of the information used in the field of sports medicine has been gleaned from studies of men; however, there is new information being obtained that relates specifically to active women. Examples of these issues are exercise in pregnancy and the **female athlete triad,** which includes menstrual dysfunction, eating disorders, and osteoporosis (see Chapter 8, Eating Disorders and Chapter 19, Osteoporosis).

Putukian M: The female triad. Eating disorders, amenorrhea, and osteoporosis. Med Clin North Am 1994;78:345. [PMID: 8121215]

Putukian M, McKeag DB: The preparticipation physical examination. In: *Sports Medicine and Physical Examination: A Sport-Specific Approach.* Buschbacher RM, Braddom RL (editors). Hanley & Belfus, 1994.

PREPARTICIPATION PHYSICAL EXAMINATION

The preparticipation physical examination for girls in school is different from that of women, and health care providers need to be familiar with the problems and issues that face each age group. In addition, different activities have different demands, which must be taken into account when making recommendations. For example, the demands on a competitive cross-country runner are different from those on a soccer player and certainly different from those on an obese individual who wants to initiate an exercise program, such as walking. To be effective, the health care provider needs to understand the goals of the individual, attain a thorough medical history, and perform a complete physical examination. At that point, recommendations regarding activity can be individualized and allow for safe and enjoyable participation in sport.

The preparticipation physical examination is one of the most important responsibilities for physicians, yet in many instances it receives little attention. School-age children often are seen in a group setting where loud gymnasium rooms do not allow for appropriate cardiac examinations or discussions of personal health issues such as sexuality, drug use, and weight control. On the other hand, individual examinations with a physician who is not familiar with the demands of the contemplated activity are not adequate either. Both office and group (or "station") settings for the preparticipation examination have their advantages and disadvantages, but both can be effective if done properly.

The timing of the preparticipation examination is also important. It should be done early enough to allow for follow-up tests, rehabilitation, and consultations, if necessary, yet close enough to the start of participation to be relevant. In general, a time frame of 2–6 weeks before the beginning of the activity is recommended. For school-age athletes, repeat examinations often are performed when a new level of school is reached, eg, middle school, high school, or college. In addition, a repeat examination is indicated if there is a new medical problem, significant injury has occurred, or the student has requested one.

History

The history component of the preparticipation physical examination should target the cardiovascular, neurologic, and musculoskeletal systems. The history also should obtain information about any ongoing or previous medical problems, prior surgery, medications, and allergies; emergency contacts should be noted. Additional questions are often helpful in targeting issues that pertain to specific age groups. For older girls and women, questions that relate to menstrual function, osteoporosis, pulmonary and cardiovascular risk factors, medical problems, and medications are important. For younger girls, questions that relate to sexuality, recreational drug use, and the components of the female athlete triad are important. For many athletes, the preparticipation physical examination can serve as an introduction to the health care system and provide the basis of a physician-patient relationship that can help foster the behaviors of a healthy lifestyle.

Other areas of importance in the preparticipation physical examination include history of an absent organ that is supposed to be paired (ie, 1 kidney, 1 ovary), seasonal allergies, medication use, and medical problems that may have an impact on the proposed exercise regimen. For example, exercise can be beneficial in the management of diabetes and asthma, but precautions are necessary to optimize participation. It is important to emphasize the benefits of being involved. At times, people have exercise goals that are not realistic, such as an older patient with degenerative arthritis and osteoporosis who wants to start roller-blading because her grandchildren enjoy it. The recommendations given to the patient must be individualized, realistic, and geared to the person's goals.

Tailoring the preparticipation physical examination to female athletes requires an understanding of the issues that are important and unique to this group, such as nutrition as it relates to health and performance, the effect of exercise on the menstrual cycle, and the high incidence of eating disorders among athletes.

A. NUTRITION

The field of sports nutrition has gained increased interest. Athletes are seeking the advice of nutritionists in an attempt to maximize their performance, and a great deal of research is going on in the area. The specific nutritional needs of women should be addressed in the preparticipation physical examination, including total caloric intake and intake of calcium, protein, fat, and iron. It is also important to consider nutrition when an athlete presents with symptoms of fatigue, burnout, and recurrent minor injuries. Constant dieting unfortunately has become acceptable for girls and women, and athletes often attempt to lose weight to improve performance. Numerous studies have demonstrated the poor eating behavior of athletes, particularly female athletes.

Ideally, nutritional intake should include 6–10 g of carbohydrate per kilogram of body weight, 0.8–1.5 g of protein per kilogram, and the rest of the calories from fat. These levels translate into a diet of 60–70% carbohydrate, 10–15% protein, and 25–30% fat. More recently, the protein recommendation has been increased to 20–25% and the fat decreased to 10–15%. In general, this translates to more than 1500 calories a day from a variety of foods. This should meet most nutritional needs with the exception of iron. This information is important to relay to female athletes, especially young girls, who may restrict their intake and attempt to meet their nutritional needs by supplementation. The use of a daily multivitamin preparation, and for some individual iron and calcium supplements, is reasonable; however, female athletes should understand that no supplement can take the place of proper food selection.

1. Iron—Iron deficiency is common entity in young athletes, especially female athletes. Iron deficiency or decreased iron stores can occur without anemia in as many as 9.5–57% of this population. Girls take in significantly less than the recommended daily allowance (RDA) of 18 mg of iron. Because there is often an increase in plasma volume of 6–25% with training, the hemoglobin and hematocrit levels can appear falsely low with resultant "pseudoanemia." A screening hemoglobin level with follow-up ferritin determination is reasonable for assessing iron deficiency in female athletes. Ferritin is the storage form of iron, and its determination can be helpful in differentiating pseudoanemia from true iron deficiency. In some situations, such as acute infection, the level of ferritin can be increased; additional studies, as well as clinical correlation, are then necessary. Iron loss can be caused by hemolysis with hemoglobinuria, gastrointestinal losses, and loss of iron through excessive sweating. Female athletes are at increased risk because of the additional iron loss that occurs with menses. Correction of iron deficiency anemia can improve performance, and therapy should include intake of iron-rich foods and adequate vitamin C and supplementation.

2. Calcium—Another important nutritional concern for female athletes is calcium intake; as with iron, the intake is often far less than the RDA. Various studies of female athletes have demonstrated that 40% of gymnasts, 42% of ballet dancers, and 51% of cross-country runners consume less than two thirds of the RDA for calcium. Calcium, along with adequate estrogen, is necessary for normal bone acquisition; if calcium stores are depleted, a lower bone density may result. Because peak bone density is reached early in life, in the 20s and 30s, ensuring adequate intake is especially important in early childhood and adolescence. Poor acquisition of bone density contributes to the development of stress fractures and premature osteoporosis, which is one of the final outcomes of the female athlete triad (see Chapter 19, Osteoporosis).

3. Calories—One of the most important nutritional concerns for young female athletes is ensuring adequate total caloric intake. Many athletes do not consume adequate calories to meet their energy needs. In an attempt to "eat healthy," many athletes restrict their fat intake such that the fat-soluble vitamins are at risk for being deficient. Risks of a diet that contains less than 10% fat include low energy intake and low levels of protein, iron, zinc, and vitamin E. Deficiencies also have been noted in zinc; magnesium; folate; and vitamins B_6, C, A, and B_{12}. Many athletes experiment in restricting their intake, often as part of a "diet" plan to lose weight, even though they may not be overweight. Distorted body image and the displeasure that young women often have with their body can result in pathogenic weight control behavior.

B. PATHOGENIC EATING BEHAVIORS

The combination of disordered eating, menstrual dysfunction, and osteoporosis has become known as the female athlete triad; it is probably one of the biggest challenges facing the sports medicine community. Pathogenic eating behavior is especially difficult to treat for several reasons: (1) weight and body image are sensitive issues to discuss; (2) it is difficult to detect normal from abnormal behavior; and (3) the individual often denies there is a problem. Although most commonly seen in sports such as figure skating, gymnastics, cross-country running, and swimming, eating disorders are present in every sport. Sports that select for a lean body weight or are judged subjectively put athletes at particular risk. The origins of eating disorders are multifactorial and beyond the scope of this chapter (see Chapter 8); they include issues of identity, self-esteem, family dynamics, control, and alterations in body image. Often there is a history of sexual or physical abuse and a sense of self-worth based on appearance. Unfortunately, societal pressures are such that a thin body is considered desirable, and constant dieting is the norm. Some of the characteristics associated with the best athletes—perfectionism, goal-setting, overachievement—may put the athlete at additional risk for developing eating disorders. Some of the features that can help distinguish athletes from people with disordered eating are shown in Table 43–1.

Table 43–1. Characteristics of anorectics and athletes.

	Anorectics	Athletes
Distinguishing features	Aimless physical activity Poor or decreasing exercise performance Poor muscle development Flawed body image Body fat below normal level Electrolyte abnormalities if abusing laxatives or diuretics Cold intolerance Dry skin Cardiac arrhythmias Lanugo hair Leukocyte dysfunction	Purposeful training Increased exercise tolerance Strong muscular development Accurate body image Body fat level within defined normal range Increased plasma volume Increased extraction from blood Efficient energy metabolism Increased high-density lipoprotein–2
Shared features	Dietary faddism Controlled caloric consumption Specific carbohydrate avoidance Low body weight Resting bradycardia and hypotension Increased physical activity Amenorrhea or oligomenorrhea Anemia (sometimes)	

Reproduced, with permission, from McSherry JA: The diagnostic challenge of anorexia nervosa. Am Fam Physician 1988;29:144.

Because eating disorders are difficult to identify, a team approach is often necessary for proper treatment. The treatment team usually includes a physician, a psychiatrist, and ultimately, a nutritionist. Others involved with treatment include the family, the athletic trainer, the team, and the coach. The fact that treatment is often unsuccessful highlights the importance of early identification and prevention. Education is one of the most important tools in preventing eating disorders, and the preparticipation physical examination is an appropriate time to start the process.

C. MENSTRUAL FUNCTION AND DYSFUNCTION

Menstrual dysfunction is another common entity for the female athlete. The exact mechanisms through which exercise-associated menstrual dysfunction occur are not well known. Most athletes understand that their menses can be affected by their exercise patterns, yet many do not understand that oligomenorrhea and amenorrhea may have long-standing, harmful consequences. A shortened luteal phase, anovulation, oligomenorrhea, and amenorrhea all have been demonstrated to occur in response to chronic exercise and in association with decreased bone mineral density. These disorders are associated with an increased risk for both stress fractures and premature osteoporosis. It is important for athletes, parents, and coaches to understand the significance of menstrual dysfunction, the risks involved with amenorrhea, and the importance of complete evaluation of symptoms. Because athletes are not immune from other medical problems, one cannot assume that the menstrual cycle has stopped because of exercise. Again, the preparticipation examination offers the opportunity to discuss this issue.

The effects of the menstrual cycle on performance have been reviewed, and the data remain controversial. In 37–63% of the studies to date, no change in performance has been found during different phases of the cycle. In 13–29% of the studies, an improvement in performance was noted during menstruation. The best performances occurred shortly after menstruation while the worst performances occurred just before. There appear to be no changes in strength during various phases of the menstrual cycle when assessed by isokinetic knee extension and flexion.

There are many variables to consider when evaluating for menstrual dysfunction in an athlete. Exercise-related changes in the stress and sex hormones, nutrition, body composition changes, and "energy drain" have been proposed as important factors that warrant consideration. Exercise-related increases in estradiol, progesterone, testosterone, prolactin, catecholamines, and cortisol all occur with acute exercise. β-Endorphin and β-lipotropin levels also increase. If an individual is amenorrheic or oligomenorrheic, careful assessment including gynecologic examination; pregnancy test; and work-up to rule out prolactin-secreting tumors, hypothyroidism, and adrenal or ovarian dysfunction should be pursued. An algorithm for work-up of amenorrhea is given in Chapter 47.

If menstrual dysfunction is discovered to be secondary to exercise, treatment includes decreasing training intensity or quantity if possible, weight gain if appropriate, and estrogen and progesterone therapy. There are some researchers who believe that progesterone, not estrogen, is the important factor in bone acquisition and that optimal therapy includes progesterone for this reason and to protect against the risks of unopposed estrogen therapy. Because estrogen therapy in postmenopausal women has been shown to protect the bone loss that normally occurs, estrogen therapy is used also in exercise-associated amenorrhea (EAA). Prior et al revealed a positive effect on bone density as measured by dual-energy x-ray absorptiometry in patients with EAA treated with progesterone. The extremely low estrogen levels appear to warrant treatment, and one of the easiest therapeutic interventions is the use of the oral contraceptive pill along with calcium supplementation. This approach is especially useful in sexually active women, and because of its few side effects, it often yields a higher compliance than other forms of estrogen. If patients do not wish to take hormones, bisphosphonates are now another option to treat osteopenia and osteoporosis.

It is important to address the issues of menstrual function, stress fractures, nutrition, and body image. Questions about dysmenorrhea, missed periods, and amenorrhea are important in detecting abnormalities but also in opening up discussion concerning the importance of maintaining a normal menstrual cycle, including the relationship to bone health. Asking questions about anemia, fatigue, burnout, and depression can highlight the relationship of proper nutrition to performance enhancement. Questions regarding stress fractures, family history of osteoporosis, smoking, and alcohol consumption can help young athletes to understand how these risk factors relate to the risks of eating disorders and menstrual dysfunction. Many young athletes do not understand the consequences of low bone density or osteoporosis. However, they may have friends who have had eating disorders, and they understand the effect of stress fractures on their ability to train and perform. Explaining the components of the female triad in a positive manner that relates to the young athlete is the key to combating the increasing incidence of the triad.

D. CARDIOVASCULAR SYSTEM

Sudden cardiac death occurs in 1 in 200,000 athletes, and studies have shown that exercise increases the risk.

The major causes for sudden death in athletes age 30 or younger and in those older than 40 years are given in Table 43–2. In individuals younger than 30, hypertrophic cardiomyopathy, anomalous coronary arteries, and ruptured aorta secondary to Marfan's syndrome are important congenital disorders to consider, whereas in athletes older than 40, the leading cause of sudden death is atherosclerotic heart disease. It is important to attempt to identify individuals with hypertrophic cardiomyopathy during the preparticipation examination because sudden death is often the presentation. However, Maron et al found that preparticipation screening was of limited value in identifying this disorder. Because hypertrophic cardiomyopathy is an autosomal dominant disorder, family history is important. Maron found that 25% of the patients with sudden death secondary to hypertrophic cardiomyopathy had a family history of sudden nontraumatic death in at least 1 parent or sibling younger than 50 years of age.

Table 43–2. Causes of sudden death in athletes.

Age 30 or Younger	
Condition	**Total (%)**
Hypertrophic cardiomyopathy	20 (24)
Coronary artery abnormalities	15 (18)
Coronary artery disease	12 (14)
Myocarditis	10 (12)
Marfan's syndrome	3 (4)
Dysrhythmias	2 (2)
Mitral valve prolapse	3 (4)
Other (include idiopathic concentric cardiac hypertrophy or rheumatic heart disease)	9 (11)
No cause identified	10 (12)

Adapted from McAffrey et al: Sudden cardiac death in young athletes; A review. AJDC, 1991;14:177.

Age 40 or Older	
Condition	**Incidence (%)**
Coronary artery disease (CAD)	88.7
Anomalous coronary arteries	4.2
Myocardial infarction without CAD Hypetrophic cardiomyopathy Myocarditis Mitral valve prolapse Mitral stenosis with left ventricular hypertrophy	7.1

Adapted from Chillags et al: Sudden Death; Myocardial infarction in a runner with normal coronary arteries. Phys and Sportsmed 1990;18(3):89.

Marfan's syndrome, another autosomal dominant disorder, also is a cause of sudden cardiac death, and family history is important in detecting those at risk. A family history is present in 85% of patients with Marfan's syndrome, and it is 1 of the 4 criteria needed to make the diagnosis. The major features of Marfan's syndrome are given in Table 43–3.

Questions should be asked about a history of chest pain, dizziness, syncope, presyncope, and extreme fatigue or shortness of breath with exertion. Any history of a heart murmur, rheumatic fever, or structural heart disease is important. If there are any symptoms, a careful history often can differentiate between benign and pathogenic causes. If an athlete has had syncope after completion of exercise at rest, or on standing quickly, the symptom is more likely to be neurocardiogenic in origin. If a syncopal episode occurs during intense exercise, there should be concern for hypertrophic cardiomyopathy or another form of outflow obstruction, some form of dysrhythmia, or seizure. The patient may warrant immediate evaluation by echocardiography and other tests before clearance is given for participation in an exercise program.

Other cardiac concerns that do not relate specifically to sudden cardiac death include arrhythmias, atherosclerotic heart disease, and hypertension. Previous or family history of arrhythmia, hypertension, or hyper-

Table 43–3. Major features of Marfan's syndrome.

1. **Family history**
2. **Cardiovascular abnormalities**
   Cystic medial necrosis
   Aortic dilatation
   Aortic aneurysm
   Aortic dissection
   Aortic insufficiency
   Mitral valve prolapse
   Mitral regurgitation
3. **Musculoskeletal abnormalities**
   Kyphoscoliosis
   Anterior thorax deformities: pectus excavatum, pectus carinatum
   Tall, with limb length greater than trunk length
   Arachnodactyly
   Spina bifida
   Spondylolisthesis
4. **Ocular disorders**
   Ectopia lentis
   Myopia
   Iridodonesis

cholesterolemia and diabetes are important to ascertain. If there are multiple cardiac risk factors, additional testing may be necessary before the patient begins an unsupervised exercise regimen. (See Chapter 29, Risk Factors for Coronary Artery Disease & Their Treatment.)

Determining eligibility for sports participation given underlying cardiovascular disease was discussed in detail at the 1994 Bethesda Conference.

E. NEUROLOGIC SYSTEM

Important questions for the neurologic history include any history of concussion, neck or spinal injury, or epilepsy. If an individual has had any of these conditions, obtaining detailed information is important. For head concussions, it is useful to determine the mechanism, whether there was loss of consciousness, results of any diagnostic tests performed, and the presence of persistent symptoms. If there is a history of spinal injury, one should obtain diagnostic tests results and information concerning treatment. A history of seizure or family history of epilepsy, along with treatment, medication use, and control of seizure activity should be obtained. This information can be useful in providing risk stratification for the various exercise activities in which the patient is interested.

The natural history of head concussions and other neurologic injuries in sport has yet to be elucidated fully. The guidelines used to treat individuals with head injuries are based on anecdotal and common sense practices, with few objective data to support them. Nonetheless, it is important to quantitate previous head injuries and the exact details of each event, as well as when they occurred. After a player sustains a first concussion, the chance of incurring a second one is more than 4 times greater than in a player who has never sustained a concussion. In addition, the "second impact syndrome" is always a concern; this phenomenon involves the occurrence of a second brain impact before recovery from a previous one is complete, which can lead to edema of the brain and sometimes death.

For individuals who have had previous spinal injury, careful assessment is important in determining the risk for further injury. In addition, ensuring that proper rehabilitation has occurred is important, although this is often difficult to ascertain. Conditions such as disk degeneration with herniation, spondylolysis or spondylolisthesis, and prior fracture or fusion may require further diagnostic studies. On determining that any of these abnormalities is present, the health care provider should make recommendations for exercise that will not put the individual at risk for further injury.

A seizure disorder that is under control should not prevent an individual from participating in an exercise program; participation in all sports, including contact sports such as football and soccer, is possible. There is debate concerning at what point a seizure disorder is considered controlled, however; this determination often is an individual matter. Epilepsy should be differentiated from other causes of seizure including febrile seizures associated with infection, seizures associated with tumor, seizures secondary to vascular abnormalities, and seizures secondary to alcohol withdrawal or cocaine toxicity.

After testing is done and diagnosis has been made, careful monitoring of medication is important. The recommended time before return to activity remains controversial; it ranges from 1 month to 1 year. There is additional concern for individuals who wish to engage in underwater sports such as snorkeling. These individuals should be given information regarding the severity of the risk if seizure occurs, and they should not be instructors in these sports.

F. MUSCULOSKELETAL SYSTEM

There are aspects of the preparticipation physical examination of the musculoskeletal system that relate specifically to women. Although upper extremity injuries are similar in men and women, lower extremity injuries appear to be slightly different. Women tend to have a wider pelvis than men, femoral neck anteversion, and varus at the hip and valgus at the knee. The result may be compensatory external rotation of the tibial tubercle with pronation at the hindfoot. These factors contribute to an increase of the Q angle, which is the angle between the femoral shaft and a line drawn from the center of the patella to the tibial tubercle. Women also have a lower center of gravity than men; it is at 56.1% of height in women and 56.7% in men.

It is important to obtain information regarding prior musculoskeletal problems, their treatment, and their rehabilitation. It is not uncommon to detect ligamentous laxity in athletes who never sought medical attention for what they thought was a minor injury. It is important to screen for the presence of scoliosis, alignment abnormalities, and general ligamentous laxity, strength, and flexibility. This process can help identify areas for which exercise recommendations can be made specific to the individual's goals.

Beard JL: Iron requirements in adolescent females. J Nutr 2000; 130:440S. [PMID: 10721923]

Chillag S et al: Sudden death: Myocardial infarction in a runner with normal coronary arteries. Phys Sports Med 1990;18:89.

Drinkwater BL et al: Bone mineral density after resumption of menses in amenorrheic athletes. JAMA 1986;256:380. [PMID: 3723725]

Grinspoon S et al: Prevalence and predictive factors for regional osteopenia in women with anorexia nervosa. Ann Intern Med 2000;133:790. [PMID: 11085841]

Hord JD: Anemia and coagulation disorders in adolescents. Adolesc Med 1999;10:359. [PMID: 10611933]

Lebrun CM: Effect of the different phases of the menstrual cycle and oral contraceptives on athletic performance. Sports Med 1993;16:400. [PMID: 8303141]

Lucas AR et al: Long-term fracture risk among women with anorexia nervosa: a population-based cohort study. Mayo Clin Proc 1999;74:972. [PMID: 10918862]

Maron BJ et al: Sudden death in young competitive athletes. Clinical, demographic, and pathological profiles. JAMA 1996; 276:199. [PMID: 8667563]

Maron BJ, Pelliccia A, Spirito P: Cardiac disease in young trained athletes. Insights into methods for distinguishing athlete's heart from structural heart disease with particular emphasis on hypertropic cardiomyopathy. Circulation 1995;91:1596. [PMID: 7867202]

Myburgh KH et al: Low bone density is an etiologic factor for stress fractures in athletes. Ann Intern Med 1990;113:754. [PMID: 1978620]

Prior JC et al: Cyclic medroxyprogesterone treatment increases bone density: a controlled trial in active women with menstrual cycle disturbances. Am J Med 1994;96:521. [PMID: 8017450]

Rowland TW et al: The effect of iron therapy on the exercise capacity of nonanemic iron-deficient adolescent runners. Am J Dis Child 1988;142:165. [PMID: 3341317]

Rowland TW, Kelleher JF: Iron deficiency in athletes. Insights from high school swimmers. Am J Dis Child 1989;143:197. [PMID: 2916491]

Zehender M et al: ECG variants and cardiac arrhythmias in athletes: Clinical relevance and prognostic importance. Am Heart J 1990;119:1378. [PMID: 219578]

Zipes DP, Garson A Jr: 26th Bethesda conference: recommendations for determining eligibility for competition in athletes with cardiovascular abnormalities. J Am Coll Cardiol 1994; 24:892. [PMID: 7523472]

Physical Examination

The areas of particular interest are the cardiovascular, neurologic, and musculoskeletal systems. Height and weight measurements, assessment of vital signs, and evaluation of visual acuity are important also. Attention to preexisting pupil size asymmetry can be useful in evaluating later head concussions.

The preparticipation physical examination should be sport-specific. Otitis can be a particular problem for swimmers, whereas it presents only minor problems for tennis players. A skin abnormality such as herpes gladiatorum is more important to recognize in someone who plays a contact sport such as basketball than in a golfer. The thyroid should be palpated, and any thyromegaly assessed. If the individual has given any history of exercise-induced cough, wheezing, or shortness of breath (consistent with exercise-induced asthma), attention to the lung examination is helpful; often, provocative testing is necessary. The abdominal examination is important for detecting hepatosplenomegaly, polycystic kidney disease, or other organomegaly or gastrointestinal disorders. The examination should include instruction regarding self-examination of the breast. A gynecologic examination may be indicated, such as in an athlete with menstrual dysfunction or amenorrhea.

The cardiovascular examination begins with an assessment of blood pressure and heart rate and rhythm. The health care provider should be familiar with **athlete's heart,** which results from the physiologic adaptations to exercise that allow the heart to work more effectively. Functional murmurs and extra heart sounds are not uncommon in athletes and must be differentiated from those seen in pathologic conditions. The changes seen in association with athlete's heart depend on the type of exercise performed; they can include enlargement of the ventricle and thickening of the ventricular walls. The electrocardiogram (ECG) and chest radiograph can demonstrate changes that correspond to athlete's heart. Sinus bradycardia, junctional rhythms, and first-degree and type I second-degree heart block all have been seen more frequently in athletes than in sedentary individuals; voltage changes and ST-segment and T-wave abnormalities also are common in athletes. Premature ventricular contractions, ventricular couplets, and bigeminy are common, although most of these benign rhythm disturbances tend to disappear with the onset of exercise. The history is crucial in determining whether these findings are functional or pathologic. It is often difficult to determine whether a murmur is pathologic or not. A murmur that increases on going from the standing to the squatting position is likely to be physiologic, because the increased venous return augments functional murmurs. If the murmur increases when going from squatting to standing, however, concern for hypertrophic cardiomyopathy or other outflow obstruction is raised. Further testing is indicated if there is any doubt about the nature of a murmur, if there is a history of cardiac symptoms with exertion, or if there is a family history of sudden cardiac death or premature atherosclerotic disease. Physical findings that are associated with some of the major causes of sudden cardiac death in athletes are given in Table 43–4.

Further diagnostic testing is based on the results of the history and physical examination. An echocardiogram is a useful and noninvasive tool to assess wall motion, chamber size, ejection fraction, valvular abnormalities, and wall thickness. It is probably the most important tool in assessing for the presence of hypertrophic cardiomyopathy, ruling out aortic dilatation, and assessing murmurs and other structural abnormalities. In thin individuals, echocardiography may help detect anomalous coronary arteries. For conduction and rhythm disturbance, an ECG in conjunction with 24- to 48-hour Holter or event monitoring and exercise

Table 43–4. Physical examination findings in conditions causing sudden cardiac death.

Condition	Finding
Hypertrophic obstructive cardiomyopathy (HOCM) or idiopathic hypertrophic subaortic stenosis (IHSS)	Jugular venous pulse with prominent a wave Carotid pulse: short duration, brisk upstroke, often bifid (67%) Double or triple apical impulse Systolic ejection murmur at left lower sternal border (classic); murmur increases with standing, expiration, and second and third phases of Valsalva; murmur decreases with squatting and inspiration Fourth heart sound at apex
Marfan's syndrome	Early ejection sound Aortic regurgitant murmur at right upper sternal border Mitral valve prolapse with mitral regurgitant murmur
Aortic stenosis (AS)	Large a wave with severe AS Narrow pulse pressure (late) Systolic thrill at base of heart Apex beat displaced inferiorly and laterally (left ventricular hypertrophy) Early systolic ejection murmur (crescendo-decrescendo) Paradox splitting S_2 (severe AS) Fourth heart sound
Anomalous coronary artery	Mitral regurgitation sometimes present secondary to papillary muscle ischemia or infarction Examination often normal

treadmill testing with monitoring are useful. For more complicated preexcitation disturbances, an ECG and electrophysiologic study may be necessary. Exercise stress testing is often helpful in assessing for anomalous coronaries and papillary dysfunction; in conjunction with echocardiography or thallium, it can be even more sensitive and specific. These procedures may reduce the need for angiography, which is a more invasive test. Angiography remains the gold standard for assessing for anomalous coronaries, however.

One of the newest tests available for evaluation of syncope is tilt table testing, which has been used to assess for neurocardiogenic syncope. There has been debate, however, concerning the usefulness of tilt table testing in athletes, in whom there may be a high rate of false-positive results because of the high vagal tone often seen. If the echocardiogram, ECG, and stress testing are all negative but tilt testing is positive in an athlete with syncope, the origin is most likely neurocardiogenic. If syncope occurs during exertion, however, further evaluation is indicated.

The neurologic examination is important is evaluating general strength, reflexes, and sensory abnormalities. Pain along the spinous processes, pain with atlantoaxial compression, and any deficit in motion or strength of the cervical spine should be assessed to rule out instability or preexisting neurologic injury. For older individuals, it is also important to assess balance, stability, and proprioception. Deficits secondary to prior concussion, injury, or cerebrovascular accident are important to assess in ensuring that the contemplated exercise regimen is realistic and safe.

The musculoskeletal examination must be done in an organized fashion. Different areas of the musculoskeletal system are more important for different activities. For example, swimming is often an excellent exercise for an older individual who may be at risk of falling and for whom knee osteoarthritis is a problem. If such a patient plans to begin rock climbing, however, careful assessment of the hip, leg, spine, and shoulders becomes more important. General strength and flexibility should be assessed, along with gait and alignment abnormalities. Scoliosis is always a concern, especially for younger athletes. Leg length discrepancies should be sought. Ligamentous laxity in the knee, shoulder, and ankle is important to assess, especially if there is a history of previous injury with little or no rehabilitation. In these situations, a careful examination can detect laxity that may put the athlete at risk for further injury. The identification of deficits can lead to the institution of a rehabilitation program before the season begins or may lead to disqualification until some kind of intervention is made. Surgery may be necessary prior to participation if rehabilitation alone is not sufficient. In making these difficult decisions, it is important to consider the risks of the sport involved and the patient's risk of injury.

CLINICAL MUSCULOSKELETAL PROBLEMS

In recent years, there have been advances in the training regimens and fitness levels and increases in the opportunities available for girls and women in sport. No longer can clinical differences between men and women be attributed to inferior strength or training; it is important for thorough assessment to be made so that problems can be detected early and rehabilitation initiated.

Iliotibial friction syndrome, patellofemoral dysfunction (PFD), reflex sympathetic dystrophy, greater trochanteric bursitis, and ankle and anterior cruciate ligament (ACL) sprains appear to occur more commonly in women than men. It remains unclear whether these clinical differences arise from differences in biomechanics and musculoskeletal structures, muscle imbalances, or unknown factors. More studies are needed of girls and women who are active in sport; the data are sparse and do not represent women who are active at increasingly competitive levels.

PFD is potentiated by an increased Q angle, genu valgum, and genu recurvatum. PFD is characterized by anterior knee pain, often made worse by climbing or descending stairs or prolonged sitting (the "theater sign"). Individuals with PFD often have deficient vastus medialis obliquus (VMO) musculature or tight vastus lateralis musculature; these conditions can combine to cause an abnormal tracking pattern of the patella with resultant patellofemoral irritation and pain. The static and dynamic orientation of the patella are important for an understanding of the biomechanics of the PFD and to plan rehabilitation. The presence of an effusion is also important; a grade 2 effusion has been shown to adversely affect the strength of the quadriceps muscle complex by as much as 10–40% by isokinetic testing. The presence of an effusion should expand the differential diagnosis to include meniscal lesions, ligamentous injury, articular surface defects, and osteochondral defects.

Strengthening of the VMO is one of the mainstays of therapy for PFD. Various taping techniques have been developed to allow the patella to track more normally and facilitate pain-free strengthening of the VMO. Closed-chain kinetic exercises, such as partial squats or one-legged squats, are excellent rehabilitative exercises. Newer rehabilitative tools include a harness system that can decrease an individual's body weight while doing exercises or running on a treadmill. As the athlete's condition improves, more weight is gradually added until they are carrying all of the their body weight again. This system allows an athlete to continue the sport-specific nature of her exercise as part of her rehabilitation. Open-chain kinetic exercises such as knee extensions and straight leg raises are used less often because they are not sport-specific; however, they may play an important role in sports such as soccer and karate that use open-chain kinetic skills.

Another clinical problem commonly seen in female athletes is trochanteric bursitis. Although it is unclear why this condition occurs more commonly in women than men, it may be because of structural differences. Tightness of the lateral structures often compress the bursa and cause an irritative force to occur with repetitive sliding of the iliotibial band over the greater trochanter. Pain is elicited with both passive and active abduction of the leg as the bursa is compressed but not with resisted abduction at the neutral position (unless there is a concomitant tendonitis or strain). Treatment with a nonsteroidal anti-inflammatory agent, ice massage, iliotibial band stretching, and, occasionally, phonophoresis or iontophoresis usually suffices. Corticosteroid injection can be useful. It is also important to assess for biomechanical problems or leg length discrepancies as a potential cause, along with training pattern errors.

An area of increasing concern is the higher number of ACL injuries in women than in men. In almost every sport that is represented in the National Collegiate Athletic Association (NCAA), women have more ACL injuries than men. A 2-year study of knee injuries in NCAA soccer and basketball athletes showed a higher ACL injury rate in women than in men. These statistics are demonstrated in Table 43–5. The female basketball and soccer players had an ACL injury rate 6 times greater and 2 times greater, respectively, than the men. These statistics are worrisome given the increased number of girls and women participating in both sports.

The explanation for this increased incidence of ACL injuries remains unclear. An initial idea was that women lacked the muscular development necessary to supplement joint stability. However, another study looked at ACL injuries in Olympic-caliber male and female basketball players and found a much higher inci-

Table 43–5. Knee injuries in collegiate basketball and soccer athletes.

Basketball (more than 400,000 A-E)	Men	Women
Knee injuries (% all injuries)	12%	19%
Knee injury requiring surgery (% all injuries)	20%	39%
Knee injury rate (per 1000 A-E)	0.7	1.0
ACL injury rate (per 1000 A-E)	0.05	0.3[1]
Soccer (more than 180,000 A-E)	Men	Women
Knee injuries (% all injuries)	16%	18%
Knee injury requiring surgery (% all injuries)	15%	22%
Knee injury rate (per 1000 A-E)	1.3	1.3
ACL injury rate (per 1000 A-E)	0.14	0.29[1]

A-E = athlete-exposure: one athlete participating in one practice or game.
[1]Significantly greater than M value ($P < .05$).
Reproduced, with permission, from Arendt EA, Dick RW: Gender Specific Knee Injury Patterns in Collegiate Basketball and Soccer Players. National Collegiate Athletic Association: NCAA Injury Surveillance System. NCAA, 1991–1992.

dence of injuries in women compared with men (53% vs 13%). In addition, the severity of injuries and the need for surgery were higher in women than men. Other factors that might explain the increased incidence of ACL injuries include muscle imbalances, trochlear groove size or configuration, biomechanical differences in jumping and landing technique, and alignment differences. More information is needed to answer this question.

As women have begun to excel in sport, the field of sports medicine has grown and more research is being done on issues related to women. Primary care physicians are often "team physicians." As more information is gained about the physiologic adaptations that occur with exercise and the risk factors for health, efforts at prevention of injury and disease will be improved.

Bennell KL et al: A 12-month prospective study of the relationship between stress fractures and bone turnover in athletes. Calcif Tissue Int 1998;63:80. [PMID: 9632851]

Messier SP et al: Etiology of iliotibial band friction syndrome in distance runners. Med Sci Sports Exerc 1995;27:951.

Thomee R et al: Patellofemoral pain syndrome in young women. I. A clinical analysis of alignment, pain parameters, common symptoms, and functional activity level. Scand J Med Sci Sports 1995;5:237. [PMID: 7552769]

Relevant Web Site

[American College of Sports Medicine]
www.acsm.org

Autoimmune Rheumatic Diseases & Arthritis

44

Jan L. Hillson, MD & Mandy D. Henderson Robertson, MD

Arthritis refers to any disorder of the articular cartilage, joint space, or synovial lining. The autoimmune rheumatic diseases (ARDs), also termed "connective tissue diseases," comprise several different multisystem disorders. They are grouped because all are thought to reflect harmful activity of the immune system, with persistent inflammation and damage to tissues. ARDs are distinguished from the many other autoimmune disorders (eg, Hashimoto's thyroiditis, Crohn's disease) partly because many have prominent joint or muscle involvement, but partly by convention.

OSTEOARTHRITIS

Osteoarthritis (OA) is joint pain, stiffness, and/or deformity caused by degeneration of cartilage. It is characterized by progressive loss of joint space, variable inflammation of the adjacent synovial lining, and often osteophytes, sclerosis, and/or cysts in surrounding bone.

ESSENTIALS OF DIAGNOSIS

- *History of progressive joint pain that increases with activity.*
- *Findings of bony hypertrophy at any joint (but especially interphalangeal (IP) or first carpal-metacarpal (CMC) joints), crepitus, reduced range of motion.*
- *Radiographic evidence of loss of joint space, sometimes with osteophytes, subchondral sclerosis, or bony cysts.*

General Considerations

Radiographic evidence of cartilage loss increases with age and is nearly universal by 75 years. However, only about 12% of the population has sufficient symptoms to be said to have clinical OA. Early symptomatic disease occurs in families with heritable factors that lead to frag-

ile cartilage (eg, mutations in collagen) or poor cartilage repair. This form is termed "primary OA" and is more often clinically significant in women than in men. Early joint damage is also seen with congenital factors that increase load on joints, such as hip deformities, hypermobility syndrome, malalignment of the patella within the intercondylar groove, which leads to chondromalacia patella, or varus deformity of the first metatarsal, which leads to degenerative change and bunions at the first metatarsophalangeal (MTP) joint. OA is termed "secondary" when it is caused by trauma, by increased load due to obesity, neuropathy, or repetitive activities, or follows ARDs, infection, gout, or metabolic disorders, such as hemochromatosis, that damage cartilage.

Clinical Findings

A. SYMPTOMS AND SIGNS

Patients report intermittent and gradually increasing pain that is made worse with use of the affected joint. Symptoms are often most severe at the end of the day and may interrupt sleep. The pattern of joint involvement varies with the type of OA. Patients with primary OA often have characteristic nodules due to hypertrophy at the distal IP joints (Heberden's nodes) and proximal IP joints (Bouchard's nodes). This pattern is sometimes called **nodal OA.** When inflammation and joint destruction at these sites are severe, patients are said to have **primary erosive OA.** The term "generalized OA" is applied to patients who exhibit most or all of a distinctive pattern of symptomatic cartilage damage, with involvement of IP and first CMC joints of the hands, cervical and lumbar discs, the first MTP joint, and sometimes knees and hips. Arthritis of the first CMC joint is distinctive and helps establish the diagnosis of OA. Patients describe difficulty opening jars or using shears and later note loss of grip strength and difficulty writing. Joint involvement in secondary OA depends on the specific precipitating events.

B. LABORATORY FINDINGS

Blood chemistries and serologies are not affected by OA. Effusions may be present, especially in the knee.

Fluid is usually clear, colorless to amber, with fewer than 2000 cells/mm². Conventional radiography reveals loss of joint space, often with sclerosis, cysts, or osteophytes of underlying bone. Magnetic resonance imaging (MRI) more clearly defines the structure of the cartilage and surrounding tissues and is often used in the knee to find meniscal tears and in the shoulder to define tears of the rotator cuff.

Differential Diagnosis

In primary erosive OA, joints are often inflamed with erythema, tenderness, synovial thickening, and effusion. When the proximal interphalangeal (PIP) joints are involved, it may suggest rheumatoid arthritis (RA). When the distal interphalangeal (DIP) joints are affected, it may resemble psoriatic arthritis. When there is simultaneous involvement of DIPs, PIPs, and the first CMC, the diagnosis can often be made by appearance alone. Other distinguishing features include the lack of synovitis at the metacarpal-phalangeal joints (MCPs), wrists, or other joint areas together with the presence of osteophytes and lack of erosions or periarticular osteopenia on radiography.

In practice, it is usually fairly easy to detect OA. The problem is in knowing whether to attribute pain to the recognized OA or to other articular or periarticular processes. For example, calcium pyrophosphate crystal deposition disease (CPPD) often accompanies OA and may cause exacerbation of pain and swelling, often in the knee or wrist. It is detected as calcifications in the cartilage on radiograph or, less reliably, as crystals in the joint fluid. Anserine bursitis arises from altered joint mechanics in patients with knee OA, while trochanteric bursitis and subacromial bursitis often create pain near the hip and shoulder, respectively. These are detected as tenderness on palpation of the bursa and by cessation of the pain following injection of local anesthetic. The pain of avascular necrosis may mimic OA and should be considered in patients at risk due to history of trauma, high-dose corticosteroids, alcoholism, renal failure, lupus, or radiation exposure. Plain films show alterations in trabecular patterns, with subchondral lucency and, late in disease, collapse of bone. MRI is sensitive for detecting lesions earlier. Any of the ARDs may produce pain that is initially attributed to OA, especially when the onset is insidious, oligoarticular, and asymmetric.

Treatment

Management focuses on joint protection, pain relief, and maintenance of function. Joint protection, at present, is largely limited to reduction or redistribution of load through weight loss, careful choice of activities, strengthening muscle groups that stabilize involved joints, and use of devices such as trekking poles, canes, cushioned shoes, braces, and shoe wedges to redistribute load. There is currently an effort to identify medications that retard cartilage degradation. Glucosamine sulfate may be the first such "chondroprotective agent;" 500 mg taken 3 times daily has been reported to reduce the rate of joint space narrowing in patients with OA of the knee. There are early reports that hyaluronate injections may also be chondroprotective. The tetracycline antibiotics inhibit metalloproteinases, including collagenases, a property that may contribute to their effectiveness in RA. Other metalloproteinase inhibitors are under investigation for possible use in OA. Because current therapies are not satisfactory, a number of naturopathic supplements have been marketed for OA, including methylsulfonylmethane (MSM), collagen, and omega-3 fatty acids, among others.

Pain relief is sometimes achieved with rest, topical therapies (eg, heat, ice, capsaicin creams), and non-narcotic analgesics (acetaminophen). Nonsteroidal anti-inflammatory drugs (NSAIDs) are often effective, although toxicity may limit use (Table 44–1). Intra-articular injection of corticosteroids can provide dramatic relief, which is consistent with the understanding that inflammation contributes to pain in OA. Injection of hyaluronate into the knee weekly for 3–5 weeks is associated with sustained analgesia when compared with placebo. Night pain may respond to tricyclic antidepressants. Patients with intractable pain, excessive narcotic requirement, or loss of function may consider arthroplasty, osteotomy, or joint fusion. There is active interest in resurfacing joints with biologic tissues. Small defects have been patched with autologous chondrocytes, and subchondral drilling has been used to stimulate growth of fibrocartilage to replace full- and partial-thickness cartilage defects.

CRYSTAL-INDUCED ARTHROPATHIES

Crystals produce joint disease through several mechanisms. Crystals directly interact with cells of the immune system and induce acute inflammatory response, as in podagra and pseudogout. Crystal deposits contribute to chronic inflammation, granulomatous reactions, and tissue damage similar to that of RA, as can be seen in CPPD, Milwaukee shoulder, and polyarticular gout. Deposits bulky enough to induce compression atrophy or to interfere with joint motion sometimes occur in tophaceous gout and scleroderma-associated calcinosis. Monosodium urate, calcium pyrophosphate, and apatite are common, but crystals of other minerals, lipids, and proteins have also been linked to arthropathy.

Table 44–1. Guidelines for monitoring medications used to treat autoimmune rheumatic diseases.

Drug	Toxicity to be monitored	Laboratory monitoring
NSAIDs	Gastrointestinal bleeding, hepatic toxicity, renal toxicity, hypertension	CBC, creatinine, AST, ALT at baseline and at least yearly; repeat creatinine after initiation in patients at risk
Corticosteroids	Osteoporosis, fluid retention, cataracts, osteonecrosis, agitation, infection, hypo-kalemia, elevations in weight, glucose, lipids, blood pressure	Baseline and yearly bone densitometry, glucose, potassium, cholesterol, triglycerides
Hydroxychloroquine	Macular damage	Yearly fundoscopy and visual fields
Sulfasalazine	Myelosuppression	CBC every 2–4 months for first 3 months, then quarterly
Methotrexate	Myelosuppression, hepatic fibrosis, pulmonary infiltrates, infection	Baseline chest radiograph, HIV and hepatitis serology; CBC, AST, albumin, creatinine every 1–3 months
Leflunomide	Myelosuppression, hepatic toxicity	CBC, AST, creatinine monthly
Azathioprine	Myelosuppression, hepatotoxicity, lymphoproliferative disorders, infection	CBC 1–2 weeks after dose change and every 1–3 months thereafter; creatinine, AST at baseline and yearly
Cyclosporine	Renal insufficiency, anemia, hypertension	Creatinine every 2 weeks after dose change then monthly; quarterly CBC, potassium, and AST
D-Penicillamine	Myelosuppression, proteinuria	CBC, UA every 2 weeks after dose change then every 1–3 months; creatinine quarterly
Mycophenylate mofetil	Myelosuppression, infection	CBC, creatinine 1–2 weeks after dose change then monthly; quarterly AST, UA
Intramuscular gold	Myelosuppression, proteinuria	CBC, UA at the time of each injection
Cyclophosphamide	Myelosuppression, malignancy, infection, hemorrhagic cystitis, infertility	Weekly CBC, UA, creatinine during dose adjustment then monthly; yearly urine cytology and Pap tests
Etanercept Infliximab	Myelosuppression, infection, drug-induced lupus	CBC after dose adjustment and quarterly; in patients at high risk (elevated ANA, overlap syndromes), consider UA, anti-DNA antibodies, and C3

NSAIDs, nonsteroidal anti-inflammatory drugs; CBC, complete blood cell; AST, aspartate transaminase; ALT, alanine transaminase; UA, urinalysis; Pap, Papanicolaou; ANA, antinuclear antibody.

ESSENTIALS OF DIAGNOSIS

Gout *is pain and swelling caused by inflammatory response to monosodium urate crystals. Diagnosis requires:*

- *Monosodium urate crystals in aspirates from synovial fluid or tophus, or*
- *The presence of at least 6 of the following features: (1) acute monoarticular arthritis, (2) hyperuricemia, (3) inflammation peaks within 1 day, (4) negative culture of joint fluid, (5) history of at least 2 attacks, (6) radiographic finding of asymmetric joint swelling or subcortical cysts without erosion, (7) involvement of first MTP, (8) unilateral*

attack involving either first MTP or tarsal joint, (9) suspected tophus, (10) joint erythema.

Pseudogout *is acute pain and swelling caused by inflammatory response to calcium pyrophosphate crystals. Diagnosis is supported by:*

- *Characteristic calcium pyrophosphate crystals in joint aspirate.*
- *Chondrocalcinosis on radiograph.*
- *Self-limited inflammation that peaks within 1 day.*

Chronic CPPD *is chronic pain, stiffness, synovitis, and functional impairment associated with calcium pyrophospate crystal deposition. Diagnosis is supported by:*

- *Radiographic evidence of chondrocalcinosis.*

- *Radiographic evidence of OA but not of RA.*
- *Patient often elderly and female.*

Apatite deposition disease *is pain, stiffness, or functional impairment associated with deposition of basic calcium phosphate (BCP) crystals of various chemical compositions.*

- *Crystal deposits often apparent by radiograph but not visible by light microscopy.*
- *Periarthritis, tendinitis, and bursitis.*
- *Destructive shoulder arthropathy; Milwaukee shoulder occurs in elderly females.*

General Considerations

A. Gout

The prevalence of hyperuricemia is 5%, while the prevalence of gout is 1%. Female:male ratio is 1:2–7. Uric acid is produced during purine metabolism and is cleared by the kidney and liver. Production is increased with ingestion of protein rich foods, in high cell-turnover states including malignancy, and in families with inherited defects of purine metabolism. Excretion is reduced in those with chronic renal failure, dehydration, and hypertension, and in the presence of diuretics, alcohol, low-dose salicylates, cyclosporine, and other drugs. Overproduction or underexcretion raises serum uric acid, promoting deposition of crystals in joints and other tissues. Hyperuricemia is often asymptomatic, and it is recognized that local factors act to promote or inhibit crystal growth. Once formed, naked crystals are highly inflammatory but are also highly adsorptive and become coated with protein that may inhibit or enhance inflammation, depending on the nature of the protein.

B. Pseudogout and Chronic CPPD

Calcification of cartilage, termed "chondrocalcinosis," is seen in 5–8% of adults and increases with age. Female:male ratio is 2–7:1. Crystal deposition is increased in damaged cartilage, as occurs with OA, neuropathy, aging and, less commonly, hemochromatosis or amyloidosis. Deposition is also favored by elevated calcium and pyrophosphate levels, as occurs with hyperparathyroidism, hypocalcuria, and hypophosphatasia. Pseudogout attacks are thought to occur when crystals "shed" deposits in cartilage and are taken up by neutrophils.

C. Apatite Deposition Diseases

Prevalence data are limited. Radiodense deposits were observed in 3% of shoulder films among working adults, and BCP crystals can be demonstrated in the synovial fluid of nearly all joints affected by OA. Dia-betes, renal failure, hyperthyroidism, parathyroid disease, scleroderma, and dermatomyositis are associated with increased risk of calcinosis. However, most deposits occur in the absence of recognized disease and the causes are not well understood. The extent to which BCP crystals contribute to pathogenesis of OA is not known, although cases of destructive arthropathy have been described, and there is speculation that BCP crystals may contribute to the inflammation seen in primary erosive OA.

Clinical Findings

A. Gout

Half of first attacks involve the first MTP joint (podagra) and another 30% involve ankle, tarsus, or knee. Wrists, fingers, elbows, and periarticular structures including bursa and tendon sheaths may also become involved. Joints are warm, swollen, and tender, and there is often sufficient periarticular swelling and erythema to suggest bacterial cellulitis or septic joint. Initial attacks are usually self-limited and resolve in 3–10 days. Chronic polyarticular inflammation that resembles RA or the reactive spondyloarthropathies develops in some patients with long-standing untreated disease. Tophaceous deposits occur only with prolonged very high uric acid levels, as is seen with inherited disorders of purine metabolism abnormalities or long-standing treatment with diuretics or cyclosporine.

Diagnosis depends on finding urate crystals in synovial fluid, synovial biopsy, or tophus aspirate. Crystals are identified by polarized light microscopy as bright, negatively birefringent needles of 5–25 μm. Synovial fluid is inflammatory, with 2000 to > 50,000 cells/μL, predominately neutrophils. Finding crystals *within* cells confirms the diagnosis. Fluid should be sent for Gram's stain and culture, since bacterial infection is in the differential diagnosis and can coexist with gout. Average uric acid levels are elevated, but isolated levels are normal in up to 40% of patients during attacks. Radiographs are normal in early disease, but in more prolonged disease, characteristic marginal erosions, which are described as "punched out" with sclerotic borders and an overhanging shelf of cortical bone, may be seen. Occasionally, tophaceous gout leads to widespread erosions and synovitis that resembles RA.

B. Pseudogout

Pseudogout presents as attacks of synovitis lasting a few days to weeks, often following illness or surgery. The knee is affected in 50% of cases, followed by the wrist, shoulder, ankle, and elbow. Chronic CPPD presents as chronic, progressive pain and swelling, usually affecting the knees, but often occurring in wrists, second and third MCPs, and sometimes in the spine, hips, ankles, shoulder, and elbows. CPPD is often discovered radiographically, as punctate or linear densities in fibrocartilage. Common sites include the menisci of the knees, triangular fibrocartilage of the radioulnar joint, symphysis pubis, intravertebral discs, and shoulder. In pseudogout flares, synovial fluid is inflammatory, usually with > 90% neutrophils. Crystals may be difficult to detect. They differ from urate crystals, in that they are short rhomboids or rods rather than needles, and exhibit weak positive birefringence. Again, fluids should be sent for Gram's stain and culture.

Usually BCP deposition is asymptomatic. **Calcific periarthritis** presents with sudden onset of severe pain, followed by swelling, erythema, and warmth. The shoulder is affected most often, followed by the hip, knee, elbow, wrist, and ankle. Milwaukee shoulder usually presents in older women, with pain and loss of range of motion. Examination reveals a large effusion that is readily palpable due to destruction of the rotator cuff. Fluid is often blood-tinged, with low numbers of cells, predominantly monocytes. Similar destructive synovitis is occasionally reported in the knees, hips, elbows, and other joints. Diagnosis of calcific periarthritis is aided by the presence of radiodense deposits. Deposits in intra-articular disease are usually too small to be seen on radiographs and are not visible in synovial fluids. Thus, the diagnosis is made on the clinical presentation.

Differential Diagnosis

As discussed above, acute crystal-associated disease can be difficult to distinguish from cellulitis and septic joint. Polyarticular gout and chronic CPPD may appear similar to RA, especially when MCPs are involved. Radiographs are often helpful: chondrocalcinosis or involvement of the spine tends to support CPPD, while periarticular demineralization and marginal erosions suggest RA. CPPD may also be difficult to distinguish from OA, and the 2 disorders often coexist.

Treatment

A. GOUT

Treatment has 3 goals: (1) to treat acute flares, (2) to reduce uric acids levels so that no further crystals form and existing crystals dissolve, and (3) to prevent flares while waiting the several months required for crystals to dissolve.

Intra-articular steroids (eg, methylprednisolone acetate, triamcinolone acetonide) combined with local anesthetics (eg, lidocaine and marcaine) are effective for acute pain and inflammation. However, gout is so painful that most patients want something to use immediately should an attack occur away from the physician's office. NSAIDs (eg, indomethacin 25–50 mg 3 times daily) are preferred when not contraindicated by gastrointestinal intolerance, age, or renal insufficiency. Oral corticosteroids (eg, prednisone 20–40 mg, with repeat every 8–12 hours until flare is resolved, then rapid taper) are usually well tolerated. Intramuscular steroids or adrenocorticotropic hormone (ACTH) can also be used. High dose colchicine is effective but leads to excessive gastrointestinal distress and is usually not required.

Patients with multiple attacks, tophaceous deposits, or very high serum uric acid levels should consider long-term therapy to reduce the levels of serum uric acid. Options include avoiding precipitating factors (eg, diuretics, ethanol, and purine-rich foods), increasing renal excretion with uricosuric agents, or reducing uric acid production by inhibiting xanthine oxidase. Uricosurics are relatively ineffective in patients with impaired renal function; they should be avoided in patients who overproduce urate because hyperuricosuria may lead to urolithiasis. When considering a uricosuric agent, first obtain a 24-hour urine for uric acid to be certain the patient is an underexcreter. Begin with a low dose of drug (eg, probenecid 500 mg/d or sulfinpyrazone 50 mg twice daily) and gradually increase (eg, probenecid to 1–2 g/d, or sulfinpyrazone to 50–400 mg twice daily) until uric acid is less than 6 mg/dL. Allopurinol may be used in both overproducers and underexcreters. It is usually started at 100 mg/d and gradually increased to 300–600 mg/d to maintain a serum uric acid less than 6 mg/dL. Although allopurinol is usually well tolerated, elevations of transaminases are common, rashes occur in 2% of patients, and an exfoliative dermatitis that can be life-threatening can develop in 1 of 1000 patients. Dose must be reduced in renal insufficiency. The dose of purine analogues (eg, azathioprine) must be reduced when allopurinol is started.

Allopurinol and uricosuric agents mobilize crystals, making acute attacks more likely for some time after initiation. Concomitant colchicine, usually at 0.6 mg twice daily, reduces the frequency of gout flares. Dose should be decreased in renal failure and when nausea or diarrhea occurs. Some patients can use only very low doses (eg, 0.3 mg every other day) yet still report benefit.

B. PSEUDOGOUT

Like gout, acute pseudogout attacks can be treated with intra-articular or systemic corticosteroids. Colchicine may be useful for prophylaxis. There is no specific therapy for chronic CPPD. Underlying metabolic disease should be treated, but treatment does not reverse joint damage. Management of pain and stiffness is the same as that outlined for OA.

RHEUMATOID ARTHRITIS

RA is a chronic progressive systemic inflammatory disorder characterized by polyarticular synovitis; often with systemic features such as fatigue, and sometimes associated with vasculitis, inflammatory lung disease, and involvement of other tissues.

 ESSENTIALS OF DIAGNOSIS

The American College of Rheumatology criteria for classification of RA requires that 4 or more of the following be observed at any time:

- *Morning joint stiffness lasting at least 1 hour.*
- *Simultaneous arthritis in 3 or more of 14 possible joint areas (right or left PIPs, MCPs, wrist, elbow, knee, ankle, MTPs).*
- *Arthritis in the PIPs, MCPs, or wrist joints.*
- *Simultaneous involvement of the same joint area on both right and left sides.*
- *Rheumatoid nodules.*
- *Elevated serum rheumatoid factor (RF).*
- *Periarticular osteopenia or erosions on radiographs of hands or wrists.*

General Considerations

The prevalence of disease is 1% in most populations, reaching 5% in some Native American groups. Female:male ratio is 3:1. Incidence peaks at 35–50 years of age. The factors that precipitate disease are unknown. However, genetic predisposition has been demonstrated, both through twin studies (monozygotic concordance is approximately 25%) and through linkage to specific major histocompatability locus (MHC) class II alleles. RA is characterized by chronic inflammation of the lining of the joint cavity (synovium), with infiltrating leukocytes, new blood vessels, active fibroblasts, and other cells. While early inflammation may be reversible, prolonged disease produces a chronically altered synovium that is immunologically and metabolically active, and leads to destruction of cartilage and thinning and erosion of periarticular bone.

Clinical Findings

The onset of RA is usually insidious, with gradual addition of joints over weeks to months. However, 10–15% of patients present with rapid onset of fulminant disease. A smaller percentage of patients exhibit fever and migratory rash, termed "adult Still's disease." Some pa-

tients report intermittent attacks of pain and swelling that involve 1 or a few joints and suggest gout. This presentation, termed "palindromic rheumatism" often resolves spontaneously, but may evolve into more typical RA.

Joints are tender and swollen, and may exhibit warmth and erythema. Later findings include chronically thickened synovium called pannus, reduced range of motion, joint deformity, subluxation, and ankylosis. MCPs are most commonly involved (> 85%), followed by wrists, PIPs, knees, MTPs, and ankles (> 75%); followed by shoulders, elbows, midfoot and hips (> 50%); and followed by cervical spine, temporomandibular joints, and sternoclavicular joints (> 30%). Patients often report fatigue, low-grade fever, and other constitutional symptoms. Rheumatoid nodules occur in about 30% of patients, usually over the olecranon, fingers, or Achilles tendon. Less common problems include vasculitis, serositis, autoimmune neutropenia (Felty's syndrome), interstitial lung disease, scleritis, episcleritis, and corneal ulcers.

Diagnosis is based largely on joint examination. RF is elevated in 75% of patients. However, RF is also elevated in 5% of young healthy individuals, and high titers may be seen with hepatitis C, dysproteinemias, and other ARDs. High titers lend support to the clinical impression of RA and predict more aggressive disease. Diagnosis is also supported by inflammation on synovial fluid analysis, elevations in acute phase reactants (erythrocyte sedimentation rate (ESR), C-reactive protein (CRP), platelets), anemia and typical radiographic appearance of involved joints.

Differential Diagnosis

Acute polyarticular RA resembles arthritis that follows viral infections, vaccination, or bacterial infections. Streptococcal antigens and antibodies to parvovirus B19, Epstein-Barr virus, hepatitis B and C viruses, and *Borrelia burgdorferi* infection should be obtained when indicated by history. Chronic disease may be difficult to distinguish from the reactive spondyloarthropathies, articular onset of the other systemic connective tissue diseases (eg, systemic lupus, polymyositis, scleroderma), polyarticular crystalline disease, or the more inflammatory forms of primary erosive OA.

Treatment

Treatment has several goals: to control pain, suppress the inflammatory process in the synovium, prevent destruction of cartilage, prevent erosion and thinning of bone, correct deformity, and reduce disability. Table 44–2 summarizes available approaches for each of these objectives.

Table 44–2. Treatment of rheumatoid arthritis.

Goal	Therapy
Control pain	Acetaminophen, NSAIDs, narcotic analgesics Topical agents, including capsaicin Tricyclic antidepressants, gabapentin, carbamazepine Splints, joint rest
Alleviate fatigue	Serotonin reuptake inhibitors, rarely stimulants such as modafinil, pemoline, or methylphenidate
Suppress inflammation	Corticosteroids, tetracycline antibiotics, hydroxychloroquine, sulfasalazine, methotrexate, leflunomide, entanercept, infliximab, anakinra, adalimumab, azathioprine, cyclosporine, mycofenylate mofitil, D-penicillamine, injectable gold salts, cyclophosphamide, tacrolimus, prosorba columns, and other agents that suppress or modify the immune response
Slow cartilage destruction (chondroprotection)	Tetracycline antibiotics inhibit collagenases. Their benefit in rheumatoid arthritis may be mediated in part through this activity.
Inhibit periarticular osteopenia	Bisphosphonates and other antiresorptive agents may inhibit bone changes in rheumatoid arthritis. These agents are always indicated when corticosteroids are used.
Correct joint deformity	Splints, physical therapy, joint reconstruction
Avoid disability	Physical therapy, occupational therapy, adaptive devices

NSAIDs, nonsteroidal anti-inflammatory drugs.

The first principle of treatment is that inflammation must be controlled rapidly and aggressively. Irreversible changes in synovium may occur within a few weeks of disease onset, and erosions are often well established by 6 months. Aggressive early treatment may permit long-term control with milder, less-toxic agents. In practice, this means that only the mildest cases, if any, should be treated with NSAIDs alone, and that rapidly acting agents (eg, corticosteroids, etanercept, antibodies to tumor necrosis factor, interleukin-1 receptor antagonists) should be used while waiting to evaluate the efficacy of slower-acting agents (eg, hydroxychloroquine, sulfasalazine, methotrexate, leflunomide, azathioprine, and others).

The course of RA is variable and is characterized by flares and remissions. Response to therapy is also variable and may change over time. Most therapeutic agents and combinations carry significant risks of adverse events, especially in pregnant women (Table 44–3). For all these reasons, patients require frequent monitoring and adjustment of therapy, and most should be managed in coordination with a provider who has specialized experience in rheumatic diseases.

REACTIVE SPONDYLOARTHROPATHIES

The reactive spondyloarthropathies are a group of disorders characterized by enthesitis, synovitis that is often asymmetric and oligoarticular, frequent involvement of the axial skeleton, and association with HLA-B27. They include psoriatic arthritis, ankylosing spondylitis, enteropathic arthritis, reactive arthritis, and undifferentiated or incomplete syndromes.

 ESSENTIALS OF DIAGNOSIS

Psoriatic Arthritis

- *Psoriasis.*
- *Asymmetric oligoarticular arthritis, axial arthritis, enthesopathy, or symmetric polyarthritis.*

Ankylosing Spondylitis

- *Radiographic evidence of sacroiliitis and/or ankylosis of spine.*
- *Chronic low back pain and stiffness that improves with exercise.*
- *Reduced motion of lumbar spine in sagittal and frontal planes.*
- *Limited chest expansion.*

Enteropathic Arthritis

- *Crohn's disease or ulcerative colitis.*
- *Migratory or additive, asymmetric, oligoarticular arthritis.*

Reactive Arthritis

- *Classic triad, following bacterial gastrointestinal or genitourinary infection.*
  - *Nongonoccal urethritis.*
  - *Conjunctivitis.*
  - *Arthritis that is asymmetric, oligoarticular, often lower limbs.*

Undifferentiated Spondyloarthropathies

- *Any disorder not included above, with inflammatory spinal pain, or synovitis that is asymmetric or*

Table 44–3. Risks associated with medications used to treat RA in pregnancy and lactation.

Drug	US FDA Category[1]	Lactation	Risks
Sulfasalazine	B	Excreted in breast milk	Crosses the placenta. No adequate, well-controlled studies. Of pregnant women who have taken it, incidence of fetal morbidity and mortality was comparable to untreated women. Exercise caution as it may cause kernicterus. Animal studies at 6 times the human dose show no harm to the fetus.
Etanercept	B	Unknown	No studies in pregnant women. In animal studies using 60–100 times higher dose, no harm to fetus due to drug.
Anakinra	B	Unknown	Unknown. No human or animal data.
Penicillamine	B	Controversial safety	Skeletal abnormalities, varicosities, and fetal death have occurred.
NSAIDs	B/C	Excreted in breast milk	Known human fetus effects during third trimester: heart malformations, platelet dysfunction, intracranial bleeding, renal dysfunction or failure, oligohydramnios, gastrointestinal bleeding or perforation. Not recommended because of cardiovascular effects on infant. Animal studies have shown cardiac malformation, increased delivery length, embryo lethality, and stillbirth. Some decrease in fertility and can cause preterm labor.
Hydroxychloroquine	C	Excreted in breast milk	Frequency of congenital anomalies not observed to be higher than in normal population. No known health compromises in follow up. In pregnant mice, deposited in fetal eyes. Controversial safety.
Infliximab	C	Unknown	Unknown. No human or animal data.
Mycophenolate	C	Excreted in breast milk	No adequate, well-controlled human studies. In animal studies, fetal malformations have occurred during organogenesis.
Cyclosporine A	C	Excreted in breast milk	Avoid. Premature births and low birth weight have consistently occurred. Malformation, neonatal complications, preeclampsia, eclampsia, abruptio placentae, premature labor, and fetoplacental dysfunction have also occurred. In animal studies, at 2–5 times the human dose, embryo toxic and fetal toxic events occurred.
Gold	C	Excreted in breast milk	Crosses the placenta. Reports of both healthy and congenital abnormalities, stillborn or premature infants. If pregnant, recommend discontinuation. In small animals, teratogenic effects, congenital abnormalities, and increased abortions. Controversial safety.
Cortisone	C/D	Excreted in breast milk	It crosses the placenta. Long-term ingestion has 1% incidence of cleft palate in human fetuses. Must monitor infants for hypoadrenalism. Animal studies show large doses early in pregnancy produce cleft palate, stillborn fetuses, and small size. Not recommended, but studies suggest long-term low doses or short periods or high doses likely do not harm infants.
Cyclophosphamide	D	Excreted in breast milk	During first and second trimesters, skeletal, cardiac, and central nervous system abnormalities have been reported. During third trimester, there does not seem to be a risk of congenital defects. Not recommended. Unknown risk on physical and mental growth abnormalities. **Paternal** use during conception has been associated with cardiac and limb abnormalities.
Minocycline	D	Excreted in breast milk	Crosses the placenta. May retard skeletal development. Permanent discoloration of teeth if used during the second or third trimester. In animal studies, evidence of embryo toxicity. Controversial safety.
Methotrexate	X	Excreted in breast milk	Causes fetal death or teratogenic effects. Exclude pregnancy before starting. Avoid pregnancy if **either partner** is receiving the drug, during and for a minimum of 3 months after discontinuation for males and 1 cycle after discontinuation for females. Controversial safety.

(continued)

Table 44–3. Risks associated with medications used to treat RA in pregnancy and lactation. (Continued)

Drug	US FDA Category[1]	Lactation	Risks
Leflunomide	X	Not recommended	No human studies. Animal studies show teratogenic effects or fetal death. Exclude pregnancy before starting. If pregnancy occurs while on medication and decision to keep pregnancy, then institute drug elimination procedure per manufacturer instructions.

RA, rheumatoid arthritis. NSAIDs, nonsteroidal anti-inflammatory drugs.

[1]US FDA Pregnancy Category Definitions:

A: Controlled studies in women fail to demonstrate a risk to the fetus in the first trimester, and the possibility of fetal harm appears remote.

B: Animal studies do not indicate a risk to the fetus and there are no controlled human studies, or animal studies do show an adverse effect on the fetus but well-controlled studies in pregnant women have failed to demonstrate a risk to the fetus.

C: Studies have shown that the drug exerts animal teratogenic or embryocidal effects, but there are no controlled studies in women, or no studies are available in either animals or women.

D: Positive evidence of human fetal risk exists, but benefits in certain situations (eg, life-threatening situations or serious diseases for which safer drugs cannot be used or are ineffective) may make use of the drug acceptable despite its risks.

X: Studies in animals or humans have demonstrated fetal abnormalities or there is evidence of fetal risk based on human experience, or both, and the risk clearly outweighs any possible benefit.

(Data from Drug Facts and Comparisons, 2002; Physicians Desk Reference. 55th ed. Medical Economics Company, Inc., 2001; and Micromedex Healthcare Series: Micromedex, Greenwood Village, Colorado.)

predominantly in lower limbs, and 1 or more of the following: positive family history; buttock pain, alternating right and left gluteal regions; enthesopathy; sacroiliitis; urethritis, cervicitis, or acute diarrhea within 1 month of onset.

General Considerations

The prevalence of reactive spondyloarthropathies, including undifferentiated spondyloarthropathies, is estimated at 1.9%. The spondyloarthropathies are characterized by familial aggregation and association with HLA class 1 antigens, especially B27, which is expressed by 25–90% of patients. The disorders are most common in populations with high frequencies of HLA-B27 (eg, Native Americans of the Haida Nation 50%, white of European ancestry 7–20%) and less common among blacks, of whom only 1–2% expresses the allele. Family studies indicate that other genes contribute risk, and that environmental factors are important. The importance of bacterial infection is clear in reactive arthritis and suspected in other disorders in this group. There are rough correlations between skin and joint activity in psoriatic arthritis and between intestinal and joint activity in enteropathic spondyloarthropathy. Animal studies indicate that the HLA class 1 molecules play a direct role in pathogenesis, perhaps by failing to eliminate organisms or by presenting "arthritogenic" peptides.

Psoriatic arthritis has a prevalence of 0.1%, affecting 5–10% of patients with psoriasis. Female:male ratio is 1:1. Incidence peaks at 30–55 years. A strong genetic basis for the disease is supported by a twin concordance rate of 70%.

Ankylosing spondylitis has prevalence of 0.1% in the African population, 0.5–1% in whites, and 6% in Haida Native Americans. Female:male ratio is reported as 1:5, although many observers believe this ratio underestimates disease in women.

Peripheral arthritis occurs in 10–20% of patients with Crohn's disease or ulcerative colitis. Women and men are affected equally and there is no association with HLA-B27. Spinal arthritis occurs in 10% of patients with ulcerative colitis, female:male ratio is 1:3, and 50% of patients express HLA-B27.

Reactive arthritis following venereal infections has a male to female ratio of 9:1. Reactive arthritis following gastrointestinal infections or respiratory infection with *Chlamydia pneumoniae* affects both sexes equally. Individuals who have gastroenteritis with arthritogenic strains of bacteria have a 5% risk of developing arthritis if they are B27 negative and a 20% risk if B27 positive.

Clinical Findings

Psoriatic arthritis usually follows the onset of rash by several years, but in 15% of cases skin and joint disease present concurrently and in 15% joint disease precedes rash. Joint involvement presents in several patterns; 30–50% exhibit oligoarthritis with enthesitis as seen in reactive arthritis, 30–50% have symmetric polyarthritis similar to RA, and 5% have predominantly axial disease resembling ankylosing spondylitis. DIP joint involvement, sacroiliitis, conjunctivitis, and spondylitis each occur in one third of patients. Osteolysis of phalanges with telescoping of the digits (arthritis mutilans) occurs in about 5% of patients. Inflammation at the site of attachment of tendons and ligaments to bones (enthesitis) often leads to symptomatic Achilles tendonitis and plantar fasciitis. Less common features include uveitis and pulmonary fibrosis. Several radiographic features are characteristic for this disease, including fusiform soft tissue swelling with normal bone mineralization (sausage digits), erosion of the proximal phalanx with proliferation of the distal phalanx (pencil in cup deformity), osteolysis of phalanges and metacarpals (arthritis mutilans), and dramatic joint space loss of the IPs with ankylosis. Spondylitis and sacroiliitis are often evident but do not distinguish psoriatic arthritis from the other spondyloarthropathies.

Ankylosing spondylitis presents with back pain or stiffness, often with sacroiliitis, costochondritis, plantar fasciitis, and Achilles enthesitis. Sacroiliitis is essential to diagnosis and may be detected early by MRI if not apparent on plain films. Enthesitis in the spine initially produces osteopenia, but later reactive bone forms leading to fusion. Fusion begins in the lumbosacral spine and proceeds upward. Clinical disease is usually evident by age 15 to 30. Thirty percent of patients have peripheral synovitis that is usually asymmetric, oligoarticular, and often involves the hip. Extra-articular manifestations include unilateral uveitis (30%), prostatitis, and salpingitis and, rarely, serositis, IgA nephropathy, and amyloidosis. Aortitis leading to aortic insufficiency occurs in 1% of patients, as does pulmonary fibrosis. Late physical findings include diminished spinal range of motion and limited chest expansion. Lumbar spine mobility can be assessed with the Schober's test: With the patient upright, a 10-cm span is marked from the 5th lumbar vertebra cephalad. The distance between the marks in measured again during maximal forward flexion. Normal is 15 cm or more. Chest expansion is recorded as the difference in circumference between inspiration and expiration, with normal at least 5 cm. Women often have a milder disease, with later onset, less hip involvement, more peripheral arthritis and osteitis pubis. Axial disease may be limited to cervical spine. Sacroiliitis may produce pain during pregnancy and limit progress during childbirth.

Enteropathic arthritis can present as migratory arthralgias or synovitis, as oligoarticular asymmetric synovitis involving joints of the lower extremity, and as axial disease with sacroiliitis and/or spinal arthritis. Extra-articular manifestations include erythema nodosum in Crohn's disease and pyoderma gangrenosum in ulcerative colitis. Fever, weight loss, fatigue, oral ulcers, and anterior uveitis can occur. Anemia, leukocytosis, thrombocytosis, antibodies to lactoferin, and elevated acute-phase reactants are common during flares.

Control of gastrointestinal disease is associated with improvement in arthritis.

Reactive arthritis begins 2–4 weeks after gastroenteritis or venereal infections. Urethritis is often the initial symptom, followed by conjunctivitis, and later by an additive, asymmetric, oligoarticular synovitis, usually involving joints of the lower extremity. Enthesitis often produces heel pain and may cause pain at ischial tuberosities, iliac crests, tibial tuberosities, and ribs. Buttock pain occurs in 50% of patients, and ankylosing spondylitis develops in 10%. Extra-articular manifestations may also include keratoderma blennorrhagicum, a form of pustular psoriasis that may involve soles and palms. Circinate balanitis may present as shallow ulcers surrounding the meatus. Anterior uveitis is seen in 20% of patients and aortitis in 1%. Amyloidosis and renal involvement are rare complications. Laboratory and radiographic features are similar to those in psoriatic arthritis and ankylosing spondylitis. Disease is self-limited over 3–12 months in most patients, but chronic disease develops in 15%.

Often patients present with enthesitis or asymmetric oligoarticular arthritis, but do not meet the full criteria for reactive arthritis and are not associated with ankylosis, rash, or inflammatory bowel disease. These features may develop later, or patients may remain undifferentiated throughout the course of their disease.

Differential Diagnosis

Psoriatic arthritis is distinguished from RA and erosive OA by skin rash, dactylitis, and characteristic radiographic changes including lack of osteopenia. However, some patients meet criteria for both disorders. HIV can present as psoriatic arthritis and should be excluded before treatment is started.

Ankylosing spondylitis is distinguished from diffuse idiopathic skeletal hyperostosis (DISH) and spinal osteoarthritis by radiography.

Enteropathic arthritis shares many features with Behçet's syndrome, and prominent ocular symptoms should prompt evaluation to exclude posterior uveitis. Treatable conditions of joint and gastrointestinal system should also be excluded, including Whipple's disease, intestinal bypass syndrome, familial Mediterranean fever, and infectious colitis.

Reactive arthritis must be differentiated from septic arthritis. Cultures are indicated to rule out ongoing infection, especially following genitourinary tract disease.

Treatment

Therapy of the spondyloarthropathies is based on the sites and severity of disease. The peripheral joints are treated according to the principles that apply to RA.

Mild disease may respond to NSAIDs. Oligoarticular disease can often be managed with intra-articular corticosteroids alone. Destructive polyarticular disease, as may occur in psoriatic arthritis, requires early aggressive therapy. Controlled trials have demonstrated some benefit from sulfasalazine and methotrexate and significant efficacy with etanercept. Uncontrolled trials report responses to antibodies to tumor necrosis factor (TNF), antimarials, gold, azathioprine, cyclosporine, mycophenolate mofetil, leflunomide, psoralen plus ultraviolet light of A wavelength (PUVA), and retinoids. PUVA is not effective for spinal disease, and retinoids are contraindicated in spinal disease because they may induce ligamentous calcification.

In the treatment of spinal disease, general measures include physical therapy to maintain range of motion, use of chest belts, head supports, and airbags while driving, and avoidance of high-risk sports. Bone antiresorptive agents reduce osteopenia. Spinal pain and stiffness may respond to NSAIDs and short courses of corticosteroids. Trials of sulfasalazine and methotrexate have been disappointing. Uncontrolled trials of etanercept and anti-TNF antibodies have been very promising, and controlled trials are underway. In contrast to peripheral disease, it is not yet known whether early intervention changes the ultimate outcome in spinal arthritis. Several years of observations of the effects of the newer biologic agents will be required to answer this question.

Iritis requires prompt referral to ophthalmology for local and/or systemic treatment. Pain from sacroiliitis that is refractory to NSAIDs often responds to corticosteroid injection performed with fluoroscopic guidance. Urethritis caused by *Chlamydia* infection should be treated with antibiotics (eg, azithromycin 1 g as a single dose, doxycycline 100 mg twice daily for 7 days). There is some data supporting antibiotic treatment in the absence of positive cultures for patients with chronic reactive arthritis following urethritis but not for patients in whom joint disease followed gastroenteritis.

PRIMARY SJÖGREN'S SYNDROME

Sjögren's syndrome is a systemic inflammatory disorder characterized by lymphocytic infiltration of exocrine glands, leading to dryness of eyes and mouth, often of the skin, and of the urogenital, respiratory, and gastrointestinal tracts.

 ESSENTIALS OF DIAGNOSIS

Diagnosis requires at least 1 of the following:
- *Characteristic histopathologic features: focus score 1 or greater on minor salivary gland biopsy*

(a focus is an agglomeration of at least 50 mononuclear cells, score is the number of foci per 4 mm² tissue.)
- *Autoantibodies to SSA/Ro, SSB/La antigens or both. Plus 2 additional objective findings or 3 additional criteria from among the following:*
  - *Ocular symptoms: dryness, sensation of foreign body, use of lubricants*
  - *Ocular signs: abnormal Schirmer's or rose bengal tests*
  - *Oral symptoms: dryness, swollen salivary glands, need for liquids with dry food*
  - *Oral signs: abnormal salivary scintigraphy, sialography, or salivary flow study*
  - *Histopathology or autoantibodies as defined above.*

General Considerations

The prevalence of Sjögren's syndrome has been reported as 0.05% to 4.8%, with the wide range reflecting variations in definitions and populations. Female:male ratio is 9:1, with incidence peaking in middle age. Sjögren's syndrome is associated with focal mononuclear cell infiltrates in exocrine tissues and with the presence of autoantibodies. Causes remain unknown, but it is speculated that viruses or other environmental factors trigger disease in genetically susceptible individuals. Exocrine glands are destroyed, but dryness is often greater than would be expected for the degree of tissue destruction, and other mechanisms are thought to contribute to exocrine dysfunction.

Clinical Findings

Sjögren's syndrome usually presents with oral and ocular sicca. Some patients do not experience a dry sensation but report inability to wear contact lenses, difficulty reading for long periods, increased dental carries or periodontal disease, or dysphagia. Tear production may be evaluated by performing a Schirmer's test, in which standardized strips of filter paper are placed under the lower lid. Wetting of less than 5 mm over 5 minutes is evidence of sicca. A punctate pattern of staining by rose bengal or lissamine green indicates keratoconjunctivitis sicca. Oral dryness may be audible in speech. The tongue often appears dry and furrowed, salivary pooling is diminished, and tooth erosions or candida may be observed. The parotid and other salivary glands may be visibly or palpably enlarged. Dryness of skin, vagina (dyspareunia), respiratory tract (cough), and gastrointestinal tract (dysphagia) are often reported. Constitutional symptoms are common, as is mild synovitis, often at the MCP joints. Less common features are leukocytoclastic vasculitis, interstitial lung disease, renal tubular acidosis with hypokalemia, glomerulonephritis, peripheral neuropathy, and, rarely, central nervous system disorders similar to those described in systemic lupus erythematosus (SLE). Sjögren's syndrome imparts a 44-fold increase in frequency of B-cell lymphomas, usually involving salivary glands and cervical nodes. Anti-SSA/Ro antibodies increase the risk of fetal heart block, although the frequency remains low. RFs are elevated in about 90% of patients. Antinuclear antibody (ANA) and antibodies to Sjögren's syndrome A (SS-A) and Sjögren's syndrome B (SS-B) are elevated in 50–90% of patients.

Differential Diagnosis

Sicca can accompany normal aging and is a side effect of many medications including antihistamines, antihypertensives, and tricyclic antidepressants. Abnormal blink, lacrimal gland obstruction, and other disorders may contribute to ocular dryness. The diagnosis of Sjögren's syndrome should not be made when there is a history of head and neck radiation, hepatitis C, AIDS, preexisting lymphoma, sarcoidosis, graft-versus-host disease, or use of anticholinergic drugs. Sjögren's syndrome may occur together with other ARDs, especially RA, SLE, and scleroderma, in which case it is termed "secondary Sjögren's." Patients should be evaluated for these disorders when Sjögren's syndrome is first recognized and should be reevaluated at intervals.

Treatment

Ocular symptoms are treated with preservative-free solutions containing 0.3% to 1% hydroxypropyl methylcellulose. Pellets (lacrisert) provide longer benefit, and ointments can be used at night. When lubricants fail, lacrimal outflow tracts can be blocked permanently or with removable silicone plugs (punctal occlusion). Oral symptoms are treated with water, artificial salivas, and gentle dentifrices (eg, the Biotene products). Muscarinic agonists (eg, pilocarpine 5 mg 4 times daily, cevimeline 30 mg 3 times daily) have been approved for treatment of xerostomia and probably also increase other secretions. Topical immunomodulatory medications are under investigation, including ophthalmic preparations of corticosteroids and cyclosporine, and interferon-containing oral troches. Oral candidiasis is treated with oral suspensions or troches containing antifungal agents (eg, nystatin, clotrimazole). Parotitis is treated with warm compresses, massage and, if necessary, antibiotics. Renal tubular acidosis is treated with

alkalinizing agents (sodium and potassium citrate at 1–2 mEq/kg/d) and potassium supplementation. Synovitis is usually mild and is treated similarly to mild RA, often with NSAIDs and hydroxychloroquine. Systemic inflammatory disease may require more aggressive immunosuppression.

SYSTEMIC LUPUS ERYTHEMATOSIS

SLE is a term applied to a group of disorders characterized by production of antibodies to components of the cell nucleus and by inflammation in multiple organ systems.

 ESSENTIALS OF DIAGNOSIS

Patients may be classified as having SLE if at least 4 of the following 11 criteria have been present at any time:
- Malar rash.
- Discoid rash.
- Photosensitivity.
- Oral ulcers.
- Arthritis.
- Serositis.
- Persistent proteinuria (> 0.5 g/d) or cellular casts.
- Neurologic disorder (seizures, psychosis).
- Hemolytic anemia, leukopenia, or thrombocytopenia.
- Increased titers of antibodies to DNA or Smith antigen or a positive LE cells preparation.
- Increased titers of ANA.

General Considerations

The prevalence of SLE is 1 in 2000, with higher prevalence among blacks and other ethnic groups. Incidence peaks between 15 and 40 years of age. In this age group, the female:male ratio is about 10:1, dropping to 2:1 when disease onset is in childhood or in older adults. The causes of SLE are only partly understood. There are multiple factors that must vary among individuals, given the heterogeneity of the disorders grouped as SLE. Twin concordance is 25–50%, implying both genetic and environmental or stochastic factors. Associations with HLA alleles and deficiencies in complement components C4, C1q, and C2 have been described. SLE-like diseases occur in animal models with lesions that interfere with immune clearance, including complement deficiency, or with immune regulation, including altered apoptosis. The presence of alleles encoding a specific antibody is associated with the development of nephritis in 1 model of lupus-prone mice. In human disease, elevated levels of some antibodies are clearly pathogenic. Specifically, antibodies to DNA and nucleosomes localize in the kidney, forming immune complexes that promote glomerulonephritis. Antiphospholipid antibodies promote thrombosis. Pathogenic roles are less well established for other antibodies, but their presence is associated with risk of disease manifestations. Specifically, anti-ribonucleoprotein (RNP) is associated with Raynaud's, myositis, and interstitial lung disease, Anti-ribosomal P is associated with psychosis and depression, and anti-SSA/Ro and anti-SSB/La are associated with sicca syndrome, subacute cutaneous lupus, neonatal lupus, and photosensitivity.

Clinical Findings

Presentations are diverse, manifestations accumulate over time, and the disease activity flares and remits, all features that make description of the disorder difficult.

Table 44–4 summarizes clinical manifestations of SLE, together with approximate frequency based on a North American cohort. ANA are often ordered as a screening test for lupus. Elevated ANA is sensitive for disease but is not specific. Elevated levels of dsDNA and Smith antigen are more specific but are not always present. Diagnosis often requires observation over time.

Differential Diagnosis

A review of Table 44–4 provides a reminder that SLE is in the differential diagnosis of a great many disorders, and the reverse is also true. Work-up is guided by the specific presentations.

Treatment

The goals of management are (1) to control acute inflammation that threatens organ systems, (2) to detect such threats early enough to allow intervention and prevent damage, (3) to reduce pain and fatigue, and (4) to limit side effects associated with therapy. This requires frequent evaluation, laboratory monitoring, and medication adjustment and is best done in coordina-

Table 44–4. Clinical manifestations of systemic lupus erythematosus.

System	Percentage of cases	Manifestation
Constitutional	80%	Fever, malaise, fatigue, weight loss
Hematologic	80%	Hemolytic anemia (< 10%), anemia of chronic disease (80%), leukopenia (50%), lymphadenopathy (30%), thrombocytopenia, splenomegaly, thrombophilia associated with antiphospholipid antibodies (ACL, LAC, antiB2GP1)
Joint	> 90%	Arthralgias (85%), nondeforming synovitis (63%), Jaccoud's arthropathy, osteonecrosis (10%)
Musle	5%	Myositis (check creatine phosphokinase)
Mucocutaneous	90%	Malar rash (30–60%), discoid rash (15–30%), mucosal ulcerations (50%), alopecia, vasculitic urticaria, purpura, digital ulcerations (50%)
Renal	75%	Glomerulonephritis; tubulointerstitial inflammation; inflammation of ureters, bladder, urethra
Vascular	60%	Raynaud's phenomenon (60%), hypertension, vasculitis
Cardiac	25%	Pericarditis (25%), myocarditis (< 10%), endocarditis, increased risk of coronary artery disease
Pulmonary	30%	Pleurisy (30%), pneumonitis, hemorrhage, pulmonary hypertension, shrinking lung (all < 10%), pulmonary embolism
Gastrointestinal	45%	Peritonitis, hepatitis (< 10%), pancreatitis (2%), vasculitis
Neuropsychiatric	65%	Headache, fatigue, cognitive dysfunction, depression, psychosis, seizures, chorea, cranial neuropathy, vasculitis, cerebral vascular accidents, transverse myelitis, mononeuritis multiplex, peripheral neuropathy
Ocular	< 5%	Cytoid bodies (3%), uveitis, scleritis

tion with a specialty center. Rest, antidepressants, and occasionally stimulants (eg, modafinil, pemoline, methylphenidate) help control fatigue. NSAIDs are often useful for arthralgias, headache, and serositis. Antimalarials (eg, hydroxychloroquine 200–400 mg/d, quinacrine 100 mg/d) may improve constitutional symptoms, rashes, joint disease, and serositis. Corticosteroids are effective for many disease manifestations. Topical and intralesional preparations are used for mucocutaneous lesions; intraarticular or modest oral doses (eg, prednisone 5–20 mg/d) are effective for joint symptoms. Very high doses (eg, prednisone 1–2 mg/kg/d in divided doses, sometimes preceded by intravenous boluses of 1 g of methylprednisolone daily for 3 days) may be required for severe flares of systemic vasculitis, pneumonitis, thrombocytopenic purpura, nephritis, or cerebritis. Corticosteroids are often used to achieve control, then tapered with addition of slower-acting agents. Most agents used in RA have been applied to patients with SLE with reports of success. Azathioprine (50–200 mg/d) and cyclophosphamide are often used as steroid-sparing agents in severe disease. Mycophenylate mofetil (500–2000 mg/d) shows promise as an alternative to cyclophosphamide for nephritis. Cyclosporine (2.5–5 mg/kg/d) may be of benefit for membranous nephritis. Methotrexate (7.5–20 mg/wk) is often used to control musculoskeletal disease and shows promise in vasculitis. Thalidomide (25–50 mg/d) and dapsone have proved beneficial for discoid lupus. Retinoids have been used with success for cutaneous disease. Danazol (400–1200 mg/d) has been effective in controlling thrombocytopenia and hemolytic anemia. Bromocriptine and dehydroepiandrosterone (DHEA) have been suggested for management of constitutional symptoms. Intravenous immunoglobulin (400 mg/kg/d for 5 days) has been used for refractory thrombocytopenia. Biologic agents that bind to TNF-alpha have been reported to control SLE-associated synovitis resistant to other therapy, but they may be associated with increased risk of rash and may induce DNA antibodies and thus increase the risk of nephritis. Several biologic agents are currently under investigation for treatment of SLE.

Patients with SLE are monitored at intervals for declining complement levels and rising levels of antibodies to DNA, as these are often associated with pending flares of renal disease and vasculitis. They are also monitored for evidence of ongoing organ system involvement, usually by complete blood cell count, urinalysis, serum creatinine, transaminases and, if indicated, creatine phosphokinase, as well as for toxicities associated with medications (see Table 44–1). Patients with SLE are at higher risk for coronary artery disease and osteoporosis, therefore hypertension, dyslipidemia, obesity, smoking, and osteopenia should be treated aggressively.

Women with SLE have normal fertility, except when acutely ill. Although some series have reported high rates of SLE flare during pregnancy, most flares are not severe and overall exacerbation rates are now estimated at < 15%. The rate of fetal loss and prematurity is higher than normal, and correlates with at least 3 factors: (1) active nephritis, (2) hypertension, and (3) elevated titers of antiphospholipid antibodies. Patients should be counseled to delay pregnancy, if possible, until clinical remission has been achieved for 6–12 months. In addition, hypertension should be treated, and patients with antiphospholipid antibodies should be referred to specialty centers to consider anticoagulation therapy before conception. Neonatal lupus is a rare complication, affecting 1–2% of fetuses of mothers with anti-SSA/Ro antibodies. Skin, hepatic, and hematologic manifestations are transient, regressing as maternal antibodies leave the circulation. Damage to the cardiac conduction system is not reversible, usually requires pacing, and carries a mortality rate of about 20%.

ANTIPHOSPHOLIPID SYNDROME

Antiphospholipid syndrome (APS) is recurrent arterial or venous thrombosis and/or fetal losses associated with anticardiolipin antibodies and/or the lupus anticoagulant.

 ESSENTIALS OF DIAGNOSIS

Preliminary criteria for diagnosis of definite APS requires at least 1 clinical and 1 laboratory criteria from the following:

- *Vascular thrombosis: at least 1 episode of arterial, venous, or small vessel thrombosis confirmed by imaging, Doppler, or histopathology and not associated with vessel inflammation.*
- *Pregnancy morbidity: 1 unexplained second- or third-trimester loss of a morphologically normal fetus or 1 premature birth prior to 35 weeks due to severe preeclampsia or placental insufficiency, or 3 unexplained spontaneous abortions in the first trimester.*
- *Lupus anticoagulant or anticardiolipin antibody of IgG and/or IgM isotype in medium or high titer on at least 2 occasions at least 6 weeks apart.*

General Considerations

The prevalence of antiphospholipid antibodies in the general population is not well established. The prevalence of APS among individuals with characteristic antibodies is estimated at < 1–9%. When the above criteria are used, women are affected more often than men. This may change, however, as the role of antiphospholipid antibodies in vascular disease are elucidated. Suggested mechanisms by which antibodies may promote thrombosis include activation of endothelial cells, platelet aggregation, or selective inhibition of the protein C anticoagulant pathway.

Clinical Findings

Venous thrombosis usually involves the deep veins of the legs, but thrombosis of superficial vessels, inferior vena cava, and pulmonary, hepatic, renal, axillary, optic, and sagittal veins is reported. Arterial thrombosis usually presents as stroke or transient ischemic attack. Ischemia of extremities, heart, bowel, liver, adrenal gland, and other organs occurs less often. Fetal loss can occur at any stage of gestation and is thought to reflect thrombosis of placental vessels. Other clinical features are variably present. A partial list includes thrombocytopenia, hemolytic anemia, livedo reticularis, Libman-Sacks endocarditis, headaches, and neuropsychiatric complications. APS may be primary or secondary to other ARDs, usually SLE.

Differential Diagnosis

Patients with unexplained venous thrombosis should be screened for other recognized causes of thrombophilia, including factor V Leiden; G2021A mutation of prothrombin; deficiencies of protein-S, protein-C, or antithrombin 3; elevated homocysteine; dysfibrogenemias; polycythemia; and oral contraceptive use. Unexplained arterial thrombosis warrants evaluation for vasculitis, sickle cell disease, dyslipidemias, hypertension, diabetes, smoking, and other vasculopathies. Patients with recurrent fetal losses should be evaluated for chromosomal abnormality, anatomic abnormalities of the uterus, and other systemic diseases of the mother.

Treatment

Patients with a history of thrombosis are treated with warfarin, with a target international normalized ratio of 3.0. Risk of fetal loss can be reduced with subcutaneous heparin at 5000 to 10,000 units twice daily plus 80 mg aspirin. Other heparin regimens, high-dose corticosteroids, and intravenous immunoglobin have also been used with success. The efficacy of platelet inhibitors and hydroxychloroquine is less well established, but these agents are often used when more aggressive therapy in contraindicated.

SYSTEMIC SCLEROSIS

Systemic sclerosis is a group of multisystem disorders characterized by fibrosis of the skin and internal organs, functional and structural abnormalities of small blood vessels, and immune system dysregulation.

 ESSENTIALS OF DIAGNOSIS

Systemic Sclerosis

- *Proximal scleroderma: thickening of skin proximal to MCPs, or 2 of the following: sclerodactyly (skin changes limited to fingers), digital pitting scars (history of ischemic injury to fingers), bibasilar pulmonary fibrosis.*

Limited Cutaneous Systemic Sclerosis

- *Scleroderma limited to face, and skin distal to elbows and knees.*
- *Often complicated by pulmonary artery hypertension.*
- *Often associated with anti-centromere antibodies.*

Diffuse Cutaneous Systemic Sclerosis (DcSSc)

- *Scleroderma proximal to elbows and knees.*
- *Often complicated by pulmonary fibrosis.*
- *Often associated with ANA and anti-SCL70 antibodies.*

Mixed Connective Tissue Disease (MCTD)

- *Overlap syndrome, often with scleroderma, myositis, synovitis, and features of SLE.*
- *Often complicated by pulmonary fibrosis.*
- *Associated with anti-RNP antibodies.*

General Considerations

When defined by the criteria above, prevalence is estimated at 0.05%. Prevalence of milder disease, with sclerodactyly and Raynaud's, may be as high as 0.4%. Incidence peaks between ages 35 and 65 years. Female:male ratio is 7–12:1. Pathologic features include vasculopathy, fibrosis, and autoimmunity. The vasculopathy is usually not inflammatory, but it is characterized by damage and dysfunction of endothelial cells with secondary proliferation of smooth muscle, vasospasm, luminal narrowing, and thrombosis. Fibrosis occurs with increased production of matrix collagen, fibronectin, and glycosaminoglycans. Inflammatory infiltrates are often present in skin and lung, and elevated titers of autoantibodies are present and may contribute to endothelial damage. Etiology in unknown. Genetic factors that confer risk have been described, including mutation of the fibrillarin-1 gene and certain HLA class 1 alleles. However, concordance rates are similar for monozygotic and dizygotic twins; thus environmental and stochastic factors are important. Factors that may play a role in some patients include exposure to silica dust, appetite suppressants, organic solvents and other agents, viruses that share homology with self-antigens, and the nature of the HLA mismatch between mother and fetus. The latter determines how long fetal cells persist in maternal circulation and tissues, a state termed "microchimerism" that may influence immune tolerance or induce graft-versus-host type responses.

Clinical Findings

Limited cutaneous systemic sclerosis (LcSSc) usually presents with a history of Raynaud's phenomenon (reversible digital vasospasm) for several years, followed by puffiness or tightness of the skin in the fingers and hands. Skin disease can progress to involve face, and upper and lower distal extremities, with flexion contractures, ulcers, and digital infarcts requiring amputation. Features of CREST syndrome often develop, including esophageal dysmotility leading to reflux and strictures, telangiectasias on the face, mucous membranes, and hands, and subcutaneous calcinosis on fingers, forearms, and pressure points. Interstitial lung disease is rare, but a progressive pulmonary vasculopathy characterized by vascular remodeling that is pathologically similar to primary pulmonary hypertension develops in about 50% of patients. Ten-year survival is greater than 70%. Diagnosis depends on identifying the typical skin changes. Capillaries at the nailfold are often abnormal. Examination at 40× to 100× magnification reveals dilation of some loops, and loss of normal capillaries. Titers of ANA and anti-centromere antibodies are often elevated, the latter associated with increased risk of lung disease. Early lung disease is detected by periodic pulmonary function testing including flows, volumes, and carbon monoxide diffusing capacity. Pulmonary hypertension may be detected by Doppler echocardiography.

Diffuse cutaneous systemic sclerosis (DcSSc) often presents with simultaneous onset of Raynaud's and skin changes. Scleroderma is more widespread than in LcSSc, with involvement of proximal limbs and trunk. Skin is initially edematous, with pruritus and erythema, but later becomes sclerotic and atrophic, with hyperpigmentation and hypopigmentation. Constitutional symptoms, including fatigue, depression, and arthralgias are common. Lung disease is the leading cause of mortality. Most patients have pulmonary fibrosis with varying degrees of inflammation; a smaller number have primary pulmonary hypertension–type vasculopathy as seen in LcSSc. Esophageal dysmotility is common, and reflux may lead to esophagitis, Barrett's metaplasia, or aspiration pneumonia. Gastric antral vascular ectasia (GAVE or watermelon stomach) can produce chronic blood loss and anemia. Dysmotility of the small intestine can cause pain, distention, malabsorption, and pseudo-obstruction. Myocardial fibrosis is often asymptomatic but can lead to diastolic dysfunction. Inflammatory cardiomyopathy and pericarditis occur more rarely. Scleroderma renal crisis is a potentially life-threatening event characterized by hypertension and rapidly progressive renal failure with proteinuria and microscopic hematuria. Overall, 10-year survival is 50%. Diagnosis depends on recognition of characteristic skin changes. Elevated titers of ANA and anti-SCL antibodies are often present. Pulmonary function testing should be done at 6–12 month intervals to detect early lung disease. High-resolution lung computed tomography is sensitive for interstitial lung disease and increased neutrophils in lavage fluids obtained at bronchoscopy indicate inflammation and predict progression of fibrosis.

Mixed connective tissue disease (MCTD) is a controversial term used to describe patients with elevated titers of anti-RNP antibodies, scleroderma, and an overlap syndrome, often with inflammatory myopathy, synovitis, and features of SLE. Patients in this category, especially those of African heritage, are at high risk for pulmonary fibrosis and should have early lung studies.

Differential Diagnosis

Skin changes that resemble scleroderma are seen in several disorders. Eosinophilic fasciitis is differentiated by tissue eosinophilia on biopsy and by a characteristic pattern of skin involvement that often includes the limbs, but spares the hands, feet, and face. Diabetes can cause skin thickening (scleredema) and hand tightness (cheiroarthropathy) that resemble scleroderma. Scleroderma-like skin changes are sometimes seen with carcinoid, myeloma, porphyria cutanea tarda, hypothyroidism, and lipodystrophies.

Treatment

No treatment is known to reverse the underlying pathologic processes of scleroderma, although there is hope that prostacyclin (eg, epoprostenol) and endothelin-1 inhibitors (eg, bosentan) may slow or reverse vascular remodeling and that antibodies to tumor growth factor may improve fibrosis. Initial reports of efficacy for skin disease have been overturned by controlled trials of penicillamine, chlorambucil, interferon-α, photopheresis, and relaxin. Controlled trials of methotrexate for skin disease returned conflicting results. Raynaud's may be treated with warm clothing, calcium channel blockers (eg, slow-release nifedipine 30–240 mg), and probably with sildenafil and bosentan. Severe digital ischemia may respond to intravenous prostaglandin, coumadin, or sympathectomy. Antireflux measures and proton pump inhibitors are indicated for management of reflux; esophageal strictures may require dilation; and GAVE is treated with laser coagulation. Promotility agents (eg, metoclopramide, octreotide) may improve gastroparesis, and rotating courses of broad-spectrum antibiotics often improve symptoms associated with small bowel dysmotility. Patients with lung disease should be evaluated for inflammatory alveolitis. Controlled trials are ongoing, but current consensus favors treating alveolitis with cyclophosphamide or azathioprine and steroids. Patients with pulmonary hypertension should be considered for treatment with epoprostenol, bosentan, and warfarin. Early introduction of angiotensin-converting enzyme inhibitors and aggressive control of hypertension has markedly reduced mortality associated with renal crisis. Methotrexate and corticosteroids are used for management of synovitis and myositis in patients with MCTD.

IDIOPATHIC INFLAMMATORY MYOPATHY

Idiopathic inflammatory myopathies are a group of disorders characterized by proximal muscle weakness and inflammation. They include polymyositis (PM), dermatomyositis (DM), inclusion body myositis (IBM), and myositis associated with other ARDs.

 ESSENTIALS OF DIAGNOSIS

- *Proximal muscle weakness.*
- *Elevated serum levels of skeletal muscle enzymes (eg, creatine kinase, aldolase).*
- *Myopathic changes on electromyography.*
- *Muscle biopsy evidence of inflammation.*
- *For DM, characteristic skin rash.*

General Considerations

These disorders are rare, and prevalence figures are not available. Incidence is estimated at 0.5 to 8.4 cases per million, with peak incidence at 10- to 15-years-old in children, and 45- to 60-years-old in adults. Female:male ratio is 2:1 for DM and PM, and 1:2 for IBM. Like the other ARDs, the myopathies are thought to be triggered by environmental factors, likely viruses, in genetically susceptible individuals. PM and IBM are characterized by CD8+ infiltrates that appear directed against antigens on the surface of muscle cells. Humoral immunity appears more prominent in DM, with perivascular infiltrates of CD4+ T cells, and deposits of immunoglobulins and complement.

Clinical Findings

Patients present with muscle weakness that is symmetric and proximal. Laboratory findings include elevated serum levels of enzymes derived from skeletal muscle, including creatine kinase, aspartate transaminase, alanine transaminase, lactate dehydrogenase, and aldolase. Electromyography (EMG) demonstrates myopathic changes. Biopsies are diagnostic, but negative biopsies are common due to the patchy nature of the disease. Abnormalities on MRI or EMG can help direct biopsy and improve yield. Diagnosis is supported by elevated ESR or CRP. Antibodies specific to myositis are observed in about 50% of patients. These include antibodies to antisynthetase antibodies, anti-Mi-2 antibodies, and anti-SRP antibodies.

Onset of polymyositis is usually insidious, beginning in the shoulder and hip girdle. Pulmonary fibrosis and alveolitis are common and should be evaluated in the same manner as in SSc. Antisynthetase antibodies occur often. Among these, anti-Jo-1 is most common and is associated with interstitial lung disease, synovitis, Raynaud's phenomenon, and darkened fissures on the palmar aspects of the fingers (mechanic's hands). Anti-SRP antibodies are less common, and predict rapid onset of disease and poor response to treatment.

Dermatomyositis rash may precede myopathy or may occur in the absence of myopathy (amyotrophic dermatomyositis). Typical features include violaceous macules or papules on the dorsal aspect of IPs, elbows, patellae, and/or medial malleoli (Gottron's papules); edema and violaceous discoloration of the eyelids (heliotrope rash); macular erythema of the shoulders and neck (shawl sign) or of the anterior neck and chest (V sign), or face and forehead. Anti-Mi-2 antibodies are often observed and predict a good response to treatment.

IBM usually affects older individuals. Myopathy may be proximal but may also be focal, asymmetric, or distal. EMG often shows mixed neurogenic and myopathic changes. Diagnosis depends on finding typical intracellular vacuoles on biopsy.

Differential Diagnosis

The differential diagnosis of muscle weakness is large and includes many endocrinologic, neuromuscular, metabolic, infectious, and other disorders as well as functional disorders, and other ARDs including poly-myalgia rheumatica (PMR). Elevations of creatine kinase should be confirmed, as spurious elevations due to minor trauma are common. Hypothyroidism should be excluded early in work-up.

Treatment

Early corticosteroids are indicated to prevent irreversible damage (eg, prednisone at 1 mg/kg/d, tapering over several weeks.) When oral corticosteroids fail, patients may be treated with high-dose intravenous methylprednisolone, intravenous immunoglobulin, or plasmapheresis. Patients who respond to oral prednisone but are unable to taper to well-tolerated doses are usually treated with methotrexate (5–30 mg/wk) or azathioprine (50–150 mg/d). Hydroxychloroquine is often used to treat skin lesions. Active alveolitis is treated with cyclophosphamide or azathioprine.

POLYMYALGIA RHEUMATICA & GIANT CELL ARTERITIS

PMR is a syndrome of limb girdle stiffness in the elderly, often with associated constitutional symptoms and signs of inflammation. Giant cell arteritis (GCA) is inflammation of the second- to fifth-order branches of the aorta, usually involving the extracranial arteries of the head. GCA and PMR are linked by a common epidemiology. Both disorders may occur in the same person.

 ESSENTIALS OF DIAGNOSIS

Polymyalgia Rheumatica

- *Pain and stiffness in muscles of neck, shoulder girdle, and hip girdle.*
- *Age older than 50, usually Northern European ancestry.*
- *ESR usually greater than 60 mm/h.*
- *Marked response to low to medium doses of corticosteroids.*

Giant Cell Arteritis

- *PMR often accompanies or precedes vasculitis.*
- *Symptoms of cranial artery insufficiency, including:*
  - *Headache (often temporal or occipital)*
  - *Scalp tenderness*
  - *Ischemic optic neuropathy*
  - *Jaw claudication*
  - *Central nervous system ischemia.*
- *ESR usually greater than 60 mm/h.*

General Considerations

The prevalence of PMR is not known, but the incidence among persons over age 50 of Northern European ancestry is estimated at 50 per 100,000 per year. Incidence of GCA is as high as 15–25 per 100,000 in the same population. Female:male ratio is 2:1. Etiology is not known, although associations with HLA alleles and Northern European ancestry suggest genetic factors, and the rapid onset and self-limited nature of the disease suggests an infectious process. Inflammation is systemic. In patients with PMR, activated monocytes can be demonstrated in blood, and highly sensitive imaging techniques demonstrate vascular involvement. GCA is characterized by a mononuclear cell infiltrate that penetrates all layers of the arterial wall.

Clinical Findings

Patients with PMR report abrupt or insidious onset of pain and stiffness in the limb girdles. Constitutional signs may include weight loss, fatigue, and depression. Elevation of ESR and prompt response to corticosteroids support the diagnosis.

Often, GCA presents with nonspecific signs of inflammation as in PMR. Fever is common. GCA is often not recognized, however, until there are signs of vascular insufficiency. Most patients present with headaches. Thickening and reduced pulses in the temporal arteries may be evident on examination. History of jaw pain when eating or findings of scalp tenderness support the diagnosis. Fleeting visual blurring may precede vision loss, but patients may present with irreversible blindness. ESR and CRP are usually increased, but there are case reports of blindness in patients with normal ESR. Diagnosis depends on finding characteristic histopathology on biopsy of the superficial temporal artery. The rate of false-negatives can be reduced by taking long samples, examining serial sections, and repeating the biopsy on the contralateral artery if biopsy results are negative.

Differential Diagnosis

PMR is differentiated from PM by the normal creatine kinase, and from fibromyalgia by laboratory abnormalities. The differential diagnosis includes malignancy, other ARDs, and infections. A complete evaluation is indicated. GCA must be differentiated from other vaso-occlusive disorders including atherosclerosis and thromboembolic disease, and other vasculitides.

Treatment

PMR usually responds to 20 mg prednisone per day, and most patients can taper the dose by 2.5 mg every 2 weeks to 7 mg/d and by 1 mg every 2 weeks thereafter. Initial dose and taper schedule must be adjusted based on both clinical features and laboratory findings. Many patients are able to wean off steroids in a few months, but some require low doses for a number of years.

GCA is treated with high doses of steroids, usually 60 mg/d, followed by a taper of 10% every 1–2 weeks, following clinical and laboratory findings. Symptoms often recur, and taper schedule must be adjusted accordingly. Patients presenting with acute blindness or stroke are treated with very high doses of parenteral steroids (eg, 1 g of methylprednisolone per day for 3 days, followed by prednisone 1 mg/kg/d). Methotrexate has been evaluated as a possible steroid-sparing agent with mixed results. The role of biologic agents is under active investigation.

Patients should be evaluated for osteopenia and should receive prophylactic calcium, vitamin D, and antiresorptive agents.

Additional reading: The Arthritis Foundation publishes *Primer on The Rheumatic Diseases* (John H. Klippel, editor), available at www.arthritis.org or by writing to The Arthritis Foundation, 1330 West Peachtree Street, Atlanta, Georgia 30309. Another excellent resource is *Primary Care Rheumatology* by John H Klippel, Paul A Dieppe and Fred F Ferri (Mosby International Limited: London, 1999).

Relevant Web Sites

[The Arthritis Foundation]
www.arthritis.org

SECTION XVI

Gynecologic Disorders

Dysmenorrhea, Endometriosis, & Pelvic Pain

45

Alan B. Rothblatt, MD

DYSMENORRHEA

ESSENTIALS OF DIAGNOSIS

- *Primary dysmenorrhea is a crampy lower abdominal and pelvic pain caused by the release of prostaglandin $F_2\alpha$ from normal endometrium.*
- *Secondary dysmenorrhea is a menstrually related pelvic and lower abdominal pain caused by disease states of the pelvic organs.*

General Considerations

The incidence of primary dysmenorrhea in women of reproductive age is approximately 50–75%. It is greatest in women in their late teens to early twenties and declines with age. Primary dysmenorrhea is commonly seen in young women who have just begun having regular ovulatory menses. Parity has a variable effect. The degree of discomfort is related directly to the amount of menstrual flow which correlates to the amount of prostaglandin $F_2\alpha$ produced in the endometrium. Use of oral contraceptives and nonsteroidal anti-inflammatory drugs (NSAIDs) can reduce the severity of dysmenorrhea. Intrauterine devices (IUDs) can worsen it. The incidence of secondary dysmenorrhea is unknown. Women with secondary dysmenorrhea are usually in their 30s and 40s when the symptoms begin and will often have abnormal findings on pelvic examination.

Prevention

Use of oral contraceptives for contraception or regulation of menses will have the additional benefit of reducing dysmenorrhea. NSAIDs taken just prior to the onset of symptoms may also be helpful. Exercise and elimination of caffeine and alcohol from the diet along with adequate calcium may confer some benefit.

Clinical Findings

A. SYMPTOMS AND SIGNS

Patients with primary dysmenorrhea typically complain of painful cramping in the central lower abdomen or pelvis beginning just before or at the onset of menses and usually lasting for the first 1–3 days of flow. The pain can be severe and may radiate to the back or down the medial thighs. Symptoms related to systemic prostaglandin excess, such as diaphoresis, tachycardia, headache, nausea, vomiting, and diarrhea, may be present. The pelvic examination may reveal mild uterine tenderness to palpation at or just before the time of menses.

The symptoms of secondary dysmenorrhea can be similar to those of primary dysmenorrhea, but they usually begin after the teenage years and progress with age. The symptoms can be suggestive, but they are not diagnostic, of an underlying pathologic condition. These symptoms include pelvic heaviness or bloating, menorrhagia, deep dyspareunia, and more generalized pelvic pain. Pelvic examination may reveal an enlarged and irregularly contoured fibroid uterus or the diffusely enlarged, globular and tender uterus of adenomyosis. IUD strings may no longer be visible if migration has occurred. Cervical stenosis will have findings of a pinpoint os with inability to pass a small dilator or a visibly scared closed os from a prior cervical surgery. The presence of an adnexal mass may be a uterine anomaly, an old tuboovarian complex, an endometrioma, or a cornual leiomyoma.

B. Imaging Studies

Radiographic testing most commonly uses pelvic ultrasonography with both transabdominal and transvaginal studies for diagnosis of most causes of secondary dysmenorrhea. Sonohysterograms can increase the accuracy of diagnosis of intrauterine masses and uterine anomalies. The diagnosis of adenomyosis can be accurately made about 60–70% of the time with pelvic magnetic resonance imaging (MRI). MRI is also helpful in diagnosing uterine anomalies including those with outflow obstructions that could be missed on sonohysterogram.

C. Special Examinations

Hysteroscopy and laparoscopy are commonly performed diagnostic procedures to help characterize and treat the cause of secondary dysmenorrhea.

Differential Diagnosis

The differential diagnosis for dysmenorrhea should include endometriosis, adenomyosis, cervical stenosis, müllerian anomalies, uterine fibroids, endometrial polyps, acute and chronic pelvic inflammatory disease (PID), and IUD-related issues.

Treatment

A. Medical

The treatment of primary dysmenorrhea is aimed at decreasing prostaglandin production and release in the endometrium. NSAIDs are an effective first-line approach (Table 45–1). The patient should begin taking the medication at the onset of menses or just before her expected menses. The medication should be continued for the first 2–3 days of flow. A systematic review of NSAIDs for dysmenorrhea has found that naproxen, ibuprofen, and mefenamic acid are all effective treatment. However, naproxen caused more adverse effects such as nausea, dizziness, and headache.

For patients who desire contraception or who have contraindications to or intolerance of NSAIDs, combination oral contraceptives are also an excellent first-line management choice. They can diminish the amount and duration of flow and may decrease the frequency of menses in women with a short menstrual interval. Patients who have not obtained sufficient relief may benefit from the use of continuous oral contraceptives (without the usual 7-day hiatus) for 3 months at a time to reduce menstrual frequency significantly. The use of other hormonal contraceptive methods such as implantable or injectable progestins is not well documented in the treatment of dysmenorrhea; these methods could be expected to provide relief through ovulation suppression and possible amenorrhea.

It is best to avoid the use of narcotic analgesics. If NSAIDs and oral contraceptives treatment regimens are unsuccessful in relieving the woman's pain, then the diagnosis of primary dysmenorrhea should be questioned and further evaluation (including laparoscopy) should be initiated.

If the patient with secondary dysmenorrhea has an obvious underlying cause, such as cervical stenosis or an IUD, treatment should address that cause. IUD-associated dysmenorrhea may respond to NSAID therapy. If the symptoms are not severe and the patient is willing, a trial of NSAIDs or oral contraceptives should be attempted. This treatment may provide adequate relief and avoid the expense and risk of invasive procedures.

B. Surgical

If the patient is unwilling to undertake symptomatic treatment or it does not provide sufficient relief, a de-

Table 45–1. Nonsteroidal anti-inflammatory drugs (NSAIDs) for the treatment of dysmenorrhea.

Drug	Dose	Frequency	Maximum Daily Dosage
Etodolac[1]	200–400 mg PO	q6–8h	1200 mg
Ibuprofen[2]	400–800 mg PO	q6–8h	3200 mg
Ketoprofen	25–50 mg PO	q6–8h	300 mg
Meclofenamate	100 mg PO	q8h	400 mg
Mefenamic acid	500, then 250 mg PO	q6h	Unavailable
Naproxen sodium[2]	550, then 275 mg PO	q6–8h	1375 mg
Ketorolac[1]	30 mg IM	q6h	120 mg

[1]Not approved for use in dysmenorrhea.
[2]Available over the counter in lower doses.

finitive diagnosis is warranted. When intrauterine disease such as submucosal fibroids or uterine polyps is suspected, the next step in evaluation is a sonohysterogram or hysteroscopy. Not only is a hysteroscopy diagnostic, but it is also therapeutic because it allows resection of fibroids and large polyps. Dilation and curettage is used to remove multiple small polyps. When endometriosis is suspected or hysteroscopy fails to confirm the diagnosis, laparoscopy is performed. Hysteroscopy and laparoscopy are often done as combined procedures in the operating room. Treatment of endometriosis or lysis of pelvic adhesions can be initiated at the time of laparoscopy.

Severe cases of dysmenorrhea that are unresponsive to conservative medical therapy with examination or MRI findings suggestive of adenomyosis require hysterectomy. This is only in women who do not wish to preserve their fertility. Hysterectomy also is performed to manage advanced endometriosis that is not responding to other treatment options. Endometrial ablation has been used successfully in the treatment of menorrhagia; it may reduce or alleviate dysmenorrhea in patients with menorrhagia and no other treatable cause for pain.

C. COMPLEMENTARY THERAPY

Herbal remedies, yoga positions, acupuncture, transcutaneous electrical nerve stimulation (TENS), relaxation techniques, exercise, and nutritional supplements have all been tried as alternative methods to treat and prevent dysmenorrhea. At this time, only TENS units, acupuncture, and 100 mg/d of thiamine have demonstrated effectiveness in clinical studies.

When to Refer to a Specialist

When medical management of dysmenorrhea fails or symptoms are too severe to allow time for a trial of medications, the patient should be referred to a gynecologist capable of performing operative laparoscopy and hysteroscopy for diagnosis and treatment.

Prognosis

About 80% of patients with primary dysmenorrhea respond to medical treatment, and those who do not should be reevaluated for the causes of secondary dysmenorrhea. Medical treatment for secondary dysmenorrhea is less successful; however, an underlying cause usually can be identified and treated. Hysterectomy is the definitive treatment, but it should be reserved for severe and refractory cases.

Davis AR, Westhoff CL et al: Primary dysmenorrhea in adolescent girls and treatment with oral contraceptives. J Pediatr Adolesc Gynecol 2001;14:3. [PMID: 11358700]

Gelbaya TA, El-Halwagy HE et al: Focus on primary care: Chronic pelvic pain in women. Obstet Gynecol Surv 2001;56:757. [PMID: 11753178]

Granot M et al: Pain perception in women with dysmenorrhea: Obstet Gynecol 2001;98:407. [PMID: 11530120]

Hu J: Acupuncture treatment of dysmenorrhea. J Tradit Chin Med 1999;19:313. [PMID: 10921141]

Mehlisch DR: Comparison of bromfenac and naproxen sodium in the management of primary dysmenorrhea. Prim Care Update Ob Gyns 1998;5:195. [PMID: 10838369]

ACUTE PELVIC PAIN

 ESSENTIALS OF DIAGNOSIS

- *Duration is less than 6 months.*
- *Source may be gynecologic, pregnancy-related, gastrointestinal, or urologic.*

General Considerations

Acute pelvic pain is a common reason that women seek urgent gynecologic evaluation. The woman with acute pelvic pain is usually in her reproductive years and may be pregnant at time of presentation.

Young women in the 15- to 19-year-old age group have the greatest incidence of PID, which affects 1 million women each year. Ectopic pregnancy is a life-threatening cause of pelvic pain that occurs in 2% of all pregnancies. Causes of acute pelvic pain such as appendicitis or adnexal torsion also occur most commonly in the 20- to 40-year-old age range (Table 45–2).

Prevention

There are no preventive measures for many causes of acute pelvic pain. However, the use of condoms can lower the incidence of PID and pregnancy. Screening for sexually transmitted infections (STIs) will reduce the number of episodes of PID (see Chapter 34). In addition, many episodes of ruptured ovarian cysts will be prevented by the use of combination oral contraceptives that usually suppress ovulation.

Clinical Findings

A. SYMPTOMS AND SIGNS

The patient may complain of fever, anorexia, emesis, dysuria, hematuria, dyspareunia, abnormal vaginal discharge, or irregular or absent menses in addition to pain originating in the pelvis, lower abdomen, flank, or periumbilically. The timing of the onset of her pain can

Table 45–2. Causes of acute pelvic pain.

Gynecologic
  Adnexal torsion
  Endometriosis
  Infection
    Pelvic inflammatory disease
    Tuboovarian abscess
  Ovarian
    Corpus luteum cyst
    Endometrioma
    Mittelschmerz
    Neoplasm
    Ruptured cyst
  Uterine
    Fibroids: degeneration, torsion
    Dysmenorrhea
Pregnancy-related
  Abortion: septic, spontaneous
  Ectopic pregnancy
Gastrointestinal
  Appendicitis
  Constipation
  Diverticulitis
  Gastroenteritis
  Inflammatory bowel disease
Urologic
  Acute cystitis
  Renal calculi

---

be varied in relation to her menstrual cycle. The initial severity of the pain can range from mild to severe with associated peritoneal signs. The level of pain may then increase or diminish depending on the cause for the pain. A detailed history is invaluable in differentiating the various causes of acute pelvic pain.

The woman with an ectopic pregnancy may have unilateral sharp or spasmodic pain that is constant or intermittent. When a hemoperitoneum develops, rebound and guarding on abdominal examination are common along with posterior shoulder pain referred from diaphragmatic irritation. The patient's vital signs often develop postural changes at this point. The patient's last menses is often irregular in regard to timing or flow. On pelvic examination, there is adnexal tenderness and occasionally a palpable mass. Cervical motion tenderness may be present especially in more advanced stages. (See Chapter 57, Early Pregnancy Loss.)

Women with PID will have symptoms and signs that range in severity from lower abdominal/pelvic tenderness with cervical motion tenderness and adnexal tenderness to severe findings such as rebound and guarding. The onset of the pain is commonly in the early part of the cycle and tends to progress over several days to weeks. Mucopurulent vaginal discharge can be present along with fever and nausea and vomiting. A tender adnexal mass may be palpable on pelvic or rectal examination. (See Chapter 34, Sexually Transmitted Infections & Pelvic Inflammatory Disease.)

The classic presentation of appendicitis is poorly localized umbilical pain that in 1–12 hours localizes to the right lower quadrant; in many cases, however, the right lower quadrant is the first site of pain. The pain location can vary with the location of the appendix, and the occurrence in a long appendix may suggest an adnexal source. The pain is typically moderate to severe and constant, and it increases with movement. The classic complaint on directed questioning is anorexia, which precedes the onset of pain. Although anorexia can occur with other sources of pain, its absence makes appendicitis unlikely. Vomiting frequently follows the onset of pain, but it is rarely prolonged and is not necessary for the diagnosis. Other gastrointestinal symptoms such as constipation or diarrhea are variable in occurrence.

The patient presenting with acute appendicitis is often afebrile but may have a low-grade fever. A temperature of greater than 38°C may represent perforation if the abdominal findings are confirmatory. The abdominal examination classically reveals tenderness at McBurney's point (located one third of the distance above the anterior iliac spine on a line between that spine and the umbilicus), but as noted, the site varies with the location of the appendix. Rebound tenderness is often present at the site of pain as is voluntary guarding.

Adnexal torsion can occur with normal ovaries, an ovarian mass, or a paraovarian cyst; it involves the right side more often than the left. Acute onset of severe, progressive, unilateral pain that may have been preceded by mild intermittent pain for days or weeks is usually the presenting complaint. In advanced cases, there may be generalized pain with guarding and rebound, and nausea and vomiting are often present. In the pregnant patient, the most common time for torsion is during the immediate postpartum period when rapid uterine involution is occurring or during the first trimester after ovarian hyperstimulation with ovulation induction medications.

Passage of a kidney stone is associated with a severe colic type pain that radiates from the flank around to the lower pelvic region and groin. The pain can mimic pain from a gynecologic source especially when the distal ureter is inflamed and distended from the stone passing in the region near the uterus and cervix. Gross hematuria is occasionally noted by the patient. Nausea and deep dyspareunia are also common complaints regardless of the cause of the pain. Anorexia, vomiting, and fever, however, are more specific to the underlying problem. A thorough history often helps narrow the differential diagnosis; pertinent aspects are outlined in Table 45–3.

B. Laboratory and Radiographic Findings

Quantitative serial levels of βHCG in conjunction with transvaginal ultrasound can detect an intrauterine pregnancy (IUP) as early as 3 weeks post conception. βHCG levels increase at least 66% over a 48-hour period in most normal IUPs. Similar βHCG rises are seen in 17% of ectopic pregnancies. At times, the ultrasound information obtained will not confirm an IUP (no yolk sac or fetal pole seen), but no ominous findings exist to diagnose an ectopic. It is important to continue to consider the diagnosis of ectopic pregnancy until a follow up ultrasound can make a definitive diagnosis. (See Chapter 57, Early Pregnancy Loss.)

Laboratory data plays a much smaller role in the diagnosis of PID. Cervical cultures may identify a specific pathogen such as *Chlamydia*, but often this test is negative. Acute elevations of the white blood cell (WBC) count or the erythrocyte sedimentation rate (ESR) may be seen, but these tests are not specific for PID. Ultrasonography can confirm the presence of a tuboovarian abscess.

Women with appendicitis usually have laboratory findings of an elevated WBC count with increased polymorphonuclear neutrophils and bands. No radiographic procedure consistently makes an accurate diagnosis of appendicitis, although many surgeons use the results of computed tomography (CT) scans to aid clinical decision-making.

Patients with a ruptured ovarian cyst or adnexal torsion of a mass will often have an elevated WBC count. Ultrasonography will often detect ascites or bloody fluid. Careful assessment of blood flow to the ovary using color Doppler ultrasonography may help rule out complete torsion of the ovary. This can be misleading when the ovary is not the structure undergoing torsion or if the torsion is of the ovary but is intermittent.

Microscopic urinalysis shows hematuria and at times crystal formation in patients with kidney stones. Finding stone material in the strained urine is the best way to confirm the diagnosis. Ultrasonography may visualize the stone if it is large, but an intravenous pyelogram or CT scan with contrast remains the best diagnostic radiographic options. The increased solute load may also help tiny stones pass.

C. Special Examinations

The vast majority of causes of acute pelvic pain can be differentiated by laparoscopic evaluation of the pelvis and abdomen. Treatment can often be initiated via the laparoscope.

Differential Diagnosis

The most common conditions that are included in the differential diagnoses of acute pelvic pain are ectopic pregnancy, PID, ruptured ovarian cyst, ovarian torsion, appendicitis, and passage of kidney stones (see Table 45–2).

Pregnant women with pelvic pain deserve special consideration. All causes of acute pelvic pain discussed above can occur in pregnant patients. The confusion with normal pregnancy-related symptoms, alterations in abdominal anatomy, and the reluctance to perform invasive or other potentially risky procedures all can lead to a delay in diagnosis and the risk of pregnancy loss.

Adnexal torsion can present in the second trimester and early postpartum period when the uterus undergoes a rapid change in size. As pregnancy advances, the appendix may rotate into the right upper quadrant, confusing the diagnosis of appendicitis. PID rarely occurs in early pregnancy; it usually requires termination of pregnancy for adequate treatment.

Complications

An incorrect diagnosis in the setting of acute pelvic pain can be fatal in the case of a ruptured tubal pregnancy or ruptured appendix. Other serious complications can include loss of a tube and ovary from torsion. Infertility can result from even mild cases of PID.

Table 45–3. Patient history for pelvic pain.

Menstrual: frequency, duration, dysmenorrhea, association with pain, changes since onset of pain

Sexual: orientation, contraception, age at first coitus, number of partners, most recent coitus, dyspareunia

Psychosocial: rape, incest, sexual or physical abuse, depression, alcohol or drug abuse

Infection: pelvic inflammatory disease, sexually transmitted disease (in self or partner)

Surgical: abdominal or pelvic surgery, documented endometriosis

Obstetric: parity, abortions (spontaneous, induced), ectopic pregnancy, desire for current pregnancy if applicable, desire for fertility

Current pain complaint:

  Description: location, quality, intensity, duration, frequency, radiation, changes since onset, factors that ameliorate and exacerbate, association with menstrual cycle

  Associated symptoms: breast tenderness, fever, nausea, vomiting, change in bowel habits, dysuria, vaginal bleeding

  Use of pain medications

  Patient's concerns and fears regarding the cause

Treatment

Medical and surgical treatment options for ectopic pregnancies are discussed in Chapter 57, Early Pregnancy Loss.

Outpatient treatment of mild PID as per the Centers for Disease Control recommendations include 400 mg of oral ofloxacin twice daily for 14 days and 500 mg of oral metronidazole twice daily for 14 days. Alternative regimens are detailed in Chapter 34. All patients must be reevaluated in 48–72 hours and hospitalized if they are not improved. In all cases of PID, the patient's partner should have a culture taken, if possible, and should be treated whether or not symptoms or signs are present. If the presenting symptoms and signs are severe, additional criteria should be used to aid in the differential diagnosis: a temperature greater than 38°C, leukocytosis, positive test for cervical *Chlamydia trachomatis* or *Neisseria gonorrhoeae,* elevated C-reactive protein, elevated ESR, or presence of inflammation on endometrial biopsy. Inpatient therapy should be initiated for the patient with moderate or severe findings, a tuboovarian abscess, who is pregnant, who has not responded to outpatient therapy, or one in whom compliance is questionable. Parenteral treatment regimens are 2 g of intravenous cefotetan every 12 hours with 100 mg of intravenous or oral doxycycline every 12 hours. Alternatives are listed in Chapter 34. Inpatient treatment should lead to improvement in 3–5 days and should be continued for 48 hours after significant clinical improvement is seen. Patients in whom treatment fails require laparoscopy to confirm the diagnosis and evacuate abscesses.

Surgical treatment is required for removal of the adnexal structure that has undergone torsion if the tissue is nonviable. If the tissue is viable, relieving the torsion laparoscopically can be attempted.

A ruptured ovarian cyst may require laparoscopic evaluation if a drop in hematocrit continues to progress indicating ongoing bleeding. Otherwise, the treatment is focused on pain management for the 4–5 days required for resolution in the majority of cases.

When to Refer to a Specialist

Most patients with acute pelvic pain can be managed by a primary health care professional. If the patient is severely ill and the diagnosis is unclear, however, an appropriate consultation is imperative. Any diagnosis with the potential need for surgery requires a consultation; the need for surgery may develop on an emergent basis. The availability of a gynecologic or general surgeon is crucial for cases of ectopic pregnancy, adnexal torsion, and appendicitis; the surgeon should be notified as soon as the diagnosis is considered.

Pregnant patients with unusual abdominal or pelvic pain should be evaluated by a provider who has a firm understanding of the alterations the condition may impose on the patient's presentation.

Prognosis

Despite conservative surgery or medical treatment for ectopic pregnancy, the likelihood of recurrence is about 20%. There is also an increased likelihood of infertility. The prognosis for immediate cure in PID, when diagnosed and treated early, is excellent; however, there is also a long-term risk of infertility. In advanced cases, there is a high risk of subsequent development of infertility, ectopic pregnancies, and chronic pelvic pain (CPP).

The prognosis is excellent for an uncomplicated recovery if appendicitis is treated prior to rupture. A ruptured appendix is a serious condition that can lead to abscess and extensive adhesion formation with subsequent chronic pain and infertility. The consequences of rupture warrant a low threshold for diagnosis and a willingness to err on the side of removing normal appendixes.

Bau A, Atri M et al: Acute female pelvic pain: ultrasound evaluation. Semin Ultrasound CT MR 2000;21:78. [PMID: 10688069]

Hewitt G, Brown RT: Acute and chronic pelvic pain in female adolescents. Med Clin North Am 2000;84:1009. [PMID: 10928199]

ENDOMETRIOSIS

 ESSENTIALS OF DIAGNOSIS

- *Endometrial glands and stroma are present in locations outside the uterine cavity.*
- *Dysmenorrhea, dyspareunia, or CPP commonly is present.*
- *Often, infertility is the only presenting symptom.*

General Considerations

Endometriosis has an estimated incidence of 7% in the general female population. In infertility patients, the prevalence is 38%, and approximately 70% of patients with CPP have endometriosis. The patient whose sister or mother had endometriosis will have a significant increased risk of developing endometriosis herself. Other well-known risk factors fall in the category of outflow obstruction of menstrual blood, such as cervical stenosis or müllerian tract anomalies. Lastly, women with excessive menstrual flow are also at greater risk.

Prevention

A menopausal or hypoestrogenic state will significantly reduce the likelihood of developing endometriosis.

Clinical Findings

A. SYMPTOMS AND SIGNS

The patient with endometriosis may complain of a variety of symptoms. The most common are dysmenorrhea, deep dyspareunia, low back pain, CPP, and infertility. When endometriosis is present, acute onset of severe pain can indicate ovarian torsion or rupture. Deeply infiltrating implants of endometriosis are strongly associated with pelvic pain. Findings on pelvic examination in the patient with endometriosis commonly include nodularity and tenderness on palpation of the uterosacral ligaments or cul-de-sac. Less frequently, the uterus is positioned in fixed retroversion or an adnexal cystic mass will be palpable.

B. LABORATORY FINDINGS

CA-125 levels are often elevated in advanced stage endometriosis. Cases of minimal and mild endometriosis do not show the same statistical correlation with serum CA-125 levels.

C. IMAGING STUDIES

Ultrasound findings of a complex adnexal mass with low level homogeneous internal echoes is often consistent with an endometrioma. Superficial implants of endometriosis cannot be imaged with ultrasound or any other technique currently available. MRI of the pelvis may be helpful in diagnosing deeply infiltrating endometriosis of the cul-de-sac or rectovaginal septum.

D. LAPAROSCOPY

The diagnosis and staging of endometriosis (revised American Society of Reproductive Medicine staging) is done by laparoscopic evaluation and often by biopsy of questionable lesions. Often, there is poor correlation between staging of disease at laparoscopy and the patient's severity of symptoms.

There is some debate whether laparoscopic evaluations for pelvic pain should include random biopsies of peritoneum if no implants are seen. Histologic findings of endometriosis are seen in approximately 20% of these biopsies.

Differential Diagnosis

The differential diagnosis for endometriosis includes PID, adenomyosis, pelvic adhesions, interstitial cystitis, and functional bowel disease. When an endometrioma is present, the differential diagnosis also includes both benign and malignant ovarian tumors.

Complications

Given the invasive nature of endometriosis, deeply infiltrating disease of the intestinal and urinary tracts and secondary obstruction of those viscera occur in advanced endometriosis. Endometriomas can rupture leading to episodes of acute pain and formation of dense scar tissue. Infertility remains the major complication caused by endometriosis. Women with stage I and stage II endometriosis and infertility who underwent laparoscopic resection and ablation of their endometriosis had statistically significant enhanced fecundity compared with similarly matched controls who only had diagnostic laparoscopy.

Stage III and stage IV endometriosis clearly impair fertility because of severe adhesions that significantly distort anatomy and block fallopian tubes. Many of these women with advanced endometriosis eventually need assisted reproductive technologies to conceive.

Treatment

At the time of laparoscopic diagnosis of endometriosis, treatment should be initiated surgically via electrocautery, laser, or excision. Sixty-two percent of women with stage I to stage III endometriosis who underwent laparoscopic surgical therapy had relief of pain symptoms lasting 6 months. When only diagnostic laparoscopy was performed, 22% of the patients had improvement in pain symptoms. Although medical therapy will not lead to complete resolution of endometriosis, the size of the lesions can be significantly decreased and pain symptoms can often be reduced. However, medical therapy is unlikely to be beneficial when the only symptom related to endometriosis is infertility. Medical treatments include oral contraceptives, Depo Provera, danazol, and gonadotropin releasing hormone (GnRH) agonists (Table 45–4). For stage I and II disease, starting with oral contraceptive therapy for a 3-month trial is appropriate. If symptoms do not improve on this regimen, then one of the other medical therapies should be initiated. GnRH agonists, which create a hypoestrogenic state by suppression of pituitary gonadotropins, have been shown to prolong the interval of pain reduction obtained after laparoscopic treatment for up to 18 months. The common side effects are those related to the hypoestrogenic state such as hot flushes, insomnia, decreased libido, vaginal dryness, and headache, all of which are reversible. A decrease in bone mineral density of 6–12% has been shown with the use of these agents, which may be reversible only

Table 45–4. Medical therapies for endometriosis.

Agent	Dose	Route	Frequency	Duration	Price[1]
GnRH[†] agonists					
Depot leuprolide	3.75 mg	IM	qmo	3–6 mo	$475
Nafarelin acetate	200 µg	Intranasal	bid	3–6 mo	$431
Goserelin acetate	3.6 mg	IM implant	q28d	3–6 mo	$521
Danazol	400 mg	PO	bid	3–6 mo	$444
Progestins					
Medroxyprogesterone acetate	30 mg	PO	qd	4–6 mo	$35
Megestrol acetate	40 mg	PO	qd	4–6 mo	$48
Depomedroxyprogesterone acetate	150 mg	IM	q3mo	6 mo +	$63
Oral contraceptives					
Ethinyl estradiol + levonorgestrel	30 µg + 0.15 mg	PO	qd	6 mo	$29

GnRH, gonadotropin releasing hormone.
[1]Wholesale price, USA, 2002, for 30 days of treatment.

partially. Amenorrhea usually occurs in 4–6 weeks, and treatment is continued for 6 months; however, recent reports suggest 3 months may be adequate. There are also studies showing that the addition of norethindrone and conjugated estrogens, the so-called "add-back" therapy, will reduce the side effects including bone mineral loss without compromising the reduction in pain symptoms.

Danazol is an androgen derivative that causes an inhibition of endometrial growth. The side effects reflect the hypoestrogenic state as well as the androgenic and anabolic effects of the medication. Hot flushes, vaginal dryness, emotional lability, weight gain, fluid retention, and acne are the more common side effects; there is a lower incidence of hirsutism, decreased breast size, and deepening of the voice. The drug may cause a mild elevation of liver function tests and a decrease in high-density lipoprotein levels. These side effects generally are reversible, although there are a few cases of permanent voice changes. These side effects have led to decreased patient acceptance of danazol as the GnRH agonists have become available.

Medroxyprogesterone acetate is as effective as danazol in the treatment of endometriosis, but it is used less often as other agents have gained favor. The most common side effect is breakthrough bleeding; others include weight gain, bloating, edema, and emotional lability. Depomedroxyprogesterone acetate should be considered as a cost-effective, long-term therapy especially after a course of GnRH agonists.

New therapies may focus on treating endometriosis as an autoimmune disease. Patients with endometriosis have elevated levels of cytokines, which can stimulate endometrial cell adhesion to peritoneal surfaces. Endometriotic implants produce excess amounts of proteases that allow for the endometriosis to invade the underlying cell tissue layer. The implants of endometriosis are able to escape cell death because of a modification of the apoptotic process. Of interest is that this modification can be returned to normal by GnRH analog therapy, which causes suppression of ovarian steroid formation and secondarily a hypoestrogenic state. GnRH analogs as well as progestins and danazol can all act to suppress cytokine levels. Pentoxifylline is a immunomodulatory agent that reduces the production and action of cytokines which, in turn, leads to the regression of ectopic endometrial tissue. This all occurs without the hypoestogenic state and all of its side effects. Total abdominal hysterectomy with bilateral salpingoophorectomy is reserved for advanced cases in women who do not desire future fertility. Estrogen replacement therapy can usually be initiated postoperatively. Involvement of other organs with endometriosis such as the bladder, ureter, or bowel requires surgical treatment.

Herbal remedies, yoga positions, acupuncture, relaxation techniques, and nutritional supplements have all been used to treat endometriosis and its associated symptoms.

When to Refer to a Specialist

Women in whom endometriosis is suspected are best managed by laparoscopy for diagnosis, staging, and initial therapy. Therefore, early referral to a gynecologist is indicated. The gynecologist should have expertise in complicated operative endoscopy to maximize the chances of thorough laparoscopic treatment.

Prognosis

The medical management of endometriosis leads to symptomatic improvement in approximately 80% of patients; however, the 5-year recurrence rate is 20–40%. Even after total abdominal hysterectomy and bilateral salpingo-oophorectomy, the potential exists for recurrent symptoms and disease.

In at least 2 clinical trials, laparosopy 6–12 months after placebo treatment showed spontaneous resolution of endometriosis lesions in one third of patients, deterioration in about one half, and no change in the remainder.

Revised American Society for Reproductive Medicine classification of endometriosis: 1996. Fertil Steril 1997;67:817. [PMID: 9130884]

American College of Obstetricians and Gynecologists. Medical Management of Endometriosis. ACOG Practice Bulletin #11. ACOG, 1999.

Azem F et al: Patients with stages III and IV endometriosis have a poorer outcome of in vitro fertilization-embryo transfer than patients with tubal infertility. Fertil Steril 1999;72:1107. [PMID: 10593389]

Berube S et al: Fecundity of infertile women with minimal or mild endometriosis and women with unexplained infertility. The Canadian Collaborative Group on Endometriosis. Fertil Steril 1998;69:1034. [PMID: 9627289]

Franke HR et al: Gonadotropin-releasing hormone agonist plus "add-back" hormone replacement therapy for treatment of endometriosis: a prospective, randomized, placebo-controlled, double-blind trial. Fertil Steril 2000;74:534. [PMID: 10973651]

Harada T, Iwabe T, Terakawa N: Role of cytokines in endometriosis. Fertil Steril 2001;76:1. [PMID: 11438312]

Kettel LM et al: Preliminary report on the treatment of endometriosis with low-dose mifepristone (RU 486). Am J Obstet Gynecol 1998;178:1151. [PMID: 9662295]

Kwok A, Lam A, Ford R: Deeply infiltrating endometriosis: implications, diagnosis, and management. Obstet Gynecol Surv 2001;56:168. [PMID: 11254153]

Lebovic DI, Mueller MD, Taylor RN: Immunobiology of endometriosis. Fertil Steril 2001;75:1. [PMID: 11163805]

Lessey BA: Medical management of endometriosis and infertility. Fertil Steril 2000;73:1089. [PMID: 10856462]

Marcoux S, Maheux R, Berube S: Laparoscopic surgery in infertile women with minimal or mild endometriosis. The Canadian Collaborative Group on Endometriosis. N Engl J Med 1997; 337:217. [PMID: 9227926]

Muzii L: Atypical endometriosis revisited: clinical and biochemical evaluation of the different forms of superficial implants. Fertil Steril 2000;74:739. [PMID: 11020516]

Nothnick WB: Treating endometriosis as an autoimmune disease. Fertil Steril 2001;76:223. [PMID: 11476764]

Olive DL, Pritts EA: Treatment of endometriosis. N Engl J Med 2001;345:266. [PMID: 11474666]

Tulandi T, al-Took S: Reproductive outcome after treatment of mild endometriosis with laparoscopic excision and electrocoagulation. Fertil Steril 1998;69:229. [PMID: 9496333]

Walter AJ: Endometriosis: correlation between histologic and visual findings at laparoscopy. Am J Obstet Gynecol 2001;184: 1407. [PMID: 11408860]

CHRONIC PELVIC PAIN

 ESSENTIALS OF DIAGNOSIS

- *Noncyclic pelvic or lower abdominal pain greater than 6 months in duration.*
- *Underlying disease processes associated with CPP syndrome may be from diseases of gynecologic, gastrointestinal, urologic, musculoskeletal, rheumatologic. and/or psychiatric origin.*
- *Women with CPP have higher rates of sexual, physical, and emotional abuse than do women without pain.*

General Considerations

Approximately 10% of outpatient gynecologic office visits, 25–40% of diagnostic laparoscopies, and 13% of hysterectomies are for CPP. CPP syndrome is most commonly seen in women between the ages of 25 and 35 years. In some cases, there has been a specific surgery or acute illness that has preceded the development of CPP syndrome. Often, there is a history of sexual trauma, child abuse, depression, relationship and sexual dysfunction, and other chronic pain syndromes.

Clinical Findings

A. SYMPTOMS AND SIGNS

The location, quality, intensity, and timing of the pain varies significantly as would be expected given the tremendous number of diseases that can give rise to CPP. Findings of dyspareunia and protracted dysmenorrhea (beginning well before and lasting long after the menses), and menorrhagia are very common. Urinary complaints and irritable bowel symptoms also frequently overlap with the gynecologic symptoms. The psychological component of CPP only recently is becoming understood. It is not clear whether this component is the result of a psychological disorder preceding the onset of pain and exacerbated by it, or the result of the patient's response to her chronic pain. Differentiation is unnecessary; the psychological component of the patient's condition needs to be addressed for an adequate chance of treatment success.

When a complete physical examination is performed (especially focusing on the back, abdominal, pelvic, and rectal areas), a variety of findings may be elicited. Palpation of the abdominal wall with the patient in a half sitting position tenses the rectus muscle and helps differentiate pain within the wall from that of a deeper source. If the patient complains of vaginal pain or dyspareunia, palpation with a cotton swab may reveal trigger points. The pelvic floor muscles (levators and piriformis) should be examined for tenderness, and an attempt to duplicate deep dyspareunia should be made with the bimanual examination. (See Chapter 46, Management of Chronic Pelvic Pain: Musculoskeletal & Psychological Considerations.) It should be remembered that the physical examination results correlate only infrequently with the patient's pain symptoms.

B. LABORATORY FINDINGS

Blood work may include a complete blood cell count, ESR, antinuclear antibodies, thyroid-stimulating hormine, and creatinine. Cervical cultures for STIs and urinalysis with microscopic analysis should also be obtained.

C. IMAGING STUDIES

In the presence of an adequate examination with normal findings, ultrasonography rarely reveals new findings of significance. When the patient has gastrointestinal complaints along with her CPP, a barium enema and a CT scan can be used for more detailed evaluation. Intravenous pyelogram and/or CT scan can delineate whether pathologic findings of the urinary tract are present. MRI may identify deeply infiltrating endometriosis of the cul-de-sac or rectovaginal septum as well as adenomyosis.

D. SPECIAL EXAMINATIONS

Laparoscopy has been considered the ultimate diagnostic test for CPP. In light of the recent understanding of the disease, laparoscopy may not always be indicated.

Laparoscopy remains an excellent diagnostic tool if the history is suggestive of endometriosis or adhesions, examination suggests pelvic disease, or the pain is well localized and reproducible. However, it should be used judiciously not routinely. Studies have shown that approximately 28% of patients with CPP have endometriosis, and 25–50% have adhesions found at the time of laparoscopy. How these factors relate to the patient's pain is not well understood because many asymptomatic patients also have these findings. The location and extent of disease in patients with CPP rarely explains their pain, and treatment of the pathologic condition alone has limited success. Other studies have shown a 47% incidence of occult somatic disease (eg, urethral syndrome, irritable bowel syndrome, abdominal wall trigger points) in patients with CPP and a negative laparoscopic evaluation. Overall, it is estimated that about 39% of patients have no abnormal findings with laparoscopy.

Cystoscopy may find evidence of interstitial cystitis and colonoscopy provides an opportunity to evaluate the colonic mucosa for evidence of inflammatory bowel disease.

Differential Diagnosis

The following disease states can contribute to the formation of CPP:

Gastrointestinal—Irritable bowel disease, inflammatory bowel disease, and colorectal cancer.

Gynecologic—Endometriosis, adenomyosis, PID, malignancies, chronic vaginitis, pelvic/abdominal adhesions, ovarian remnant syndrome.

Rheumatologic—Fibromyalgia and regional pain syndromes.

Urologic—Interstitial cystitis, urethral syndrome, kidney stones.

Psychiatric—Depression, prior sexual trauma, somatization.

Musculoskeletal—Abdominal wall defects, incisional neuroma, and lumbar disc disease.

Treatment

Psychological issues are present in at least 50% of patients with CPP. It is therefore essential to address these issues initially with the patient and give referral to mental health specialists as well as to the specialists who are most appropriate to evaluate and treat the patient's symptoms.

Multispecialty pain management clinics offer a range of therapies that usually are administered by an anesthesiologist and physical medicine specialist. Nerve blocks, trigger point injections, intrathecal morphine pumps are used with a variety of medications that affect the pain nerve pathways. These include selective serotonin reuptake inhibitors, tricyclic antidepressants, gabapentin, and as a last resort long-term narcotic administration.

Even when documented pathology is found, surgery may lead to improvement in the patient's pain symptoms in only select cases. In 1 study, an improvement in pain at 1 year following laparoscopic lysis of pelvic adhesions was found in 75% of patients without CPP and in only 40% of patients with CPP. This speaks to the multifactorial cause of CPP syndrome and to the fact that the pain from the original problem may have lasted long enough to cause the CPP syndrome itself. In cases of "residual ovary syndrome" or "ovarian remnant syndrome," surgical treatment is necessary to remove the ovarian tissue, but not all patients have resolution of their CPP syndrome postoperatively. Laparoscopic presacral neurectomy and laparoscopic uterine nerve ablation have helped some patients with CPP who had very well-defined midline pain.

Based on treatment for endometriosis, GnRH agonists have been employed with some success in patients who also have CPP syndrome. In one study, more than 70% of patients with CPP felt significantly better with GnRH agonist therapy, even when laparoscopy failed to find endometriosis.

It is important to begin an integrated approach to the patient with CPP syndrome at the onset of evaluation. This approach decreases the risk of somatic fixation on the part of the patient and decreases the pursuit of inappropriate treatment such as "definitive surgery." The patient should be advised that in many cases of CPP an underlying cause is not found; regardless of the presence or absence of an organic cause, however, she needs to be aware of the role the psychological component plays. The clinician should explain the relationship of significant past or present stressors to the patient's ability to cope with pain. It is best to mention at the first visit that the diagnostic work-up may involve a psychiatrist, psychologist, social worker, physical therapist, and nutritionist, among others. Most patients with CPP require more than diagnosis and treatment of underlying disease. Addressing the psychological component from the beginning may help the patient understand the depth of the problem and the lack of an immediate cure. Reassurance that her physical findings are not life-threatening and that removal of her uterus and adnexa will not cure her pain may help her to accept a treatment plan. Frequently scheduled visits for emotional support and to monitor treatment may decrease the pain-reinforcing behavior of emergency visits. Psychological and sometimes musculoskeletal considerations are key to a long-term treatment plan (see Chapter 46, Management of Chronic Pelvic Pain: Musculoskeletal & Psychological Considerations).

When to Refer to a Specialist

The primary care provider is in an excellent position to treat patients with CPP. These patients require extensive education and counseling as well as coordination of specialty consultations with psychologists, gynecologists, or physical therapists. A physical therapy consultation should be considered when musculoskeletal components are suspected or identified or when biofeedback is a consideration for treatment. CPP is a complex, poorly understood process that in many cases requires skilled, long-term treatment. Severely disabled patients are best managed in multispecialty pain clinics or by providers who have appropriate resources available.

American College of Obstetrics and Gynecology. Adult Manifestations of Childhood Sexual Abuse. ACOG Educational Bulletin #259. ACOG 2000.

Ling FW: Randomized controlled trial of depot leuprolide in patients with chronic pelvic pain and clinically suspected endometriosis. Pelvic Pain Study. Obstet Gynecol 1999;93:51. [PMID: 9916956]

Zondervan KT et al: Chronic pelvic pain in the community—symptoms, investigations, and diagnoses. Am J Obstet Gynecol 2001;184:1149. [PMID: 11349181]

Relevant Web Sites

[American College of Obstetricians & Gynecologists All publications and educational material can be ordered.]

www.acog.com

[American Society of Reproductive Medicine]

www.asrm.org

[Centers for Disease Control and Prevention]

www.cdc.gov/mmwr

[Healthwell.com provides alternative health care and nutritional and herbal therapies for a multitude of medical problems. Limited by the lack of good studies supporting many of the therapies.]

www.healthwell.com

[The Endometriosis Association is an international organization that provides education and support for women with endometriosis.]

http://www.endometriosisassn.org

Management of Chronic Pelvic Pain: Musculoskeletal & Psychological Considerations

46

Mitchell Levy, MD & Kathe Wallace, PT

Chronic pelvic pain (CPP), a condition spanning the domain between organic dysfunction and psychological distress, poses a challenge to practitioner and patient alike. The scope of the problem is extensive: studies estimate CPP may represent 2–10% of outpatient gynecologic referrals. Over 50% of these patients lack an etiologic diagnosis and of those, nearly 60% experience lost work time or reduced productivity. Women seeking medical treatment for this condition often report dissatisfaction with their care and doctor-patient communication. Management of CPP involves appropriate and thorough assessment for treatable causes of pain and awareness of underlying or occult conditions (see Chapter 45, Dysmenorrhea, Endometriosis, & Pelvic Pain). Conversely, management also must address the suffering of those patients with clear organic disease (eg, endometriosis) in whom a complex and CPP syndrome develops. Assembling a program aimed at alleviating a persistent pain problem often shifts clinical focus from "cure" to improving psychosocial function and relieving disability.

Not all women who experience CPP feel it is severe enough to seek medical help; some live productive lives with persistent, low-level pain. The development of disability appears to be an important factor in the establishment and maintenance of CPP, and it is predictive of high levels of medical care use and poor treatment outcome.

Musculoskeletal factors have been frequently overlooked in a traditional biopsychological model of CPP. The musculoskeletal origin of CPP must be considered in a comprehensive evaluation of and treatment plan for patients with CPP.

In addition, physical therapy addresses the physical and functional changes brought on by the vicious cycle of chronic pain.

MUSCULOSKELETAL CONSIDERATIONS

ESSENTIALS OF DIAGNOSIS

- *Chronic tension in the pelvic floor muscles can result from a variety of musculoskeletal, psychogenic, genitourinary or iatrogenic causes and can result in CPP.*
- *Musculoskeletal examinations for CPP should include a postural assessment, range of motion and strength testing, and pelvic floor muscle examination.*
- *A pelvic floor muscle examination can localize specific muscle problems including pelvic floor hypertonus, tenderness, or trigger points.*

General Considerations

In patients with CPP, identification of any musculoskeletal dysfunction is important. A chronic pain-tension cycle can develop from orthopedic malalignment, postural abnormalities, pelvic floor muscle dysfunction, urogynecologic and colorectal disease, or psychological dysfunction.

Specifically, lumbar, sacroiliac, or hip joint malalignment or disease can affect the pelvic muscles, causing limitations in range of motion, strength, muscle length, posture, and functional activities. In 1 study, 75% of patients with CPP were found to have a typical pattern of faulty posture. Myofascial pain and dysfunction have been identified in specific muscles of the pelvic region by Travell and Simons. The coccygeus, levator ani, obturator internus, adductor magnus, piriformis, and oblique abdominal muscles can have trigger points that refer pain to the pelvic region.

Psychological causes of pain can lead to changes in posture as well as chronic muscle tension. Although psychological causes of pain frequently are difficult to separate from musculoskeletal causes, patients often consider musculoskeletal causes of pain more tangible and acceptable.

Painful visceral or systemic medical conditions such as endometriosis or interstitial cystitis can cause tension to be held in the pelvic floor musculature. Chronic tension in these muscles can lead to pain in the pelvic region. This condition is called a **hypertonus dysfunction of the pelvic floor.** Frequently, such a dysfunction may be caused by any of the following factors:

1. Musculoskeletal—Postural dysfunction, joint or soft tissue restrictions of the musculoskeletal system
2. Psychogenic—Sexual abuse, muscle tension in pelvic floor and abdomen caused by stress
3. Visceral or systemic—Pelvic inflammation, infection, or disease
4. Iatrogenic—Surgeries with urogenital or rectal approaches or episiotomy
5. Neurologic factors—Entrapment of the pudendal nerve.

Clinical Findings

A. SYMPTOMS AND SIGNS

Pelvic floor tension myalgia is a diagnostic term used to describe a wide variety of syndromes of pelvic floor muscle hypertonus. These syndromes include levator ani syndrome, levator spasm syndrome, coccygodynia, vaginismus, and piriformis syndrome. Often, pelvic floor hypertonus problems are labeled **levator ani syndrome.** The primary symptom is pain that is usually poorly localized in the perivaginal area, perirectal region, lower abdominal quadrants, or pelvis. In addition, suprapubic, coccygeal, posterior thigh, vulvar, or clitoral localization of pain is sometimes present.

Other conditions that may have a component of pelvic floor hypertonus dysfunction include chronic low back pain, urethral syndrome, vulvodynia, sphincter dyssynergia, and fibromyalgia.

A musculoskeletal screening examination is indicated in patients who complain of pelvic and abdominal pain, suprapubic pressure, or urogenital symptoms. Key factors in a patient's history include symptom alteration caused by stress, activity, or position changes. It is important to screen for a history of spinal or lower

extremity trauma, injury, or pathologic conditions. Musculoskeletal examinations include a postural assessment, range of motion and strength testing, and pelvic floor muscle examination.

Pelvic floor muscle examinations should be a routine part of the screening evaluation. In a pelvic examination, the speculum covers the pelvic floor musculature, and its examination frequently is overlooked. Internal and external palpation of the pelvic floor can locate and isolate specific muscle problems including increased tone (pelvic floor hypertonus), tenderness, or trigger points. One component of this examination is the specific palpation of the pelvic musculature. When performed externally, it is called the **pelvic clock examination,** which is illustrated in Figure 46–1. With the patient in a lithotomy position, an external palpation examination is performed to assess muscle tone, tenderness, or trigger points of the perineum. The individual muscles of the perineum can be assessed clockwise, starting from the symphysis pubis and moving to the ischial tuberosities, and the perineal body. Each number on an imaginary clock is palpated to identify the muscle that may be contributing to the pain or hypertonus dysfunction. The urogenital triangle is represented by the 1, 2, 3, 9, 10, 11, and 12 o'clock positions. The deeper levator ani muscles in the anal triangle are represented by the 4, 5, 7, and 8 o'clock positions. The 1 and 11 o'clock positions represent the ischiocavernosus muscle. The 2 and 10 o'clock positions represent the bulbocavernosus muscle. The 3 and 9 o'clock positions represent the superficial transverse perineal muscle. The 4, 5, 7, and 8 o'clock positions represent the levator ani muscles. The 6 o'clock position represents the perineal body. The 12 o'clock position represents the boney landmark of the pubic symphysis.

B. SPECIAL TESTS

Surface electromyography (SEMG) biofeedback evaluation with anal or vaginal electrodes can objectify muscle activity and monitor skeletal muscle tension of the pelvic floor and the related musculature.

C. SPECIAL EXAMINATIONS

Positive findings in the initial screening examination warrant a comprehensive musculoskeletal evaluation by a physical therapist.

This evaluation should include a patient interview and a review of the patient's medical history. During the interview, the patient's functional limitations are outlined, and a list is made of the patient's present techniques of pain management. The physical examination includes a neurologic scan examination and an assessment of trunk and lower extremity muscle strength, active and passive range of motion, joint mobility, and myofascial and scar tissue restrictions. Static and dy-

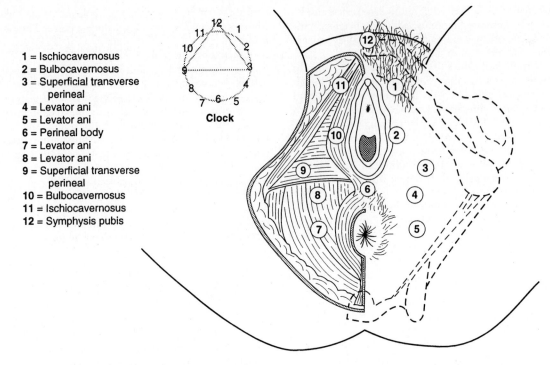

1 = Ischiocavernosus
2 = Bulbocavernosus
3 = Superficial transverse
    perineal
4 = Levator ani
5 = Levator ani
6 = Perineal body
7 = Levator ani
8 = Levator ani
9 = Superficial transverse
    perineal
10 = Bulbocavernosus
11 = Ischiocavernosus
12 = Symphysis pubis

Clock

Figure 46–1. Pelvic clock examination. Muscles of perineum are palpated in order, according to corresponding numbers of superimposed clock face. (Reproduced, with permission, from Herman H, Wallace K: *The APTA Section on Obstetrics and Gynecology, Pelvic Floor Seminar Manual.* American Physical Therapy Association, 1993.)

namic postural alignment in standing, sitting, and walking also is assessed. In addition, specific muscle palpation in the pelvic floor (the pelvic clock examination), trunk, and hip musculature can identify the muscles that may be referring pain to the pelvic region.

Treatment

The physical therapy evaluation identifies musculoskeletal problems requiring treatment. Goals of treatment include management and reduction of musculoskeletal factors that could contribute to or cause CPP and its frequent sequelae of dyspareunia.

Herman (2000) outlines how orthopedic malalignment should be treated with manual therapy techniques. Functional and postural limitations should be treated with specific exercise programs for the pelvic floor and abdominal wall.

Chronic pain and muscle guarding require patient education in the physiology of pain and instruction on muscle relaxation techniques. Therapeutic interventions include specific pelvic floor exercises, scar mobilization, myofascial release, and trigger point treatment.

Physical therapy modalities such as heat, cold, and electrotherapy may provide pain relief and physiologic quieting. The emphasis should be on introducing treatment that is aimed at reducing the musculoskeletal factors of CPP and breaking the CPP using physical therapy interventions and biofeedback. An additional home program of relaxation and key therapeutic exercises is also beneficial.

Biofeedback can be used to facilitate self-regulation of pain and to assist with the diagnosis of hypertonus dysfunction and treatment of CPP. The desired outcome is to shape a self-management response to pain. The goal of biofeedback is to learn control of typical physiologic responses to pain and dysfunction through the use of SEMG, electrodermal response, respiration, and skin temperature.

Computer-assisted equipment is available to enhance the quality of the feedback provided. Visual and audio signals assist the patient in learning self-regulation of pain. Typical relaxation training such as diaphragmatic breathing, Jacobson relaxation techniques, imagery, and autogenic training all are enhanced by the use of biofeedback.

SEMG biofeedback is a training device that assists the patient in identifying the difference between a contracted and a relaxed muscle. This training helps the patient identify chronic muscle tension holding patterns and assists with performance of pelvic floor exercises. Patients learn to detect changes in muscle tension that can occur from increased pain. Specific vaginal and rectal electrodes are available to treat pelvic floor muscles with SEMG; they are particularly useful because the pelvic floor muscles are frequently difficult to identify and exercise properly.

For the symptom of dyspareunia a common sequelae of CPP and vulvodynia, Glazer reports the use of pelvic floor SEMG biofeedback evaluation and home SEMG treatment. This approach was based on examination of the pelvic floor, which showed hyperirritability of the pelvic floor with local tenderness when compressed. SEMG biofeedback demonstrated abnormally high or unstable resting baseline levels. Treatment consisted of two 20-minute sessions of pelvic muscle exercises with 10 seconds of work and 10 seconds of rest for 60 repetitions. This protocol was designed to "break" the tension level with active exercise. This protocol produced an average of 83% reduction in subjective pain reports in women with vulvovaginal pain.

The goals of biofeedback treatment are to encourage behavioral changes in pain management and to learn and practice normal use of the pelvic floor muscles. As part of a comprehensive treatment program using a biopsychosocial model, biofeedback treatment can provide a nonpharmacologic approach to relaxation and pain management.

When to Refer to a Specialist

A musculoskeletal screening examination, including a pelvic floor muscle examination can be done by the primary care provider. Abnormal findings should prompt referral to a physical therapist. The American Physical Therapy Association has a specialty Section on Women's Health. This subgroup of physical therapists specializes in obstetric and gynecologic evaluation and treatment.

Baker PK: Musculoskeletal origins of chronic pelvic pain. Diagnosis and treatment. Obstet Gynecol Clin North Am 1993; 20:719. [PMID: 8115087]

Glazer HI et al: Treatment of vulvar vestibulitis syndrome with electromyographic biofeedback of pelvic floor musculature. J Reproduct Med 1995;40:283. [PMID: 7623358]

Herman H: Conservative management of female patients with pelvic pain. Urol Nurs 2000;20:393.

Markwell SJ: Physical therapy management of pelvi/perineal and perianal pain syndromes. World J Urol 2001;19:194. [PMID: 11469607]

Meadows E: Treatments for patients with pelvic pain. Urol Nurs 1999;19:33. [PMID: 10373990]

Kasman GS, Cram JR, Wolf SL: *Clinical Applications in Surface Electromyography: Chronic Musculoskeletal Pain.* Gaithersburg, Md: Aspen Publishers, 1998.

King PM et al: Musculoskeletal factors in chronic pelvic pain. J Psychom Obstet Gyneaecol 1991;12:87.

Simons D, Travell J, Simons L: Myofascial pain and dysfunction. *The Trigger Point Manual.* 2nd ed, vol 1. Baltimore, Md: Williams & Wilkins, 1999.

Sinaki M, Merrit J, Stillwell GK: Tension myalgia of the pelvic floor. Mayo Clin Proc 1977;52:717. [PMID: 926848]

PSYCHOLOGICAL CONSIDERATIONS

ESSENTIALS OF DIAGNOSIS

- *A history of childhood or adult sexual victimization, physical abuse, or emotional abuse is more likely in women with CPP than in those without symptoms.*
- *Alternate between biomedical and psychosocial emphases in the evaluation and use the term "stress" as a common explanatory mode.*

General Considerations

Management of multifactorial conditions such as CPP strains medical models, dividing problems into strictly "body" or "mind" related. Acknowledging patient and provider frustration with understanding chronic pain that has evolved beyond the sum of its apparent parts can be an important first step in treatment. Nonetheless, studies of CPP have highlighted relevant psychosocial associations. These include current and lifetime psychiatric disorders and depression; somatization; and prior emotional, sexual, and physical trauma.

When compared with women undergoing laparoscopy for tubal ligation and infertility, women with CPP are significantly more likely to have current and lifetime episodes of major depression, somatization disorder, sexual dysfunction, and medically unexplained physical symptoms in several organ systems without significant objective laparoscopic findings. High rates of relationship and sexual dysfunction have also been uncovered in these patients for whom the presence of underlying organic pathology is often unclear after diagnostic studies.

Associated complex medical conditions, including dysmenorrhea, dyspareunia, and irritable bowel syndrome (IBS) frequently coexist in CPP. Nearly 40% of women in 1 study of IBS reported prior or current pelvic pain, distinct from their gastrointestinal discomfort. Women with histories of both IBS and CPP were more distressed than women with IBS alone or pain-free controls. Patients with both disorders showed the highest rates of current and lifetime psychiatric disorders, somatization, dissociation, and gynecologic disorders including dysmenorrhea and dyspareunia as well as having higher rates for hysterectomy.

Several studies have found significantly higher rates of sexual, physical, and emotional abuse in patients with CPP compared with women who did not report pelvic pain. Prevalence rates for childhood rape or incest as well as adult sexual victimization are frequently documented as higher than for women without pain, particularly in those women suffering sexual abuse before age 15 years. Physical and emotional abuse as well as neglect are also significantly more common in these patients. Indeed, psychological distress, early and recent sexual and physical abuse, and lifetime psychiatric disorders may be better predictors than physical diagnostic techniques of whether pelvic pain is functional or organic. These factors also may be important predictors of which patients will go on to develop chronicity through disability.

Disability

Recent studies have investigated the relationship of syndromes of chronic pain to functional disability. Studies of other chronic abdominal pain disorders such as inflammatory bowel disease (IBD) have shown that most patients continue to function remarkably well despite the stress of repeated surgeries, parenteral nutrition, and recurrent episodes of diarrhea and pain. Despite the long-term medical and surgical distress endured by patients with IBD, they do not display psychiatric disorder or abuse prevalence rates that are much higher than comparable medical clinic patients. On the other hand, patients with chronic abdominal pain syndromes such as CPP and IBS experience an apparently more benign course of illness and do not undergo such extreme treatments but show far greater levels of distress. Studies comparing CPP with vulvodynia, another genitourinary pain syndrome, have noted higher rates of physical and psychiatric distress and disability in those patients with CPP.

One of the important differences appears to be disability. People who are not disabled perceive themselves to be primarily healthy with occasional periods of illness. People with disability, on the other hand, perceive themselves as ill, with occasional periods of health. The view of oneself as disabled often is found in people with somatization, and both somatization and disability can

occur in those patients with early experiences of abuse or neglect. It is not surprising, therefore, that patients with CPP, with their higher prevalence rates of psychiatric disorders and developmental stressors, should have an increased risk for disability. Once disability has been established firmly, it is very difficult to return the patient to the prior, nondisabled state.

Although abdominal disease frequently is associated with acute pelvic pain, the relationship of physical findings to CPP recently is unclear (see Chapter 45, Dysmenorrhea, Endometriosis, & Pelvic Pain). Several controlled studies have shown no association between laparoscopic findings and severity of pain. Laparoscopies of women with CPP are frequently normal, whereas abnormal findings often are discovered unexpectedly in pain-free women undergoing laparoscopy for tubal ligation or infertility.

Chronic pain syndrome and its associated disability can develop in patients with known organic pelvic disease. This comorbidity can occur because the relatively benign pathophysiologic findings of CPP are likely to be distinct from the more severe organic disease. The risk of procedure-related complications is also present, and some have even advocated an entirely empiric approach to treatment.

Clinical Findings

A patient with CPP frequently endures a long biomedical work-up only to hear her doctor announce that no explanation can be found for her incessant pain. Not only is this finding unbelievable intellectually, it is unsatisfying emotionally. Fears of abandonment, of a lifetime of pain, and of overlooked disease such as cancer can engender a range of emotions from hopelessness to rage. The serial process of performing a systematic biomedical evaluation before pursuing psychosocial factors may be problematic.

Several techniques can help maintain a therapeutic liaison with the patient. It is imperative for the clinician to make the patient aware that he or she believes the pain to be real regardless of cause. The clinician should insist on an integrated biopsychosocial model that considers the interaction of physical and psychosocial factors from the beginning of the evaluation to demonstrate the importance of considering all aspects of her pain. This task can be carried out by alternating between biomedical and psychosocial emphases in the evaluation and using the term **stress** as a common explanatory model for the pain.

Hearing the cause of her problem described as stress may assist the patient who is ambivalent about making links between her pain and depression, anxiety, and psychosocial vulnerabilities. Education about a vicious cycle of pain (ie, pain leads to stress, which leads to worsening pain) may help the patient see that stress is a factor in the worsening of all forms of pain. Many patients have discovered that narcotic analgesics are of minimal value; helping patients to understand the differences between functional and nociceptively derived pain may be useful. All the above factors point toward the complex nature of chronic types of pain. Research in this area increasingly indicates a physiologic process influenced by multiple factors. This had originally been framed in pain research as the "gate control" model of pain: factors such as stress and cognition influencing the degree of pain "gated" by the nervous system. Increasingly, the degree to which nervous system "memory" for unpleasant stimuli plays a role in pain highlights the processes underlying syndromes of pain "without obvious pathology."

Treatment

The treatment plan focuses on the reframing of pain as a stress symptom. Techniques aimed at changing pain behavior rather than understanding it may be more effective than those therapies requiring insight (eg, psychoanalysis). The provider should focus on coping and should not promise a cure. Reduction of disability by restoration of adaptive coping skills is a far better goal than the possibly unreachable outcome of elimination of pain. These strategies may better reflect the degree to which affecting change in multiple chronic pain components may be required to reduce a physiologic chronic pain process.

A. BIOPSYCHOSOCIAL MODEL

It is useful to employ the biopsychosocial model as a guide to care. This model can be divided conveniently into biomedical, psychological, and social components. Each of these aspects has a separate diagnostic and treatment formulation. Careful alternation between a graded, judicious biomedical investigation (including musculoskeletal factors) and a rational, progressive psychosocial evaluation should result in a treatment plan that is efficient, cost-conscious, and effective.

In many patients who have chronic pain, these biologic, social, and developmental forces form interlocking, mutually reinforcing maladaptive patterns that need to be modified together. Interventions that do not address all of these areas are likely to have limited effectiveness. Multidisciplinary pain treatment centers that emphasize integrated and empirically validated multimodal treatment strategies have been successful. Their goal is to break the chronic pain cycle and return the patient to a functional level.

Although many patients resist the biopsychosocial model as an explanation of their pain, most readily accept that their physical illness causes them stress, which worsens their pain. Although these stress factors may be causal in the development of pain, it is better not to press this point at the beginning. The acceptance that stress is an object of treatment in pain reduction is enough. Open communication between a mental health provider and the primary care clinician is essential in gradually moving the patient away from a disease-oriented model to one that includes treatment of disability and psychological factors as primary goals.

B. SPECIFIC TREATMENT STRATEGIES

Although a thorough biomedical evaluation may have been accomplished previously with few positive findings, several biologically based strategies can be used. Patients who have been dependent on narcotics require careful withdrawal. Antidepressants have demonstrated efficacy in many patients with other forms of chronic pain. Although trials of antidepressants for CPP alone have not demonstrated efficacy, the high comorbidity with both major and minor forms of depression warrants having a low-threshold for initiating an antidepressant trial.

Physical therapy evaluation and interventions including biofeedback should be used for all patients with CPP. These interventions may provide a nonpharmacologic alternative to the management of chronic pain. They should be considered even when the primary cause of pain is believed to be psychological. In addition, patients often find biofeedback and physical therapy interventions more acceptable than therapy to address a psychological cause directly. Beginning with the more easily understandable physical conditions can open a pathway to the patient's final understanding of the mind-body connection. This approach may allow for an introduction of the psychological component of CPP into the treatment plan.

Patients may live in situations that reinforce or maintain their pain. Attention to support structures and family and work dynamics may suggest social and lifestyle interventions that provide benefits similar to those attained by using pain behaviors. For example, a woman who is in a physically abusive relationship may experience less abuse when her partner perceives her chronic illness. Many pain behaviors are reinforced by financial, emotional, or situational factors that provide essential benefits to the patient while the pain is present but disappear when the pain subsides. Learning to "live despite the pain" is often the first step in restructuring the world of the patient with chronic pain. Collaborative interaction between the mental health and primary care providers leads to earlier psychosocial evaluation and treatment as well as better outcomes for these highly distressed patients.

When to Refer to a Specialist

Inquiring about early family experiences of abuse or neglect may raise issues that need to be dealt with in psychotherapy. Many women need to understand that experiences of early sexual or physical victimization as well as emotional abuse or neglect can have long-lasting emotional and medical sequelae and may be important factors in maintaining their pain. This understanding should be reached in the context of psychotherapy. If psychotherapy is unavailable, the clinician can recognize and empathically support the patient as she struggles with these issues. Patients with high levels of physical and psychological distress or disability should be referred to a center with multimodal treatment strategies.

Duffy S: Chronic pelvic pain: defining the scope of the problem. Int J Gynaecol and Obstetrics 2001;74(suppl 1):S3. [PMID: 11549393]

Grace VM: Pitfalls of the medical paradigm in chronic pelvic pain. Bailleirs Best Pract Res 2000;3:525. [PMID: 10962640]

Grace VM: Problems women patients experience in the medical encounter for chronic pelvic pain: a New Zealand study. Health Care Women Int 1995;16:509. [PMID: 8707686]

Lampe A et al: Chronic pelvic pain and previous sexual abuse. Obstet Gynecol 2000;96:929. [PMID: 11084180]

Mathias SD et al: Chronic pelvic pain: prevalence, health-related quality of life and economic correlates. Obstet Gynecol 1996;87:321. [PMID: 8598948]

Nitsch W: Chronic Pelvic Pain in Women: Etiology and Intervention. A Review of the Literature and its Implications for Physical Therapists. Journal of the Section on Women's Health. 2001;25:3, 7–12.

Reed BD et al: Psychosocial and sexual functioning in women with vulvodynia and chronic pelvic pain. A comparative evaluation. J Reprod Med 2000 Aug;45:624. [PMID: 10986680]

Reiter RC: A profile of women with chronic pelvic pain. Clin Obstet Gynecol 1990:33:130. [PMID: 2178832]

Reiter RC: Evidenceñbased management of chronic pelvic pain. Clin Obstet Gynecol 1998;41:422. [PMID: 9646974]

Savidge CJ, Slade P: Psychological aspects of chronic pelvic pain. J Psychosom Res 1997;42:433. [PMID: 9194016]

Stones RW, Mountfield J: Interventions for treating chronic pelvic pain in women (Cochrane Review). In: *The Cochrane Library* 2001:4.

Walker EA et al: Medical and psychiatric symptoms in women with childhood sexual abuse. Psychosom Med 1992;54:658. [PMID: 1454959]

Walker EA et al: Psychiatric diagnoses and sexual victimization in women with chronic pelvic pain. Psychosomatics 1995;36:531. [PMID: 7501783]

Walker EA et al: The prevalence of chronic pelvic pain and irritable bowel syndrome in two university clinics. J Psychosom Obstet Gynecol 1991;12(Suppl):65.

Walker EA, Stenchever M: Sexual victimization and chronic pelvic pain. Obstet Gynecol Clin North Am 1993;20:795. [PMID: 8115092]

Winkel CA: Role of a symptom-based algorithmic approach to chronic pelvic pain. Int J Gynaecol Obstet 2001;74(Suppl 1):S15. [PMID: 11549395]

Zondervan KT et al: Chronic pelvic pain in the community—symptoms, investigations, and diagnosis. Am J Obstet Gynecol 2001;184:1149. [PMID: 11349181]

Relevant Web Sites

[American Academy of Family Physicians Patient information website]

http://familydoctor.org/handouts/033.html

[American Physical Therapy Association]

http://www.apta.org

http://www.womenshealthapta.org

Disorders of Menstruation: From Amenorrhea to Menorrhagia

47

Gerard S. Letterie, MD

The pendulum for managing abnormal uterine bleeding has historically swung between medical and surgical therapies. For the first half of the 20th century, the options for medical management were few and usually included therapies with ergot alkaloids (Figure 47–1). When this failed, a broad range of more aggressive therapies was tried. Over this period, pelvic radiation (1930s) and cryosurgery of the intrauterine cavity (1970s) were used with variable success. Hysterectomy was reserved for refractory cases with considerable variation in the threshold for making this decision. Fortunately, progress has been made since Frank in 1931 described whole pelvic radiation in the management of abnormal uterine bleeding. An array of options now exist, ranging from nonsteroidal anti-inflammatory drugs (NSAIDs) to hormonal therapies including intrauterine delivery devices for potent progestins. Surgical options are also now considerably greater than the single option of hysterectomy in the past.

NORMAL PHYSIOLOGY

Menstruation is the physiologic shedding of the endometrium that occurs at approximately monthly intervals from menarche to menopause. Menarche occurs between 11 and 14 years of age, with a mean of 13 years. From that time, the cycles continue at 28-day intervals (± 7 days). The average length of flow is 4 (± 2) days. Volume may vary from 30 to 60 mL of blood (equivalent of 10 pads per menses). Ninety-five percent of women bleed less than 60 mL.

The normal phases of the menstrual cycle are characterized by distinct physiologic changes in the ovary and endometrium that correspond to fluctuations in gonadotropins, follicle-stimulating hormone (FSH) and luteinizing hormone (LH) and the gonadal steroids estradiol and progesterone (Figure 47–2). The preovulatory part of the cycle is called **proliferative** (referring to the endometrium) or **follicular** (referring to the ovary). The postovulatory part of the cycle is called **secretory** (referring to the endometrium) or **luteal** (referring to the ovary). The secretory, or luteal, phase is followed by the menstrual phase of the cycle. The luteal phase is consistently 14 days, based on the normal life

span of the corpus luteum. The proliferative and menstrual phases may vary and contribute any perceived variability of cycle length (Figure 47–2).

Complicated neuroendocrine changes occur each month to ensure the regularity of the cycle. These changes involve endocrine and paracrine events in the hypothalamic-pituitary-ovarian axis and may be summarized in the following manner (Figure 47–3): The low estradiol level during menstruation stimulates pulsatile gonadotropin-releasing hormone (GnRH) production in the hypothalamus. GnRH stimulates FSH and LH release from the pituitary. FSH and LH cause folliculogenesis and ovulation, respectively. The ovary produces primarily estradiol in the follicular phase, which stimulates the development of the endometrium in preparation for implantation. An estradiol peak followed by a midcycle LH surge provides the trigger for ovulation. The corpus luteum, which develops from the site on the ovary where ovulation occurred, now produces both estradiol and progesterone to maintain the endometrial lining. Without a pregnancy and secretion of human chorionic gonadotropin (HCG), the corpus luteum degenerates after 14 days and progesterone levels fall rapidly. Within 1–2 days, this drop in progesterone causes the organized shedding of the endometrium. If all these events do not occur in a sequential fashion, abnormal uterine bleeding can occur. These irregularities may occur at any time during reproductive life but appear clustered during the first 2 years after menarche and the 3 years before menopause, when anovulatory cycles are more frequent (Figure 47–4).

AMENORRHEA & OLIGOMENORRHEA

ESSENTIALS OF DIAGNOSIS

- *Exclude pregnancy.*
- *Rule out endometrial neoplasia, hormonal abnormalities, or anatomic abnormalities with appropriate biopsy, laboratory study, and ultrasonography.*

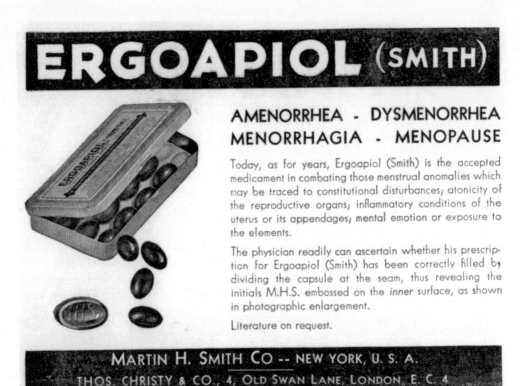

Figure 47–1. Advertisement circa 1935 for ergot alkaloid product for diverse menstrual disorders.

- *Oligomenorrhea: infrequent menses (interval greater than 35 days).*
- *Premature ovarian failure (premature menopause): cessation of menses due to follicular exhaustion before the age of 40 years.*
- *Primary amenorrhea: lack of secondary sexual characteristics and no menses before age 14 or no menses before age 16 regardless of development of secondary sexual characteristics.*
- *Polycystic ovarian syndrome: complex array of symptoms of infrequent or absent menses, hirsutism, and/or acne.*
- *Exclude hypothalamic causes: anorexia, exercise, or stress.*

General Considerations

Amenorrhea can occur in up to 5% of the general population, excluding pregnant women. In an unselected adolescent population, the figure may be as high as 8.5%. Between 10% and 20% of vigorously exercising women and perhaps as many as 40–50% of long distance runners and professional ballet dancers are amenorrheic. Absent or infrequent menses may be interpreted by patients as a sign of serious illness and prompt their request for evaluation.

Pathogenesis

The absence of regular menstrual cycles either absolute (amenorrhea) or relative (oligomenorrhea) may result from changes in either the hypothalamic-pituitary-ovarian axis or from structural changes in the uterus. Any event that leads to alterations in the pulse frequency of secretion of GnRH by the hypothalamus will cause changes in menstrual frequency (hypothalamic amenorrhea). For regular secretion of FSH by the pituitary, GnRH must be secreted within a range of 1 pulse every 90–180 minutes. Stress, excessive physical activity, or anorexia change menstrual frequency by altering GnRH pulse frequency. Any changes in ovarian responsiveness such as follicular depletion will also lead to changes in menstrual frequency (premature ovarian fail-

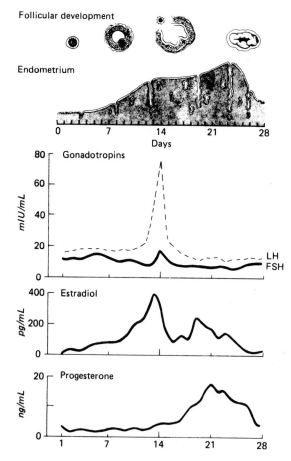

Figure 47–2. The menstrual cycle, showing pituitary and ovarian hormones and histologic changes in the endometrium. (Reproduced, with permission, from Katzung BG (editor): *Basic & Clinical Pharmacology,* 8e. Mc-Graw-Hill, 2001.)

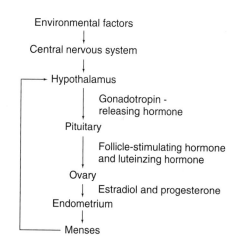

Figure 47–3. Endocrinologic factors of normal menstruation.

ure). Any instrumentation of the uterus such as a dilatation and curettage may damage the delicate endometrium and render it unresponsive to the cyclic secretion of estrogen and progesterone by the ovary. Systemic illnesses, such as hypothyroidism, may result in absent or infrequent menses.

Clinical Findings

A. Symptoms and Signs

Amenorrhea refers to the absence of menses and can be categorized as primary or secondary. **Primary amenorrhea** refers to lack of menses before 14 years of age in the absence of growth and development of secondary

sexual characteristics or the lack of menses before 16 years of age regardless of the presence of normal growth and development of secondary sexual characteristics.

Secondary amenorrhea is defined as 6 months or longer without menses or lack of menses for a length of time equivalent to a total of the duration of at least 3 previous cycles. For example, if the woman normally has a 30-day cycle, absent menses for longer than 3 months would establish the diagnosis of secondary amenorrhea.

Oligomenorrhea refers to infrequent menses occurring at intervals greater than 35 days. Although these intervals can represent a normal pattern, several abnormalities should be excluded before that assumption is made. Because there is a great deal of overlap in the causes and treatment of secondary amenorrhea and oligomenorrhea, these 2 conditions are dealt with together in the following sections.

In taking the patient's history, several issues should be addressed that may help direct the evaluation. The

CYCLE CHARACTERISTICS

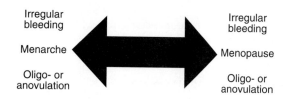

Figure 47–4. Spectrum of reproductive life at risk for menstrual disorders.

possibility of pregnancy should be considered regardless of contraceptive history. Exercise habits, any sudden weight changes, and eating habits should be reviewed. Symptoms of hypothyroidism such as weight gain or hair changes should be sought. Any history of galactorrhea, headaches, or visual field defects may suggest a pituitary adenoma. Long-standing hirsutism suggests polycystic ovarian syndrome (PCOS), but an androgen-secreting tumor should be considered if hirsutism suddenly appeared or worsened. Any history of hot flashes, night sweats, vaginal dryness, or sleep disturbances could identify the rare patient with premature ovarian failure.

A careful physical examination should be performed. General appearance may suggest an eating disorder. Height and weight should be measured. Percentage of body fat can be estimated or measured with calipers. The distribution and amount of hirsutism present at the time of examination should be noted as well as other signs of androgen excess such as acne or temporal balding. The neck examination should exclude thyromegaly. At the time of the breast examination, the nipples should be squeezed gently to demonstrate galactorrhea. If secretions are present, they should be examined microscopically to confirm the presence of fat globules. One third of parous patients have expressible galactorrhea. In this setting, it is not abnormal. On pelvic examination, attention should be focused on excluding atrophic vaginitis and adnexal masses.

B. Laboratory Findings

Initial laboratory evaluation should include a urine pregnancy test and levels of thyroid-stimulating hormone (TSH), prolactin (PRL), FSH, and estradiol. Determination of FSH and estradiol expedites the evaluation and avoids missing the diagnosis of premature ovarian failure. Figure 47–5 is an algorithm that combines laboratory testing and treatments for amenorrhea.

A sensitive urine pregnancy test can detect low levels of BHCG in the range of 25–50 mIU/mL, which correspond to a pregnancy approximately 12–14 days from ovulation. These levels of sensitivity are available in most home pregnancy kits. Thus, most pregnancies may be detected by this method at or just before the missed menses. If the patient has a positive pregnancy test and is having abnormal bleeding, the possibility of a spontaneous abortion, ectopic pregnancy, or gestational trophoblastic disease should be considered. Serial quantitative serum BHCG levels and gynecologic consultation are recommended.

Hypothyroidism can be associated with a modest elevation of the PRL level (ie, 20–40 ng/mL). The elevated level of thyrotropin-releasing hormone (TRH) associated with hypothyroidism stimulates PRL release from the pituitary. Treatment of hypothyroidism normalizes the PRL in most cases. Any concern over a pituitary microadenoma is resolved. The combination of an elevated PRL level (above 20 ng/mL) and a normal TSH level warrants a repeat PRL in the morning, in the early follicular phase, and in the fasting state as well as a gynecologic consultation.

The interpretation of the FSH level can be confusing. If the woman has amenorrhea and an elevated FSH, it is helpful to recheck this level 2 weeks later if she does not have a menses within 2 weeks. The FSH level is increased at mid cycle and can mimic menopause if tested on only 1 occasion (see Figure 47–2). If the woman has oligomenorrhea and is perimenopausal, the FSH may be elevated on some occasions but normal at other times.

If there has been recent-onset or rapidly progressive hirsutism, levels of serum testosterone and dehydroepiandrosterone sulfate (DHAS) should be drawn to exclude an androgen-producing tumor, and ultrasonography should be performed to evaluate the ovaries. If the level of testosterone is greater than 200 ng/dL or DHAS is greater than 700 µg/dL, a tumor should be suspected and a referral initiated.

PCOS has been referred to classically as the Stein-Leventhal syndrome. However, given the broad clinical spectrum of hormonal, cardiovascular, and neoplastic changes, the broader term PCOS is used. The diagnosis of PCOS usually can be established by history and physical examination.

Currently, any woman with chronic anovulation and hyperandrogenemia (by clinical or laboratory findings) satisfies the clinical criteria for PCOS if related diagnoses have been excluded. PCOS usually presents a clinical picture of obesity, hirsutism, oligomenorrhea, and enlarged ovaries with multiple tiny cysts in the cortex. However, some patients with PCOS are lean, and those with markedly elevated androgen levels are amenorrheic.

C. Imaging Studies

Pelvic ultrasound examination remains a mainstay of evaluating any abnormality of menstruation. This evaluation is directed at assessing the degree of follicular development and checking for any structural abnormalities of the ovary and uterus. Ovarian morphology with multiple (8 to 12) follicular units in a 2-dimensional plane is strongly suggestive of PCOS. Endometrial thickness may also be measured as an indication of estrogen status. Magnetic resonance imaging is the technique of choice in evaluating the pituitary gland for any adenoma and is occasionally useful to evaluate pelvic anatomy when ultrasound imaging is unclear. Hysterosalpingography (HSG) is the simplest and most

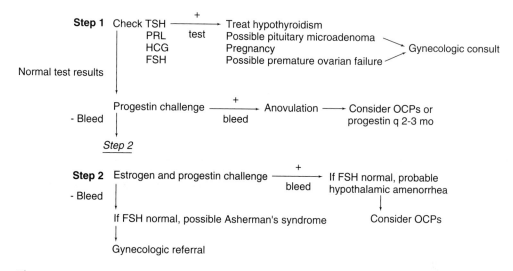

Figure 47–5. Algorithm for the evaluation and treatment of secondary amenorrhea. TSH, thyroid-stimulating hormone; PRL, prolactin; HCG, human chorionic gonadotropin; FSH, follicle-stimulating hormone; OCPs, oral contraceptives.

cost-effective technique to rule out intrauterine adhesions.

D. Hormone Challenges

There are 2 steps in evaluating amenorrhea and oligomenorrhea (Figure 47–5):

Step 1: If the TSH, PRL, and FSH levels are normal and the BHCG is negative, a progestin challenge test is given. Medroxyprogesterone acetate (MPA), 10 mg, given for 10 days should induce a withdrawal bleed within 2–7 days of completing the course if there are adequate levels of endogenous estrogen to stimulate the development of an endometrial lining.

If a withdrawal bleed occurs, amenorrhea is most likely a result of anovulation, either due to disordered hypothalamic function or PCOS. No other studies are necessary. Medical therapy should be considered to prevent endometrial neoplasia, especially in patients with PCOS. The patient should be offered oral contraceptive pills (OCPs) or MPA every 2–3 months if the amenorrhea continues. Although the appropriate frequency of progestin administration is unknown, this regimen will most likely protect against neoplasia.

Step 2: If the progestin challenge does not produce a withdrawal bleed, a trial using estrogens followed by progestin may be initiated. This therapy supplements an inadequate production of endogenous estrogen. OCPs for 1 month or 2.5 mg/d of conju-

gated estrogens for 21 days plus 10 mg of MPA for the final 10 days, (days 12–21) should be given.

If a withdrawal bleed occurs this time, the cause of the amenorrhea probably is related to the low endogenous estrogen levels associated with hypothalamic-pituitary dysfunction. Assessment of FSH and estradiol levels may be insightful. If serum FSH is low or normal, the absent or infrequent menses most likely is due to hypothalamic amenorrhea. If there is no obvious reason for a patient's hypothalamic amenorrhea, consultation is recommended. Further evaluation may include magnetic resonance imaging of the pituitary to rule out an adenoma.

If the patient does not have a withdrawal bleed to the estrogen and progestin challenge and if the FSH level is normal, there may be an end-organ problem with the uterus, such as Asherman's syndrome. This condition is associated with intrauterine scarring usually related to a prior endometrial curettage. Gynecologic consultation is recommended, especially if the patient is interested in pregnancy.

Differential Diagnosis

When evaluating patients for amenorrhea or oligomenorrhea, it is important to consider several possible causes: (1) pregnancy, (2) hypothyroidism, (3) prolactin-secreting pituitary tumor, (4) hyperprolactinemia without tumor (medications, breast trauma, damaged pituitary stalk), (5) pituitary tumor with normal PRL level (rare), (6) chronic anovulation, (7) PCOS, (8) hypothalamic dysfunction, (9) Asherman's syndrome, and (10) ovarian failure.

Primary amenorrhea may be due to hormonal, genetic, or anatomic abnormalities. Gonadal dysgenesis—frequently called Turner's syndrome—is an abnormality in or an absence of one of the X chromosomes (45X) and accounts for 30–40% of cases of primary amenorrhea. It is a diagnosis made with karyotyping. All patients presenting with primary amenorrhea should have a karyotype performed. This is particularly important in patients with elevated gonadotropins, even in those patients who do not have typical phenotypic findings of Turner's syndrome. Premature ovarian failure accounts for approximately 10% of cases of primary amenorrhea with an unknown etiology. In these circumstances, the FSH and LH are extremely high, the estradiol is less than detectable (ie, less than 20 pcg/mL), and the karyotype is normal 46XX. Anatomic findings associated with primary amenorrhea include müllerian agenesis (Mayer-Rokitansky-Küster-Hauser syndrome), androgen insensitivity (testicular feminization) and its variants, and a transverse vaginal septum. In patients with vaginal or müllerian agenesis, the karyotype is 46XX. There is a blind vaginal pouch with no uterus present. The ovaries and ovarian function are normal with ovulatory cycles but no menses secondary to an absence of the uterus and vagina. In androgen insensitivity syndrome, the karyotype is 46XY and the phenotype is female. It is inherited as a maternal X-linked recessive and is also associated with a 5% incidence of gonadal tumors. These findings result from an inability of androgen-sensitive tissues to respond to normal levels of testosterone. This failure results in a completely female phenotype. In patients with a transverse vaginal septum, the karyotype is 46XX. There is completely normal pelvic anatomy; ie, uterus, fallopian tubes, and ovaries, with a vaginal septum usually at the junction of the upper one third and lower two thirds of the vaginal vault. In patients with primary amenorrhea, it is extremely important to obtain appropriate karyotyping and appropriate psychological evaluation for these patients. Depending on age, any abnormalities in reproductive anatomy may challenge sexual identity and should be dealt with delicately.

Complications

In any patient with amenorrhea, especially of long duration, the possibility of osteoporosis exists. Depending on history, a bone mineral density study may be appropriate to determine bone status prior to initiating therapy. In premature ovarian failure, evaluation for autoimmune diseases is essential. In this group, a concerted search for multiple endocrinopathies should be made to rule out Addison's disease, hypothyroidism, and hyperparathyroidism.

Treatment

Pituitary microadenomas are generally slow growing and do not always require dopamine-agonist therapy. Therapy is required if the patient has significant galactorrhea or wishes to conceive. Aggressive evaluation and therapy is required for any patient with visual field changes. Conservative approaches, however, are appropriate. Menstrual abnormalities associated with hyperprolactinemia usually can be treated with OCPs. If a specific disorder such as hypothyroidism is diagnosed, the appropriate therapy should be initiated, as outlined in Chapter 17, Thyroid Disorders. Consultation with a specialist is recommended when treating hyperprolactinemia with a dopamine agonist.

Treatment of the patient with PCOS depends on the specific manifestations. Contemporary treatments for anovulation, hirsutism, and insulin resistance are described in Chapter 20. Women with PCOS are at risk for endometrial neoplasia. They have increased estrone levels from peripheral conversion of androgens to estrogen as well as low or absent progesterone production. Both of these problems contribute to excessive estrogenic stimulation of the endometrium. Use of OCPs or oral MPA (10 mg/d for 10 days at least every 2–3 months) should prevent endometrial neoplasia.

OCPs are a convenient method to provide estrogen replacement to prevent the increased risk of osteoporosis and lipid changes associated with hypoestrogenism. Occasionally, bone mineral density studies show early osteoporosis, and this documentation may help convince a patient to use OCPs. In select circumstances, addition of one of the bisphosphonates to augment bone remodeling may be indicated.

If the FSH is persistently elevated (greater than 30 mIU/mL), the diagnosis of ovarian failure should be entertained. A gynecologic consultation is in order. Premature ovarian failure may be associated with organ-specific autoimmune diseases. The evaluation of premature ovarian failure should include screening for autoimmune disorders and, if onset before age 30, a karyotype. In these patients, hormone replacement therapy (HRT) should be initiated to prevent osteoporosis and cardiovascular disease. Continuous HRT with conjugated estrogens (0.625 mg) or 17-β-estradiol (1 mg/d) and MPA (2.5 mg/d) is adequate to maintain bone integrity and eliminate bothersome symptoms. Patients with premature ovarian failure also can be treated with OCPs. If pregnancy is desired, referral to a reproductive endocrinologist is indicated to discuss options. Recommended doses of estrogen to prevent osteoporosis in the postmenopausal patient are well defined. However, in the premenopausal patient with hypothalamic amenorrhea, higher doses of estrogen may be needed. Oral contraceptives with monitoring of bone density may be needed.

When to Refer to a Specialist

An adolescent with primary amenorrhea should be referred to a pediatrician with an interest in this area, a pediatric endocrinologist, a general gynecologist with an interest in adolescent gynecology, or a reproductive endocrinologist. If the differential diagnosis includes hyperprolactinemia, premature ovarian failure, elevated androgens, Asherman's syndrome, or pregnancy, referral to a gynecologist with an interest in the specific disorder, to a reproductive endocrinologist, or sometimes to a medical endocrinologist should be made. If the patient has PCOS or premature ovarian failure and desires pregnancy, referral to a reproductive endocrinologist is appropriate.

Prognosis

If the cause of the amenorrhea or oligomenorrhea is identified, appropriate replacement therapy may be initiated and the long-term prognosis is excellent. It is important to identify the patient with premature ovarian failure, normal menopause, or hypothalamic amenorrhea so that hormonal therapy can be initiated early to prevent osteoporosis. The risk of endometrial neoplasia in patients with chronic anovulation is increased throughout their life span. Any excessive vaginal bleeding in these women, even when they are younger than 40 years, needs to be evaluated with transvaginal ultrasound and possibly with an endometrial biopsy.

Patients with PCOS have associated increased risks of cardiovascular disease, hypertension, and diabetes, and they should be monitored appropriately. Preventive health changes such as diet and exercise modifications may be especially beneficial in these patients, because they often are identified at a young age.

Alzubaidi NH et al: Meeting the needs of young women with secondary amenorrhea and spontaneous premature ovarian failure. Obstet Gynecol 2002;99:720. [PMID: 11978278]

Crow SJ et al: Long-term menstrual and reproductive function in patients with bulimia nervosa. Am J Psychiatry 2002;159:1048. [PMID: 12042197]

Falsetti L et al: Long-term follow-up of functional hypothalamic amenorrhea and prognostic factors. J Clin Endocrinol Metab 2002;87:500. [PMID: 10519605]

Fitzpatrick LA, Good A: Micronized progesterone: clinical indications and comparisons with current treatments. Fertil Steril 1999;72:389. [PMID: 10519605]

Glueck CJ et al: Metformin to restore normal menses in oligo-amenorrheic teenage girls with polycystic ovary syndrome (PCOS). J Adolesc Health 2001;29:160. [PMID: 11524214]

Kondoh Y et al: A longitudinal study of disturbances of the hypothalamic-pituitary-adrenal axis in women with progestin-negative functional hypothalamic amenorrhea. Fertil Steril 2001;76:748. [PMID: 11591409]

Vegetti W et al: Premature ovarian failure. Mol Cell Endocrinol 2000;161:53. [PMID: 10773392]

Warren MP: Clinical review 40: Amenorrhea in endurance runners. J Clin Endocrinol Metab 1992;75:1393. [PMID: 1464637]

Warren MP, Shantha S: Uses of progesterone in clinical practice. Int J Fertil Womens Med 1999;44:96. [PMID: 10338267]

MENORRHAGIA & METRORRHAGIA

 ESSENTIALS OF DIAGNOSIS

- *Exclude pregnancy.*
- *Quantify amount of bleeding with a hematocrit.*
- *Menorrhagia: menstrual bleeding for longer than 7 days or excessive flow (greater than 80 mL) at regular intervals.*
- *Metrorrhagia: bleeding at irregular intervals or intermenstrual bleeding.*
- *Evaluate neoplasia, hormonal abnormalities, or anatomic abnormalities when present.*
- *Rule out coagulopathy in adolescents with menorrhagia.*
- *Discuss herbal therapies in use (if any).*

General Considerations

Excessive bleeding is a common and at times debilitating problem. Abnormal menstrual bleeding in the United States is among the most common gynecologic complaints affecting approximately 2.5 million women aged 18 to 50. Thirty-one percent of these women describe spending approximately 10 days in bed annually secondary to disorders of their menstrual cycle. The cost of menstrual disorders to the US industry has been estimated to be approximately 8% of the total wage bill. However, aggravating symptoms of menstruation extend far beyond the economics. There are a variety of catamenial abnormalities or events that impact the quality of life for millions of women.

A variety of terms and definitions are used to describe abnormalities associated with excessive bleeding. The various definitions can be confusing. Abnormal uterine bleeding refers to heavier than normal bleeding due to anatomic abnormalities. The term **"abnormal uterine bleeding"** should be qualified with stipulation of what anatomic abnormality is causing the bleeding.

Dysfunctional uterine bleeding (DUB) is used to describe bleeding of an endocrine origin. It is a diagnosis frequently associated with anovulation. **Menorrhagia** refers to menstrual bleeding for greater than 7 days or excessive flow; ie, greater than 80 mL (equivalent of 6 saturated pads per day) at regular intervals. The term **metrorrhagia** refers to heavier than normal bleeding at irregular intervals or intermenstrual bleeding. These last 2 terms are frequently combined into the term **menometrorrhagia,** referring to heavier than normal bleeding at irregular intervals. DUB is frequently a diagnosis of exclusion; ie, demonstrating no neoplastic or anatomic cause of the bleeding. In these circumstances, it is usually due to subtle hormonal/endocrine changes. One clinical definition of excessive menstrual bleeding is passing quarter-sized or larger clots or the need to change a saturated tampon or sanitary pad more than 6 times daily. The perception of bleeding can vary considerably between patients. What is irregular and excessive bleeding to one patient may not warrant reporting by another. There is also considerable divergence between a patient's perception of the degree of bleeding and the actual amount that the patient bleeds (Figure 47–6).

Pathogenesis

A variety of metabolic, endocrine, and gynecologic factors may contribute to abnormal uterine bleeding. Medical risk factors include a history of coagulation disorders, such as von Willebrand's disease, idiopathic thrombocytopenia, or liver disease. Approximately 20% of adolescents with menorrhagia have a coagulation disorder. Anovulatory cycles and disorders of menstruation are most common just after menarche and just before menopause. Women taking anticoagulants or undergoing chemotherapy can develop excessive bleeding. Thyroid disorders can present with abnormal bleeding.

Gynecologic risk factors include any event of pregnancy including intrauterine and ectopic, neoplasia, and uterine abnormalities. If there has been a long interval since the patient's last Papanicolaou (Pap) smear, suspicion of cervical neoplasia is increased. If the patient has a history of diabetes, hypertension, obesity, or chronic anovulation, she could be at increased risk for endometrial neoplasia. Uterine leiomyoma and endometrial polyps should be ruled out. Leiomyoma can cluster in families; leiomyoma occurs in about 1 in 4–5 white women and in about 1 in 3 black women. Leiomyoma can be a common cause of malignant menorrhagia, although infrequently (less than 0.1%). Adenomyosis is a condition in which endometrial tissue is located within the myometrium and is associated with menorrhagia in 40–50% and dysmenorrhea in 25–30% of patients.

Clinical Findings

A. Symptoms and Signs

When taking the woman's history, eliciting the amount and pattern of bleeding is important. Is the frequency

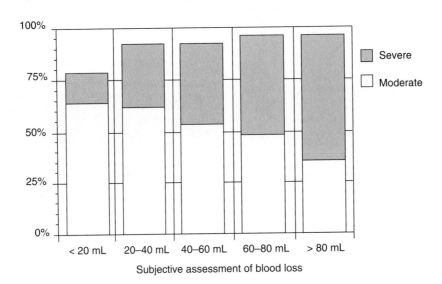

Figure 47–6. Subjective assessment versus quantitative measurement of blood loss.

regular or irregular, and what is the exact amount of flow? As noted above, perceptions of heavy bleeding can vary considerably. What may seem excessive to 1 patient may be within an acceptable range when compared with other women. Often a "bleeding calendar" is helpful to define the pattern and to record the number of pads or tampons used each day. Postcoital bleeding suggests a cervical problem such as an endocervical polyp or cervical neoplasia. Midcycle spotting is usually normal and is related to the physiologic drop in estradiol levels at the time of ovulation. Screening for symptoms of iron deficiency anemia, such as fatigue, dizziness, or headaches, is also important. Any history of uterine leiomyomas or uterine or endocervical polyps can indicate recurrent problems from these anatomic abnormalities.

B. LABORATORY FINDINGS

Laboratory evaluation should include a hematocrit, cervical cytology, and a urine pregnancy test. Rarely, thyroid disorders can be associated with menorrhagia or metrorrhagia, and the TSH should be checked. Coagulation tests, such as prothrombin time (PT), partial thromboplastin time (PTT), and bleeding time, should be checked, especially in the adolescent with menorrhagia.

It is important to exclude pregnancy. The possibility of a spontaneous abortion, gestational trophoblastic disease, or ectopic pregnancy always should be considered. Even if the woman has had a tubal ligation, ectopic or intrauterine pregnancy is possible. If the patient is pregnant, her blood type should be determined; if she is Rh-negative, Rh immune globulin should be given (see Chapter 56, Preconception Counseling & Care of Common Medical Disorders in Pregnancy). Gynecologic consultation should be obtained.

C. IMAGING STUDIES

Transvaginal ultrasonography is useful in determining endometrial thickness, especially after menopause. There have not been extensive studies on its use in premenopausal women. The hyperechoic endometrium is measured in 2 layers from 1 adjacent inner myometrium to the other adjacent inner myometrium. It is normal for there to be a small fluid collection in a premenopausal woman. Biopsy of an asymptomatic premenopausal patient based on the thickness measurement is still unclear, but a thickness of more than 15 mm is grounds to suspect neoplasm. This test can be especially helpful in the evaluation of women in whom the office endometrial sampling cannot be accomplished easily. In a menopausal patient, an endometrial thickness of 4 mm effectively rules out endometrial hyperplasia. A thin lining (less than 4 mm) may spare this patient a dilatation and curettage procedure.

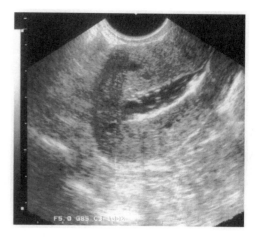

Figure 47–7. Sonohysterogram of normal endometrial cavity. Note smooth endometrial walls. Speckled pattern represents air bubbles.

Sonohysterography is a useful technique for evaluating the endometrial cavity and for ruling out anatomic contributions to abnormal uterine bleeding (Figures 47–7 and 47–8). Sterile saline is used as a distending media and an insemination catheter is carefully passed into the endometrial cavity. Under direct transvaginal imaging, saline is injected into the endometrial cavity and the cavity examined in the longitudinal and coronal planes for any anatomic defects such as submucosal leiomyoma or endometrial polyp.

D. ENDOMETRIAL BIOPSY

In a setting where transvaginal ultrasound imaging suggests a thickened endometrium (greater than 15 mm

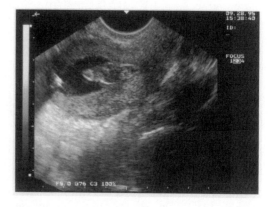

Figure 47–8. Sonohysterogram of submucous fibroid (far right of image).

and 4 mm in premenopausal and postmenopausal women respectively), an endometrial biopsy is indicated; it is also indicated for any patient regardless of age if the cause of the bleeding is unclear. Office endometrial biopsy is performed by many primary care providers. Its use has eliminated the need for many outpatient dilatation and curettage procedures. The following describes the technique for obtaining an endometrial biopsy:

1. Premedicate the patient with 600 mg ibuprofen 1 hour before the procedure.

2. Perform a bimanual examination to determine the size and direction of the uterus.

3. Insert the speculum and clean the cervix with antibacterial solution.

4. Provide a paracervical block if needed for patient comfort, especially if the cervix is stenotic. Ten milliliters of 1% lidocaine is administered using a 22-gauge spinal needle.

5. Place a single-tooth tenaculum on the anterior lip of the cervix.

6. Using sterile technique, gently insert the endometrial suction curette into the cervical os while placing traction on the tenaculum. A "release" should be felt on entering the endometrial cavity and some resistance should be felt at the top of the fundus. If there is no release, the curette may still be within the cervical canal. If there is no fundal resistance, perforation may have occurred; suction should not be applied, and the curette should be removed. The depth of the uterus should be noted; in a premenopausal woman, it is unlikely the cavity has been entered if the depth of the sound is less than 5 cm.

7. If the cavity is not clearly entered, make a single attempt to dilate the cervix gently with the smallest available dilator. A paracervical block can be placed at this time.

8. Apply suction with the curette, and while maintaining traction on the tenaculum, obtain circumferential sampling of the endometrium from the fundus to the internal os for 15 seconds.

9. After confirming hemostasis of the anterior cervix, remove all instruments from the vagina and place the specimen in formalin. Bleeding points on the cervix usually can be controlled with silver nitrate applicator sticks.

Most patients can undergo the procedure successfully in the office and tolerate it well with premedication with NSAIDs. The sensitivity of the test for diagnosis of endometrial carcinomas is in the range of 95–97%. If the endometrial biopsy is abnormal or inadequate or if the result is normal but the bleeding continues, gynecologic referral for hysteroscopy should be considered. A report of "inadequate tissue" can be reassuring in a postmenopausal woman, if the biopsy curette clearly entered the uterus and atrophic endometrium is strongly suspected. Correlation with transvaginal ultrasound results is essential in this case. However, inadequate tissue is not an acceptable diagnosis in the premenopausal or perimenopausal woman with excessive bleeding, and further diagnostic procedures are warranted.

Endometrial biopsy should be performed to exclude neoplasia in any woman over age 40 who is experiencing abnormal excessive vaginal bleeding. Even if the patient has a leiomyoma, she could also have endometrial hyperplasia or carcinoma; one should not assume that the bleeding is related to the leiomyoma without excluding neoplasia first. If the patient has had a normal biopsy within the past year, a repeat test is probably not necessary. If the patient has risk factors such as diabetes, obesity, chronic anovulation, or a family history of endometrial neoplasia, endometrial biopsy should be performed even if she is in her 30s.

Differential Diagnosis

An approach that evaluates hormonal and structural causes of excessive bleeding is designed to detect (1) pregnancy, (2) cervicitis or endometritis, (3) endometrial or endocervical polyps, (4) leiomyoma, (5) endometrial hyperplasia or carcinoma, and (6) cervical dysplasia or carcinoma.

Complications

Obesity poses the greatest risk to health and well being. Patients whose irregular bleeding is associated with obesity are at risk for diabetes, cardiovascular disease, and endometrial hyperplasia/carcinoma. These patients require an aggressive approach with counseling, dietary restrictions, exercise and, if necessary, medications and surgery for weight loss. These patients also require monitoring of glucose, insulin, and lipids on a regular basis.

Treatment

A. MEDICAL

Figure 47–9 and Table 47–1 present a systematic approach to evaluating and treating excessive bleeding. Any patient with iron deficiency anemia should be treated with iron therapy.

If the patient does not require an endometrial biopsy, initial therapy includes 10 mg/d of MPA for 10 days each month (days 19–28 of the cycle), monophasic OCPs, or NSAIDs. The OCPs promote atrophy of

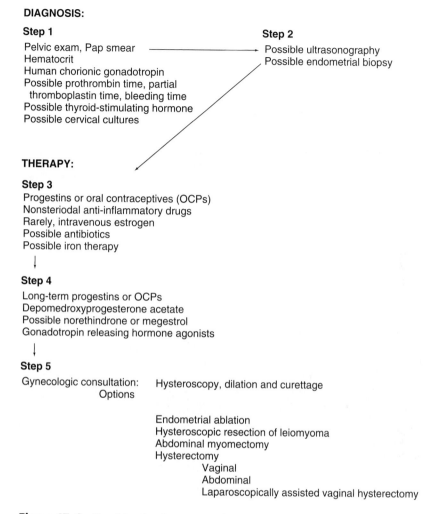

DIAGNOSIS:

Step 1

Pelvic exam, Pap smear
Hematocrit
Human chorionic gonadotropin
Possible prothrombin time, partial
  thromboplastin time, bleeding time
Possible thyroid-stimulating hormone
Possible cervical cultures

Step 2

Possible ultrasonography
Possible endometrial biopsy

THERAPY:

Step 3

Progestins or oral contraceptives (OCPs)
Nonsteriodal anti-inflammatory drugs
Rarely, intravenous estrogen
Possible antibiotics
Possible iron therapy

Step 4

Long-term progestins or OCPs
Depomedroxyprogesterone acetate
Possible norethindrone or megestrol
Gonadotropin releasing hormone agonists

Step 5

Gynecologic consultation: Hysteroscopy, dilation and curettage
                  Options

Endometrial ablation
Hysteroscopic resection of leiomyoma
Abdominal myomectomy
Hysterectomy
            Vaginal
            Abdominal
            Laparoscopically assisted vaginal hysterectomy

Figure 47–9. Algorithm for diagnosis and treatment of excessive vaginal bleeding.

the endometrial lining to decrease menorrhagia and provide the progestin lacking when anovulation is the cause of metrorrhagia. NSAIDs also have been shown to decrease the endometrial blood flow by their antiprostaglandin effect. Alone, they may reduce blood loss by 30%.

NSAIDs are effective methods of medical management. These drugs are cyclooxygenase inhibitors and inhibit prostacyclin. With continued use, there is a gradual reduction in blood flow. They appear most effective in the management of ovulatory abnormal uterine bleeding.

If the patient is having an acute hemorrhage and is not pregnant, estrogens are often helpful initially. With hemorrhage, much of the endometrium is shed, and rebuilding it initially with estrogen halts the bleed from

the denuded spiral arterioles of the basalis layer. OCPs are given twice daily for 1 week, then once daily for the next 2 weeks. Conjugated estrogens, 1.25 mg twice daily for 1 week, then MPA, 10 mg/d for another 2 weeks also can be used. Rarely, if this regimen is not successful, intravenous estrogens and gynecologic consultation may be needed. After the acute hemorrhage is controlled, further diagnostic studies can be performed and a long-term plan formulated. In those patients who do not respond to either nonsteroidal therapy or hormonal therapy, the insertion of a levonorgestrel (LNG) intrauterine device (IUD) is an effective technique for long-term management of abnormal uterine bleeding. In comparative studies, LNG IUDs are an extremely effective method resulting in amenorrhea thus avoiding any surgical intervention.

Table 47–1. Summary of management.

Hormonal
Estrogens (conjugated estrogens)
Acute: 10 mg PO qid/25 mg IV q4–6h
Chronic: 1.5–5 mg daily
Oral Contraceptives
Acute: tid × 7–10 days/bid × 7–10 days/once daily × 7
days
Chronic: one tablet daily
Progestins
Acute: 20–30 mg MPA daily
Chronic: 10 mg MPA daily
GnRH Analog
Acute: no indication
Chronic: daily with/without supplemental estrogen
("add-back") therapy

In some circumstances, treatment can be directed by the results of the endometrial biopsy. Not only can the biopsy exclude neoplasia, but it also provides some information on the present hormonal status of the endometrium and what therapy is appropriate. The diagnoses of menstrual or secretory endometrium are helpful only in excluding neoplasia and any obvious hormonal imbalance. Such patients often can benefit from monophasic OCPs. Proliferative endometrium in the presumed secretory phase of the cycle or disordered proliferative endometrium often responds to progestin supplementation in the last 10 days of the cycle (days 19–28).

Acute or chronic endometritis is an easily treated cause of abnormal bleeding in a premenopausal patient. Antibiotic therapy with doxycycline, 100 mg twice daily for 7 days, should be successful. In a postmenopausal patient, there can be hyperplasia or carcinoma underneath the endometritis. Postmenopausal patients should be given antibiotic therapy, and repeat biopsy should be performed within 1–3 months to exclude any neoplasia.

Simple or cystic hyperplasia can be treated with MPA, 10 mg daily 10 days each month for 3 months; repeat biopsy is needed 3 months later to assess the efficacy of treatment. Atypical adenomatous hyperplasia, which is considered premalignant, requires higher progestin dosing, dilatation and curettage, or both. Referral to a gynecologist or gynecologic oncologist may be necessary. Carcinoma needs immediate consultation.

Long-term hormonal therapy for DUB includes monophasic OCPs, monthly luteal-phase MPA, depot MPA (150 mg intramuscularly every 3 months), LNG IUD, or GnRH analogs. Initially, some patients taking depot MPA have abnormal bleeding, but approximately 50% achieve amenorrhea after 1 year of use. This treatment may be a satisfactory nonsurgical option for women who can be patient with the lack of results in the initial months of therapy. Women who have side effects of depression, headache, or nausea from the MPA may do better with norethindrone, 0.35–0.7 mg daily. If the patient does not respond to oral hormonal therapy, an option to be considered should be the insertion of the levonorgestrel IUD. A GnRH analog is another option for the long-term management in select patients, especially those with uterine fibroids. GnRH analog therapy should be viewed as a temporary measure. Its use beyond 6 months should be in conjunction with estrogen replacement therapy as "add-back therapy."

B. SURGICAL

Endometrial ablation with a resectoscope ("roller-ball" ablation) may be performed if future fertility is not desired. Endometrial ablation may be performed with or without hysteroscopic guidance. There is an increasing body of evidence that supports the non-hysteroscopic endometrial approach as equally effective therapy with fewer complications. In comparative studies, endometrial resection has shown to be more cost-effective than an abdominal hysterectomy and is the first surgical option to be exercised in patients who have no anatomic distortion of the uterus. If the patient has no leiomyoma and no adenomyosis, this procedure results in amenorrhea in about 50% and hypomenorrhea in another 30–40% of women. This procedure is performed as outpatient surgery and may prevent a future hysterectomy and the need for hospitalization.

If the patient has leiomyomas, many treatment alternatives exist. Gynecologic consultation is recommended for leiomyomas that are larger than 6 cm in size or a uterus that is greater than 15 cm in its largest dimension or has rapidly enlarging leiomyomas, or significant anemia (hematocrit less than 30). Hydronephrosis can occur with larger leiomyomas. If the patient is not having any of these problems, expectant management is best initially. If the patient is older than 40 years and having abnormal bleeding, endometrial biopsy should be performed to exclude neoplasia. One should not assume leiomyomas are the cause of the abnormal bleeding without further investigation. If the patient has menorrhagia caused by the leiomyoma, progestins or OCPs may promote atrophy of the endometrial lining and improve the bleeding pattern. There is a theoretic concern regarding estrogenic stimulation of leiomyomas with combination OCPs, but this is not often a problem. The risk of this stimulation needs to be weighed against that of continued menorrhagia if progestins alone are not helpful.

If the woman does not respond to hormonal therapy, submucous leiomyomas can be resected hysteroscopically. Ablation procedures can be done at the same time and may augment the resection, if future fertility is not desired. An abdominal myomectomy can be considered by the consulting gynecologist if future fertility is desired. These patients sometimes are treated with GnRH agonists preoperatively to decrease the size of the leiomyomas and reduce intraoperative blood loss. GnRH therapy is associated with bone loss if continued longer than 6 months; therefore, it is generally used preoperatively and not for long-term therapy.

As a final treatment option, hysterectomy can be considered for the patient who does not respond to medical therapy or conservative surgical options. Less invasive options, if appropriate, may be considered in conjunction with this procedure. If the patient has large leiomyomas or significant anemia and does not desire future fertility, hysterectomy may be the best option. Vaginal hysterectomy is preferred, if feasible, because hospitalization and recovery time are usually shorter and less pain medication is required than with an abdominal approach. Laparoscopically assisted vaginal hysterectomy is a newer procedure that may convert an abdominal approach to a vaginal approach, with a faster recovery.

Medical management is the first option and is usually successful. However, in refractory cases or when anatomic abnormalities exist, surgery may be necessary.

C. COMPLEMENTARY THERAPY

Evaluations may be performed using basal body temperature monitoring, evaluation of cervical mucus, and determination of estrogen and progesterone secretion using salivary assays. A variety of herbal remedies are available that contain forms of estrogen, progestin, and related gonadal steroids. These formulations are available as oral preparations, creams, ointments, and suppositories. They may have a role in treating amenorrhea/oligomenorrhea and are useful in alleviating bothersome symptoms. However, what is not clear at present are the doses and duration of use to prevent both osteoporosis and endometrial hyperplasia. Although useful, these herbal and hormonal remedies remain complementary.

When to Refer to a Specialist

When a woman's bleeding affects her lifestyle and the interventions by the primary care provider are not effective, gynecologic consultation is recommended. If the patient has normal results on endometrial biopsy and does not respond to hormonal therapy, a referral to a gynecologist for sonohysterography or hysteroscopy

to exclude polyps or submucosal leiomyomas is appropriate. If the endometrial biopsy shows atypical hyperplasia or carcinoma, a referral to a gynecologist or gynecologic oncologist is needed. If the patient is pregnant and is having abnormal bleeding, obstetric consultation may be helpful. If the patient is having an acute hemorrhage and is hemodynamically compromised, acute interventions by a gynecologist may be lifesaving. If the woman has symptomatic leiomyomas and has infertility or recurrent pregnancy losses, she should see a gynecologist or reproductive endocrinologist for possible myomectomy.

Prognosis

Overall, most patients with menorrhagia/metrorrhagia may be successfully managed without a hysterectomy. Early endometrial carcinomas usually can be treated successfully with total abdominal hysterectomy and bilateral salpingo-oophorectomy without adjuvant therapy. Leiomyomas are frequently asymptomatic, but they may increase in size with age and during pregnancy with the added estrogenic stimulation. Any woman who chooses a conservative procedure for the treatment of leiomyomas, such as a myomectomy, should understand that there is a risk of recurrence depending on a variety of factors. Endometrial ablation results in amenorrhea or hypomenorrhea in about 90% of patients, with failures usually associated with multiple leiomyomas or undiagnosed adenomyosis.

Bevan JA et al: Bleeding disorders: a common cause of menorrhagia in adolescents. J Pediatr 2001;138:856. [PMID: 1139129]

Corson SL: A multicenter evaluation of endometrial ablation by Hydro ThermAblator and rollerball for treatment of menorrhagia. J Am Assoc Gynecol Laparosc 2001;8:359. [PMID: 11509774]

Dutton C et al: Outcomes after rollerball endometrial ablation for menorrhagia. Obstet Gynecol 2001;98:35. [PMID: 1143093]

Epstein E et al: Transvaginal sonography, saline contrast sonohysterography and hysteroscopy for the investigation of women with postmenopausal bleeding and endometrium > 5 mm. Ultrasound Obstet Gynecol 2001;18:157. [PMID: 11529998]

Gebauer G et al: Role of hysteroscopy in detection and extraction of endometrial polyps: results of a prospective study. Am J Obstet Gynecol 2001;184:59. [PMID: 11174480]

Goodman-Gruen D et al: The prevalence of von Willebrand disease in women with abnormal uterine bleeding. J Womens Health Gend Based Med 2001;10:677. [PMID: 11571097]

Hurskainen R et al: Quality of life and cost-effectiveness of levonorgestrel-releasing intrauterine system versus hysterectomy for treatment of menorrhagia: a randomised trial. Lancet 2001;357:273. [PMID: 11214131]

Istre O et al: Treatment of menorrhagia with the levonorgestrel intrauterine system versus endometrial resection. Fertil Steril 2001;76:304. [PMID: 11476777]

Jones K et al: Endometrial laser intrauterine therapy for the treatment of dysfunctional uterine bleeding: the first British experience. BJOG 2001;108:749. [PMID: 11467703]

Jones K et al: The feasibility of a "one stop" ultrasound-based clinic for the diagnosis and management of abnormal uterine bleeding. Ultrasound Obstet Gynecol 2001;17:517. [PMID: 11422975]

Kaunitz AM: Menstruation: choosing whether...and when. Contraception 2000;62:277. [PMID: 11239613]

Mousa HA et al: Medium-term clinical outcome of women with menorrhagia treated by rollerball endometrial ablation versus abdominal hysterectomy with conservation of at least one ovary. Acta Obstet Gynecol Scand 2001;80:442. [PMID: 11328222]

Munro MG: Dysfunctional uterine bleeding: advances in diagnosis and treatment. Curr Opin Obstet Gynecol 2001;13:475. [PMID: 11547028]

Nagata C et al: Soy product intake and premenopausal hysterectomy in a follow-up study of Japanese women. Eur J Clin Nutr 2001;55:773. [PMID: 11528492]

Rannestad T et al: Are the physiologically and psychosocially based symptoms in women suffering from gynecological disorders alleviated by means of hysterectomy? J Womens Health Gend Based Med 2001;10:579. [PMID: 11559455]

Stewart EA: Uterine fibroids. Lancet 2001;357:293. [PMID: 11214143]

Subramanian S et al: Outcome and resource use associated with myomectomy. Obstet Gynecol 2001;98:583. [PMID: 11576571]

Willet C et al: Guidelines for healthy weight. N Engl J Med 1999; 341:427. [PMID: 10432328]

Relevant Web Sites

Health information by National Institute of Child Health & Human Development

www.NICHD.nih.gov/publications/pubs/uterine.htm

Women's Health Information by Jacob Institute of Women's Health

www.jiwh.org

Review article on abnormal uterine bleeding by Postgraduate Medicine online

www.postgradmed.com/issues/2001/01_01/kilbourn.htm

Diseases of the Vulva & Vagina 48

Raymond H. Kaufman, MD & Dale Brown, Jr, MD

Before any attempt at therapy is undertaken in the management of the patient with disease involving the vulva or vagina, it is imperative that a correct diagnosis be made. One of the major problems associated with conditions affecting these areas is the fact that often the patient has received multiple treatments prior to the establishment of an accurate diagnosis, making it difficult for the clinician to evaluate and treat the patient. This is often the case in patients complaining of vaginal discharge or vulvar pruritus and pain. Often therapy is prescribed over the phone on the basis of an initial diagnosis made years before.

VULVAR DISEASES

ESSENTIALS OF DIAGNOSIS

- *Visual examination of the vulva can be aided with a magnifying glass or colposcope.*
- *Vulvar biopsy is a simple office procedure that should be performed liberally since accuracy of diagnosis is essential for treatment.*
- *Vaginitis and cervicitis should be excluded.*

Examination of the Vulva

In the majority of cases, visual examination of the vulva allows the clinician to define clearly the changes that are present. Often, the use of a handheld magnifying glass allows the physician to inspect the vulva in greater detail. The use of a colposcope also may valuable, especially in defining possible changes related to human papillomavirus (HPV) infection. Frequently, washing the vulva and vestibule with 3–5% acetic acid highlights lesions, especially those related to HPV infection and those representing intraepithelial neoplasia, particularly on the mucosal surfaces of the vulva, ie, inner labia minora and vestibule.

It is also advisable to inquire about and inspect other areas of the body to look for the presence of dermatologic problems that may involve the glabrous skin as well as the vulva. For example, the individual with erosive lichen planus of the vulva often has lesions involving the buccal mucosa. The changes of psoriasis that may be classic elsewhere on the body may be present in an atypical fashion on the vulva because of the local environment of warmth and moisture. Thus, a clue to the cause of the vulvar disease may be found by careful inspection of the skin and mucosal surfaces elsewhere on the body.

The vagina and cervix should also be evaluated for the presence of vaginitis or cervicitis. Often, the patient with a candidal infection of the vagina has secondary manifestations present on the vulva or may have an associated cutaneous candidiasis involving the vulva. The irritating discharge associated with trichomoniasis frequently results in secondary changes on the vulva. The diagnosis of vaginal infection often is made easily in the office on the basis of saline and potassium hydroxide (KOH) wet mount preparations obtained from vaginal secretions. When the vaginal pH is normal (3.8–4.4), it is highly unlikely that the patient has a bacterial vaginosis or trichomonal infection. Cultures are rarely necessary to establish a diagnosis; when they are necessary, the laboratory should be advised specifically concerning the suspected organism so that the appropriate culture media can be used. Obtaining a culture for *Candida* is worthwhile in most cases because the culture is often positive even when the wet mount preparation is negative. The use of Sabouraud's medium is recommended. Numerous patients presenting with a complaint of recurrent candidal infection of the vagina do not in fact have such an infection. Verification by appropriate culturing of the vulva and vagina avoids incorrect treatment and overtreatment.

Technique of Vulvar Biopsy

A liberal biopsy specimen of the vulva should be obtained in the office because adequate therapy is based on a correct diagnosis. This simple office procedure is virtually free from complications and is essentially painless when local anesthesia is used. Small, discrete lesions are best handled by excisional biopsy. Larger lesions or widespread skin lesions can be biopsied easily using the Keye's cutaneous dermal punch biopsy instrument. A sharp, disposable cutaneous biopsy instrument is also available and has the advantage of not requiring periodic sharpening as is necessary with the Keye's punch (Figure 48–1). In most instances, a 4-mm instrument is sufficient to obtain the biopsy.

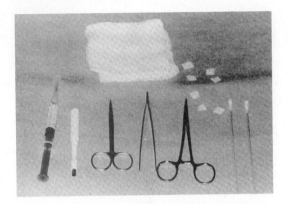

Figure 48–1. Vulvar biopsy tray with disposable 4-mm cutaneous punch instrument.

The area from which the specimen will be obtained is infiltrated with 1% lidocaine solution using a small-gauge (30-mm) needle. The sharp edges of the dermal punch are then twisted up and back into the site of the biopsy. After the epithelium and dermis have been cut through, the circular portion of tissue is lifted with small tissue forceps, and the base of the specimen is severed with small scissors. The small area of the biopsy site obviates the need for sutures. Hemostasis is easily accomplished by the application of Monsel's solution (ferric subsulfate) or by cautery with a silver nitrate applicator. The tissue specimen should be placed on a small piece of filter paper or paper towel with the epithelial surface on top. This allows for proper orientation of the tissue when sections are cut. Poorly oriented tissue specimens often result in tangential cutting, which occasionally can lead to an erroneous diagnosis. Washing the vulva with 3–5% acetic acid highlights mucosal lesions such as intraepithelial neoplasia, which often turn acetowhite after the application of this solution. Similar changes are seen in the presence of an HPV infection.

When multifocal or diffuse lesions are present, it is advisable to obtain biopsy specimens from several different locations. When an erosive lesion involves the vulva, the differential diagnosis is often confusing.

Immunofluorescent staining often is valuable in establishing the diagnosis. Direct immunofluorescent testing using the patient's own tissue is most often employed. This type of study is of value in distinguishing among the different chronic "vesiculobullous" diseases such as pemphigus, pemphigoid, lupus erythematosus, and leukocytic vasculitis. If immunofluorescent staining is to be performed, it is important that the biopsy specimen not be taken directly from the lesion but rather from the normal-appearing tissue adjacent to it. The specimen must be examined in the "fresh" state and should be kept in either a special "holding" solution or transported in phosphate-buffered normal saline. The location of various immunoglobulins (ie, IgG) is often valuable in clarifying the diagnosis.

Clinical Findings & Treatment

There are several disease processes that can present with different appearances; for example, vulvar intraepithelial neoplasia (VIN) may be seen as a white, red, or pigmented lesion or as all of the preceding.

A. WHITE LESIONS

1. Nonneoplastic epithelial disorders—The International Society for the Study of Vulvar Disease has established a classification for the nonneoplastic epithelial disorders. Unlike the prior classification, which was based purely on histopathologic findings, the current classification is based on a combination of gross appearance and histopathologic changes. The classification is as follows:

- Squamous cell hyperplasia (formerly hyperplastic dystrophy).
- Lichen sclerosus.
- Other dermatoses (eg, psoriasis, eczematoid dermatitis, lichen planus).

Squamous cell hyperplasia represents changes for which no specific cause has been established and in which significant squamous cell hyperplasia is noted in the biopsy specimen. These changes probably represent lichen simplex chronicus and are related to persistent rubbing or scratching of the vulva as a result of pruritus from any cause. Lichen sclerosus is a specific dermatologic problem that may involve other areas of the body in addition to the vulva. It was formerly classified as a mixed dystrophy when associated with squamous cell hyperplasia. When these 2 changes are associated, the current recommendation is to report both lichen sclerosus and squamous cell hyperplasia. The other specific dermatoses, such as psoriasis and lichen planus, should be diagnosed specifically. Lesions with associated squamous cellular atypia should be classified under VIN. When intraepithelial neoplasia is associated with a nonneoplastic epithelial disorder, both diagnoses should be listed separately.

a. Squamous cell hyperplasia—As already indicated, most examples of squamous cell hyperplasia probably represent lichen simplex chronicus. Hyperplastic lesions are usually associated with epithelial thickening and hyperkeratosis. Moisture, scratching, and rubbing, as well as the application of medications, may cause variation in the appearance of lesions in the same patient.

Squamous cell hyperplasia may be localized, elevated, well demarcated, or poorly demarcated (Figure 48–2). The vulvar tissues may appear red, or if a thick keratin layer is seen on the surface, they appear white. Lichenification, an accentuation of the skin markings, frequently occurs. Fissures and excoriations may result from chronic scratching. The latter requires careful evaluation because a carcinoma may appear first as a minute ulcer.

The microscopic findings consist of a variable degree of acanthosis with associated elongation and blunting of the epithelial folds. The granular layer is frequently prominent, and a thick keratin layer is often seen on the surface. An inflammatory infiltrate consisting primarily of lymphocytes and plasma cells is often seen in the upper dermis.

b. Lichen sclerosus—The vulva is a common site of lichen sclerosus (Figure 48–3). Occasionally, however, lichen sclerosus is found exclusively in nongenital areas. It may involve any or all areas of the vulva, including the perineal skin, the skin folds adjacent to the thighs, and the inner buttocks. Often, the changes extend around the anus in a figure-of-eight or keyhole fashion. The hood of the clitoris is frequently involved as well. Hart et al observed extragenital lesions in 5% of a group of patients they monitored.

In lichen sclerosus, the skin frequently has a crinkled or parchment-like appearance. At times, edema of the clitoral foreskin completely hides the clitoris. Phimosis of the clitoris may be seen late in the course of the disease. Often, the labia minora fuse to the labia majora and are not seen as distinct entities. Fissures often develop in the natural folds of the skin and in the posterior fourchette. The introitus may become stenotic and preclude sexual relations. Small areas of ecchymosis and telangiectasia are often noted.

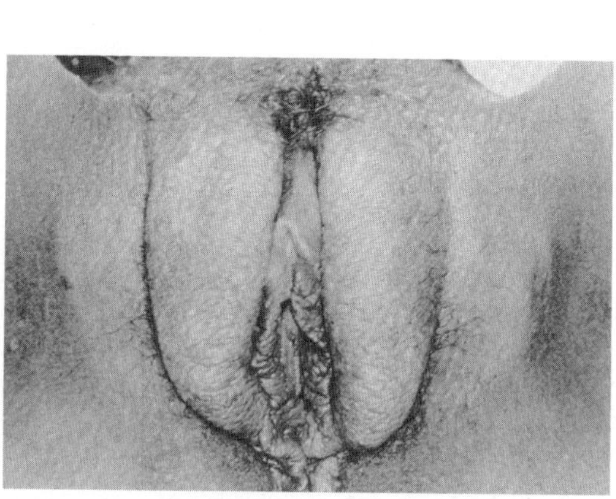

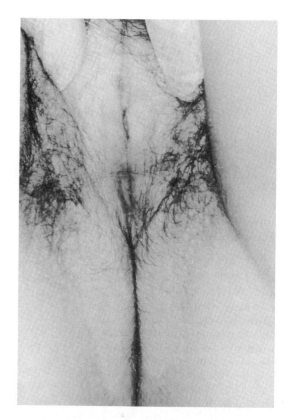

Figure 48–3. Lichen sclerosus. The tissues have a crinkled white appearance. Phimosis is evident.

The microscopic features of lichen sclerosus consist of epithelial thinning with flattening of the pegs, hyperkeratosis, cytoplasmic vacuolation of basal cells, and follicular plugging. Beneath the epidermis, a characteristic homogeneous pink-staining, relatively acellular zone is seen. An inflammatory infiltrate of lymphocytes and plasma cells is often seen deep to this acellular zone. Not uncommonly, areas of squamous cell hyperplasia are seen in association with lichen sclerosus. These changes probably represent a secondary response of the epithelium to chronic scratching of the tissues.

Occasionally, lichen sclerosus may be seen in a child. It has the same gross and microscopic features as noted in the adult.

Pruritus is the primary complaint of most individuals with squamous cell hyperplasia and lichen sclerosus. Occasionally, vulvar pain is the primary complaint. In individuals with introital stenosis, dyspareunia may be an associated complaint as well.

The likelihood of invasive squamous cell carcinoma developing in a patient with pure squamous cell hyperplasia is quite low. In the presence of lichen sclerosus,

Figure 48–2. Squamous cell hyperplasia. Marked lichenification of the labia majora is evident.

this probability increases to between 3% and 5% over a prolonged period of time. Cancer is seen most commonly in persons with persistent pruritus with associated scratching in whom squamous cell hyperplasia along with the lichen sclerosus develops. Although the likelihood that vulvar squamous cell carcinoma will develop in a patient with squamous cell hyperplasia or lichen sclerosus is low, the risk is higher than in the general population. Thus, these patients require careful management and follow-up.

Prior to undertaking therapy, a correct diagnosis should be established. This can best be accomplished by biopsy. Any aggravating factors such as candidiasis or other vaginitis, allergy, or contact irritants should be looked for and, if found, treated accordingly. Attention subsequently can be directed to specific control of the patient's symptoms, primarily pruritus.

The hyperplastic lesions are best treated with topical corticosteroids. The use of 0.025 or 0.01% fluocinolone acetonide, 0.01% triamcinolone acetonide, 1% or 2.5% hydrocortisone cream, or similar preparations 2–3 times daily usually relieves pruritus. One of the newer superpotent steroids, clobetasol 0.05%, may be successful in relieving pruritus when the preceding preparations are not successful. Long-term topical treatment with mid- and high-potency steroids should be used with caution because atrophy of the treated tissue may result. Once pruritus is brought under control, these potent steroids should be discontinued and replaced with a medication containing hydrocortisone. Warm sitz baths 2–3 times daily offer temporary relief of pruritus.

Clobetasol ointment or cream (0.05%) is extremely effective in the management of lichen sclerosus. When compared with topical testosterone and topical progesterone, clobetasol has been shown to be the most effective drug for relief of symptoms and improvement of objective and histopathologic findings. One study demonstrated relief of pruritus in over 95% of patients treated. Clobetasol should be applied twice daily for 1 month, once daily for 2 months, and twice weekly for an additional 3 months. After completion of this regimen, the medication may be used as needed once or twice a week.

On occasion, vulvar pruritus may persist despite medical therapy. Under these circumstances, the subcutaneous injection of triamcinolone may be used. Five milligrams of triamcinolone suspension is diluted in 2 mL of saline. A 3-inch spinal needle is inserted just below the mons pubis and passed subcutaneously through the labium majus to the perineum. As the needle is slowly withdrawn, the suspension is fanned out into the subcutaneous tissue. This process is repeated on the opposite side. The tissue should be gently massaged to disperse the suspension. If this approach does not offer lasting relief from pruritus, the subcutaneous injection of absolute alcohol may relieve the symptoms. This treatment requires hospitalization and anesthesia. Aliquots of 0.1–0.2 mL of alcohol are injected subcutaneously at 1-cm intervals over the vulva. After injection of the alcohol, the vulva should be gently massaged to disperse the alcohol.

The treatment of lichen sclerosus in a child is directed toward the relief of pruritus. This can often be accomplished with intermittent use of topical corticosteroids. Clobetasol (0.5%) ointment has been used effectively to manage this problem.

c. Dermatoses—The characteristic findings of many dermatoses on the glabrous skin often are not observed when these changes involve the vulva. The local environment of moisture and warmth may alter the gross appearance of these lesions. For this reason, whenever changes are observed on the vulva that are not easily diagnosable, the remaining skin of the body should be carefully examined, looking for lesions that may give a clue to the changes seen on the vulva. The characteristic papular hyperemic scaly lesions of psoriasis may present as diffuse, well-demarcated, hyperemic areas on the vulva. Likewise, the violaceous papular lesions often associated with lichen planus are rarely seen involving the vulva. The most common manifestation of lichen planus involving the vulva is that of erosive lichen planus. Under these circumstances, the changes seen on the vulva consist of hyperemic eroded areas primarily involving the inner labia minora and vestibule. The lacy, white Wickham's striae also may be seen adjacent to these changes. Well-demarcated, hyperemic, eroded areas also are often seen within the vagina in such individuals. Approximately two thirds of patients with erosive lichen planus involving the vulva have or eventually develop similar erosive lesions involving the gums. The management of the various dermatoses involving the vulva is complex and in most cases should be left to an experienced dermatologist.

2. Vulvar intraepithelial neoplasia—The International Society for the Study of Vulvar Disease has proposed a classification for intraepithelial neoplasia involving the vulva; the diseases of squamous cell type have been grouped under a single heading. Paget's disease and melanoma also may present as intraepithelial lesions, but they have distinctly different histopathologic appearances, histochemical characteristics, and natural history. Therefore, they have been listed separately in this classification. The vulvar intraepithelial neoplasia (VIN) classification is as follows:

1. Squamous cell (may include HPV change)
   a. VIN I (mild dysplasia)
   b. VIN II (moderate dysplasia)

c. VIN III (severe dysplasia, carcinoma in situ)
2. Other
   a. Paget's disease (intraepithelial)
   b. Melanoma in situ (level 1)

a. VIN I and II—The appearance of these lesions is often quite distinct; they can be distinguished from hyperplastic lesions that do not show cellular atypia. The majority of lesions are well delineated, white, slightly elevated, and irregular. Occasionally, pigmented and red areas may be noted. Microscopic examination demonstrates mild cellular atypia beginning in the deeper portion of the epithelium with cell maturation occurring as the cells move toward the surface. The size and shape of the nuclei vary, and they are often hyperchromatic. Scattered atypical mitoses may be seen. The microscopic changes noted in VIN I and II must be distinguished from those observed in a "flat condyloma." In the latter, the nuclei may be hyperchromatic, large, and irregular, and multinucleated cells often are observed. Koilocytosis is a prominent feature of the flat condyloma, but it also may be seen in association with VIN. The lack of significant pleomorphism and atypical mitotic figures distinguishes the flat condyloma from VIN.

b. VIN III (squamous carcinoma in situ)—No specific gross or microscopic feature is characteristic of VIN III. The changes seen grossly may vary from a localized, white, slightly raised lesion (Figure 48–4) to one that is diffuse (Figure 48–5) and involves labia majora, hood of the clitoris, labia minora, and perineum and may extend into the anal canal, vagina, and distal urethra. Lesions may at times appear red, moist, and crusted, and on other occasions, hyperpigmentation is the predominant finding. Not uncommonly, lesions may have a white, red, and pigmented appearance. Areas of ulceration, induration, and granularity should

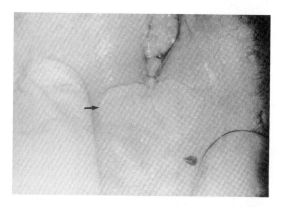

Figure 48–4. Vulvar intraepithelial neoplasia (VIN) III. A sharply demarcated, white lesion is noted (**arrow**).

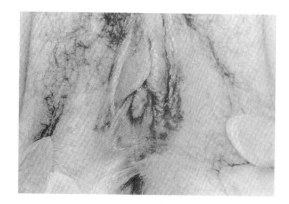

Figure 48–5. Vulvar intraepithelial neoplasia (VIN) III. Diffuse, confluent, pigmented lesions are seen.

arouse suspicion of invasive carcinoma. Biopsy provides a definitive diagnosis.

Multifocal lesions are quite common, especially in individuals under 40 years of age. In studies by Bornstein et al and Barbero et al at least one third of the patients with VIN III had multifocal lesions.

The histopathologic features associated with VIN III include the presence of hyperchromatic, irregular nuclei arranged in a disorderly fashion. Multinucleated epidermal cells are occasionally present, and periodically, cytoplasmic vacuoles may be seen. Atypical mitoses are seen scattered throughout the epithelium. These changes may extend through the full thickness of the epithelium, or there may be a few layers of a superficial granular or hyperkeratotic layer. Occasionally, a well-differentiated form of VIN III may be seen. These lesions are believed to be unusually aggressive with a high propensity to progress to invasive squamous cell carcinoma.

c. Paget's disease—Extramammary Paget's disease is a slowly progressive intraepithelial carcinoma containing typical vacuolated Paget cells. The overwhelming majority of cases are intraepithelial in location, and when recurrences occur, they are usually intraepithelial. Rarely does primarily intraepithelial Paget's disease progress to invasive Paget's disease. However, it may be seen primarily as invasive disease and may, in a small percentage of instances, be associated with underlying sweat gland adenocarcinoma. Paget's disease also may be associated with a primary carcinoma of the anus or rectum, urethra, or bladder, especially when it involves the perianal region.

The typical appearance of Paget's disease is that of an erythematous, eczematoid lesion with scales and crusts scattered over the surface. It may also present as a white lesion or as a hyperemic lesion with scattered white plaques. The histopathologic changes are typical but occasionally can be confused with squamous cell carcinoma in situ and melanoma. Large, irregular Paget's cells containing clear vacuolated cytoplasm are characteristic. The nuclei are vesicular, vary in size and shape, and may exhibit hyperchromatosis. The Paget's cells often are seen in clusters in the deeper portions of the epithelial folds, and scattered cells may be distributed throughout the epithelium above. Occasionally, Paget's cells may be seen in the underlying skin appendages; this does not represent invasive carcinoma or a primary underlying adnexal carcinoma. The intraepidermal migration of Paget's cells is common, and often these cells extend well beyond the grossly visible disease. The latter accounts for incomplete excision and so-called recurrence of the tumor.

Histochemical staining should confirm the diagnosis of Paget's disease and rule out such lesions as melanoma and squamous cell carcinoma in situ. The finding of acid or neutral mucopolysaccharides within the cells is pathognomonic of the disease. Various monoclonal antibodies also have been used in distinguishing the cells of Paget's disease from those of intraepithelial squamous cell carcinoma and melanoma. The monoclonal antibodies KA-4 and GCDFP-15 can be used to distinguish the cells of Paget's disease from other intraepithelial disorders. In addition, Paget's cells almost invariably are positive with immunohistochemical staining for CEA.

d. Treatment of VIN—The most commonly used treatment for intraepithelial neoplasia of the vulva is that of wide local excision of the lesion. This is easily accomplished in the presence of unifocal lesions; however, when multifocal disease is present, the wide local excision may consist of a "skinning" vulvectomy. The latter allows for the preservation of the normal anatomy of the vulva yet permits removal of extensive lesions. On occasion, the surgical defect must be covered with a skin graft. The carbon dioxide laser also has been found to be extremely effective in treating intraepithelial neoplasia of the vulva, especially for unifocal disease. Some clinicians avoid use of laser therapy when disease involves hair-bearing areas of the vulva. The intraepithelial neoplasia often extends down into the hair shafts, making it necessary to carry the laser destruction down to a depth of approximately 3 mm if all potential disease is to be eradicated. This often results in a prolonged, painful period of healing and resulting scarring.

In the presence of disease involving the clitoris, the vulvar lesions can be excised by wide local excision, and disease involving the clitoris can be eradicated using the carbon dioxide laser. This method allows for preservation of the clitoris. When local excision is used, it is advisable to obtain frozen sections of the excised margins of tissue to be sure that the disease has been adequately excised. If margins are positive, additional tissue should be excised.

Paget's disease of the vulva should be treated somewhat more aggressively because of the occasional association of an underlying skin-appendage adenocarcinoma. In addition, the intraepidermal migration of Paget's cells requires that a wide margin of normal tissue be removed when the primary lesion is excised. Even in the latter instance, recurrence of disease is not uncommon.

3. Vitiligo—Vitiligo is an autoimmune disease resulting in lack of pigmentation of the skin. The overwhelming majority of patients with vitiligo involving the vulva also demonstrate areas of vitiligo elsewhere on the body. Thus, the remaining glabrous skin should be carefully examined when these changes are noted on the vulva. In the presence of vitiligo, the tissues have a white, "nonpigmented" appearance. The skin appears perfectly normal in all other respects (Figure 48–6). Because of the white appearance of the skin associated with vitiligo, the condition may be confused with other white lesions involving the vulva. No effective therapy is available for the treatment of this condition.

B. RED LESIONS

1. Contact irritant dermatitis—This condition is one of the more common, yet often unrecognized, problems involving the vulva. Often, patients have clinical symptoms related to a specific disease process such as candidiasis. Treatment of these conditions may result in a contact irritant or contact allergic dermatitis. Unfortunately, with the exacerbation of symptoms, it is assumed that the patient is not responding adequately to the treatment of the originally diagnosed disease. Other medications are prescribed, which often exacerbate the symptoms.

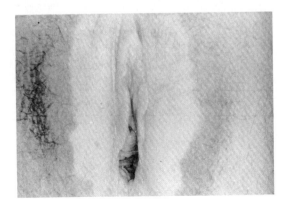

Figure 48–6. Vitiligo. Lack of pigmentation of the vulvar tissue is noted. In contrast to lichen sclerosus, the texture of the skin is normal.

On inspection of the vulva, the tissues often have an erythematous, edematous appearance (Figure 48–7). Occasionally, vesiculation may occur with rupturing of the vesicles being accompanied by a moist "weeping" appearance. It is important that the clinician recognize the underlying cause of the patient's complaints, because the most appropriate treatment is to discontinue all local therapy and allow the tissues to undergo healing spontaneously. Warm sitz baths are of value in alleviating symptoms, and occasionally, the use of a topical 1% hydrocortisone cream helps alleviate the pruritus. An oral antihistamine may be of some value in reducing symptoms.

2. Candidiasis—Erythema of the vulvar vestibule and inner labia minora is common in association with vaginal candidiasis. Not uncommonly, however, patients also have a cutaneous candidiasis, which is associated with significant, diffuse hyperemia of the outer labia minora, the labia majora, and often the inner aspect of the thighs (Figure 48–8). Peripheral pustules also are often seen in the presence of cutaneous candidiasis. These patients usually complain of severe pruritus. The diagnosis is easily established by obtaining a scraping from the lesion, which is placed on a slide with 15% KOH. The slide should be gently heated over a flame to help dissolve the keratinized cells, and the specimen is examined under the microscope. The presence of typical spores and mycelia establishes the diagnosis.

Cutaneous lesions can be treated effectively with topical 1% clotrimazole or 2% ketoconazole cream. Any one of a variety of antifungal medications can be used intravaginally to treat any vaginal infection present.

3. Invasive squamous cell carcinoma—Invasive squamous cell carcinoma most often presents as a raised, red, granular lesion (Figure 48–9). When seen early, these lesions may vary from 0.5 to 1 cm in diameter. In long-standing cases, however, the entire vulva may be replaced by an ulcerated, necrotic, indurated mass. Biopsy of the lesion confirms the diagnosis of invasive squamous cell carcinoma.

The treatment of invasive squamous cell carcinoma consists of wide local excision of the lesion. In the presence of large lesions, an extensive deep vulvectomy and an inguinal femoral lymph node dissection should be performed on the side of the tumor. If the carcinoma involves the midline or both sides of the vulva, bilateral inguinal femoral groin dissection should be carried out. The sentinel lymph nodes can be identified using injection of isosulfan blue or lymphoangiography. If frozen section of these nodes is negative, further removal of additional lymph nodes is not required. If nodes are positive on the side of the neoplasm, the nodes on the

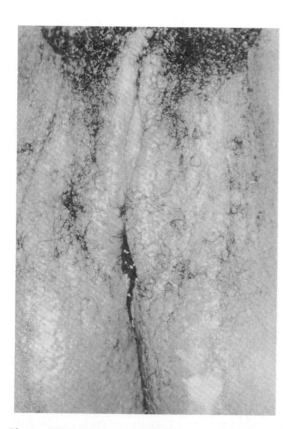

Figure 48–7. Severe contact irritant vulvitis. Long-term vulvitis secondary to topical use of various medications. (Reproduced, with permission, from Kaufman RH, Faro S: *Benign Diseases of the Vulva and Vagina.* Mosby-Yearbook, 1994.)

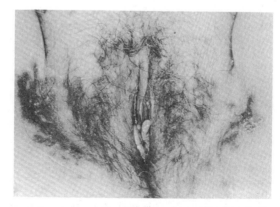

Figure 48–8. Cutaneous candidiasis. Diffuse erythema involving the labia majora and crural folds is seen.

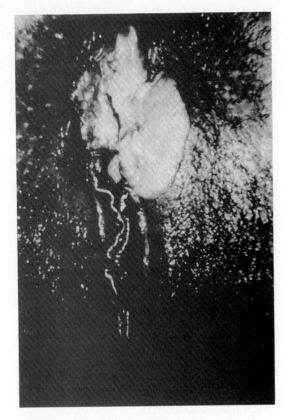

Figure 48–9. Invasive squamous cell carcinoma. A raised, red granular lesion is apparent involving the upper labia majora, labia minora, and clitoris.

opposite side should be surgically removed followed by radiotherapy to the deep pelvic lymph nodes.

4. Dermatophytoses—The dermatophytoses are superficial fungal infections that involve the skin and its appendages. The fungi thrive best on softened skin such as that found in the groin area, where the environment of warmth and moisture predisposes to the growth of these organisms.

Tinea cruris is a fungal infection of the genitocrural area. The etiologic agents are *Epidermophyton floccosum, Trichophyton mentagrophytes,* and *Trichophyton rubrum.* These organisms do not invade the tissue, and thus the lesions remain superficial and limited to the stratum corneum of the epidermis.

Infection begins as a small, erythematous patch with crusting or scale formation. The lesions spread peripherally and coalesce as they enlarge, with clearing occurring at the center of the lesion. The infection usually occurs on the upper, inner aspects of the thighs and may spread to the groin, perineum, and buttocks. The lesions are well circumscribed and have sharply defined

margins that are erythematous and slightly elevated. They may vary in color from slightly pigmented to fiery red. Pruritus is the chief complaint.

The gross appearance of these lesions is characteristic enough to suggest the diagnosis strongly. Final diagnosis, however, depends on confirmation by smear or culture. The hyphae of the fungus can be found in marginal scrapings suspended in 10–20% KOH solution. On gentle heating over a light bulb for 15–20 seconds, the keratinized, cellular debris dissolves, and the organisms are easier to find. The fungi also can be cultured on Sabouraud's medium.

The identification of hyphae alone on KOH smear helps distinguish tinea cruris from cutaneous candidiasis. Both hyphae and spores are formed in the presence of the latter infection.

Erythrasma is similar to tinea cruris in appearance, although it lacks an active border. It is associated with minimal or no itching and is fluorescent under Wood's light.

Miconazole nitrate cream, clotrimazole liquid or cream, and ketoconazole cream are specific therapeutic agents for most of the fungi causing the superficial mycoses. Any of these creams can be applied twice daily for a period of 2–3 weeks.

Erythrasma is effectively treated with oral erythromycin, 200 mg 4 times daily for 7 days. Scrubbing the affected area twice daily with an antibacterial soap also results in a cure in most patients.

5. Seborrheic dermatitis—Seborrheic dermatitis most commonly involves the scalp, mid portion of the face, and presternal and interscapular regions. However, the pubic, genital, and perianal regions also may become involved. The diagnosis of seborrheic dermatitis of the vulva is usually confirmed following identification of seborrheic dermatitis involving other areas of the body. The typical lesions of seborrheic dermatitis are pale to yellowish red and may be covered with dull, greasy, nonadherent scales and crusts. They are usually superficial and poorly defined. The lesions often take on an eczematoid appearance in the vulvar area because of the local environment of moisture and friction. The primary complaint is of mild to moderate pruritus.

Seborrheic dermatitis must be differentiated from psoriasis, cutaneous candidiasis, tinea cruris, and squamous cell hyperplasia (lichen simplex chronicus). Examination of scrapings from the lesion mixed in 10–20% KOH usually helps distinguish seborrheic dermatitis from candidiasis and tinea cruris.

Treatment of seborrheic dermatitis consists of the local application of a corticosteroid lotion or cream.

C. PIGMENTED LESIONS

1. Nevus—Nevi may be found on the vulva as well as other areas of the body. Their chief significance lies in their distinction from and possible development into melanoma. More than 50% of melanomas arise from preexisting nevi. Certain types of nevi carry a greater risk for the development of melanoma than others; these types are the dysplastic nevus and the congenital nevus. Individuals with dysplastic nevi usually have many lesions in contrast to the solitary or occasional lesion of the common nevus. The common nevus usually appears in young adulthood, whereas the dysplastic nevus appears in adolescence and may continue to appear in adulthood. Nevi are usually described as flat, slightly elevated, papillomatous, dome-shaped, and pedunculated. The flat nevus is usually junctional, whereas the other types are usually compound or intradermal.

The pigmented nevi vary in color from light tan to dark brown and vary considerably in size from 1 to 2 cm. The diagnosis is established by biopsy of the lesion.

Treatment of vulvar nevi consists of local excision. All pigmented lesions of the vulva should undergo biopsy, which can be accomplished easily by local excision.

2. Melanosis—Melanosis of the vulva is often confused with junctional nevi and melanoma. It usually presents as a pigmented patch that is flat and smooth (Figure 48–10). It may be focal or may present as a large, diffuse, macular, pigmented area. Biopsy of the area reveals the presence of increased numbers of typical melanocytes arranged in solitary units at the dermoepidermal junction of a hyperpigmented epidermis. These lesions are asymptomatic, and their significance lies in their confusion with other pigmented vulvar lesions

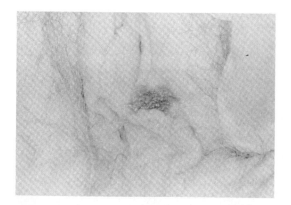

Figure 48–10. Melanosis. A sharply demarcated, pigmented area is seen on the outer aspect of the labium minus extending to the inner labium majus. (Reproduced, with permission, from Kaufman RH, Faro S: *Benign Diseases of the Vulva and Vagina.* Mosby-Yearbook, 1994.)

such as VIN III or melanoma. Once the diagnosis is established, no therapy is required.

3. Melanoma—Approximately 1% of deaths from neoplasia are from melanomas. One percent to 3% of all malignant vulvar neoplasms are melanomas. Prevalence and associated mortality of melanoma make the early diagnosis extremely important. Any pigmented lesion demonstrating an increase in size, deepening of color, ulceration, or pigment incontinence along the edges should arouse suspicion of melanoma. Melanomas may be seen as superficial spreading or nodular lesions. The superficial type usually has a better prognosis than the nodular melanoma. Biopsy is necessary to confirm the diagnosis. The prognosis is directly related to the depth of invasion of the melanoma. Disease limited to the epithelium or dermal papillae has an excellent prognosis, whereas melanoma cells that extend to the reticular dermis or subcutaneous fat have an extremely poor prognosis.

Treatment for melanoma consists of wide, deep excision of the lesion (partial deep vulvectomy) with removal of the ipsilateral inguinal and femoral lymph nodes. In the presence of metastasis to the regional lymph nodes, supplemental radiation therapy to the inguinal and femoral areas on both sides, as well as the deep pelvic lymph nodes should be carried out.

4. Seborrheic keratosis—Seborrheic keratosis is most commonly found on the trunk, face, neck, and arms of postmenopausal women. On occasion, however, lesions may appear on the vulva either as a solitary tumor or in association with similar growths elsewhere in the body.

Seborrheic keratoses are sharply demarcated, raised lesions that are usually papular but may appear flat. They vary in diameter from 1 to several centimeters and may appear singly or in groups. Most often, they are flesh-colored to brown, but they may appear black. The lesions often have a scaly appearance.

Treatment of seborrheic keratosis involves local excision. The lesion is limited in its growth potential and does not become malignant.

5. VIN III—VIN may present as a pigmented lesion or lesions. Often, multiple pigmented papules may be seen covering the labia majora and perineum. The term **bowenoid papulosis** has been used to designate such lesions; morphologically, however, they demonstrate the changes of VIN III.

D. Erosive and Ulcerated Lesions

1. Herpes simplex viral infections—Clinical manifestations of herpes simplex virus (HSV) infection never develop in the majority of persons. It is a sexually transmitted infection, and most infections involving the vulva are caused by HSV II (see Chapter 34). HSV infections of the lips are usually caused by HSV I. When clinical manifestations develop, they present as an initial primary, nonprimary, or recurrent infection. An initial primary infection develops in an individual who has never been exposed and developed antibodies to HSV I or II. An initial nonprimary infection is defined as the first occurrence of clinical symptoms in an individual who already has antibodies to HSV I or II. Recurrent infection is defined as clinical manifestation in an individual with prior documented clinical manifestations of infection and with antibodies to the virus recovered on culture.

Herpes genitalis infection is acquired through sexual contact. The symptoms of a primary infection occur within 3–7 days after exposure. Mild paresthesia and burning may be experienced before lesions become visible. Occasionally, the patient may complain of a neuralgic pain radiating to the back or hips or down the legs. When lesions develop, the patient reports severe pain and tenderness in the affected tissues. She also may complain of dysuria as well as inguinal and pelvic pain. The lesions seen in primary infections are often extensive and may involve the entire vulva, perineal skin, vestibule, vagina, and ectocervix. Initially, multiple vesicles may be seen, but these rupture rapidly and leave shallow, pink, ulcerated areas (Figure 48–11). Lesions may coalesce to form bullae that ultimately lead to large ulcerations. Superficial ulcerations may be seen on the ectocervix and within the vagina. Occasionally, a fungating necrotic mass may cover the entire ectocervix and be confused with invasive carcinoma of the cervix. The lesions seen in primary infection may persist for 2–6 weeks. After healing, no residual scarring or induration is noted.

Occasionally, meningitis and encephalitis may be associated with a primary infection. The recovery rate following meningitis is excellent; however, the mortality associated with HSV II encephalitis is quite high.

The symptoms associated with recurrent genital herpes viral infections are milder than those associated with primary infections. Frequently, prodromal symptoms of burning and tingling occur. These are followed by the formation of vesicles, which quickly rupture, leaving superficial ulcerated lesions (Figure 48–12). Healing usually occurs within 7–10 days after the onset of recurrences and leaves the vulva completely normal in appearance. Pain with recurrent infection may last from 5–7 days.

Before any patient is labeled as having genital herpes, the diagnosis should be confirmed by both clinical and laboratory evaluation. This task is best accomplished by viral culture. The virus can be readily isolated from sterile cotton-tipped swab specimens taken from ulcers or recently ruptured vesicles. The swab should be placed in Eagle's medium containing 2% fetal bovine serum and antibiotics. The specimen

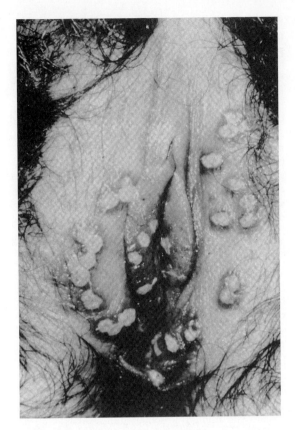

Figure 48–11. Primary herpes. Multiple ulcerated areas are scattered over the labia majora, labia minora, and perineum. A red area is noted around many of the ulcerations. (Reproduced, with permission, from Kaufman RH, Faro S: *Benign Diseases of the Vulva and Vagina.* Mosby-Yearbook, 1994.)

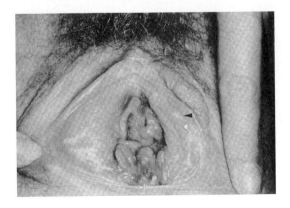

Figure 48–12. Recurrent herpes. Several superficial ulcers following rupture of the vesicles are noted (**arrow**).

should be transported rapidly to the virology laboratory. If rapid transport is not possible, the culture tube should be kept in a refrigerator at 4°C until it can be sent to the laboratory. A positive culture result can be established within 48–72 hours after inoculation of the culture medium. Viral cultures should be obtained as soon as possible after the onset of clinical symptoms because viral titers quickly begin to diminish 48 hours after the onset of lesions.

Acyclovir, valacyclovir and famciclovir are all effective in the management of genital HSV infection. For primary lesions, treatment should be instituted as soon as possible with valacyclovir, 500–1000 mg twice daily; acyclovir, 200 mg 5 times daily; or famciclovir, 250 mg 2–3 times daily for a period of 7–10 days or until symptoms have disappeared. In the presence of severe primary infection, meningitis, or encephalitis, intravenous therapy should be instituted.

Treatment of recurrent infection should be instituted as soon as prodromal symptoms begin. Acyclovir, 400 mg twice daily; valacyclovir, 500 mg once or twice daily; or famciclovir, 125 mg twice daily should be given orally for a period of 5 days or until the lesions regress. In the individual with frequently recurring episodes, long-term suppressive therapy with the same regimens as above is effective in preventing recurrences.

The side effects from long-term suppressive therapy are minimal, and laboratory studies including complete blood cell count, liver enzymes, and creatinine remain consistently normal.

2. Chancroid—The annual incidence of chancroid has increased in the United States over the last 40 years. However, its occurrence among women in the United States is still uncommon. Chancroid is responsible for 25–60% of genital ulcers in Asia and Africa, making it an important consideration when evaluating patients from these areas with a genital ulcer.

The lesion usually begins as a tender papule surrounded by erythema. Within 48 hours, it develops a pustular center that rapidly erodes and becomes ulcerated. The ulcer is extremely tender in contrast to the chancre of syphilis. Approximately one third of the patients have multiple lesions, and closely approximated ulcers may fuse to form large ulcers. Inguinal lymphadenopathy is a common characteristic of this infection and occurs in approximately 50% of cases.

Diagnosis is based on history, clinical findings, symptoms, and the exclusion of other ulcerative diseases of the vulva. A Gram-stained smear is often diagnostic; diagnosis is based on the morphologic features and the arrangement of the bacilli causing this infection. The bacterium is a short, plump, coccobacillus and is gram-negative. Organisms may be seen intracellularly, but more often they are found in clusters out-

side polymorphonuclear leukocytes and arranged in groups often referred to as a "school of fish" arrangement. Obtaining a culture from the base of the ulcer or following aspiration of a suppurative bubo often confirms this infection. However, selective media must be used for culturing this organism, and the laboratory should be informed of the clinical diagnosis that is suspected.

Systemic antibiotic therapy with trimethoprim-sulfamethoxazole is effective in eradicating the causative organism, *Haemophilus ducreyi*. The recommended dose is 1 tablet (160 mg trimethoprim and 800 mg sulfamethoxazole) every 12 hours for 7–10 days. (See Table 34–8 for alternative regimens.)

3. Syphilis—Both the primary and secondary lesions of syphilis may present as ulcerative vulvar lesions. If this infection is undiagnosed and left untreated, the long-term consequences are devastating. The causative agent, *Treponema pallidum,* is transmitted by intimate contact of an infected individual with another. The chancre, the lesion of primary syphilis, usually appears approximately 3 weeks after inoculation, although it may not appear for up to 3 months. It usually begins as an erythematous macule, following which a papule develops, which erodes in the center forming an ulcer. The ulcer has a clean, smooth base with a well-defined border (Figure 48–13). The chancre is painless unless it becomes secondarily infected. Approximately 1 week after the appearance of the chancre, unilateral or bilateral regional lymphadenopathy may occur. The chancre lasts for 2–8 weeks and then spontaneously disappears.

The diagnosis of primary syphilis is made by darkfield examination. The specimen should be obtained from the clean surface of a chancre by gentle rubbing of

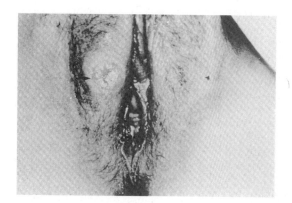

Figure 48–13. Chancre of primary syphilis (**arrow**). Darkfield examination revealed motile *Treponema pallidum.*

the ulcer. The serous exudate, free of red blood cells and cellular debris, is then examined using darkfield microscopy to identify the motile *T pallidum*. Lesions of secondary syphilis begin to appear approximately 6 weeks after the chancre first appears. Vulvar manifestations include the development of papulosquamous, macular, and maculopapular lesions. These may coalesce to form large plaques and often are seen as moist, slightly raised, eroded, nontender areas. Inguinal lymphadenopathy is frequently seen.

The diagnosis of secondary syphilis commonly is missed because the physician fails to consider syphilis in the differential diagnosis. The diagnosis can be confirmed on darkfield examination. At this stage of the disease, serologic tests also are positive. Benzathine penicillin, 1.2 million units intramuscularly into each buttock, is the usual treatment with both primary and secondary syphilis.

4. Granuloma inguinale—This condition is a chronic, progressively destructive infection if left untreated. The initial lesion is a papule that undergoes central necrosis to form a clean, granulomatous, sharply defined ulcer. The lesions have a beefy red base of granulation tissue and bleed easily on contact. The ulcers often are multiple because of auto-inoculation, and these eventually may become confluent. The organism *Calymmatobacterium granulomatis* causes the infection. Secondary infection of the regional lymph nodes results in the development of bubos. The diagnosis of this infection is easily established by the demonstration of Donovan bodies in scrapings, tissue smears, or histopathologic specimens. Smears can be performed easily by taking a scraping from the lesion or by placing a small piece of tissue from the base of the lesion on a slide, crushing it between 2 slides, allowing it to air dry, and staining with Wright's or Giemsa stain. The Donovan bodies are seen as dark organisms that resemble a safety pin. They are frequently found within the numerous histocytes seen within the tissue.

Treatment of this infection is usually effective; it consists of tetracycline, 500 mg orally every 6 hours for 3 weeks or until the lesion has disappeared completely. Trimethoprim-sulfamethoxazole, 2 tablets twice daily for 14–21 days, is also effective therapy.

5. Erosive lichen planus, pemphigus, pemphigoid, and Behçet's disease—A number of autoimmune-related diseases may affect the vulva. These also are frequently associated with oral lesions, and in Behçet's disease, there are ocular manifestations. Erosive lichen planus may present as diffuse, eroded areas involving the inner labia minora, vulvar vestibule, and vagina. When the vagina is involved, a profuse seropurulent exudate may be present. In approximately two thirds of patients, similar oral lesions are found or ultimately de-

velop. Biopsy of the edge of an eroded area frequently demonstrates a characteristic band-like infiltrate of lymphocytes approximating the epithelium or the eroded surface. The use of intravaginal hydrocortisone suppositories (half of a 25-mg suppository) inserted into the vagina twice daily has proved to be the most effective therapy for the vulvovaginal lesions.

Pemphigus vulgaris is a rare autoimmune blistering disease that usually affects older people. The mouth is often the first site to be affected, and the vulva is involved in approximately 10% of women with the disease. The changes are noted most often on the inner labia minora and vulvar vestibule. Bullae quickly rupture and present as shallow, red ulcerations with serpiginous borders. Immunofluorescent staining of a biopsy taken from the border of an eroded area (to include normal-appearing tissue) distinguishes this lesion from other erosive lesions. Pemphigoid is similar to pemphigus in that it is autoimmune in nature and is characterized by the formation of bullae with subsequent ulceration. Once again, immunofluorescent staining of a biopsy taken adjacent to a lesion allows for a specific diagnosis to be made. Both pemphigus and pemphigoid are treated most effectively using systemic corticosteroids although topical corticosteroids are often of benefit in managing pemphigoid.

Behçet's disease is characterized by genital and oral ulceration as well as ocular inflammation. In the more severe form of this disease, systemic manifestations involving the central nervous system, intestines, and kidneys are noted. The vulvar ulcers begin as small vesicles or papules that ulcerate and become crater-like. These ulcers tend to heal and recur at irregular intervals. Biopsy of a lesion often demonstrates findings that are suggestive but not diagnostic of Behçet's disease. No specific treatment has been successful; the best results have been obtained using 40 mg of triamcinolone injected intramuscularly 2 or 3 times at 10- to 14-day intervals.

Occasionally, vulvar manifestations may be seen in association with Crohn's disease. These may include perineal and vulvar abscesses, rectoperineal and rectovaginal fistulas, sinus tracts, and characteristic "knife cut" ulcers in the inguinal, genitocrural, and inner labial folds. Management is aimed at treatment of the intestinal disorder, although Millar has suggested the use of a local injection of triamcinolone suspension into the affected vulvar areas.

6. Basal cell carcinoma—Approximately 2–4% of the neoplasms involving the vulva are basal cell carcinomas. Typically, the vulvar tumors are slightly raised, slowly growing nodules with central ulceration and pearly rolled borders (Figure 48–14). The base of the ulcer may be covered with small amounts of necrotic debris

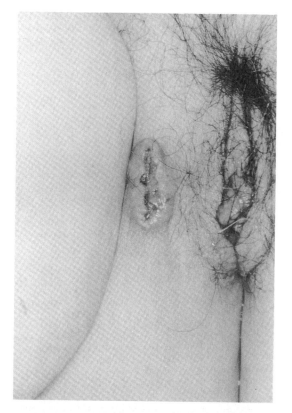

Figure 48–14. Basal cell carcinoma. Raised border and central ulceration are noted. (Reproduced, with permission, from Kaufman RH, Faro S: *Benign Diseases of the Vulva and Vagina.* Mosby-Yearbook, 1994. Courtesy of Dwayne Townsend, MD.)

or small crusts. If left untreated, the tumor may erode deeply into the underlying tissues and even into the bone of the symphysis pubis. These are locally destructive tumors that rarely metastasize. Biopsy confirms the diagnosis. Treatment is directed toward wide, local excision of the lesion.

E. Benign Tumors

A wide variety of benign cystic and solid tumors may involve the vulva. They may be classified as shown in Table 48–1. The majority of these tumors can be diagnosed easily on gross inspection. The most important factors to consider are whether or not the lesion appears to be malignant and whether or not it is symptomatic. If even the slightest doubt exists concerning the correct diagnosis or potential malignancy of such a tumor, it should be either removed or biopsied.

F. Vulvodynia

Vulvodynia is the chronic burning pain of the vulva that may be local or generalized and may be characterized as stinging, irritation, or rawness. This symptom must be distinguished from the complaint of pruritus. Occasionally, minimal or no physical findings will be found to associate with the patient's symptoms.

The patient may have a specific problem associated with vulvodynia or she may have "vulvar dyesthesia" which is independent of recognizable disease. Vulvar vestibulitis is the most common associated problem; gross physical findings are limited to vestibular erythema.

1. Physical examination—In many instances, vulvar burning is associated with specific gross changes; therefore, it is important that, in addition to a careful history regarding the intensity of burning, cyclicity of symptoms, and relationship to contact with medications, a careful physical examination of the vulva and vagina should be carried out. Not infrequently colposcopic visualization is indicated. It is important to define specifically in what areas of the vulva the symptoms occur. Does it involve primarily the labia majora and mons pubis, the region of the vulvar vestibule, or both? The following list shows several of the problems that may be associated with vulvodynia:

1. Dermatoses (erosive lichen planus or lichen sclerosus)
2. Behçet's syndrome, bullous dermatoses (ie, pemphigus vulgaris)
3. Contact irritant dermatitis (periorificial dermatitis)
4. Cyclic candidiasis
5. Herpes genitalis (postherpetic neuralgia)
6. Vulvar vestibulitis (HPV infection)
7. Referred nerve root pain
8. Pudendal neuralgia
9. "Essential or dysesthetic vulvodynia."

Vulvar dysesthesia is defined as vulvar pain either generalized or local occurring independently of recognizable relevant disease. Objective evaluation may be difficult in that scratching may provoke erythema and excoriations.

A careful history and physical examination often demonstrate obvious gross findings that give a clue to the correct diagnosis. The following steps should be carried out during the course of the examination:

1. Culture of vulva and vagina for candidal organisms.
2. Culture for presence of altered vaginal flora, both aerobic and anaerobic organisms.

Table 48–1. Classification of benign solid and cystic tumors.

Solid tumors	Cystic tumors
Epidermal origin	Epidermal origin
Condyloma acuminatum	Epidermal inclusion cysts
Molluscum contagiosum	Pilonidal cysts
Acrochordon	Epidermal appendage origin
Seborrheic keratosis	Sebaceous cysts
Nevus	Hidradenoma
Keratoacanthoma	Fox-Fordyce disease
Epidermal appendage origin	Syringoma
Hidradenoma	Embryonic remnant origin
Sebaceous adenoma	Mesonephric (Gartner's) cysts
Basal cell carcinoma	Paramesonephric (müllerian) cysts
Mesodermal origin	Urogenital sinus cysts
Fibroma	Cysts of canal of Nuck (hydrocele)
Lipoma	Adenosis
Neurofibroma	Cysts of supernumerary mammary glands
Leiomyoma	Dermoid cysts
Granular cell tumor (myoblastoma)	Bartholin's gland origin
Hemangioma	Duct cysts
Pyogenic	Abscesses
Lymphangioma	Urethral and paraurethral origin
Vulvovaginal polyp	Paraurethral (Skene's duct) cysts
Bartholin's and vestibular gland origin	Urethral diverticula
Adenofibroma	Miscellaneous origins
Mucous adenoma	Endometriosis
Urethral origin	Cystic lymphangioma
Caruncle	Liquefied hematoma
Prolapse of urethral mucosa	Vaginitis emphysematosa

3. Biopsy of any abnormalities noted.

4. Washing the vulva with 4–5% acetic acid looking for acetowhite change. Special attention should be directed toward the vestibule.

5. In the presence of erosive or bullous disease, biopsy with appropriate immunofluorescent staining (IgG, IgA, IgM, CIII) of biopsy.

With full knowledge the resolution of symptoms in the majority of cases is slow. The following steps should be followed in treating the patient with vulvodynia:

1. A correct diagnosis must be made.

2. Prior treatment must be stopped, especially if it is not relevant to the clinical impression or findings.

3. Steroids may be used for specific processes (local or systemic).

4. Long-term candidal therapy may be prescribed for persons with chronic or cyclic candidiasis.

5. Acyclovir is given to the patient with herpes genitalis or possible postherpetic neuralgia.

6. Antidepressants, eg, amitriptyline or desipramine, may be helpful.

7. Emotional support is important.

8. Biofeedback of pelvic floor musculature.

2. Vulvar vestibulitis—One of the most perplexing and confusing problems related to vulvodynia is vulvar vestibulitis. The largest subset of patients with vulvar pain is composed of patients suffering from this problem. Vestibulitis is associated with an exquisitely painful inflammatory process (vestibulodynia) involving the vulvar vestibule. The symptoms and dyspareunia usually will be encountered after a period of sexual intercourse without dyspareunia.

Woodruff and Parmley reported a group of cases with vestibular pain and speculated that the disease represented infection of the minor vestibular glands. Friedrich termed this disorder "vulvar vestibulitis syndrome" and defined the diagnostic criteria as follows:

1. Severe pain on vestibular touch or attempted vaginal entry.

2. Tenderness to pressure localized within the vulvar vestibule.

3. Gross physical findings limited to vestibular erythema.

By definition patients must have had the symptoms of moderate to severe intensity for at least 6 months. Most patients, however, had symptoms lasting for months to years and have seen many physicians in an attempt to obtain relief. Many patients report an absence of sexual lubrication, with a feeling that the vulvar tissues are being rubbed with sandpaper during intercourse. Many also have a history of recurrent vaginal candidiasis and condylomata acuminata. An association between vulvar vestibulitis and HPV infection has been reported. In a subset of patients with vulvar vestibulitis, HPV DNA has been identified in biopsy specimens taken from the vestibule.

Vestibulitis is best identified by careful history and careful inspection of the vulvar vestibule and vagina. Palpation of the vestibule with a moist cotton-tipped applicator usually elicits a sensation of severe pain. Not infrequently, areas of hyperemia are seen in the vestibule, especially around the openings of the Bartholin's and Skene's ducts (Figure 48–15). After the vestibule is washed with 5% acetic acid, an acetowhite change often is demonstrated covering either large areas of the vestibule or focal areas where tenderness is most pronounced. Findings have shown a high concordance rate between vulvar vestibulitis syndrome and interstitial cystitis, a condition that mimics the symptoms of a urinary infection in the absence of bacteria.

Traditional therapy for vestibulitis has been perineoplasty. This procedure encompasses surgically removing the vulvar vestibule and undermining the vaginal mucosa, which is brought down to cover the defect. Perineoplasty results in relief of symptoms in approximately 70–75% of cases. The intralesional injection of interferon has proved effective in treating these patients with evidence of HPV. One million units of recombinant alpha-interferon II is injected submucosally at a different location in the vestibule 3 times weekly for a total of 12 injections until the entire vestibule is injected with interferon in a clockwise fashion. The therapeutic success using this form of treatment has been reported as 50% or higher. No success was found in those women who were HPV-negative. One advantage is the fact that it is a noninvasive approach to management. The use of a low-oxalate diet along with the ingestion of calcium citrate tablets has been reported to relieve the symptoms of vestibulitis, success with this treatment has not been consistent.

Treatment of patients with vulvar vestibulitis syndrome by electromyographic (EMG) biofeedback of the pelvic floor musculature appears to be a promising, noninvasive behavioral treatment. Studies have reported significant decreases of introital pain with resumption of sexual activity.

VAGINITIS

 ESSENTIALS OF DIAGNOSIS

- *Diagnosis can usually be made in the office by examination, saline and KOH wet mount, and pH determination.*
- *Bacterial vaginosis and trichomoniasis are unlikely when the pH is normal.*
- *Mucopurulent endocervicitis may present as a vaginal discharge; cultures for chlamydia, gonorrhea, and HSV infection are indicated.*

General Considerations

The symptoms of leukorrhea, vulvar pruritus, malodor, irritation, and burning frequently are associated with one of several vaginal infections. The 3 most common types of vaginitis encountered by the clinician include candidiasis, bacterial vaginosis, and trichomoniasis. In the presence of a mucopurulent discharge coming from the cervix or a hyperemic friable-appearing cervix, cultures should be taken from this area to test for *Chlamydia* and *Neisseria gonorrhoeae* and HSV infection. These organisms may result in a profuse discharge coming from the cervix, which presents to the patient as a vaginal discharge.

Clinical Findings & Treatment

Careful inspection of the vulva and vagina often leads to a presumptive diagnosis; however, treatment should

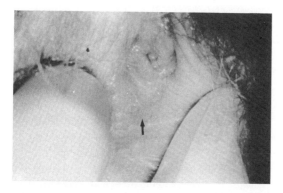

Figure 48–15. Vulvar vestibulitis. Hyperemic areas are noted in the posterior vestibule (**arrow**). (Reproduced, with permission, from Kaufman RH, Faro S: *Benign Diseases of the Vulva and Vagina.* Mosby-Yearbook, 1994.)

not be instituted until laboratory confirmation of the cause of the infection has been established. In the presence of a candidal infection, the vestibule often appears hyperemic as may the vulva. The characteristic white, cheesy, thrush-like patches are seen uncommonly; more often, a white, cheesy, or even creamy discharge is present. In the presence of trichomoniasis, the vulvar inner labia majora, labia minora, and vestibule frequently appear hyperemic with an associated greenish yellow discharge that occasionally is frothy and malodorous. The discharge associated with bacterial vaginosis appears grayish-tan (slate-colored) and is frequently not noticeable by the patient. Often the patient complains of a disagreeable odor. Rarely are there any irritative signs noted in association with bacterial vaginosis.

In the overwhelming majority of instances, a specific diagnosis is made on the basis of wet mount preparations and examination of the vaginal pH. The vaginal pH probably provides the best objective evidence regarding the vaginal ecosystem. The normal vaginal pH varies between 3.8 and 4.4. In the presence of a pH in this range, it is almost certain that trichomoniasis or bacterial vaginosis is not present. Candidal vaginitis, however, may be found when the vaginal pH is within the normal range. Bacterial vaginosis usually is associated with a pH higher than 4.5. Trichomoniasis is seen in the presence of a vaginal pH that is often 6.0 or higher. The saline and KOH wet mounts allow the clinician to make a specific diagnosis of the cause of the vaginitis in most instances. Not uncommonly, more than 1 infection may be diagnosed. A small amount of vaginal secretion is obtained on a cotton-tipped applicator and mixed with several drops of normal saline on a glass slide. A cover slip is added, and the secretion is examined under the microscope at both low and high powers. The presence of motile trichomonads, "clue" cells, or the hyphae and spores of *Candida* allow for a correct diagnosis. It is usually not necessary to perform cultures to establish a diagnosis. Furthermore, the finding of a predominant organism in a vaginal culture does not necessarily mean that this organism is the cause of the patient's symptoms. When symptoms are strongly suggestive, obtaining cultures from the vagina for *Candida* is of value. Because in a significant number of cases, the saline and KOH wet mount preparations are negative in the presence of a positive culture for *Candida*.

A. Vaginal Candidiasis

Candida albicans is the organism that is most often associated with this infection. Other organisms that occasionally result in clinical vaginitis include *Candida glabrata* (approximately 8%), and *Candida tropicalis*. Other species are occasionally recovered from the vagina, but these only rarely give rise to vaginitis.

1. Symptoms and signs—It should be noted that lower genital tract candidal infections involve both the vagina and vulva. Vulvar pruritus is the primary symptom of candidiasis. The itching may vary from slight to severe and may interfere with the individual's normal activities and rest. Patients often complain of a burning sensation, especially on urination. Dyspareunia is not uncommon. Leukorrhea is not a predominant symptom of candidiasis, although the majority of women with this infection complain of a slight discharge at some stage of the infection. Examination often reveals an abnormal redness of the vagina, although it is unmistakably present in only a small percentage of infected women. Typical thrush-like patches are not often seen, but when present, they consist of loosely adherent creamy or yellow curdy-appearing material (Figure 48–16). The vaginal secretions in most nonpregnant women with candidiasis are essentially normal in consistency, color, volume, and odor.

2. Diagnosis—Diagnosis depends on a demonstration of the *Candida* species and the presence of clinical symptoms compatible with the disease. As indicated, the vaginal pH usually remains within the normal range. Microscopic examination of vaginal material mixed with physiologic saline often reveals the spores and hyphae of the candidal organisms (Figure 48–17). Often, it is easier to identify the candidal organisms using 20% KOH rather than saline because the former usually causes dissolution of the epithelial cells present in the smear. In the absence of identification of the organisms on KOH preparations, a culture should be taken using Sabouraud's medium.

3. Treatment—The most commonly used medications for treating candidal vaginitis include the various imi-

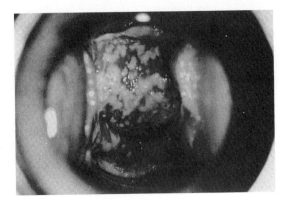

Figure 48–16. Candidiasis. "Thrush" patches are seen adherent to the vaginal wall. (Reproduced, with permission, from Kaufman RH, Faro S: *Benign Diseases of the Vulva and Vagina.* Mosby-Yearbook, 1994.)

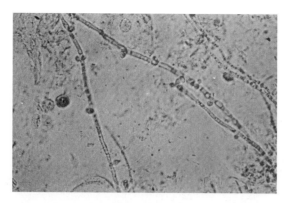

Figure 48–17. Candidiasis. Hyphae and conidia are seen using saline wet mount preparation.

dazole compounds (Table 48–2). These act by interfering with the demethylation steps in ergosterol synthesis, which is found within the yeast membrane wall, thus preventing the formation of normal yeast cell walls. Dosage recommendations vary from drug to drug; however, clotrimazole, miconazole, butoconazole, tioconazole, and ketoconazole intravaginally all appear to be equally effective. Depending on the medication and dosage used, treatment lasts from 3 to 7 days. With recurrent or persistent infections, fluconazole can be taken orally. In severe cases, 2 doses of fluconazole taken 72 hours apart has been shown to have a higher cure rate.

B. Trichomoniasis

Trichomoniasis is caused by infection with the organism *Trichomonas vaginalis.* It is a unicellular protozoan flagellate that usually can be identified easily by morphologic findings and movement characteristics in a saline wet mount preparation.

1. Symptoms and signs—Trichomoniasis exhibits a wide variety of clinical patterns. The symptoms associated with acute infection differ significantly from those seen in the individual with long-standing infection. The typical manifestations are a copious vaginal discharge, pruritus, and burning. Although the characteristics of this discharge are variable, usually there is a profuse, frothy discharge that is greenish in color and foul smelling. In the presence of a chronic infection, the discharge is usually slight to moderate, may be slight gray to tan in appearance, and is homogeneous. Generalized erythema is the only gross change noted within the vagina of some patients with acute infection. Pruritus of the vulva is found frequently in association with trichomoniasis. Erythema of the vulvar vestibule and inner labia minora are not uncommon. The diag-

Table 48–2. Recommended regimens for the treatment of vulvovaginal candidiasis.

Intravaginal agents
  Butoconazole 2% cream 5 g intravaginally for 3 days
    Or
  Butoconazole 2% cream 5 g B1-BSR, single intravaginal application
    Or
  Clotrimazole 1% cream 5 g intravaginally for 7–14 days
    Or
  Clotrimazole 100 mg vaginal tablet for 7 days
    Or
  Clotrimazole 100 mg vaginal tablet, 2 tablets for 3 days
    Or
  Clotrimazole 500 mg vaginal tablet, 1 tablet in a single application
    Or
  Miconazole 2% cream 5 g intravaginally for 7 days
    Or
  Miconazole 100 mg vaginal suppository, 1 suppository for 7 days
    Or
  Miconazole 200 mg vaginal suppository, 1 suppository for 3 days
    Or
  Nystatin 100,000 units vaginal tablet, 1 tablet for 14 days[1]
    Or
  Tioconazole 6.5% ointment 5 g intravaginally in a single application
    Or
  Terconazole 0.4% cream 5 g intravaginally for 7 days
    Or
  Terconazole 0.8% cream 5 g intravaginally for 3 days
    Or
  Terconazole 80 mg vaginal suppository, 1 suppository for 3 days
Oral agent
  Fluconazole 150 mg oral tablet, 1 tablet in a single dose[1]

[1]Only agents not over-the-counter

nosis is established following identification of the motile trichomonads on a saline wet mount preparation (Figure 48–18). A culture is rarely necessary to identify the organism.

2. Treatment—Metronidazole is currently the standard for the treatment of this infection. A single dose, of 2 g of the medication may be used. Other approaches to therapy include a regimen of 250 mg, 3 times daily for 7 days, or 500 mg, twice daily for 5 days. However, the single 2-g oral dose appears to be as effective as the other approaches to treatment. The sexual partner of the patient also should be treated.

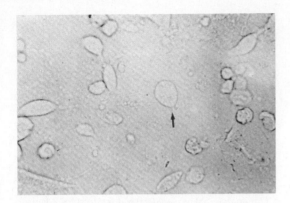

Figure 48–18. Trichomoniasis. Wet mount preparation with physiologic saline reveals multiple motile trichomonads (**arrow**).

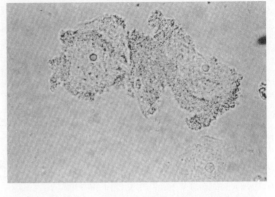

Figure 48–19. Bacterial vaginosis. Clue cells are evident. (Reproduced, with permission, from Kaufman RH, Faro S: *Benign Diseases of the Vulva and Vagina.* Mosby-Yearbook, 1994.)

C. BACTERIAL VAGINOSIS

Bacterial vaginosis is a polymicrobial syndrome occurring as the result of a synergism between *Gardnerella vaginalis* and anaerobic bacteria, including mobiluncus species and *Bacteroides*. The altered vaginal flora is a result of various factors causing a lessening of hydrogen peroxide-producing lactobacilli and, therefore, increasing vaginal pH. In some instances this may be sexually transmitted.

1. Symptoms and signs—The predominant symptom is malodor with an associated discharge. Examination reveals a normal-appearing vulva with a slate-gray, homogeneous discharge present within the vagina. The vaginal mucosa appears normal, and there is none of the inflammatory response noted with candidal or trichomonal infections. The vaginal discharge usually has an offensive odor.

2. Diagnosis—The diagnosis usually can be established on careful examination of the patient, measurement of vaginal pH, and examination of a wet mount preparation. The vaginal pH is elevated above 4.5. The discharge usually has a foul odor, but if this is not readily noticeable, the addition of a few drops of 20% KOH to some of this discharge results in an offensive odor (Whiff test). Wet mount preparation demonstrates the presence of characteristic "clue" cells (Figure 48–19). These are squamous epithelial cells covered by adherent, rod-like bacteria. In addition to the clue cells, the absence of lactobacilli is another essential feature seen in association with this infection.

3. Treatment—Several topical agents have been found to be extremely effective in treating bacterial vaginosis (see also Table 34–2). Clindamycin 2% cream used once daily for 7 days and metronidazole gel applied twice daily for 5 days have proved to be effective agents in eradicating the infection. If there is recurrent infection, metronidazole may be administered 500 mg twice daily for 7 days. Patients who are at high risk for preterm labor are treated with clindamycin 2% cream or augmentin (Amoxicillin with clavulanic acid).

When to Refer to a Specialist

The primary care provider should be able to examine the vulva, perform a vulvar biopsy, and manage many of the problems described in this chapter. When the diagnosis is unclear or treatment is unsuccessful, referral to a dermatologist or to a gynecologist with an interest in vulvar diseases is indicated.

Many metropolitan areas have at least 1 gynecologist with a special interest in vulvar diseases, including vulvodynia. Surgical procedures require referral to a gynecologist. Referral to a gynecologic oncologist is necessary when a vulvar malignancy has been diagnosed. When vaginitis fails to respond to recommended treatments, referral to a gynecologist, particularly one that specializes in infectious diseases, is recommended.

Barbero M et al: Vulvar intraepithelial neoplasia. A clinical pathologic study of 60 cases. J Reprod Med 1990;35:1023. [PMID: 2177508]

Bornstein J et al: Multicentric intraepithelial neoplasia involving the vulva. Clinical features and association with human papillomavirus and herpes simplex virus. Cancer 1988;62:1601. [PMID: 2844383]

Bracco GL et al: A critical evaluation of clinical and histologic effects of topical treatment of lichen sclerosus with 2% testosterone, 2% progesterone, and 0.05% clobetasol and cream base. Proceedings of The International Society for the Study of Vulvar Disease, September 1991.

De Cesare SL et al: A pilot study utilizing intraoperative lymphoscintigraphy for identification of the sentinel lymph nodes in vulvar cancer. Gynecol Oncol 1997;66:425. [PMID: 9299256]

Eckert LO et al: Vulvovaginal candidiasis: clinical manifestations, risk factors, management algorithm. Obstet Gynecol 1998; 92:757. [PMID: 9794664]

Friedrich EG Jr: Vulvar vestibulitis syndrome. J Reprod Med 1987;32:110. [PMID: 3560069]

Goldberg LH et al: Long-term suppression of recurrent genital herpes with acyclovir. A 5-year benchmark. Acyclovir Study Group. Arch Dermatol 1993;120:582. [PMID: 8481018]

Hart WR, Norris, HJ, Helwig EB: Relation of lichen sclerosus et atrophicus of the vulva to the development of carcinoma. Obstet Gynecol 1975;45:369. [PMID: 1091897]

McKay M et al: Vulvar vestibulitis, and vestibular papillomatosis. Report of the ISSVD Committee on Vulvodynia. J Reprod Med 1991;36:413. [PMID: 1650839]

Kaufman RH, Faro S: *Benign Diseases of the Vulva and Vagina,* 4th ed. Mosby-Yearbook, 1994.

Levenback C et al: Potential applications of intraoperative lymphatic mapping in vulvar cancer. Gynecol Oncol 1995;59: 216. [PMID: 7590476]

Lever WF, Schaumburg-Lever G: *Histopathology of the Skin,* 7th ed. Lippincott, 1990.

Lorenz B, Kaufman RH, Kutzner K: Lichen sclerosis. Therapy with clobetasol propionate. J Reprod Med 1998;43:790. [PMID: 9777618]

Mann MS, Kaufman RH: Erosive lichen planus of the vulva. Clin Obstet Gynecol 1991;34:605. [PMID: 1934713]

Mann MS et al: Vulvar vestibulitis: Significant variables in treatment outcome. Obstet Gynecol 1992;79:122. [PMID: 1370123]

McKay E et al: Treating vulvar vestibulitis with electromyographic biofeedback of pelvic floor musculature. J Reprod Med 2001; 46:337. [PMID: 11354833]

Millar D: Crohn's disease of the vulva. J R Soc Med 1992;85:305. [PMID: 1433106]

Solomons CC, Melmed MH, Heitler SM: Calcium citrate for vulvar vestibulitis. A case report. J Reprod Med 1991;36:879. [PMID: 1816400]

Sobel JD et al: Treatment of complicated candida vaginitis: comparison of single and sequential doses of fluconazole. Am J Obstet Gynecol 2001;185:363. [PMID: 11518893]

Turner ML, Marinoff SC: Association of human papillomavirus with vulvodynia and the vulvar vestibulitis syndrome. J Reprod Med 1988;33:533. [PMID: 2841460]

Umpierre SA et al: Human papillomavirus DNA in tissue biopsy specimens of vulvar vestibulitis patients treated with interferon. Obstet Gynecol 1991;78:693. [PMID: 1717908]

Woodruff JD, Parmley TH: Infection of the minor vestibular gland. Obstet Gynecol 1983;62:609. [PMID: 6621951]

Woodruff JD, Thompson B: Local alcohol injection in the treatment of vulvar pruritis. Obstet Gynecol 1972;40:18. [PMID: 5044933]

Relevant Web Sites

[National Vulvodynia Association. Disseminates information on treatment options for vulvodynia.]
http://www.nva.org
[Vulvar Pain Foundation. Publishes newsletter for patients with vulvodynia.]
http://www.vulvarpainfoundation.org

Cervical Cancer Screening & Management of the Abnormal Papanicolaou Smear

49

Howard G. Muntz, MD

ESSENTIALS OF DIAGNOSIS

- *Most women with abnormal Papanicolaou smears are asymptomatic.*
- *Early cytologic detection of preinvasive lesions or minimally invasive cancers in asymptomatic women allows effective treatment without significant morbidity and usually with preservation of fertility.*
- *Colposcopy is essential to the diagnosis and management of preinvasive and microinvasive cervical neoplasia because it shows the changes in color, vascular pattern, and surface contour that identify neoplastic regions on the cervix.*
- *Women with deeply invasive cervical cancer usually report abnormal vaginal bleeding or discharge, and a gross cervical tumor is seen on pelvic examination.*
- *Signs of advanced cervical cancer include replacement of the cervix and upper vagina by a large friable tumor mass, erosion into the bladder or rectum, ureteral obstruction, and metastatic spread to the liver, lungs, and retroperitoneal lymph nodes.*

General Considerations

In developed countries with Papanicolaou (Pap) smear cytologic screening programs, there has been a dramatic fall in cervical cancer incidence and mortality rates and an increase in the incidence of cervical carcinoma in situ (CIS). In the United States in 2002, there were an estimated 50,000 cases of CIS, but only 13,000 cases of invasive cervical cancer, resulting in 4100 deaths. These favorable ratios are related to the high proportion of patients with preinvasive or early-stage cervical neoplasia detected by Pap smear screening. Overall, cervical cancer ranks as only the seventh cause of cancer mortality among women in the United States. In underdeveloped countries with inadequate Pap smear screening programs, cervical cancer is still the leading cause of cancer deaths among women.

The age-specific incidence of cervical CIS and invasive cancer (Figure 49–1) affects the rational approach to Pap smear screening. The incidence of cervical CIS peaks between ages 25 and 35, whereas invasive cervical cancer rates increase with age. In some populations, preinvasive cervical lesions occur at a very early age, perhaps related to sexual practices among young teenagers. At the opposite end of the age spectrum, epidemiologic data indicate a problem with controlling cervical cancer in elderly women.

The overall incidence of Pap smear abnormalities has risen rapidly over the last 2 decades. Currently, in a typical screening program, up to 5% of all Pap smears may be interpreted as abnormal, although the exact proportion varies widely. A major challenge in women's health care is to provide cost-effective yet reliable evaluation of a large number of abnormal smears.

Pathogenesis

Molecular biologic studies have now linked almost all cervical cancers with human papillomavirus (HPV) infection. More than 30 types of this common—often sexually transmitted—infection have been identified, of which approximately 10–15 have been categorized as "high-risk" due to association with cervical cancer (Table 49–1). It is now known that the E6 and E7 gene products of high-risk HPV types interact with the retinoblastoma and p53 factors, resulting in deregulation of cell proliferation. Presence of cofactors such as exposure to carcinogens in cigarette smoke are also important.

The previously established epidemiologic risk factors for cervical cancer (Table 49–2) can be accounted for by high-risk HPV infection, with or without interaction with carcinogens. Unfortunately, many of these factors, such as early age at first intercourse and expo-

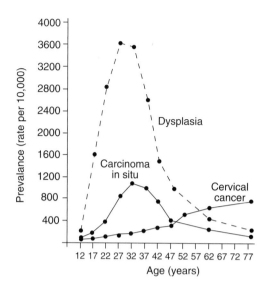

Figure 49–1. Age-specific incidence of cervical dysplasia, carcinoma in situ (CIS), and invasive cancer. The incidence of cervical dysplasia and CIS rises sharply at approximately age 20 and peaks between ages 25 and 35. Invasive cervical cancer rates have a more gradual rise, with the highest incidence from age 50 through senescence. (Reproduced, with permission, from Reid R, Fu YU: In: *Banbury Report 21: Viral Etiology of Cervical Cancer.* Peto R (editor). Cold Spring Harbor Laboratory Press, 1986.)

sure to a "high-risk" male partner, are beyond the province of the health care provider. While HPV vaccine research is promising, dissemination of HPV in a sexually active population is probably not currently preventable. Although the use of condoms and other safe sex practices should be encouraged on general principles, they are ineffective against transmission of HPV, which has a large reservoir in genital tract skin and mucous membranes. Clinicians must be aware that, based

Table 49–1. Common types of human papillomavirus (HPV) and association with different clinical conditions.

HPV Type	Association
1–4	Common skin wart
6, 11, 42, 43, 44	Benign condylomata of lower genital tract
16, 18, 31, 33, 35, 39, 45, 51, 52, 56, 58, 59, 68	Invasive cancers and high-grade dysplasia of the cervix

Table 49–2. Risk factors associated with cervical cancer.

Early age at first intercourse
Multiple sex partners
"High-risk" male consort
Low socioeconomic status
Black race
Early age at childbearing
Intrauterine diethylstilbestrol (DES) exposure
Human papillomavirus (HPV) infection
Herpes simplex virus (HSV II) infection
Compromised immunity, including HIV infection
Deficiency in vitamins A and C
Cigarette smoking

on epidemiologic data, almost all women in the United States are at risk for cervical cancer.

Schlecht NF et al: Persistent human papillomavirus infection as a predictor of cervical intraepithelial neoplasia. JAMA 2001; 286:3106. [PMID: 11754676]

Walboomers JM et al: Human papillomavirus is a necessary cause of invasive cervical cancer worldwide. J Pathol 1999;189:12. [PMID: 10451482]

Screening

A. GUIDELINES

There is universal agreement that an effective Pap smear screening program can dramatically reduce cervical cancer incidence and mortality. However, the optimal interval for obtaining smears remains controversial. The theoretic benefit of annual screening is supported by a number of case-control studies that demonstrate progressively decreasing cervical cancer incidence and mortality rates as screening intervals are shortened. However, most of the benefit from Pap smear screening can be achieved with intervals of 2–3 years, which is more cost-effective than shorter intervals. New consensus guidelines for cervical cancer screening were released in 2002 by the American Cancer Society (Table 49–3). These guidelines endorse annual screening, but allow longer screening intervals after 3 consecutive negative smears for patients who are at low risk for cervical cancer.

Whether elderly women require Pap smear screening is also controversial. The 2002 consensus guidelines permit low-risk women to halt Pap smear screening after age 70. Other organizations (including the Canadian and US Preventive Services Task Forces) have recommended that Pap smear screening cease at age 60, on the assumption that a woman with serial normal smears in her younger and middle-aged years will have

Table 49–3. Recommendations for cervical cancer screening.[1]

- Papanicolaou (Pap) smear screening should begin approximately 3 years after a woman becomes sexually active or reaches age 21.
- Screening should be performed every year (or every 2 years with liquid-based tests).
- After age 30, women with 3 consecutive normal Pap smears can be screened every 2–3 years in the absence of other risk factors for cervical dysplasia.
- After age 70, women who have had 3 or more normal Pap smears and no abnormal smears in the last 10 years may choose to stop screening.
- Screening after total hysterectomy (with removal of the cervix) is usually not indicated, unless the hysterectomy was performed for treatment of cervical dysplasia or dysplasia, or the patient has a history of in utero DES exposure.

DES, diethylstilbestrol.
[1]From the 2002 American Cancer Society guidelines. For complete guidelines see http://CAonline.AMCancerSoc.org or CA Cancer J Clin 2002;52:342.

a negligible risk of developing cancer as an older woman. As noted previously, however, the incidence and mortality rates in the United States for cervical cancer are highest among older women, which is evidence that this population is currently underscreened. Primary care practitioners must ensure that their older patients have had several documented normal smears before Pap smear screening is halted solely on the basis of age. After that time, routine inspection of the female genital tract to screen for pelvic tumors and gynecologic problems should continue.

A related issue is vaginal apex Pap smear screening of post hysterectomy patients. Any woman who underwent a supracervical hysterectomy still has a cervix and thus needs to have Pap smears. Because vaginal cancer is so rare, vaginal apex Pap smear screening after a hysterectomy is not necessary for most women. However, there is risk of vaginal cancer for women previously treated for lower genital tract cancer or who were exposed to diethylstilbestrol (DES) in utero; Pap smear screening should continue indefinitely for those two groups of women. Women who have had a hysterectomy for cervical dysplasia or endometrial cancer also should have vaginal apex Pap smears performed for several years until consecutive normal smears are documented.

B. Pap Smear Technique

Most cervical dysplasias arise in the transformation zone. This region is usually located at or near the cervical os and represents the junction between the squa-

mous epithelium of the vagina and exocervix and the columnar epithelium of the endocervix and endometrium (Figures 49–2 and 49–3).

Most false-negative Pap smears are due to sampling error by the clinician rather than faulty interpretation by the cytologist. The specimen should not be contaminated by lubricant and should be obtained before samples are acquired for cervical cultures. Large amounts of vaginal discharge, if present, should be removed gently. With care taken to avoid excessive bleeding, the clinician scrapes a wooden or plastic spatula circumferentially over the exocervix; this step is followed by a gentle, partial rotation of an endocervical brush within the cervical canal. An additional circumferential smear of the upper two thirds of the vagina should be obtained in DES-exposed women. The material obtained should be smeared on a glass slide and fixative rapidly applied. Air drying, which can occur within seconds, renders the sample uninterpretable.

The adequacy of the specimen should be described in the report from the cytologic laboratory. Smears should be repeated when considered unsatisfactory for evaluation because of too few endocervical cells, excessive blood, or inflammation. In the latter situation, a repeat smear can be delayed until after treatment for any infectious cause of cervicitis or vaginitis. The clinician should recognize that the intense inflammation and bloody discharge associated with an occult cancer could be the underlying reason for the inadequate smear.

C. New Technologies

Preparation of cytology slides from a suspension of cells in a liquid medium allows easier interpretation, since the cells are dispersed in a monolayer rather than lumped together as on a conventional Pap smear. Cellular detail is also less likely to be obscured by blood, inflammatory cells, or other debris, which can improve the accuracy of the Pap smear report. Commercially available fluid-based cytology systems include Cytec's ThinPrep and AutoCyte's SurePath System. Many health insurance companies are now covering the additional expense of these monolayer cytology slides.

Computer-based automated systems use a neural network processor to help select abnormal cells from the thousands of cells in a typical Pap smear. Early studies reported up to a 12% improvement in the detection of dysplasia with computerized screening. However, skepticism about the cost of computerized screening systems has probably hampered both the acceptance of this new technology by clinicians and the success of the companies that developed the systems.

Several commercially available tests have also been developed to detect HPV on cervical samples. Hybrid Capture II, provided by Digene Corp., detects the

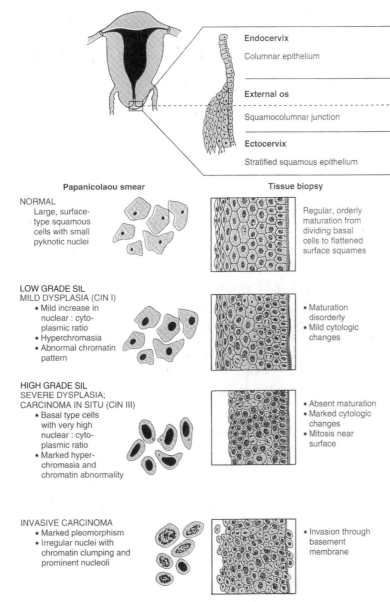

Figure 49–2. Squamous epithelial abnormalities and carcinoma of the cervix, showing criteria used to grade dysplasia. (Reproduced, with permission, from Chandrasoma P, Taylor CR: *Concise Pathology.* Appleton & Lange, 1991.)

DNA of most of the known high-risk HPV types. The clinical usefulness of HPV assays is probably limited to women with borderline abnormal smears, as discussed in the following Evaluation section.

Together, these new technologies do have the ability to improve slightly the sensitivity of cervical cytology. However, the cost-effectiveness of these more expensive tests does need to be considered carefully.

Mark DH: Visualizing cost-effectiveness analysis. JAMA 2002; 287:2428. [PMID: 11988064] (Excellent editorial explaining

cost-effectiveness analyses for cervical cancer screening strategies.)

Pap Smear Classification Systems

A. BACKGROUND

Figure 49–2 illustrates the spectrum of cervical disease, ranging from normal squamous epithelium to microinvasive squamous carcinoma. Progressive replacement of the epithelium by dysplastic cells defines the worsening degrees of dysplasia. Table 49–4 provides an overview

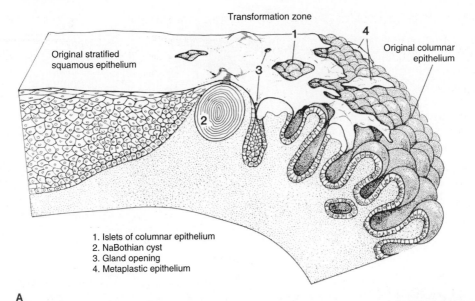

Transformation zone

Original stratified
squamous epithelium

Original columnar
epithelium

1. Islets of columnar epithelium
2. NaBothian cyst
3. Gland opening
4. Metaplastic epithelium

A

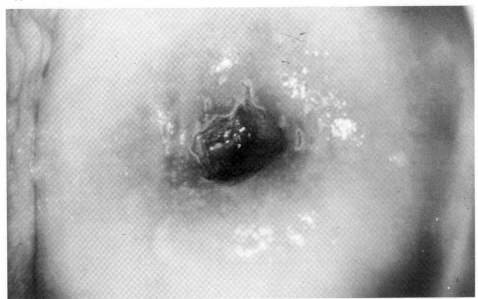

B

Figure 49–3. The transformation zone and the physiologic squamocolumnar junction. At birth, the squamocolumnar junction usually is located on the exocervix. Beginning in adolescence, it gradually migrates into the cervical canal as columnar epithelium undergoes metaplasia and matures into squamous epithelium. **A:** Schematic diagram. **B:** Colpophotograph of normal transformation zone. Note the squamocolumnar junction and gland openings. (Reproduced, with permission, from Burke L, Antonioli DA, Ducatman BS: *Colposcopy: Text and Atlas.* Appleton & Lange, 1991.)

Table 49–4. Overview of classification systems for Papanicolaou smears.[1]

Original "class" system	Modifications (1960s, 1970s)	Bethesda system[2] (1988–2001)
Class I—normal	Normal	Normal
Class II—slightly suspicious for malignancy	Atypical cells, but below the level of cervical neoplasia	Atypical squamous cells of undetermined significancer (ASCUS)
Class III—moderately suspicious for malignancy	Dysplastic cells present consistent with intraepithelial neoplasia; often graded as cervical intraepithelial neoplasia (CIN) I–III	Low-grade squamous intraepithelial lesion (LSIL); equivalent to changes associated with human papillomavirus (HPV) and CIN I
Class IV—highly suspicious for malignancy	Carcinoma in situ (CIN III)	High-grade squamous intraepithelial lesion (HSIL); equivalent to CIN II–III
Class V—diagnostic for malignancy	Invasive cancer	Invasive cancer

[1]These systems are not directly interchangeable.
[2]Table 49–5 contains additional details of the Bethesda system.

of the different classification systems for Pap smears, including the "class" system, the dysplasia and cervical intraepithelial neoplasia (CIN) nomenclature, and the modern Bethesda system.

B. THE BETHESDA SYSTEM

Although the dysplasia and CIN nomenclatures have been used for several decades, variability in reporting results from different laboratories has hampered effective clinical management. A national interdisciplinary group was convened in 1988 to standardize the interpretation of cervical Pap smears and biopsies, leading to the current Bethesda system (Table 49–5). The most sweeping change was the use of only 2 terms, **low-grade squamous intraepithelial lesion (LSIL)** and **high-grade squamous intraepithelial lesion (HSIL),** to encompass the entire spectrum of squamous cell carcinoma precursors. The LSIL category includes CIN I (mild dysplasia) as well as HPV-associated changes (koilocytosis). The Bethesda system recognizes the linkage of HPV infection with cervical neoplasia and the practical difficulty in distinguishing koilocytosis from mild dysplasia by cytologic or histologic criteria. The HSIL category includes CIN II and III (moderate dysplasia, severe dysplasia, and carcinoma in situ). The Bethesda system also sought to define more precisely the term "atypia," which in the past had become so overused it was clinically meaningless. The category **atypical squamous cells of undetermined significance (ASCUS)** should be applied to relatively few cases. Glandular cell abnormalities also are reported more precisely in the 2001 Bethesda systems. Specifically, the term "atypical glandular cells of undetermined significance" (AGCUS) is no longer used. **Atypical glandular cells (AGCs)** are more ominous than

atypical squamous cells and should prompt referral to an experienced gynecologist.

Solomon D et al: The 2001 Bethesda System: terminology for reporting results of cervical cytology. JAMA 2002;287:2114. [PMID: 11966386]

Evaluation

A. INDICATIONS FOR COLPOSCOPY

An abnormal Pap smear report merely identifies a patient who needs additional evaluation. The severity of the cervical lesion and its precise topographic location can be determined best by colposcopically directed cervical biopsies. Any woman with a Pap smear diagnosis of HSIL or AGC should undergo colposcopic evaluation promptly. With few exceptions, colposcopy is also now recommended to evaluate an LSIL Pap smear, in contrast to earlier recommendations that allowed repeat cytologic testing.

Significant controversy persists concerning the evaluation of the ASCUS Pap smear, however. Earlier series have identified high-grade dysplasia in 3–77% of patients within this Pap smear category. The wide disparity can be attributed to variable definitions of atypia and to dissimilar patient populations. Table 49–6 lists acceptable management options for different clinical situations. Under the 2001 Bethesda system, there should be a very low rate of occult dysplasia among smears classified in the new ASCUS category. Because dysplasia is detected at a higher rate when the cytologist cannot exclude HSIL (eg, ASC-H category), colposcopy is recommended for those patients.

Current guidelines have been influenced by new information from the ongoing ASCUS/LSIL Triage

Table 49–5. 2001 Bethesda system for reporting cervical and vaginal cytologic diagnoses.[1]

SPECIMEN TYPE
  Conventional Pap smear versus liquid-based versus other
ADEQUACY SPECIMEN
  Satisfactory for evaluation
  Unsatisfactory for evaluation
GENERAL CATEGORIZATION
  Negative for intraepithelial lesion or malignancy
  Epithelial cell abnormality: see Interpretation/Result (specify "squamous" or "glandular" as appropriate)
  Other: see Interpretation/Result
AUTOMATED REVIEW
  If case examined by automated device, specify device and result
ANCILLARY TESTING
  Provide a brief description of the test (e.g., HPV typing) and report the result so that it is easily understood by the clinician.
INTERPRETATION/RESULT
  NEGATIVE FOR INTRAEPITHELIAL LESION OR MALIGNANCY
  ORGANISMS
    Trichomonas vaginalis
    Fungal organisms morphologically consistent with *Candida*
    Shift in flora suggestive of bacterial vaginosis
    Bacteria morphologically consistent with *Actinomyces*
    Cellular changes consistent with herpes simplex virus
  OTHER NONNEOPLASTIC FINDINGS (LIST NOT INCLUSIVE)
    Reactive cellular changes associated with inflammation (includes typical repair)
    Radiation
    Intrauterine contraceptive device (IUD)
    Glandular cells status post hysterectomy
    Atrophy
  OTHER
    Endometrial cells (in a woman 40 years of age or older) (specify if "negative for squamous intraepithelial lesion")
SQUAMOUS CELL ABNORMALITIES
  Atypical squamous cells of undetermined significance (ASCUS) cannot exclude HSIL (ASC-H)
  Low-grade squamous intraepithelial lesion (LSIL) encompassing: HPV/mild dysplasia/CIN I
  High-grade squamous intraepithelial lesion (HSIL) encompassing: moderate to severe dysplasia and CIS/CIN II and CIN III
  With features suspicious for invasion
  Squamous cell carcinoma
GLANDULAR CELL ABNORMALITIES
  Atypical glandular cells (AGC)
  Atypical glandular cells, favor neoplastic (specify endocervical, endometrial, or NOS)
  Endocervical adenocarcinoma in situ
  Adenocarcinoma (Specify endocervical, endomatrial, extrauterine, or NOS)
OTHER MALIGNANT NEOPLASMS: (specify)
EDUCATIONAL NOTES AND SUGGESTIONS (optional)
  Suggestions should be concise and consistent with clinical follow-up guidelines published by professional organizations
    references to relevant publications may be included).

NOS, not otherwise specified.
[1]Complete 2001 Bethesda System is available at www.bethesda2001.cancer.gov. See also JAMA 2002;287:2114.

Study (ALTS), in which approximately 7200 women with these Pap smear results were randomly assigned to (1) immediate colposcopy, (2) HPV testing, with colposcopy if high-risk HPV was detected, or (3) repeat cytology, with colposcopy if repeat cytology was also abnormal. Early analysis indicates that HPV testing is not useful when evaluating women with LSIL. But a positive test for high-risk HPV can be used to select women with ASCUS cytology for colposcopy.

The American Society for Colposcopy and Cervical Pathology (ASCCP) 2001 guidelines include HPV DNA testing as the preferred approach for triaging women with ASCUS when liquid-based cytology is used for the initial Pap smear. In this situation, the

Table 49–6. Management options[1] for the diagnosis of atypical squamous cells of uncertain significance (ASCUS) on Papanicolaou (Pap) smear.[2]

Immediate referral for colposcopy
    Patients at significant risk for occult dysplasia or cancer
        High risk HPV type
        HSIL cannot be excluded (ASC-H)
        Persistently atypical smears
        Prior treatment for dysplasia
        Epidemiologic high risk (see Table 49–2)
        AIDS or HIV-seropositive
    Patient considered unreliable for long-term monitoring
Antibiotic therapy for cervicitis,[3] followed by repeat Pap in
    6–12 wk
    Yeast, *Chlamydia*, or *Trichomonas* infections
Estrogen therapy for atrophy, followed by repeat Pap in 3 mo
    Postmenopausal women with lower genital tract atrophy
Repeat Pap smear in 4–6 mo
    All other patients[4]

HSIL, high-grade squamous intraepithelial lesion; HPV, human papillomavirus.

[1]Accurate information about the patient's clinical history and close dialogue between the primary practitioner and laboratory are essential for optimal management of patients in this Pap smear category.

[2]Patients with atypical glandular cells (AGC) detected on Pap smears should be referred to an experienced colposcopist for evaluation.

[3]Inflammation can be associated with normal metaplasia, so in the absence of cytologic atypica is not necessarily abnormal; severe inflammation may mask invasive cancer.

[4]Women with *negative* assay for high-risk HPV type can delay next Pap smear for 1 year; otherwise, persistent ASCUS requires colposcopy.

original cytology specimen can be used for "reflex" HPV DNA testing, and the 40–60% of women with a negative test for high-risk HPV DNA can be spared an unnecessary colposcopy. But the "best" management strategy is still being debated. Many women (up to 75%) who test positive for high-risk HPV do not have colposcopic evidence of high-grade dysplasia. And the potential value of inexpensive Pap smear surveillance can be determined only after long-term follow-up information is known from the ALTS trial.

B. Technique of Colposcopy

Colposcopic evaluation relies on stereoscopic magnification to visualize the changes in color, vascular pattern, and surface contour that identify neoplastic regions on the cervix (Figure 49–4). The vagina and vulva also should be evaluated carefully because vulvovaginal dysplasias and cancers may coexist with cervical

lesions. The application of 3% acetic acid causes neoplastic regions to appear white as the result of transient dehydration. Abnormal vascularity, usually recognized as mosaic or punctate patterns, is seen more easily when viewed with a green light filter. Dense acetowhitening, unusual surface contour changes, and marked vascular changes are hallmarks of occult invasive cancer. Determining the extent of the dysplastic lesions is necessary in planning subsequent therapy. Colposcopy is considered satisfactory when the entire transformation zone and any associated abnormalities can be visualized fully. An unsatisfactory colposcopic examination is dangerously inaccurate because occult carcinoma may escape detection. Areas demonstrating colposcopic changes consistent with neoplasia can be biopsied with minimal discomfort (Figure 49–5). In general, an endocervical curettage (ECC) also should be performed. HSIL Pap smears should not be ignored if biopsies are negative or show only LSIL. Although possible "over-call" of the original Pap smear should be addressed by the cytopathologist, the more likely explanation of this discrepancy is an error by the colposcopist. Repeat colposcopy should be performed promptly. A diagnostic cervical conization may be necessary.

C. Cervical Conization

As a diagnostic procedure, cone biopsy of the cervix (Figure 49–6) should be performed when any of the following 4 clinical situations is present: (1) the colposcopic examination is unsatisfactory, (2) the ECC is positive for neoplasia, (3) the cytologic diagnosis is significantly more severe than shown by the colposcopically directed biopsies; or (4) biopsies suggest a microinvasive cancer or adenocarcinoma in situ.

Herbst AL et al: The management of ASCUS cervical cytologic abnormalities and HPV testing: a cautionary note. Obstet Gynecol 2001;98:849. [PMID: 11704181] (Respected authors question the role of routine HPV testing in clinical practice.)

Kaufman RH: Is there a role for human papillomavirus testing in clinical practice? Obstet Gynecol 2001;98:724. [PMID: 11704159] (Respected authors question the role of routine HPV testing in clinical practice.)

Solomon D, Schiffman M, Tarone R: ASCUS LSIL Triage Study (ALTS) conclusions reaffirmed: response to a November 2001 commentary. Obstet Gynecol 2002;99:671. [PMID: 12039132] (With rebuttal by lead investigators in the ALTS group.)

Wright TC Jr et al: 2001 Consensus Guidelines for the management of women with cervical cytological abnormalities. JAMA 2002;287:2120. [PMID: 11966387]

Psychosocial Concerns

It is very stressful for a woman to receive an abnormal Pap smear report. She must confront the possibility of

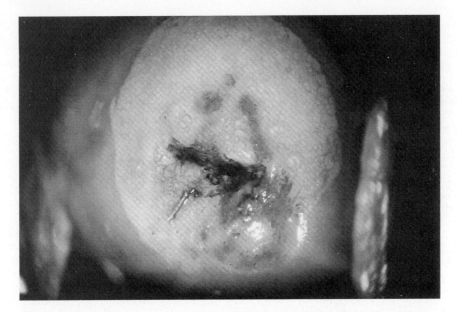

Figure 49–4. Colpophotograph after application of 3% acetic acid demonstrating acetowhitening and a mosaic vascular pattern. Biopsies revealed high-grade squamous intraepithelial lesions (HSIL). The broad area of dysplasia in this case is best treated with carbon dioxide laser vaporization rather than cryocautery. (Reproduced, with permission, from Burke L, Antonioli DA, Ducatman BS: *Colposcopy: Text and Atlas.* Appleton & Lange, 1991.)

malignancy while at the same time dealing with a disease process and necessary treatments that threaten core elements of her sexual, reproductive, and gender identities.

It is imperative that the patient be provided with complete and accurate information about her Pap smear abnormality. Women often complain that they were notified of their abnormal Pap result by inexperienced office staff. In addition, every effort should be made to avoid stigmatizing cervical cancer as a sexually transmitted disease.

Treatment of Cervical Dysplasia

A. ROLE OF EXPECTANT MANAGEMENT

Women with HSIL should undergo prompt treatment because of the risk of progression to invasive cancer. Although progression is not a certainty and it may take several years, there is a subset of patients in whom cancer rapidly develops. Furthermore, early treatment of preinvasive neoplasia can be accomplished by any of several procedures outlined in the following section, with preservation of fertility. The only reason to delay treatment of HSIL is a concurrent pregnancy.

On the other hand, the observation that over 50% of all mildly dysplastic lesions may resolve spontaneously has prompted some practitioners to defer therapy for these lesions. Surveillance is most appropriate for a young woman found to have koilocytotic atypia bordering on mild dysplasia who agrees to at least semiannual Pap smears and colposcopic examinations. Certainly, many women classified in the new Bethesda system with LSIL have only HPV-associated changes, and most experts currently recommend that such patients not be treated.

B. TREATMENT METHODS

A variety of techniques may be used to treat preinvasive neoplasia of the cervix. These include ablative therapy (electrocoagulation diathermy, cryocautery, carbon dioxide laser vaporization) and excisional procedures (scalpel or laser conization, loop excision). The choice of therapy depends on the severity, size, and distribution of the lesion. It is of paramount importance that, before the initiation of any ablative therapy, there is histologically proven dysplasia consistent with the cytologic diagnosis and no evidence of endocervical involvement or occult invasion. Up to half of invasive cervical

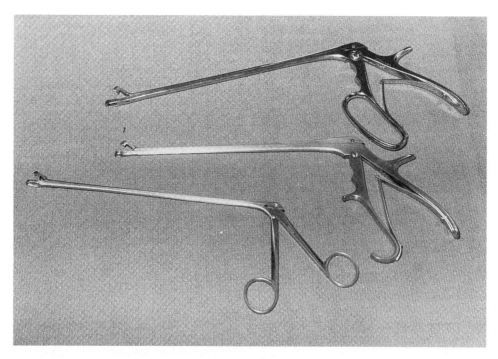

Figure 49–5. Biopsy instruments used during colposcopy. From top to bottom: Tischler, Burke, and Eppendorfer biopsy forceps. (Reproduced, with permission, from Burke L, Antonioli DA, Ducatman BS: *Colposcopy: Text and Atlas.* Appleton & Lange, 1991.)

cancers occurring after ablative therapy for dysplasia are due to errors by the colposcopist, usually because an indication for excisional conization was not recognized.

Cryocautery with a liquid nitrogen or carbon dioxide–cooled probe is effective therapy for small, low-grade lesions of the exocervix. Cryocautery is most effective when applied in two 3-minute freezings with a 5-minute period for thaw between applications. Using the double-freeze technique, 94–97% of mildly or moderately dysplastic lesions occupying less than 25% of the surface of the cervix are treated effectively.

There are a number of disadvantages to the use of cryocautery in all cases. First, its success rate depends on the degree of dysplasia. Failure rates in the treatment of CIS range from 18% to 39%. In addition, regardless of the grade of dysplasia, lesions occupying more than half of the cervical surface (see Figure 49–4) or involving endocervical glands may have a 20–50% failure rate. Another disadvantage to cryocautery is that it may cause migration of the squamocolumnar junction into the endocervical canal, rendering all subsequent colposcopic examinations unsatisfactory.

Vaporization of the abnormal cervical epithelium to a depth of 7–8 mm with a **carbon dioxide laser** has

significant advantages over cryocautery. Over 90% of women can be treated successfully with laser therapy, and unlike cryocautery, cure rates are not related to lesion size or degree of dysplasia. In addition, healing is rapid, with less posttreatment vaginal discharge. When this treatment is performed properly, the transformation zone remains visible. The major disadvantages of laser vaporization are its cost and technical complexity.

Although primarily a diagnostic procedure, **scalpel conization** may be therapeutic if the lesion is excised completely with negative margins. If the lesion is resected completely, the recurrence rate following conization of squamous lesions is 2% or less. Management of the less common, adenocarcinoma in situ lesions is more controversial, although carefully selected young women can be treated safely by conization alone.

The **loop electrosurgical excision procedure (LEEP)** is a common office technique for the treatment of cervical dysplasia (Figure 49–7). It allows histologic evaluation without the cost of performing a scalpel conization in the operating room. Removal of the entire transformation zone to a depth of 7–8 mm is termed "large loop excision of the transformation zone" (LLETZ) and is equivalent to laser vaporization of the

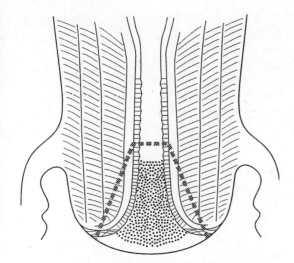

Figure 49–6. Schematic of traditional broad, deep cervical conization. Smaller, more precise conizations under colposcopic guidance can be performed now for most women in an office setting with the carbon dioxide laser or the loop electrosurgical excision procedure (LEEP). (Reproduced, with permission, from Berek JS, Hacker NF: *Practical Gynecologic Oncology*, 2nd ed. Williams & Wilkins, 1994.)

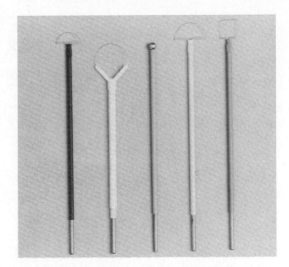

Figure 49–7. Selection of electrodes used for loop electrosurgical excision procedures (LEEP). Large loop excision of the transformation zone (LLETZ) usually can be done in a single pass with a loop that is 15 mm wide and 7 mm deep. Narrow loops can excise portions of the endocervical canal, and large loops are useful for office conizations. Ball electrodes are used for hemostasis. (Courtesy of Virginia Mason Medical Center Medical Art and Photography.)

exocervix. A larger loop can be used to perform office cone biopsies.

Hysterectomy has little role in the treatment of women with cervical squamous intraepithelial lesions. In general, hysterectomy is advised only for women who have completed childbearing and have dysplasia at the endocervical margin of an adequate cone biopsy. When fertility is important and dysplasia involves a cone margin, a careful colposcopic examination, Pap smear, and ECC should be repeated after 3 months. If dysplasia is detected again, reconization can be considered before a hysterectomy is recommended.

C. POSTTREATMENT SURVEILLANCE AND PROGNOSIS

After treatment for cervical dysplasia, the first follow-up Pap smear should be done in 3–4 months; repeat colposcopy and endocervical curettage are generally advised when monitoring patients after treatment for HSIL or endocervical dysplasia. Patients should be monitored subsequently with Pap smears and selective colposcopic examinations every 4–6 months for 2 years, during which time almost all recurrences (or treatment failures) will occur. Long-term annual follow-up is required, nonetheless, because recurrences can occur years later and involve any portion of the lower genital tract. Fortunately, lifetime risk of developing invasive cancer

is low (less than 3%) after appropriate management of preinvasive lesions.

Gold M et al: Loop electrocautery excisional procedure: therapeutic effectiveness as an ablation and a conization equivalent. Gynecol Oncol 1996;61:241. [PMID: 8626140]

Hildescheim A et al: Risk factors for rapid-onset cervical cancer. Am J Obstet Gynecol 1999;180:571. [PMID: 10076130]

Holowaty P et al: Natural history of dysplasia of the uterine cervix. J Natl Cancer Inst 1999;91:252. [PMID: 10037103]

When to Refer to a Specialist

Gynecologic oncologists and obstetrician-gynecologists who have received specialized training currently perform most colposcopic examinations in the United States. Considering the increasing number of women with abnormal Pap smears, it is appropriate for primary care clinicians with an interest in women's health care to become proficient in colposcopy. Similarly, although most patients who require treatment are referred to a specialist, some primary care providers may choose to learn techniques of cryotherapy, laser therapy, or loop excision. This circumstance is most appropriate in rural or other areas underserved by gynecologic specialists. Some clinical situations that may require consultation

Table 49–7. Evaluation of the abnormal Papanicolaou (Pap) smear: indications for specialty referral.

A. Suspicion of cancer, based on 1 or more of the following:
   1. Malignant cells on Pap smear
   2. Colposcopically directed biopsies
   3. Colposcopy suggestive of cancer, even if not confirmed by biopsy
B. Unsatisfactory colposcopy or other situation requiring cervical conization
C. Unexplained discrepancy between cytologic and histologic findings[1]
D. Pregnancy complicated by abnormal Pap smear
E. Nonsquamous lesions, including cytologic findings consistent with atypical glandular cells, adenocarcinoma in situ, or adenocarcinoma; and unusual diagnoses (lymphoma, sarcoma)

---

[1]Review by a gynecologic pathologist may be required in addition to referral to a clinical specialist.

with a specialist in obstetrics and gynecology, gynecologic oncology, or gynecologic cytopathology are listed in Table 49–7.

Relevant Web Sites

[American Society for Colposcopy and Cervical Pathology]
   www.asccp.org
[Bethesda System (2001)]
www.bethesda2001.cancer.gov
[Gynecologic Cancer Foundation]
www.wcn.org/gcf/
[Society of Gynecologic Oncologists]
www.sgo.org
[Women's Cancer Network]
www.wcn.org
[2002 American Cancer Society Guidelines for Pap smear screening]
http://Caonline.AmCancerSoc.org

Evaluation of Adnexal Masses & Screening for Ovarian Cancer

50

Susan P. Kupferman, MD & Kathryn F. McGonigle, MD

ESSENTIALS OF DIAGNOSIS

- *Adnexal masses can be found in women of all age groups.*
- *Determining the cause of an adnexal mass depends on patient's age and menstrual status.*
- *The primary role of the clinician is to exclude those adnexal masses that are malignant.*

General Considerations

Ovarian cancer is the most common cause of death due to gynecologic cancer; it is the fifth most common cancer in women and the third most common cause of overall cancer death in women. The American Cancer Society estimates that there will be 23,300 cases and 13,900 deaths from ovarian cancer in 2002. This figure exceeds the number of deaths in the United States from cervical and endometrial cancer combined.

The lifetime risk of ovarian cancer developing in a woman is about 1 in 70, or 1.4%. The risk varies with age groups. In the 20- to 29-year-old group, the risk is 4 in 100,000; in the 40- to 44-year-old group, it is 15 in 100,000; and in the 75- to 79-year-old group, it is 54 in 100,000.

Although the cause of ovarian cancer is unknown, several potential risk factors have been identified. Ovarian cancer tends to be a disease of Western industrialized countries and of nulliparous white women. Other known risk factors include family history of ovarian cancer and the presence of BRCA1 or BRCA2 gene mutations. Associated but unproven risk factors include a history of severe mumps, increased fat in the diet, increased coffee or caffeine intake, late menopause, exposure to fertility drugs, alcohol consumption, and exposure to talc or asbestos.

To date, the data regarding the role of hormone replacement therapy (HRT) and ovarian cancer remain controversial. Population studies by Weiss and Cramer have described relative risks of 1.3 (95% CI 0.9, 1.8) and 1.5 (95% CI 0.85, 2.87). More recently, this positive association was shown by Risch as well. Conversely, other researchers have reported either no effect or a protective effect on the risk of ovarian cancer among patients using HRT. Whittemore et al analyzed 12 case-control studies done over a 30 year period and described a relative risk of 1.1 (95% CI 0.59–2). They concluded that data provided no evidence of an altered risk for the development of ovarian cancer among women using HRT over the age of 40.

Multiparity, breast-feeding, and the use of oral contraceptives seem to be protective, possibly by decreasing the number of lifetime ovulatory events. Tubal ligation and prior hysterectomy also are associated with a decreased risk of ovarian cancer. The protection provided by oral contraceptives appears to be strong and increases as the duration of pill use increases. A reduction in risk of up to 60% may occur with oral contraceptive use for 6 or more years. A protective effect is present for even short-term users (3–6 months) and increases with longer-term use, persisting for many years after discontinuation of oral contraception. A significant reduction in risk of ovarian cancer among woman with a genetic mutation in the BRCA1 or BRCA2 gene who used oral contraceptives has also been found. The reduction in risk was 20% for up to 3 years of use, rising to 60% for 6 or more years of use.

The most probable cause of an adnexal mass differs depending on the patient's age. Less than 5% of ovarian malignancies occur in children and adolescents, with the incidence of ovarian malignancy being lower among adolescents than among younger children. The incidence of adnexal masses in the reproductive age group is difficult to determine since many nongynecologic etiologies are confused with gynecologic ones (Table 50–1). The chance of an adnexal mass being malignant in a women younger than 45 years is less than 1 in 15. The incidence of ovarian cancer increases with age, with the median age of diagnosis being 63 years. In postmenopausal patients, the chance at laparotomy of a primary adnexal mass being malignant is much higher.

Table 50–1. Nongynecologic sources of pelvic masses.

Organ or System	Disorder
Urinary tract	Distended bladder (urinary retention)
	Bladder diverticulum
	Pelvic kidney
	Polycystic kidney disease
	Urachal cyst
	Carcinoma of the bladder
Gastrointestinal tract	Cecum, redundant
	Sigmoid, redundant
	Appendiceal abscesses or tumors
	Diverticular disease
	Mesenteric cysts
	Carcinoma of the colon or small bowel
Spleen	Splenic cysts
	Enlarged spleen or malaria
	Accessory spleen
Others	Abnormal, asymmetric, or hypertrophic pelvic musculature
	Aneurysms of the pelvic vessels

Pathogenesis

Incessant ovulation, increased gonadotropin levels, and local chemical carcinogenesis are possible causes of ovarian cancer although the specific etiology is unknown. The most significant risk factor for the development of ovarian cancer, other than age, is family history. Although a strong family history on the maternal side has been recognized for a number of years as being important, recent data have shown that paternal history may be equally important.

The risk of developing ovarian cancer increases with the number of affected family members. Having 1 affected first-degree family relative increases a woman's lifetime risk from 1.4% to as high as 3% to 3.5%. In women with 2 or more affected first-degree relatives, the lifetime risk may be as high as 50%. The current theory is that germ-line inheritance of a mutant gene, which is transmitted in an autosomal dominant fashion with variable penetrance, increases the susceptibility to ovarian cancer. It is estimated that up to 10% of all epithelial ovarian cancers result from a hereditary predisposition.

Three different syndromes fall under the heading of familial ovarian cancer. First, there is the site-specific, **hereditary ovarian cancer syndrome,** in which only ovarian cancer is recorded. One study shows that essentially all families with site-specific ovarian cancer syndrome are linked to BRCA1 gene. More common is the hereditary breast-ovarian cancer syndrome, in which there is a mixture of both diseases, both often occurring in the same patient. The majority of these cases are associated with mutations of BRCA1 locus, with some involving the BRCA2 locus. Last, there is what used to be called the Lynch II syndrome, in which there are breast, ovarian, colon, endometrial, and other cancers presenting throughout the pedigree. This is now referred to as the **hereditary nonpolyposis colorectal cancer syndrome.** Recent information indicates that penetrance of the BRCA1 mutation is not as high as initially thought and that modifying genetic loci may affect penetrance. Current estimates suggest a lifetime ovarian cancer risk of 16% for carriers of either BRCA1 or BRCA2 gene mutations, in a group of Ashkenazi Jewish women.

One of the characteristics of these familial syndromes is that the ovarian cancers tend to occur at a younger age in successive generations. It is recommended that prophylactic oophorectomy be considered in women in these families between the ages of 30 and 35 or after childbearing is completed. These families also have a significantly increased incidence of benign neoplasms of the ovary, such as cystadenomas. The malignant potential of these processes is unknown.

Screening for Ovarian Cancer

There is great interest in early detection of ovarian cancer in the hopes that this would be a method of decreasing mortality of the disease. An acceptable screening test for ovarian cancer should be accurate with sensitivity > 75%, specificity > 99.6%, and positive predictive value > 10%. It should also be safe, inexpensive, and widely available.

The lack of symptoms in its early stages has led to a high fatality-to-case ratio. Advanced stage disease is diagnosed in 75% of women with the disease; these women have a 5-year survival of about 28%.

There are 3 screening techniques available at this time: 1) pelvic examination, 2) transvaginal ultrasound 3) CA-125 level. However, no single test or combination of these modalities has been shown to translate into a reduction in ovarian cancer mortality. Research studies continue in an attempt to identify an acceptable screening strategy.

The usefulness of a pelvic examination as a tool to detect ovarian cancer is limited. There is a greater than 30% inaccuracy level in the physical assessment of pelvic disease compared with that found with ultrasonography, laparoscopy, or laparotomy. Masses as large as 8–10 cm are missed by experienced examiners. It has been estimated that it would take approximately 10,000 pelvic examinations to detect 1 case of ovarian cancer in the general female population. Furthermore, there is no evidence that ovarian cancer detected in asymptomatic women based on abnormal pelvic examination alters their morbidity or mortality. While frequent pelvic examinations for women over 40 continue to be recommended, the benefit of using these examinations as a screening method has not been established. Transvaginal sonography (TVS) has been investigated as a noninvasive screening tool. It is preferred over transabdominal sonography because of its increased resolution, which is capable of detecting small morphologic changes in the ovary. In a recent study, TVS scans were done on 57,214 patients of which 180 were subjected to surgery. The investigators found 17 ovarian cancers; of these 11 were stage I, 3 were stage II, and 3 were stage III. This study showed TVS to have an 81% sensitivity and 98% specificity, with a positive predictive value of 9.4%. These investigators found that the survival of patients with ovarian cancer in the annually screened population was 93% at 2 years and 83.6% at 5 years. However, both the monetary cost of annual TVS and the personal cost of subjecting an unacceptable number of patients to surgery limits the usefulness of TVS as a single screening modality.

Color Doppler imaging coupled with TVS has been used in an effort to improve the accuracy of ultrasound. This procedure detects intra-ovarian vascular changes. It is hypothesized that neovascularization and changes in impedance of blood flow can be used to determine benign from malignant ovarian tumors. To date the ability of color-flow Doppler to differentiate benign from malignant processes is unknown and requires further investigation to determine its accuracy.

The most extensively studied tumor marker for ovarian cancer is CA-125 (see the following section, Laboratory Findings). The use of CA-125 to detect early ovarian cancer is limited by its lack of sensitivity and poor specificity in early disease. Furthermore, this marker may be elevated in a number of benign as well as malignant

conditions (Table 50–2). Serum CA-125 levels have been demonstrated to be elevated in 82% of women with advanced ovarian cancer, compared with less than 1% in healthy women. Intervention would most likely have an impact on mortality by detecting ovarian cancer in stage I or II. However, CA-125 levels were elevated in only 50% of women with these earlier stages. One of the larger studies to date is a study from Sweden, which measured CA-125 annually in 5550 women over the age of 40. The investigators found that of 175 women with elevated CA-125 levels, there were 6 cases of ovarian cancer, with cases evenly distributed among stages I, II, and III. In those women with normal CA-125 levels, 3 developed ovarian cancer. For women older than 50 years, CA-125 had a specificity of 99% in this study. The specificity is extremely poor for premenopausal women because CA-125 levels are often elevated as a result of benign disease. The results of this and other recent studies suggest that CA-125 does not have sufficient specificity to warrant its use in routine screening for ovarian cancer.

Other serum markers to be used alone or to complement CA-125 are being studied. Lysophosphatidic acid is a new marker that was found in a preliminary study to be present in 9 of 10 cases of early ovarian cancer. Additional studies are under way to determine the sensitivity and specificity of this marker.

In an attempt to improve the accuracy of the serologic screening, other tumor-associated markers have been combined in "panels." Many of these panels are commercially available, but their usefulness remains to be proved. These include CA-15-3, TAG 75, CA-19-9, NB/70K, CA-195, CST-1, and others. To date, no combination of tests has proved to be an accurate, consistent screening tool.

More recently, studies are focusing on a multimodal approach. A large, prospective, randomized trial of asymptomatic postmenopausal women was undertaken. These women were either randomized to no screening or to annual multimodal screening, which included annual CA-125, TVS, and a gynecologic examination when appropriate. The authors found a positive predictive value of 21% and found that those women who were screened and in whom cancer developed had a longer survival rate compared with those that were unscreened and in whom cancer subsequently developed. The mortality rates between the 2 groups did not significantly differ. Although combined modalities have improved sensitivity and specificity, overall effectiveness in detecting ovarian cancer has not yet been confirmed. These authors were encouraged that a multimodal approach to screening is feasible and recommended a larger randomized trial to determine effects on mortality.

Based on the high false-positive rate of screens that lead to an unacceptably large number of negative laparotomies in the above studies, the National Cancer

Table 50–2. Elevations of CA-125.

Benign	Malignant
Normal variation with menstrual cycle	Ovarian cancer
Endometriosis	Endometrial cancer
Adenomyosis	Cervical cancer
Pelvic inflammatory disease	Tubal cancer
Pancreatitis	Biliary tract cancer
Renal failure	Liver cancer
Leiomyomas	Pancreatic cancer
Early pregnancy	Breast cancer
Liver disease	Lung cancer
Cirrhosis	Colon cancer
Peritonitis	
History of abdominal or pelvic radiation	

Institute at its 1994 consensus conference concluded that there is no evidence that screening with CA-125 and/or TVS can be used to effectively decrease ovarian cancer mortality or morbidity. Thus, these tests are not recommended for routine screening in average risk patients.

The appropriate screening strategy for women at high risk based on family history or genetic studies is debated. The ability of screening to detect earlier stage cancer or affect mortality from the disease even in this group is unknown. However, given the increased risk in this population, it seems prudent to advocate multimodal screening. Although unproven, the American College of Obstetricians and Gynecologists recommends that women with documented BRCA1 or BRCA2 mutations or genetic predisposition to ovarian cancer should undergo serial testing, including transvaginal ultrasound studies and CA-125 levels until childbearing is complete or to the age of 35 at which time they recommended considering a prophylactic oophorectomy.

Screening has other limitations. There is strong evidence that at least some cases of so-called advanced ovarian cancer are not ovarian in origin but multifocal, arising de novo on peritoneal surfaces. These cases may represent as many as 9–10% of "ovarian" cancers and have been reported to occur in patients who have had their ovaries removed. Clearly, screening the pelvis for ovarian disease has no effect on the early detection of peritoneal cancer in these patients. Optimal management of women in high-risk families remains controversial. However, it is prudent to refer a woman with these genetic mutations to established genetic research programs for evaluation and discussion of options.

Clinical Findings

It is often diagnostic clues such as history, physical, and sonographic findings as well as the results of laboratory studies such as tumor markers that help the clinician determine the etiology of an adnexal mass.

A. SYMPTOMS AND SIGNS

Most cases of ovarian cancer are diagnosed when the disease has already spread through the peritoneal cavity. Nonspecific symptoms such as ascites, abdominal distention, vague gastrointestinal symptoms, pelvic or abdominal masses, or pain are often the presenting complaints. Earlier stage disease is often diagnosed serendipitously while the clinician is looking for something else. It is not unusual for ovarian cancer to be detected in women undergoing laparoscopy as part of an infertility evaluation. Therefore, it is necessary for providers of women's health care to consider ovarian neoplasms when any of these vague symptoms persist unexplained.

Patients with an adnexal mass may present with 1 or multiple symptoms. The severity and nature of the symptoms are important. It is important to ascertain if the patient is asymptomatic, if she is having acute symptoms such as pain and bleeding, or if her symptoms are more chronic. Midcycle pain may be consistent with a physiologic cyst. Acute pelvic pain associated with nausea and vomiting raises the possibility of adnexal torsion. Severe dysmenorrhea suggests endometriosis, and menorrhagia suggests fibroids.

During the pelvic examination, it is important to note not only the presence of a pelvic mass but also such details as size, bilaterality, mobility (fixed vs mobile), consistency (solid vs cystic), tenderness, contours (smooth vs irregular), and location. Associated symptoms such as fever, peritoneal signs, ascites, or pleural effusion are also important.

Ascites in the presence of a pelvic mass should suggest malignant disease until proved otherwise. **Meigs' syndrome,** a benign solid ovarian fibroma associated with ascites and a right-sided pleural effusion, is rare. Alcoholic patients with cirrhosis can present with ascites and elevated CA-125 levels. This clinical picture with or without an associated pelvic mass can be confusing and sometimes lead to unnecessary and life-threatening surgical interventions.

B. LABORATORY FINDINGS

A complete blood cell count with differential can be useful in sorting out inflammatory processes. A mildly elevated white blood cell count with a slight shift can be associated with salpingitis, diverticulitis, or torsion of the ovary. A normal white blood cell count, however, does not exclude any of these disease processes; many patients with significant inflammatory processes including peritonitis and even sepsis can present with normal counts.

Alpha-fetoprotein and carcinoembryonic antigen, lactate dehydrogenase (LDH), human chorionic gonadotropin can be elevated in germ cell tumors of the ovary and tend to occur in younger women. They are not useful as screening tests for pelvic masses.

CA-125 is a high-molecular-weight surface glycoprotein expressed by coelomic epithelium. This antibody was found to be elevated in some cases of epithelial ovarian cancer; when elevated, its level is somewhat proportional to the amount of tumor present. Therefore, in patients with epithelial ovarian cancers with elevated CA-125 levels, the test can be used to monitor progress of the disease that is under treatment or in remission. However, even in patients with documented ovarian cancer, a normal CA-125 does not exclude the presence of disease. Ninety-nine percent of normal women have a level of CA-125 below 35, and 99.8% have a level below 65. A CA-125 level of 35 is considered the upper limits of normal. Approximately 80–85% of patients with epithelial ovarian cancer have elevated CA-125 levels. This antibody is elevated in a large number of both benign and malignant processes (Table 50–2). In ovarian malignant disease, it tends to be elevated mainly in serous tumors. Mucinous tumors have a lower incidence of elevated CA-125 levels. In the postmenopausal patient with an adnexal mass, determination of a CA-125 level may be more useful, because the incidence of false-positive results in this group is significantly less.

C. IMAGING STUDIES

Once a pelvic mass has been found on examination, the next step is to select 1 or more of the available imaging studies to help formulate a diagnosis and a treatment plan. The pelvic ultrasound is the best radiologic test available to evaluate adnexal masses. Other currently available techniques include magnetic resonance imaging (MRI), computed tomography (CT), as well as the more conventional intravenous pyelography, barium enema, upper gastrointestinal (GI) series, and cystography.

CT generally is less helpful in diagnosing diseases of the pelvis than ultrasonography or MRI, although CT scans are probably more cost-effective in detecting diseases of the upper abdomen. MRI is particularly useful in differentiating leiomyomas, dermoids, and endometriomas from other pelvic masses.

Ultrasonography, especially transvaginal, is the most valuable diagnostic tool for most adnexal and uterine diseases, particularly in the asymptomatic patient. The transvaginal approach provides better resolution and less artifact and does not require the patient to have a full bladder. The transabdominal approach will add information regarding other abdominal processes. The normal ovary measures $3.5 \times 2.1 \times 1.5$ cm in the premenopausal patient and shrinks to $1.5 \times 0.7 \times 0.5$ cm by 2–5 years after menopause. In premenopausal women, a single ovarian follicle can enlarge in volume by up to 3 cm during the mid- to late-follicular phases of the menstrual cycle. These follicular cysts normally resolve spontaneously. However, a corpus luteum cyst may persist and findings on ultrasound may be consistent with hemorrhage or clot formation. These cysts ordinarily regress within 2 months, so a follow-up ultrasound to document regression is all that is usually required. Ultrasound will differentiate whether a mass is cystic or solid. Those masses that are of greater concern are those that have septations, excrescences, papillae, and all masses that contain both a solid and cystic component. Doppler ultrasound can also be used to help differentiate malignant from benign masses. Malignant cysts tend to have more neovascularization than do benign masses.

The availability and possible overuse of some tests has led to some dilemmas. This is especially evident in postmenopausal women in whom it appears that ovarian cysts are far more common than was previously known. At one time, it was clinical dogma that any enlargement in an ovary in a postmenopausal patient was an indication for surgical removal. Although this is still true for solid enlargement, increased use of pelvic ultrasonography and CT has taught clinicians that small unilocular cysts in postmenopausal patients may be stable or transient.

There is no reason to do an upper GI series or a small-bowel follow-through study in patients who present with a pelvic mass but do not have any upper tract symptoms. When GI symptoms are present, an evaluation of the colon may be worthwhile.

Differential Diagnosis

Adnexal masses occur in women of all ages. In considering a differential diagnosis for an adnexal mass, the clinician must first determine whether the etiology is gynecologic or nongynecologic and then distinguish whether the process is neoplastic or nonneoplastic (Tables 50–1 and 50–3). One of the most important diagnostic clues is the patient's age. Differential diagnosis for adnexal masses may be considered in terms of menstrual status.

The differential diagnosis of an adnexal mass in the premenarchal female includes primary neoplastic and nonneoplastic ovarian masses, Wilm's tumor, neuroblastoma, and abnormalities of the GI system. In newborns and infants, pelvic masses are most likely of ovarian origin, and are most likely due to nonneoplastic follicular cysts. These cysts occur in response to excessive stimulation of the fetal ovary by either placental or maternal hormones. The large majority of these regress spontaneously within 3–6 months after birth. The most common neoplastic ovarian mass in this age category is the benign cystic teratoma. The most common malignant ovarian masses for this age group are germ cell tumors, and of these dysgerminomas are the most common. Dysgerminomas are bilateral in 10–15% of cases. They may produce LDH, which may be used in the diagnosis and follow-up of this tumor. The major presenting symptoms are abdominal pain and a palpable mass.

The differential diagnosis of an adnexal mass in women of reproductive age is broad. However, the most common adnexal mass in the nonpregnant menstruating female is the physiologic (follicular and corpus luteum) ovarian cyst. Ninety percent of ovarian growths are benign. In the nonneoplastic category of adnexal masses, the most common is the functional ovarian cyst. Most ovarian cysts are no more than 8–10 cm in diameter.

Table 50–3. Ovarian and non-ovarian causes of adnexal masses.

Ovarian
  Neoplastic
    Benign
      Cystic teratoma
      Ovarian fibroma
      Cystadenoma
    Malignant
      Epithelial ovarian cancer
      Germ cell tumor
      Stromal tumor
      Metastatic tumors
  Nonneoplastic
    Functional
      Follicular cysts
      Corpus luteum cysts
      Hemorrhagic cysts
    Inflammatory
      Pelvic inflammatory disease
      Tuboovarian abscess
    Other
      Endometrioma
      Tuboovarian adnexal torsion
      Polycystic ovaries
      Paraovarian cyst
Non-ovarian
  Tubes
    Ectopic pregnancy
    Pyosalpinix
    Hydrosalpinix
    Tuberculosis endosalpingitis
    Malignant disease of tubes
    Endometriosis of tubes
  Uterus
    Pedunculated leiomyoma
    Mullerian malformation (bicornuate, unicornuate)
    Hematometria
    Malignant tumor (fundal, cervical)

Other nonneoplastic causes of adnexal masses such as endometriomas, polycystic ovaries, and tuboovarian abscesses must be considered in addition to both benign and malignant neoplasms. The overall risk of ovarian malignancy in the menstruating female is about 5%, but the risk increases depending on the complexity of the mass. Pregnancy should be excluded in all premenopausal patients with an adnexal mass. Ectopic pregnancy is a major cause of maternal mortality even in the 21st century and therefore must be excluded immediately. Once this has been ruled out, the clinician can then proceed with the appropriate work-up.

Endometriosis is suspected by a history of infertility, increasing dysmenorrhea, and premenstrual spotting. Endometriomas are suspected in the differential of a benign neoplasm that presents as an adnexal mass. They arise from ectopic endometrial tissue growth outside the uterus. They can often cause pelvic pain and dyspareunia. Endometriomas may appear as a complex mass on ultrasound and may be associated with an elevated CA-125.

Leiomyomas (fibroids) are a benign neoplasm of smooth muscle origin that may arise from the uterus or broad ligament. These masses are very common, occurring in 30% of premenopausal women. They are more common in black women. Patients often present with pelvic pain and pressure, urinary frequency, menorrhagia, and dysmennorhea. Cystic degeneration of a fibroid may present as a complex mass on ultrasound and fibroids can cause an elevated CA-125, raising suspicion of a malignancy during preoperative work-ups. A pedunculated uterine myoma may appear as a solid adnexal mass on physical examination and on radiologic studies.

Inflammatory etiologies are also an important consideration in nonneoplastic etiologies of a pelvic mass. Acute salpingitis usually is associated with fever, peritoneal signs, adnexal tenderness, purulent cervical discharge, and cervical motion tenderness. There may be a history of prior episodes, but the clinician should not be lulled into making a diagnosis of pelvic inflammatory disease (PID) just because the patient has had that diagnosis in the past. The prior diagnosis may have been in error. Tuboovarian abscess and hydrosalpinx and/or pyosalpinx are sequelae of chronic PID that should be considered in the differential diagnosis of an adnexal mass.

The presence of an adnexal mass in a postmenopausal female is concerning since the mass is more likely to be an ovarian malignancy. The older woman with an infectious process in the pelvis is more likely to have diverticular disease than PID. In a postmenopausal woman, any change in GI, urinary, or bowel habits needs to be investigated. Colonoscopy or barium enema combined with flexible sigmoidoscopy can be used to exclude diverticular disease or colon cancer.

Treatment

The differential diagnosis and management of an adnexal mass depends on the patient's age and menstrual status.

A. PREPUBESCENT FEMALE

The suspicion of a mass in a prepubescent female warrants an ultrasound. If the mass is cystic and asymptomatic, it can be followed safely. The presence of a solid mass in this age group should prompt a thorough work-up and surgical evaluation by a gynecologic oncologist.

B. Reproductive Age

1. Endometriosis—Laparoscopy is still the gold standard for diagnosing endometriosis, although its presence can be suspected from the history, physical examination, and ultrasonographic findings suggestive of an endometrioma. Elevated CA-125 levels up to 200 have been reported. Endometriomas and associated endometriosis can usually be removed adequately and safely with laparoscopic operative techniques.

2. Ovarian cysts—Ultrasonography is helpful in determining which cysts can be monitored and which cannot. In the premenopausal patient, cysts of less than 8 cm can be monitored for 1 or 2 cycles with the expectation that they are functional and will resolve. Clinicians can expect about 25–35% of these to persist. Cysts greater than 8 cm, even if considered functional, usually do not resolve spontaneously and are subject to rupture, bleeding, or torsion and infarction. Also, cysts less than 8 cm that persist beyond 1 to 2 menstrual cycles tend not to be functional and may need to be investigated surgically, especially if they are multilocular or septate. Hemorrhagic cysts such as corpora lutea should resolve, whereas endometriomas do not.

It is common practice to "suppress" suspected functional cysts by prescribing oral contraceptives for 2–3 months. Currently, there are no data that support the contention that oral contraceptives accelerate the resolution of functional ovarian cysts.

C. Postmenopausal Female

In the postmenopausal patient, the guidelines are different. Any solid enlargement of an ovary must be investigated and considered to be cancer until proved otherwise. However, numerous studies have demonstrated that unilocular cysts less than 5 cm in diameter may be observed. This is true only if there are no other associated risk factors such as ascites; in this situation, a CA-125 serum test might be useful because false-positive results are less common in the postmenopausal patient. If observation is chosen, the cyst should be monitored with serial ultrasound examinations. Many of these cysts resolve under observation. In 1 study of unilocular cysts, 40% were in postmenopausal women. If there is any increase in size during follow-up, the ovary needs to be removed expeditiously and its histologic structure examined.

Once it has been determined that an ovarian cyst is not likely to be functional, surgical intervention via laparoscopy is a viable option, particularly in the premenopausal patient. The use of this method in postmenopausal patients remains somewhat controversial, although there are reliable studies available that indicate its safety when correctly applied.

When to Refer to a Specialist

When and to whom to refer the patient once an adnexal mass has been detected can be challenging. If studies suggest that the mass is benign or a complication of pregnancy, referral to a general gynecologist, particularly one with expertise in laparoscopy, is appropriate. If there is any question that the mass may be malignant, early referral to a gynecologic oncologist may avoid unnecessary testing and can provide the patient with the best possible surgical intervention. Often a phone call to a specialist can guide the practitioner along the proper route of investigation and possibly save the patient from the expense and stress of unnecessary invasive procedures.

Prognosis of Ovarian Cancer

The prognosis of ovarian cancer is related directly to the stage of the disease at the time of diagnosis. Although there is greater than 90% 5-year survival rate in patients who have a low-grade ovarian cancer confined to 1 ovary, this situation is seldom encountered except by accident while investigating the patient for something else. Patients with stage II carcinomas of the ovary have a 5-year survival rate of approximately 60%; however, the rate for stage III and IV ovarian cancer is in the 15–28% range. Unfortunately, because of the insidious nature of the disease, most tumors are stage III or IV when first detected.

Cramer DW et al: Determinants of ovarian cancer risk. I. Reproductive experience and family history. J Natl Cancer Inst 1983;71:711. [PMID: 6578366]

Drake JG, Londono J, Hoffman MS: Evaluation of the adnexal mass. Up to date, www.uptodate.com, 2002.

Hankinson SE et al: A prospective study of reproductive factors and risk of epithelial ovarian cancer. Cancer 1995;76(No 2):284. [PMID: 8625104]

Hempling RE et al: Hormone replacement therapy as a risk factor for epithelial ovarian cancer: results of a case control study. Obstet Gynecol 1997;89:1012. [PMID: 9234929]

Jemal A et al: Cancer Statistics, 2002. CA Cancer J Clin 2002;52: 23. [PMID: 11814064]

Morgan A: Adnexal mass evaluation in the emergency department. Emerg Med Clin North Am 2001;19(No 3):799. [PMID: 11554288]

Narod SA et al: Oral contraceptives and the risk of hereditary ovarian cancer. N Engl J Med 1998;339:424. [PMID: 9700175]

Parazzini F et al: The epidemiology of ovarian cancer. Gynecol Oncol 1991;43:9. [PMID: 2066215]

Partridge EE, Barnes MN: Epithelial ovarian cancer: prevention, diagnosis, and treatment. CA Cancer J Clin 1999;49:297. [PMID: 11198956]

Ozols RF: Update of the NCCN ovarian cancer practice guidelines. Oncology 1997;11:95. [PMID: 9430180]

Paley PJ: Screening for the major malignancies affecting women: current guidelines. Am J Obstet Gynecol 2001;184:1021. [PMID: 11303215]

Risch HA: Estrogen replacement therapy and the risk of epithelial ovarian cancer. Gynecol Oncol 1996;63:254. [PMID: 8910636]

Weiss NS et al: Noncontraceptive estrogen use and the occurrence of ovarian cancer. J Natl Cancer Inst 1982;69:95. [PMID: 6948131]

Whittemore AS et al: Personal and environmental characteristics related to epithelial ovarian cancer. II. Exposures to talcum powder, tobacco, alcohol, and coffee. Am J Epidemiol 1988; 128:1228.

Relevant Web Sites

[National Cancer Institute]
www.nlm.nih.gov/medlineplus/ovariancancer.html

The Victim of Rape

51

Bonnie J. Dattel, MD

ESSENTIALS OF DIAGNOSIS

- *Screen and treat all victims for sexually transmitted infections.*
- *Offer pregnancy testing and emergency contraception to all victims.*
- *Consider a history of sexual assault when patient complaints cannot be clinically substantiated.*

Sexual violence remains a significant social and public health problem that disproportionately affects women. Survivors of this trauma frequently experience short- and long-term sequelae that can impact their lives. These symptoms often prompt women to seek medical care.

Primary care providers will see women with symptoms that may be associated with a history of sexual violence. These symptoms often do not respond to routine treatment, which can be frustrating for both physician and patient. An understanding of the magnitude and impact of sexual violence—along with knowledge about screening and intervention—can help providers offer appropriate care and support to patients.

General Considerations

Violence against women is not a new problem; it has been recognized since the recording of time. There are references to rape in biblical passages, works of art, and literature. Universally, girls and women continue to live with the reality of gender-based violence, selective abortion, murder, food deprivation, honor killing, and bride burning.

In 2000, The National Violence Against Women Survey released estimates that 302,091 women are raped each year. Research finds that most victims do not file police reports, making rape and sexual assault the most underreported violent crime. While the true prevalence of rape is unknown, it is clear that it affects primarily women. According to the Bureau of Justice Statistics report, rape and sexual assault are the only violent crimes that have not decreased in recent years.

Victims come from every socioeconomic, racial, and age group. Therefore, all practitioners of women's health are likely to see patients with a history of sexual assault or abuse. Most victims do not seek care immediately after the acute assault but rather days or weeks later.

A national survey conducted by the Department of Justice and the Centers for Disease Control and Prevention found that 18% of female respondents reported sexual assault at some time in their lives. Of note, 54% of these assaults occurred before the age of 18 years and 22% before the age of 12 years. Similar studies confirm that college-aged women are at high risk for sexual assault. Recent data suggest that nearly 5% of all college-aged women are victimized in any give calendar year. Most victims know their assailants. Classmates, friends, boyfriends or ex-boyfriends, and acquaintances have been identified as assailants.

Other issues may increase a woman's risk for sexual assault. Women who have been previously assaulted or abused are at increased risk. This increased risk is the result of negative self-perceptions developed secondary to abuse by a trusted adult or caregiver. A child may come to believe that she caused the abuse to occur. As a result, during adolescence and adulthood many individuals can exhibit what might be termed "loose boundaries" that can result in problematic relationships. In addition, it is not uncommon for women with such a history to use risky coping behaviors such as abuse of alcohol or drugs. All of these factors contribute to an increased vulnerability to victimization. Similarly, women with disabilities are at increased risk for victimization.

It is important to recognize that sexual assault is a violent crime of aggression, power, and control. Regardless of the gender of the victim, sexual assault offenders are most often male and are known to the victim. They are not "sex-crazed" maniacs hiding in the bushes. Rather, offenders are frequently enabled by other male friends who either support negative attitudes or who are passive bystanders to offender behavior. Compared with other violent convicted criminals, sex offenders are more likely to have suffered physical or sexual abuse as a child. However, two thirds of offenders report that they were not abused. Offenders will often exhibit or endorse other antisocial behaviors and attitudes as well as accept interpersonal violence as a way to solve problems (Table 51–1).

Table 51–1. Offender characteristics.

Offenders are NOT "sex-starved" maniacs
One third of convicted offenders suffered physical or sexual abuse as a child
Offenders often exhibit and/or endorse the following:
  Sexism, homophobia, heterosexism
  Anger and hostility toward women
  Acceptance of rape myths
  Rigid gender roles, hypermasculinity
  Lack of empathy

Definitions

In order to fully understand the issues surrounding sexual assault, it is imperative to have a working definition of **sexual assault.** There are no uniform definitions. Laws vary from state to state, as does the language surrounding the issue of sexual assault. In general, sexual assault is a term that can be defined as any unwanted sexual act. This can range from exhibitionism to penetration and must involve threats, physical force, intimidation, and/or deception. This can occur at any stage of a woman's life. During childhood, it is referred to as **sexual abuse.**

The legal definition of **rape** differs somewhat. It generally has 3 separate components: 1) sexual penetration; 2) force, intimidation, or lack of consent; and 3) threat of harm. The issue of consent is one of the most contentious during litigation. Lack of consent may be due to a variety of factors. These include disability, illness, or ingestion of drugs or alcohol (as in drug-facilitated sexual assault [DFSA]).

It is important to realize that rape per se is not the only form of sexual violence that can impact a woman's health. There is a wide range of sexual acts that can result in long-term consequences. This is particularly true with childhood sexual abuse. Sexual abuse can be defined slightly differently. It can be defined as engaging a child in sexual activities for which she is developmentally unprepared and therefore cannot give informed consent. It may not involve intercourse but instead such acts as fondling or being forced to watch sexual acts. Such acts may be as emotionally traumatic as penetration, especially since the perpetrator is most often a close male relative or family friend. All states have laws requiring health care providers to report suspected childhood sexual abuse.

Rape is usually used to describe an attempted or completed act of oral, anal, or vaginal penetration without obtaining consent. There are a variety of different "types" of rape:

Acquaintance rape: Attempted or completed nonconsensual sexual acts committed by someone known to the victim. The victim and the perpetrator have met previously in some kind of informal way. Date rape is a form of acquaintance rape.

Marital rape: Attempted or completed nonconsensual sexual acts committed in the context of a marriage or intimate live-in relationship.

Gang rape: Two or more perpetrators may or may not be known to the victim.

Statutory rape: State-defined and generally governs sexual relationships between adults and minors, regardless of whether the minor believes the relationship is consensual.

Drug-facilitated sexual assault: Refers to a rape perpetrated on a victim who is mentally and/or physically incapacitated by drugs and/or alcohol (see below).

Stranger rape: Attempted or completed nonconsensual sexual acts committed by a person unknown to the victim. This is the least common form of sexual assault.

DFSA has emerged in recent years as a more common form of acquaintance rape. Victims may consume alcohol and/or drugs voluntarily, as does the offender. Alcohol is the substance most frequently associated with sexual assault. In the last several years, rape crisis centers have had increasing reports of drugs being administered to the victim without her knowledge or consent. These drugs can be either illicit or over-the-counter substances. Whether the victim was given the drugs or took them voluntarily, the offender has still engaged in sexual activity without consent. Victims of DFSA often report having been in a social situation with a feeling of inebriation that does not correspond with the amount of alcohol consumed. There may be unexplained trauma and/or gaps in memory. There may be no knowledge of who or how many perpetrators existed. This is frustrating for the victim. In addition, the usual support systems such as friends and family minimize the trauma secondary to the victim's lack of memory. This can serve to exacerbate her feelings of powerlessness. The role of the health care provider is not to determine the truth but to respond to the patient's concerns with appropriate treatment and referrals.

Prevention

As part of a greater community, health care providers should participate in sexual assault prevention efforts. In order to do so effectively, it is best to understand the various types of prevention. The 3 basic types follow:

1. Primary: education, change in societal violence
2. Secondary: risk reduction strategies
3. Tertiary: prevention of adverse long-term consequences of sexual assault and abuse for individuals.

Historically, prevention efforts have been directed at women to prevent rape or sexual assault. This is a type of secondary prevention. It focuses on teaching young girls and women how to avoid potentially dangerous situations and use self-defense techniques. However, this may perpetuate the notion that girls and women can prevent sexual assault from happening. It unintentionally stigmatizes victims by implying they are to blame if an assault does occur. Naturally, this does little to reduce the prevalence of sexual assault or abuse.

The role of the health care providers has been mainly in tertiary prevention, working with the woman to help her overcome the trauma from the sexual violence.

Newer efforts focus on societal beliefs about power, sexuality, and violence. Primary prevention attempts to promote healthy relationship skills. It teaches alternative, nonviolent means of communication. Organizations such as the American College of Obstetricians and Gynecologists have developed prevention materials for adolescents. This type of prevention effort more appropriately focuses on perpetrators or potential perpetrators.

Consequences of Sexual Assault

In addition to the acute fears surrounding pregnancy and sexually transmitted infections (STIs) after sexual assault, there are a variety of short- and long-term sequelae. Women are likely to present to their health care provider with a variety of symptoms or complaints, many of which can be related to the traumatic experience. Usually, women do not associate these symptoms with the assault.

A. SHORT-TERM CONSEQUENCES

Short-term responses to sexual assault are physical, emotional, and behavioral (Table 51–2). The process of recovery from sexual assault generally follows a pattern. This is often called "rape trauma syndrome" and is similar in many respects to posttraumatic stress disorder (PTSD) (Table 51–3). Most providers of women's health care will not see victims in the acute phase but are more likely to see women in the stages of denial, reorganization, or integration and recovery. It is helpful to know as much as possible about these stages, in order to be most responsive to the patient. It is important to note that while most victims do not seek immediate medical care, or follow up after forensic examination, they do use the health care system at increased rates compared with women who have not experienced sexual violence. There is an 18% increase in health care utilization in the first year following assault. There is a 56% increase in the second year and a 31% increase in the third year after the assault. Thus, women who have experienced sexual violence do seek medical attention from their health care providers, underscoring the need to understand the presenting symptoms and appropriate interventions.

B. LONG-TERM CONSEQUENCES

Long-term health effects in victims of sexual assault can result directly from injuries sustained during the assault or abuse and/or from conversion symptoms secondary to the abuse. It is possible for any symptom to be referable to the assault, but common complaints include gynecologic problems, chronic pain, anxiety or depression, cardiac symptoms, gastrointestinal complaints, headaches, or multiple medical symptoms without apparent physical basis. In addition to the physical problems that can arise from assault or abuse, certain behaviors with potential adverse health consequences are more common in sexual assault victims. These risky behaviors may be coping mechanisms used to relieve emotional symptoms. Some survivors believe that something about them caused the abuse to happen or that they somehow deserve to be abused.

C. POSTTRAUMATIC STRESS DISORDER

Many of the short- and long-term consequences suffered by victims of abuse are directly related to PTSD.

Table 51–2. Short-term responses and consequences of rape.

Physical	Emotional	Behavioral
Injury	Depression	Risk taking
STI	PTSD	Substance use and abuse
Pregnancy	Rape trauma	Health care use
Somatization	Eating disorders	Avoidance of pelvic examination
	Sleep disorders	
	Suicide thoughts	
	Panic attacks	

STD, sexually transmitted diseases; PTSD, posttraumatic stress disorder.

Table 51–3. Rape trauma syndrome.

Acute phase
  Fear, physical symptoms
  Flashbacks, anxiety, mood swings
Denial phase
  Avoidance
Reorganization
  Life changes, recurrent symptoms
Integration and recovery
  Appropriate placement of blame
  Healing, advocacy

This can be of significant help to health care providers in caring for women suffering from sexual assault. There are 3 main reactions associated with PTSD: avoidance, hyperarousal, and reexperiencing. Most sexual assault victims experience emotional reactions to their victimization. However, if these symptoms persist beyond 6 months, PTSD may be diagnosed.

Fortunately, PTSD is treatable with medication, psychotherapy, or both. Being aware of PTSD and having the ability to make the appropriate referrals for long-term therapy is very reassuring to the patient.

Evaluation & Treatment of Victims of Sexual Violence

Screening and treating a patient who has been a victim of sexual violence can result in a stressful situation for the health care provider and staff as well as the patient. For providers who are also survivors, this can be particularly unsettling. It is important to remember that self-care is important to every provider, and debriefing skills can be an important part of the health care provider's professionalism. Ways to debrief include talking to colleagues or other support persons, exercise, relaxation, meditation, or prayer.

A. SCREENING FOR SEXUAL VIOLENCE

In order to provide comprehensive health care for women, it is important to screen for sexual violence. All women should be screened for such a history. Tips for screening include asking questions in a natural way. This allows for normalization of the experience while giving the patient control over the act of disclosure. This is not dissimilar to screening for domestic violence or sexual dysfunction. Over time, the practitioner develops his or her own style regarding the phrasing of questions of a sensitive nature. Perhaps the best method for screening is to ask direct questions:

> "Has anyone forced you or tricked you into having sexual activity that made you feel uncomfortable?"
>
> "When you had sex for the first time, was it something that you wanted to do?"
>
> "Has a sexual partner(s) ever forced you to have sex when you didn't want to? Has any other person?"
>
> "Will you have difficulty abstaining from sex?"

One of the first steps in conducting screening of any nature is to create an environment conducive to disclosure. This can be accomplished through artwork such as posters as well as patient education pamphlets or buttons. Materials of a sensitive nature can also be left in the restrooms so that women may access them confidentially. By making such screening a regular part of practice, the stigma associated with sexual victimization is lessened.

Despite best efforts to facilitate disclosure and assistance to victims, there will still be barriers to reporting sexual assault (Table 51–4). In addition, the sexual violence may be occurring or have occurred in the context of an intimate relationship. This type of violence may result in unintended pregnancies as well as inability to comply with medical recommendations.

Health care providers, too, may have barriers to screening. A busy provider may avoid screening because of the time that it may take to respond appropriately to disclosure of sexual assault. The provider may fear that the victim will "break down" once the disclosure is made. In fact, it is unlikely that this will happen, since most survivors of sexual assault have been dealing with the trauma for a long time. At the time of disclosure, the victim usually believes that this history is essential to receive appropriate health care.

Before screening is instituted, it is important to know the laws of the particular state in which the health care provider practices. The provider can then inform the patient of reporting requirements as well as fulfill legal obligations. For example, some states require that a report be filed even when an adult patient discloses that a sexual assault occurred during her childhood. In this situation, it is unlikely that social services or law enforcement will take action.

B. EMERGENCY SEXUAL ASSAULT EXAMINATION AND TREATMENT

Victims of sexual assault are often reluctant to report the occurrence of the sexual assault for a variety of reasons. They may have blacked out and are not sure what happened, or they might blame themselves—especially if they were using drugs or alcohol. Many women also have a cynical view of the medical and legal processes involving sexual assault, based on media portrayals and past experiences or anecdotal stories from other women. This means that many women may not seek medical care until days or weeks after the incident. When a patient calls requesting emergency contracep-

Table 51–4. Barriers to reporting rape.

Fear of retribution, stigmatization
Self-blame, embarrassment, shame
Unwillingness to label experience as rape
Lack of faith in the legal system
Limited access to care
Do not think they need medical attention
Confidentiality issues
Disclosure of victim's behaviors
Fear of insensitivity of police and health professionals
Fear of going through the court process
Ongoing abuse

tion, STI testing, HIV or pregnancy testing, it is important to consider that sexual victimization may have occurred and prompted these requests. The health care provider can open the door to disclosure by asking why the patient is requesting these tests or medications.

While the purpose of this chapter is not to provide a comprehensive guide to emergency sexual assault examinations, it is important to know local protocols and laws for such medical care. In general, if the patient discloses that she has been sexually assaulted within the last 72 hours, she should be referred for a forensic examination. Gently advise her that there is a limited amount of time during which evidence can be collected. It is, of course, her decision whether or not she chooses to proceed with such an examination. If she is so inclined, the physician or office staff can offer to help in arranging transportation or a patient advocate to accompany her throughout the examination.

Patients may also request testing for the presence of drugs if they suspect a DFSA. While it may still be possible to test for substances after the 72-hour period, it is critical that the patient understands the pros and cons of drug testing, since it may affect legal proceedings regarding the sexual assault.

Emergency contraception should be offered if the victim is at risk for pregnancy (see Chapter 52, Contemporary Contraception Practices in Clinical Care). The risk of pregnancy after a sexual assault is approximately 5%. There are 2 dedicated emergency contraception products. (Table 51–5). Both of these products require 2 doses. The first dose is administered as soon as possible following unprotected intercourse, and the second dose is given 12 hours later. Antinausea medications should be prescribed with ethinyl estradiol plus levonorgestrel (Preven). Other oral contraceptives may be used as emergency contraception. Dosages vary and in most cases antinausea medications should be used.

Another concern in the aftermath of sexual assault is the risk of exposure to STIs. The rate of acquiring gonorrhea, syphilis, or chlamydia after sexual assault ranges from 3.6–30%. This is highly dependent on the prevalence of the disease in the community as well as whether or not condoms were used during the assault. Because of the high risk of acquiring an STI, it is recommended that all women receive prophylaxis directed against gonorrhea, syphilis, and chlamydia after a sexual assault (see Chapter 34, Sexually Transmitted Infections & Pelvic Inflammatory Disease).

There is growing concern over the possible acquisition of viral STIs, especially HIV. The risk for HIV transmission during a sexual assault is estimated to be 1:500. This can be reassuring to victims, and at present, there are no standard recommendations for postexposure antiretroviral therapy in cases of sexual assault where the perpetrator's status is unknown. In cases where the perpetrator is known to be HIV positive, recommendations are to offer prophylaxis similar to post–needle stick exposure for health care workers. This is best coordinated with an infectious disease specialist so that the appropriate antiretroviral therapy can be instituted and follow-up arranged.

For all victims of sexual assault, an appointment should be scheduled for a follow-up evaluation of both physical and emotional needs.

Other Principles of Intervention

Once a woman has disclosed sexual trauma, it is critical to acknowledge the experience by letting her know the following:

- That you are sorry that his has happened to her
- That she is not alone; many women have experienced similar trauma
- That she did not do anything to deserve the assault
- That she is not to blame.

It is important to evaluate all victims for stage of emotional recovery and for the possible diagnosis of PTSD. This assessment can be made by a series of questions (Table 51–6). An answer of "yes" to any of these questions should prompt referral to a specialist in PTSD or victims of sexual assault.

In addition to the emotional assessment, the patient should be asked if she has any health concerns related to the trauma. The patient may not be able to relate her health complaints to her experience, and it may be appropriate to make that connection for her.

While it is necessary to know what to say, how to say it, and what to do, it is equally as important to know what **not** to say. Inappropriate statements such as "Why didn't you . . ." "You shouldn't have . . ." "You should have . . ." and "What did you do to lead him on?" may contribute to the guilt or shame felt by the victim as a result of the sexual assault. Similarly, the

Table 51–5. Emergency contraception therapies.

Drug	First Dose[1]	Second Dose[1]	Antinausea Therapy Recommended
(Plan B) ethinyl estradiol plus levonorgestrel	1 white	1 white	No
(Preven) Levonorgestrel	1 blue	1 blue	Yes

[1]The first dose should be administered as soon as possible, and the second dose should be given 12 hours later.

Table 51–6. Assess the patient's emotional recovery.

Have you ever talked to anyone about this? Would you like to?

Do you have flashbacks or avoid things that remind you of what happened?

Are your relationships (work or school) or day-to-day activities effected?

Do you want referral information?

---

physician or other health care provider must acknowledge their limitations. The provider cannot fix the situation but may help the patient regain control over her life through interactions with her both verbally and during examination.

To avoid re-traumatization, all procedures during an examination must be explained to the patient (Table 51–7). She has the right to decline procedures or ask them to be stopped if she is uncomfortable proceeding. Checking in with the patient during the examination (eg, "Are you okay with this?" or similar phraseology) gives the patient control over her body and allows the examination to proceed at her pace. Whenever possible, the patient should be allowed to suggest ways to minimize her fears during the examination. She may wish to have a friend, partner, or specific office staff person present with her during her examination. Before inviting an outside person into the examination room, it is imperative to ask the patient if you may speak freely in front of that person to maintain her confidentiality.

Regardless of the time between the assault and your interaction with the patient, providers should respond to disclosures by offering supportive statements, providing good referral information, and by modifying clinical practice to avoid re-traumatization.

Recently assaulted patients should be informed about some of the typical responses she may experience. She should be encouraged to be aware of any possible maladaptive behaviors that may occur, especially substance abuse, self-destructive activities, or mental health symptoms (eg, panic, depression, anxiety). This is a

Table 51–7. Avoid re-traumatization.

Explain each procedure in advance and during

Ask her permission to begin examination

Help her retain control during procedure

    Let her dictate pace of examination

    Maintain eye contact and conversation

    Provide a mirror if wanted

    Have patient assist

Tell her that she can stop examination if necessary

---

time when the clinician can assist in the process of recovery by educating patients. Explanations about the physiologic changes can help the woman understand her symptoms.

Finally, is important to realize that common life event "triggers" exist that can prompt a woman to seek care or develop difficulties because of the sexual assault. Knowing in advance what may "trigger" such an experience can be helpful for understanding the patient's reactions and concerns (Table 51–8).

When to Refer to a Specialist

It is of utmost importance for clinicians to provide appropriate referrals for women who have experienced sexual assault. It is especially helpful to identify a specific purpose for the referral, not only for the referring professional but for the woman as well. This reinforces the notion that her complaints are not just psychological but rather a real manifestation of her traumatic experience. It is the choice of the woman to accept or reject the referral.

Rape crisis centers are excellent resources for physicians, women, and the community. These centers offer a wide range of services including individual and group counseling, support systems, and referral lists. The woman must give her authorization before the referral is made. The ability for the professionals to speak to one another regarding the patient allows for a collaborative practice that is of great benefit to the patient. However, it is the patient who must decide if she wishes this information to be shared among the health professionals.

Traumatized patients generally benefit from mental health care. Women who disclose a history of sexual assault should be asked if they have ever had the opportunity to discuss this with anyone else. For patients who have not sought such assistance, the women's health care provider can be a powerful ally in the healing process by offering both referral and support. Since not

Table 51–8. Common life events that may act as "triggers."

Pregnancy or childbirth

Gynecologic or pelvic examinations

Key "anniversary" dates

Survivor's child is same age as survivor at time of abuse onset

Illness or injury of survivor's child

Sexual stimuli

Family reunions, illness or death of parent or perpetrator

Workplace situation mirrors a relationship with abuser

Viewing movies or television programs with abuse content

Sights, sounds, or smells

---

all mental health professionals are experienced in treating women survivors of sexual assault, it is helpful to compile a list of such individuals to have available in the office. These lists can be developed through a variety of sources such as State Boards, Rape Crisis Centers, battered women's shelters, medical schools or universities, and Veteran's centers. The appropriate crisis hotline numbers for the community should also be available for both physicians and staff.

Increasingly, communities are responding to sexual assault through the establishment of Sexual Assault Response Teams (SARTs). These are multidisciplinary by nature and seek to establish coordination and collaboration within the community. The goal of the teams is to establish a working protocol as well as investigative strategies and to serve as an information resource for the community. By participating in a SART or knowing SART members, clinicians facilitate the treatment process for women. Many communities do not have a large enough population to support a SART. There are, however, national resources available to assist in providing the best care possible for the sexual assault victim.

American College of Obstetricians and Gynecologists: Adolescent victims of sexual assault, ACOG Technical Bulletin #252. ACOG, 1998.

Bradley F et al: Reported frequency of domestic violence: cross sectional survey of women attending general practice. BMJ 2002; 324:271. [PMID: 11823359]

Centers for Disease Control and Prevention. 1998 Guidelines for treatment of sexually transmitted disease. MMWR 1998; 47(RR-1):108. [PMID: 9461053]

Gupta GR: How men's power over women fuels the HIV epidemic. BMJ 2002;324:183. [PMID: 11809629]

Holmes MM et al: Rape-related pregnancy: estimates and descriptive statistics from a national sample of women. Am J Obstet Gynecol 1996;175:320. [PMID: 8765248]

Irwin KL et al: Urban rape survivors: characteristics and prevalence of human immune deficiency virus and other sexually transmitted infection. Obstet Gynecol 1995;85:330. [PMID: 7862367]

Richardson J et al: Identifying domestic violence: cross sectional study in primary care. BMJ 2002;324:271. [PMID: 11823360]

Stewart FH, Trussell J: Prevention of pregnancy resulting from rape: a neglected preventive health measure. Am J Prev Med 2000;19:228. [PMID: 11064225]

Relevant Web Sites

[American College of Obstetricians and Gynecologists]

www.acog.org

[American College of Emergency Physicians. Guidelines for evaluation and management of sexually assaulted or abused patients available to all users.]

www.acep.org

[National Center for Victims of Crime]

www.ncvc.org

[American College Health Association]

www.acha.org

[National Sexual Violence Prevention Resource Center]

www.cdc.gov/ncipc/dvp/dvp.htm

[Violence Against Women Office—Domestic Violence coalitions of States and Territories]

www.ojp.usdoj.gov/vawo/state.htm

[Rape, Abuse & Incest National Network (RAINN)]

http://feminist.com/rainn.htm

[National Organization for Victim Assistance]

www.try-nova.org

[National Coalition Against Domestic Violence]

www.ncadv.org

SECTION XVIII

Reproductive Health Issues

Contemporary Contraceptive Practices in Clinical Care

52

Gerard S. Letterie, MD

No discussion of politics and practice of contraception would be complete without comment about its origins. The contemporary birth control movement can be traced to the efforts of 2 women on either side of the Atlantic. The early efforts of an American nurse named Margaret Sanger (1879–1965) (Figure 52–1) led to the establishment of the Birth Control League and its successor Planned Parenthood Federation of America. Marie Stopes (1880–1958), a British paleontologist, established the first clinic for contraceptive counseling and distribution of contraceptive devices in England.

Contraceptive research was slow to develop from the 1920s to the 1950s. This disinterest was influenced in part by an unreceptive social and political climate and in part by a rudimentary understanding of reproductive physiology. Primarily through the efforts of Margaret Sanger, sufficient funds were finally raised in the 1950s for formal investigations of contraceptive techniques. These studies came approximately 50 years after the initial description of hormonal contraceptives was made by Halverstadt in Vienna.

In 1959, after clinical trials demonstrated efficacy and effectiveness, the Searle Company launched Enovid E, an oral contraceptive with 150 μg of ethinyl estradiol (3 to 6 times the concentration of estrogen of contemporary preparations). The systematic investigations into oral contraceptives and their marketing represent landmark achievements in the cooperation between commercial and scientific endeavors in response to a clear-cut social need. However, the need continues unabated as the unintended pregnancy rates surge and world population growth continues. Alternative forms of contraception are needed, and wider dissemination to both male and female populations appears to be crucial.

CONTRACEPTION COUNSELING

The cornerstone of effective contraceptive practice is counseling. Unfortunately, the widespread availability of contraceptive techniques has not been matched by widespread dissemination of accurate information about these techniques. Misunderstandings among patients persist and, in some circumstances, contribute to a failure to use contraception. According to a 1993 survey of females from 15 to 45 years, only 73% of those who wished to avoid pregnancy used contraception. The remainder, primarily adolescents and women older than 40 years, stated that they did not use any contraception because of fears regarding side effects and health risks. Fears concerning oral contraceptives included a suspicion of increased cardiovascular disease and various types of cancer. These misconceptions have changed little since a 1985 Gallup Poll found that 75% of women thought oral contraception caused cancer. It is essential for clinicians to dispel such fears and concerns. This goal is best achieved through detailed one-on-one discussion regarding contraceptive options, a difficult task in clinical settings in which appointments are brief.

Several groups are at risk for unintended pregnancy and need intensive counseling (Table 52–1). Adolescents emerge as an at-risk group in particular need of counseling regarding contraceptive options. Approximately 1 million teenagers become pregnant each year, and 80% of these pregnancies are unintended. Com-

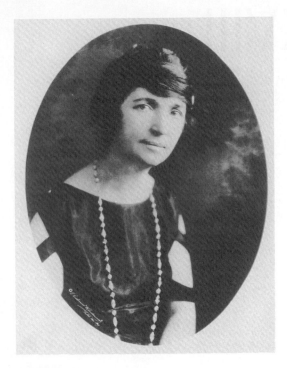

Figure 52–1. Portrait of Margaret Sanger (1879–1965).

pared with other industrialized countries, the adolescent pregnancy rate in the United States is 2 times as high as that in England, Wales, and Canada and more than 9 times as high as that in The Netherlands and Japan (in spite of Japan's relatively late approval of oral contraceptives in 1999). Twenty-five percent of adolescents practice no form of contraception. This failure risks not only pregnancy, but also exposure to sexually transmitted infections (STIs). Pregnancy in an adolescent is also an established sign of potential sexual abuse, with 66% of pregnant adolescents relating a history of such. Teenage mothers are significantly less likely to receive a high school diploma and more likely to live in poverty and receive public assistance.

Every patient has contraceptive needs that are personally and medically unique. These needs may change

Table 52–1. Populations at risk for unintended pregnancy.

Adolescents
Females over 40 years
History of multiple negative tests
History of frequent requests for emergency contraception
History of noncompliance with any medication

during her reproductive life depending on age, health, relationship status, and fertility plans. Discussions should match these needs with the safest and most effective method of contraception. In discussing contraceptive effectiveness, the best estimate (method effectiveness) should be explained and compared with the usual field experience for a particular contraceptive method (use effectiveness) (Table 52–2). A range of effectiveness that incorporates both the lowest possible number and an expected number should be cited. For example, patients may be advised that National Survey of Family Growth estimated overall failure rates for oral contraception at approximately 5% in the first year, decreasing thereafter to less than 1%.

Once a contraceptive method has been chosen, detailed explanations should be given describing how the technique works; the risks, benefits, contraindications, and alternatives of the method; the amount of follow-up and the timing of follow-up visits; the signs of potential complications; and the need for condom use in some circumstances. The last factor is particularly important when discussing protection from STIs. To prevent transmission of HIV and other STIs, patients should be counseled that oral contraceptives, implantable and injectable contraceptives, intrauterine devices (IUDs), and natural membrane condoms do not protect against STIs. Use of a latex condom should be advised when appropriate.

All patients, regardless of contraceptive choice, should be informed of emergency contraceptive measures in case a primary method fails. One option is to prescribe an emergency contraceptive regimen at the counseling session to have on hand at home should the primary technique fail or if compliance is questionable.

Hapangama DK, Glasier AF, Baird DT: Noncompliance among a group of women using a novel method of contraception. Fertil Steril 2001;76:1196. [PMID: 11730750]

Henshaw SK: Unintended pregnancy in the United States. Fam Plann Perspect 1998;30:24. [PMID: 9494812]

Horbacher D, Grimes DA: Noncontraceptive health benefits of intrauterine devices: a systematic review. Obstet Gynecol Surv 2002;57:120. [PMID: 11832788]

Potts M, Walsh J: Making Cairo work. Lancet 1999;353:315. [PMID: 9929040]

CONTRACEPTIVE TECHNIQUES

Hormonal Contraception

A. COMBINATION ORAL CONTRACEPTIVES

1. Background—Oral contraceptive pills (OCPs) are the most commonly used reversible form of contraception. Currently, approximately 15 million women in the United States use OCPs. These preparations consist

Table 52–2. Failure rates for contraceptive methods.[1]

Method	Percentage of Women with Pregnancy	
	Lowest (Method Effectiveness)	Typical (Use Effectiveness)
Combination pill	0.1	3.0
Progestin-only pill	0.5	3.0
Intrauterine device (IUD)		
Progesterone IUD	2.0	< 2.0
Copper T 380A	0.8	< 1.0
Implantable agents	0.2	0.2
Female sterilization	0.2	0.4
Male sterilization	0.1	0.15
Depot medroxyprogesterone	0.3	0.3
Spermicides only	3.0	21.0
Withdrawal	4.0	18.0
Cervical cap	6.0	18.0
Sponge		
Parous women	9.0	28.0
Nulliparous women	6.0	18.0
Diaphragm and spermicides	6.0	18.0
Condom and spermicides	2.0	12.0

[1]Failure rates are the lowest expected and typical pregnancy rates for first year of use.

of a combination of a synthetic estrogen and a progestin. The estrogenic component is either ethinyl estradiol or mestranol. While first-generation progestins were weak and ineffective, second-generation progestins are synergistic with ethinyl estradiol and effective orally. Second-generation progestins include norethindrone, norethindrone acetate, norethynodrel, ethynodiol diacetate, and norgestrel. These progestins are 19-nortestosterone derivatives and maintain a small and variable aspect of their androgenic heritage. Androgenic actions may be manifested at times by adverse side effects such as mild acne and unfavorable changes in lipoprotein profiles. A third generation of progestins has become available recently, including desogestrel, gestodene, and norgestimate. This group of compounds has a marked reduction in androgenicity. Such a favorable profile has positive implications for both long-term use and use in .patients older than 40 years. The newest progestin drospirenone is an analog of spironolactone and exhibits antimineralocorticoid activity.

Concerns persist regarding cardiovascular risks in spite of significant improvements in formulations. Users of OCPs have a 3-fold increased risk of venous thromboembolism when compared with nonusers or never-users. Inherited defects in certain anticoagulation factors may increase this susceptibility. The identification of a common (up to 7% of the general population) hereditary clotting factor disorder (factor V Leiden or activated protein C resistance) has raised some concerns regarding the potential contribution of this thrombophilia to cardiovascular complications associated with oral contraceptive use. There is a suggestion that patients with a factor V Leiden abnormality may be at highest risk for cardiovascular complications with oral contraceptives or perhaps with any steroidal hormonal preparation. To date, the data are unclear. There are no current recommendations to routinely screen potential oral contraceptive users for this abnormality. A study by the Royal College of General Practice showed no increased risk of myocardial infarction and ischemic stroke in nonsmokers using OCPs with less than 50 μg ethinyl estradiol.

The improved safety profile for OCPs may be traced to a reduction in the estrogen and progestin content of the pills and the introduction of the newer progestin compounds. The 1960s saw the introduction of OCPs with estrogen concentrations more than 3–6 times those of the currently available agents. Initial efforts at improved formulations in the 1970s and 1980s focused on a gradual reduction in the estrogen concentration to as low as 20 μg/tablet.

There are 3 different classes of combination oral contraceptives available. Monophasic oral contraceptives contain a fixed dosage of ethinyl estradiol and a progestin. Biphasic oral contraceptives contain a fixed dose of ethinyl estradiol during the cycle, but a variable concentration of the progestin. Triphasic oral contraceptives contain various amounts of ethinyl estradiol and a progestin with 3 separate phases throughout the cycle. The rationale behind the triphasic preparations is to more closely mimic the natural menstrual cycle and minimize side effects such a breakthrough bleeding and amenorrhea. Current formulations have estrogen concentrations that range from 20–50μg of ethinyl estradiol or mestranol (Table 52–3). The 1980s and 1990s have seen marked changes in the type and concentration of the progestins. The introduction of biphasic and triphasic combination pills (Table 52–4) and the second-generation progestins has led to a marked improvement in the profile of the currently available pills.

2. Mechanism of action—Oral contraceptives achieve their contraceptive effect primarily at the level of the

Table 52–3. Monophasic combination oral contraceptives.

Commercial Name	Estrogen (μg)	Progestin (mg)
Norinyl 1+50	mestranol, 50	norethindrone, 1
Ortho-Novum 1/50	mestranol, 50	norethindrone, 1
Ovcon-50	ethinyl estradiol, 50	norethindrone, 1
Norinyl 1+35	ethinyl estradiol, 35	norethindrone, 1
Ortho-Novum 1/35	ethinyl estradiol, 35	norethindrone, 1
Brevicon	ethinyl estradiol, 35	norethindrone, 1
Modicon	ethinyl estradiol, 35	norethindrone, 0.5
Ovcon 35	ethinyl estradiol, 35	norethindrone, 0.4
Loestrin (Fe) 1/20	ethinyl estradiol, 20	norethindrone acetate, 1
Loestrin (Fe) 1.5/30	ethinyl estradiol, 30	norethindrone acetate, 1.5
Demulen 1/50	ethinyl estradiol, 50	ethynodiol diacetate, 1
Demulen 1/35	ethinyl estradiol, 35	ethynodiol diacetate, 1
Ovral	ethinyl estradiol, 50	norgestrel, 0.5
Lo/Ovral	ethinyl estradiol, 30	norgestrel, 0.3
Levlen	ethinyl estradiol, 30	levonorgestrel, 0.15
Nordette	ethinyl estradiol, 30	levonorgestrel, 0.15
Ortho-Cyclen	ethinyl estradiol, 35	norgestimate, 0.25
Desogen	ethinyl estradiol, 30	desogestrel, 0.15
Ortho-Cept	ethinyl estradiol, 30	desogestrel, 0.15

Table 52–4. Bi- and tri-phasic combination oral contraceptives.

Commercial Name	Estrogen (μg)	Progestin (mg)
Ortho-Novum 10/11[1]	35/35	0.5/1
Tri-Norinyl[1]	35/35/35	0.5/1/0/5
Ortho-Novum 7/7/7[1]	35/35/35	0.5/0.75/1
Jenest 28[1]	35/35/35	0.5/1/1
		Norgestimate
Ortho Tricyclin[1]	35/35/35	0.18/0.21/50.25
		Desogestrel
		20/10
		Levonorgestrel
Triphasil[2]	30/40/30	.05/.075/.125
Tri-Levlen[2]	30/40/30	.05/.075/.125

[1]Variable dose of progestin only.
[2]Variable dose of both estrogen and progestin.

hypothalamic-pituitary axis. The estrogenic and progestational components suppress follicle-stimulating hormone and luteinizing hormone, respectively. Secondary effects are changes in tubal motility and ovum transport, sperm penetration and implantation, and cervical mucus, all significant factors contributing to contraceptive efficacy.

3. Clinical management—Oral contraceptives are extremely well tolerated and safe medications. OCPs may be prescribed to patients without absolute contraindications or risk factors (Table 52–5). Absolute contraindications preclude pill use. Relative contraindications are guidelines under which oral contraceptives may be prescribed cautiously, with close follow-up.

Table 52–5. Relative and absolute contraindications to combination oral contraceptive use.

Relative	Absolute
Migraine headaches	Thromboembolic disease or thrombophlebitis, cerebral vascular disease, coronary artery disease, or history of these conditions
Hypertension	Known or suspected carcinoma of the breast
Uterine leiomyoma	Known or suspected estrogen-dependent neoplasia
Epilepsy	Undiagnosed abnormal genital bleeding
Varicose veins	Known or suspected pregnancy
Gestational diabetes	
Elective surgery	

An initial evaluation should include a general examination with blood pressure determination and cervical cytologic study. In patients at risk, the initial evaluation also may include screening for lipoprotein profiles, fasting serum glucose level, and liver function. Follow-up visits may be scheduled at 12-month intervals and should include, at a minimum, blood pressure determination, pelvic examination, and cervical cytologic study. For some patients, a follow-up visit at 3 or 6 months may be advantageous for further discussion to answer any questions about troublesome side effects or worries, to ensure compliance, and evaluate blood pressure.

The oral contraceptive that provides adequate contraception with the fewest side effects at the lowest possible dose and cost should be used. Multiphasic preparations usually fulfill these criteria, but any low-dose pill may be used. None has a distinct advantage over another. Matching an OCP to a patient may require trial and error.

Compliance is essential for successful use of OCPs. Adequate counseling has been shown to improve compliance, especially in adolescents. Patients should be carefully counseled regarding when to start. Pills may be initiated on either the first day of the menstrual cycle or as a "Sunday start." Effective contraception is ensured when the medications are taken on the first day of the menstrual cycle; should the patient elect to initiate a Sunday start, the effectiveness of the oral contraceptives for that cycle may be questioned if the Sunday start is not within a day or 2 of the first day of the patient's menstrual cycle. If this scenario applies, the first pill cycle should be considered at risk, and a reliable alternative method should be used for 1 month.

In the postpartum setting, oral contraceptives should be prescribed within 3 weeks after delivery, because ovulation may occur as early as the third week postpartum. Low-dose preparations may be used in breast-feeding patients with little influence on either the quantity or quality of the milk or the growth of the infant. After an elective termination of pregnancy, oral contraceptives may be started on the day of the procedure.

Guidelines regarding use should be given to patients when OCPs are first prescribed. If 1 pill is missed, the dose should be doubled for the next day. If 2 pills are missed, 2 pills on 2 successive days should be taken until the patient is back in phase with her package. If more than 2 pills are missed, the patient should be considered at risk for pregnancy, and an alternative form of contraception should be used until the onset of menses. Repeated compliance problems suggest an alternative form of contraception should be discussed.

Oral contraception is an extremely safe method of birth control, but bothersome side effects do exist. Side effects commonly experienced are breakthrough bleeding, weight gain, and mild acne, and oily skin. Breakthrough bleeding appears to be the most troublesome and may compromise compliance. It may be managed with the use of supplemental estrogen, either 1.25 mg of conjugated estrogens or 20 µg of ethinyl estradiol at the time of the irregular bleeding.

Benefits of OCPs include a reduction in the risk for iron deficiency anemia, pelvic inflammatory disease, ovarian cysts, ovarian cancer, dysfunctional uterine bleeding, rheumatoid arthritis, and endometrial and colorectal cancer.

Data from 54 epidemiologic studies demonstrated that the characteristics of contraceptive use, estrogen and progestin doses, type of progestin or duration of use do not increase the risk of breast carcinoma with one exception. Among women who have a first-degree relative (sister, mother) with breast cancer, the oral contraceptive-associated breast cancer risk is 3-fold higher for those who ever used OCPs before 1975 (greater than 50 µg estrogen). Women with similar family histories using formulations after 1975 (less than 50 µg estrogen) had the same risk as nonusers.

Contraceptive choices for women over the age of 35 were few until recently. Data evaluating oral contraceptives have shown that these agents may be used safely throughout reproductive years. If no contraindications exist, such as smoking or hypertension, oral contraceptives may be used until menopause for excellent contraceptive efficacy with good tolerance and virtual lack of side effects. These agents in this age group has the added benefit of cycle control with no apparent pill-related changes in lipoprotein patterns or coagulation parameters. Frequency of surveillance remains yearly. Screening may also include lipoprotein profiles (for possible age-related changes) and mammography.

Controversy continues to surround the issue of increased breast cancer with any estrogen-containing substance, including oral contraception.

B. PROGESTIN-ONLY PILLS (MINIPILLS)

The progestin-only oral contraceptive contains a small dose, less than 0.5 mg, of norethindrone or norgestrel (Table 52–6). Unlike combination oral contraceptives containing both estrogen and progestin, the minipill must be taken every day at the same time continuously. Compared with combination OCPs, progestin-only tablets account for a small portion of oral contraceptive use (0.2% in the United States). These agents are associated with more irregular bleeding than the combination pills; hence, their acceptability to patients is considerably less. These side effects can be troublesome. Women contemplating use of a progestin-only contraceptive method need to be counseled about alterations to the menstrual cycle but can be reassured that the

Table 52–6. Progestin-only
(minipill) contraceptives.

Commercial Name	Estrogen (μg) Ethinyl estradiol	Progestin (mg) Norethindrone	Cost
Nor QD	0	0.35	$34.25
Micronor	0	0.35	$38.06
		Norgestrel	
Ovrette	0	0.075	$33.62

total blood loss will usually be much less than a normal menstrual cycle. Breakthrough bleeding is experienced by 20–30% of patients who use progestin-only pills. This incidence decreases with continued use. The non-menstrual side effects from the use of these pills are few. Progestin-only pills have a slightly increased pregnancy rate, possibly secondary to a failure of the method itself but possibly secondary to poor compliance because of the side effects. Failure rates appear to be higher in heavier women, as may be the case with most other progestin-containing contraceptives. Progestin-only pills were initially prescribed in patients who had a contraindication to estrogen use, such as breast-feeding or age greater than 35 years. Their role has been markedly decreased in view of the safety of combination OCPs in both of these clinical circumstances.

C. Long-Acting Implantable Contraceptive Agents

1. Background—Contraception with an implantable device was initially described in the mid-1960s. These early studies sought to devise a means of passive hormonal contraception with a prolonged duration of action. A delivery system for the progestin, norgestrel, became available in 1967. The Norplant system was approved by the US Food and Drug Administration (FDA) in December 1990. Since its introduction, it has been the focus of litigation related in part to difficulty localizing and removing the rods. There has also been a recall of this product from the market. The Norplant system was removed from availability in the United States and Canada in September 2001. This decision was related to issues of possible diminished effectiveness in 7 lots of the product. The manufacturer plans to make the system or a similar system available again at a later date.

Since the initial introduction of the Norplant system, implantable contraceptive agents have undergone a number of revisions and refinements. Newer delivery systems contain fewer implants, shorter-acting systems, biodegradable capsules, and different progestins. Uni-plant, Norplant II, and Implanon are implantable systems containing megestrol, norgestrel and desogestrel, respectively. These changes are intended to improve the ease of insertion and removal as well as to increase safety and compliance. None are available for use in the United States.

2. Mechanism of action—The Norplant system achieves a constant serum level of norgestrel. The mechanism of action of the norgestrel is identical to that of all progestin-only contraceptives. These agents act primarily by altering ovulation, cervical mucus, and endometrial receptivity. Suppression of ovulation occurs in approximately 50% of cycles.

3. Clinical management—Norplant consists of 6 silastic capsules that are placed subcutaneously. These capsules are easily placed under local anesthesia using a trocar supplied by the manufacturer (Figure 52–2). Removal has been more problematic. In 1 series, the time required to remove the capsules ranged from 4 to 215 minutes, with approximately 50% of the removals completed in less than 30 minutes and approximately 20% requiring longer than 1 hour. Localization of the rods may be difficult. Plain radiography, film screen mammography, and magnetic resonance imaging have been effective tools for identification. The 1-year removal rate in the United States has been 13%, with the rate in other countries ranging from 1.25% to 10%.

Key aspects to the use of implantable contraception appear to be patient selection and provision of adequate counseling. The patient's ability to tolerate the 2 most significant side effects—irregular bleeding and weight gain—appears to be related to the adequacy of counseling prior to insertion. A patient's experience with previous methods of contraception does not predict satisfaction or dissatisfaction with implantable agents. If contraception is for spacing of pregnancies, a shorter acting agent should be considered. Most important, pregnancy should be excluded at the time of insertion. Two related issues are of importance in long-term management: annual examinations and condom use have been less than ideal after insertion. Especially among adolescents, appropriately timed reminders for routine annual care and condom use are recommended.

D. Long-Acting Injectable Contraceptive Agents

The concept of an injectable contraceptive was initially introduced in 1950. Long-acting injectable agents provide a passive means of contraception that must be renewed at 1-month or 3-month intervals. These agents have the advantage of requiring little daily involvement by the user and are ideal for patients with problems in compliance. Two agents are available in the United States.

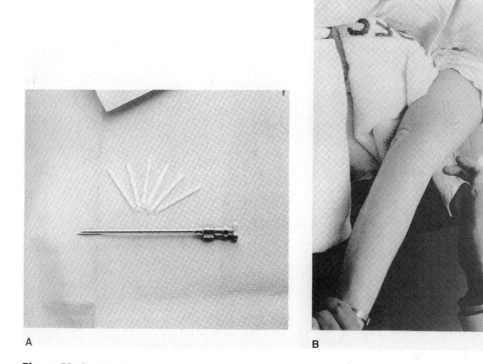

Figure 52–2. Norplant system (**A**) and outline of pattern of insertion on the medial aspect of the brachium (**B**).

Depot medroxyprogesterone acetate (DMPA) is the most commonly used injectable contraceptive; it has been in use in more than 90 countries. This agent attracted considerable controversy because initial studies in beagle dogs suggested an association between long-acting progestational agents and breast cancer. Subsequent studies did not confirm this finding, and the agent was approved in 1992 by the FDA as a contraceptive agent. DMPA has been used for more than 20 years in 90 countries and has an excellent safety record. It is a highly effective contraceptive with failure rates less than 1%.

DMPA is used as a single 150-mg dose repeated at 3-month intervals. The most common side effects are irregular bleeding and weight gain. After a 150-mg injection of DMPA, the mean interval for return of ovulation is 4–5 months. There is no correlation between the number of injections and the length of time for return of ovulatory function. Seventy percent of DMPA users conceive within the first 12 months following discontinuation and 90% within 24 months. The efficacy

rate of DMPA is similar to that cited for oral contraceptives. Clinicians are encouraged to begin DMPA within 5 days of the onset of menses to ensure that the patient is not pregnant and to prevent ovulation during the first month of use. It has been demonstrated to prevent ovulation when administered as late as day 9 of the menstrual cycle. In addition to contraception, DMPA has been shown to reduce the risk of endometrial cancer, pelvic inflammatory disease, and endometriosis. There is controversy regarding a possible reduction in bone mineral density in long-term users, but the data are unclear.

The second long-acting injectable is a monthly combination of estrogen and progestin. The combination of medroxyprogesterone acetate (25 mg) and estradiol cypionate (5 mg) is the first new contraceptive option approved by the FDA in 5 years. This monthly combination injection is a safe and effective option for patients who prefer a passive form of contraception with failure rates of less than 1%. It has several similarities to oral contraceptives, including similar indications and contraindications and side effects. The monthly combination injection offers an acceptable option for patients who have difficulty with compliance and experience bothersome side effects with progestin only preparations.

Continuation rates among patients using this preparation were 68% at 6 months among new users and 84% among patients switching from another form of contraception to the combination injection. There appears to be a higher failure rate in low income women and those under the age of 25, possibly related to the timing of the injections.

E. CONTRACEPTIVE PATCH

A new transdermal contraceptive patch was approved for use by the FDA in 2001. It is a 20 cm^2, 3-layer system consisting of an outer protective layer, a medicated adhesive layer, and a clear release liner that is removed before patch application. The components are ethinyl estradiol 20 µg/d and norelgestromin 150 µg/d. Recommended use is one patch applied once weekly for 3 consecutive weeks (21 days) followed by a patch-free interval of 1 week. The patch appears to be effective regardless of location (arm, abdomen, buttock) and a variety of climates and conditions (humidity, exercise, heat, cold and water submersion). It is readily reversible. Data from more than 3000 subjects and 27,000 cycles show a favorable profile and one similar to oral contraceptives. Side effects and contraindications are similar to that for oral contraceptives. It appears to have a higher failure rate for patients weighing greater than 90 kg.

Burkman RT et al: Current perspectives on oral contraceptive use. Am J Obstet Gynecol 2001;185:54. [PMID: 11521117]

Croxatto HB et al: Mechanism of action of hormonal preparations used for emergency contraception: a review of the literature. Contraception 2001;63:111. [PMID: 11368982]

French RS et al: Levonorgestrel-releasing (20 microgram/day) intrauterine systems (Mirena) compared with other methods of reversible contraceptives. BJOG 2000;107:1218. [PMID: 11028571]

Glasier AF, Smith KB, Cheng L: An international study on the acceptability of a once-a-month pill. Hum Reprod 1999;14: 3018. [PMID: 10601090]

Mira Y et al: Congenital and acquired thrombotic risk factors in women using oral contraceptives: clinical aspects. Clin App Thromb Hemost 2001;6:162. [PMID: 10898277]

Petta CA et al: Timing of onset of contraceptive effectiveness in Depo-Provera users. II. Effects on ovarian function. Fertil Steril 1998;70:817. [PMID: 9806559]

Price DT, Ridker PM: Factor V Leiden mutation and the risks for thromboembolic disease: a clinical perspective. Ann Intern Med 1997;127:895. [PMID: 9382368]

Rivera R, Yacobson I, Grimes D: The mechanism of action of hormonal contraceptives and intrauterine contraceptive devices. Am J Obstet Gynecol 1999;181:1263. [PMID: 10561657]

Schwartz JL et al: Predicting risk of ovulation in new start oral contraceptive users. Obstet Gynecol 2002;99:177. [PMID: 11814492]

Intrauterine Devices

Through the late 1960s and early 1970s, IUDs were used by 10% of women as contraceptive devices. However, the initial descriptions of severe pelvic inflammatory disease and maternal death when pregnancy occurred with the Dalkon shield (Figure 52–3) in situ led to an expanding investigation of the Dalkon shield and of IUDs in general regarding their safety and efficacy.

In an increasingly litigious atmosphere, concerns regarding product liability led to a dramatic decrease in IUD use. When the public was polled regarding the safety of IUDs, no distinction was made by respondents between Dalkon shields and other IUDs. All IUDs were withdrawn from the market in the early 1980s, which left a substantial gap in choices of passive types of contraception. The debate persists regarding the exact association between infertility and pelvic inflammatory disease and IUD use. It is only in the case of the Dalkon shield that this association appears unquestionable. With further scrutiny of the past data and recent well-designed studies, the IUD appears to offer an effective and safe contraceptive method to monogamous couples. A new generation of IUDs is now available; these IUDs are distinct from their predecessors. These devices offer contraception that is as safe as other contraceptive methods with no greater complication rate. However, despite a favorable profile, IUD use accounts for only 1% of contraception in the United States.

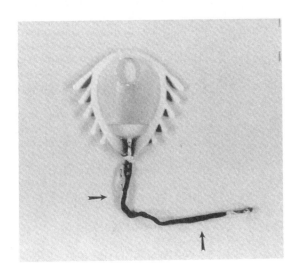

Figure 52–3. Dalkon shield intrauterine device (IUD). Note multifilament tail (arrow).

There are currently 3 IUDs available in the United States: a copper-containing device, the T380, marketed as the Paragard; the Progestasert, a progesterone-containing intrauterine device; and Mirena, a levonorgestrel-containing device. A frameless IUD implant (GyneFix) and intrauterine drug delivery system (FibroPlant) are effective and well tolerated but not available in the United States.

A. MECHANISM OF ACTION

Copper-containing IUDs act by the induction of a sterile inflammatory reaction within the uterine cavity. This reaction fosters a milieu unsuitable for implantation; data suggest there is also interference with fertilization. The copper in the devices may contribute to the interference by increasing the inflammatory reaction, decreasing the viability of sperm, and limiting the transport of ovum.

Progesterone- and levonorgestrel-containing IUDs combine the potential advantages of an IUD as a passive means of contraception and hormonal contraceptives known to decrease the risk of pelvic inflammatory disease. These devices are designed to release a fixed amount of a progestin per day. Their primary activity appears to be at the level of the endometrium and cervix. These devices release progesterone or levonorgestrel from the vertical stem of the T-shaped frame. The effectiveness of the Progestasert decreases markedly after 1 year, and annual replacement is essential. The levonorgestrel IUD has an effective life of 5 years. Data suggest that in addition to its efficacy as a contraceptive agent, the local effect of the progestin results in less blood loss during menstruation and a decrease in the incidence of dysmenorrhea. Levonorgestrel-containing IUDs have been shown to be effective contraceptive agents in addition to reducing the incidence of pelvic inflammatory disease, probably secondary to a local progesterone effect.

Users of IUDs may be at risk for colonization with actinomyces gram-positive non–acid-fast anaerobic bacteria. These may be detected in cervical cytology of women using any IUD. The incidence appears to depend on the type of IUD used, ranging from 3% for levonorgestrel IUD users to approximately 20% in copper-containing IUDs. The concern regarding the detection of actinomyces-like organisms on a Papanicolaou (Pap) smear in an otherwise asymptomatic patient centers on the possibility of acute pelvic inflammatory disease developing in these patients secondary to these organisms. When detected on cervical cytology, the patient should be counseled regarding the possible need for antibiotic therapy. In extreme circumstances or when the bacteria persists on repeated Pap smears removal of the IUD should be considered.

B. CLINICAL MANAGEMENT

The cornerstone to safe IUD use is patient selection. Patients are not candidates for IUD use if there is a history of pelvic inflammatory disease or ectopic pregnancy, undiagnosed dysfunctional uterine bleeding, multiple sexual partners, or if they are unable to assess string placement. Caution should be exercised in patients who have structural abnormalities of the uterine cavity, such as fibroids or a history of in utero exposure to diethylstilbestrol (DES), a history of valvular heart disease, an allergy to copper, or a history of impaired fertility.

Placement may occur at any time in the cycle if the woman is reliably using other contraception or if 2 sensitive pregnancy tests are negative at least 10 days apart. Infection and expulsion rates appear lower if the placement occurs on a nonmenstruating day in the cycle. In the immediate postpartum period, placement is associated with higher expulsion rates and is best avoided. The IUD should be placed 6 weeks postpartum if the woman is breast-feeding, is not sexually active, is reliably using contraception, or has had negative pregnancy testing as just described.

The patient must be well informed regarding the signs and symptoms of infection, perforation, ectopic pregnancy, and expulsion. She should be counseled to seek immediate care in such instances. Past unfavorable publicity of IUDs has created an emotionally charged atmosphere. It is essential that adequate counseling take place before IUD insertion. Preplacement counseling to minimize the fears and complications of this method cannot be overemphasized. Informed consent materials are distributed with the IUDs and provide an opportunity for this discussion. It is essential for the physician or clinic representative to review and sign these documents with each patient.

Menorrhagia may occur during the first 2–3 months after placement of any IUD (copper- or progestin-containing). If this symptom persists, the patient should undergo further evaluation to rule out infection or pregnancy and transvaginal ultrasound to verify the location of the IUD. A common and at times desirable side effect of the levonorgestrel IUD is amenorrhea. Patients should be advised of this possibility. Nonsteroidal antiinflammatory drugs may be used in an attempt to decrease the amount of monthly bleeding; dysmenorrhea also may be managed with these drugs. Should the pain become severe, culture and appropriate treatment for possible STIs or pelvic infection should be considered.

Dardano KL, Burkman RT: The intrauterine contraceptive device: an often-forgotten and maligned method of contraception. Am J Obstet Gynecol 1999;181:1. [PMID: 10411781]

Hubacher D et al: Use of copper intrauterine devices and the risk of tubal infertility among nulligravid women. N Engl J Med 2001;345:561. [PMID: 11529209]

Barrier Methods

A. MALE CONDOMS

1. Background—The demonstration that the transmission of the virus responsible for AIDS could be prevented by appropriate barrier contraceptive techniques brought condom use to the forefront of contraceptive technology after some period of dormancy. Concomitant use of condoms and spermicidal agents cannot be overemphasized. Condoms are not only a technique of contraception, but also a necessary adjunct to other contraceptive techniques that do not prevent the spread of STIs.

Male condoms may be lubricated, textured, tinted, contoured, or equipped with a spermicidal jelly or a reservoir tip. Regardless of options, male condoms are all basically the same design, measuring 19 cm in length and 2.5 cm in width. The effectiveness of condoms is enhanced when combined with the use of spermicidal agents, which have the additional benefit of activity against a variety of viruses, *Chlamydia,* and gonorrhea, and efficacy in the reduction of pelvic inflammatory disease in the female partner.

2. Mechanism of action—Placement of a condom is intended to prevent sperm from entering the female reproductive tract and as a barrier against STIs and HIV transmission. A spermicidal gel or foam may increase effectiveness by reducing viable sperm and is recommended routinely. These agents also afford a degree of protection against AIDS and STIs. Spermicidal condoms became available in the early 1980s. This addition has been shown to reduce the motile sperm detected 60 seconds after ejaculation from 50% without spermicide to 4% with spermicide.

3. Clinical management—The male condom is used by 15% of couples as a sole method of contraception. Its over-the-counter availability is a distinct advantage over some of the other methods. The rate of breakage varies widely depending on the study population. The average rate per act of intercourse is approximately 1 in 100. It is part of routine counseling to encourage all couples in the early phases of a new relationship to use condoms and spermicide until there is certainty that neither partner is HIV-positive. Latex condoms, as opposed to those made of natural products, offer the greatest protection against HIV. Those impregnated with spermicide appear to be particularly protective.

Regular use of male condoms presents unique social aspects not found with other techniques. Both men and women may report some degree of dissatisfaction with this method, owing to decreased sensation during intercourse, lack of spontaneity, and irritation. Although most users prefer a prelubricated condom, any additional lubricants should be water-based. Mineral-based lubricants may weaken the latex at body temperature and predispose to breakage when used. Surgical jelly such as K-Y lubricant jelly is preferred. Mineral and vegetable oil, cold cream, and petroleum jelly are to be avoided.

B. FEMALE CONDOMS

1. Background—Approval by the FDA in 1993 has brought the female condom to the marketplace. Reality® is the first dual protection barrier method that is used at the initiation of women. It is inexpensive ($3.50) and available over the counter. This device offers women for the first time the opportunity to be autonomous in condom use; no participation from a male partner is required. The female condom is a long polyurethane pouch 7.8 cm wide and 17 cm long that is designed to line the vagina. It has 2 rings: an inner ring fitted over the cervix (similar to a diaphragm) and an outer ring to anchor the pouch outside the vagina (Figure 52–4). The sheath lines the vagina, extends outside the vagina once inserted and is prelubricated with dimethicone, a medical grade silicone lubricant. Data

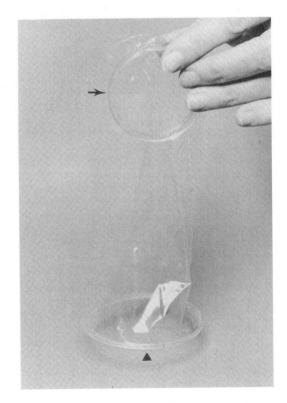

Figure 52–4. Female condom demonstrating the inner cervical ring (arrow) and outer vaginal ring (arrowhead).

on effectiveness are limited, but the use effectiveness failure rate at 1 year has been estimated at 15%.

2. Clinical management—The female condom is a reasonable alternative to the male version. Because it is relatively new in use, the ability to describe the "ideal" user is difficult. Physical sensation does not appear to be compromised for either the male and female partners. In 1 study, male users described the sensation of the female condom to be more acceptable than that of the male condom. However, it is also reported to be more troublesome to use than other barrier methods. It can be pushed entirely into the vagina or fall completely out of the vagina. The outer ring can irritate the external genitalia of both the male and female partner. It is also a concern that vaginal penetration may occur outside of the condom (between the pouch and the vaginal wall).

C. DIAPHRAGM

1. Background—Margaret Sanger established the first diaphragm manufacturing firm in 1925, thus bringing contemporary contraceptive techniques to the United States. With FDA approval as a medical device, the diaphragm received an early initial endorsement and found widespread use. This early endorsement and approval by the FDA led to a distinct advantage over the cervical cap, which was not endorsed until 1988.

The diaphragm has unique advantages in that it is a woman-controlled method useful for women who have only intermittent needs for contraception. The diaphragm has been shown to confer protection against pelvic inflammatory disease and tubal infertility resulting from STIs. It is unevaluated in its ability to protect against HIV.

2. Mechanism of action—The diaphragm provides a vaginal barrier method to prevent viable sperm from entering the upper female reproductive tract. In addition to providing a physical barrier, the diaphragm also provides a vehicle for the administration of spermicidal jelly. These agents have been shown to increase markedly the use effectiveness of the diaphragm.

3. Clinical management—The diaphragm is a soft dome of latex on a flexible rim, allowing for its insertion in the vagina and expansion to cover the cervix. It should be used in conjunction with spermicidal jelly to maximize its contraceptive effectiveness and as a further guard against infectious disease. The diaphragm must be inserted prior to intercourse, left in place for at least 6 hours after intercourse and taken out at least every 24 hours. It should not be removed if doing so would cut short the 6 hours required after intercourse. If the couple has intercourse more than once or if the diaphragm is inserted more than 6 hours in advance of intercourse, it is suggested that an extra applicator of spermicide be inserted without removing the diaphragm.

The diaphragm needs to be fitted to each woman. Diaphragms should be fitted to accommodate the largest diameter possible for a patient without any discomfort. Sizes are numbered according to the diameter of the rim. The rims may be made of a flat spring, a coil spring, an arching spring, or a wide-seal rim. The diaphragm may be inserted by folding it in half after placement of the spermicidal jelly and sliding it into the vagina. Adequate positioning should be verified after placement. For patients who have difficulty with the vaginal insertion of the diaphragm, a plastic introducer is available that may facilitate placement. The patient should demonstrate to a provider her ability to use it properly.

The inconvenience of insertion in advance of sex, although not different from other over-the-counter methods, has been cited as altering the spontaneity of the sex act. Education in its proper use is essential to maximize its effectiveness. The woman who uses this method has to be motivated and informed. The continuation rate for 1 year is between 50% and 80%. A diaphragm should not be fitted within 6 weeks of delivery and should not be used in patients with a history of toxic shock syndrome.

A common complaint is recurrent candidal infection. Switching to a different spermicidal preparation may be of some benefit. Continued irritation should prompt consideration of other methods of contraception. In some cases, a change to the cervical cap may reduce the irritation because there is significantly less spermicide used for this method.

D. CERVICAL CAP

1. Background—The cervical cap is a barrier method similar to the diaphragm. It is snugly fitted over the cervix, unlike the arching dome of the diaphragm, which covers the anterior portion of the vagina and includes the cervix (Figure 52–5). The cap, perhaps more than any other barrier method, requires a highly motivated woman to learn the appropriate use. This subset of women report high satisfaction with this method, especially when there have been problems with other methods in the past. The cap must be inserted prior to intercourse.

2. Mechanism of action—The mechanism of action of the cap is multifold and is somewhat different from other barrier forms. First, it is a barrier between sperm and egg. When the cap is inserted, it is filled approximately one third full with spermicide, thus providing the second mechanism of action. The most significant mechanism of action involves sequestration of cervical secretions within the cap. In this fashion, vaginal secretions predominate and create an acidic environment. This alteration of the pH creates an environment that is naturally spermicidal. The woman has to wear the cap

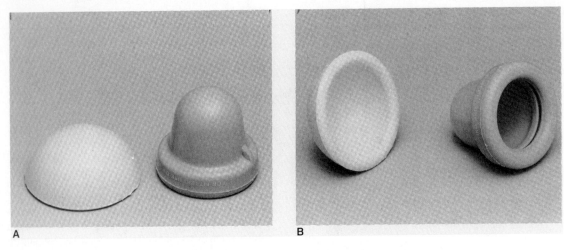

Figure 52–5. Prentif and Dumas cervical caps, vaginal side (**A**) and cervical side (**B**).

for at least 8 hours after intercourse to maintain this environment and ensure the maximal effectiveness.

3. Clinical management—The cervical cap may be considered an alternative barrier technique for couples who find that condoms, the diaphragm, or spermicidal agents inhibit sexual responsiveness. For some couples, sexual responsiveness may be more favorable with the cap. The fact that the cervix is within the cap may heighten the awareness of the uterine contractions at climax. Male partners, who may be able to feel the cap, have described its use both positively and negatively. Because the cap may be placed hours to a day or more in advance of intercourse, it does not have to interfere with the spontaneity of sex. It is significantly less cumbersome than the diaphragm, because the required amount of spermicide is much less, and the spermicide is contained within the vessel of the cap. The contraindications for the use of the cap include a history of DES exposure, a history of toxic shock syndrome, and untreated cervical dysplasia.

The cap is approved for use for 48 hours, a potential advantage over the 24-hour limit of the diaphragm. It should be removed for a few hours every other day. Extra spermicide should not be inserted if intercourse occurs more than once when the cap is in place or if the cap is inserted hours in advance of intercourse. To insert extra jelly or cream may alter the manner in which the cap is secured onto the cervix.

It is essential that the placement of the cap be checked both before and after intercourse because of the possibility of dislodgment during intercourse. The placement is checked by running a finger around the top edge of the cap to make sure that the cervix is fully contained within the cap. The person who is not able

to do this check is probably not a candidate for the cap. The clinician and the patient should feel confident that she can identify both appropriate and inappropriate placement in the subsequent checking for accurate insertion.

It is recommended that the new cap wearer use a backup method for the first month while gaining proficiency with the cap. If the woman has been taking oral contraceptives, she should continue for 1 month. A routine follow-up appointment is recommended at that time to ensure proper fit and technique.

Vaginal Spermicides

A. BACKGROUND

Spermicidal preparations have been available for some time. The 2 agents most commonly used are nonoxynol 9, which is the active ingredient in most spermicidal jellies, and octoxynol 9. Their relative ease of use and affordability make them an important over-the-counter method of contraception. Benefits of the spermicides include activity against a wide range of viruses and bacteria, which appears to provide additional protection against STIs. They are available in a variety of forms, such as foams, jellies, and creams. These agents may be considered for patients who have infrequent intercourse and in whom compliance is not an issue.

B. MECHANISM OF ACTION

Spermicidal preparations are surface active agents that destroy the sperm cell membrane. This is the most important mechanism of action of nonoxynol 9 and octoxynol 9. Other spermicidal agents with surface active properties include menfegol and benzalkonium chloride, which are available in other parts of the world. Enzymatic inhibition is a second mechanism of action in these agents. In addition to their inhibitory action on sperm, these agents may be active also in preventing STIs. Data suggest that there is significant protection against gonorrhea and *Chlamydia* when nonoxynol 9 products are used, although 1 randomized controlled trial failed to show an effect. This agent also has been shown to be effective against the herpes virus, *Trichomonas,* syphilis, and HIV. The protection against STIs and HIV appears to be enhanced when the spermicidal agents are used in conjunction with a barrier method.

C. CLINICAL MANAGEMENT

The failure rate for the first year of use for the spermicidal agents as sole contraception is extremely high at 21%, probably because of nonuse. When used reliably, however, vaginal spermicides provide an effective means of contraception, with failure rates of 3%. Their greatest disadvantage is the need for absolute compliance. There are no data to suggest that the use of 1 agent over the other is more effective. Each product appears to offer comparable contraception. If foams, films, or suppositories are used, adequate time must be factored into the use of these agents to permit dissolution and dispersion of the agent within the vagina. A barrier method in conjunction with the spermicide markedly increases the effectiveness. In the absence of a barrier method, reliable and consistent use is absolutely essential. Accurate placement using an applicator high in the vagina is required. Spermicides for vaginal douching after intercourse as a contraceptive is not acceptable. If an individual wishes to douche following vaginal intercourse and is reliably using a vaginal spermicidal jelly, she should wait 6–8 hours after intercourse.

Hatcher RA, Warner DL: New condoms for men and women, diaphragms, cervical caps, and spermicides: overcoming barriers to barriers and spermicides. Curr Opin Obstet Gynecol 1992;4:513. [PMID: 1504271]

Natural Family Planning

A. BACKGROUND

Natural family planning (also known as the rhythm method) focuses on observable and measurable changes in a woman's body at the time of ovulation. These changes serve as signals to the couple to avoid intercourse during the times that are considered to be high risk for pregnancy. The World Health Organization estimates worldwide use of this method to be as high as 11%. Women may choose this method because of religious preferences, availability and low cost, complete absence of drugs, or the desire to have a sense of control over their body. The method requires a significant commitment to identify the physical changes specific

for ovulation, which can be subtle. The pregnancy rate with this method is between 10 and 25 per 100 woman years.

B. MECHANISM OF ACTION

Natural family planning has as its underpinning the definition of a "fertile zone." The exact definition of this interval is essential in determining both the earliest and latest possible times of fertility. Implicit in this method is abstinence or other contraceptive use during the fertile interval.

C. CLINICAL MANAGEMENT

Detailed instruction in temperature charting, definition of time of ovulation, and awareness of events of the menstrual cycle are essential prerequisites for natural family planning. The woman who participates in this technique, sometimes referred to as the *Billings* method, is instructed in the distinct features of the cervical secretions during each phase of the cycle. The critical phases suggesting fertility are identified, and intercourse is avoided during these phases. Fertile days are those in which the secretion is changing from watery to a consistency resembling raw egg white and for 3 days thereafter.

Data suggest that the cervical mucus method alone is not as effective as a combined use of temperature charting, menstrual calendar tracking, and monitoring other symptoms of ovulation. Basal body measurements that are taken and charted correctly provide useful visual data for the prediction of ovulation. To maximize the accuracy of this method, the woman measures her temperature each day on awakening and before engaging in any activity. The reading is plotted on a graph so that the marked increase in temperature that occurs with ovulation is apparent. Intercourse should be avoided 3 days prior to ovulation and the 3–4 days following ovulation, although cycle variation may occur.

Patients who are candidates for use of natural family planning are highly motivated women with an understanding of the menstrual cycle and the subtleties of the cyclic changes in their body. Irregular cycles or any menstrual disorder seriously limits the applicability of this technique. Essential to natural family planning is a skilled instructor who is readily available to the user. It is consistent with the teachings of certain religious groups and thereby appeals to the large segment of the world population that strictly follows these teachings. The most obvious shortcomings are a high failure rate in certain populations, particularly among women who are not motivated or do not fully understand the method, and the need for intensive instruction sessions and instructors available for consultation.

EMERGENCY CONTRACEPTION

Background

What has come to be known as a "morning after" pill is now labeled "emergency contraception." It is essential that patients understand that this form of contraception may be used after an interval greater than 1 day after unprotected intercourse. Hence the term "morning after" is misleading and inaccurate. Different forms of emergency contraception may be reliably used for up to 5 days (and perhaps longer) after an episode of unprotected intercourse. Patients frequently have the impression that emergency contraception would be ineffective if used in the late afternoon or evening on the day after an episode of unprotected coitus. The data simply do not support this. Emergency contraceptive techniques may be used effectively as late as 72 hours for hormonal emergency contraception and as late as 5 days for IUD insertion to avoid an unwanted pregnancy. Hence, the term *morning after pill* is an unfortunate misnomer and should be avoided in most circumstances.

Mechanism of Action

Emergency contraception appears to act primarily through an alteration in the endometrial receptivity. The mechanism of action for the IUD appears to be the inhibition of implantation by the sterile reaction initiated by the IUD and the cytotoxic effects of the copper in the IUD.

Clinical Management

Emergency contraception should be part of any counseling session regardless of the primary contraceptive technique chosen. Two regimens are available, Preven and PlanB (Table 52–7). These agents may be used any time within 72 hours, and there are no data to suggest that if used earlier or later they are more or less efficacious. After administration of these agents, it is prudent to wait 2–3 weeks for the onset of menses and, if no

bleeding occurs, to order a pregnancy test. During this interval, the patient must either abstain from intercourse or use a barrier method of contraception such as condoms or foam to avoid the possibility of a second episode of unprotected intercourse. Should the patient have a second episode of unprotected intercourse, this regimen should be repeated. The failure rate is approximately 3% for this method. Should the patient become pregnant secondary to failed emergency contraception, there is no evidence to suggest that the pregnancies are in any way affected adversely.

Contraindications to these regimens are identical to those for oral contraceptives. The indications for emergency contraception include unprotected intercourse during the critical midcycle window in patients with regular monthly menses or at any time in patients with an uncertain first day of last menstrual period or irregular cycles; in patients who have missed 2 pills and did not use an alternative contraceptive technique; when a diaphragm becomes dislodged earlier than expected; and when the interval since depot medroxyprogesterone (Depo-Provera) injection exceeds 15 weeks.

Insertion of a copper-containing IUD may be considered emergency contraception in multiparous patients in the following circumstances: if there have been multiple unprotected exposures during the critical time of ovulation; if the patient wants to opt for an IUD as her method of contraception; and if the patient presents for evaluation and therapy at a time after intercourse that exceeds the 72-hour time limit for hormonal emergency contraception.

In a novel approach to increasing access and availability to emergency contraception, the Washington State legislature passed revisions to the Pharmacy Practice Act and enabled prescribing pharmacists in collaboration with practitioners to prescribe emergency contraception. The rationale was to have emergency contraception easily available 24 hours a day, 7 days a week. The program has been very successful. It was estimated that from 500 to 2000 unintended pregnancies were prevented in the first year by increasing availability of emergency contraception through this protocol.

Emergency contraceptive users appear to be older, better educated, and more often in stable relationships than nonusers. Women should be encouraged to seek consultation as quickly as possible after unprotected intercourse. The usual time limit for emergency contraception is 72 hours. However, use after 72 hours may still be considered with a favorable outcome and a pregnancy rate that is significantly lower than would be expected if no contraception were prescribed.

Table 52–7. Two emergency contraceptive regimens.

Commercial Name	Estrogen	Progestin	Cost
Plan B	—	Levonorgestrel 0.75 mg	$21.95
Preven	Ethinyl estradiol 50 μg	Levonorgestrel 0.25 mg	$19.94

Piaggio G et al: Timing of emergency contraception with levonorgestrel or the Yuzpe regimen. Lancet 1999;353:721. [PMID: 10073517]

Ward G: Community pharmacy supply of emergency contraception. Collaboration is vital. BMJ 2001;323:752. [PMID: 11675728]

FEMALE STERILIZATION

Background

There has been a 3- to 4-fold increase since the early 1970s in the number of women who undergo sterilization. The original descriptions of the procedure involved a transabdominal approach with ligation and resection of the tube in what is commonly referred to as a **Pomeroy tubal ligation.** The advent of sophisticated endoscopic equipment in the early 1970s made possible the performance of tubal ligations through the laparoscope. This approach was facilitated by the widespread use of safe electrical generators for electrocoagulation in the early 1970s and the subsequent development of spring-loaded clips and Silastic rings in the mid-1970s. The availability of an operating laparoscope has enabled this procedure to be performed through a single infraumbilical incision. Postpartum tubal ligations had been described as early as 1903. This procedure has remained relatively unchanged and involves an infraumbilical incision and Pomeroy tubal ligation.

Mechanism of Action

Tubal ligations interrupt the fallopian tube and exert their contraceptive effect simply by mechanical interruption of tubal continuity. A tubal ligation does not appear to compromise ovarian function or result in irregular bleeding after the procedure.

Clinical Management

The cornerstone for management of patients requesting a tubal ligation is adequate counseling. Concomitant with the increase in tubal ligations has been a definition of the legal rights of individuals seeking sterilization and the legal responsibilities of the practitioners performing them. Contemporary legal doctrine is explicit in describing the expectations that patients may have and the duties that are incumbent on the practitioner performing the tubal ligation. Informed consent is essential. Patients should be aware that, although the procedure is considered permanent, there are failure rates inherent to the procedure. Adequate counseling of patients regarding these points of management will reduce the likelihood of litigation should a pregnancy occur in the future. Average failure rates for all types of tubal ligations may be quoted to patients in the range of 1 in 250 to 1 in 500. Although the procedure is considered safe, there is a case fatality rate of 4 in 100,000 procedures.

Preoperative laboratory screening should be kept to a minimum, but a hematocrit and urinary pregnancy test are essential. Other tests should be ordered only as indicated by history. Extensive preoperative laboratory screening is not beneficial or cost-effective. Patients should be counseled to continue their method of reversible contraception until the time of the procedure. For patients using oral contraceptives, the procedure may be performed at any time. In these circumstances, the patients should be counseled to continue their oral contraceptives until they have completed a full cycle. For patients who are not using a reliable form of contraception, the tubal ligation may be performed either at the time of menses or after 2 negative urinary pregnancy tests obtained 10 days apart while the patient uses reliable contraception in the interim.

Patients frequently inquire regarding the reversibility of a tubal ligation. The procedure should not be performed on any patient who is even remotely considering a reversal. If the patient does harbor such hopes, a reversible form of contraception is a better choice.

SPECIAL NEEDS GROUPS

Two groups in particular emerge as having special contraceptive needs: those with chronic disease and those with severe mental disabilities. Ten percent of all women of reproductive age have experienced a serious chronic physical disorder or disease by 18 years of age. In this group of patients, particular care must be taken to adequately counsel the patient and match her needs to a technique compatible with her primary disease. In the second group of patients, special needs groups may have not only contraceptive needs but also hygienic issues. Counseling may also be an issue depending on the degree of understanding. Regardless of the circumstances, every attempt should be made to extend to this group of patients all contraceptive options. If full understanding is not possible, appropriate parental and/or legal counsel should be sought. Only under extreme cases and when adequate legal safeguards have been observed should sterilization be considered.

When to Refer to a Specialist

The majority of complications from the use of any contraceptive agent can usually be managed by simple intervention. Techniques for managing these complications are outlined for each type of contraception in this chapter. However, there are unusual circumstances that may require further evaluation and referral to a specialist.

Patients with irregular and persistent bleeding while taking low-dose OCPs that does not respond to supplemental estrogen therapy should be referred to a specialist for evaluation to rule out anatomic abnormalities such as endometrial polyps. This evaluation may be done through sonohysterography or hysteroscopy.

Patients with medical problems such as diabetes or migraine headaches may take OCPs. Should their medical problems become exacerbated in association with OCPs, they should be evaluated further by a specialist prior to discontinuing the OCPs. If a patient is pleased with the reliability of an oral contraceptive, the patient should be evaluated to make sure that there are not other factors contributing to the symptoms.

Patients who use implantable devices should be referred to a specialist if there is extreme difficulty in removing the implants or if not all the implants can be retrieved. Patients who have used long-acting, injectable contraceptive agents should be referred for evaluation if their menses have not begun 12 months after discontinuation.

If IUDs cannot be removed easily or if the string is not immediately evident, patients should be referred for evaluation. In select circumstances, an IUD may be retrieved during pregnancy by hysteroscopic means without interrupting the pregnancy.

PREGNANCY & FAILED CONTRACEPTION

Contemporary contraceptive techniques, in spite of their high reliability, are occasionally associated with failure. When a patient becomes pregnant while using any contraceptive, the immediate priority should be to verify the location of the pregnancy. There is an increase in the incidence of ectopic pregnancies in patients who use either a progestin-only contraceptive or an IUD or who have had a tubal ligation. In these circumstances, early transvaginal ultrasonography to verify an intrauterine location of the pregnancy is warranted.

There is no evidence to suggest that conception while taking a hormonal contraceptive has a higher incidence of birth defects. The original suspicion that pregnancies occurring while patients were using OCPs resulted in more birth defects—specifically limb bud defects—has not been verified by larger studies. Patients who continue to term in whom emergency hormonal contraceptive measures failed similarly do not have a higher incidence of birth defects. Data published in 1981 suggested a potential association between spermicide use at the time of conception and a broad range of congenital anomalies. Subsequent studies failed to confirm this association.

Special circumstances apply when a patient becomes pregnant and an IUD is in place. This situation requires careful management. Approximately 30% of IUD-related pregnancies are associated with inadvertent expulsion of the IUD. The management of a pregnancy complicated with an IUD in place is dictated by the patient's interest in maintaining or aborting the pregnancy. If the patient requests termination, the IUD should be removed at the time of the abortion. However, it is essential prior to performing the abortion, to attempt to locate the IUD by ultrasonography, because it may have been expelled or may have perforated the uterus. If the patient wishes to maintain the pregnancy and the IUD string is visible, the IUD should be removed and an early transvaginal ultrasonographic examination performed to determine the location of the pregnancy. If the patient is interested in maintaining the pregnancy and the IUD string is not visible, management depends on the presence or absence of signs and symptoms of infection. Any suggestion of an infection necessitates evacuation of the uterus and appropriate treatment using intravenous antibiotic therapy. Aggressive treatment of serious pelvic infections cannot be overemphasized. If there are no signs of infection, the patient should be informed of her options and managed conservatively. Since the discontinuation of Dalkon shields and the recommendation to remove IUDs in the event of pregnancy, no deaths have been reported among pregnant women with an IUD in situ.

Five percent of women who are pregnant with an IUD in place have an ectopic pregnancy. Data further suggest that progesterone-containing IUDs are associated with a 6- to 10-fold increase in the ectopic rate over other IUDs. When an event of pregnancy has been verified, early testing for serum human chorionic gonadotropin concentrations and a transvaginal ultrasonographic examination should be performed.

COMPLEMENTARY & ALTERNATIVE THERAPIES

There are no alternative therapies for reliable contraception. Suppression of sperm counts with androgens and linseed oil extracts have been investigated but are not reliable in either their effectiveness or reversibility.

Relevant Web Sites

[Discussion of emergency contraceptive techniques]
http://www.contraception.net/
[Planned Parenthood Federation of America]
http://www.plannedparenthood.org/library/birthcontrol/emergcontra.htm
[The Emergency Contraception Hotline]
http://www.not-2-late.com/

Infertility

53

Lorna A. Marshall, MD

ESSENTIALS OF DIAGNOSIS

- *Evaluation should be initiated after a couple has had unprotected intercourse for 12 months or sooner if the woman is older than 35 years, has a history of oligomenorrhea or amenorrhea, has known endometriosis or tubal disease, or has a partner known to be subfertile.*
- *Semen analysis must be done during the initial evaluation.*
- *Ovarian reserve testing should be performed when the female partner is older than 35 years.*
- *Diagnostic testing is unable to evaluate all potential fertility defects. Fifteen to 25 percent of couples have unexplained infertility after an evaluation has been completed.*

General Considerations

Since the 1980s, infertility has become an increasingly visible problem. There are greater numbers of women in the reproductive age group. Career demands and contraceptive availability have resulted in delayed conception, increasing the incidence of age-related infertility. Couples are anxious to build their families in a shorter period of time, increasing the use of the health care profession for assistance. The media have focused on the dramatic aspects of the reproductive technologies. Finally, alternative routes to parenting such as adoption have become more difficult. Fewer infants are available for adoption, possibly because of legalization of abortion and a greater acceptance of single parents.

Surveys to determine the prevalence of infertility have been taken of married women and sometimes of married couples. However, surveys do not include such groups as single women desiring childbirth. These surveys estimate that 8–15% of married couples in the United States are infertile.

Advanced age of the female partner is a strong risk factor for infertility. The risk for infertility is doubled for women ages 35–44 compared with women 30–34.

It is estimated that one third of women who delay pregnancy until their mid to late 30s have an infertility problem. This finding is believed to be related to the effect of aging on egg quality and ovulatory function as well as to an increased chance of disorders such as endometriosis. In addition, the risk of pregnancy loss increases substantially with age, to greater than 30% in women in their early 40s.

Other risk factors for infertility include a history of menstrual abnormalities, extremes of body weight, sexually transmitted infections (STIs) or pelvic inflammatory disease (PID), cigarette smoking, ruptured appendix, in utero diethylstilbestrol (DES) exposure to male or female partner, and mumps orchitis in the male partner.

Prevention

The primary care provider is in an excellent position to take steps toward the prevention of infertility. To lower the risk of STIs, condoms should be advised for contraception, and limitation of the number of sexual partners should be encouraged strongly. STIs should be treated promptly to prevent PID and subsequent tubal infertility. Patients with progressive dysmenorrhea and pelvic pain should be evaluated aggressively to exclude endometriosis.

Couples should be encouraged strongly to conceive before the female partner reaches her mid 30s. Older women have an increased chance of infertility as well as a shorter period of time during which conception can occur.

When a couple is considering conception, they should be counseled about lifestyle factors that may diminish their chances of conception. Smoking and recreational drug use and, possibly, high caffeine and alcohol intake, may diminish the fertility of either partner. The female partner should scale down a vigorous exercise program, especially if her menstrual periods are abnormal.

The male reproductive system is probably more sensitive to environmental influences than the female system. Nevertheless, both partners should be encouraged to minimize occupational exposures. The male partner should avoid prolonged exposure to heat, such as in hot tubs or saunas or in wearing tight briefs. Anabolic steroids can act as a contraceptive in men. Many lubricants are spermicidal; if a lubricant is necessary, vegetable oil is advised.

Preconception counseling should include a discussion of the menstrual cycle and of the appropriate frequency and timing of intercourse. In general, the optimal frequency of intercourse is every 36–72 hours from 3–4 days before until 2 days after ovulation. Few couples have intercourse too frequently for conception to occur, and daily intercourse in the periovulatory period should not reduce the chance of conception. Ovulation usually occurs about 14 days before the subsequent menses, or on about day 14 of a 28-day cycle. Normal sperm can fertilize eggs for 72 hours or longer after ejaculation, but an egg can be fertilized for only about 6–12 hours after ovulation. Couples need to understand that it is important for sperm to be available before ovulation. When the basal body temperature (BBT) has begun to climb, ovulation usually has already occurred. Rigorous attention to timing of intercourse should not be encouraged when a couple first attempts pregnancy, however, because of the potential for adversely affecting a couple's sexual relationship.

Finally, couples who are at high risk for infertility should be identified, and an evaluation or referral should be initiated earlier than the 1-year mark. When the female partner is older than 35 years, an evaluation should be initiated after 6 months of unprotected intercourse and should proceed more quickly than for younger women.

Wilcox AJ, Weinberg CR, Baird DD: Timing of sexual intercourse in relation to ovulation. Effects on the probability of conception, survival of the pregnancy, and sex of the baby. N Engl J Med 1995;333:1516. [PMID: 7477165]

Clinical Findings

It is a common misconception that infertility is a woman's problem. In fact, a male factor is involved in 35–45% of cases. Accordingly, an infertility evaluation should involve both the male and female partners.

Considerable controversy exists about what constitutes a basic and complete fertility evaluation. Cost-effectiveness is an important part of decision-making, since many insurance plans cover little or none of the evaluation and treatment of infertility. The current trend is to minimize testing and to move more quickly through a treatment plan. A laparoscopy was once a standard part of a fertility evaluation; now its expense is often avoided in favor of using resources for treatments such as reproductive technologies.

A. Symptoms and Signs

When possible, the male and female partner should present together for the initial interview. A careful menstrual history should be taken, with attention to the recent pattern of menstrual flow and dysmenorrhea. A history of contraceptive practices, STIs, pelvic surgery, and pregnancies should be taken. For the male partner, the history should include any testicular injury or surgery, mumps orchitis, heat exposures, environmental exposures, smoking, alcohol use, recreational drug use including anabolic steroids, and in utero exposure to DES.

An initial evaluation for infertility gives the provider a chance to provide preconception counseling (see Chapter 56). Medical, genetic, and medication histories (including dietary supplements and herbal preparations) should be reviewed; appropriate laboratory testing should be performed; and vaccinations should be given if indicated.

Physical examination of the female partner should include attention to lean body mass, abnormal hair growth, and galactorrhea as well as a careful pelvic examination. A fixed, retroverted uterus or tender nodularity in the cul-de-sac could suggest endometriosis and should be evaluated before the infertility evaluation progresses further.

The male partner can be examined at the initial visit or later if semen abnormalities are present.

B. Laboratory Findings

A semen analysis should be one of the first tests conducted in the infertility evaluation. Neither a history of past paternity nor a normal postcoital test replaces the semen analysis. The specimen should be collected by masturbation into a clean container after 2–3 days of abstinence. If the specimen is collected at home, it should be brought to the laboratory within 1 hour, preferably within 30 minutes, of collection. The man may use a silicone condom during intercourse if obtaining a specimen by masturbation is unsuccessful or too stressful. Normal semen parameters defined by the World Health Organization are listed in Table 53–1. Some laboratories perform a strict, or Kruger, assessment of sperm morphology on a routine basis because this method may be more predictive of sperm dysfunction. Fourteen percent of sperm should be normal when using this strict assessment.

A clinician should not designate a male as infertile based on a single semen analysis because there may be variation from sample to sample. The time for spermatogenesis is about 72 days, so that a second specimen should be requested after 2–3 months has elapsed. If the second specimen is abnormal, further diagnostic procedures in the female partner should be delayed until decisions are reached concerning the male partner. The semen analysis is so crucial to the evaluation of an infertile couple that no treatment, such as ovulatory medications, should be prescribed without the results.

Table 53–1. Normal values for semen analysis by WHO standards.

Factor	Values
Volume	≥ 2 mL
Viscosity	Liquefaction in 1 h
pH	7–8
Concentration	≥ 20 million/mL
Motility	≥ 50% (25% with rapid progressive motility) within 60 min of ejaculation
Morphologic factors	≥ 30% forms normal[1]
White blood cell count	< 1 million/mL

[1]Currently, each laboratory determines its own reference range for morphology. Multicenter, population-based studies by WHO are in progress.

If the semen analysis is normal, the couple should be reassured. However, it should be made clear that this test is only a screening test for male factor fertility and that abnormalities of sperm function may be identified later. The couple should be discouraged from assigning responsibility to either partner.

Ovulation may be evaluated in many ways. If the menstrual interval is greater than 35 days, anovulation is likely, and the patient should not be asked to do BBT charting. In women with normal menses, the BBT chart may give indirect evidence of ovulation. Temperature is taken immediately on awakening with either a BBT or digital thermometer. This constant vigilance of the menstrual cycle can cause significant stress to the couple, so many fertility specialists no longer recommend routine BBT charting. Usually, 2–3 cycles should be sufficient to establish whether or not and when ovulation occurs. Since ovulation usually occurs before the first temperature elevation, a rise in the BBT should not be used by the infertile couple as a signal to have intercourse.

Ovulation predictor tests are readily available and are accurate means to detect the luteinizing hormone (LH) surge, which begins about 36 hours before ovulation. These tests are useful in timing intercourse for couples with busy schedules and infrequent intercourse. Careful recording of the day of onset of a menstrual cycle, the day of the LH surge, and the first day of the subsequent cycle gives the clinician as much information as BBT charts do and may be less stressful for the patient. Ovulation can be confirmed with a midluteal (usually day 21) progesterone level of > 5 ng/mL.

Other laboratory tests should be used sparingly. Oligomenorrheic and amenorrheic women should have thyroid-stimulating hormone, follicle-stimulating hormone (FSH), and prolactin measured. Many clinicians measure thyroid-stimulating hormone and prolactin levels on all infertile women, even with normal menses. Anovulatory women in whom polycystic ovary syndrome (PCOS) is suspected should have fasting insulin and glucose levels and sometimes androgen measurements performed (see Chapter 20).

Ovarian reserve testing should be performed for women older than 35 years and for younger women with a history of multiple pelvic surgeries or unexplained infertility. FSH levels are most useful when drawn on day 3 of the menstrual cycle, when estradiol levels are usually low. In general, a day-3 FSH level higher than 10 mIU/mL and an estradiol > 50 pg/mL are predictive of poor results with assisted reproductive technologies (ART) except egg donation, and probably also with other fertility treatments. A variety of other hormonal challenges to test ovarian reserve can be used, with the most common being the clomiphene citrate challenge test (CCCT). In this test, a cycle 3 day FSH and estradiol are measured, clomiphene citrate is prescribed day 5–9, and FSH is measured again on day 10. FSH values should be low, usually less than 10 mIU/mL on both days 3 and 10. The combination of a female partner being older than 40 years and an abnormal FSH level on day 3 or an abnormal CCCT result is a particularly poor prognostic factor. The patient should be so informed to avoid large expenditures or substantial risk for potentially futile treatment.

C. Imaging Studies

Hysterosalpingography (HSG) is an excellent screening tool to evaluate the uterine cavity and the patency of the fallopian tubes and should be offered in the initial evaluation (Figure 53–1). Several studies suggest that pregnancy rates are enhanced in the subsequent months when the results are normal. False-negative and false-positive rates for patency are about 15%. An HSG cannot detect pelvic adhesions or endometriosis. The risk of serious PID after HSG in women with a history of previous PID is 3%; therefore, some specialists recommend laparoscopy instead of HSG to evaluate the fallopian tubes in these women. No studies support the ability of prophylactic antibiotics to prevent these infections. However, about 50% of reproductive endocrinologists prescribe prophylactic doxycycline routinely, and most others prescribe antibiotics when the examination shows abnormal tubes or when there is a possible history of PID.

Some clinicians perform transvaginal ultrasonography at the initial evaluation for all patients to exclude significant ovarian or uterine pathology. Selective use of sonography is the most practical option for most primary care providers. Serial ultrasounds to study follicu-

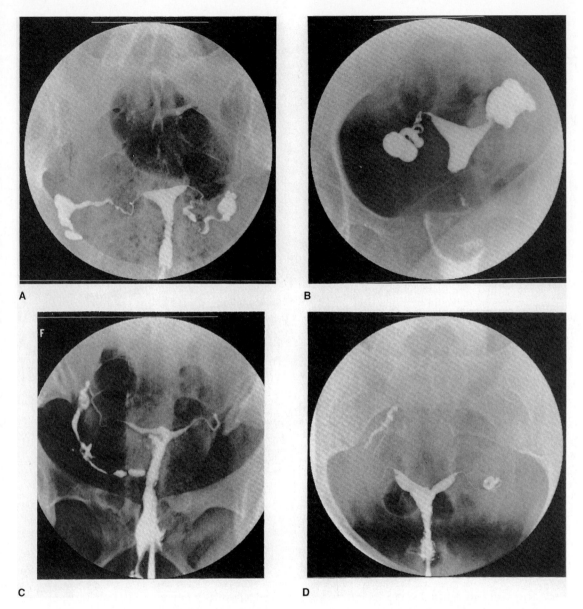

Figure 53–1. **A:** Normal hysterosalpingogram demonstrates a normal cavity and oil droplets seen exiting from patent tubes. **B:** Fallopian tubes markedly dilated from bilateral hydrosalpinges. **C:** Filling defect in uterine cavity caused by Asherman's syndrome. **D:** Abnormal uterine cavity, found at hysteroscopy/laparoscopy to be a midline uterine septum.

lar development and ovulation add considerable expense and rarely influence decision-making.

D. Other Tests

The postcoital test was once a standard test for infertility, but its utility and predictive value are low, and it is now rarely part of an initial fertility evaluation. A normal test is reassuring, but there are many reasons for an abnormal test, the most important being poor timing. Routine use of this test may lead to more tests and treatments but has not been shown to improve pregnancy rates.

A postcoital test may be useful to exclude a significant antiestrogen effect on the cervical mucus in women on clomiphene citrate, or to evaluate mucus production in women who have had cervical surgery. The test is intended to measure the ability of sperm to reach and survive in the cervical mucus. The test usually is scheduled about 2 days before ovulation is anticipated, and 2–8 hours after the couple has had intercourse. The physician and office staff need to be sensitive to the "sex on demand" aspect of this test. A specimen of mucus is obtained with nasal polyp forceps or a tuberculin syringe. The cervical mucus should be clear and hypocellular, with 6–10 cm of elasticity (spinnbarkeit). At least 5 motile sperm with forward progression should be seen for the test results to be considered acceptable.

Once ovulation has occurred, the mucus is no longer receptive to sperm. If the test result is abnormal and excessive numbers of white blood cells are seen, cervical cultures should be obtained for *Chlamydia trachomatis* and *Neisseria gonorrhoeae,* and antibiotic treatment should be initiated, if indicated.

A luteal phase (10–12 days after ovulation) endometrial biopsy can be performed and the endometrium dated by the pathologist to exclude a luteal phase defect. This test will document normal ovulation, but it is expensive and uncomfortable and rarely influences decision-making.

Other tests that are often useful in the evaluation of infertile couples include sperm antibody testing, sperm penetration assay, strict (Kruger) assessment of sperm morphology, sonohysterography, laparoscopy, and hysteroscopy. These tests may add considerable expense to the evaluation, and their use should be considered carefully. Often, it is more cost-effective to refer the patient to a specialist at this time so that the remainder of the evaluation can be integrated into the overall treatment plan.

Forti G, Krausz C: Clinical review 100: Evaluation and treatment of the infertile couple. J Clin Endocrinol Metab 1998;83: 4177. [PMID: 9851748]

Rosene-Montella K et al: Evaluation and management of infertility in women: the internists' role. Ann Intern Med 2000;75;191. [PMID: 10858181]

Sharara FI, Scott RT Jr, Seifer DB: The detection of diminished ovarian reserve in infertile women. Am J Obstet Gynecol 1998;179:804. [PMID: 9757994]

van Zonneveld P et al: Diagnosis of subtle ovulation disorders in subfertile women with regular menstrual cycles: cost-effective clinical practice? Gynecol Endocrinol 1999;13:42. [PMID: 10368797]

World Health Organization: WHO laboratory manual for the examination of human semen and sperm-cervical mucus interaction. 4th ed. Cambridge University Press, 1999.

Differential Diagnosis

A male factor is involved in a couple's infertility in 35–45% of cases. Male factors include abnormalities recognized in the semen analysis, as well as functional abnormalities of sperm such as antisperm antibodies, poor penetration of the zona pellucida, or failed in vitro fertilization (IVF). In about 15% of men where the semen analysis is normal, the sperm may be unable to fertilize an egg.

Disorders of ovulation are present in 20–32% of couples and include polycystic ovarian syndrome (see Chapter 20), hypothalamic amenorrhea, ovarian failure, and hyperprolactinemia (see Chapter 47, Disorders of Menstruation). The importance of subtle ovulatory disorders such as a luteal phase defect is often overstated and probably occurs in less than 5% of infertile women with normal menses.

Other causes include endometriosis, tubal disease, and other female factor; the estimated frequency of occurrence is 5%, 15%, and 5%, respectively. Multiple factors may be present, involving both the female and male partners.

When an initial evaluation is normal, possible diagnoses include subtle ovulation disorders, abnormalities of sperm function, minor tubal abnormalities, diminished ovarian reserve, and endometriosis. Often, a treatment plan can be initiated without further diagnostic tests to identify the causes of infertility. Costs of additional testing should be discussed with the patient so that she can make choices about the use of her resources.

The term **unexplained infertility** refers to the couple that has completed an infertility evaluation, and no abnormalities have been uncovered. Its incidence is 15–25%, depending on what is thought to constitute a complete evaluation. Unexplained infertility is more common when the female partner is in her late 30s or early 40s; it may be termed **age-related infertility** in this group of women.

Complications

There are short- and long-term complications of infertility, fertility treatments, and nulliparity.

The most significant unique complication of ovulation induction medications is ovarian hyperstimulation. Severe hyperstimulation is an unusual complication of gonadotropin therapy and IVF, resulting from an excessive response of the ovaries to stimulation. It can be associated with adult respiratory distress syndrome, hypercoagulability with thromboembolic sequelae, multiple organ failure, or even death. However, outpatient management is usually possible and involves fluid management and often paracentesis.

Women who have been infertile have a higher chance of ectopic pregnancy, spontaneous pregnancy loss, and multiple pregnancies when they conceive. The risk of pregnancy loss may as much as 3 times that of the general population, and some studies have shown especially high rates in women with PCOS. The increased rate of multiple gestations associated with ovulation induction medications and assisted reproductive technologies is of great concern. In 2000, 36% of clinical pregnancies resulting from IVF involved multiple gestations. Triplets or more accounted for 8% of clinical pregnancies, and the remainder were twin gestations. This can be compared with the multiple birth rate of less than 3% in the general population.

The primary care provider should consider long-term sequelae of nulliparity and infertility treatments. Women with PCOS have a higher risk of type II diabetes as well as gestational diabetes. Anovulatory infertility is associated with an increased risk of endometrial cancer, and care should be taken to ensure that these patients have adequate progesterone throughout their reproductive years. Nulliparous women with a history of infertility are probably at higher risk for ovarian cancer than the general population, but there is currently no good evidence that the use of fertility drugs alters that risk. The data are inconsistent regarding the relationship between infertility, fertility treatments, and breast cancer. At this time, no changes in screening are recommended for ovarian, endometrial, or breast cancer in women with a history of infertility or fertility treatments.

Fluker MR, Copeland JE, Yuzpe AA: An ounce of prevention: outpatient management of the ovarian hyperstimulation syndrome. Fertil Steril 2000;73:821. [PMID: 10731547]

Whelan JG, Vlahos NF: The ovarian hyperstimulation syndrome. Fertil Steril 2000;73:883. [PMID: 10785212]

Treatment

If initial tests are normal, a younger couple may be advised to continue timed intercourse for an additional 3–6 months before further testing or treatment is initiated. Some treatments are offered before a complete evaluation has been performed in an effort to allow the couple to conceive in the most cost-effective manner. However, it should be kept in mind that many couples have several factors preventing conception. If one problem has been corrected, but pregnancy does not occur, other problems should be considered.

A. CLOMIPHENE CITRATE

If the female partner is anovulatory or oligomenorrheic (cycle interval greater than 35 days), treatment with clomiphene citrate is usually the first step. It is essential that other causes for anovulation such as hyperprolactinemia and ovarian failure be excluded before ovulation induction is initiated. Clomiphene citrate is a nonsteroidal medication that binds to the estrogen receptor and can initiate ovulation in women who have some endogenous estrogen. Generally, it is given orally in doses of 50–100 mg for 5 days, beginning on day 3, 4, or 5 of a menstrual cycle. It also can be given after a menstrual bleed has been induced with 10 mg of medroxyprogesterone acetate for 5–10 days. Ovulation usually occurs 5–10 days after the last day of medication. BBT charts provide the most cost-effective method for monitoring ovulation in a patient taking clomiphene citrate. Clomiphene should be started at a dose of 50 mg and increased to 100 mg if ovulation does not occur or occurs later than 10 days after the last dose of the medication. If ovulation occurs but pregnancy does not, there is no reason to increase the dose of clomiphene citrate. After the first cycle of treatment, and about every 2 months thereafter if pregnancy does not occur, the woman should have her BBT chart reviewed and her ovaries examined to exclude persistent ovarian cysts. If large ovarian cysts are present, no more clomiphene citrate should be administered until the cysts resolve.

Because of the long half-life of the drug, antiestrogenic effects such as endometrial thinning may worsen until a 1-month hiatus in treatment is taken. No more than 3 consecutive cycles should be prescribed.

A referral should be initiated if ovulation does not occur on a regimen of 100 mg of clomiphene or if pregnancy does not occur after 3–6 months of treatment. Ultrasonographic monitoring generally is recommended if doses greater than 100 mg are used.

About 80% of anovulatory women ovulate after taking clomiphene, and approximately 40% conceive. The multiple pregnancy rate is about 5–8%; the multiple births are almost entirely twins. No increased risk of birth defects has been reported.

Side effects of clomiphene include vasomotor symptoms, mood changes and, less commonly, headache, visual symptoms, and ovarian enlargement. Some reports have raised the question of an increased risk of ovarian cancer in infertile women who have taken fertility drugs, but the majority of studies have not supported a causative association between clomiphene citrate or other fertility treatments and ovarian cancer.

There is little evidence that clomiphene alone is beneficial to women who have normal menstrual cycles; in some cases, its antiestrogenic effect on cervical mucus and on the endometrial lining may prevent conception. For couples with unexplained infertility, a limited number of cycles of clomiphene with intrauterine insemination may be beneficial (see next section).

Special considerations for ovulation induction in women with PCOS are outlined in Chapter 20. In some cases, the addition of insulin-sensitizing agents such as metformin may facilitate ovulation and pregnancy in these patients and avoid referral for gonadotropin therapy.

B. INTRAUTERINE INSEMINATIONS

In couples with male factor infertility, intrauterine inseminations of processed sperm of the male partner doubles the chance of pregnancy compared with natural intercourse. The likelihood of pregnancy is maximized when more than 4 million motile sperm are available after processing. Inseminations may also be indicated when a woman on clomiphene has poor postcoital tests, when semen volume is low, or in conjunction with gonadotropins or clomiphene citrate for the management of unexplained infertility. In addition, intrauterine inseminations are generally more successful than intravaginal inseminations when donor sperm is used. Usually, inseminations are performed best at an office that has access to a laboratory for the preparation of sperm and can perform inseminations 7 days of the week. Inseminations usually are performed 24 hours after the LH surge is detected or HCG is administered. A variety of catheters can be used, including the sheath of an 18-gauge intravenous catheter. A tenaculum may be used if intrauterine placement of the catheter is difficult.

C. ASSISTED REPRODUCTIVE TECHNOLOGIES

Since the birth of the first child resulting from IVF in 1978, the reproductive technologies have evolved into important and efficient treatments for tubal disease, male factor infertility, endometriosis-related infertility, and unexplained infertility. According to the Center for Disease Control and Prevention, 99,639 ART cycles were performed in the United States in 2000, resulting in over 25,228 live birth deliveries and 35,025 babies. Unfortunately, these procedures are not available to most couples who could benefit from them, primarily because of their high cost and the failure of most insurance plans in this country to cover even a limited number of cycles.

It is important that the primary care provider understand the options available and their approximate success rates. In 2000, about 25.4% of IVF cycles started in the United States and Canada resulted in a live birth delivery. Each reproductive technology program is now required by law to report outcome data to the Centers for Disease Control and Prevention. This information is available online to the public and may help guide appropriate referrals.

IVF is the most commonly performed assisted reproductive procedure today. It was developed initially to bypass the function of the fallopian tube for women with severe tubal disease. After stimulation of oocyte development with gonadotropins, the eggs are retrieved under transvaginal ultrasonographic guidance. Insemination with the partner's sperm occurs in the laboratory, and the fertilized and cleaving embryo is transferred transcervically into the uterus 3–6 days after the retrieval. Culture of embryos to the blastocyst stage, 5–6 days after retrieval, may allow fewer, more highly selected embryos to be transferred. The availability of embryo cryopreservation allows embryos to be saved for future transfer after the initial placement of a limited number of embryos in the uterus.

Gametes or embryos can be replaced to the ampullary portion of the fallopian tubes, usually by laparoscopy, in gamete intrafallopian transfer (GIFT) and zygote intrafallopian transfer (ZIFT) procedures. Enthusiasm for these procedures has diminished with time, so that less than 2% of ART procedures were GIFT or ZIFT in 2000.

Microinjection techniques have allowed couples with sperm counts too low for conventional IVF to reconsider the option. With intracytoplasmic sperm injection (ICSI), a single sperm is placed into the cytoplasm of the egg. Sperm can be retrieved from the epididymis or testes of men with obstructive, or sometimes nonobstructive, azoospermia to allow conception using ICSI.

Biopsy of the preimplantation embryo can be performed and a single cell analyzed to exclude a chromosomal or single gene defect, to perform HLA antigen typing, or to determine the sex of the embryo. In some circumstances, preimplantation genetic diagnosis may be a useful adjunct to infertility treatment.

Third party or collaborative reproductive options are being chosen more frequently. Women with ovarian failure, even those with primary ovarian failure from Turner's syndrome, can conceive with donated eggs, fertilized in vitro with the husband's sperm. Ovum donation is frequently the best option for couples when the female partner is older than 40, when ovarian reserve testing is abnormal, or when a couple has undergone multiple cycles of IVF with poor embryo quality. Live birth rates after IVF fall dramatically with increasing age of the female partner, while birth rates after ovum donation remain high regardless of the age of the female partner (Figure 53–2). Unused frozen embryos can be donated from one couple to another. In some states, surrogate arrangements are used to allow a couple in which the female partner lacks a normal uterus to use a "host uterus" to carry their genetic child. The complex ethical and legal issues of collaborative reproductive arrangements are addressed continually through professional societies such as the American Society for Reproductive Medicine.

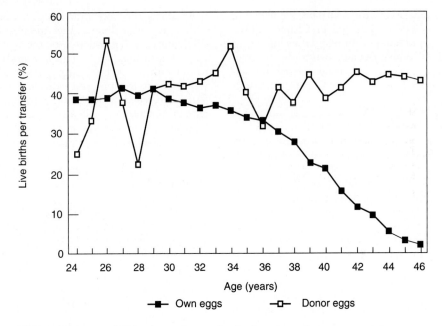

Figure 53–2. Live birth per transfer rate for fresh embryos from own and donor eggs (by age of recipient), 1999. (Reproduced from Centers for Disease Control and Prevention: 1999 Assisted Reproductive Technology Success Rates.)

D. OTHER TREATMENTS

Other therapeutic options depend on the problems identified, the age of the female partner, and the couple's emotional and financial resources. Most reproductive surgery, including microsurgical tubal repair, is performed using the laparoscope or hysteroscope. Proximal tubal obstruction often can be treated with cannulation of the tube under fluoroscopic or hysteroscopic guidance. Gonadotropins are used with or without inseminations for the treatment of most ovulatory disorders that are unresponsive to clomiphene and also are useful for the treatment of unexplained infertility. Bromocriptine, cabergoline, and progesterone are useful in the treatment of selected ovulatory disorders. Insulin-sensitizing agents such as metformin may be prescribed with clomiphene after the patient with PCOS does not conceive with clomiphene alone, or it may sometimes be used as a first-line agent to induce ovulation (see Chapter 20). Varicocele repairs can sometimes improve semen quality and function in carefully selected men.

Many couples who are infertile want to be as informed as possible about the treatment process, and the primary care provider can complement the educational services provided by the specialist. Patient brochures about the evaluation and treatment of infertility are available from a variety of professional organizations (see following section, Relevant Web Sites).

E. COMPLEMENTARY THERAPY

Infertile couples frequently seek the assistance of alternative medicine before, during, or after they undergo a traditional evaluation and treatment for infertility.

The perception that stress is a causative factor for infertility has prompted infertile individuals to seek out massage, acupuncture, and other complementary medicine in an effort to reduce stress. Stress reduction techniques have entered traditional fertility programs in the form of "mind/body" programs.

A variety of dietary supplements, including vitamin E and para-aminobenzoic acid, and herbal treatments, including *Vitex* and dong quai, have been recommended to treat the infertile female. The provider should recognize that many herbal treatments are mildly estrogenic, so they may interact with ovulation induction medications. In addition, some may lower cycle day-3 FSH levels without improving ovarian reserve, so may result in false-negative test results of ovarian reserve.

Many dietary supplements have been recommended for the male partner to improve sperm counts and fertility. These include zinc, vitamins C, E, and B$_{12}$, L-arginine, coenzyme Q10, selenium, and L-carnitine. The male partner should be cautioned to avoid supplements and herbal treatments that contain testosterone or other androgenic agents because they may suppress spermatogenesis.

Acupuncture has been proposed as a way to improve sperm counts and function in the male partner and to induce ovulation or improve implantation in the female partner. Clinical trials are underway to evaluate the effectiveness of this method.

Hughes E, Collins J, Vandekerckhove P: Clomiphene citrate for unexplained subfertility in women. Cochrane Database Syst Rev 2000;3:CD000057. [PMID: 10908459]

Karande VC et al: Prospective randomized trial comparing the outcome and cost of in vitro fertilization with that of a traditional treatment algorithm as first-line therapy for couples with infertility. Fertil Steril 1999;71:468. [PMID: 10065784]

Mol BW et al: Cost-effectiveness of in vitro fertilization and embryo transfer. Fertil Steril 2000;73:748. [PMID: 10731536]

Paulus WE et al: Influence of acupuncture on the pregnancy rate in patients who undergo assisted reproduction therapy. Fertil Steril 2002;77:721. [PMID: 11937123]

Steptoe PC, Edwards RG: Birth after implantation of a human embryo. Lancet 1978;2:366.

Stone BA et al: Determinants of the outcome of intrauterine insemination: analysis of outcomes of 9963 consecutive cycles. Am J Obstet Gynecol 1999;180:1522. [PMID: 10368500]

When to Refer to a Specialist

The primary provider for male and female partners is in an excellent position to treat infertile couples. The provider may play a vital role in the prevention of infertility, including preconception counseling to maximize a couple's chance of conception. Providers choose variable involvement in infertility evaluations and treatments. It is important to have a general understanding of the available treatments and processes involved so that appropriate referrals can be made and emotional support given.

The timing of referral depends on the provider's training, interest, and office organization, as well as on the availability of infertility specialists in the area. Infertility is a rapidly changing field, with reproductive technology services becoming more available and successful. Patients are increasingly aware of the services available and often seek out a specialist to initiate an evaluation.

The best option for referral of the female partner is a board certified reproductive endocrinologist, who can guide a couple from a basic evaluation to consideration of ARTs. Many gynecologists who have a special interest in infertility can perform a basic evaluation and initiate treatments other than the reproductive technologies.

If semen abnormalities are identified on 2 specimens, a referral to an urologist is recommended to evaluate the male partner further, treat any pyospermia, and recommend therapy. An urologist also should be seen if impotence might be affecting fertility. If a varicocele is present, repair may improve sperm parameters and increase the chance of pregnancy. The decision whether or not to fix a varicocele is sometimes difficult and requires input from both the urologist and the provider who is managing the female partner's evaluation.

Many couples, especially those with an older female partner, express frustration that referrals were not made soon enough. It is important for the provider to identify couples who require an early referral to a specialist.

Prognosis

It is often difficult to evaluate the success of each treatment because of a significant spontaneous conception rate. Approximately half of couples who are evaluated after 1 year of infertility and have a normal evaluation will achieve pregnancy in the next year without treatment. There are few randomized, controlled trials that are large enough to give accurate chances of conception for most infertility treatments. In general, most treatments other than some ARTs do not exceed the monthly conception rate in normal couples, which is about 20%. All treatments including IVF become significantly less successful as the female partner ages. In fact many treatments have not been evaluated in women over 40 because of their low success rates.

Outcome data for all ARTs are collected by each program that provides these services. The Centers for Disease Control and Prevention reports national and clinic-specific data yearly, although with a lag of 2–3 years.

When treatments are not successful, the provider can help the patient understand the limitations of treatment. In addition, decisions about adoption or living without children should be reinforced when appropriate.

Relevant Web Sites

[American Society for Reproductive Medicine. All practice guidelines and patient information sheets from ASRM are available online]

http://www.asrm.org

[Centers for Disease Control Assisted Reproductive Technology Success Rates. National and program-specific success rates for reproductive technologies are published yearly by the CDC.]

http://www.cdc.gov/nccdphp/drh/art.htm

[Resolve. Patient information and referrals to providers including counselors.]

http://www.resolve.org

[American Infertility Association. Patient information and support.]

http://www.americaninfertility.org

Emotional Aspects of Infertility

54

Mary Ann Draye, ARNP, MPH, FNP

Infertility has been described as a developmental crisis; as such, it has the potential to disrupt the progression of adult development. According to Erickson's theory of development, **generativity,** or guiding the next generation, is a major developmental task of adulthood. Most often in society, the task of generativity is translated into bearing and raising children. Failure to achieve generativity can lead to stagnation and self-absorption.

Reproduction is a basic expectation and couples often think of themselves as potential parents long before children arrive. Infertility may result in a developmental crisis by defying the cultural norm (despite some support for child-free living) and the individual's own goal of parenthood. If parenthood is viewed as the primary means of role fulfillment, the threat of failure is significant, resulting in a sense of despair and loneliness. Components of generativity include creativity and productivity as well as nurturing. Parenthood is the primary, although not exclusive, means of accomplishing these adult development tasks.

The chronicity of infertility adds to the disruptive nature of the experience and necessitates consideration. Infertility brings one crisis after another (eg, negative pregnancy tests and monthly disappointments as new treatments are tried and failed). As time goes on, certain events such as birthdays or holidays may mark the attempts and failures at becoming pregnant.

The steps of resolution used in crisis and grief models do not always hold for infertility. Rather, the ongoing nature of infertility contributes to a chronic sorrow and mourning. The emotional pain is cyclic; it is experienced periodically as one is reminded of one's losses. In addition, the sorrow that accompanies infertility is not only for what is perceived as lost, but also for the current distress.

Common Responses to Infertility

Infertility is exhausting for all those involved. Extensive treatment and testing over time, the experience of hopes rising only to be shattered, and the expenditure of resources exact an emotional toll. Increasingly, the emotional aspects of infertility have been acknowledged in the literature. Common feelings associated with infertility are anger, denial, guilt, depression, isolation, grief, and decreased self-esteem. In addition, a patient may feel profoundly out of control. Perceived powerlessness, coupled with decreased self-esteem, leads to feelings of inadequacy.

A. ANGER AND FRUSTRATION

The patient's anger results primarily from feeling out of control and from the perceived unfairness of infertility. Many patients feel angry when they encounter parents who seem unfit, children who are abused, or news accounts of unwanted pregnancies. Frustration accompanies anger, because the demands and sacrifice associated with treatment are upsetting but must be tolerated to increase the chance of achieving pregnancy. Also, the inability to comfort one's partner is a source of extreme frustration for some (see the section following, Gender Differences).

Anger can be rational, if it is directed at the situation, or irrational. Anger may be projected onto providers, one's partner, family and friends, or a stranger who has children. Anger also can be turned inward resulting in depression.

B. DENIAL

Denial is one of the early feelings associated with infertility. Most individuals assume they are fertile, especially when they are healthy. Reluctance to participate in certain procedures or refusal to accept a negative result may indicate some denial on the part of patient. Denial serves as a protective mechanism until a person can comprehend the magnitude of the crisis. However, denial is appropriate and effective only as a short-term coping mechanism.

C. GUILT

In trying to explain infertility, cause and effect relationships often are sought. Past thoughts and actions are reviewed as possible causes of infertility. Issues that commonly produce guilt include premarital sex, masturbation, previous abortion, contraceptive use, sexually transmitted diseases, divorce, and even ambivalence about parenting. Self-blame over these events leads to feelings of guilt or of being punished.

D. ANXIETY

Feelings of impending doom, worry, and uncertainty about the future all contribute to anxiety. In addition, treatment procedures may contribute to anxious feelings. Waiting for tests, worrying about how the partner will react, financial worries, and deciding how to tell others what is happening are dominant concerns.

E. ISOLATION

Often, infertile patients experience the loss of friends who become parents. For some, the pain of being around friends with children is too much to bear. If information regarding infertility is not shared, the person may be the recipient of pressure, well-meaning advice, and worse—bad jokes. If the information is shared with others, even more advice may be forthcoming along with stories of cures, others' successes, unwelcome sympathy, and uncomfortable silence. Whether or not the information is shared, the result may be that gatherings with family and friends become so painful that the infertile couple withdraws. Many infertile couples report feeling alone in a fertile world. They often turn to each other for their support, which can put further strain on a relationship that is already stressed. Although frequent communication is necessary, a common complaint of couples is that infertility is all they ever talk about anymore.

F. GRIEF

The grief associated with infertility has some unique characteristics. **Grief** is defined as a response to loss. For infertile couples, the grief process is different because they feel a potential loss rather than the concrete loss experienced with the death of a child. There is nothing tangible to mourn, and there are no rituals of support to help bear this loss. Moreover, the loss may be trivialized by well-meaning people who point out the benefits of being free of parenting responsibilities.

Simultaneously, couples experience grief over painful and costly treatments, strained relationships, and an uncertain future. The pain and loss are not forgotten but experienced repeatedly as patients cycle through treatments.

G. DEPRESSION

Feelings of sadness, despair, pessimism, and fatigue accompany infertility. Apathy and loss of pleasure also can characterize the normal depression of infertility. However, most infertility patients with mild depression are able to continue to function and do not use maladaptive coping strategies for extended periods of time. Patients with more severe depression have intense symptoms that significantly affect their functioning over time.

Worsening persistent sadness (depression), extreme changes in sleep and eating patterns, anxiety, increased use of alcohol and drugs, feeling out of control, persistent thoughts of suicide and death, and obsessive behavior all indicate more than the normal depression associated with infertility; referral to a mental health professional is indicated for patients with these symptoms.

H. DECREASED SELF-ESTEEM

Infertile patients are at risk for decreased self-esteem. Both women and men report feeling that their sexuality has been attacked by infertility. Women report feeling incomplete, less feminine, or a failure as a woman. Men report feeling defective and less virile. Consequently, both men and women may feel less desirable sexually or less confident about their sexuality. In addition, some medications used in fertility treatment may decrease sexual desire and pleasure.

Loss of self-confidence may occur in other areas of life as well. Pursuing treatment and working through the feelings involved take precedence over other activities. Competence in other areas of life such as career and partner relationships is minimized. Infertility can become the central focus of life. When one's central view of oneself is associated with failure, as in the inability to achieve pregnancy, one's self-esteem suffers.

Erikson EH: Childhood and Society. Norton, 1993.

Gonzalez LO: Infertility as a transformational process: a framework for psychotherapeutic support of infertile women. Issues Ment Health Nurs 2000;6:619. [PMID: 11271137]

Woods NF, Olshansky E, Draye MA: Infertility: Women's experiences. Health Care Women Int 1991;12:179. [PMID: 2022528]

Gender Differences

Infertility and its treatment affect women and men differently. Initially, women seem to be more vulnerable to the infertility crisis than their male partners. Women appear to experience more distress, regardless of the medical cause. They report disruption in their personal lives, worries over role failure, decreased self-esteem, and a significant sense of loss. Women may seek care from both medical and mental health professionals, whereas men may be less inclined to use such services. Commonly, the woman is the initiator of all types of treatment and has the most interactions with the health care system.

When the cause for infertility is a male medical factor, men report more feelings of loss and decreased self-esteem than men without a medical factor. However, these men do not report the same degree of disruption as their female counterparts. Women without a medical factor feel the loss of childbearing as strongly as those with such a factor. Men without a medical factor feel loss because of their inability to help their partner.

A. COPING PATTERNS

Women and men cope differently in response to infertility (Table 54–1). Women typically use a greater variety of coping methods. Social coping includes talking,

Table 54–1. Common responses to infertility by gender.

Area	Male Response	Female Response
Communication	Less need or desire to discuss infertility	Needs and desires to discuss repeatedly
	Use of conversation primarily to problem-solve or compete	Use of conversation primarily to connect, relax, and discuss feelings
Coping	Private coping	Social coping
	Primarily problem-focused	Primarily emotion-focused, variety of strategies
Isolation	Some; generally able to compartmentalize infertility	Often significant; infertility pervades all areas of life; feels separate from other women
Frustration	Major source of frustration is feeling helpless to comfort partner; cannot seem to "make it better"	Major source of frustration is childlessness; lack of "success"
Options for parenting	Often able to consider child-free life earlier	Usually strong drive for motherhood

seeking support, reading, and attending lectures. Emotion-focused coping, eg, wishing, hoping, and escaping is also used although not to the exclusion of purposeful problem-solving coping.

Men are less likely to use social coping. Rather they use a more private, problem-solving style of coping. Problem-focused coping implies developing and following an action plan. Men often substitute other activities for those lost, and they are more likely than women to continue to find pleasure in those other activities.

B. COMMUNICATION PATTERNS

It has been suggested that if women and men talked through interpreters, they might have a better chance of staying together. Differing communication styles present a challenge to all couples, but they are of greater magnitude for partners facing infertility. During the course of treatment, many decisions need to be made including those concerning options for parenthood and expenditure of resources. These decisions require effective communication between partners. Furthermore, the emotions associated with infertility need to be shared with the partner.

Couples need to be open and honest in their communication and avoid making assumptions about their partner. To assume one knows what the partner thinks about an issue or feels in response to a loss is dangerous. These assumptions can be wrong and lead to resentment and hurt feelings.

Another danger in communication is to judge the value of a communication style. For example, women tend to cope with infertility by verbalizing. It is helpful for them to talk about how they feel and review the dilemma of infertility. The male partner, on the other hand, may tire of hearing the same words over and over. To him, to communicate is to problem-solve and sometimes to be assertive and show what he knows. Therefore, he offers a solution to her verbalizing when a solution is not what she desires. She simply wants to express herself and be listened to empathically. The deleterious effect occurs when value judgments are ascribed to the styles. He thinks she is overemotional, compulsive, and obsessive. She thinks he is uninterested, less caring, and detached. He tends to withdraw and feel nagged. She feels alone and unsupported. In truth, they are merely using different styles of communication.

Studies indicate that when communication becomes difficult or upsetting, men feel threatened and less equipped to handle their partner's expressions of negative emotions. This reaction contributes to frustration. He may express himself as follows: "I try to help her but nothing seems to work, so I just quit and wait it out, but it's getting tiring." "I wish I could be more in touch with my feelings like she is, but I'm not—that's just the way I am." Repeatedly and poignantly, men have shared their profound sense of frustration at (1) not being recognized for trying to communicate and (2) inability to comfort their partner no matter how hard they try.

The existence of these differing styles does not mean that women and men do not communicate successfully concerning infertility or that women never problem-solve and men never support. Rather, these are some of the prevailing patterns and pitfalls that can be difficult for some partners.

Jordan C, Revenson TA: Gender differences in coping with infertility: a meta-analysis. J Behav Med 1999;4:341. [PMID: 10495967]

Kowalcek I: Coping with male infertility: Gender differences. Arch Gynecol Obstet 2001;3:131. [PMID: 11561741]

Woods NF, Olshansky E, Draye MA: Infertility: Women's experiences. Health Care Women Int 1991;12:179. [PMID: 2022528]

Assisted Reproductive Technologies

The advancing technologies of assisted reproduction (see Chapter 53, Infertility) bring new hope to couples who previously had none. Although changes occur in technology, the emotional aspects of infertility are not changed. When patients consider the wide range of treatment options, however, additional dynamics related to the "high tech" nature of treatments are added to the emotional aspects of infertility. It is worth considering the blessings as well as the burdens of these new technologies.

The assisted reproductive technologies (ART) offer patients more hope than ever before, sometimes making it hard for patients to stop treatment. Many patients report that they feel compelled to try ART to "close the door" on infertility treatment. For some patients, ART represents the next logical step in treatment. ART often is viewed as the last chance for a biologic child, and chances for success may be overestimated. Taking advantage of the reproductive technologies usually requires significant expenditure of resources, not only financial but emotional and physical as well. In addition, a significant amount of time is required for clinic appointments and procedures. Life is rearranged around the demands of the treatment protocols.

Issues common to ART patients include expenditure of resources, confidentiality, ethics and values, handling loss, informed consent, and coping with the intrusion of technology into their lives. These issues may become even more compelling when surrogacy or the use of donor gametes or embryos is being considered. These treatments may mean that one or both partners will not be genetically related to the child. It is imperative that the rights and welfare of all parties are considered: potential parents, donor or surrogate, and child. Balancing hope with realism proves to be a significant task for most patients. Worry for the welfare of the woman and normalcy of a child conceived through ART is also present (despite data showing that these pregnancies and outcomes are no different from spontaneous pregnancies). The rigors of ART treatment can have significant impact on patients. Daily monitoring and complex physical procedures can be stressful. Moreover, patients undergo these treatments with the knowledge that the chances for success are relatively low. This can contribute to worry and anxiety. For some couples the strain of waiting can be more difficult than the physical aspects of treatment (eg, "Did the eggs fertilize?" "Did pregnancy occur?"). When ART fails, the feelings of loss and sadness are profound. Although most couples eventually work through their grief, the emotional stress surrounding a failed ART cycle is significant.

Treatment: Strategies for Helping

Primary care providers can play a valuable role in helping infertility patients. It may be the primary care provider who first discovers or hears about fertility problems. The relationship with the patient that has already been established can be helpful even as specialty care is being considered.

The primary care provider should inform patients of various options and services available and facilitate an appropriate referral. This includes a transfer of records and assistance as patients move from a familiar provider to the care of a specialist. Even while patients are being seen by specialists, the primary care provider may play a role in ongoing support. Obtaining feedback from specialists is important also, especially if the provider continues to see these patients for support, counseling, and other areas of primary care. Being accessible to provide information or discuss feelings in the office or by phone is important.

A. EMPATHY

The principal component of each interaction with patients should be empathy. **Empathy** is defined as an emotional sensitivity; it implies an understanding of the other person's thoughts and feelings. Empathic listening involves sincerely hearing what the patient is saying in a nonjudgmental way. Sometimes merely interacting with an empathic provider is immensely helpful to patients.

B. EMPOWERMENT

A second role of the provider is to facilitate the empowerment of infertility patients. Clinicians do not directly empower patients because that connotes a hierarchy of power. Rather, clinicians provide information and choices and support patients in their decision-making. When recommendations are made by the health care team, patients are encouraged to weigh them in light of their life goals, values, and resources. For example, the recommendation may be to undertake another cycle of in vitro fertilization (IVF) when the patient's present goal is to stop treatment and reevaluate.

Another part of facilitating empowerment is helping patients redefine the concepts of success and failure. Surely, taking home a baby is defined as success. Although facing adversity with courage, redefining life goals, and planning for the future are components of successful maturity; such qualities are rarely affirmed or acknowledged in the course of infertility treatment. Providers should use every opportunity to acknowledge the significant emotional work being done by infertility patients.

C. ANTICIPATORY GUIDANCE

Providing information is another way to facilitate empowerment in patients. When patients understand the treatment protocol, they usually feel more in control. Potentially serious errors can be avoided, and patient anxiety can be reduced. Anticipatory guidance helps prepare patients for the future stages of treatment. For example, outlining the steps for obtaining a hystero-salpingogram helps the patient to know what to expect. Providing such guidance usually reduces fear of the unknown.

A part of anticipatory guidance includes information regarding community resources, including patient support groups, relaxation training, or a RESOLVE chapter if available. (RESOLVE is a national, nonprofit organization that offers information and support for infertile patients.) Crisis phones and professional therapists may be needed for a small percentage of patients. In addition, primary care providers can recommend reputable Internet sources that may be helpful to patients.

Klonoff-Cohen H et al: A prospective study of stress among women undergoing in vitro fertilization or gamete intrafallopian transfer. Fertil Steril 2001;76:675. [PMID: 11591398]

Van Horn AS, Reed SA: Medical and psychological aspects of infertility and assisted reproductive technology for the primary care provider. Mil Med 2001;11:1018. [PMID: 11725314]

When to Refer to a Specialist

If patients are feeling anxious, depressed, out of control, or overwhelmed for prolonged periods of time, they may benefit from a referral to a mental health professional. Primary care providers should continually assess for depressive symptoms. In addition, a mental health provider may provide insight into feelings and clarify thinking when the patient is considering alternative options for building a family, is having difficulty making a treatment decision, or is considering closure of treatment. Primary care providers should maintain a referral network of mental health providers with an expertise in infertility. Local RESOLVE chapters often maintain lists of experienced counselors.

Prognosis

In general, patients survive their infertility crisis as they conceive, build their family by alternate means, or choose to remain childfree. Some studies indicate that pregnancy after infertility can lead to increased anxiety especially in the first trimester. Studies show no differences in parenting between fertile and infertile, biologic or adoptive parents. Research findings are also reassuring for families formed after ART, with multiple births as a major continuing issue. However, issues of secrecy and anonymity are major dilemmas for families built using donor gametes.

Domar AD et al: Impact of group psychological interventions on pregnancy rates in infertile women. Fertil Steril 2000;73:805. [PMID: 10731544]

Relevant Web Sites

[American Infertility Association. A national nonprofit lay organization dedicated to assisting patients facing infertility and reproductive health issues. The site contains information, advocacy issues, support line, and links to other relevant sites.]

www.americaninfertility.org

[American Society for Reproductive Medicine. A professional nonprofit organization with information for patients and professionals. Some information in Spanish.]

www.asrm.org

[Resolve is a lay organization that provides advocacy, support, and education. Information is available to patients, family and friends, and health professionals. The site offers a helpline, referrals, information on coping, treatments, and data on chapters nationwide.]

www.resolve.org

Pregnancy Termination

55

Susan P. Kupferman, MD

General Considerations

Since the 1973 United States Supreme Court decision of *Roe v Wade,* a woman may elect to terminate her pregnancy during the first trimester for her own reasons. During the second and third trimesters, each state may regulate the abortion procedures in ways that are reasonably related to maternal health.

Elective abortion, or voluntary termination of pregnancy, is the interruption of pregnancy before fetal viability at the woman's request. **Therapeutic abortion** is the termination of pregnancy before viability to protect maternal health or because the fetus is affected by disease or deformity. Certainly, the vast majority of abortions currently performed in the United States are elective.

It is estimated that approximately 25% of pregnancies worldwide are terminated by induced abortion, rendering this perhaps the most common method of birth control. The most recent statistics from the Centers for Disease Control and Prevention (CDC) provide information through 1997 (Figure 55–1). These indicate that the number of legal abortions performed in the United States rose steadily from 1973 to 1981, and then began to decrease slightly each year from 1990 to 1995. In 1997, the number of abortions was the lowest it has been since 1978. In 1997, there were 1.18 million abortions in the United States, or 305 induced abortions per 1000 live births.

The ratio of abortions to live births was highest for members of ethnic minority groups and women younger than 15 years of age. In 1997, 20% of women obtaining legal abortions were younger than 19 years old, and 32% were between the ages of 20 and 24.

In general, women obtaining abortions were young, white, and unmarried (21% were married), had no previous live births, and were having the procedure for the first time. Approximately 54% of abortions in 1997 were performed at 8 weeks or less gestational age, and 86% before the 13th week. Four percent of abortions were performed at 16–20 weeks of gestation, and 1.4% at greater than 21 weeks. Information on medical abortions is not yet available by CDC.

Prevention

Almost all abortions can be prevented by encouraging the avid use of contraception. Contraception should be discussed before performing any abortion technique and should be reviewed again immediately after the termination. If desired, contraception can be initiated the day of the procedure. It is important for patients to realize that ovulation can occur as soon as 2 weeks after a first trimester abortion. Of contraceptive methods available, all are appropriate for immediate use with the exception of intrauterine devices after a second trimester termination. In this case, the chance of expulsion is higher and placement of an intrauterine device should be delayed after a second trimester procedure.

Clinical Findings

As in any procedure, it is essential to obtain informed consent. The nature, risks, alternatives, benefits, and indications for the proposed procedure or treatment need to be discussed in detail with the patient. All of her questions should be answered satisfactorily. The clinician should feel certain that the patient requests this procedure of her own volition. It is prudent to mention other options for unplanned pregnancies such as adoption but important to respect the woman's right to self-determination.

A. History

The preoperative evaluation should include a medical history with particular attention paid to previous surgical problems, gynecologic disease, allergies, possible coagulopathy, and perceived pain tolerance. All of these factors may influence the planning and performance of the procedure.

B. Physical Examination

Physical examination should include heart, lung, abdominal, and pelvic examinations. It is essential to establish gestational age, because this generally determines the type of procedure to be performed. If the patient is uncertain of gestational age or if there is dis-

577

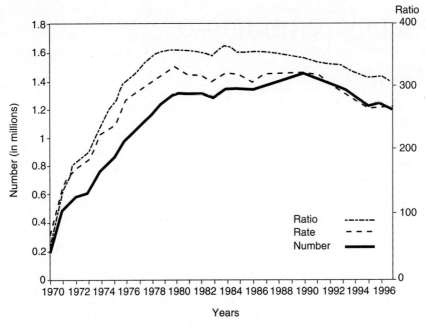

Ratio
Rate
Number

* Number of abortions per 1,000 live births.
† Number of abortions per 1,000 women aged 15-44 years.

Figure 55–1. Number (in millions), ratio (per 1000 live births), and rate (per 1000 women ages 15–44) of legal abortions in the United States between 1970 and 1997. (Reproduced, with permission, from Koonin et al: Abortion Surveillance. Centers for Disease Control and Prevention/US Department of Health and Human Services 1997;49:1.)

cordance between reliable dates and pelvic examination, it is wise to obtain an ultrasonographic scan to guide therapy decisions. Ultrasonography also may be appropriate if there has been abnormal bleeding to identify a molar or ectopic pregnancy.

C. LABORATORY TESTS

Routine laboratory tests include a pregnancy test, hematocrit, and Rh typing and antibody screen. Controversy exists over the need for screening for sexually transmitted infections (STIs) and cervical neoplasia (see Chapter 34). Rho (D) immune globulin should be administered to women who are Rho (D) negative without Rh antibodies. Fifty micrograms should be given when the gestational age is 12 weeks or less, and 300 μg should be given when the gestational age is greater than 12 weeks.

Techniques

There are 4 main methods for performing an abortion: medical abortion, instrumental evacuation vaginally, stimulation of uterine contractions, and major surgical procedures. Generally speaking, gestational age determines the technique.

A. MEDICAL ABORTION

Medical abortion offers an alternative to surgical termination of pregnancy for women with early pregnancies. More than 3 million women worldwide have had medical abortions over the last 10 years. In China and Europe, medical abortion has been offered since 1988. However, the US Food and Drug Administration (FDA) only granted approval to mifepristone as of July 1996.

The history of medical abortion dates back to the 1950s when folic acid antagonists were used. These regimens caused intolerable nausea, vomiting, diarrhea, and fever. In the early 1980s French scientists developed RU-486 (mifepristone) a compound that bound strongly to the progesterone receptor without activating it and as such acts as an antiprogestin. During early pregnancy, mifepristone alters the endometrium by affecting the capillary endothelial cells of the decidua. This results in separation of the trophoblast and the decidua and declining levels of secretion of human chorionic gonadotropin (hCG) secretion. As a result of these events bleeding occurs. In addition, mifepristone will soften the cervix. Initially, investigators tried to use mifepristone alone as an abortifactant and found that at best, only 80% of women (< 49 days gestational age) had complete abortions. In 1988, France became the first country to license the use of mifepristone in combination with a prostagladin for early abortion treatment.

Methotrexate is a substance that blocks dihydrofolate reductase, an enzyme required for the production of thymidine during DNA synthesis. Methotrexate used in combination with misoprostol has been shown to have the same overall efficacy as mifepristone and a prostaglandin analogue. However, the methotrexate regime takes a longer time interval to cause abortion and so is used far less frequently.

The standard regimen recommended by the FDA is 600 mg of mifepristone followed by 400 μg of oral misoprostol 48 hours later. For pregnancies of fewer than 49 days, the efficacy of this regime is 95–96%, beyond 49 days the efficacy falls to 85%. Studies have shown that there is no significant difference in the rate of abortion completion with a single versus multiple doses of mifepristone and that regimens using lower doses of mifepristone (200 μg) may yield similar results to those using the conventional 600 μg.

In the United States the synthetic prostaglandin E_1 (PGE_1) used with mifepristone is misoprostol (Cytotec). This drug, unlike some of the other prostaglandins used, is inexpensive and can be stored at room temperature. Regimens using varying amounts of misoprostol or multiple doses have been tested. These studies have shown that a second dose of misoprostol does not increase overall efficacy. In addition, they have shown that intravaginal use of 800 μg misoprostol decreases time to expulsion and side effects. Investigators have reported higher rates of success with the 800 μg intravaginal dosing for pregnancies between 49 and 63 days. Acceptability of the methods to both providers and patients has been high. In 1 study, only 9% of women who received a medical abortion said they would opt for surgical therapy in the future.

The current FDA regimen requires that mifepristone be prescribed by physicians in a 3-visit program. On day 1, mifepristone is given as a single oral dose. On day 3, patients return to the clinic and are assessed, usually by ultrasonography, for completion of the termination. If abortion has not occurred at this point, an oral dose of misoprostol is administered, and the patients are then watched in the clinic for 4 hours. Patients return on day 15 to ensure that the abortion is completed.

Medical abortion needs to be performed by a health care professional who can provide services in the case of a method failure or excessive bleeding. Contraindications to a medical abortion include ectopic pregnancy, intrauterine device in place, chronic adrenal failure, current long-term use of systemic corticosteriods, allergy to mifepristone or misoprostol, and hemorrhagic disorders or current anticoagulation therapy. The abortion provider must confirm that the woman is amenable to having a surgical abortion in the event of failure of the medical abortion.

Side effects include bleeding, nausea, vomiting, pain, and diarrhea. After expulsion of the conception product, bleeding will occur for a median of 9 to 13 days, but in the majority of women bleeding tapers off quickly.

B. Menstrual Extraction

Menstrual aspiration or extraction is early suction curettage of the endometrium; it may be performed up to 50 days after the last menstrual period. A flexible plastic cannula is used, 4–6 mm in diameter, with a self-locking syringe to provide suction. Menstrual aspiration has the advantage that anesthesia and cervical dilation often are not required. If a chosen cannula cannot be passed, a smaller one of the set might serve as a dilator. After the appropriate size cannula is inserted, the syringe is attached and the pinch valve released to begin suction. Uterine contents flow into the syringe. The procedure is done by radial passes starting at the fundus and moving to the lower uterine segment, covering all of the uterine cavity until the gritty feel of the endometrium is present and bubbles appear in the syringe. Two cautions should be emphasized: (1) the cannula must not be removed while a vacuum exists in the syringe and (2) the plunger of the syringe should not be advanced while the cannula is connected within the uterus because an air embolism could result.

Because this procedure is performed so early in pregnancy, it could be done unnecessarily on a nonpregnant woman. It should not be performed unless a positive result on a pregnancy test is obtained. There exists a higher failure rate in terminating a pregnancy before 6 weeks of gestation, perhaps because the target is so small. Microscopic examination of the products of conception, plus careful follow-up, can reduce the likelihood of a persistent pregnancy going unrecognized.

C. Suction Curettage

This procedure has proved to be the most effective surgical technique for pregnancy termination during the first trimester. Its advantages over sharp curettage include less blood loss, shorter procedure time, and lower incidence of uterine perforation. The use of a strong vacuum (50–60 mm Hg) quickly shears the products of conception away from the uterine wall, evacuates them from the uterine cavity, and induces uterine contractions. This process minimizes blood loss.

Preoperatively, the patient is instructed to consume only a clear liquid diet. Preoperative medications include a nonsteroidal anti-inflammatory agent such as ibuprofen, 600 mg (for cramps); diazepam 10 mg (for anxiety); and tetracycline 250 mg, all taken 1 hour before the procedure begins.

After the procedure, ibuprofen is continued every 6 hours as needed. The patient is instructed to call the physician if she experiences fever, chills, vaginal bleeding heavier than a normal menses, severe abdominal or pelvic pain, or persistent nausea and vomiting.

Patients report less discomfort when preoperative cervical laminaria tents are used. Laminaria are hygroscopic, long, thin aggregates of desiccated, sterilized seaweed. Although the mechanism of action may be multifactorial, the principal mechanism seems to be desiccation of the cervix, causing it to soften and dilate. The use of laminaria greatly reduces cervical trauma and laceration, as well as the incidence of uterine perforation.

To place a laminaria, the cervix is cleaned antiseptically, and the cervical lip is grasped with a Jacobs tenaculum (which tears the pregnant cervix less than a single tooth) to render the endocervical canal parallel to the vagina. The anterior lip is grasped on an anteflexed uterus and the posterior lip on a retroflexed uterus (Figure 55–2), and steady traction is applied. Using ring or packing forceps, the appropriate width laminaria is placed gently through the cervix just past the level of the internal os (Figure 55–3). Its position is maintained with a gauze sponge.

At the time of the evacuation procedure, the vaginal sponge and laminaria are removed and a bimanual examination is performed again to guide the physician in determining the cannula size and direction of its passage. Exposure of the upper vagina and cervix is obtained with a bivalve speculum, generally the Graves. Some physicians prefer the Moore modification, in which the blades are 1 inch shorter, which allows the cervix to be drawn closer to the introitus. The cervix and upper vagina are cleansed antiseptically.

In the United States, most abortions are done with local anesthesia, which is quicker, cheaper, and safer than general anesthesia. However, its use is predicated on patient cooperation and relaxation. If these criteria cannot be met or if the informed patient requests it, general anesthesia is used.

The paracervical block is effective in decreasing pain, but the patient should be informed that the placement itself may be uncomfortable. Most physicians use 1% lidocaine because it is effective and inexpensive. The clinician should anesthetize the tenaculum site. It is important to wait 3 minutes after injection for the block to be most effective.

The tenaculum is used to apply traction on the cervix, thereby aligning the cervical canal parallel to the

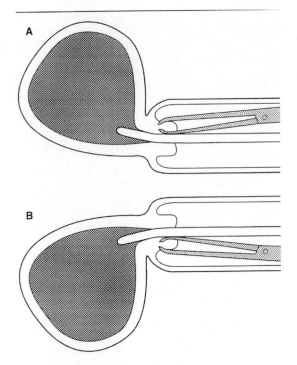

Figure 55–2. Traction on cervix during dilation. **A:** The tenaculum is placed vertically on the anterior lip. **B:** The tenaculum is placed vertically on the posterior lip for a retroverted uterus. (Reproduced, with permission, from Thompson JD, Beck JA: *Te Linde's Operative Gynecology*, 7e. Lippincott, 1997.)

vagina (Figure 55–4). Tapered mechanical dilators, eg, Pratt, are associated with easier dilation and a lower perforation rate than nontapered dilators, eg, Hegar. The fourth and fifth fingers of the dilating hand are maintained against the patient's buttocks and perineum to minimize excessive force and perforation (Figure 55–4). The cervix is dilated until the appropriate-size cannula can be placed.

Should the clinician find the cervix difficult to dilate to the desired width, 2 options are available: (1) using a smaller cannula or (2) packing the os with laminaria and returning to complete the operation several hours later.

Next the cannula is inserted into the uterus. Rigid or soft cannulas are available. The cannula size generally is 1 less than the gestational age in weeks from the last menses. If the slightly angled type of cannula is used, the cannula is placed just above the internal os at the level of the lower uterine segment. If the straight type of cannula is selected, it is placed gently just below the level of the fundus. In either case, suction of 50–60

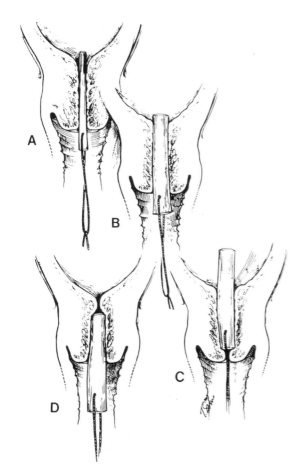

Figure 55–3. Insertion of laminaria. **A:** Laminaria immediately after being placed appropriately with its upper end just through the internal os. **B:** The swollen laminaria and dilated, softened cervix about 18 hours later. **C:** Laminaria inserted too far through the internal os; the laminaria may rupture the membranes. **D:** Laminaria not inserted far enough to dilate the internal os. (Reproduced, with permission, from Cunningham FG et al (editors): Abortion. In: *Williams Obstetrics,* 19e. Appleton & Lange, 1993.)

mm Hg is generated, and the cannula is rotated 360 degrees slowly, multiple times, until bubbles are seen in the cannula. A gentle, sharp curettage can confirm that the cavity is empty, and a subsequent quick pass with the suction removes any clots or tissue that might promote excessive postoperative bleeding. The tenaculum is removed and direct pressure applied for a few minutes to stop any bleeding from the puncture sites.

It is critical to examine the aspirated tissue to confirm completion of the procedure, to identify a molar pregnancy, and to exclude the possibility of an ectopic pregnancy. If the uterus seems empty after the procedure but the tissue appears insufficient or atypical, the specimen should be submitted for pathologic examination, and gynecologic consultation should be sought.

D. DILATION AND EVACUATION

In 1997, the percentage of second-trimester (greater than 13 weeks) abortions performed by dilation and evacuation (D&E) was 98.6%, whereas the percentage performed by intrauterine instillation was approximately 0.2%. The increasing use of D&E may have resulted from the improved technology, especially ultrasonographic guidance, and the lower risk of complications associated with the procedure. Younger women account for a higher percentage of these advanced procedures.

D&E differs from suction curettage in 2 ways: (1) D&E requires greater cervical dilation, usually accomplished by placing multiple laminaria the afternoon before the procedure, and (2) forceps are needed to evacuate the more advanced pregnancies. From 13 to 16 weeks, vacuum aspiration alone is sufficient; thereafter, specialized forceps extraction is needed. Confirmation of completeness of uterine evacuation is accomplished with gentle, sharp curettage or ultrasonography. In D&E, the skill and expertise of the surgeon determines in large part the safety of the procedure.

E. STIMULATION OF UTERINE CONTRACTIONS

This technique is used predominantly for more advanced pregnancies, usually over 16–17 weeks of gestation. In 1997, less than 1% of legal abortions were accomplished by intrauterine saline or prostaglandin instillation, with the latter technique being more prevalent. Intrauterine saline or urea generally results in fetal death, with labor following thereafter. The prostaglandin directly activates myometrial fibers, inducing labor. In the United Kingdom and Sweden, use of the antiprogesterone mifepristone (RU-486) with vaginal and intracervical prostaglandins has resulted in a shorter time from induction to abortion.

F. HYSTEROTOMY AND HYSTERECTOMY

These methods should not be considered primary methods for abortion. They carry undue risk, expense, and pain when compared with the aforementioned techniques. Indeed, less than 0.9% of abortions were performed by these methods in 1997. Hysterectomy should be performed only as dictated by preexisting disease.

Complications

Morbidity is determined largely by gestational age and abortion method. The safest interval has been reported to be 7–10 weeks of gestation (Table 55–1). Suction

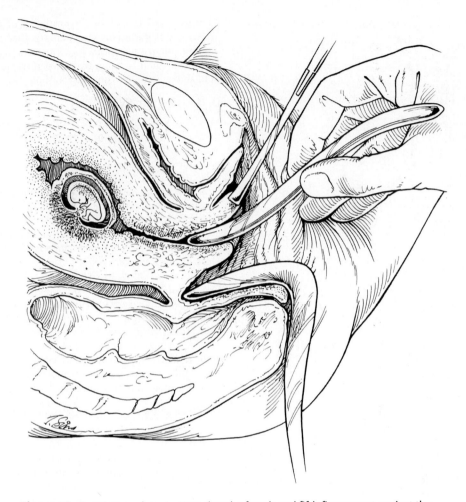

Figure 55–4. Dilation of cervix. Note that the fourth and fifth fingers rest against the perineum and buttocks, lateral to the vagina, to lower the risk of perforation of the uterus. (Reproduced, with permission, from Cunningham FG et al (editors): Abortion. In: *Williams Obstetrics*, 19e. Appleton & Lange, 1993.)

curettage appears to be the safest surgical method available (Table 55–2).

Immediate complications of suction abortion include hemorrhage (0.05–4.9%), cervical laceration (0.01–1.6%), uterine perforation (0.2%), and acute hematometra (0.2–1%). The latter condition is characterized by severe cramping within 2 hours of the procedure; less than expected vaginal bleeding; weakness; perspiration; and a tender, enlarged uterus. Treatment involves prompt reevacuation. Often neither anesthesia nor dilation is necessary. Removal of the liquid and clotted blood gives prompt relief.

Retained tissue often is expelled with vaginal bleeding. Otherwise, it manifests itself by cramping and bleeding several days after the procedure in less than 1% of abortions. Reevacuation is indicated if symptom severity persists, ultrasonographic findings demonstrate persistent tissue, or a fever occurs.

Postabortal infection occurs in less than 1% of suction dilation and curettage (D&C) procedures and in 1.5% of D&E procedures. The organisms usually responsible are group B β-hemolytic streptococci, *Bacteroides* species, *Neisseria gonorrhoeae*, *Escherichia coli*, and *Staphylococcus aureus*. Treatment consists of appro-

Table 55–1. Serious complication rates for legal abortion by gestational age, United States, 1975–1978.[1]

Gestational Age (wk)	Rate[2]
≤6	0.4
7–8	0.2
9–10	0.1
11–12	0.3
13–14	0.6
15–16	1.3
17–20	1.9

[1]For women with follow-up and without concurrent sterilization or preexisting conditions; serious complications include fever of 38 °C or higher for 3 d or more, hemorrhage requiring blood transfusion, and any complication requiring unintended surgery (excluding curettage). (Reproduced, with permission, from Thompson, JD, Beck JA: *Te Linde's Operative Gynecology,* 7/e. Lippincott, 1997)
[2]Per 100 abortions.

priate antibiotics and careful follow-up. Curettage is indicated if the infection is associated with retained tissue.

The incidence of Rho sensitization should be minuscule if the health care provider follows standard care guidelines for Rho (D) immune globulin administration.

More than 1 million abortion procedures were performed in 1992, with 10 maternal deaths, which is equivalent to a case-fatality rate of 0.7 in 100,000. Deaths from legal abortions have declined between 1973 and 1992 from 3.3 to 0.7 deaths per 100,000 procedures, reflecting increased physician education

Table 55–2. Serious complication rates for legal abortion by method, United States, 1975–1978.[1]

Method	Rate[2]
Suction curettage	0.2
Dilation and evacuation	0.7
Saline instillation	2.1
Prostaglandin, instillation	2.5
Urea and prostaglandin instillation	1.3

[1]For women with follow-up and without concurrent sterilization or preexisting conditions; serious complications include fever of 38 °C or higher for 3 d or more, hemorrhage requiring blood transfusion, and any complication requiring unintended surgery (excluding curettage). (Reproduced, with permission, from Thompson, JD, Beck JA: *Te Linde's Operative Gynecology,* 7/e. Lippincott, 1997)
[2]Per 100 abortions.

and skills, improvements in medical technology, and earlier termination of pregnancy. Risk factors for maternal death include ethnic minority group, age greater than 35 years, and increasing gestational age. There is no evidence that a single vacuum aspiration procedure increases the risk of subsequent infertility, ectopic pregnancy, or other complications of pregnancy. Insufficient data are available for women who have had multiple or second-trimester procedures.

When to Refer to a Specialist

Many primary care providers choose to refer all patients desiring an abortion to providers or clinics that perform large numbers of these procedures. Most providers who are comfortable with endometrial biopsies and D&C procedures can perform first-trimester abortions safely in their office.

Patients requesting second-trimester abortions should be referred to providers who perform large enough numbers of them to demonstrate a low complication rate. Not all gynecologists who perform first-trimester abortions fall into this category.

When the products of conception are absent or abnormal at the time of suction curettage, a gynecologist should be consulted. In addition, any indication of an ectopic, molar, or cornual pregnancy at the time of preprocedure ultrasonography should prompt a referral. Women with significant medical problems such as von Willebrand's disease, unstable cardiovascular disease, or pulmonary hypertension should be referred for medical consultation, and the abortion usually should be performed in the operating room with an anesthesiologist present.

Creinin MD: Medical abortion regimens: historical context and overview. Am J Obstet Gynecol 2000;183:S3. [PMID: 10944364]

Creinin MD: Medical management of abortion. ACOG Practice Bulletin #26. American College of Obstetrics and Gynceology, Washington DC, 2001.

Council on Scientific Affairs, American Medical Association: Induced termination of pregnancy before and after *Roe v Wade.* Trends in the mortality and morbidity of women. JAMA 1992;268:3231. [PMID: 1433765]

Koonin LM et al: Abortion surveillance—United States, 1997. MMWR Morb Mortal Wkly Rep CDC Surveill Summ 2000;49(SS11):1. [PMID: 11130580]

Newhall EP, Winikoff B: Abortion with mifepristone and misoprostol: regimes, efficacy, acceptability and future directions. Am J Obstet Gynecol 2000;183:S44. [PMID: 10944369]

Shulman LP, Frank WL: Termination of pregnancy first trimester. UpToDate web site www.UpToDate.com 2002.

Spitz IM et al: Early pregnancy termination with mifepristone and misoprostol in The United States. N Engl J Med 1998; 338:1241. [PMID: 9562577]

Spitz IM: Mifepristone for medical termination of pregnancy. UpToDate web site www.UpToDate.com 2002.

Relevant Web Sites

[Emergency Contraception]
http://ec.princeton.edu

[American College of Obstetricians and Gynecologists]
http://www.acog.org
[Planned Parenthood]
http://www.plannedparenthood.com

Preconception Counseling & Care of Common Medical Disorders in Pregnancy

56

Roberta Haynes de Regt, MD

GENETIC COUNSELING & RISK ASSESSMENT

A vital segment of the preconception counseling visit is genetic risk assessment. Identification of factors that place the pregnancy at increased risk is important for preconception as well as pregnancy management. Identifying risk factors prior to pregnancy allows time for reduction or elimination of risk as well as consideration of alternative pregnancy choices. Genetic counselors help women understand difficult obstetric issues so that they can make informed decisions about pregnancy.

The American Society of Human Genetics has adopted the following definition of genetic counseling: Genetic counseling is a communication process that deals with human problems associated with the occurrence, or risk of occurrence, of a genetic disorder in a family. This process involves an attempt by 1 or more appropriately trained person(s) to help the individual or family

1. Comprehend the medical facts, including the diagnosis, probable course of the disorder, and the available management.
2. Appreciate the way heredity contributes to the disorder and the risk of recurrence in specified relatives.
3. Understand the options for dealing with the risk of recurrence.
4. Choose the course of action that seems appropriate to them in view of their risk, and the family goals, and act in accordance with that decision.
5. Make the best possible adjustment to the disorder in an affected member and/or to the risk of recurrence of that disorder.

RISK IDENTIFICATION

Part of the preconception intake should include the patient completing a preliminary family and personal history as shown in Figure 56–1. A standard list of indications for referral by the provider is seen in the Box, Recommendations for Prenatal Services. Positive responses to any of these questions indicate an increased risk; such families should see a geneticist, genetic counselor, or maternal-fetal medicine subspecialist. These professionals are able to give nondirective information regarding individual risks, carrier screening, and options for prenatal diagnosis as well as to counsel and support these families.

An essential part of prenatal risk assessment is the development of a family pedigree. The pedigree should contain at least 3 generations and should include all the children of a sibship, whether abnormal or normal, living or dead. A multigenerational pedigree is mandatory in the assessment of the inheritance pattern of a disorder in a particular family. This is important because of the possibility of generation skipping in disorders such as X-linked recessive or autosomal dominant disorders in which reduced penetrance is present. Basic information should include age and cause of death. Specific questions should be asked about congenital malformations, mental retardation, genetic conditions, infant deaths, stillbirths, and pregnancy losses. If accurate information is unobtainable, such as the age or cause of death of an individual, this ambiguity should be included in the pedigree. It is imperative to obtain medical records for confirmation of diagnosis as well as clarification of unclear or inaccurate information. For example, if a patient reports a family history of hemophilia and prenatal diagnosis is offered for that condition, an incorrect diagnosis of the fetus may be given if it was hemophilia B, and not hemophilia A, that was present in this family. Pedigree terminology is reviewed in Figure 56–2.

Advanced Maternal Age

An increasing number of women aged 35 to 49 years will have live births; in 1997, 12.6% of women were in this age group. It is considered the standard of care in this country and is the recommendation of the American College of Obstetricians and Gynecologists

Genetic History Questionnaire for Prenatal Patients

- **The answers to these questions will help in the care of your pregnancy.**
- **All answers will remain part of your private confidential medical record.**
- **Please answer these questions as well as you can. If you need help answering the questions, please ask.**

Patient Name: _____   Date: _____

1. When your baby is born, will you be 35 years of age or older?   ☐ No ☐ Yes

---

Where your ancestors came from may sometimes give us important information about the health of your baby.

---

2. Is your family or your baby's father's family . . .

    a. from Southeast Asia, Taiwan, China, or the Philippines?   ☐ No ☐ Yes ☐ Not sure

    b. from Italy, Greece or the Middle East?   ☐ No ☐ Yes ☐ Not sure

3. a. Was there ever a baby (or unborn baby) in your family or your baby's father's family born with an opening in the back or spine, also called spina bifida?   ☐ No ☐ Yes ☐ Not sure

    b. Was there ever a baby (or unborn baby) in your family or your baby's father's family who had an opining in the head, also called anencephaly?   ☐ No ☐ Yes ☐ Not sure

4. Were you, or was anyone in your family or your baby's father' family born with a heart defect?   ☐ No ☐ Yes ☐ Not sure

5. Have you, or has anyone in your family or your baby's father' family had an unborn baby or a child who had Down syndrome (some call it trisomy 21)?   ☐ No ☐ Yes ☐ Not sure

6. Is your family or your baby's father's family Eastern European (Ashkenazi) Jewish or Cajun?   ☐ No ☐ Yes ☐ Not sure

7. If your family or your baby's father's family African-American (Black)?   ☐ No ☐ Yes ☐ Not sure

Figure 56–1. Questionnaire detailing personal and family history for the preconception counseling visit. (From Pacific Southwest Regional Genetics Network.)

(ACOG) to inform women age 35 or older of the availability of prenatal counseling and testing. Genetic counseling for discussion of age-related chromosomal abnormalities such as Down syndrome and other nondisjunctional events resulting in fetal aneuploidy as well as the sensitivity and specificity of available screening and diagnostic tests should precede any testing. The relevant prenatal diagnostic procedures should be explained, and the possible risks should be detailed. The maternal age of 35 years has been established as the cut-off point at which pregnant women are referred for prenatal diagnosis for fetal aneuploidy. Since 1978, amniocentesis has routinely been offered to women over

age 35; however, some investigators are now recommending maternal serum marker screening as the first line of surveillance. When the criteria for prenatal diagnosis were established in the 1970s, the risk of having an aneuploid fetus outweighed the risk of procedure-related miscarriage at the maternal age of 35 years. Studies of complications from amniocentesis indicated that 35 was the age when the risk of having an aneuploid fetus equaled or was greater than the risk of losing the pregnancy as the result of complications from the procedure (approximately 0.5%). In fact, procedure-related risk may be as high as the 1% risk quoted in a classic Danish randomized trial. Chorionic villus sam-

Do you, or does your baby's father, or any blood relative have . . .

8. hemophilia or other bleeding disorders? ☐ No ☐ Yes ☐ Not sure

9. muscular dystrophy? ☐ No ☐ Yes ☐ Not sure

10. cystic fibrosis (CF)? ☐ No ☐ Yes ☐ Not sure

11. Huntington disease? ☐ No ☐ Yes ☐ Not sure

12. a. Is any blood relative in your family or your baby's father's family mentally retarded or developmentally delayed?
☐ No ☐ Yes ☐ Not sure

   b. Do you, or does your baby's father, or any blood relative have fragile X syndrome?
☐ No ☐ Yes ☐ Not sure

13. Do you, or does your baby's father, or any blood relative have any other chromosome problems?
☐ No ☐ Yes ☐ Not sure

14. a. Do you have diabetes? ☐ No ☐ Yes ☐ Not sure

   b. Do you have phenylketonuria (PKU) or other metabolic condition requiring special foods or other treatment? ☐ No ☐ Yes ☐ Not sure

15. Were you, or was your baby's father, or any blood relative born with . . .

   a. a cleft lip or palate? ☐ No ☐ Yes ☐ Not sure

   b. any other birth defects? ☐ No ☐ Yes ☐ Not sure

16. Have you ever had . . .

   a. two or more miscarriages? ☐ No ☐ Yes

   b. a still born baby and one or more miscarriage(s)? ☐ No ☐ Yes

17. During this pregnancy, have you taken . . .

   a. a doctor's prescription or medications from a drug store? ☐ No ☐ Yes

   b. alcohol? ☐ No ☐ Yes

   c. recreational or street drugs? ☐ No ☐ Yes

18. Do you, or does your baby's father, or any blood relative have any other birth defect, disease or health problem that is inherited (runs in the family)? ☐ No ☐ Yes ☐ Not sure

   If you marked yes or not sure, then please describe: _____

   _____

19. Is there a possibility that you and the baby's father could be related by blood (e.g., cousins)?
☐ No ☐ Yes ☐ Not sure

   Completed by: _____ Date: _____ / _____ / _____

   Reviewed by: _____ Date: _____ / _____ / _____

Figure 56-1. Continued

RECOMMENDATIONS FOR PRENATAL SERVICES[1]

1. Advanced maternal age (35 or over at delivery).
2. Abnormal serum marker screening test results (multiple marker screening).
3. Either parent or other family member with a chromosomal rearrangement.
4. Previous child or family history of a chromosomal abnormality (eg, Down syndrome, trisomy 18, fragile X syndrome).
5. Either parent or previous child with a known or suspected inborn error of metabolism (eg, phenylketonuria, maple syrup urine disease, galactosemia, Hurler syndrome, lactic acidosis, Tay-Sachs disease).
6. Previous child with a significant personal history of a major structural abnormality (eg, neural tube defect, congenital heart disease, cleft lip and palate).
7. Parent or previous child with a known genetic abnormality (eg, osteogenesis imperfecta, neurofibromatosis, myotonic dystrophy, tuberous sclerosis).
8. Fetus with anomalies suspected on ultrasound (eg, single or multiple malformations, hydrops, oligohydramnios, growth retardation without a known etiology, neural tube defect).
9. Women exposed to known or suspected teratogen in pregnancy (eg, alcohol, parvovirus, anticonvulsant, Accutane).
10. Women with a condition known or suspected to affect fetal development and/or outcome (eg, diabetes, alcoholism, collagen vascular disease, phenylketonuria).
11. Parent is a known carrier, has a family history of, or is in an at-risk ethnic or racial group for a disorder for which prenatal testing may be available (eg, Tay-Sachs, cystic fibrosis, sickle cell disease, alphathalassemia).
12. Consanguinity/incest.
13. Multiple pregnancy losses (equal or greater than 2); recurrent abortion and/or stillbirths.

[1]These guidelines were prepared by the Pacific Southwest Regional Genetics Network (http://www.psrgn.org).

pling (CVS) offers an earlier diagnosis, although the risk of pregnancy loss from this procedure appears to be slightly higher (approximately 1%). It has been suggested that a maternal serum test called the "quad screen" (see the section following, Types of Prenatal Diagnosis) be offered as an alternative screen to try to reduce age-related risks for women over age 35. ACOG has not yet adapted serum screening as the primary form of surveillance because the screening tests have neither the sensitivity nor the specificity of fetal karyotype analysis. Some investigators have suggested that the cutoff age for amniocentesis should be lowered or, at least, amniocentesis should be offered to younger women who are pregnant with multiple gestation. Table 56–1 lists age-related risks for Down syndrome and all chromosomal abnormalities.

Previous Child With a Chromosomal Abnormality

Parents who have had a child with an extra chromosome (aneuploidy) such as trisomy 21 (Down syndrome), trisomy 13, or trisomy 18, have an empiric recurrence risk of 1–2%. When a child has a chromosomal transloca-

tion, deletion, or duplication, the parental chromosomes should be tested to determine whether the parents are balanced translocation carriers. If 1 of the parents is found to be a balanced translocation carrier, there is an increased risk to future pregnancies, and prenatal diagnosis should be offered in all subsequent pregnancies. Elevated risks to future pregnancies include delivery of a live-born child with an unbalanced translocation as well as stillbirth, spontaneous abortion, and infertility.

Structural Chromosomal Rearrangement

Although parents who are carriers of balanced chromosomal rearrangements do not have any medical or physical problems related to this rearrangement, they are at increased risk for having a child with an unbalanced rearrangement. The risk of having a child with an unbalanced chromosomal rearrangement varies with the type of parental balanced translocation as well as the gender of the parent carrying the translocation. The overall risk is 10–12%. Robertsonian translocations (the fusion of 2 acrocentric chromosomes, such as 14 and 21) carry a transmission risk of 15% if the mother carries the

Female   Male

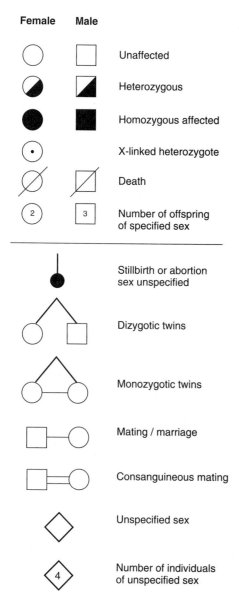

Unaffected

Heterozygous

Homozygous affected

X-linked heterozygote

Death

Number of offspring of specified sex

Stillbirth or abortion sex unspecified

Dizygotic twins

Monozygotic twins

Mating / marriage

Consanguineous mating

Unspecified sex

Number of individuals of unspecified sex

Figure 56–2. Terms and symbols used in family pedigrees.

Table 56–1. Age-related risks of chromosomal abnormalities (live births).[1]

Maternal Age	Down Syndrome	All Chromosomal Abnormalities
20	1/1667	1/526[2]
21	1/1667	1/526
22	1/1429	1/500
23	1/1429	1/500
24	1/1250	1/476
25	1/1250	1/476
26	1/1176	1/476
27	1/1111	1/455
28	1/1053	1/435
29	1/1000	1/417
30	1/952	1/384
31	1/909	1/384
32	1/769	1/322
33	1/635	1/317
34	1/500	1/260
35	1/385	1/204
36	1/294	1/164
37	1/227	1/130
38	1/175	1/103
39	1/137	1/82
40	1/106	1/65
41	1/82	1/51
42	1/64	1/40
43	1/50	1/32
44	1/38	1/25
45	1/30	1/20
46	1/23	1/15
47	1/18	1/12
48	1/14	1/10

[1]Reproduced with the permission of the American College of Obstetrics and Gynecology from Hook EB: Rates of chromosome abnormalities at different maternal ages. Obstet Gynecol 1981;58: 282.
[2]47, XXX excluded for ages 20 to 32 (Data not available).

child or identification in a relative is 20%; if the abnormality is ascertained by a history of multiple miscarriages, the risk falls to 2–5%. Genetic counseling for individual risk assessment and prenatal diagnosis, such as CVS or amniocentesis, to determine fetal karyotype should be offered to the couple at risk.

Previous Child With an Isolated or Multiple Congenital Anomalies

The delivery of a child with a birth defect, such as a congenital heart defect, increases the risk that siblings may be born with a similar problem. Recurrence risk counseling depends on the mode of inheritance as well

translocation and 2–4% if the translocation is paternal. The risk of having an offspring with unbalanced translocation to a couple who carries a reciprocal translocation (the transference of chromosomal material between 2 nonhomologous chromosomes) depends on the ascertainment of the abnormality. The risk to a carrier couple ascertained by delivery of an affected as the relationship of the affected individual to the couple. For example, the parents of a child with a congenital heart defect would have a recurrence risk of 1–4%, but a second-degree relative would have a risk of approximately 1% that their child would also be affected. Many birth defects follow a multifactorial pattern of inheritance. In these cases, a collection of factors, some known, most unknown, have to combine to reach a threshold before a child is affected. Common isolated defects have known empiric risks of recurrence based on large population studies. However, children with multiple congenital anomalies should be evaluated by a geneticist for a pattern of defects that might lead to a diagnosis. If a definitive diagnosis is made, it could alter the risk for the parents of having a second affected child especially if it is a syndrome with autosomal recessive inheritance (Table 56–2). If there is a known environmental agent that increases the risk of having a child with a particular birth defect, this agent can be avoided in future pregnancies. Also, some agents have been discovered that can be protective. For example, couples who have had a previous child with a neural tube defect (NTD) (eg, spina bifida or anencephaly) have a 3–5% risk of recurrence. Recent studies have shown, however, that if folic acid supplementation is given to the mother prior to neural tube closure (21–28 days postconception), the risk for a second affected child may be reduced by as much as 70%.

Previous Stillborn

Parents with a previous pregnancy resulting in a stillbirth of unknown cause may be at increased risk for a second stillbirth. Proper evaluation of a stillbirth may determine the cause of fetal death and therefore help assess risks to future pregnancies; 8% of stillbirths have chromosomal abnormalities and 20% have dysmorphic features or skeletal abnormalities. Maternal evaluation also is indicated to establish maternal causes of pregnancy loss. If no cause for stillbirth is found, couples who have experienced 1 stillbirth have an empiric recurrence risk of 3%; in families with 2 previous stillbirths, the overall risk to subsequent pregnancies is about 15%.

Family History of Mendelian Disorder

A family history of a Mendelian disorder may put a couple at risk for having a child with that disorder. Risks to the pregnancy vary depending on both the type of inheritance of the condition in the family as well as which members of the family are affected. Carrier screening before pregnancy may reassure a couple that they are not at increased risk for having a child with a specific genetic disorder. If an increased risk is identified preconceptionally, however, more time is available for the couple to discuss options in pregnancy such as prenatal diagnosis. Early risk identification also gives the couple sufficient time to discuss pregnancy management with their physician. Couples who are identified prenatally as being at increased risk for having a child with a Mendelian disorder also have the option to discuss and choose alternatives to conventional pregnancy including in vitro fertilization, preimplantation genetic diagnosis, artificial insemination by donor, surrogacy, or adoption.

Table 56–2. Common congenital abnormalities.

Type	Incidence in Newborns	Recurrence Risks
Congenital heart disease	8/1000, 0.8%	1–4%
VSD: ventricular septal defect	1/532, 0.19%	1.7–4.2%
ASD: atrial septal defect	1/1548, 0.6%	0.7–2.9%
PDA: patent ductus arteriosis	1/1340, 0.75%	1–3.5%
Neural tube defects	1–2/1000	3–5%
Clubfoot	3/1000	3%
Diaphragmatic hernia	1/2000–1/3000	0–2%
Cleft lip and palate	1/1000	4%
Dislocation of hip	1/1400	6%
Tracheoesophageal fistula	1/3000	1%
Gastroschisis	1/10,000	1/10,000
Omphalocele	1/4000	1/4000, some inherited
Duodenal atresia	1/10,000	
Nonimmune hydrops	1/1500–1/4000	
Down syndrome	1/700	1% (all aneuploidies)

Ethnic Background & General Population Screening

Each ethnic group has genetic disorders that are more common within the ethnic group than in the general population (Table 56–3). For example, cystic fibrosis (CF) and phenylketonuria (PKU) are more common in the Northern European population, and Tay-Sachs disease is more common in the Ashkenazi Jewish and French Canadian populations.

By determining the disorders for which the couple is at risk, carrier screening, if available, can be performed before conception. Some screening tests, such as for Tay-Sachs and hemophilia, are more accurate prior to conception than during pregnancy.

Population screening for identification of heterozygote carriers is offered to individuals of Jewish ancestry for Tay-Sachs disease, CF, and Canavan's disease; to blacks for sickle cell anemia and alpha-thalassemia; and to individuals of Mediterranean or Southeast Asian descent for the thalassemias. In 1997, there was a National Institutes of Health Consensus for Development Conference and subsequent workshop recommending that CF screening be offered to individuals with family history of CF, reproductive partners of persons affected with CF, and couples in whom 1 or both partners are white and are planning a pregnancy or who are in the first or second trimesters of pregnancy. ACOG and the American College of Medical Genetics have been working together to develop educational materials that were first made available in 2001 to aid the generalist in determining who may best benefit from being offered CF screening as well as patient education booklets to supplement their own explanations.

History of Multiple Miscarriages

It is estimated that approximately half of all recognized pregnancies that result in miscarriage involve chromosomal abnormalities. Recurrent miscarriages occur in approximately 2% of pregnant women. Couples who have recurrent miscarriages have a 6% risk that 1 partner has a balanced chromosomal rearrangement. Karyotype analysis of parental blood determines whether or not this couple is at an increased risk for having a child with an unbalanced karyotype. If a balanced rearrangement is identified in 1 of the parents, a probable cause of the spontaneous abortion has been identified. However, if the parental chromosomes are normal, further investigation into the cause of the miscarriages is indicated (see Chapter 57, Early Pregnancy Loss).

ACOG Committee Opinion: Screening for Canavan disease. Number 212 November 1998. Committee on Genetics. American College of Obstetricians and Gynecologists. Int J Gynaecol Obstet 1999 Apr; 65:91. [PMID: 10390111]

American College of Medical Genetics College Newsletter, ACMG Position Statement on Multiple Marker Screening in Women 35 and Older. 1994;2. Addendum 1996.

American College of Obstetricians and Gynecologists and American College of Medical Genetics: Preconception and Prenatal Carrier Screening for Cystic Fibrosis Clinical and Laboratory Guidelines 2001, Oct.

Table 56–3. Ethnic distribution of mendelian disorders.

Ethnic Group	Disorder
Northern European	Phenylketonuria
	Cystic fibrosis
African	Sickle cell anemia
	Alpha-thalassemia
	Glucose-6-phosphatase dehydrogenase deficiency
Mediterranean	Beta-thalassemia
	Glucose-6-phosphatase dehydrogenase deficiency
Southeast Asian	Alpha-thalassemia
	Glucose-6-phosphatase dehydrogenase deficiency
Ashkenazi Jewish	Tay-Sachs disease
	Gaucher's disease
	Familial dysautonomia
Quebec French	Tay-Sachs disease
	Morquio's syndrome
	Agenesis of the corpus callosum
Sephardic Jewish	Congenital adrenal hyperplasia
	Cystinosis

TYPES OF PRENATAL DIAGNOSIS

Chorionic Villus Sampling

CVS is performed early in pregnancy, typically at 9–12 weeks of gestation. CVS involves a placental biopsy of the chorionic villi to obtain tissue for chromosomal analysis. Depending on the placement of the placenta, which is determined by ultrasonography, villi are obtained either transcervically or transabdominally. Approximately 10–20 mg of tissue is obtained during the procedure. Occasionally, a second procedure is necessary for failure to obtain the necessary tissue sample. This tissue is suitable also for enzyme or molecular analysis if the family is known to be at risk for a specific genetic disorder. The major complication from CVS is spontaneous abortion, which occurs less than 1% of the time. This risk is in addition to the 3–10% loss rate at this stage of pregnancy. In experienced centers, complications are probably no higher for CVS than amniocentesis. Results of the chromosomal analysis are available in 10–14 days. Because of about a 1% incidence of confined placental mosaicism (abnormality present in the placenta but not the fetus), a confirmatory second test may be necessary in the face of an abnormal cytogenetic result.

There has been some controversy concerning the safety of the CVS procedure. CVS performed prior to 10 menstrual weeks seemed to be associated with increased risk of limb reduction defects. However, the CVS registry indicates that fetal defects of all anatomic locations are similar in frequency to those of the base population and that CVS is safe if performed by an experienced clinician after the 10th week of gestation.

Amniocentesis

Amniocentesis is a procedure used to obtain a sample of amniotic fluid for karyotypic and alpha-fetoprotein (AFP) analysis. Amniocentesis for prenatal diagnosis is performed in the second trimester of pregnancy (between 15 and 20 weeks of gestation). Under direct ultrasound guidance, 20 mL of amniotic fluid is aspirated directly. Procedure-related risk of miscarriage is estimated to be between 1 in 100 and 1 in 200. The results of the AFP screen are ready in approximately 1 week, and the chromosome results are typically available in 10–14 days. In situations where a rapid karyotype is requested for trisomy 21, 18, or 13 or abnormality in number of sex chromosomes, or in a select number of specific abnormalities like a deletion leading to DiGeorge syndrome, FISH (fluorescence in situ hybridization) can be performed. This is a chromosome specific probe with high specificity and good sensitivity. FISH will frequently be ordered in the face of a high probability of a common aneuploidy or in a situation where gestational age is advanced. A negative result is reassuring, but final culture result would be awaited to exclude some of the less common abnormalities of chromosome number or even a deletion.

Some programs have used early amniocentesis, which is performed prior to 15 weeks of gestation, as an alternative form of prenatal diagnosis. The technique for early amniocentesis is similar to that of traditional amniocentesis except that less fluid is aspirated, usually 1 mL for each completed week of gestation. In the Canadian Early and Mid-Trimester Amniocentesis Trial (CEMAT), patients who had an early amniocentesis (11 to 12 gestation weeks 6 days gestational weeks) had more fetal losses, an increase in talipes equinovarus, and more postprocedure amniotic fluid leakage than patients who had an amniocentesis during 15 to 16 gestation weeks and 6 days. It is unclear whether there is

an increase in complications if amniocentesis is done between 13 and 15 weeks, so many centers are only offering CVS and traditional amniocentesis.

Ultrasonography

Ultrasonography can visualize fetal anatomy during pregnancy and can help rule out some congenital anomalies that cannot be detected by CVS or amniocentesis. Patients must be counseled that ultrasonography is not infallible and structural abnormalities as well as underlying genetic disorders, eg, beta-thalassemia, can be missed. The best time during pregnancy to obtain a complete scan of the fetal anatomy is at 18–20 weeks of gestation. The incidence of karyotypic abnormalities in a population of fetuses ascertained by ultrasonography to have a single structural abnormality is 15–22%; in fetuses ascertained to have multiple anomalies, the incidence is approximately 33%. The frequency of chromosomal abnormalities is greater with certain anatomic abnormalities, such as cardiovascular anomalies (approximately 35%), central nervous system (CNS) anomalies (approximately 22%), and omphalocele (30–55%) (Table 56–4).

Targeted ultrasound performed at 15 to 20 weeks has been used to screen for trisomy 21. Subtle markers have been identified (nuchal translucency in the first trimester and a panel of second trimester findings including mild pyelectasis, increased nuchal thickening, short limbs, and echogenic bowel) that can be used to increase or decrease a woman's baseline risk. The training, experience, and general or referral population risk of an ultrasound laboratory influence the validity of the results.

Multiple Marker Screening-Prenatal Risk Profile (PRP)

Multiple marker screening of maternal blood has improved the efficiency of Down syndrome detection. First trimester testing of pregnancy associated plasma protein A (PAPP-A) can be combined with NT ultrasound to help women determine the need for CVS in the first trimester. The quad screen measures second trimester levels of human chorionic gonadotropin, estriol, inhibin, and AFP. Based upon the pattern of these analyses with about a 5% false-positive rate, a woman can be a given a numerical risk for open spina bifida, trisomy 21, and trisomy 18. Better than 50% of fetuses with Down syndrome can be detected using the quad screen as a primary screen. A combination of first trimester nuchal translucency measurement and PAPP-A with second trimester quad screen and targeted ultrasound is called the integrated screen, yielding in some studies an 85% detection rate for trisomy 21.

Table 56–4. Risk of abnormalities related to ultrasonographic findings.

Ultrasonographic Finding	Risk of Aneuploidy	Risk of Other Abnormalities
Omphalocele	30–55%	50%
Gastroschisis	0–3%	4–25%
Duodenal atresia	33%	48–78%
Nonimmune hydrops	34%	64%
Nuchal folds	33%	—
Cystic hygroma	50%	—
Intrauterine growth retardation	2–5%	10–30%
Congenital heart disease	22%	5.2%
ASD: atrial septal defect	14%	
VSD: ventricular septal defect	8%	4.7%
Renal abnormalities		
Urethrovesical junction	23%	—
Urethropelvic junction	4%	—
Central nervous system		
Neural tube defects	8–33%	—
Holoprosencaphaly	40–60%	37% intracranial
Hydrocephalus	3–9%	63% extracranial
Agenesis of the corpus callosum	14%	—
Choroid plexus cysts	1%	—
Diaphragmatic hernia	6–25%	50–57%
Single umbilical artery	0–5%	21%
Cleft lip or palate	0.15%	13%
Clubfoot	25–31%	77%
Esophageal atresia	19%	50–70%

Access to all of these screening tests is not available in all locations although most pregnant women are now offered quad screen testing in the second trimester.

Although the risk of having a fetus with trisomy 21 does increase with age, the majority (80%) of babies with trisomy 21 are born to women under the age of 35. If a woman's PRP result indicates an increased risk for aneuploidy, genetic counseling and prenatal testing should be offered. It is not yet recommended that the PRP be used as a substitute for prenatal diagnosis for women over the age of the 35. However, it may be offered to help define the risk for fetal aneuploidy if amniocentesis or CVS is declined.

A study by Haddow et al investigated the effectiveness of the PRP through the triple marker screen as an alternative to amniocentesis in women age 35 or older. Using a risk cutoff of 1 in 200 and a false-positive rate of 25%, 89% of fetuses with Down syndrome would have been identified. However, only 47% of other autosomal trisomies and 44% of gender aneuploidies were identified using these criteria. Haddow concluded that triple marker screening can provide a basis for decision making in the cases of women older than 35 as well as younger women. Egan estimated that 12.6% of women were in the advanced maternal age group in 1997; a cutoff of age 35 resulted in high false-positive rates and

was less effective based on likelihood ratio and positive predictive value. Egan concluded that serum testing of all pregnant women would reduce the number of amniocenteses and decrease procedure-related losses.

Canadian Early and Mid-Trimester Amniocentesis Trial (CEMAT) Group: Randomised trial to assess safety and fetal outcome of early and midtrimester amniocentesis. Lancet 1998;351:242. [PMID: 9457093]

Haddow JE et al: Prenatal screening for Down's syndrome with use of maternal serum markers. N Engl J Med 1992;327:588. [PMID: 1379344]

Papantoniou NE et al: Risk factors predisposing to fetal loss following a second trimester amniocentesis. Br J Obstet Gynecol 2001;108:1053. [PMID: 11702837]

Tabor A et al: Randomised controlled trial of genetic amniocentesis in 4606 low-risk women. Lancet 1986;1:1287. [PMID: 2423826]

Wald NJ, Watt HC, Hackshaw AK: Integrated screening for Down's syndrome based on tests performed during the first and second trimesters. N Engl J Med 1999;341:461. [PMID: 10441601]

PRECONCEPTION COUNSELING

Ideally, any woman considering pregnancy would have preconception counseling. In addition to a family history, an extensive maternal medical history should be obtained at all preconception intake interviews. Use of an extensive medical history checklist helps ensure that all potential risks are identified. Nutrition; exercise; adverse habits such as smoking, drinking, and drug abuse; and physical disorders should be discussed. The patient should be encouraged to eliminate all avoidable hazards to a pregnancy with the appropriate social and medical support, eg, counseling for weight loss or eating disorder, or referral to social services programs for substance abuse and smoking cessation. Women should be counseled to abstain from alcohol once pregnant. Occupational hazards should be eliminated, and any preexisting medical condition should be controlled with appropriate therapy, including a review of all medications and treatments that may have an impact on the pregnancy, ie, potential teratogens. All diabetics should be encouraged to achieve euglycemia preconceptually. The risks and benefits of therapy must be compared with the risk of untreated disease; for example, untreated hyperthyroidism is far more dangerous to the mother and fetus than the potential negative effects of propylthiouracil or methimazole. Some medications such as anticonvulsants might be able to be discontinued during the periods of organogenesis if the patient has been seizure free for a prolonged period. Encouraging women to document a menstrual diary will help determine probable conception date.

Appropriate laboratory tests may include the following:

Rubella antibodies

Varicella antibodies

Toxoplasmosis antibody

Cytomegalovirus antibody

Hepatitis B and C screening

Parvovirus antibody

HIV

Glucose testing

Rh and antibody screening

Hemoglobin electrophoresis (Asian and black patients)

Tuberculosis testing

CF screening (in white patients)

Patients who require vaccinations (rubella or varicella nonimmune, tetanus toxoid) should receive them preconception; those who are susceptible to high-risk perinatal infections (cytomegalovirus, toxoplasmosis) should be counseled regarding prophylaxis and avoidance of high-risk situations.

All women considering pregnancy should start taking 400 μg/d of folic acid preconceptually to reduce the rate of NTDs. The Centers for Disease Control and Prevention recommends all women who have had an infant affected by NTD take 4 mg/d of folic acid for at least a month prior to pregnancy. Recently, Wald suggested all women who are planning a pregnancy take 5 mg/d of folate.

In addition to the genetics issues related to maternal age over 35 years, these patients are prone to the development of chronic disease. Medical illnesses that are more prevalent in these women include diabetes, hypertension, renal disease, and heart disease. The incidence of (superimposed) preeclampsia increases with age as does the severity of the condition. Gestational diabetes is 3-fold more common in older women, as is overt diabetes. Other complications of pregnancy that develop with increasing frequency include miscarriage (2- to 3-fold increase), preterm labor and premature rupture of membranes (2-fold increase), fetal macrosomia (related to the increase in gestational diabetes and postterm pregnancies), multiple gestations, fetal intrauterine growth retardation (related to the increase in vascular disease), placental abruption and placenta previa, and ectopic pregnancy. These issues should be discussed thoroughly.

The following is a list of signs that should alert the primary physician to high-risk pregnancies:

Advanced maternal age (older than 35)

Grand multiparity (greater than 4)

Small stature (less than 5 feet tall)

Low maternal weight (less than 55 kg)

Obesity (more than 20% over ideal weight)

Preexisting medical disorders

Abnormal uterine bleeding

History of infertility

History of sexually transmitted infection (increased risk of ectopic pregnancy)

Prior poor pregnancy outcome (fetal or neonatal loss, prematurity)

Table 56–5 lists high-risk medical conditions that could affect the mother and fetus.

Wald NJ et al: Quantifying the effect of folic acid. Lancet 2001;358:2069. [PMID: 11755633]

TERATOGEN EXPOSURE

A **teratogen** is an agent that produces abnormality or anomaly in a fetus that is exposed to it during organogenesis. There are 3 defined developmental periods in the fetus. The first is commonly known as the "all or none" period, which exists from the day of conception

Table 56–5. High-risk medical conditions.

Diabetes mellitus
    Type 2, controlled by diet or with oral medication[1]
    Type 1 or 2, insulin-dependent[1]
Malignant disease
Hypertension
    Chronic[1]
    Pregnancy-induced hypertension
        Mild
        Severe
Heart disease
    Class[1]
    Class 2, 3, 4[2]
Pulmonary disease
    Asthma, well-controlled
    Unstable asthma[2]
Gastrointestinal problems
Hepatitis
    HIV infection[1]
    Antiphospholipid antibody syndrome[1]
    Prior thromboembolic episode or inherited thrombophilia[1]

[1]Consultation with subspecialty physician in maternal-fetal medicine is advised.
[2]Care by maternal-fetal medicine subspecialist is advised.

to day 9–13. During this period, the pregnancy is either lost because of the exposure or it is unaffected. The next period extends to approximately day 70 and is considered the period of **organogenesis** or **embryogenesis.** During this period, exposure to a teratogen affects individual organ systems. The period of fetal growth is from day 70 to term. During this time, teratogens can impact on fetal growth and development and can affect the organs that are still in the process of development, specifically the eyes, ears, and CNS. The major teratogenic agents are listed in Table 56–6.

COMMON MEDICAL DISORDERS IN PREGNANCY

Diabetes

Diabetes affects 3–5% of all pregnant women, making it one of the most common medical complications of pregnancy. Diabetes is a heterogeneous disorder with a wide spectrum of manifestations ranging from insulin-dependent diabetes mellitus (IDDM) to gestational diabetes. Glucose intolerance detected in pregnancy is called **gestational diabetes mellitus (GDM).** GDM is one of the most frequent and significant risks for adverse maternal and fetal outcome in pregnancy; it accounts for 90% of cases of diabetes in pregnant women,

whereas IDDM and noninsulin-dependent diabetes mellitus (type I and type II diabetes) account for the remainder. Diabetes will develop in approximately 30–50% of patients with GDM. GDM has been viewed by some as the extreme end of a spectrum of carbohydrate intolerance, whereas others consider it to be of major pathologic significance. It is clear that the effects of maternal hyperglycemia include fetal hyperinsulinemia, which results in fetal macrosomia and increases the chance of birth injury or cesarean delivery, fetal metabolic disorders, neonatal complications including severe hypoglycemia, and possible long-term complications for both fetus and mother. Neonatal morbidity and mortality in well-controlled gestational diabetes is equivalent to that of nondiabetic pregnancies. Generally, universal GDM screening of all pregnant women is offered, usually in the form of a 1-hour 50 g glucose tolerance test. Women with abnormal results are followed up with a definitive 3-hour 100 g glucose tolerance test.

A. RISKS AND MEDICAL COMPLICATIONS OF IDDM

The medical management of the woman with IDDM or GDM is complex. A major key is the involvement of an entire team: the patient and her partner, a diabetes nurse educator, nutritionist, endocrinologist, obstetrician, ultrasonographer, and pediatrician. Optimal management includes normal glycemia prior to conception with maintenance throughout the pregnancy and throughout the antepartum and intrapartum periods.

Medical preconception counseling with intensive diabetic management has resulted in a reduction in the incidence of congenital malformations. The most frequent fetal malformations are found in the cardiovascular system and the CNS. High levels of glycosylated hemoglobin in the first trimester during the critical period for organogenesis have been correlated with an increased number of malformations. Recent studies in the United States using programs that have developed preconception counseling and strict metabolic control in the first trimester of pregnancy have shown a reduction to the baseline background population risk for congenital malformations.

The risk of early abortion has also been shown to diminish with tight control prior to and in the first month of pregnancy. Long-term effects on the offspring are beginning to be evaluated in extended studies; prospective evaluation of aberrant maternal metabolism has been associated with poorer intellectual and psychomotor development, obesity, and impaired glucose tolerance among the offspring. The maternal vascular complications of pregnancy (including the manifestations of hypertension, proliferative retinopathy, renal disease, and neuropathy) should be assessed and

Table 56–6. Teratogenic agents.

Agent	Effects	Comments
Alcohol	Growth restriction before and after birth, mental retardation, microcephaly, midfacial hypoplasia producing atypical facial appearance, renal and cardiac defects, various other major and minor malformations	Nutritional deficiency, smoking, and multiple drug use of confound data. Risk due to ingestion of 1 to 2 drinks per day is not well defined but may cause a small reduction in average birth weight. Fetuses of women who ingest 6 drinks per day are at a 40% risk of developing some features of the fetal alcohol syndrome.
Androgens and testosterone derivatives (eg, danazol)	Virilization of female, advanced genital development in males	Effects are dose dependent and related to the stage of embryonic development at the time of exposure. Given before 9 weeks of gestation, labioscrotal fusion can be produced; clitoromegaly can occur with exposure at any gestational age. Risk related to incidental brief androgenic exposure is minimal.
Angiotensin-converting (enzyme (ACE) inhibitors (eg, enalapril, captopril)	Fetal renal tubular dysplasia, oligohydramnios, neonatal renal failure, lack of cranial ossification, intrauterine growth restriction	Incidence of fetal morbidity is 30%. The risk increases with second- and third-trimester use, leading to in utero fetal hypotension, decreased renal blood flow, and renal failure.
Coumanin derivatives (eg, warfarin)	Nasal hypoplasia and stippled bone epiphyses are most common; other effects include broad short hands with shortened phalanges, ophthalmologic abnormalities, intrauterine growth restriction, developmental delay, anomalies of neck and central nervous system	Risk for a seriously affected child is considered to be 15–25% when anticoagulants that inhibit vitamin K are used in the first trimester, especially during 6–9 weeks of gestation. Later drug exposure may be associated with spontaneous abortion, stillbirths, central nervous system abnormalities, abruptio placentae, and fetal or neonatal hemorrhage.
Carbamazepine	Neural tube defects, minor craniofacial defects, fingernail hypoplasia, microcephaly, developmental delay, intrauterine growth restriction	Risk of neural tube defect, mostly lumbosacral, is 1–2% when used alone during first trimester and increased when used with other antiepileptic agents.
Folic acid antagonists (methotrexate and aminopterin)	Increased risk for spontaneous abortions, various anomalies	These drugs are contraindicated for the treatment of psoriasis in pregnancy and must be used with extreme caution in the treatment of malignancy. Cytotoxic drugs are potentially teratogenic. Effects of aminopterin are well documented. Folic acid antagonists used during the first trimester produce a malformation rate of up to 30% in fetuses that survive.
Cocaine	Bowel atresias; congenital malformations of the heart, limbs, face and genitourinary tract; microcephaly; intrauterine growth restriction; cerebral infarctions	Risks may be affected by other factors and concurrent abuse of multiple substances. Maternal and pregnancy complications include sudden death and placental abruption.
Diethylstilbestrol	Clear-cell adenocarcinoma of the vagina or cervix, vaginal adenosis, abnormalities of cervix and uterus, abnormalities of the testes, possible infertility in males and females	Vaginal adenosis is detected in more than 50% of women whose mothers took these drugs before 9 weeks of gestation. Risk for vaginal adenocarcinoma is low. Males exposed in utero may have a 25% incidence of epididymal cysts, hypotrophic testes, abnormal spermatozoa, and induration of the testes.
Lead	Increased abortion rate, stillbirths	Fetal central nervous system development may be adversely affected. Determining preconceptional lead levels for those at risk may be useful.
Lithium	Congenital heart disease, in particular, Ebstein anomaly	Risk of heart malformations due to first-trimester exposure is low. The effect is not as significant as reported in earlier studies. Exposure in the last month of gestation may produce toxic effects on the thyroid, kidneys, and neuromuscular systems.

Agent	Effects	Comments
Organic mercury	Cerebral atrophy, microcephaly, mental retardation, spasticity, seizures, blindness	Cerebral palsy can occur even when exposure is in the third trimester. Exposed individuals include consumers of fish and grain contaminated with methyl mercury.
Phenytoin	Intrauterine growth retardation, mental retardation, microcephaly, dysmorphic craniofacial features, cardiac defects, hypoplastic nails and distal phalanges	The full syndrome is seen in less than 10% of children exposed in utero, but up to 30% have some manifestations. Mild to moderate mental retardation is found in some children who have severe physical stigmata. The effect may depend on whether the fetus inherits a mutant gene that decreases production of epoxide hydrolase, an enzyme necessary to decrease the teratogen phenytoin epoxide.
Streptomycin and kanamycin	Hearing loss, eighth-nerve damage	No ototoxicity in the fetus has been reported from use of gentamicin or vancomycin.
Tetracycline	Hypoplasia of tooth enamel, incorporation of tetracycline into bone and teeth, permanent yellow-brown discoloration of deciduous teeth	Drug has no known effect unless exposure occurs in second or third trimester.
Thalidomide	Bilateral limb deficiencies, anotia and microtia, cardiac and gastrointestinal anomalies	Of children whose mothers used thalidomide between 35 and 50 days of gestation, 20% show the effect.
Trimethadione and paramethadione	Cleft lip or cleft palate; cardiac defects; growth deficiency; microcephaly; mental retardation; characteristic facial appearance; ophthalmologic, limb, and genitourinary tract abnormalities	Risk for defects or spontaneous abortion is 60–80% with first-trimester exposure. A syndrome including V-shaped eyebrows, low-set ears, high arched palate, and irregular dentition has been identified. These drugs are no longer used during pregnancy due to the availability of more effective, less toxic agents.
Valproic acid	Neural tube defects, especially spina bifida; minor facial defects	Exposure must occur prior to normal closure of neural tube during first trimester to produce open defect (incidence of approximately 1%).
Vitamin A and its derivatives (eg, isotretinoin, etretinate, and retinoids)	Increased abortion rate, microtia, central nervous system defects, thymic agenesis, cardiovascular effects, craniofacial dysmorphism, microphthalmia, cleft lip and palate, mental retardation	Isotretinoin exposure before pregnancy is not a risk because the drug is not stored in tissue. Etretinate has a long half-life and effects occur long after drug is discontinued. Topical application does not have a known risk.

Infections

Agent	Effects	Comments
Cytomegalovirus	Hydrocephaly, microcephaly, chorioretinitis, cerebral calcifications, symmetric intrauterine growth restriction, microphthalmos, brain damage, mental retardation, hearing loss	Most common congenital infection. Congenital infection rate is 40% after primary infection and 14% after recurrent infection. Of infected infants, physical effects as listed are present in 20% after primary infection and 8% after secondary infection. No effective therapy exists.
Rubella	Microcephaly, mental retardation, cataracts, deafness, congenital heart disease; all organs may be affected	Malformation rate is 50% if the mother is infected during first trimester. Rate of severe permanent organ damage decreases to 6% by midpregnancy. Immunization of children and nonpregnant adults is necessary for prevention. Immunization is not recommended during pregnancy, but the live attenuated vaccine virus has not been shown to cause the malformations of congenital rubella syndrome.
Syphilis	If severe infection, fetal demise with hydrops; if mild, detectable abnormalities of skin, teeth, and bones	Penicillin treatment is effective for *Treponema pallidum* eradication to prevent progression of damage. Severity of fetal damage depends on duration of fetal infection; damage is worse if infection is greater than 20 weeks. Prevalence is increasing; need to rule out other sexually transmitted diseases.

(continued)

Table 56–6. Teratogenic agents. (Continued)

Agent	Effects	Comments
Toxoplasmosis	Possible effects on all systems but particularly central nervous system: microcephaly, hydrocephaly, cerebral calcifications. Chorioretinitis is most common. Severity of manifestations depends on duration of disease.	Low prevalence during pregnancy (0.1–0.5%); initial maternal infection must occur during pregnancy to place fetus at risk. *Toxoplasma gondii* is transmitted to humans by raw meat or exposure to infected cat feces. In the first trimester, the incidence of fetal infection is as low as 9% and increases to approximately 59% in the third trimester. The severity of congenital infection is greater in the first trimester than at the end of gestation. Treat with pyrimethamine, sulfadiazine, or spiramycin.
Varicella	Possible effects on all organs, including skin scarring, chorioretinitis, cataracts, microcephaly, hypoplasia of the hands and feet, and muscle atrophy	Risk of congenital varicella is low, approximately 2–3% and occurs between 7 and 21 weeks of gestation. Varicella-zoster immune globulin is available regionally for newborns exposed in utero during last 4–7 days of gestation. No effect from herpes zoster.
Radiation	Microcephaly, mental retardation	Medical diagnostic radiation delivering less than 0.05 Gy[1] to the fetus has no teratogenic risk. Estimated fetal exposure of common radiologic procedures is 0.01 Gy or less (eg, intravenous pyelography, 0.0041 Gy).

[1]1 gray = 100 rad.

treated and reevaluated frequently throughout the pregnancy. A thorough ophthalmologic examination with treatment of proliferative retinopathy should be performed prior to pregnancy. Management of normal glycemia during pregnancy involves cooperation between the medical team and the nutritionist. Strict dietary management and self-monitoring of capillary blood glucose should be thoroughly explained to the patient prior to conception with frequent reviews. Glycosylated hemoglobin values below approximately 6.9% (each laboratory establishes its own ranges of normal) should be the ultimate goal, preferably prior to conception. The majority of investigators consider normal test results to be a fasting blood glucose level of below 95 and a 1-hour postprandial level of below 140 mg. Gestational diabetes often can be managed by dietary control and exercise alone. Many investigators have reported a decrease in the incidence of macrosomia and neonatal metabolic disturbances, the most common complications of gestational diabetes, with the use of insulin and most recently with glyburide after the first trimester. Best results appear to have been achieved with multiple daily home capillary fasting and postprandial blood glucose measurements.

B. Obstetric Management of Diabetes

The intense medical management and strict metabolic control have decreased both the maternal and perinatal morbidity and mortality in the pregnancies of women with IDDM over the last decade. Complications such as polyhydramnios, macrosomia, intrauterine growth retardation, hypertensive disorders, preterm labor, and intrauterine fetal demise occur with much less frequency, but they are present in women with type I diabetes with inadequate glycemic control. In the first trimester, spontaneous abortion or fetal embryopathy are the most frequent complications. Fetal malformations can be detected by a combination of second-trimester surveillance techniques such as the quad screen and targeted ultrasonographic evaluation with fetal echocardiography at 16–20 weeks of gestation. Sonography is also the method of choice for detection of polyhydramnios and growth abnormalities in the fetus and should be performed every 4–8 weeks. Antepartum testing in the form of nonstress tests or biophysical profiles will be performed regularly in the third trimester in diabetics requiring insulin or oral medications. Diabetic women used to give birth early for fear of fetal death, now patients may await spontaneous labor unless there are worrisome maternal or fetal complications. Any elective delivery prior to 39 weeks should have documentation of fetal lung maturity by amniocentesis first. In addition to being watched closely for a reduction in insulin need in the postpartum period, women with type 1 diabetes have a 25% risk of developing postpartum thyroid dysfunction.

Urinary Tract Disorders

A. Asymptomatic Bacteriuria

Asymptomatic bacteriuria occurs in as many as 10% of all pregnant patients; if untreated, its presence increases the risk of acute urinary tract infection and pyelonephritis 10-fold. Diagnosis is made from culture of a midstream clean catch with a count of greater than 10^5 per milliliter of urine. All pregnant women should have a culture at the first prenatal visit.

Diabetes mellitus and sickle cell trait increase the risk of asymptomatic bacteriuria. Patients with increased parity and black patients have a higher risk than patients who are white or of low parity.

Asymptomatic bacteriuria requires therapy with a sensitive agent (see the following section, Acute Pyelonephritis). After drug treatment is complete, a repeat culture should be performed to confirm the effectiveness of the treatment.

B. Cystitis

Cystitis is a symptomatic urinary tract infection. Inflammation or infection of the bladder or bladder wall is common in pregnancy. Symptoms include abdominal discomfort, dysuria, frequency, and urgency. The diagnosis is made in the same manner as for asymptomatic bacteria. A symptomatic patient with urinalysis showing pyuria accompanied by positive leukocyte esterase or nitrite tests has a presumptive diagnosis of cystitis. More than 10^5 bacteria on a midstream clean catch specimen confirms the diagnosis. *Escherichia coli* is present in more than 75% of patients diagnosed with cystitis. *Chlamydia trachomatis* and *Staphylococcus saprophyticus* are other common pathogens. The patient can be treated effectively with the appropriate oral medications. A "test of cure" culture should be performed after completion of therapy. Recurrence or incomplete response to treatment occurs in 15% of patients so follow-up culture is important.

C. Acute Pyelonephritis

The presence of fever, chills, costovertebral angle tenderness, and low abdominal pain in combination with frequency, dysuria, and urgency is consistent with the diagnosis of acute pyelonephritis. The diagnosis is confirmed when a symptomatic patient has a midstream clean catch urine with greater than 10^5 bacteria per milliliter of urine, with the presence of numerous white blood cells. *E coli* is the most frequent organism. Other organisms that can be seen include enterococci, staphylococci, *Proteus,* and *Klebsiella.* The distinction between lower and upper tract disease is largely clinical. Acute infection of the lower urinary tract should not be associated with systemic symptoms. There is no consistent laboratory technique to differentiate between the two.

The treatment of pyelonephritis is hospitalization and intravenous antibiotics until the patient has been afebrile for 24–48 hours, followed by oral antibiotics for 10–14 days. As in both asymptomatic bacteriuria and cystitis, antibiotic therapy is aimed at sensitivities. Ampicillin has been the traditional drug of first choice; however, the increase in resistance of *E coli* to ampicillin may dictate the use of an aminoglycoside or cephalosporin in conjunction with or in place of ampicillin. Oral medications for the renal infectious disorders include the sulfonamides, ampicillin, amoxicillin plus clavulanate, and trimethoprim-sulfamethoxazole. Choice of antibiotics will be dictated by gestational age since sulfa is avoided in the late third trimester and trimethoprim is avoided in the first trimester. If a patient has pyelonephritis or recurrent urinary tract infections, suppression therapy using nitrofurantoin can be maintained at a dose of 100 mg/d throughout the rest of the pregnancy.

It is important to remember that appropriate therapy of pyelonephritis is critical. Reports over the last 5–7 years have indicated that inadequately treated pyelonephritis may result in acute respiratory distress syndrome. This extremely serious complication can be avoided by appropriate and timely therapy.

D. UROLITHIASIS

Urolithiasis, or urinary calculus, is an infrequent occurrence in pregnancy. Smooth-muscle relaxation caused by increases in progesterone concentration and the mechanical obstruction of the uterus caused by its increasing size predispose pregnant women to both infection secondary to urinary stasis and the formation of renal calculi.

Urolithiasis, which occurs in 0.02–0.05% of pregnancies, has potentially disastrous implications for the fetus and mother. Because urolithiasis can be confused with other abdominal or pelvic disorders during pregnancy, serious consideration must be given to this diagnosis in pregnant women with abdominal or flank pain, hematuria, or unresolved bacteriuria. Urinary tract infection is the most common presentation of this disorder in pregnancy. When antibiotic therapy is unsuccessful in resolving urinary tract infection or pyelonephritis in the patient in whom culture reveals a susceptible organism, the diagnosis of urolithiasis should be suspected.

The diagnosis of urolithiasis is critical. Ultrasonography can be surprisingly useful. Diagnosis of urinary tract calculi may be made in greater than 70% of patients with urolithiasis, even in the third trimester.

Noninvasive testing always should be attempted initially. In the presence of complications that may require invasive intervention, pregnancy should not deter appropriate roentgenographic evaluation. Limited intravenous pyelography and, more recently, magnetic resonance urography or noncontrast helical computed tomography have all been used with limited radiation exposure. Treatment includes allowing spontaneous passage of the stone (75%), ureteral stent placement, nephrostomy tube insertion or, rarely, ureteral laser lithotripsy.

Thyroid Disease

A. HYPOTHYROIDISM

Symptomatic hypothyroidism in pregnancy is an uncommon phenomenon. The most common causes include Hashimoto's disease, subacute thyroiditis, thyroidectomy, radioactive iodine treatment, and iodine deficiency. Many cases are subclinical and difficult to detect. Symptoms include obesity or hypometabolism; dry, coarse hair and skin; cold intolerance; and gastrointestinal dysfunction. It is diagnosed by an increase in thyroid-stimulating hormone (TSH) with or without below normal levels of T_4 and T_3.

Complications of hypothyroidism include infertility, which serves as a partial explanation for the decreased incidence in pregnancy. In patients who become pregnant, hypothyroidism is associated with an increased risk of intrauterine growth retardation, stillbirth, placental abruption, and preeclampsia. There is also a 4- to 5-fold increase in miscarriage. Women with iodine-deficient hypothyroidism are at increased risk of having a child with congenital cretinism.

Patients who are diagnosed with hypothyroidism should be treated with levothyroxine. The initial dosage is 50 μg daily. Since it may take 4 weeks for thyroxine therapy to alter TSH, the dosage should be increased every 3–4 weeks based on the impact of the therapy on TSH levels (normal levels: below 6 μU/mL). Most patients can treated adequately during pregnancy with a maintenance dose of 100–150 μg daily. Because hormone requirements tend to increase throughout pregnancy, TSH levels should be checked each trimester.

B. HYPERTHYROIDISM

Hyperthyroidism is relatively common in pregnancy, occurring in approximately 1–2 pregnancies per 1000. The most common cause is Graves' disease, although Hashimoto's thyroiditis, hyperemesis, and trophoblastic disease also occur in association with this condition.

Symptoms of hyperthyroidism include hyperdynamic cardiovascular function (tachycardia, palpitations, tremor), increased appetite with weight loss, heat intolerance, nervousness, weakness, fatigability, and insomnia. There may be diffuse enlargement of the thyroid or, in the presence of a tumor, a thyroid nodule. A bruit may be heard over the organ.

The diagnosis of hyperthyroidism is made clinically and by laboratory tests. An elevation of T_4, T_3, or both, and an increased free thyroxine index are generally present. Treatment of hyperthyroidism in pregnancy is described in Chapter 18, Thyroid Disorders.

Hypertensive Disorders of Pregnancy

Hypertension associated with pregnancy is a common complication of primigravid pregnancies in the United States, occurring in 6–8% of the population. The etiology of this condition has yet to be determined. Chesley showed an increased incidence of the disorder in the daughters of women who had a history of pregnancy-induced hypertension (PIH) that was consistent with an autosomal recessive mode of inheritance. Other investigators have postulated an autoimmune cause, suggested by the preponderance of primiparous women who acquire the disease. An increased vasoreactivity has been reported by Gant et al; pregnant women in whom PIH developed had a greater reaction to infused angiotensinogen, which persisted until delivery. Patients in whom PIH or intrauterine growth retardation developed have been shown by placental biopsy to have reduced trophoblastic invasion and thickening of smooth muscle arterioles compared with the normal low resistance placental bed. Doppler flow studies of the uterine artery vascular resistance at 24 weeks have a high positive predictive value for development of PIH and third trimester complications. Interestingly, Easterling suggests that patients at risk for PIH can be identified in the second trimester by a significant increase in cardiac output over pregnancy baseline. Ultimately, hypertension is a balance between increased resistance from vasospasm and increased cardiac output. Classification of hypertension has been problematic due to shifting terminology. It is most important to distinguish between chronic hypertension and PIH (see Box, Criteria for Diagnosing Chronic Hypertension in Pregnancy).

The presence of preexisting hypertension, any intrinsic vascular or autoimmune disease, diabetes, multiple gestation, trophoblastic disease, or a hydropic fetus increases the risk of coincident PIH. A diagnosis of chronic hypertension mandates evaluation of renal, cardiac, and ophthalmologic function early in pregnancy. There has been no improvement in maternal or perinatal outcome by treating mild hypertension. Therefore, antihypertensives such as methyldopa and labetalol are reserved for severe hypertension. Calcium channel blockers and diuretics are occasionally used whereas angiotensin-converting enzyme inhibitors are contraindicated in pregnancy. ACOG recommends against pre-

---

CRITERIA FOR DIAGNOSIS OF CHRONIC HYPERTENSION IN PREGNANCY

- Mild: Systolic blood pressure ≥ 140 mm Hg
  Diastolic blood pressure ≥ 90 mm Hg

- Severe: Systolic blood pressure ≥ 180 mm Hg
  Diastolic blood pressure ≥ 110 mm Hg

- Use of antihypertensive medications before pregnancy.

- Onset of hypertension before 20th week of gestation.

- Persistence of hypertension beyond the usual postpartum period

(Taken from ACOG Practice Bulletin No. 29 Chronic Hypertension in Pregnancy July 2001.)

---

scribing atenolol because of reports of small for gestational age infants, but Easterling believes that it is useful if the mother's cardiac output and resistance are monitored. Preeclampsia usually can be distinguished from chronic hypertension because preeclampsia typically appears after the 20th week of pregnancy in a woman who was normotensive prior to pregnancy. PIH can be subgrouped depending on specific end-organ effects. Preeclampsia implies hypertension with proteinuria secondary to renal effect. Eclampsia connotes seizures related to CNS effect. The syndrome of hemolysis, elevated liver function, low platelets (HELLP) is a multiorgan subgroup of severe preeclampsia.

Diagnosis of Severe Preeclampsia

Preeclampsia is considered severe if 1 or more of the following criteria is present:

- Blood pressure of 160 mm Hg systolic or higher or 110 mm Hg diastolic or higher on 2 occasions at least 6 hours apart while the patient is on bed rest.

- Proteinuria of 5 g or higher in a 24-hour urine specimen or 3+ or greater on 2 random urine samples collected at least 4 hours apart.

- Oliguria of less than 500 mL in 24 hours.

- Cerebral or visual disturbances.

- Pulmonary edema or cyanosis.

- Epigastric or right upper quadrant pain.

- Impaired liver function.

- Thrombocytopenia.

The management of PIH is defined by the severity of the disorder. Ultimately, only delivery of the fetus cures the disease. However, fetal well-being and maternal well-being both must be considered. In the case of extreme prematurity, maternal risks of conservative therapy must be balanced against severe immaturity. Usually, consultation with a maternal-fetal medicine specialist would be indicated.

In a near-term pregnancy, in the absence of severe preeclampsia, amniocentesis for lung maturity may be indicated. If the lungs are immature, corticosteroids and conservative management for the mother are appropriate. Bed rest (at home if patient is compliant and stable) is vital. Hospitalization is necessary for patients who cannot remain on bed rest at home or whose blood pressure is sustained above 140/90 mm Hg despite rest.

Cardiac Disease

Maternal cardiac disease is a serious complication of pregnancy and can lead to increased morbidity and mortality in both the mother and fetus. The incidence of these disorders is relatively low in pregnancy. However, the physiologic changes that occur in pregnancy may exacerbate an underlying cardiac abnormality or may make the diagnosis difficult.

An increase in cardiac output occurs early and maximizes at 30–50% of normal values by the beginning of the third trimester. It is recognized that the red blood cell mass does not increase to the same extent that plasma volume expands, creating the so-called "physiologic anemia" that is seen in the gravid female. Excessive iron utilization may result in iron deficiency anemia. Cardiac output increases 30–40% above nonpregnant values by mid pregnancy. The increase begins as early as 6–8 weeks and reaches its peak at 26–28 weeks. Stroke volume is increased 15–20%, and the maternal heart rate is increased 10–15 beats in the average pregnant woman.

Other physiologic parameters and hemodynamic changes in pregnancy can make the diagnosis of a pathologic condition difficult. Physical examination of a pregnant woman often reveals a systolic flow murmur (greater than 90%), a venous hum, S_3 90%, S_4 (less than 10%), tachycardia, cardiomegaly, prominent jugular veins, and peripheral edema. Changes may occur in the electrocardiogram. The average pregnant female evidences a shift of the main QRS, with minor ST depression and T-wave flattening or inversion often seen in leads 3 and aVF. Small Q waves also are sometimes present. Tachycardia is seen in more than 90% of pregnant women and is atrial in origin; extrasystoles and premature ventricular contractions are also common.

It is vital that a woman with a history of cardiac disease discuss the ramifications of the disease and pregnancy with her physician prior to pregnancy. The risk to the mother during pregnancy varies with the type of preexisting disease. Functional status traditionally has been measured by the New York Heart Association classification as follows:

- Class I—asymptomatic
- Class II—symptoms with greater than normal activity
- Class III—symptoms with normal activity
- Class IV—symptoms at bed rest

In patients with preexisting heart disease, a careful search for diagnosis and a thorough evaluation of cardiac function should be performed before the risks of pregnancy are discussed. Cardiac condition is evaluated by the traditional methods of physical examination, echocardiography, and electrocardiography; the more invasive procedures such as cardiac catheterization and evaluation of pulmonary pressure are performed only in more serious cases. The information gathered by appropriate diagnosis and definition of functional status is useful in counseling the patient regarding risks of pregnancy to herself and her fetus.

Specific risk factors for maternal mortality resulting from a pregnancy with preexisting maternal congenital heart disease are listed Table 56–7. This table can be used to approximate the risk to a woman with known congenital heart disease. The risk level of the first category is acceptable to most pregnant women, and these patients may be followed by a generalist in obstetrics and gynecology. Women in group 2 require specific counseling by a specialist familiar with cardiac disease (preferably a subspecialist in maternal-fetal medicine) and appropriate follow-through in the event of pregnancy. Patients in group 3 should be counseled by a subspecialist in maternal-fetal medicine; the high risk to the mother requires discussion of pregnancy termination.

Counseling must include discussion of the risk to the fetus. The incidence of congenital cardiac defects in the fetus of an affected mother ranges from 5% to 10%; the defect is concordant in less than 50%. The perinatal outcome of affected pregnancies depends on the severity of the maternal disease. In general, maternal hypoxemia (PO_2 below 70%) and hyperemia (hematocrit greater than 65%) are associated with poor perinatal outcome. Increased risks of intrauterine growth retardation; preterm labor; and birth, stillbirth, and miscarriage are seen in affected pregnancies.

American College of Obstetricians and Gynecologists: Gestational Diabetes Practice Bull No. 30, Sept 2001.

Table 56–7. *Maternal risk associated with pregnancy.*

Group I: Minimal risk of complications
Atrial septal defect[1]
Ventricular septal defect[1]
Patent ductus arteriosus[1]
Pulmonic/tricuspid disease
Corrected tetralogy of Fallot
Bioprosthetic valve
Mitral stenosis, New York Heart Association (NYHA)
  classes I and II
Marfan syndrome with normal aorta

Group II: Moderate risk of complications
Mitral stenosis with atrial fibrillation[1]
Artificial valve[1]
Mitral stenosis, NYHA classes III and IV
Aortic stenosis
Coarctation of aorta, uncomplicated
Uncorrected tetralogy of Fallot
Previous myocardial infarction

Group III: Major risk of complications or death
Pulmonary hypertension
Coarctation of aorta, complicated
Marfan syndrome with aortic involvement

---

[1]If anticoagulation with heparin, rather than coumadin, is elected.
(Reproduced, with permission, from Clark SL et al (editors): Critical
Care Obstetrics, 3rd ed. Blackwell

American College of Obstetricians and Gynecologists: Diabetes
  and Pregnancy Technical Bull No. 200, Dec 1994.

American College of Obstetricians and Gynecologists: Thyroid disease in pregnancy. Practice Bull No. 32, Nov 2001.

American College of Obstetricians and Gynecologists: Chronic Hypertension in Pregnancy Practice Bulletin No. 29, July 2001.

American College of Obstetricians and Gynecologists: Diagnosis
  and Management of Preeclampsia and Eclampsia, Practice
  Bulletin No. 33, Jan 2002.

Clark SL et al (editors): *Critical Care Obstetrics,* 3rd ed. Blackwell
  Scientific Publications, 1997.

Easterling TR et al: Treatment of hypertension in pregnancy:
  effect of atenolol on maternal disease, preterm delivery,
  and fetal growth. Obstet Gynecol 2001;98:427. [PMID:
  11530124]

Langer O et al: A Comparison of glyburide and insulin in women
  with gestational diabetes mellitus. N Engl J Med 2000;343:
  1134. [PMID: 11036118]

Lees C et al: Individualized risk assessment for adverse pregnancy
  outcome by uterine artery Doppler at 23 weeks. Obstet Gynecol 2001;98:369. [PMID: 11530114]

Locksmith G, Duff P: Infection, antibiotics, and preterm delivery.
  Semin Perinatol 2001;25:295. [PMID: 11707017]

Ramsey PS, Ramin KD, Ramin SM: Cardiac disease in pregnancy.
  Am J Perinatol 2001;18:245. [PMID: 11552178]

When to Refer to a Specialist

General recommendations regarding referral from primary care physician to subspecialist for at least 1 consultation and decision for further management follow:

1. At the preconception intake appointment, any patient with a positive response to questions in Figure 56–1 should be referred to a geneticist, genetic counselor, or maternal-fetal medicine specialist for counseling.

2. Any patient at high risk for cesarean birth should be referred for consultation to an obstetrician-gynecologist during the pregnancy. Patients at risk for cesarean include those who have had a Prior cesarean section, whose fetus is in the breech position after 34 weeks, and those who have placenta previa after 32 weeks.

3. Patient with significant medical problem probably requiring extra antepartum testing should be referred to an obstetrician-gynecologist during the pregnancy:

   Severe intrauterine growth retardation with fetal weight < 10 percentile

   Medical complication of pregnancy (eg, hypertension, renal disease, epilepsy, asthma) requiring additional medication

   Decrease in fetal movement accompanied by any other complication

   Diabetes requiring medication (either glyburide or insulin)

   Oligohydramnios defined as amniotic fluid index < 8
   Placental abruption

   Abnormal prenatal risk profile with elevated human chorionic gonadotropin, inhibin, or MSAFP

4. Patients who desire prenatal diagnosis because of maternal age, family history of birth defect or genetic abnormality, abnormal prenatal risk profile, or abnormal ultrasound should be referred to an obstetrician-gynecologist or directly to a maternal-fetal medicine program (includes genetic counseling and perinatologist).

5. Fetal anomalies that may affect the management of the pregnancy mandate referral to a maternal-fetal medicine program.

6. Severe medical problems that place patient at increased risk for maternal death or worsening of disease (eg, serum creatinine above 1.8, severe cardiac disease—class III, IV, and class F, R, or H insulin-dependent diabetes) mandate referral to maternal-fetal medicine specialist.

7. Patients at high risk for recurrent preterm birth (eg, uterine didelphys, prior preterm birth) bene-

fit from consultation at least with an obstetrician-gynecologist, and preferably with a maternal-fetal medicine specialist.

8. All multiple gestation patients should have consultation with an obstetrician-gynecologist; all triplets or higher order multiples should be managed by maternal-fetal medicine specialist.

Relevant Web Sites

[TERIS]
http://www.depts.washington.edu/~terisweb/teris/

[REPROTOX]
http://reprotox.org/
[American College of Genetics general information website]
www.acmg.net
[Another useful genetics based website for patients/providers]
geneclinics.org
[American College of Obstetrics & Gynecology]
[Individual technical bulletins/committee opinions]
www.acog.org
[Ob Gyn general overview for patients]
www.medem.com

Early Pregnancy Loss

57

Susan C. Conway, MD

ESSENTIALS OF DIAGNOSIS

- *Bleeding or pelvic pain during the first 20 weeks of pregnancy. Any pregnancy with abnormal bleeding or pain must be considered ectopic until its location is determined.*
- *Positive human chorionic gonadotropin*
  —β subunit (βHCG).
- *Ultrasound at ≥ 6 weeks gestation*
  –Spontaneous abortion: intrauterine gestational sac without fetal cardiac activity.
  –Ectopic pregnancy: absence of intrauterine gestational sac and/or adnexal mass suggestive of ectopic gestation.

A **spontaneous abortion** is any intrauterine pregnancy that ends before the 20th week of gestation. A **missed abortion** is defined by lack of fetal cardiac activity after 7 gestational weeks in the absence of bleeding or cramping. A **threatened abortion** occurs when there is vaginal bleeding or cramping and the cervical os is not dilated. **Inevitable abortion** is diagnosed when bleeding and cramping occur and either the cervical os is dilated or tissue is present in the cervical canal. An **ectopic pregnancy** is located outside the endometrial cavity and may be life-threatening.

General Considerations

A. Spontaneous Abortion

The process of human reproduction is inherently inefficient. Nearly 70% of conceptions are lost shortly after implantation and do not interfere with the onset of menses. About 15–20% of clinically recognized pregnancies end in spontaneous abortion. About 80% of clinical abortions occur before 12 weeks gestation. Most occur during the embryonic period (up to 8 weeks) and two thirds of these are due to chromosomal abnormalities. The incidence of spontaneous abortions rises with advancing maternal age, approaching 50% by age 40. Table 57–1 describes the incidence of spontaneous pregnancy loss as a function of maternal age.

When embryonic cardiac activity is present sonographically between 6 and 12 weeks gestation, the incidence of subsequent pregnancy loss is between 2% and 8%. Most embryonic deaths take place several days or weeks prior to uterine bleeding, cramping and expulsion of products of conception.

The most frequent cause of spontaneous abortion is a genetic abnormality, independent of maternal age. Cytogenetic studies reveal abnormalities in 50–85% of abortions, depending on the technique used. The majority of the abnormal karyotypes are numeric abnormalities as a result of errors in gametogenesis, fertilization, or the first cell division of the fertilized oocyte. Only 5% are due to structural chromosome defects, such as translocation. The most common defect identified is autosomal trisomy, a risk directly related to maternal age. Euploid losses tend to occur somewhat later in gestation, most commonly around 12–13 weeks. For unknown reasons, this incidence also increases with maternal age, starting at age 35 and rising to more than 30% of clinical conceptions among women older than 40.

Other contributing factors to first trimester pregnancy loss are less frequent or of a more controversial nature, including congenital uterine anomalies, acquired uterine defects (fibroids, intrauterine adhesions), endocrine abnormalities (progesterone deficiency, hypersecretion of luteinizing hormone [LH]), medical illnesses (thyroid disease, diabetes mellitus), immunologic factors (HLA sharing, lupus anticoagulant, antiphospholipid antibodies) and environmental factors (tobacco, alcohol, caffeine, toxins, radiation).

B. Ectopic Pregnancy

The incidence of ectopic pregnancy has been steadily increasing over the past 40 years. In 1992, the estimated number of ectopic pregnancies occurring in the United States was 108,000 for a rate of 19.7 per 1000 reported pregnancies. Thus, approximately 2 of every 100 women known to have conceived had an ectopic gestation. The increased incidence is thought to be due to both the increased incidence of salpingitis from infection with sexually transmitted infections (STIs), primarily *Chlamydia trachomatis,* and improved diagnostic techniques leading to earlier and more frequent detection.

Table 57–1. Risk of pregnancy loss by maternal age.

Age of Mother	Percent Spontaneous Abortions (CI)[1]
19 or younger	10.8 (9.0–12.7)
20–29	9.7 (9.2–12.7)
30–34	11.5 (10.6–12.6)
35–39	21.4 (19.2–23.7)
40 or older +	42.2 (35.1–47.4)

[1]Figures in brackets are 95% confidence intervals (CIs) drawn from a sampling of study patients.
(From Knudsen UB et al: Eur J Obstet Gynecol Reprod Biol 1991;39:31.)

Most ectopic pregnancies (97.7%) occur in the oviduct; approximately 1.4% implant in the abdominal cavity and less than 1% implant on the ovary. Of the tubal pregnancies, 81% are located in the ampullary portion, 12% in the isthmus, 5% in the fimbrial region, and 2% in the interstitial region. Despite the trend toward earlier diagnosis and treatment over the past 15–20 years, ectopic pregnancy is still the most common cause of maternal death in the first half of pregnancy. Profound blood loss is the major cause of death (88%) followed far behind by infection (3%), and anesthesia complications (2%). Eighty percent of fatal ectopic gestations occur in the tube while 20% are interstitial or abdominal gestations. Given the low overall incidence in extratubal locations, interstitial and abdominal pregnancies carry a 5 times greater risk of mortality. Delay in consultation after development of symptoms account for 30% of the deaths and treatment delay from misdiagnosis contributes to 50%. More than half die of hemorrhage without emergency surgery.

The majority (50%) of initial episodes of ectopic pregnancy are the result of the morphologic sequelae of acute salpingitis. *C trachomatis* infection is the leading pathogen. In 10%, other morphologic factors are identified, such as scarring or adhesions from previous abdominal surgery, sterilization or tubal reversal procedures, as well as anatomic abnormalities associated with in utero diethylstilbestrol (DES) exposure. In 40%, the causes cannot be identified and are thought to be due to migration delays in the passage of the embryo into the uterine cavity. Such delays could be due to intratubal hormonal imbalances or abnormalities of embryonic development. Thus, a history of multiple partners, STIs, pelvic inflammatory disease (PID), tubal surgery, or ruptured appendix increases the risk of tubal damage. Among women with tubal ligation for sterilization, the risk of failure up to 10 years after the procedure is approximately 2%. Of the pregnancies occurring in such women, 50% are ectopic. Progestin-only birth control pills and progestin-releasing intrauterine devices (IUDs) alter normal tubal contractility, which may impede the progress of the early embryo through the tube. Iatrogenic, physiologically increased levels of estrogen and progesterone occur after ovulation induction with clomiphene citrate or gonadotropins and has been associated with increased rates of ectopic gestation. One third of tubal gestations are aneuploid, suggesting chromosomal abnormalities can cause ectopic implantation. Several epidemiologic studies show cigarette smoking is an independent factor for a 2-fold increased risk of ectopic pregnancy, rising to a 4-fold increase among women who smoked 30 or more cigarettes a day.

Any pregnant woman with a history of previous ectopic pregnancy should be assumed to have another until proved otherwise. About 25% of subsequent pregnancies are ectopic among women who conceive after having 1 ectopic pregnancy.

Clinical Findings

A. SYMPTOMS AND SIGNS

The most common signs and symptoms of early pregnancy are missed menstrual period, nausea, breast tenderness, fatigue, occasional irregular uterine cramping, and intermittent adnexal pain caused by tension and strain of the round ligaments or a corpus luteum cyst. There is a great deal of overlap between symptoms of normal and abnormal pregnancies. Some women with normal intrauterine pregnancies deny any symptoms at all, and some women with ectopic pregnancies describe symptoms consistent with normal pregnancy. Any pregnancy with abnormal bleeding or pain must be considered ectopic until its location is determined.

1. Threatened abortion—Bleeding occurs during the first 20 weeks of pregnancy in about 30–40% of gestations. Half will end in spontaneous abortion; the other half are said to be threatened abortions. The risk of abortion is greater if the bleeding persists for 3 or more days. The bleeding may range from bright red and brisk to light, brownish spotting. Women with threatened abortions who do not go on to abort usually do not have cramps.

2. Inevitable, incomplete, and complete abortions—If uterine cramping and cervical dilation accompany uterine bleeding, the abortion is **inevitable.** Large clots and brisk bleeding is usually noted in the vagina on examination. The abortion is **incomplete** if only a portion of the products of conception has been expelled and the cervix remains dilated. If all fetal and placental tissue has been expelled, the cervix is closed, and bleeding and cramping is waning, the abortion is complete. Complete abortions commonly occur before 6 weeks and after 14 weeks of gestation; those occurring between 6 and 14 weeks are usually incomplete and are accompanied by profuse uterine bleeding.

3. Missed abortion—If the uterus fails to enlarge with or without associated bleeding, a **missed** abortion is suspected. Decreasing or suddenly absent symptoms of breast tenderness, nausea, and fatigue are also clues that the pregnancy may not be progressing normally. Pain is *not* usually present. The term "missed" is less relevant in this era of early ultrasonographic diagnoses of anembryonic gestations (the so-called "**blighted ovum**") or fetal death. If no expulsion or removal of the uterine contents occurs beyond 5 weeks after fetal death, consumptive coagulability and hypofibrinognemia may occur.

4. Septic abortions—Approximately 1–2% of all spontaneous abortions may have associated infection, the incidence increasing markedly if the abortion was induced with nonsterilized instruments (eg, "self-instrumented" attempted terminations). Fever, leukocytosis, lower abdominal tenderness, cervical motion tenderness, and a foul uterine discharge are the hallmark signs. Septic abortion may be threatened, inevitable, or incomplete and should be considered a life-threatening emergency due to the high risk of septic shock.

5. Ectopic pregnancy—It is frequently possible to diagnose ectopic pregnancy before the onset of symptoms among women with risk factors. The use of transvaginal ultrasonography and early βHCG levels facilitate early diagnosis and medical management (see following section, Treatment). Symptoms develop as the gestational age increases and intraperitoneal bleeding occurs as blood extrudes through the fimbriated end of the tube or from tubal rupture. The most common symptoms are abdominal pain, absence of menses, and irregular vaginal bleeding. The nature of the universally present abdominal pain may be vague and colicky prior to rupture and the location may be generalized, unilateral, or bilateral. During rupture, the pain may intensify. Shoulder pain indicates diaphragmatic irritation from hemoperitoneum in 25% of cases. Syncope occurs in 33% of tubal ruptures. Other symptoms include dizziness and rectal pain or an urge to defecate. About 5–10% of women will note passage of a decidual cast, so a report of passage of tissue does not specifically rule out ectopic pregnancy. Findings on examination include tachycardia, orthostatic hypotension, rebound, guarding, and localized adnexal pain upon palpation.

B. LABORATORY FINDINGS

1. Human chorionic gonadotropin–β subunit—βHCG is produced by placental villi and can be mea-sured in both serum and urine. For quantitative serum levels, most laboratories use either a radioimmunoassay (RIA) or an enzyme-linked immunosorbent assay (ELISA) with sensitivities to 5–10 mIU/mL. Qualitative urine pregnancy tests measure a minimum of 25–50 mIU/mL.

During the first 6 weeks of gestation, the βHCG approximately doubles every 48 hours, but there can be wide variations from this pattern in both normal and abnormal pregnancies. A minimum 67% rise every 48 hours is considered acceptable. Pregnancies that do not maintain this doubling curve may be abnormal, ie, ectopic or failing pregnancies. βHCG increases more rapidly in multiple gestations and molar pregnancies.

In normal intrauterine pregnancies, βHCG levels have generalized temporal thresholds. By the day of missed menses (day 29 of the usual 28-day cycle), the βHCG level is around 100 mIU/mL. By 33 days from the last menstrual period, it is between 1000 and 1500 mIU/mL. By 39–43 days, the βHCG is usually more than 13,000 mIU/mL. These thresholds correspond to ultrasonographic findings (see following section, Imaging Studies).

Serial βHCG measurements can aid in the differentiation between normal and abnormal gestation in otherwise asymptomatic women in early pregnancy. However, differentiation between ectopic and failing intrauterine pregnancies cannot be made with this technique because the rates of increasing βHCG are similar in both groups.

2. Progesterone—Since isolated βHCG levels do not provide sufficient laboratory information to diagnose ectopic pregnancy, many investigators have incorporated progesterone levels into the diagnostic algorithm. Many have shown that serum progesterone levels in women with ectopic pregnancies are significantly lower than in women with viable or nonviable intrauterine pregnancies. One study showed that at 4 weeks gestation a threshold progesterone level of 5 ng/mL was able to differentiate ectopic from intrauterine gestations with 100% sensitivity and 97% specificity. At 5 weeks, the threshold increased to 10 ng/mL and at 6 weeks to 20 ng/mL, but the sensitivity and specificity decreased. Obviously, the usefulness of the progesterone level decreases with advancing gestational age. Given that "stat" progesterone levels are not widely available and that ultrasound findings (see following section, Imaging Studies) combined with βHCG are sufficiently diagnostic, their value in differentiating normal from abnormal pregnancies is controversial.

3. Other laboratory tests—Hematocrit, blood type and screen (to determine whether the patient needs Rh immune globulin (RhoGAM), should be ordered. Cross-match is indicated when suspicion of ruptured ectopic is high. Cultures of the cervix for gonorrhea and *C trachomatis* can be considered, but the cultures are not valid when there is significant bleeding, nor do they alter treatment recommendations.

C. IMAGING STUDIES

The development of transvaginal ultrasonography has made it possible to accurately diagnose abnormalities of early pregnancy, especially when used in conjunction with quantitative serum βHCG levels (see above section, Laboratory Findings). In normal intrauterine pregnancies, a 3-mm gestational sac can be seen as early as 33 days gestation. Between 34 and 38 days, the sac size increases to more than 10 mm in diameter and the yolk sac is visible. Between 39 and 43 days gestation, the sac should be more than 18 mm and an embryo with cardiac activity should be visualized. If the sac measures more than 18 mm and no embryo is seen, it is an anembryonic gestation (blighted ovum).

Much attention has been given to ultrasonographic findings as prognostic factors among women with threatened abortions. Embryonic heart rates much slower or faster than the normal 100–120 beats per minute during early gestation are associated with higher loss rates. Small and irregular gestational sacs are very poor prognostic signs, with abortion rates of 80% or more. Several ultrasound series among women with threatened abortion have been reported. In two thirds of threatened abortions, a live fetus is present at ultrasound and 85% of those survive and proceed to delivery. Among the one third who do not have a live fetus present at ultrasound, half are anembryonic and the remaining half are equally divided between embryonic demise and incomplete abortion, with an occasional molar gestation.

Ultrasonography is less helpful in cases of complete abortion in which the patient does not give a history of passage of tissue. As there is no intrauterine sac, the cervix is closed, and the βHCG is often still elevated at the time of presentation, a complete abortion can be easily mistaken for an ectopic pregnancy (see below).

Using a transvaginal probe with 5.0 to 7.0 MHz scanning frequency, it is possible to identify an intrauterine gestational sac when the βHCG level exceeds 2000 mIU/mL (Third International Standard) about 5–6 weeks after the last menses. Given the extreme rarity of heterotopic (combined intrauterine and extrauterine) pregnancies, the presence of an intrauterine sac excludes an ectopic pregnancy. When no intrauterine sac is present and the βHCG is more than 2000 mIU/mL, an abnormal gestation should be suspected. An adnexal mass and/or gestational sac-like structure may be seen in the oviduct when an ectopic pregnancy produces βHCG levels greater than 2500 mIU/mL. About two thirds of women presenting with symptoms of ectopic pregnancy have βHCG levels above 2500 mIU/mL and the diagnosis can be made ultrasonographically. For the remaining one third with lower βHCG levels and no intrauterine sac, other diagnostic techniques (serial βHCG, serum progesterone) should be performed and consideration given to serial ultrasounds if the patient is clinically stable.

D. SPECIAL EXAMINATIONS

When serum βHCG levels are greater than 2000 mIU/mL, the gestational age exceeds 38 days, or the serum progesterone level is less than 5 ng/mL and no intrauterine gestational sac is seen on transvaginal ultrasonography, a curettage of the endometrial cavity may be done to determine the presence or absence of gestational tissue. Frozen section is 93% accurate in identifying chorionic villi. If no villi are present, a presumptive diagnosis of ectopic pregnancy is made.

If dilation and curettage (D&C) does not reveal chorionic villi, diagnosis via laparoscopy may be considered.

Differential Diagnosis

Any female patient of childbearing age with unexplained pelvic or abdominal pain should have a serum pregnancy test. A negative test effectively rules out abnormal intrauterine or ectopic pregnancy. Other entities that may present with similar symptoms include salpingitis, ruptured corpus luteum cyst, appendicitis, dysfunctional uterine bleeding, adnexal torsion, degenerative uterine leiomyomata, and endometriosis. A useful diagnostic algorithm is shown in Figure 57–1.

Psychosocial Concerns

Patients frequently ask "What did I do wrong?" "When can we have sex?" and "When can we try to conceive again?" It is important to dispel the concept that the pregnancy loss was caused by anything the patient did or did not do either before or during the pregnancy. It is useful to find out what the couple thinks may have caused the loss and address these issues. Stress following miscarriage and ectopic pregnancy can be enormous. Women and their partners should be told to expect that the pregnancy loss will have a strong emotional impact. The woman may cry easily or for no apparent reason. She may have a difficult time on her projected due date. Much like infertile women and their partners (see Chapter 54, Emotional Aspects of Infertility), the couple may not want to see friends who have children or who are pregnant. This is normal grieving for what might have been, and the reaction will diminish with time.

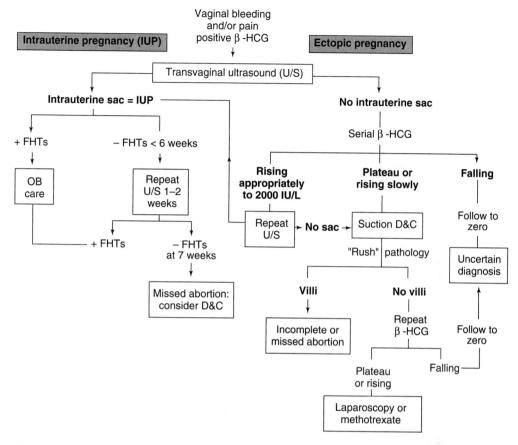

Figure 57–1. Algorithm for diagnosis and treatment of spontaneous abortion and ectopic pregnancy.

Frequently, women and their partners deal differently with a pregnancy loss. Clinicians can encourage partners to comfort each other and communicate, but it is important to realize they may not be recovering at the same rate. Women who experience miscarriage have a 3.4- to 4.3-fold greater chance of having depressive symptoms than other pregnant women or nonpregnant women. It is important to be aware of the resources in the community, especially counselors and therapists who are experienced in grief and loss therapy. The organization RESOLVE provides support to couples with pregnancy losses as well to infertile couples (see Chapter 54, Emotional Aspects of Infertility).

Traditionally, a 3-month waiting period has been advised before attempting conception. This interval is intended to allow the couple time to grieve, to let the woman's cycles become regular, and to allow the endometrial cavity or fallopian tube to heal. However, gestations that begin in the month following an early pregnancy loss have a similar outcome to those that are delayed by 3 months or more. Some couples want to attempt conception right away, whereas others decide to wait a longer time. Couples postponing pregnancy should be counseled about contraception.

Treatment

A. THREATENED ABORTION

There is no evidence that restriction of activity or active medical therapy improves the prognosis of threatened abortion. Hormonal treatments to presumably improve pregnancy retention, such as progesterone supplementation, have no effect on outcome. Nevertheless, many providers advise restriction of physical activity and pelvic rest until the bleeding ceases. If it increases and/or becomes associated with uterine cramping, it is likely that the abortion is becoming inevitable. Further ultrasonographic evaluation may reveal an anembryonic or nonviable gestation. The uterus may then be evacuated surgically via D&C or medically via an oxytocic agent, prostaglandin, or misoprostol.

B. Inevitable and Incomplete Abortion

Since most abortions occurring between 8 and 14 weeks are incomplete and are associated with heavy bleeding, surgical intervention is usually required via D&C. The procedure is usually done as an outpatient. If bleeding is profound, transfusion may be necessary. Evacuation of small amounts of retained products in incomplete abortions may be accomplished with vaginal misoprostol. Prophylactic oral oxytocics (eg, 0.2 mg of oral methergine every 8 hours for 3 days) are sometimes given postoperatively, as are iron supplements or antibiotics as indicated.

If the abortion occurs during the second trimester, it often passes spontaneously in a process identical to labor. If a second trimester abortion is "missed," it requires either dilation and evacuation (D&E) or prostaglandin induction of labor. D&E requires a highly skilled surgeon, as the uterus is easier to perforate in the second trimester and the complication rates for the procedure are higher than first trimester D&C. The longer potentially necrotic tissue remains in the uterus, the higher the risk of coagulopathy and fibrinolysis. Thus, prompt uterine evacuation is essential.

C. Complete Abortion

If the uterus is indeed empty, no further treatment is usually required. Sonographic measurement of the endometrial thickness often assists the assessment: a depth of 10 mm or less is consistent with complete evacuation of the uterus and no D&C is required.

D. Septic Abortion

Septic abortion is a potentially fatal condition and should be considered a life-threatening emergency. A complete blood cell count, urinalysis, and electrolyte panel should be obtained. If the woman is profoundly ill, blood cultures, chest radiograph, and a coagulation panel should also be obtained. Intravenous antibiotics with coverage against polymicrobial anaerobic bacteria should be started immediately. A combination of several agents is usually recommended. After adequate antibiotic blood levels are obtained, usually within 2 hours, the uterus should be evacuated as previously described. If the sepsis is severe and the uterus cannot be evacuated through the cervix, hysterectomy may become necessary. If shock develops, medical intensive care is required, including central venous pressure monitoring, oxygen therapy, and vasopressor support. The

fatality rate is estimated at 0.4–0.6 per 100,000 spontaneous abortions.

E. Ectopic Pregnancy

The clinical presentation of the patient directs therapy. Nearly all ruptured ectopic pregnancies require surgical intervention. Patients who are clinically stable and meet the criteria for medical management may avoid surgery.

1. Surgical therapy—Depending on the extent of bleeding and potential anatomic damage, surgical management may be via salpingostomy, salpingotomy, or salpingectomy. Linear salpingostomy via laparoscopy is the procedure of choice for unruptured ampullary ectopic pregnancies less than 3 cm in diameter. Persistent ectopic pregnancy occurs in 5%, usually as a result of the incision being made medially to the implantation site. This event is uncommon when the preoperative βHCG levels are less than 3000 mIU/mL. Most persistent ectopics are then treated medically. If rupture occurs, repeat surgery is necessary. Larger tubal pregnancies may be removed by partial salpingectomy. Microsurgical reanastomosis is possible in some cases after healing is complete. However, in this era of highly successful assisted reproductive technology, further surgical therapy is often not desired. Cornual resection of the uterus may be sufficient for interstitial and corneal pregnancies. All attempts at ovarian conservation should be made, especially if future fertility is desired. Fimbrial evacuation by digital expression or blunt curettage is not advisable as the rates of recurrent ectopic pregnancy after such techniques are quite high. If the bleeding and anatomic damage are profound and life-threatening, hysterectomy may be required.

2. Medical therapy—Patients that are hemodynamically stable with unruptured ectopic pregnancies less than 3.5 cm on ultrasound are considered good candidates for medical therapy. Approximately one third of women with ectopic pregnancies satisfy these criteria. Additional criteria include absence of free fluid in the pelvic cavity on ultrasound and no evidence of hepatic, hematologic, or renal disease. Absolute and relative indications and contraindications are shown in Table 57–2. Methotrexate is a potent dihydrofolic acid inhibitor used extensively for choriocarcinoma and trophoblastic disease. It has been successfully used in multi- and single-dose regimens since the first report in 1982. The most common regimen uses a single dose of 50 mg/m². βHCG levels are followed until the pregnancy is resolved. Overall success rates of 85–90% have been reported; additional doses are required in 10% and 5% ultimately require surgical intervention. About 85% of patients treated with methotrexate have a transient rise in the βHCG level 1–4 days after treatment. Levels should drop by 15% or more between 4 and 7

Table 57–2. Criteria for receiving methotrexate.

Absolute indications

Hemodynamically stable without active bleeding or signs of hemoperitoneum

Nonlaparoscopic diagnosis

Patient desires future fertility

General anesthesia poses a significant risk

Patient is able to return for follow-up care

Patient has no contraindications to methotrexate

Relative indications

Unruptured mass < 3.5 cm at its greatest dimension

No fetal cardiac motion detected

βHCG level does not exceed a predetermined level (6000–15,000 mIU/mL)

Absolute contraindications

Breast-feeding

Overt laboratory evidence of immunodeficiency

Alcoholism, alcoholic liver disease, or other chronic liver disease

Preexisting blood dyscrasias, such as bone marrow hypoplasia, leukopenia, thrombocytopenia, or significant anemia

Known sensitivity to methotrexate

Active pulmonary disease

Peptic ulcer disease

Hepatic, renal, or hematologic dysfunction

Relative contraindications

Gestational sac ≥ 3.5 cm

Embryonic cardiac motion

(From ACOG Medical Management of Tubal Pregnancy Practice Bulletin No. 3, December 1998.)

days after treatment. If this fall does not occur or there is less than a 15% decline in each subsequent week, additional doses may be given for a maximum of 3 doses. If the levels still do not decline appropriately, then surgical intervention is warranted.

3. Expectant management—In appropriately selected patients, a suspected ectopic pregnancy may be managed expectantly. The best candidates are reliable patients without symptoms, a sonographic diameter of the tubal mass less than 3 cm, an initial βHCG level less than 1000 mIU/mL, and no rise in βHCG levels during a 2-day period. If the patient remains asymptomatic and the βHCG levels subsequently fall, no other therapy is needed. Resolution rates as high as 88% have been reported. One series reported that 25% of all the patients with ectopic pregnancy at their institution during the observation period met these criteria; spontaneous resolution occurred in two thirds, or 16% of the original ectopic group. Given the potentially grave consequences of untreated ectopic pregnancy, many providers are reluctant to offer expectant management.

F. PREVENTION OF ISOIMMUNIZATION

Isoimmunization of the mother can occur during both ectopic pregnancies and abortions if fetal red blood cells enter the maternal system. Red blood cells are present in the developing embryo at approximately 6 weeks. All women who are Rh-negative and who have been treated for ectopic pregnancy or spontaneous or therapeutic abortion up to and including 12 weeks should be given 50 μg Rh immune globulin (MICRhoGAM). This dose is designed to suppress the immune response to 2.5 mL or less of blood. Losses occurring after 13 weeks should receive the full 300-μg dose of immune globulin (RhoGAM), which covers 15 mL or less. Patients who have bleeding episodes with threatened abortions also should be given immune globulin. Maternal side effects are extremely rare, but treatment should be avoided in anyone known to have had an anaphylactic reaction to any immune globulin. Some centers advocate the use of the 300-μg dose in all cases, because the amount of blood transfused is difficult to estimate with certainty, the cost differential is small, the side effects to the mother are rare, and the potential consequences to future pregnancies are great if isoimmunization should occur. The full dose offers protection against future bleeds for 2–4 months.

When to Refer to a Specialist

The skill level and knowledge base of the provider are the most important determinants of referral for specialty care. The diagnosis of ruptured ectopic pregnancy should prompt immediate referral to a gynecologic surgeon for emergency surgery. The diagnosis of possible unruptured ectopic pregnancy requires referral to a gynecologist experienced in both surgical and medical management. Women who are found to have pelvic adhesions or other abnormalities at the time of surgery for ectopic pregnancy or who have recurrent ectopic pregnancies should be referred to a reproductive endocrinologist for consultation if fertility is desired.

Only providers comfortable with the procedure and management of complications should perform D&C for incomplete or missed abortions in the first trimester. All women with molar pregnancies should be referred to a gynecologist. Not all gynecologists are skilled in second-trimester abortions; therefore, patients needing either a D&C or D&E in the second trimester should be referred to gynecologists who perform the procedure regularly and have low complication rates. Women experiencing 2 spontaneous abortions in the first trimester or 1 spontaneous abortion after 13 weeks of gestation should be referred to an obstetrician or reproductive endocrinologist for further evaluation.

All couples should be offered emotional support at each visit. If further counseling is needed, patients should be referred to mental health workers experienced in dealing with grief and loss. If suicidal ideation is elicited, immediate psychiatric evaluation is indicated.

Prognosis

The likelihood of successful pregnancy after experiencing a single intrauterine pregnancy loss is approximately 90%. The risk of subsequent pregnancy loss is higher among women with more than 1 previous loss or no previously successful pregnancies. A history of 2 or more consecutive abortions is termed **recurrent pregnancy loss** and warrants referral. Karyotyping of tissue obtained at D&C during a second loss may provide an explanation for the loss. Aneuploidy is present in 70% of cases in which aneuploidy was present in the first abortus, but in only 20% when the first abortus was chromosomally normal. However, less than 6% of couples with recurrent pregnancy loss have chromosomal abnormalities themselves.

Uterine abnormalities are identified in approximately 15% of women with recurrent pregnancy loss. These abnormalities are usually identified by hysterosalpingography. Abnormalities of coagulation associated with the antiphospholipid antibody syndrome are linked to recurrent pregnancy loss. Prophylactic heparin and low-dose aspirin has been shown to be helpful in appropriately selected patients. The relationship between autoimmune or alloimmune factors or presumptive hormonal defects and recurrent pregnancy loss is highly controversial. At this time, there is no consensus on diagnosis or treatment based on these factors. More than 50% of couples with recurrent pregnancy loss have no identifiable etiology despite extensive evaluation. Informative and sympathetic counseling appears to be useful, as up to 70% have a successful subsequent untreated pregnancy.

Second trimester losses frequently are attributed to maternal causes, but they also can be caused by genetic anomalies. Rapidly enlarging leiomyomas or other structural anomalies can lead to expulsion of the fetus. An incompetent cervix (painless dilation of the cervix) should be followed carefully during a subsequent pregnancy with possible cerclage placement. Systemic maternal disease such as diabetes, systemic lupus erythematosis, or chronic renal disease should be managed by a medical specialist and an obstetrician prior to conception of the next pregnancy.

Any woman treated for an ectopic pregnancy should be considered at increased risk for subsequent ectopic pregnancy. Approximately 50% of women have an intrauterine pregnancy with the next attempt, but 20% have a repeat ectopic pregnancy. Therefore, serial βHCGs and early ultrasonography are indicated with all subsequent pregnancies. The remaining 30% of patients are unable to conceive without in vitro fertilization.

American College of Obstetricians and Gynecologists: Compendium of Selected Publications, 2001. (www.acog.org)

American College of Obstetricians and Gynecologists: Early Pregnancy Loss Educational and Technical Bulletin No. 212, 1995.

American College of Obstetricians and Gynecologists: Management of Ectopic Pregnancy Practice Bulletin No. 3, 1998.

Cramer DW, Wise LA: The epidemiology of recurrent pregnancy loss. Semin Reprod Med 2000;18:331. [PMID: 11355791]

Lee RM, Silver RM: Recurrent pregnancy loss: summary and clinical recommendations. Semin Reprod Med 2000;18:433. [PMID: 11355802]

Knudsen UB et al: Prognosis of a new pregnancy following previous spontaneous abortions. Eur J Obstet Gynecol Reprod Biol 1991;39:31. [PMID: 2029953]

Relevant Web Sites

[American College of Obstetricians and Gynecologists]
www.acog.org

SECTION XIX

Complementary & Alternative Medicine Use

Integrative Approaches to Women's Health

58

Richard Liebowitz, MD

More than 40% of the American population use alternative medicine approaches. Demographics reveal that women are significantly more likely to use these approaches than men. Contrary to conventional wisdom, dissatisfaction with conventional medicine has not been found to be predictive of the use of alternative medicine. Rather, it is congruence with personal beliefs and philosophies regarding health and wellness that attracts patients to alternative providers. Integrative medicine seeks to be a bridge between conventional and alternative systems of care. Integrative medicine encompasses and promotes the best techniques of care regardless of the system of origin, thereby developing a "best practice" of medicine that is both centered on the patient and based on the evidence. While many modalities are included within integrative approaches, this chapter will be limited to the use of herbal products and supplements.

Any discussion concerning the use of herbal products and supplements must include the issue of the Dietary and Supplement Health Education Act. This act categorizes these over-the-counter products in a class other than drugs. Therefore, they are not subject to scrutiny by the US Food and Drug Administration (FDA) regarding content and purity as long as no specific health claims are stated. The burden is placed on the FDA to document a hazard, rather than the manufacturer to document efficacy and safety. Knowledge of which brand name products contain the stated quantity of compound and how it is standardized is essential. Consumerlab.com is an Internet site that analyzes supplements and herbal products and compares the advertised concentration to the results of their analysis. Limited information is available at no cost; otherwise, this site does have a nominal charge to gain full access, but it is highly recommended. Brand names such as Nature's Way, PhytoPharmica, and Twin Laboratories appear several times for a number of products. Care must always be exercised when herbal products and supplements are considered in pregnant women and children and when used in combination with prescription and over-the-counter drugs. Additional information that presents evidence-based reviews of herbal and supplement approaches is available at such web sites as Bandolier, Cochrane, and the National Institutes of Health.

Managing Symptoms of Menstrual Disorders

While it has been estimated that as many as 80% of women experience symptoms related to their menstrual cycle, less than half of these women have symptoms severe enough to seek treatment. A number of alternative herbal and supplement approaches have been popular with varying degrees of evidence of efficacy.

A. CHASTEBERRY

Extracts of *Vitex agnus castus* have been used traditionally for a wide variety of indications. The name chasteberry reflects the belief that extracts from *Vitex* were helpful in monk's maintaining their vows of chastity.

Recently, a double-blinded, placebo-controlled study documented its efficacy in the treatment of premenstrual syndrome (PMS). Specifically, a *Vitex* extract using 20 mg of a casticin-standardized formulation was found to significantly improve several symptoms of PMS including anger, mood alteration, irritability, headache, breast fullness, and bloating. When using the crude herb, doses range from 500 to 1000 mg of herb per day. It has been postulated that the mechanism of action likely revolves around the herb's ability to decrease prolactin levels via a dopaminergic pathway. *Vitex* has also been documented to restore progesterone levels. In Germany, it is used to treat menstrual irregularities as well as undiagnosed infertility. No significant toxicities have been reported with *Vitex* extracts when used in appropriate doses.

B. ST. JOHN'S WORT

Hypericum perforatum is most recognized as an effective treatment for mild to moderate depression. One study found that this compound, when used at a dose of 300 mg/d of a 0.3% hypericin-standardized extract, was effective in the treatment of PMS. Most herbalists, however, recommend a higher dose of 300 mg of the extract 3 times a day. When studied in PMS, St. John's Wort was used on an every day basis rather than in a cyclic fashion. While adverse reactions occur less frequently than with prescription antidepressants, care must be exercised with the use of this product. Most common side effects include gastrointestinal upset, headache, and agitation. Rare but severe phototoxicity has been reported. Because St. John's Wort induces the cytochrome P-450 complex, significant drug interactions have been recognized. Specifically, there have been reports of St. John's Wort lowering levels of birth control pills, theophylline, cyclosporine, and antiretroviral drugs in the blood. Interactions have also been described with buspirone, statins, calcium channel blockers, digoxin, and carbamezepine. There are no apparent significant interactions with coumadin. The mechanism of action for its efficacy in the treatment of PMS has not been elucidated.

C. VITAMIN B$_6$

Vitamin B$_6$ has been the subject of a number of studies investigating its efficacy in PMS. A systematic review of 9 trials indicated significant benefit over placebo for the symptoms of mastalgia, swollen breasts, pain, and depression. Doses of B$_6$ evaluated ranged from a low of 50 mg to a high of 600 mg/d. High-dose B$_6$ therapy may lead to neuropathy as well as interaction with other medications, specifically anti-Parkinson's drugs. B$_6$ is a cofactor for L-aromatic amino acid decarboxylase, and as such is intimately involved in the biosynthesis of dopamine.

D. CALCIUM AND MAGNESIUM

Supplementation with both calcium and magnesium has been proposed as treatment for PMS. Multiple studies have been conducted utilizing both elements, and the results have been inconsistent. Dosages have not been consistent, the formulations have varied, and in some studies these elements have been combined with other dietary or supplemental approaches. Calcium appears to be effective when taken in a dose of at least 1200 mg/d. During the luteal phase at this dose, calcium has demonstrated improvement in pain, food cravings, water retention, and negative affect. Magnesium as a sole agent has less evidence, although low magnesium levels have been reported in women suffering from PMS. When used in combination with 50 mg of vitamin B$_6$, 200 mg of magnesium per day led to lower levels of nervous tension, anxiety, irritability, and mood swings.

E. OMEGA-3 FATTY ACIDS

Omega-3 fatty acids are recognized as anti-inflammatory in that they shift arachadonic acid metabolism away from PgF2-alpha and increase levels of the less inflammatory PgE1. A number of studies have found that the intake of marine origin omega-3 fatty acids (such as salmon and sardines) decrease complaints of dysmenorrhea. Given the established benefits of omega-3 fatty acids in other conditions such as heart disease, high intake of these compounds can be recommended throughout the cycle. Supplementation with oils such as evening primrose oil have had uniformly negative results in alleviating the symptoms of PMS.

F. VITAMIN E

Studies performed in the 1940s suggested that vitamin E might be effective in the treatment of menstrual disorders such as PMS. Recent studies have failed to reproduce these results. These newer studies have used doses in the range of 200–600 IU, leading some to suggest that a dose as high as 1200 IU may be necessary for the therapeutic effect. Vitamin E has been noted to cause spontaneous subarachnoid hemorrhages in at least 1 study, as it has recognized anticoagulant properties.

G. GINKGO BILOBA

While *Ginkgo biloba* is best known as an herbal remedy in the treatment of memory and circulatory disorders, it also has been used in the treatment of PMS symptoms. In doses ranging from 60 to 240 mg of standardized extract per day, ginkgo has clinical efficacy in the treatment of breast pain, tenderness, and fluid retention. In at least 1 study, ginkgo has also been found to be effective in the relief of symptoms related to emotional distress. Ginkgo has been promoted as an agent that can increase libido. Studied mostly in cases of antidepressant-induced sexual dysfunction, ginkgo has produced some promising results. Significant methodologic criticism of these studies exists however, and further studies are required to better define the herb's role. Side effects include gastrointestinal upset and headache. Ginkgo also has anticoagulant activity and care must be taken when used with anti-inflammatory drugs as well as with warfarin. In patients scheduled for surgery, it is generally suggested that ginkgo be discontinued 2 weeks before surgery or other invasive procedures.

Deutch B: Menstrual pain in Danish women correlated with low omega-3 polyunsaturated fatty acid intake. Eur J Clin Nutr 1995;49:508. [PMID: 7588501]

Facchinetti F et al: Oral magnesium successfully relieves premenstrual mood changes. Obstet Gynecol 1991;78:177. [PMID: 2067759]

Schellenberg R: Treatment for the premenstrual syndrome with agnus castus fruit extract: a prospective, randomised, placebo controlled study. BMJ 2001;322:134. [PMID: 11159568]

Stevinson C, Ernst E: A pilot study of Hypericum perforatum for the treatment of premenstrual syndrome. BJOG 2000;107:870. [PMID: 10901558]

Tamborini A, Taurelle R: Value of standardized Ginkgo biloba extract (EGb 761) in the management of congestive symptoms of premenstrual syndrome. Rev Fr Gynecol Obstet 1993;88:447. [PMID: 8235261]

Thys-Jacobs S et al: Calcium carbonate and the premenstrual syndrome: effects on premenstrual and menstrual symptoms. Premenstrual Syndrome Study Group. Am J Ob Gyn 1998;179:444. [PMID: 9731851]

Wyatt KM et al: Efficacy of vitamin B-6 in the treatment of premenstrual syndrome: systematic review. BMJ 1999;318:1375. [PMID: 10334745]

Managing Symptoms of Menopause

Menopause is a time of physiologic change that is experienced differently from culture to culture and woman to woman. Many women value the use of natural products through this normal period of transition. Various herbs and supplements have been promoted both for symptomatic relief as well as potential long-term health benefits. It is critical to determine what the goal of treatment is and that recommendations be individualized based on the indications for use.

A. BLACK COHOSH

Extracts of *Cimicifuga racemosa* are undoubtedly the best studied herbal remedies for the treatment of menopausal symptoms. Taken in a dosage of 40 mg twice a day standardized to 2.5% triterpenes, most studies have documented efficacy in decreasing menopausal symptoms. While the exact mechanism of action is not clear, recent evidence indicates that *Cimicifuga racemosa* does not have estrogenic activity. The safety of black cohosh in women with a history of

breast cancer has not been established. A recent study using the herb in patients with a history of breast cancer currently taking tamoxifen revealed no significant benefit.

B. KAVA

Extracts of *Piper methysticum* are used extensively in Europe for the treatment of menopausal symptoms, most commonly in combination with other compounds such as black cohosh and valerian. When studied as a single agent, 100–200 mg up to 3 times a day of an extract standardized to contain 30% kavalactones decreases mood symptoms such as irritability and insomnia in menopausal women. Extreme caution must be exercised, as a number of recent reports have implicated kava in the development of rare but severe hepatotoxicity, leading to liver transplantation and even death. Consideration must be given to the risk-benefit ratio of continued use of this product and whether or not there are safer alternatives.

C. PHYTOESTROGENS

Many different plant-based foods contain isoflavones. These phenolic compounds are converted by the body into compounds that bind weakly to estrogen receptors. Soy products are best recognized as containing these compounds, but they are also found in multiple other food sources including lentils and chickpeas. Approximately 60 g of soy protein are needed for the resolution of hot flashes, while doses over 90 g have been documented to decrease cholesterol levels and may be protective against bone loss. Not all soy products contain the same concentration of isoflavones, with edamame (roasted soybeans) having significantly higher levels than soymilk. Many oncologists recommend against significant soy intake in patients with a history of breast cancer. While epidemiologic studies suggest a protective effect of soy with regards to the development of breast cancer in cultures with traditionally high intake of soy products, it is not clear whether initiating soy intake later in life is protective or in fact harmful. Concern also exists about the risk of childhood leukemia in the offspring of mothers with high isoflavone intake late in pregnancy.

D. RED CLOVER

Unlike black cohosh, *Trifolium pratense* has not been traditionally used as a treatment for menopausal symptoms. Red clover was discovered to have significant estrogenic activity when it was noted to cause reproductive problems in sheep grazing in fields of red clover. Studies reveal decreases in follicle-stimulating hormone levels and altered vaginal cytology consistent with an estrogenic effect. Despite its demonstrated estrogenic activity, several studies have failed to demonstrate superiority over placebo in the treatment of menopausal symptoms. It is not recommended for women with a history of breast cancer.

E. DONG QUAI

Dong quai is but one of a number of herbs commonly used in combination with other Chinese herbs by Chinese medicine practitioners in the treatment of menopausal symptoms. Studies using this herb alone have failed to demonstrate any efficacy in the treatment of hot flashes, vaginal dryness, or other menopausal symptoms. Its isolated use is therefore not recommended.

Albertazzi P: The effect of dietary soy supplementation on hot flashes. Obstet Gynecol 1998;91:6. [PMID: 9464712]

Ashton AK: Antidepressant-induced sexual dysfunction and Ginkgo biloba. Am J Psychiatry 2000;157:836. [PMID: 10784488]

Dog TL, Riley D, Carter T: An integrative approach to menopause. Altern Ther Health Med 2001;7:45. [PMID: 11452567]

Hirata JD et al: Does dong quai have estrogenic effects in postmenopausal women? A double-blind, placebo-controlled trial. Fertil Steril 1997;68:981. [PMID: 9418683]

Jacobson JS et al: Randomized trial of black cohosh for the treatment of hot flashes among women with a history of breast cancer. J Clin Oncol 2001;19:2739. [PMID: 11352967]

Liske E: Therapeutic efficacy and safety of Cimicifuga racemosa for gynecologic disorders. Adv Ther 1998;15:45. [PMID: 10178637]

Warnecke G: Psychosomatic dysfunctions in the female climacteric. Clinical effectiveness and tolerance of kava extract WS 1490. Fortschr Med 1991;109:119. [PMID: 2029982]

Zava DT, Dollbaum CM, Blen M: Estrogen and progestin bioactivity of foods, herbs, and spices. Proc Soc Exp Biol Med 1998;217:369. [PMID: 9492350]

Managing Symptoms of Depression

Depression is a widespread condition with a lifetime prevalence in women that has been estimated as high as 25%. While the treatment of depression with prescription pharmaceuticals has become better tolerated with the availability of the selective serotonin reuptake inhibitors (SSRIs) class of drugs, patients nonetheless often seek a more natural approach. It is important to note that where evidence exists for efficacy of herbs and supplements, it is in the treatment of mild to moderate and not severe depression.

A. ST. JOHN'S WORT

Extracts of *Hypericum perforatum* are the best studied and most commonly used herbal approaches for the treatment of depression. While the mechanism of action was originally believed to be as a weak monoamine oxidase inhibitor, this has been refuted and its true mechanism is not known. Standardization has also been subject to some controversy with both hypericin and hyperforin used in different preparations. St. John's Wort has documented efficacy in the treatment of mild to moderate depression after 4–6 weeks of use. Approximately 60% of patients report a beneficial effect on mood, energy, and sleep disturbances. Regardless of the compound used as the standard, the dosing is the same, with 300 mg 3 times a day being the typical dose. Higher doses do not produce better results and do increase the risks of side effects as noted above. A recent article revealed that both St. John's Wort and sertraline (Zoloft) were no more effective than placebo in the treatment of moderate to severe depression, and should not be used in these patients. There was, however, a large placebo response in the study, which may have been at least partially responsible for the apparent lack of effect.

B. 5-HYDROXYTRYPTOPHAN

5-Hydroxytryptophan (5-HTP) is an intermediate compound in the body's synthesis of serotonin, a neurotransmitter intimately involved in mood and depression. While unproven, 1 theory proposes increasing precursors necessary for the biosynthesis of serotonin will increase serotonin levels and therefore relieve the symptoms of depression. Several studies have documented the efficacy of 5-HTP. At least 1 head-to-head study comparing 5-HTP (100 mg 3 times a day for 6 weeks) with an SSRI showed equal efficacy. The maximal recommended dose is 200 mg 3 times a day. Side effects are rare, with gastrointestinal complaints the most common. A potential concern for 5-HTP is that it is chemically related to tryptophan, and significant toxicity from a contaminant found in this product resulted in tryptophan's removal from the market. There have been reports of a similar contaminant appearing in some formulations of 5-HTP.

C. S-ADENOSYLMETHIONINE

S-Adenosylmethionine (SAMe) has been used extensively for a significant period of time in the parenteral form in Europe for the treatment of depression. While it is known that SAMe serves as a donor of methyl moieties, it is not clear how this relates to its mechanism of action. Recent data have demonstrated that newer oral preparations contain SAMe in a bioavailable form and studies with the oral administration of the compound have demonstrated its efficacy. Trials comparing SAMe with both placebo and tricyclic antidepressants found the compound to be effective and that it produces fewer adverse effects than tricyclic antidepressants. The dosage for SAMe is 400 mg 3–4 times a day. It is one of the most expensive supplements commonly used.

D. GINKGO

Several small studies have evaluated ginkgo in the treatment of depression in elderly adults as well as in patients suffering from seasonal affective disorder. Results have been mixed, and there is insufficient evidence to recommend its use.

Bressa GM: S-adenosyl-l-methionine (SAMe) as antidepressant: meta-analysis of clinical studies. Acta Neurol Scand Suppl 1994;154:7. [PMID: 7941964]

Byerley WF: 5-Hydroxytryptophan: a review of its antidepressant efficacy and adverse effects. J Clin Pyschopharmacol 1987; 7:127. [PMID: 3298325]

Linde K et al: St John's wort for depression—an overview and meta-analysis of randomized clinical trials. BMJ 1996;313: 253. [PMID: 8704532]

Meyers S: Use of neurotransmitter precursors for treatment of depression. Altern Med Rev 2000;5:64. [PMID: 10696120]

Relevant Web Sites

[Bandolier]
www.jr2.ox.ac.uk/bandolier
[Cochrane Collection]
www.cochrane.org
[National Center for Complementary and Alternative Medicine]
http://nccam.nih.gov
[Site that analyzes supplements and herbal products]
Consumberlab.com
[Natural Standard]
www.naturalstandard.com

Index

NOTE: A *t* following a page number indicates tabular material and an *f* following a page number indicates a figure.

leukocytosis in, 374–375

preeclampsia and eclampsia in, 377–378

referral in, 383

sickle cell anemia in, 372–374

thrombocytopenia in, 375

von Willebrand disease in, 381t, 381–382, 383f

in systemic lupus erythematosus, 462t

venous thromboembolic disease in, 345–367

anticoagulation in special populations and, 361–362

antiphospholipid antibodies and, 347–348

complementary therapy for, 363, 363t

complications of, 358

diagnosis of, 357–358

duration of anticoagulation in, 366–367

elevated factor levels and, 348

estrogens and, 348t, 348–350, 349t

general considerations in, 345

hemorrhagic risks and reversal of anticoagulation in, 365–366

heparin for, 359t, 359–360, 360t

heparin-induced thrombocytopenia and, 364–365, 365t

hereditary hypercoagulable states and, 345–347, 346t

hyperhomocysteinemia and, 348

imaging studies for, 354–355, 355t

inferior vena cava filters for, 362–363

laboratory findings in, 355–357, 356t, 357t, 358t

malignancy and, 350

oral warfarin therapy for, 360–361

post-phlebitic syndrome and, 358–359

pregnancy and, 350

prevention of, 350–353, 351t, 352t, 353t

referral in, 367

screening for, 353–354

superficial and calf vein thrombosis in, 363

thrombolytic therapy for, 362, 362t

Hematoma, perispinal, 351–352

Hematuria, 210

lower urinary tract pain and, 197

in urologic malignancy, 199–200

Hemochromatosis, hereditary, 235–236

Hemodynamic changes in pregnancy, 292, 293t

Hemoglobin, 370, 370t

Hemorrhagic skin necrosis, 366

Heparin, 359t, 359–360, 360t

bone loss and, 158

effect on thyroid function, 142t

heparin-induced thrombocytopenia and, 364–365, 365t

for postpartum depression, 98

for superficial and calf vein thrombosis, 363

use during pregnancy, 297t, 298, 298t, 361–362

Heparin-induced thrombocytopenia, 360, 364–365, 365t

Hepatic steatosis, 237

Hepatitis

autoimmune, 234t, 234–235

chronic B, 231t, 231–232

chronic C, 232–234

in nonalcoholic steatohepatitis syndrome, 237–238

Hepatitis A vaccine, 37t, 39, 230

Hepatitis B, 231t, 231–232, 309t

Hepatitis B e antigen, 231

Hepatitis B immune globulin, 38

Hepatitis B surface antigen, 231

Hepatitis B vaccine, 37t, 38, 230

Hepatitis C, 232–234, 434t

Hepatotoxicity, 238, 238t

HER2/neu oncoprotein, 332–333

Herbal supplements

adolescent and, 12t

for chronic liver conditions, 238

for depression, 616

for fibromyalgia, 437

hepatotoxicity of, 238t

for menopause, 151, 615–616

for menstrual disorders, 613–614

for perimenopause depression, 99

for polycystic ovary syndrome, 172

for premenstrual syndrome, 95

warfarin interactions with, 363t

Herceptin. See Trastuzumab.

Hereditary breast-ovarian cancer syndrome, 533

Hereditary hemochromatosis, 235–236

Hereditary hypercoagulable states, 345–347, 346t

Hereditary nonpolyposis colorectal cancer syndrome, 533

Hereditary ovarian cancer syndrome, 533

Herpes genitalis infection, 309t, 510, 510f

Herpes simplex virus

in genital ulcer, 311–314, 313t, 314t

in HIV infection, 301

vulvar, 509–511, 510f

Heterocyclic antidepressants, 88t

High-density lipoproteins, 257, 257t

evaluation of, 252–253

hyperlipidemia and, 256–258, 258t

metabolic syndrome and, 255t

High-grade squamous intraepithelial lesion, 525

High-risk pregnancy, 594, 595t

Hip fracture

hormone replacement therapy and, 147, 148t

osteoporosis-related, 153

Hip protector, 163, 163f

Hirsutism, 419–420

amenorrhea and, 490

in polycystic ovary syndrome, 165–167

treatment of, 170–171

Hirudin, 364, 365t

HIV. See Human immunodeficiency virus infection.

HMG CoA reductase inhibitors, 254t

Homicide, domestic violence and, 101, 105

Homocysteine, 247

Hormonal contraception, 548–554

combination oral contraceptives in, 548–551, 550t

contraceptive patch in, 554

long-acting implantable agents in, 552, 553f

long-acting injectable agents in, 552–554

progestin-only pills in, 551–552, 552t

Hormonal fluctuations

mood disorders and, 80

in multiple sclerosis, 405–406, 406t

Hormonal risk factors in breast cancer, 323–324

Hormonal therapy

for breast cancer, 338–339, 341

for postpartum depression, 98

Hormonally related psychiatric disorders, 93–100

depression during pregnancy in, 95–97

perimenopause depression in, 99

postpartum depression in, 97–98

premenstrual syndrome in, 93–95

Hormone replacement therapy

cardiovascular risks and, 265

coronary artery disease and, 146, 248–249

endometrial hyperplasia and, 151

for menopause, 145–149, 148t

for menorrhagia and metrorrhagia, 498t

migraine and, 393

ovarian cancer and, 532

for perimenopause, 99